Advances in Experimental Medicine and Biology

Volume 1464

Advances in Experimental Medicine and Biology provides a platform for scientific contributions in the main disciplines of the biomedicine and the life sciences. This series publishes thematic volumes on contemporary research in the areas of microbiology, immunology, neurosciences, biochemistry, biomedical engineering, genetics, physiology, and cancer research. Covering emerging topics and techniques in basic and clinical science, it brings together clinicians and researchers from various fields.

Advances in Experimental Medicine and Biology has been publishing exceptional works in the field for over 40 years, and is indexed in SCOPUS, Medline (PubMed), EMBASE, Reaxys, EMBiology, the Chemical Abstracts Service (CAS), and Pathway Studio.

2023 CiteScore: 5.9

Therese Sørlie • Robert B. Clarke
Editors

A Guide to Breast Cancer Research

From Cellular Heterogeneity and Molecular Mechanisms to Therapy

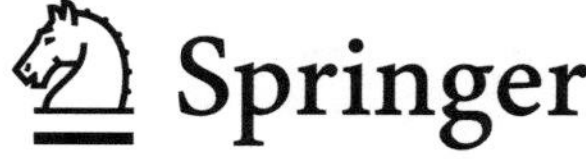

Editors
Therese Sørlie
Department of Cancer Genetics,
Institute for Cancer Research
Oslo University Hospital
Oslo, Norway

Robert B. Clarke
Manchester Breast Centre, Division of
Cancer Sciences, Faculty of Biology,
Medicine and Health
University of Manchester
Manchester, UK

ISSN 0065-2598 ISSN 2214-8019 (electronic)
Advances in Experimental Medicine and Biology
ISBN 978-3-031-70874-9 ISBN 978-3-031-70875-6 (eBook)
https://doi.org/10.1007/978-3-031-70875-6

This Springer imprint is published by the registered company Springer Nature Switzerland AG
The registered company address is: Gewerbestrasse 11, 6330 Cham, Switzerland

Foreword

A Guide to Breast Cancer Research: From Cells and Molecular Mechanisms to Therapy was conceived following an education talk on breast cancer cell lineages that Therese gave at a European Association for Cancer Research conference. Rob and Therese developed the idea into a more comprehensive guide for young investigators and postgraduate students who want an overview of the most important topics in contemporary breast cancer research. These chapters are not intended to be comprehensive literature reviews but rather to help explain the new methodologies and approaches that have led to the recent advances in studying both normal mammary gland development and breast cancer. The book begins with a description of embryonic mammary gland development and then postnatal development of the human breast. This is followed by a comparison of single-cell analyses of the mouse and human mammary gland, and the use of barcoding technologies to help elucidate the origin of various mammary cell lineages. In both cases the authors explain the various methods used as well and their advantages and disadvantages. The next section focuses on the development of new models to study early breast cancer progression, the use of patient-derived xenografts, and rediscovery and advances in the development of new rat models of breast cancer. Some of the earliest breast cancer models were the DMBA-induced rat models developed by Charles Huggins, who won the Nobel Prize in 1966. Several chapters are then devoted to the discussion of the cells of origin, the mechanisms of cell fate regulation, and the classification of breast cancer based on cell identity models. The next sections deal with the characteristics and signaling pathways present in various breast cancer subtypes including metabolic reprogramming and adaptation during progression and metastasis. This is followed by a more in-depth exposition of the role of the immune microenvironment, dormancy, and metastasis. The volume culminates in the clinical and therapeutic implications of these studies. In many ways this book mirrors many aspects of my own career beginning with our studies of hormone signaling and normal mammary gland development, the development of new preclinical models, and finally translating these studies into the clinic. I think it will be a valuable resource for new breast cancer researchers. It sets the stage for exciting ongoing studies in many laboratories using spatial transcriptomics and artificial intelligence for the analysis of breast pathology and new drug design, which ultimately will improve the outcome for patients with breast cancer.

Baylor College of Medicine
Houston, TX, USA
June 17, 2024

Jeffrey M. Rosen

Contents

Part II Development and Cancer: Model Systems and Approaches

About the Editors

Robert B. Clarke is Professor of Breast Biology at the University of Manchester and is currently Director of the Manchester Breast Centre, which comprises 40 academics active in breast research. Rob was awarded a Cancer Research Campaign Fellowship which established the Breast Biology Group that he has led for over 20 years. He is a co-founder of the European Network for Breast Development and Cancer and the EuroPDX Consortium. Rob's research achievements include the first use of Ki67 as a proliferation biomarker in neoadjuvant tamoxifen and fulvestrant studies, the discovery of the importance of paracrine signaling in normal breast epithelium including EGF and Notch pathways, and establishing the roles of stem cell signaling pathways including cytokines in breast cancer therapy resistance and metastasis. Rob has over 170 peer-reviewed publications in these areas of research.

Therese Sørlie is Head of the Department of Cancer Genetics, Institute for Cancer Research, Oslo University Hospital, and she is Associate Professor in Cancer Genetics at Oslo University. She received a young investigator grant from the Norwegian Research Council and has led her own research group since 2012. She is a member of the European Network for Breast Development and Cancer. Therese Sørlie's work includes contribution to the pioneering gene expression studies of breast tumors that has resulted in a classification scheme that is implemented in international guidelines for the treatment of breast cancer. Her research interest is in breast tumor initiation and progression: from the cell of origin in which the first oncogenic events take place, the specific pathways and processes that are deregulated in the further progression of the intrinsic subtypes, to the specific events that are essential for the transition from in situ to invasive cancer.

A Guide to Breast Cancer Research: An Introduction

1

Robert B. Clarke and Therese Sørlie

Abstract

"A Guide to Breast Cancer Research: From Cells and Molecular Mechanisms to Therapy" is designed as a comprehensive reference for early career investigators and postgraduate students. This book aims to provide a broad overview of contemporary breast cancer research. It covers key areas including development and cancer, metastasis and immunology, subtypes, signalling, therapy, and resistance. This book is organised into seven sections addressing mammary gland development, model systems, cellular origins and heterogeneity, cellular and molecular bases, signalling pathways, metastasis and immunity, and treatment and resistance mechanisms. A few topics such as specific signalling pathways, some emerging therapies, imaging technologies, and AI applications are only briefly mentioned or omitted, reflecting the ever-evolving nature of breast cancer research. This book emphasises the importance of collaboration in advancing cancer research. Initiatives like the Cancer Moonshot and Cancer Grand Challenges advocate for "radical collaboration" of researchers with shared visions and resources. We also note the significance of global efforts in breast cancer research, the need for addressing disparities in care across different regions and for equity in healthcare. Overall, this book showcases milestones and advances in breast cancer research over the past three decades, reflecting significant progress in understanding and treating the disease, which has led to improved patient outcomes.

Keywords

Breast cancer · Development · Subtypes · Signalling · Metastasis · Immunology · Therapy

The idea for a guide to breast cancer research as a primer for early career investigators grew out of

Key Points

- Concept for a guide for doctoral students, early career scientists, and clinical fellows.
- Scope of the book from development, cancer, subtypes, metastasis, immunology, and therapy.
- The next challenges in mammary gland biology and breast cancer research.

R. B. Clarke
Faculty of Biology, Medicine and Health, Division of Cancer Sciences, Manchester Breast Centre, University of Manchester, Manchester, UK
e-mail: robert.clarke@manchester.ac.uk

T. Sørlie (✉)
Department of Cancer Genetics, Institute for Cancer Research, Oslo University Hospital, Oslo, Norway
e-mail: therese.sorlie@medisin.uio.no

T. Sørlie, R. B. Clarke (eds.), *A Guide to Breast Cancer Research*, Advances in Experimental Medicine and Biology 1464, https://doi.org/10.1007/978-3-031-70875-6_1

- Cancer Team Science: adopting "radical collaboration" in which there are six "Hallmarks of Cancer Collaboration".
- Milestones in breast cancer research and treatment.

an educational talk on breast cancer cell lineages that one of the editors, Therese Sørlie, gave at the virtual European Association for Cancer Research (EACR) Congress. Through discussions that Therese held with Robert Clarke, who is co-editor of this book, the plan evolved into a more comprehensive tome with additional sections on topics we thought were essential for young scientists beginning their research careers. Thus, we aimed to create a reference book for young investigators and postgraduate students who want to get an overview of the most important topics in contemporary breast cancer research and to expand their knowledge on topics outside their own research focus. The scope is a reflection of current research on development and cancer, metastasis and immunology, subtypes, signalling, therapy, and resistance. We believe that such a book will be a unique addition to the literature. The result is "A Guide to Breast Cancer Research: From Cells and Molecular Mechanisms to Therapy", which is an introduction to the world of breast cancer research aimed at early career researchers who are developing the breadth of their knowledge in this subject.

We are tremendously grateful to the authors of the 23 chapters who devoted their time to this project and delivered expert and amazingly readable narratives on their fields. The book is organised into seven themed sections, each focusing on different aspects of breast cancer development, progression, and treatment. In Part I, it focuses on the development of the mammary gland and its connection to breast cancer. It covers topics such as mammary gland embryonic development, postnatal changes, and the use of single-cell analysis to understand mammary gland development and tumorigenesis. Part II explores model systems and approaches used to study mammary gland development and breast cancer progression. This section discusses techniques such as lineage tracing, patient-derived xenografts, and the potential of rat models for breast cancer research. In Part III, the authors describe research into the cells of origin and heterogeneity in breast cancer. They examine the regulatory mechanisms governing cell fate decisions, the classification of breast cancer based on cell identity, and the implications for targeted therapies. Part IV examines the cellular and molecular basis of breast cancer. It covers topics such as ductal carcinoma in situ, breast cancer heterogeneity, and the role of E-cadherin in invasive lobular carcinoma. In Part V, the chapters provide insights into key signalling pathways in breast cancer, including hormone signalling, the RANK pathway, and metabolic reprogramming. Part VI sheds light on metastasis and immunity in breast cancer, from cellular dormancy to the roles of myeloid cells and other immune cells in breast cancer progression. Finally, in Part VII, the authors provide insights linking breast cancer subtypes to treatment, and resistance mechanisms, addressing topics such as estrogen receptor and human epidermal growth factor receptor 2 (HER2) signalling-targeted therapies and resistance to specific inhibitors.

Overall, this book offers a holistic view of breast cancer research, covering a wide range of topics from basic cellular mechanisms to advanced therapeutic strategies, aiming to improve our understanding of breast cancer and enhance treatment outcomes. However, space in this book is limited, and there are some omissions in this edition of the book. For example, the contribution of HER2, fibroblast growth factor receptor (FGFR), phosphatidylinositol-4,5-bisphosphate 3-kinase catalytic subunit alpha (PIK3CA)/AKT/mechanistic target of rapamycin (mTOR), and many other signalling pathways are only partially described; emerging therapies such as antibody-drug conjugates, CAR T cell, and other cellular therapies are not described in detail; there is little on the spatial molecular landscape of breast tumours, imaging technologies, and the impact of artificial intelligence in research and the clinic. These are some of the known unknowns, but many other gaps in research will no doubt emerge over the coming decades (the unknown unknowns). In a recent review, we explored some of these and other known unknowns (gaps) and the next challenges in mammary gland biology and breast cancer research (van Amerongen et al. 2023).

There is an emerging belief that there is a need to exploit team science to accomplish the best and most effective cancer research, as exemplified by initiatives such as the Cancer Moonshot and the Cancer Grand Challenges for example, the current focus of some funders (Boehm and Jacks 2024). In their commentary, Boehm and Jacks propose adopting "radical collaboration" in which six "Hallmarks of Cancer Collaboration" are utilised: common vision, leaders as catalysts, aligned incentives, shared culture, resource sharing, and operational groundwork (Hanahan and Weinberg 2011) (cf. the classic "Hallmarks of cancer" review by Hanahan and Weinberg). Some of these have long been used in cancer research, and others are emerging. For example, the well-established national and international societies that promote breast cancer research, its communication, and the fostering of collaboration such as the Gordon Research Conference on Mammary Gland Biology, the San Antonio Breast Cancer Symposium, as well as the more general cancer research societies like American Association for Cancer Research (AACR), European Association for Cancer Research (EACR), American Society of Clinical Oncology (ASCO) and European Society for Medical Oncology (ESMO). We established the European Network for Breast Development and Cancer as an international grouping of labs researching in this area (https://enbdc.org/) (Chalmers et al. 2023) and the EuroPDX and PDXnet consortia for sharing patient-derived cancer models including breast (https://www.cancermodels.org/) (Hidalgo et al. 2014; Byrne et al. 2017; Woo et al. 2021).

The breast cancer research associations listed above are mainly based in North America and Europe but we must acknowledge the growing efforts of existing and nascent research groups across all six continents, including several authors of chapters within the book. Breast cancer is a global health issue and research needs to address the differences that ethnicities and disparities in income bring to susceptibility, incidence, diagnosis, and treatment capabilities. Many of these issues are discussed in the Lancet Breast Cancer Commission, which is a collaborative effort by a diverse, multidisciplinary international group of researchers and patient advocates from across all 6 continents committed to raising the standard of breast cancer care to close the equity gap that exists between and within countries (Coles et al. 2024).

Milestones in breast cancer research and advances in treatment over 30 years from 1994 to 2023 demonstrate significant progress in the understanding and management of the disease (Box 1.1). Selected key milestones include the cloning of BRCA1 and BRCA2 genes linked to breast cancer risk, FDA approvals of drugs such as anastrozole and tamoxifen for treatment and prevention, the delineation of breast cancer molecular subtypes, and the discovery of transplantable breast cancer stem cells. Clinical use of the targeted therapies trastuzumab for HER2-positive, and CDK4/6 inhibitors for ER-positive breast tumours mark important step changes that improve treatment and outcomes in the majority of patients. The timeline reflects the multidimensional approach to combating breast cancer, with advances in understanding biology leading to the development of effective targeted treatments. Remarkably, Taylor et al. (2023) report a population study of 500,000 breast cancer cases demonstrating a 66% drop in mortality between 1993 and 2015 (Taylor et al. 2023), suggesting real-world progress in treating breast cancer. This astounding progress and further future advances hinge on the quality of research that increases our understanding of breast development and cancer, which underpins and informs the development of better approaches to prevention, diagnosis, and treatment of the disease.

Box 1.1 Selected Milestones in Breast Cancer Research and Treatment from 1994 to 2023

Additional recent milestones are covered in detail in many of the chapters in this book.

1994–95: Scientists clone the tumour suppressor genes BRCA1 and BRCA2 genes for which inherited mutations predict an increased risk of breast cancer (Miki et al. 1994; Wooster et al. 1995).

1996: FDA approves anastrozole, an aromatase inhibitor of estrogen synthesis, as a treatment for breast cancer.

1997–98: Clarke and Brisken establish the paracrine signalling paradigm for normal breast epithelial proliferation in response to estrogen and progesterone (Clarke et al. 1997; Brisken et al. 1998).

1998: Tamoxifen is found to decrease the risk of developing breast cancer in at-risk women by 50%, leading to its approval by the FDA for use as a preventive therapy.

1998: Trastuzumab (Herceptin), a drug targeting cancer cells that are over-expressing HER2, is approved by the FDA.

2000–01: Perou and Sørlie delineate the molecular subtypes of breast cancer (Perou et al. 2000; Sørlie et al. 2001).

2003: Wicha and Clarke describe transplantable human breast cancer stem cells (Al-Hajj et al. 2003).

2006: Visavader and Eaves define single transplantable mouse mammary gland epithelial stem cells (Shackleton et al. 2006; Stingl et al. 2006).

2012: Approval for the mTOR inhibitor everolimus in the treatment of advanced ER+ breast cancer.

2016: Approval of the first CDK4/6 inhibitor palbociclib for the treatment of advanced ER+/HER2- breast cancer.

2018: Approval for the PARP inhibitors olaparib and talazoparib in the treatment of BRCA1/2 germline-mutated HER2-negative breast cancer.

2019: Approval for the PI3K inhibitor alpelisib in the treatment of PIK3CA-mutated advanced ER+ breast cancer.

2019: Enhertu is approved by the FDA for treating HER2-positive metastatic breast cancer.

2020: The drug Trodelvy is approved by the FDA for treating metastatic triple-negative breast cancer.

2022: Approval for the immune checkpoint PD-L1 inhibitor pembrolizumab in the treatment of advanced triple-negative breast cancer.

2023: Approval for the AKT inhibitor capivasertib in the treatment of PIK3CA- or AKT-mutated advanced ER+ breast cancer.

2023: Dodwell reports a population study of 500,000 breast cancer cases demonstrating a 66% drop in mortality between 1993 and 2015 (Taylor et al. 2023).

References

Al-Hajj M, Wicha MS, Benito-Hernandez A et al (2003) Prospective identification of tumorigenic breast cancer cells. Proc Natl Acad Sci USA 100:3983–3988. https://doi.org/10.1073/pnas.0530291100

Boehm JS, Jacks T (2024) Radical collaboration: reimagining cancer team science. Cancer Discov 14:563–568. https://doi.org/10.1158/2159-8290.CD-23-1496

Brisken C, Park S, Vass T et al (1998) A paracrine role for the epithelial progesterone receptor in mammary gland development. Proc Natl Acad Sci USA 95:5076–5081. https://doi.org/10.1073/pnas.95.9.5076

Byrne AT, Alférez DG, Amant F et al (2017) Interrogating open issues in cancer precision medicine with patient-derived xenografts. Nat Rev Cancer 17:254–268. https://doi.org/10.1038/nrc.2016.140

Chalmers SB, van der Wal T, Fre S, Jonkers J (2023) Fourteenth annual ENBDC workshop: methods in mammary gland biology and breast cancer. J Mammary Gland Biol Neoplasia 28:22. https://doi.org/10.1007/s10911-023-09549-7

Clarke RB, Howell A, Potten CS, Anderson E (1997) Dissociation between steroid receptor expression and cell proliferation in the human breast. Cancer Res 57:4987–4991

Coles CE, Earl H, Anderson BO et al (2024) The lancet breast cancer commission. Lancet 403:1895–1950. https://doi.org/10.1016/S0140-6736(24)00747-5

Hanahan D, Weinberg RA (2011) Hallmarks of cancer: the next generation. Cell 144:646–674. https://doi.org/10.1016/j.cell.2011.02.013

Hidalgo M, Amant F, Biankin AV et al (2014) Patient-derived xenograft models: an emerging platform for translational cancer research. Cancer Discov 4:998–1013. https://doi.org/10.1158/2159-8290.CD-14-0001

Miki Y, Swensen J, Shattuck-Eidens D et al (1994) A strong candidate for the breast and ovarian cancer susceptibility gene BRCA1. Science 266:66–71. https://doi.org/10.1126/science.7545954

Perou CM, Sørlie T, Eisen MB et al (2000) Molecular portraits of human breast tumours. Nature 406:747–752. https://doi.org/10.1038/35021093

Shackleton M, Vaillant F, Simpson KJ et al (2006) Generation of a functional mammary gland from a single stem cell. Nature 439:84–88. https://doi.org/10.1038/nature04372

Sørlie T, Perou CM, Tibshirani R et al (2001) Gene expression patterns of breast carcinomas distinguish tumor subclasses with clinical implications. Proc Natl Acad Sci USA 98:10869–10874. https://doi.org/10.1073/pnas.191367098

Stingl J, Eirew P, Ricketson I et al (2006) Purification and unique properties of mammary epithelial stem cells. Nature 439:993–997. https://doi.org/10.1038/nature04496

Taylor C, McGale P, Probert J et al (2023) Breast cancer mortality in 500000 women with early invasive breast cancer diagnosed in England, 1993-2015: population based observational cohort study. BMJ 381:e074684. https://doi.org/10.1136/bmj-2022-074684

van Amerongen R, Bentires-Alj M, van Boxtel AL et al (2023) Imagine beyond: recent breakthroughs and next challenges in mammary gland biology and breast cancer research. J Mammary Gland Biol Neoplasia 28:17. https://doi.org/10.1007/s10911-023-09544-y

Woo XY, Giordano J, Srivastava A et al (2021) Conservation of copy number profiles during engraftment and passaging of patient-derived cancer xenografts. Nat Genet 53:86–99. https://doi.org/10.1038/s41588-020-00750-6

Wooster R, Bignell G, Lancaster J et al (1995) Identification of the breast cancer susceptibility gene BRCA2. Nature 378:789–792. https://doi.org/10.1038/378789a0

Part I

Development and Cancer: Basic Concepts

Therese Sørlie and Robert B. Clarke

Understanding the normal mammary gland, its many cell types, their complex interactions, and the governing cellular pathways provides a fundament for understanding breast carcinogenesis.

In Chap. 2, Marja Mikkola and her colleagues at the University of Helsinki, Finland, explore the intricate process of embryonic mammary gland development. It begins with bilateral mammary line formation, progresses through stages like placode, bud, and sprout, and culminates in branching morphogenesis. Interaction between primary and secondary mammary mesenchyme drives this process, with cell influx dominating early growth and increased cell proliferation during the sprout stage. Signaling pathways like Wnt/β--catenin, Fgf, and Eda play key roles, hinting at a connection to ancestral hair follicles. Unique features include Pthlh signaling and inhibition of Hedgehog activity, alongside mechanisms like EMT and MET, crucial for development and remodeling.

In Chap. 3, Thorarinn Gudjonsson and his colleagues at the University of Iceland delve into the postnatal development and dynamic remodeling of the human breast gland, composed of branching epithelial ducts that culminate in terminal duct lobular units (TDLUs). The epithelial compartment consists of luminal epithelial cells (LEP) and myoepithelial cells (MEP), both arising from a common stem cell population. Hormonal regulation, primarily by estrogen and progesterone, plays a significant role in these processes. The chapter explores the interactions between LEPs and MEPs with the surrounding stroma in both normal and cancerous states, emphasizing the changes in the tumor microenvironment during cancer progression.

Chapter 4 by Walid Khaled and his colleagues at the University of Cambridge, UK, highlight the use of single-cell analysis to unravel the complexities of mammary gland development and tumorigenesis. The mammary gland's ability to undergo significant restructuring during pregnancy and

---

T. Sørlie
Oslo, Norway

R. B. Clarke
Manchester, UK

revert to a nearly identical resting state during involution demonstrates its remarkable plasticity. Single-cell techniques allow for a detailed examination of the cellular and molecular mechanisms at play, providing insights into the various cell types and their functions from birth through adulthood and in cancer formation. The chapter also discusses the benefits and limitations of single-cell methodologies and the relevance of mouse models in studying critical time points in human development and disease.

Understanding these developmental processes, from embryogenesis through postnatal changes and single-cell insights, provides a comprehensive view of normal mammary gland development and its links to cancer progression, offering potential pathways for therapeutic interventions.

2 Embryonic Mammary Gland Morphogenesis

Satu-Marja Myllymäki, Qiang Lan, and Marja L. Mikkola

Abstract

Embryonic mammary gland development unfolds with the specification of bilateral mammary lines, thereafter progressing through placode, bud, and sprout stages before branching morphogenesis. Extensive epithelial–mesenchymal interactions guide morphogenesis from embryogenesis to adulthood. Two distinct mesenchymal tissues are involved, the primary mammary mesenchyme that harbors mammary inductive capacity, and the secondary mesenchyme, the precursor of the adult stroma. Placode and bud stages are morphologically similar with other ectodermal appendages like the hair follicle, reflecting the mammary gland's assumed evolutionary origin from an ancestral hair follicle-associated glandular unit. The shared features extend to signalling cascades such as the Wnt/β-catenin, fibroblast growth factor (Fgf), and ectodysplasin (Eda) pathways, while pathways unique to mammary gland include parathyroid hormone-like hormone (Pthlh) signalling and Hedgehog activity suppression. Mammary gland branching is highly non-stereotypic, achieved by the dynamic use of two distinct modes of branching: tip bifurcation and side branching and stochastic branch point formation. The cellular mechanisms driving the initial morphogenetic steps are slowly beginning to be unravelled. During placode and bud stages, mammary primordium predominantly grows through cell influx, while sprouting correlates with heightened proliferation. Branch elongation is driven by directional cell migration combined with differential cell motility and proliferation supplying the reservoir of migratory cells, whereas a bifurcating tip is associated with localized repression of the cell cycle and cell motility. Numerous similarities exist between embryonic programs and breast tumorigenesis, spanning cellular plasticity, epithelial–stromal interactions, and molecular regulators. Understanding embryonic mammogenesis may provide insights into how normal developmental processes can go awry, leading to malignancy, or how they can be reversed to prevent cancer progression.

S.-M. Myllymäki
Institute of Biotechnology, Helsinki Institute of Life Science HiLIFE, University of Helsinki, Helsinki, Finland

Faculty of Medicine, Stem Cells and Metabolism Research Program, University of Helsinki, Helsinki, Finland

Q. Lan · M. L. Mikkola (✉)
Institute of Biotechnology, Helsinki Institute of Life Science HiLIFE, University of Helsinki, Helsinki, Finland
e-mail: marja.mikkola@helsinki.fi

T. Sørlie, R. B. Clarke (eds.), *A Guide to Breast Cancer Research*, Advances in Experimental Medicine and Biology 1464, https://doi.org/10.1007/978-3-031-70875-6_2

Keywords

Mammary line · Placode · Bud · Sprout · Branching · Epithelial–mesenchymal interaction · Wnt

Key Points

- Mammary gland development commences in utero with the specification of two bilateral ectodermal fields competent to give rise to mammary primordia. These primordia progress through placode, bud, and sprout stages prior to the onset of branching morphogenesis. This developmental sequence is conserved across all placental mammals, although specific details vary among species. During the placode and bud stages, the mammary primordium primarily grows through cell influx, with sprouting correlating with increased proliferation.
- Mammary gland is thought to have evolved from an ancestral hair follicle-associated glandular unit. Early stages of mammary gland development share morphological similarities with analogous steps in other ectodermal appendages, including the hair follicle. This resemblance extends to the use of conserved signalling cascades such as the Wnt/β-catenin, Fgf, and Eda pathways. Features unique to mammary glands include Pthlh signalling and suppression of Hedgehog activity.
- The development of the mammary gland relies on extensive epithelial–mesenchymal tissue interactions that guide morphogenesis from embryogenesis through puberty and into adulthood. Two distinct mesenchymal tissues play crucial roles during embryonic development: the fibroblastic primary mammary mesenchyme, condensing around the bud and providing cues supporting mammary cell identity and survival, and the secondary mammary mesenchyme, the precursor tissue of the adult stroma, regulating branching morphogenesis.
- Embryonic mammary gland branching involves two distinct mechanisms: tip bifurcation and lateral branching, resulting in a highly non-stereotypic branching pattern. Tissue recombination experiments have revealed that the dominant role of the mesenchyme is defining the growth rate and density of the ductal tree, while the mode of branching is an intrinsic property of the mammary epithelium. Paracrine factors, including Fgfs, ErbB ligands, transforming growth factor-β (Tgf-β) family members, Eda, and Insulin-like growth factor 1 (Igf-1), regulate epithelial growth and branching morphogenesis.
- The cellular mechanisms driving branching morphogenesis begin to be unravelled as methods combining *ex vivo* culture with high-resolution live imaging are developed. Ductal elongation is propelled by directional cell migration and differential cell motility, while tip bifurcation involves spatially coordinated changes at the branch point; localized repression of the cell cycle and cell motility. Nascent tips remain proliferative but split into two new streams of migratory cells. However, cell cycle activity does not drive elongation, but rather replenishes the reservoir of migratory cells.
- Numerous similarities exist between embryonic programs and breast tumorigenesis, extending from primitive cell states and cellular plasticity to epithelial–stromal interactions, molecular regulators, and cellular behaviours.

2.1 Introduction

Mammary glands represent class-defining features of mammals, believed to have evolved from an ancestral apocrine gland-pilo-sebaceous (hair follicle)-like unit (Oftedal and Dhouailly 2013). This joint evolutionary history may account for the morphological similarities observed in the early developmental stages of the mammary gland and the hair follicle, as well as other organs that develop as appendages of the surface ectoderm, such as the tooth, that all proceed through shared placode and bud stages (Mikkola and Millar 2006). The commonalities extend to the molecular level, with the early development of ectodermal appendages relying on extensive epithelial–mesenchymal tissue interactions mediated by a few key signalling cascades including the Wnt/β-catenin, Fgf, and the Eda/NF-κB pathways (Biggs and Mikkola 2014).

In all placental mammals, the embryonic mammary anlage progresses through similar developmental stages, although the details vary among taxa (Oftedal and Dhouailly 2013). The first phase involves the specification of bilateral mammary lines (or milk lines), the ectodermal fields on the surface of the foetus competent to generate mammary placodes (Spina and Cowin 2021). The mammary lines extend from the fore- to the hindlimb bud, but the position and number of mammary placodes along the mammary line, and consequently mammary glands, exhibit significant variation in mammals. In most species, their number ranges between two (e.g. human and horse) and ten (e.g. mouse and many dog breeds), but can be up to 14 in domestic pigs and 24 in multimammate mice (*Mastomys natalensis* and its closely related species) (Brambell and Davis 1941; Oftedal and Dhouailly 2013).

In this chapter, we will focus on murine embryonic mammary gland morphogenesis, as mammary gland development is best known in mice. For a comprehensive understanding of human foetal breast development, we direct the reader to several excellent reviews (Howard and Gusterson 2000; McNally and Stein 2017; Oftedal and Dhouailly 2013). It is worth noting that comparisons of gene-modified mouse models and genetic human conditions affecting breast development indicate conservation at the molecular level, suggesting that many of the findings made in mice can be extrapolated to humans. For example, in humans, heterozygous mutations in the transcriptional repressor *TBX3* underlie the ulnar-mammary syndrome (MIM 181450) characterized by hypoplasia of the breast, and in mice, *Tbx3* deficiency results in complete failure of mammary gland development (Douglas and Papaioannou 2013).

2.2 Overview of Embryonic Mammary Gland Development

Morphological development of the mammary gland begins with the formation of placodes at conserved locations of the surface of the embryo (Fig. 2.1). Placodes are stratified multilayered epithelial thickenings that in mice emerge between embryonic day 11 (E11.0) and E12.0 in an asynchronous manner, placode 3 forming first and placode 2 last (Veltmaat et al. 2004). These lens-shaped thickenings gradually grow into buds, slightly elevated from the surface of the skin. Starting from E12.5, they initiate invagination into the underlying dermis leading to the formation of 'a neck' between the skin and the bud, giving rise to a light bulb-shaped configuration (Trela et al. 2021). A more nuanced nomenclature has also been proposed for the E12.0–E14.5 stages: hillock, bud, and bulb (Propper et al. 2013). However, for simplicity, we will use 'bud' as a generic term for these stages. The bud grows slowly in size until it develops into a sprout at ~E15.5 and begins to branch ~E16.5. The onset of sprouting and branching is also asynchronous, the posterior glands 4 and 5 commencing branching at E17.5, i.e. about a day later than glands 1–3 (Satta et al. 2024a; Veltmaat et al. 2003). After several branching events, a rudimentary ductal tree with some 15 to 25 branches has formed by birth (E19-E20). Towards the end of embryogenesis, small micro-lumini emerge at the core of the

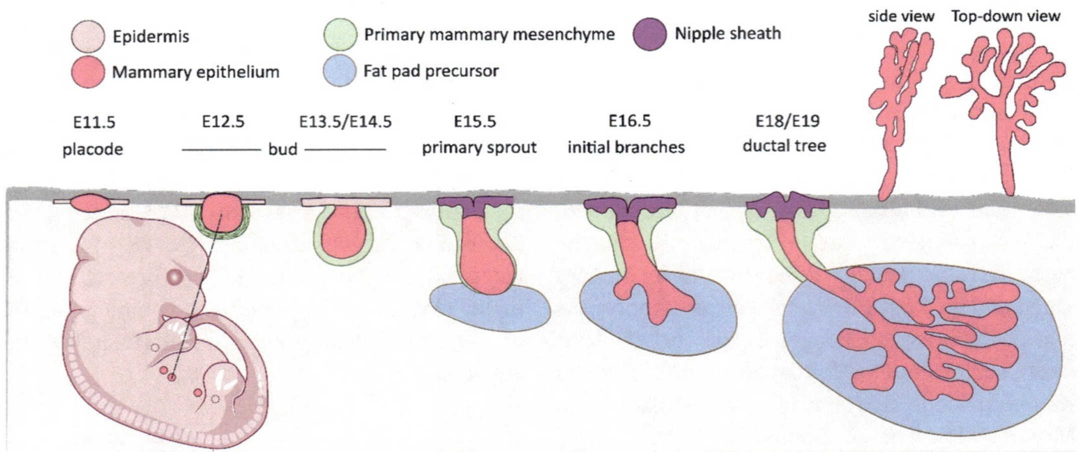

Fig. 2.1 Overview of embryonic mammary gland development. Mammary placodes become visible at E11.5 and give rise to elevated buds by E12.5, associated with the condensed primary mammary mesenchyme. The bud grows slowly while subtending to the underlying dermis. At E15.5, the epidermis overlying the bud ingresses, and the bud generates a sprout progressing towards the secondary mammary mesenchyme, the precursor of the fat pad. First branches form at E16.5, a small arborized gland with 15–25 branches forming prior to birth. The posterior glands 4 and 5 sprout and branch a day later. Lumen formation begins ~E17.5 (not depicted), marked by small micro-lumini emerging and giving rise to a continuous lumen around birth

branches (Hogg et al. 1983) and nipple formation begins. Variations to the embryonic program exist between species—e.g. in humans, several sprouts arise from the same bud such that the mammary gland has multiple ductal trees connecting to the same opening. After birth, the ductal tree undergoes slow isometric growth and branching until the onset of puberty, when ovarian hormones stimulate robust expansion that ceases when the ductal network reaches the borders of the fat pad. Of note, the growth pace and extent of branching varies substantially between wild-type mouse strains, evident already in the embryo (Satta et al. 2024a; Naylor and Ormandy 2002).

During embryogenesis, the outer and inner cells of the mammary rudiment begin to differentiate into two distinct epithelial lineages of the postnatal gland, basal (or myoepithelial) and luminal, organized as two layers around a central lumen. However, a continuous lumen only forms around birth (Hogg et al. 1983) and thus, early morphogenesis occurs almost entirely in the stratified epithelium. The outermost cells are connected to a basement membrane, beyond which lies the mesenchyme. At the bud stage, the fibroblasts beneath the mammary epithelium elongate and concentrically align around the bud generating three to five compacted cell layers referred to as the primary mammary mesenchyme (Cowin and Wysolmerski 2010; Howard 2012) (Fig. 2.1). As the mammary bud begins to sprout, it passes through these cells into a more deeply placed secondary mammary mesenchyme, termed the fat pad precursor, where embryonic branching morphogenesis commences. This precursor tissue matures into the adult stroma, the fat pad, composed of adipocytes, fibroblasts, nerve, immune, and endothelial cells, as well as the extracellular matrix that collectively support all post-natal development.

Embryonic mammary gland morphogenesis is established upon inductive epithelial–mesenchymal tissue interactions, independent of hormones (Brisken and Ataca 2015; Watson and Khaled 2020). Testosterone production; however, plays an important role in sexual dimorphism of the mouse embryonic mammary gland—the mammary rudiment undergoes apoptosis due to androgen receptor (Ar) activation in the mammary mesenchyme from E14 onward (Kratochwil and Schwartz 1976). Hence, male mice have no nipples or ductal system, or a very rudimentary one, although male mammary glands generally develop in other mammals. Post-natal morphogenesis during puberty and pregnancy is largely hormone driven, yet the effects of the hormones are mediated by locally produced paracrine and autocrine factors and epithelial-stromal crosstalk that share commonalities with the embryonic program, including the Fgf and TGF-β pathways (Brisken and Ataca 2015; McNally and Martin 2011; Rivetti et al. 2020).

2.3 From Milk Line to Mammary Buds

The prospective mammary line region is not anatomically discernible in mice but can be visualized at E10.5 by a broad band of mesenchymal *Tbx3* expression (Jerome-Majewska et al. 2005). Somewhat later, a streak of epithelial *Wnt10b* expression emerges in the region of prospective placodes 2–4, followed by the appearance of two additional ones corresponding to areas where placodes 1 and 5 will form (i.e. at regions where the limb buds connect to the trunk). These streaks fuse to a thin continuous line only after placodes have appeared but interplacodal expression disappears within the following ~24 h. As a result, expression of *Wnt10b* and other placode markers becomes confined to individual buds (Propper et al. 2013; Veltmaat et al. 2004). In addition, a fourth stripe of *Wnt10b* exists, encircling the forelimb bud dorsally, ending at its anterior edge (Veltmaat et al. 2004). A transient placode-like structure forms at this site and can be maintained and developed into a functional mammary gland upon receiving placode-promoting cues such as the tumour necrosis factor-like ligand Eda (Voutilainen et al. 2015). Collectively, these studies indicate that the mammary line does not pre-exist as a molecular continuum before placode formation but is broader than previously appreciated, extending anteriorly past mammary gland 1.

Relatively little is known about the molecular mechanisms defining the position of the mammary line, the involvement of Fgf10 being best described. *Fgf10* is expressed in the limb bud mesenchyme and the ventral extensions of thoracic somites underneath the prospective mammary line (placodes 2–4), while its receptor *Fgfr2b* is broadly expressed in the epithelium (Mailleux et al. 2002; Veltmaat et al. 2006). In *Pax3* mouse mutants, where the ventral extension of somites fails leading to a corresponding shift in the *Fgf10* expression domain, the position of mammary placodes is dorsalized (Veltmaat et al. 2006). *Ex vivo* studies where the expression of bone morphogenetic protein 4 (*Bmp4*) and *Tbx3* were manipulated imply that the dorsoventral positioning is also influenced by the mutual antagonism of Bmp4 and Tbx3 (Cho et al. 2006). Instead, the Hox code may play a role in the anterior-posterior positioning of mammary glands. Anterior misexpression of *Hoxc8*, a mid-thoracic Hox gene, expands the domain of thoracic identity, accompanied by upregulation of *Fgf10* expression in cervical somites and formation of ectopic mammary placodes anterior to mammary placode 1 (Carroll and Capecchi 2015).

Fgf10/Fgfr2b signalling is critical also for mammary placode morphogenesis. In hypomorphic *Fgf10* mutants expressing low levels of *Fgf10*, placode 3 fails to form and others are smaller, while a complete lack of Fgf10 (or Fgfr2b) results in the absence of all but placode 4 (Mailleux et al. 2002; Veltmaat et al. 2006). Wnt/β-catenin pathway is equally essential for mammary cell fate acquisition and placode formation. Deletion of transcription factor Lef1, one of the four Tcf/Lef1 proteins mediating Wnt/β-catenin signalling, leads to the absence of mammary placodes 2 and 3 (van Genderen et al. 1994), whereas transgenic overexpression of the secreted Wnt inhibitor Dickkopf 1 (Dkk1) precludes mammary placode formation altogether (Chu et al. 2004). Expression of *Wnt10b* and *Lef1* is reduced in *Fgf10* hypomorphs, while somitic expression of *Fgf10* remains unaffected in *Dkk1* transgenic mice placing Fgf10/Fgfr2b upstream of the Wnt/β-catenin pathway in placode induction (Chu et al. 2004; Veltmaat et al. 2006). How Fgf10 impinges on Wnt/β-catenin activity at the molecular level is unknown.

The Eda pathway is another example of a signalling cascade that intersects with the canonical Wnt pathway. Binding of Eda to its epithelially expressed receptor Edar leads to the activation of the transcription factor NF-κB (Lindfors et al. 2013). In humans, loss-of-function mutations in *EDA*, *EDAR*, or the essential intracellular signalling mediator *EDARADD* cause hypohidrotic ectodermal dysplasia, a rare congenital disorder characterized by impaired development of various ectodermal appendages including the breast (Clarke et al. 1987; Wahlbuhl-Becker et al. 2017). In *Eda* null mice, all mammary buds form but are smaller in size (Lan et al. 2024; Voutilainen et al. 2015), while multiple supernumerary mammary placodes (and later mammary glands) develop along the mammary line in Eda overexpressing (K14-*Eda*) mice (Mustonen et al. 2004). *Ex vivo* tissue culture experiments showed that their formation can be dose-dependently inhibited by suppressing Wnt signalling (Voutilainen et al. 2015). An unbiased screen for immediate Eda-induced genes revealed that Eda target genes are numerous, and include e.g. parathyroid hormone-like hormone-related peptide (Pthlh, a.k.a. PTHrP). Importantly, several Wnt pathway components were induced including *Wnt10a* and *Wnt10b*, suggesting a direct link between these two pathways (Voutilainen et al. 2012, 2015). However, also negative Wnt regulators such as *Dkk4* and *Lrp4* were upregulated, evidencing a complex interplay between the two pathways. These results mirror the findings from developing hair follicles where the crosstalk between Eda/Edar and the Wnt ligands and their secreted inhibitors are important for placode patterning and for defining the correct placode size, through a reaction-diffusion type of process (Biggs and Mikkola 2014; Zhang et al. 2009). The same may apply also to mammary placodes.

Another pathway with a possible link to Wnt/β-catenin signalling is the neuregulin 3 (Nrg3) pathway, which plays an inductive role in mammary placode formation (Kogata et al. 2013). Keratin 14 (K14) promoter-driven overexpression of *Nrg3* induces a supernumerary mammary primordium between placodes 3 and 4 (Panchal et al. 2007), while *scaramanga* (*Nrg3*^{Ska}) embryos carrying a hypomorphic allele of *Nrg3* are characterized by hypoplasia or aplasia of mammary placode 3 (Howard et al. 2005). In addition, mesenchymal cell condensation and expression of mesenchymal markers such as Lef1 is reduced, indicative of compromised specification of the mammary mesenchyme in *Nrg3*^{Ska} embryos (Kogata et al. 2014). However, the mesenchymal effects appear indirect, as the expression patterns of *Nrg3* and its cognate receptor *ErbB4* at this developmental stage suggest autocrine epithelial signalling (Kogata et al. 2013).

Besides Lef1, a few other transcriptional regulators have been implicated in early placode morphogenesis (Spina and Cowin 2021). Once the mammary field has been specified, *Tbx3* expression is upregulated in the nascent placodes; in its absence, mammary placodes fail to form with the exception of an occasional placode 2. A complex interplay between the Tbx3, Wnt, and Fgf10/Fgfr2b pathways, involving potential feedback mechanisms has been proposed to govern placode induction, but the details remain to be clarified (Douglas and Papaioannou 2013). Conditional K14-Cre-driven deletion of Gata3, which later marks the luminal population, leads to absent/severely hypoplastic placodes, with little to no ductal growth thereafter (Asselin-Labat et al. 2007). Placode morphogenesis is arrested at an aberrant placode stage also in compound mouse mutants lacking *Msx1* and *Msx2*, two related homeobox genes co-expressed in the mammary epithelium (Satokata et al. 2000). Transcriptional profiling of mammary bud (E13.5) and early branching stage (E16.5) epithelia from an epithelial Wnt gain-of-function mouse model expressing stabilized β-catenin revealed >30-fold upregulation of both *Msx1* and *Msx2* (Satta et al. 2024b), suggesting that Wnt/β-catenin signalling induces and/or maintains their expression.

It has long been recognized that mammary placodes and buds are much less proliferative than the surrounding epidermal cells (Balinsky 1950; Lee et al. 2011; Trela et al. 2021) and appear even less proliferative than other skin appendage placodes (Biggs and Mikkola 2014). The underlying reason has remained enigmatic, but studies on mouse mutants lacking the negative Wnt/β-catenin pathway regulator Lrp4, or its ligand Sostdc1 (a.k.a. Wise, ectodin), imply that canonical Wnt signalling plays a role (Ahn et al. 2013; Närhi et al. 2012). In *Lrp4* mutants, cell proliferation is greatly reduced in the interplacodal region, and instead of epidermal fate, these cells adopt a mammary fate leading to fused and larger mammary buds, a phenotype normalized by reducing the dose of Wnt co-receptors Lrp5/6 (Ahn et al. 2013). In addition, absence of signalling pathway activity may contribute to the observed low mitotic rate. The embryonic mammary gland is devoid of Hedgehog (Hh) signalling activity (Hatsell and Cowin 2006), a major driver of proliferation in developing hair follicles and teeth (Biggs and Mikkola 2014). Gli3 is a transcriptional regulator of the Hh pathway that generally represses Hh signalling but can also act as an activator. The importance of the Hh pathway repression in early mammary development was revealed by the analysis of *Extra-toes* (*Gli3^{xt}*) mice, where the repressor function is abrogated. As a result, placodes 3 and 5 are absent, while other buds are hypoplastic and often fail to invaginate (Hatsell and Cowin 2006; Veltmaat et al. 2006; Lee et al. 2011).

The relative quiescence of the mammary primordia implies that mechanisms other than locally enhanced proliferation drive placode morphogenesis, cell migration being the prevailing hypothesis for long (Balinsky 1950; Propper et al. 2013). However, it was only recently when high-resolution whole-mount confocal live imaging enabled visualization of placode cell behaviours that the importance of cell migration in placode formation was confirmed (Trela et al. 2021). Further analysis indicated that the placode-to-bud transition is primarily fuelled by influx of new cells, supported by (low level of) proliferation and cellular hypertrophy, the latter coinciding with basally located cells acquiring a characteristic elongated and apically constricted shape (Kogata et al. 2014; Lee et al. 2011; Trela et al. 2021). The signalling pathway(s) underlying cellular motility and hypertrophy are currently unknown, but good candidates have emerged. Epithelial cell size is reduced in *Eda* (Lan et al. 2024), and in particular *Nrg3^{Ska}* mutants (Kogata et al. 2014). In developing hair placodes—that also form by directional cell migration—Wnt/β-catenin and Eda pathways were shown to increase cell motility (Ahtiainen et al. 2014) and may have a similar function in mammary primordia.

Later stages of mammary bud morphogenesis involve additional cellular mechanisms contributing to the formation of the subtended, bulb-shaped bud. The mechanisms of this invagination process remained long elusive, but a recent study shed some light on it by revealing that thin, elongated keratinocytes form a contractile rim around the mammary bud. These cells apply force via the actomyosin network and move in a circle-like fashion to promote invagination (Trela et al. 2021). Concurrently, the 'neck' of the mature, bulb-shaped mammary bud forms. Additional cellular mechanisms contributing to bud invagination undoubtedly exist but are currently unknown.

As the transition from placodes to buds is a gradual process, it seems plausible that many of the same molecular mechanisms that regulate placode morphogenesis are important also in bud formation. For example, several mouse models in which genes positively regulating the Wnt pathway have been inactivated such as *Lrp5*, *Lrp6*, or *Pygo2*, have hypoplastic mammary buds suggesting that Wnt signalling aids in the recruitment of mammary cells and/or their survival (Spina and Cowin 2021). Likewise, in *Tbx3* heterozygous mice where all mammary buds form, their maintenance is often compromised leading to the absence of the ductal tree (Jerome-Majewska et al. 2005). In mice lacking *Fgf20*, a Wnt and Eda target gene expressed in the mammary epithelium, mammary primordia are smaller from early bud to late sprout stages, though later in embryogenesis the ductal tree appears normal (Elo et al. 2017).

As mammary placodes gradually grow and take the shape of the bud, prominent changes take place also in the adjacent mesenchyme. From E12.5 onward, the mammary bud is surrounded by condensed mesenchymal cells that express markers such as Lef1, Ar, and oestrogen receptor 1 (alpha) (Esr1) (Spina and Cowin 2021). Classic tissue recombination experiments have revealed the remarkable inductive role of the mammary mesenchyme. When E13.5 mammary mesenchyme isolated from mouse embryos was recombined with skin epidermis from rat embryos, branched epithelial structures formed which upon grafting to lactating female hosts, developed into lobulo-alveolar structures and expressed milk proteins (Cunha and Hom 1996). Given this confirmed role of the mammary mesenchyme to instruct mammogenesis, identification of the factors conferring the mesenchyme its inductive capacity is of high interest.

Two signalling pathways have well-recognized roles in the specification of the primary mammary mesenchyme, Pthlh, and Wnt/β-catenin. The role of the Pthlh pathway was discovered by the analysis of mice lacking *Pthlh*, expressed in the mammary bud, and its receptor *Pthr1*, expressed in the mesenchyme, each with an identical mammary gland phenotype (Wysolmerski et al. 1998). In their absence, mesenchymal compaction is compromised, and expression of Lef1, Esr1, Ar, and other markers of the mammary mesenchyme is either abolished or severely reduced indicating defective specification of the mammary mesenchyme (Hiremath et al. 2012). This in turn impairs epithelial–mesenchymal tissue cross-talk: mammary epithelial cells are shunted towards epidermal fate, the buds fail to sprout properly, and nipples do not form (Foley et al. 2001; Hens et al. 2009; Wysolmerski et al. 1998). In human foetuses carrying inactivating mutations in *PTHR1*, breasts and nipples are also absent (Wysolmerski et al. 2001). In mice, inactivation of mesenchymal Wnt/β-catenin activity resembles loss of *Pthlh*/*Pth1r* with respect to both fibroblast condensation and mesenchymal marker gene expression. The similarities in the phenotypes were explained when it was shown that mesenchymal Wnt activity depends on Pthlh signalling, though the underlying molecular basis remains to be clarified (Hiremath et al. 2012).

2.4 Acquisition of Branching Competency

The invaginated mammary bud grows rather slowly until branching begins and therefore the stages after E13.5 have often been called the 'rest phase' of the embryonic mammary gland (Cowin and Wysolmerski 2010). However, recent studies show that growth is slowest between E13.5 and E14.5 followed by a substantial surge thereafter, reflecting a concomitant increase in cell proliferation (Lan et al. 2024). As branching commences, the overall proliferation rate stabilizes but becomes regionalized such that the nascent tips exhibit higher proliferative activity compared to the prospective main duct (Balinsky 1950; Lan et al. 2024; Satta et al. 2024a). At the same time, expression of basal and luminal lineage markers becomes gradually segregated (Lilja et al. 2018; Van Keymeulen et al. 2011; Voutilainen et al. 2015; Wuidart et al. 2018), but whether a causal link exists between lineage commitment and onset of branching morphogenesis is currently unknown.

The mechanisms driving mammary epithelial cells from the rest phase to active branching remain poorly understood. However, while an increase in proliferation is undoubtedly a prerequisite, it alone seems not to suffice. This is suggested by the fact that only the E16.5 mesenchyme-free, intact epithelial mammary sprouts, not those from earlier stages, are capable of branching in 3D Matrigel, despite the robust increase in the proliferation rate observed already a day earlier (Lan et al. 2024). These data also underscore the essential role of epithelial–mesenchymal interactions for acquisition of branching competency. The pioneering work by Klaus Kratochwil who cultivated E12 to E16 intact mammary epithelia with E12 mammary mesenchyme *ex vivo* implies that the epithelium governs initiation of branching, as the onset of branching correlated with the epithelial age (Kratochwil 1969). In accordance with this, when E13.5 to E16.5 epithelial rudiments were cultured with mesenchymes from different developmental stages, onset of branching faithfully followed the age of the epithelium (Lan et al.

2024). In other words, mesenchymes from advanced embryonic stages fail to advance onset of branching in younger epithelia. However, only mammary mesenchyme can confer the ability to branch: E13.5 mammary epithelia remain inert when recombined with the salivary gland mesenchyme, yet upon acquiring branching ability at E16.5, they grow rigorously with salivary mesenchyme (Kratochwil 1969; Lan et al. 2024). Collectively, current knowledge suggests that mammary mesenchyme-specific cues are necessary until E16.5 to maintain mammary cell identity, support survival, and stimulate onset of proliferation. Thereafter, epithelial cells acquire the capacity to branch in a stroma-free organoid culture (Lan et al. 2024) and maintain lineage identity even when cultured with the salivary gland mesenchyme (Sakakura et al. 1976). Moreover, when dissociated into single cells, they gain the ability to reconstitute the ductal tree in the fat pad transplantation assay (Spike et al. 2012).

Of the potential pathways controlling onset of branching, Pthlh/Pth1r signalling is best studied. However, Pth1r's exclusive mesenchymal expression (Wysolmerski et al. 1998) shows that the effect is indirect. As described above, the inability of *Pthrp*- and *Pth1r*-null mammary glands to branch may reflect the failure of the epithelial cells to maintain the mammary fate rather than a direct morphogenetic effect on branching. The same mechanism may also explain the similar mammary gland phenotype observed in *Msx2* deficient mice, as *Msx2* is expressed at high levels in the mesenchyme at this developmental stage and is significantly reduced in *Pthlh* and *Pth1r* null mice (Hens et al. 2007; Satokata et al. 2000). Eda is a mesenchymal factor implicated in branching initiation: K14-*Eda* mice display precocious branching already at E14.5 (Voutilainen et al. 2012), while loss of *Eda* delays onset of branching (Lan et al. 2024; Voutilainen et al. 2012). This may be attributed to the ability of Edar to enhance cell division as the phenotypic changes observed in *Eda* loss- and gain-of-function mice correlate with temporal changes in epithelial cell proliferation (Lan et al. 2024; Voutilainen et al. 2012).

The molecular changes occurring in the epithelium that provide branching ability are poorly understood. For a long time, epithelial Wnt activity has been considered a good candidate to regulate onset of branching, supported by analysis of *Lrp6*$^{-/-}$ mice where development halts at an unbranched sprout stage (Lindvall et al. 2009). Moreover, mice overexpressing Wnt1 (MMTV-*Wnt1*) have a highly branched ductal tree at E18 (Cunha and Hom 1996), a phenotype identical to that observed in K14-*Eda* mice (Voutilainen et al. 2012), implying precocious onset of branching, though this has not been formally demonstrated. Perhaps counterintuitively, analysis of several transgenic Wnt reporter mice indicates a significant decrease in epithelial Wnt/β-catenin signalling activity when the buds progress to branching (Chu et al. 2004; Satta et al. 2024b; van Amerongen et al. 2012). This conclusion was supported by transcriptional profiling of E13.5 and E16.5 mammary epithelia revealing >90% decrease in the levels of *Axin2*, the most commonly used transcriptional readout of Wnt/β-catenin activity (Satta et al. 2024b). We have recently tested the effect of forced β-catenin activation in embryonic mammary epithelium. Although genetic stabilization of β-catenin instigated sprout-like outgrowths at E13.5, by E16.5 epithelial growth was severely impaired with limited expansion thereafter (Satta et al. 2024b). This, together with the reporter expression data, seems to suggest that after the bud stage, downregulation of epithelial Wnt activity might be a prerequisite for branching. What could explain the seemingly contradictory results of the different mouse models? One plausible explanation is that the target tissue is different: in the *Lrp6*$^{-/-}$ embryos also the fat pad is poorly developed (Lindvall et al. 2009) and in MMTV-*Wnt1* mice, the secreted ligand may also activate signalling in the mesenchyme. Hence the epithelial effects might be secondary. On the other hand, Wnts typically induce the expression of their feedback inhibitors that tune the strength and location of the signalling activity, and such processes could be important also for onset of branching when proliferation and cellular behaviours become regionalized (Myllymäki et al. 2023). Evidently, mammary epithelia expressing stabilized β-catenin are insensitive to feedback inhibition that takes place upstream in the signalling cascade.

As the bud progresses towards branching, the epithelial transcriptomes change drastically, many transcription factors being strongly downregulated while others show the opposite trend (Satta et al. 2024b). The latter are good candidates to regulate mammary epithelium's growth and branching potential, as shown by recent studies on transcription factor Sox10 (Dravis et al. 2015). Expression of Sox10 is undetectable at E13.5 but increases gradually such that at E16.5, the newly formed tips express high levels of Sox10, a finding in good agreement with a 250-fold increase at the *Sox10* transcript level (Dravis et al. 2015; Satta et al. 2024b). Remarkably, although *Sox10*$^{-/-}$ mammary buds generate initial sprouts, they fail to branch in the fat pad (Mertelmeyer et al. 2020). The normal upregulation of Sox10 fails in mice expressing stabilized β-catenin (Satta et al. 2024b), suggesting suppressed Wnt/β-catenin is necessary for Sox10 expression at late embryogenesis.

2.5 Branching Morphogenesis: Paracrine Factors at the Centre Stage

Once the mammary sprout reaches the fat pad precursor tissue, branching commences. Due to the asynchrony in the onset of branching, the anterior glands have often been regarded as 'more branched' than the posterior ones at birth. However, 3D morphometric analysis of approx. 100 E16.5 to E18.5 mammary glands revealed that, despite these temporal differences, the frequency of branching (number of branch tips generated per the total length of the ductal tree) is remarkably constant across different pairs of glands and developmental stages (Satta et al. 2024a). While this observation might imply a stereotypical branching pattern, it is not the case. Matching pairs of mammary glands differ from one embryo to another, and between the left and right sides of the same embryo (Satta et al. 2024a; Veltmaat et al. 2003). Furthermore, adjacent branch points are not evenly spaced but follow an almost random distribution, consistent with a stochastic branching regime (Satta et al. 2024a). Supporting this view, live imaging of whole mammary gland explants revealed bifurcating tips with visible clefts in branches of variable lengths (Satta et al. 2024a; Myllymäki et al. 2023).

In principle, new branches can form by two mechanisms: tip bifurcation (or splitting) and side branching (or lateral branching). For example, the kidney and salivary gland utilize tip splitting only, while both modes are observed in developing lungs (Lang et al. 2021; Myllymäki and Mikkola 2019). Early observations on cultured embryonic mammary glands suggested the architecture is asymmetric (Kratochwil 1969). Symmetric (dichotomous) patterns arise by tip bifurcation, where every branch creates two new branches in the order of n^2. This symmetry can be broken by additional side branching, which is well documented in the mammary gland during the oestrous cycle and pregnancy (Brisken and Ataca 2015). Small branches protruding from the sides of ducts have been observed also in embryonic mammary glands, commonly interpreted as side branches (Kratochwil 1969; Propper et al. 2013). However, branches may also terminate 'early', as predicted based on computational modelling on reconstructed pubertal mammary glands (Hannezo et al. 2017), and hence a small lateral bud could either represent an incipient side branch, or a branch that formed earlier through bifurcation but ceased to grow. Direct evidence of side branching was recently obtained by time-lapse imaging of cultured embryonic glands, revealing a prevalence of ~75% of all branching events (Satta et al. 2024a; Myllymäki et al. 2023). The *in vivo* architecture was formally shown to be non-dichotomous, further supporting the notion that side branching is common during embryonic mammary gland development (Satta et al. 2024a).

Pioneering tissue recombination studies have established the importance of the mesenchymal tissue in epithelial patterning, not only for mammary gland but also for other branched organs

(Lang et al. 2021). When E16.5 mammary gland epithelium was recombined with embryonic salivary gland mesenchyme, the branching pattern was described as salivary-like, leading the authors to conclude that the mesenchyme dictates the branching pattern (Kratochwil 1969; Sakakura et al. 1976). These ideas were recently tested by modern methods combining fluorescent tissues with live imaging. Although the mammary epithelium recombined with the salivary gland mesenchyme appeared salivary-like in ductal density and the speed of growth, as expected based on prior reports, time-lapse evidence revealed that branching was still mammary-like, both lateral branching and terminal bifurcation occurring at similar frequencies as in control mammary glands (Lan et al. 2024). Similar conclusions were drawn from embryonic mammary epithelial organoids cultured in 3D (Myllymäki et al. 2023). Thus, although the mesenchyme governs the growth rate and branching frequency, the mode of branching appears to be mammary epithelium-intrinsic.

Various signalling pathways play a role in branching morphogenesis, with receptor tyrosine kinase pathways serving as significant positive regulators across different branched organs. Specifically, Fgf signalling is conserved, although the conservation of downstream effects remains less clear (Goodwin and Nelson 2020; Lang et al. 2021). Several Fgf ligands are expressed in the embryonic and pubertal fat pad, most prominently Fgf2, Fgf7, and Fgf10 (Lan et al. 2024; Zhang et al. 2014), and the importance of Fgfr2b in pubertal branching morphogenesis has long been recognized (Rivetti et al. 2020). The early developmental arrest of the Fgfr2b null mammary glands precludes further analysis (Mailleux et al. 2002). Epithelial deletion of Fgfr1 reduces the number of ramifications significantly during the prepubertal period (Pond et al. 2013) and may imply a defect already during embryogenesis. In line with these findings, the pan-Fgfr inhibitor SU5402 suppresses growth of cultured embryonic mammary glands, while Fgf10 has the opposite effect (Satta et al. 2024a). When *Fgf10* is deleted from mouse embryos, the only mammary bud that develops, bud 4, forms a primary sprout but fails to branch (Mailleux et al. 2002). Also, the fat pad is underdeveloped, reflecting Fgf10's pleiotropic role, extending beyond the epithelium to adipocyte differentiation (Sakaue et al. 2002).

The ErbB pathway also promotes branching morphogenesis, likely through multiple receptors. Loss of either Egfr, or the metalloproteinase Adam17 that processes many Egf-family ligands, leads to a marked 3–4 fold reduction in the number of branches generated from the primary duct by birth (Sternlicht et al. 2005), while exogenously added Egf-family ligands amphiregulin and epigen increase the size and branch number in cultured embryonic mammary glands (Voutilainen et al. 2012). Recombination experiments on post-natal tissues suggest that Egfr activity is required in the fat pad (Wiesen et al. 1999), but whether this applies to the fat pad precursor is unknown. Inactivation of either ErbB2 or ErbB3 leads to early embryonic lethality, but fat pad transplantation assays of the embryonic mammary rudiments suggest that they may also play a role in embryonic branching morphogenesis (Jackson-Fisher et al. 2004, 2008).

Eda is an example of a mesenchymal factor regulating growth in many branched organs of ectodermal origin, likely downstream of mesenchymal Wnt/β-catenin signalling, as shown by studies in the salivary gland mesenchyme (Häärä et al. 2011). In embryonic mammary glands, in addition to its ability to induce precocious branching, the ductal trees of K14-*Eda* mice grow much faster, and by E18.5, they are about 5 times larger than in the control littermates (Voutilainen et al. 2012). Conversely, the ductal trees of *Eda*$^{-/-}$ embryos, or those with suppressed NF-κB activity, are smaller, and in K14-*Eda* background, abrogation of NF-κB activity fully inhibits the hyper-growth phenotype (Voutilainen et al. 2012). The effects of Eda are likely mediated by multiple target genes. In addition to *Pthlh* and Wnt pathway genes, Eda induces the expression of ErbB ligands and Fgfs (Voutilainen et al. 2015). Deletion of *Fgf20* in the K14-*Eda* background greatly attenuated the branching phenotype (Elo et al. 2017).

The observation that the mammary epithelium grows faster and forms a denser ductal network in the salivary gland mesenchyme, while the salivary gland epithelium exhibits poor growth in the mammary mesenchyme (Kratochwil 1969; Lan et al. 2024), suggests that differences in mesenchymal signalling molecules govern the epithelial growth rate, as well as determine whether an 'open', mammary-like or a dense salivary-like ductal tree forms. To identify potential candidates, we performed RNA-sequencing of salivary and mammary gland mesenchymes and focused on differentially expressed genes encoding paracrine factors and other extracellular molecules (Lan et al. 2024). This analysis revealed that several signalling molecules such as Eda, Fgf10, insulin-like growth factor 1 (Igf-1), and Igf-2 are expressed at higher levels in the salivary gland mesenchyme, suggesting multiple growth factors contribute to the observed growth differences. On the other hand, many negative regulators of the Wnt pathway showed the reverse pattern, suggesting that the mammary mesenchyme may represent a Wnt-suppressed milieu (Lan et al. 2024).

As discussed in the previous section, the Wnt/β-catenin pathway has a role in branching morphogenesis that might be exerted in part through the mesenchyme. However, this possibility has not obtained much attention, possibly due to the lack of suitable mouse models. Fibroblasts fail to acquire dermal fate if the Wnt/β-catenin signalling is inactivated in the embryonic mesenchyme too early, while early mesenchymal activation via stabilization of β-catenin causes embryonic lethality ~E13.5 (Biggs and Mikkola 2014). To overcome this challenge, we combined *ex vivo* organ culture, virus-vector mediated Cre delivery, and tissue recombination to achieve a mosaic β-catenin activation in the fat pad precursor tissue (Lan et al. 2024). This led to an enhancement of ductal growth implying that Wnt/β-catenin signalling induces the expression of paracrine growth factors. Igf-1 was identified as a candidate, based on a prior screen of Wnt-regulated genes in postnatal mammary fibroblasts (Wang et al. 2021). Supplementation of Igf-1 on wild-type mammary glands increased ductal growth *ex vivo*, as was expected based on Igf-1's well-described function in promoting cell proliferation and tissue growth. More surprisingly, mice lacking the cognate receptor *Igf1r* displayed a severe branching phenotype: the buds formed sprouts but very few branches if any formed by E18.5 and mammary bud 3 was missing altogether (Lan et al. 2024). *Igf1r* null embryos are about half the size of wild-type embryos at E18.5, but even after normalization to body size, the difference was highly significant and unique to the mammary gland, as salivary glands did branch and the size reduction appeared proportional to the body size (Lan et al. 2024).

The role of TGF-β signalling pathway as a negative regulator of mammary gland growth and branching was introduced already three decades ago, based on loss- and gain-of-function on studies during puberty (McNally and Martin 2011). This role can be extended to the embryo as exogenous TGF-β1 not only inhibits growth but also decreases branch point frequency in *ex vivo* cultured mammary glands. When supplemented locally as beads, ductal tips preferentially avoided TGF-β1 releasing beads (Satta et al. 2024a). The existence of an intrinsic 'spacer' that maintains the open architecture of the mammary gland has been largely attributed to TGF-β signalling activity (Nelson et al. 2006). Interestingly, one of the downstream targets of TGF-β signalling is Wnt5a – a ligand associated with the non-canonical Wnt pathway, which restricts the sites of side branch formation during puberty (Roarty and Serra 2007). However, *Wnt5a* null mice have no embryonic mammary gland phenotype (Chu et al. 2004), indicating additional targets may be at play in the embryo.

2.6 Branching Morphogenesis: Cellular Behaviours

The processes of tip bifurcation and side branching are seemingly different forms of epithelial remodelling with potentially unique cellular mechanisms. During post-natal development, they have been proposed to be separated by developmental stage and at least partially governed by different signals, although both occur simultaneously in the embryo. Cells may respond differently to morphogens based on their localization, but whether this is because tip and duct cells are somehow different or only their circumstances differ, remains unclear. Signalling pathway activity is influenced by tissue geometry, which may locally regulate new branch formation (Nelson et al. 2013).

Time-lapse imaging on *ex vivo* cultured embryonic mammary rudiments has provided evidence regarding cell behaviours involved in branching, although how these are governed by signals, remains to be elucidated. Fresh progenitors are generated at the branch tips and are channelled into the trailing duct based on a gradient of cell movement that exists along the distal branch, which together with cells' directionality forms a basis for branch elongation. Cell cycle activity does not drive elongation, but rather replenishes the reservoir of migratory cells (Myllymäki et al. 2023). Branches may also elongate by tissue rearrangements, as suggested based on progressive lengthening and narrowing of the main duct between E16 and E18, occurring without gross change in the volume. The same phenomenon could also be detected in growing branches by time-lapse imaging (Satta et al. 2024a). This may be governed by the planar cell polarity (PCP) pathway (Satta et al. 2024b; Smith et al. 2019), which is known to facilitate tissue rearrangements such as convergent extension (Butler and Wallingford 2017). Mice carrying a dominant negative missense mutation, or a null allele of *Vangl2*, a PCP component, display a stunted outgrowth phenotype (Satta et al. 2024a; Smith et al. 2019), but the great variation in the embryonic ductal trees of mutant mice makes it challenging to pinpoint the exact defect.

In contrast to elongating branches, tip bifurcation is associated with localized suppression of both cell cycle activity and cell movement at the nascent branch point, which correlates with low levels of Erk activity in contrast to daughter tips where activity is high (Myllymäki et al. 2023). Erk signalling may be involved in regulating actomyosin contractility, which is required for epithelial branching and is likewise high in branching tips. Less is known about the mechanisms of side branching in the embryo, although it occurs mainly in distal branches that have a relatively high cell cycle activity compared to branches closer to the main duct (Satta et al. 2024a; Myllymäki et al. 2023). The basement membrane remains intact, but remodelling of the adhesion components has been described, though their functional relevance is currently unknown (Howard 2012). The mesenchymal tissue may also play a mechanical role in branching beyond supplying morphogens. Evidence of this is supported by findings that mesenchymal fibroblasts facilitate branching of the mammary epithelial organoids also in the absence of exogenous growth factors based on direct contact and contractility (Sumbal et al. 2024). Furthermore, stromal extracellular matrix (ECM) deposition may contribute to stabilization of bifurcated tips (Nerger et al. 2021). Remodelling of the stromal ECM is important during post-natal development, as exemplified by the requirement of matrix metalloproteinase (MMP) activity (Feinberg et al. 2018; Wiseman et al. 2003) and that the treatment of *ex vivo* cultured embryonic mammary glands with GM6001, a broad range MMP inhibitor, also impairs growth (Hens et al. 2009). Integrins, a major family of cell adhesion receptors, are likely involved, but their global deletion often leads to embryonic lethality warranting conditional mouse models.

2.7 Concluding Remarks

While the pathways, and to some extent the cellular behaviours, governing embryonic mammary gland morphogenesis have been discovered, several questions remain unanswered. How is mammary cell identity determined? The pathways critical for placode formation such as the Wnt, Fgf, and Eda, regulate placode formation also in other ectodermal appendages, so what confers organ identity? The answer may lie in the distinct use of two pathways, the Hh and Pthlh. As described above, mesenchymal Pth1r signalling is essential for the maintenance of mammary epithelial cell identity but the molecular mechanism remains elusive, though mesenchymal Bmp has been implicated (Hens et al. 2007, Hens 2009). On the other hand, Hh signalling is repressed during embryonic mammogenesis, while it is essential for the downgrowth of hair and tooth buds (Biggs and Mikkola 2014). Intriguingly, when Hh activity was abrogated in the hair follicle epithelium by deleting Smoothened, an obligate signalling receptor, the resulting appendages gained mammary gland-like features (Gritli-Linde et al. 2007). In hair placodes, Sonic hedgehog (Shh), one of the three Hh family members, is expressed downstream of Wnts and Eda/Edar. However, *Shh* expression is undetectable in mammary buds despite active Wnt and Edar signalling in these cells. How this is achieved is unknown, but one possibility is that the level of Wnt signalling is critical. In mice where high Wnt activity was achieved via β-catenin stabilization, *Shh* and many other hair follicle-specific genes, were ectopically expressed early on in the mammary buds and along the mammary line, followed by epidermal signature genes (Satta et al. 2024b). Similarly, a hair follicle/epidermal differentiation program was observed upon sustained β-catenin activation in the adult (Lloyd-Lewis et al. 2022).

In hair follicles, Hh signalling has important functions both in the epithelium and in the condensed mesenchyme where it regulates the formation of the dermal condensate, the hair follicle-specific mesenchymal compartment (Biggs and Mikkola 2014). In *Gli3*^{xt} mammary buds, ectopic Hh activity is confined to the mesenchyme, further highlighting the importance of the mesenchyme in the maintenance of mammary cell fate. If an E13.5 mammary bud epithelium is transplanted next to a dermal condensate, it loses its identity and adopts hair follicle fate and morphogenesis (Satta et al. 2024b). In support of the idea that suppression of Hh activity together with Pthlh signalling have a pivotal role in defining mammary cell identity, a recent study reported the generation of multi-lineage mammary organoids from mouse embryonic stem cells by adapting a previously developed hair follicle-forming skin organoid model (Sahu et al. 2024). Transformation of the dermal mesenchyme into a mammary-specific type was achieved by sequential activation of Bmp4, Pthlh, and inhibition of Hh activity. These organoids reconstituted the mammary gland upon fat pad transplantation and produced milk proteins in response to lactogenic hormones (Sahu et al. 2024).

Another important question relates to the onset of branching morphogenesis. How do the quiescent mammary epithelial cells gain their outgrowth potential? Does this require epigenetic changes that either make them responsive to the cues from the fat pad or change their responses to these signals? This process is temporally associated with the emergence of basal and luminal lineages, but what initially triggers lineage segregation and how is it impacted by mesenchymal factors is poorly understood (for more discussion on this topic, see Chap. 5). While different experimental approaches will be needed to answer these questions, novel insights can be expected from single-cell RNA-sequencing (for more discussion on this topic, see Chap. 4).

The mechanisms of branching morphogenesis remain far from resolved. As introduced in previous chapters, several signalling pathways have been implicated in embryonic branching morphogenesis, typically based on examination of the number of branches at birth. However, it has remained unclear if only growth was affected (i.e. the ductal tree was smaller/larger, but branch point frequency unaltered), or if there was a genuine branching phenotype (decreased/increased branch point frequency), as these parameters are rarely reported. Some phenotypes may also simply reflect delayed development secondary to compromised bud/sprout morphogenesis. For these reasons, care should be taken when interpreting the results. In the future, further insights can be obtained by combining high-resolution time-lapse imaging with gene manipulations, but these are cumbersome experiments due to the time it takes to generate the necessary mouse crosses for fluorescent imaging and the rather challenging *ex vivo* culture methods. Some of these challenges can be overcome by applying factors of interest (signalling molecules, inhibitors, small molecule drugs) to the culture medium of *ex vivo* cultivated embryonic mammary glands. However, in these cases the effects are ubiquitous, affecting all cell types in the explant (provided that the target molecule is expressed in all cells), while *in vivo*, the activities may be more localized.

Embryonic mammary gland development lays the foundation for morphogenesis during puberty and the reproductive cycle, and many of the same principles apply to postnatal development. Importantly, embryonic mammary gland development is regulated by pathways and cellular processes with great relevance to breast cancer (Abreu de Oliveira et al. 2022; Lee 2022; Oliphant et al. 2020; Seldin et al. 2017). Embryonic development involves cellular plasticity that is often recapitulated in cancer, where cells can undergo dedifferentiation, contributing to tumour heterogeneity. Understanding how normal tissue undergoes cellular differentiation and branching morphogenesis may inform strategies to promote reversion of cancerous cells to a more differentiated state and restrain aberrant cellular behaviours that enable breaching of the basement membrane and invasion. Signalling pathways with essential functions in embryonic mammary gland development, such as Fgf and Wnt/β--catenin, are often dysregulated in breast cancer. Identifying how these pathways impact embryonic mammary progenitors may provide clues for how they contribute to cancer progression. Aberrant interactions between epithelial cells and the surrounding stroma play a role in tumour initiation, progression, and metastasis. Insights from embryonic development can inform our understanding of these interactions and their impact on cancer.

Acknowledgements We are grateful to all past and present members of the Mikkola lab for the fruitful discussions on the intricacies of embryonic mammary gland development, which never cease to amaze us. Ewelina Trela and Jyoti Satta are acknowledged for their support in preparing Fig. 2.1. The image of the E12.5 mouse embryo in Fig. 2.1 was created with the help of BioRender.

References

Abreu de Oliveira WA, El Laithy Y, Bruna A, Annibali D, Lluis F (2022) Wnt signaling in the breast: from development to disease. Front Cell Dev Biol 10:884467. https://doi.org/10.3389/fcell.2022.884467

Ahn Y, Sims C, Logue JM, Weatherbee SD, Krumlauf R (2013) Lrp4 and Wise interplay controls the formation and patterning of mammary and other skin appendage placodes by modulating Wnt signaling. Development 140(3):583–593. https://doi.org/10.1242/dev.085118

Ahtiainen L, Lefebvre S, Lindfors PH, Renvoise E, Shirokova V, Vartiainen MK, Thesleff I, Mikkola ML (2014) Directional cell migration, but not proliferation, drives hair placode morphogenesis. Dev Cell 28(5):588–602. https://doi.org/10.1016/j.devcel.2014.02.003

Asselin-Labat ML, Sutherland KD, Barker H, Thomas R, Shackleton M, Forrest NC, Hartley L, Robb L, Grosveld FG, van der Wees J, Lindeman GJ, Visvader JE (2007) Nat Cell Biol 9(2):201–209. https://doi.org/10.1038/ncb1530

Balinsky BI (1950) On the prenatal growth of the mammary gland rudiment in the mouse. J Anat 84(3):227 235

Biggs LC, Mikkola ML (2014) Early inductive events in ectodermal appendage morphogenesis. Semin Cell Dev Biol 25-26:11–21. https://doi.org/10.1016/j.semcdb.2014.01.007

Brambell FR, Davis D (1941) Reproduction of the multimammate mouse (*Mastomys erythroleucus* Temm.) of Sierra Leone. Proc Zool Soc Lond Ser B 111:1–11

Brisken C, Ataca D (2015) Endocrine hormones and local signals during the development of the mouse mammary gland. Wiley Interdiscip Rev Dev Biol 4(3):181–195. https://doi.org/10.1002/wdev.172

Butler MT, Wallingford JB (2017) Planar cell polarity in development and disease. Nat Rev Mol Cell Biol 18(6):375–388. https://doi.org/10.1038/nrm.2017.11

Carroll LS, Capecchi MR (2015) Hoxc8 initiates an ectopic mammary program by regulating Fgf10 and Tbx3 expression and Wnt/beta-catenin signaling. Development 142(23):4056–4067. https://doi.org/10.1242/dev.128298

Cho KW, Kim JY, Song SJ, Farrell E, Eblaghie MC, Kim HJ, Tickle C, Jung HS (2006) Molecular interactions between Tbx3 and Bmp4 and a model for dorsoventral positioning of mammary gland development. Proc Natl Acad Sci USA 103(45):16788–16793. https://doi.org/10.1073/pnas.0604645103

Chu EY, Hens J, Andl T, Kairo A, Yamaguchi TP, Brisken C, Glick A, Wysolmerski JJ, Millar SE (2004) Canonical WNT signaling promotes mammary placode development and is essential for initiation of mammary gland morphogenesis. Development 131(19):4819–4829. https://doi.org/10.1242/dev.01347

Clarke A, Phillips DI, Brown R, Harper PS (1987) Clinical aspects of X-linked hypohidrotic ectodermal dysplasia. Arch Dis Child 62(10):989–996. https://doi.org/10.1136/adc.62.10.989

Cowin P, Wysolmerski J (2010) Molecular mechanisms guiding embryonic mammary gland development. Cold Spring Harb Perspect Biol 2(6):a003251. https://doi.org/10.1101/cshperspect.a003251

Cunha GR, Hom YK (1996) Role of mesenchymal-epithelial interactions in mammary gland development.

J Mammary Gland Biol Neoplasia 1(1):21–35. https://doi.org/10.1007/BF02096300
Douglas NC, Papaioannou VE (2013) The T-box transcription factors TBX2 and TBX3 in mammary gland development and breast cancer. J Mammary Gland Biol Neoplasia 18(2):143–147. https://doi.org/10.1007/s10911-013-9282-8
Dravis C, Spike BT, Harrell JC, Johns C, Trejo CL, Southard-Smith EM, Perou CM, Wahl GM (2015) Sox10 regulates stem/progenitor and mesenchymal cell states in mammary epithelial cells. Cell Rep 12(12):2035–2048. https://doi.org/10.1016/j.celrep.2015.08.040
Elo T, Lindfors PH, Lan Q, Voutilainen M, Trela E, Ohlsson C, Huh SH, Ornitz DM, Poutanen M, Howard BA, Mikkola ML (2017) Ectodysplasin target gene Fgf20 regulates mammary bud growth and ductal invasion and branching during puberty. Sci Rep 7(1):5049–5049. https://doi.org/10.1038/s41598-017-04637-1
Feinberg TY, Zheng H, Liu R, Wicha MS, Yu SM, Weiss SJ (2018) Divergent matrix-remodeling strategies distinguish developmental from neoplastic mammary epithelial cell invasion programs. Dev Cell 47(2):145–160 e146. https://doi.org/10.1016/j.devcel.2018.08.025
Foley J, Dann P, Hong J, Cosgrove J, Dreyer B, Rimm D, Dunbar M, Philbrick W, Wysolmerski J (2001) Parathyroid hormone-related protein maintains mammary epithelial fate and triggers nipple skin differentiation during embryonic breast development. Development 128(4):513–525. https://doi.org/10.1242/dev.128.4.513
Goodwin K, Nelson CM (2020) Branching morphogenesis. Development 147(10). https://doi.org/10.1242/dev.184499
Gritli-Linde A, Hallberg K, Harfe BD, Reyahi A, Kannius-Janson M, Nilsson J, Cobourne MT, Sharpe PT, McMahon AP, Linde A (2007) Abnormal hair development and apparent follicular transformation to mammary gland in the absence of hedgehog signaling. Dev Cell 12(1):99–112. https://doi.org/10.1016/j.devcel.2006.12.006
Häärä O, Fujimori S, Schmidt-Ullrich R, Hartmann C, Thesleff I, Mikkola ML (2011) Ectodysplasin and Wnt pathways are required for salivary branching morphogenesis. Development 138(13):2681–2691. https://doi.org/10.1242/dev.079558
Hannezo E, Scheele C, Moad M, Drogo N, Heer R, Sampogna RV, van Rheenen J, Simons BD (2017) A unifying theory of branching morphogenesis. Cell 171(1):242–255 e227. https://doi.org/10.1016/j.cell.2017.08.026
Hatsell SJ, Cowin P (2006) Gli3-mediated repression of Hedgehog targets is required for normal mammary development. Development 133(18):3661–3670. https://doi.org/10.1242/dev.02542
Hens JR, Dann P, Zhang JP, Harris S, Robinson GW, Wysolmerski J (2007) BMP4 and PTHrP interact to stimulate ductal outgrowth during embryonic mammary development and to inhibit hair follicle induction. Development 134(6):1221–1230. https://doi.org/10.1242/dev.000182
Hens J, Dann P, Hiremath M, Pan TC, Chodosh L, Wysolmerski J (2009) Analysis of gene expression in PTHrP−/− mammary buds supports a role for BMP signaling and MMP2 in the initiation of ductal morphogenesis. Dev Dyn 238(11):2713–2724. https://doi.org/10.1002/dvdy.22097
Hiremath M, Dann P, Fischer J, Butterworth D, Boras-Granic K, Hens J, Van Houten J, Shi W, Wysolmerski J (2012) Parathyroid hormone-related protein activates Wnt signaling to specify the embryonic mammary mesenchyme. Development 139(22):4239–4249. https://doi.org/10.1242/dev.080671
Hogg NA, Harrison CJ, Tickle C (1983) Lumen formation in the developing mouse mammary gland. J Embryol Exp Morphol 73:39–57
Howard BA (2012) In the beginning: the establishment of the mammary lineage during embryogenesis. Semin Cell Dev Biol 23(5):574–582. https://doi.org/10.1016/j.semcdb.2012.03.011
Howard BA, Gusterson BA (2000) Human breast development. J Mammary Gland Biol Neoplasia 5(2):119–137. https://doi.org/10.1023/a:1026487120779
Howard B, Panchal H, McCarthy A, Ashworth A (2005) Identification of the scaramanga gene implicates Neuregulin3 in mammary gland specification. Genes Dev 19(17):2078–2090. https://doi.org/10.1101/gad.338505
Jackson-Fisher AJ, Bellinger G, Ramabhadran R, Morris JK, Lee KF, Stern DF (2004) ErbB2 is required for ductal morphogenesis of the mammary gland. Proc Natl Acad Sci USA 101(49):17138–17143. https://doi.org/10.1073/pnas.0407057101
Jackson-Fisher AJ, Bellinger G, Breindel JL, Tavassoli FA, Booth CJ, Duong JK, Stern DF (2008) ErbB3 is required for ductal morphogenesis in the mouse mammary gland. Breast Cancer Res 10(6):R96. https://doi.org/10.1186/bcr2198
Jerome-Majewska LA, Jenkins GP, Ernstoff E, Zindy F, Sherr CJ, Papaioannou VE (2005) Tbx3, the ulnar-mammary syndrome gene, and Tbx2 interact in mammary gland development through a p19Arf/p53-independent pathway. Dev Dyn 234(4):922–933. https://doi.org/10.1002/dvdy.20575
Kogata N, Zvelebil M, Howard BA (2013) Neuregulin 3 and erbb signalling networks in embryonic mammary gland development. J Mammary Gland Biol Neoplasia 18(2):149–154. https://doi.org/10.1007/s10911-013-9286-4
Kogata N, Oliemuller E, Wansbury O, Howard BA (2014) Neuregulin-3 regulates epithelial progenitor cell positioning and specifies mammary phenotype. Stem Cells Dev 23(22):2758–2770. https://doi.org/10.1089/scd.2014.0082
Kratochwil K (1969) Organ specificity in mesenchymal induction demonstrated in the embryonic development of the mammary gland of the mouse. Dev Biol 20(1):46 71. https://doi.org/10.1016/0012-1606(69)90004-9

Kratochwil K, Schwartz P (1976) Tissue interaction in androgen response of embryonic mammary rudiment of mouse: identification of target tissue for testosterone. Proc Natl Acad Sci USA 73(11): 4041–4044. https://doi.org/10.1073/pnas.73.11.4041

Lan Q, Trela E, Lindström R, Satta J, Kaczyńska B, Christensen MM, Holzenberger M, Jernvall J, Mikkola LM (2024) Mesenchyme instructsgrowth while epithelium directs branching in the mouse mammary gland. elife 13:e93326. https://doi.org/10.7554/eLife.93326

Lang C, Conrad L, Iber D (2021) Organ-specific branching morphogenesis. Front Cell Dev Biol 9:671402. https://doi.org/10.3389/fcell.2021.671402

Lee MY (2022) Embryonic programs in cancer and metastasis-insights from the mammary gland. Front Cell Dev Biol 10:938625. https://doi.org/10.3389/fcell.2022.938625

Lee MY, Racine V, Jagadpramana P, Sun L, Yu W, Du T, Spencer-Dene B, Rubin N, Le L, Ndiaye D, Bellusci S, Kratochwil K, Veltmaat JM (2011) Ectodermal influx and cell hypertrophy provide early growth for all murine mammary rudiments, and are differentially regulated among them by Gli3. PLoS One 6(10):e26242. https://doi.org/10.1371/journal.pone.0026242

Lilja AM, Rodilla V, Huyghe M, Hannezo E, Landragin C, Renaud O, Leroy O, Rulands S, Simons BD, Fre S (2018) Clonal analysis of Notch1-expressing cells reveals the existence of unipotent stem cells that retain long-term plasticity in the embryonic mammary gland. Nat Cell Biol 13(6):1. https://doi.org/10.1038/s41556-018-0108-1

Lindfors PH, Voutilainen M, Mikkola ML (2013) Ectodysplasin/NF-kappaB signaling in embryonic mammary gland development. J Mammary Gland Biol Neoplasia 18(2):165–169. https://doi.org/10.1007/s10911-013-9277-5

Lindvall C, Zylstra CR, Evans N, West RA, Dykema K, Furge KA, Williams BO (2009) The Wnt co-receptor Lrp6 is required for normal mouse mammary gland development. PLoS One 4(6):e5813. https://doi.org/10.1371/journal.pone.0005813

Lloyd-Lewis B, Gobbo F, Perkins M, Jacquemin G, Huyghe M, Faraldo MM, Fre S (2022) In vivo imaging of mammary epithelial cell dynamics in response to lineage-biased Wnt/β-catenin activation. Cell Rep 38(10):110461. https://doi.org/10.1016/j.celrep.2022.110461

Mailleux AA, Spencer-Dene B, Dillon C, Ndiaye D, Savona-Baron C, Itoh N, Kato S, Dickson C, Thiery JP, Bellusci S (2002) Role of FGF10/FGFR2b signaling during mammary gland development in the mouse embryo. Development 129(1):53–60. https://doi.org/10.1242/dev.129.1.53

McNally S, Martin F (2011) Molecular regulators of pubertal mammary gland development. Ann Med 43(3):212–234. https://doi.org/10.3109/07853890.2011.554425

McNally S, Stein T (2017) Overview of mammary gland development: a comparison of mouse and human. Methods Mol Biol 1501:1–17. https://doi.org/10.1007/978-1-4939-6475-8_1

Mertelmeyer S, Weider M, Baroti T, Reiprich S, Frob F, Stolt CC, Wagner KU, Wegner M (2020) The transcription factor Sox10 is an essential determinant of branching morphogenesis and involution in the mouse mammary gland. Sci Rep 10(1):17807. https://doi.org/10.1038/s41598-020-74664-y

Mikkola ML, Millar SE (2006) The mammary bud as a skin appendage: unique and shared aspects of development. J Mammary Gland Biol Neoplasia 11(3–4):187–203. https://doi.org/10.1007/s10911-006-9029-x

Mustonen T, Ilmonen M, Pummila M, Kangas AT, Laurikkala J, Jaatinen R, Pispa J, Gaide O, Schneider P, Thesleff I, Mikkola ML (2004) Ectodysplasin A1 promotes placodal cell fate during early morphogenesis of ectodermal appendages. Development 131(20):4907–4919. https://doi.org/10.1242/dev.01377

Myllymäki SM, Mikkola ML (2019) Inductive signals in branching morphogenesis - lessons from mammary and salivary glands. Curr Opin Cell Biol 61:72–78. https://doi.org/10.1016/j.ceb.2019.07.001

Myllymäki SM, Kaczyńska B, Lan Q, Mikkola ML (2023) Spatially coordinated cell cycle activity and motility govern bifurcation of mammary branches. J Cell Biol 222(9). https://doi.org/10.1083/jcb.202209005

Närhi K, Tummers M, Ahtiainen L, Itoh N, Thesleff I, Mikkola ML (2012) Sostdc1 defines the size and number of skin appendage placodes. Dev Biol 364(2):149–161. https://doi.org/10.1016/j.ydbio.2012.01.026

Naylor MJ, Ormandy CJ (2002) Mouse strain-specific patterns of mammary epithelial ductal side branching are elicited by stromal factors. Dev Dyn 225(1):100–105. https://doi.org/10.1002/dvdy.10133

Nelson CM, Vanduijn MM, Inman JL, Fletcher DA, Bissell MJ (2006) Tissue geometry determines sites of mammary branching morphogenesis in organotypic cultures. Science 314(5797):298–300. https://doi.org/10.1126/science.1131000

Nelson DA, Manhardt C, Kamath V, Sui Y, Santamaria-Pang A, Can A, Bello M, Corwin A, Dinn SR, Lazare M, Gervais EM, Sequeira SJ, Peters SB, Ginty F, Gerdes MJ, Larsen M (2013) Quantitative single cell analysis of cell population dynamics during submandibular salivary gland development and differentiation. Biol Open 2(5):439–447. https://doi.org/10.1242/bio.20134309

Nerger BA, Jaslove JM, Elashal HE, Mao S, Kosmrlj A, Link AJ, Nelson CM (2021) Local accumulation of extracellular matrix regulates global morphogenetic patterning in the developing mammary gland. Curr Biol 31(9):1903–1917 e1906. https://doi.org/10.1016/j.cub.2021.02.015

Oftedal OT, Dhouailly D (2013) Evo-devo of the mammary gland. J Mammary Gland Biol Neoplasia 18(2):105–120. https://doi.org/10.1007/s10911-013-9290-8

Oliphant MUJ, Kong D, Zhou H, Lewis MT, Ford HL (2020) Two Sides of the Same Coin: The Role of Developmental pathways and pluripotency factors in normal mammary stem cells and breast cancer metastasis. J Mammary Gland Biol Neoplasia 25(2):85–102. https://doi.org/10.1007/s10911-020-09449-0

Panchal H, Wansbury O, Parry S, Ashworth A, Howard B (2007) Neuregulin3 alters cell fate in the epidermis and mammary gland. BMC Dev Biol 7:105. https://doi.org/10.1186/1471-213X-7-105

Pond AC, Bin X, Batts T, Roarty K, Hilsenbeck S, Rosen JM (2013) Fibroblast growth factor receptor signaling is essential for normal mammary gland development and stem cell function. Stem Cells 31(1):178–189. https://doi.org/10.1002/stem.1266

Propper AY, Howard BA, Veltmaat JM (2013) Prenatal morphogenesis of mammary glands in mouse and rabbit. J Mammary Gland Biol Neoplasia 18(2):93–104. https://doi.org/10.1007/s10911-013-9298-0

Rivetti S, Chen C, Chen C, Bellusci S (2020) Fgf10/Fgfr2b signaling in mammary gland development, homeostasis, and cancer. Front Cell Dev Biol 8:415. https://doi.org/10.3389/fcell.2020.00415

Roarty K, Serra R (2007) Wnt5a is required for proper mammary gland development and TGF-beta-mediated inhibition of ductal growth. Development 134(21):3929–3939. https://doi.org/10.1242/dev.008250

Sahu S, Sahoo S, Sullivan T, O'Sullivan TN, Turan S, Albaugh ME, Burkett S, Tran B, Salomon DS, Kozlov SV, Koehler KR, Jolly MK, Sharan SK (2024) Spatiotemporal modulation of growth factors directs the generation of multilineage mouse embryonic stem cell-derived mammary organoids. Dev Cell 59(2):175–186.e8. https://doi.org/10.1016/j.devcel.2023.12.003

Sakakura T, Nishizuka Y, Dawe CJ (1976) Mesenchyme-dependent morphogenesis and epithelium-specific cytodifferentiation in mouse mammary gland. Science 194(4272):1439–1441. https://doi.org/10.1126/science.827022

Sakaue H, Konishi M, Ogawa W, Asaki T, Mori T, Yamasaki M, Takata M, Ueno H, Kato S, Kasuga M, Itoh N (2002) Requirement of fibroblast growth factor 10 in development of white adipose tissue. Genes Dev 16(8):908–912. https://doi.org/10.1101/gad.983202

Satokata I, Ma L, Ohshima H, Bei M, Woo I, Nishizawa K, Maeda T, Takano Y, Uchiyama M, Heaney S, Peters H, Tang Z, Maxson R, Maas R (2000) Msx2 deficiency in mice causes pleiotropic defects in bone growth and ectodermal organ formation. Nat Genet 24(4):391–395. https://doi.org/10.1038/74231

Satta JP, Lindström R, Myllymäki S-M, Lan Q, Trela E, Prunskaite-Hyyryläinen R, Kaczyńska B, Voutilainen M, Kuure S, Vainio SJ, Mikkola ML (2024a) Exploring the principles of embryonic mammary gland branching morphogenesis. Development 151(15):dev202179. https://doi.org/10.1242/dev.202179

Satta JP, Lan Q, Taketo MM, Mikkola ML (2024b) Stabilization of epithelial β-catenin compromises mammary cell fate acquisition and branching morphogenesis. J Invest Dermatol. 144(6):1223–1237. https://doi.org/10.1016/j.jid.2023.11.018

Seldin L, Le Guelte A, Macara IG (2017) Epithelial plasticity in the mammary gland. Curr Opin Cell Biol 49:59–63. https://doi.org/10.1016/j.ceb.2017.11.012

Smith P, Godde N, Rubio S, Tekeste M, Vladar EK, Axelrod JD, Henderson DJ, Milgrom-Hoffman M, Humbert PO, Hinck L (2019) VANGL2 regulates luminal epithelial organization and cell turnover in the mammary gland. Sci Rep 9(1):7079. https://doi.org/10.1038/s41598-019-43444-8

Spike BT, Engle DD, Lin JC, Cheung SK, La J, Wahl GM (2012) A mammary stem cell population identified and characterized in late embryogenesis reveals similarities to human breast cancer. Cell Stem Cell 10(2):183–197. https://doi.org/10.1016/j.stem.2011.12.018

Spina E, Cowin P (2021) Embryonic mammary gland development. Semin Cell Dev Biol 114:83–92. https://doi.org/10.1016/j.semcdb.2020.12.012

Sternlicht MD, Sunnarborg SW, Kouros-Mehr H, Yu Y, Lee DC, Werb Z (2005) Mammary ductal morphogenesis requires paracrine activation of stromal EGFR via ADAM17-dependent shedding of epithelial amphiregulin. Development 132(17):3923–3933. https://doi.org/10.1242/dev.01966

Sumbal J, Fre S, Sumbalova Koledova Z (2024) Fibroblast-induced mammary epithelial branching depends on fibroblast contractility. PLoS Biol 22(1):e3002093. https://doi.org/10.1371/journal.pbio.3002093

Trela E, Lan Q, Myllymäki SM, Villeneuve C, Lindström R, Kumar V, Wickstrom SA, Mikkola ML (2021) Cell influx and contractile actomyosin force drive mammary bud growth and invagination. J Cell Biol 220(8). https://doi.org/10.1083/jcb.202008062

van Amerongen R, Bowman AN, Nusse R (2012) Developmental stage and time dictate the fate of Wnt/beta-catenin-responsive stem cells in the mammary gland. Cell Stem Cell 11(3):387–400. https://doi.org/10.1016/j.stem.2012.05.023

van Genderen C, Okamura RM, Farinas I, Quo RG, Parslow TG, Bruhn L, Grosschedl R (1994) Development of several organs that require inductive epithelial-mesenchymal interactions is impaired in LEF-1-deficient mice. Genes Dev 8(22):2691–2703. https://doi.org/10.1101/gad.8.22.2691

Van Keymeulen A, Rocha AS, Ousset M, Beck B, Bouvencourt G, Rock J, Sharma N, Dekoninck S, Blanpain C (2011) Distinct stem cells contribute to mammary gland development and maintenance. Nature 479(7372):189–193. https://doi.org/10.1038/nature10573

Veltmaat JM, Mailleux AA, Thiery JP, Bellusci S (2003) Mouse embryonic mammogenesis as a model for the molecular regulation of pattern formation. Differentiation 71(1):1–17. https://doi.org/10.1046/j.1432-0436.2003.700601.x

Veltmaat JM, Van Veelen W, Thiery JP, Bellusci S (2004) Identification of the mammary line in mouse by

Wnt10b expression. Dev Dyn 229(2):349–356. https://doi.org/10.1002/dvdy.10441

Veltmaat JM, Relaix F, Le LT, Kratochwil K, Sala FG, van Veelen W, Rice R, Spencer-Dene B, Mailleux AA, Rice DP, Thiery JP, Bellusci S (2006) Gli3-mediated somitic Fgf10 expression gradients are required for the induction and patterning of mammary epithelium along the embryonic axes. Development 133(12):2325–2335. https://doi.org/10.1242/dev.02394

Voutilainen M, Lindfors PH, Lefebvre S, Ahtiainen L, Fliniaux I, Rysti E, Murtoniemi M, Schneider P, Schmidt-Ullrich R, Mikkola ML (2012) Ectodysplasin regulates hormone-independent mammary ductal morphogenesis via NF-κB. Proc Natl Acad Sci USA 109(15):5744–5749. https://doi.org/10.1073/pnas.1110627109

Voutilainen M, Lindfors PH, Trela E, Lönnblad D, Shirokova V, Elo T, Rysti E, Schmidt-Ullrich R, Schneider P, Mikkola ML (2015) Ectodysplasin/NF-κB promotes mammary cell fate via Wnt/β-catenin pathway. PLoS Genet 11(11):e1005676. https://doi.org/10.1371/journal.pgen.1005676

Wahlbuhl-Becker M, Faschingbauer F, Beckmann MW, Schneider H (2017) Hypohidrotic ectodermal dysplasia: breastfeeding complications due to impaired breast development. Geburtshilfe Frauenheilkd 77(4):377–382. https://doi.org/10.1055/s-0043-100106

Wang J, Song W, Yang R, Li C, Wu T, Dong XB, Zhou B, Guo X, Chen J, Liu Z, Yu QC, Li W, Fu J, Zeng YA (2021) Endothelial Wnts control mammary epithelial patterning via fibroblast signaling. Cell Rep 34(13):108897. https://doi.org/10.1016/j.celrep.2021.108897

Watson CJ, Khaled WT (2020) Mammary development in the embryo and adult: new insights into the journey of morphogenesis and commitment. Development 147(22):dev169862. https://doi.org/10.1242/dev.169862

Wiesen JF, Young P, Werb Z, Cunha GR (1999) Signaling through the stromal epidermal growth factor receptor is necessary for mammary ductal development. Development 126(2):335–344. https://doi.org/10.1242/dev.126.2.335

Wiseman BS, Sternlicht MD, Lund LR, Alexander CM, Mott J, Bissell MJ, Soloway P, Itohara S, Werb Z (2003) Site-specific inductive and inhibitory activities of MMP-2 and MMP-3 orchestrate mammary gland branching morphogenesis. J Cell Biol 162(6):1123–1133. https://doi.org/10.1083/jcb.200302090

Wuidart A, Sifrim A, Fioramonti M, Matsumura S, Brisebarre A, Brown D, Centonze A, Dannau A, Dubois C, Van Keymeulen A, Voet T, Blanpain C (2018) Early lineage segregation of multipotent embryonic mammary gland progenitors. Nat Cell Biol 20(6):666–676. https://doi.org/10.1038/s41556-018-0095-2

Wysolmerski JJ, Philbrick WM, Dunbar ME, Lanske B, Kronenberg H, Broadus AE (1998) Rescue of the parathyroid hormone-related protein knockout mouse demonstrates that parathyroid hormone-related protein is essential for mammary gland development. Development 125(7):1285–1294. https://doi.org/10.1242/dev.125.7.1285

Wysolmerski JJ, Cormier S, Philbrick WM, Dann P, Zhang JP, Roume J, Delezoide AL, Silve C (2001) Absence of functional type 1 parathyroid hormone (PTH)/PTH-related protein receptors in humans is associated with abnormal breast development and tooth impaction. J Clin Endocrinol Metab 86(4):1788–1794. https://doi.org/10.1210/jcem.86.4.7404

Zhang Y, Tomann P, Andl T, Gallant NM, Huelsken J, Jerchow B, Birchmeier W, Paus R, Piccolo S, Mikkola ML, Morrisey EE, Overbeek PA, Scheidereit C, Millar SE, Schmidt-Ullrich R (2009) Reciprocal requirements for EDA/EDAR/NF-kappaB and Wnt/beta-catenin signaling pathways in hair follicle induction. Dev Cell 17(1):49–61. https://doi.org/10.1016/j.devcel.2009.05.011

Zhang X, Martinez D, Koledova Z, Qiao G, Streuli CH, Lu P (2014) FGF ligands of the postnatal mammary stroma regulate distinct aspects of epithelial morphogenesis. Development 141(17):3352–3362. https://doi.org/10.1242/dev.106732

3 Breast Morphogenesis: From Normal Development to Cancer

Saevar Ingthorsson,
Gunnhildur Asta Traustadottir,
and Thorarinn Gudjonsson

Abstract

The human breast gland is composed of branching epithelial ducts that culminate in milk-producing units known as terminal duct lobular units (TDLUs). The epithelial compartment comprises an inner layer of luminal epithelial cells (LEP) and an outer layer of contractile myoepithelial cells (MEP). Both LEP and MEP arise from a common stem cell population. The epithelial compartment undergoes dynamic branching morphogenesis and remodelling, which expands the surface area for milk production. The epithelial remodelling that starts at the onset of menarche is largely under hormonal control, first and foremost by estrogen and progesterone from ovaries, the production of which is stimulated by pituitary-derived hormones. Menopause leads to a significant decline in estrogen and progesterone levels, resulting in involution and senescence of the breast epithelium. The branching morphogenesis involves developmental events such as epithelial-to-mesenchymal transition (EMT) and mesenchymal-to-epithelial transition (MET). EMT and MET confer plasticity to the epithelial compartment enabling the migration of epithelial cells through the stroma and restoration of the epithelial phenotype. In the normal breast, the stroma, including the basement membrane (BM), collagen-rich extracellular matrix, and various stromal cells, supports the correct histoarchitecture of the glandular tree. However, in cancer, the stroma can acquire tumour-promoting properties and is referred to as the tumour microenvironment. This chapter will explore the developmental processes including branching morphogenesis in the normal breast gland and discuss the lineage relationship between LEPS and MEPs

Saevar Ingthorsson, Gunnhildur Asta Traustadottir and Thorarinn Gudjonsson contributed equally to this book chapter.

S. Ingthorsson
Stem Cell Research Unit, Biomedical Center, School of Health Sciences, University of Iceland, Reykjavik, Iceland

Faculty of Nursing and Midwifery, School of Health Sciences, University of Iceland, Reykjavik, Iceland

G. A. Traustadottir
Stem Cell Research Unit, Biomedical Center, School of Health Sciences, University of Iceland, Reykjavik, Iceland

Department of Pathology, Landspitali University Hospital, Reykjavik, Iceland

T. Gudjonsson (✉)
Stem Cell Research Unit, Biomedical Center, School of Health Sciences, University of Iceland, Reykjavik, Iceland

Department of Laboratory Hematology, Landspitali University Hospital, Reykjavik, Iceland
e-mail: tgudjons@hi.is

T. Sørlie, R. B. Clarke (eds.), *A Guide to Breast Cancer Research*, Advances in Experimental Medicine and Biology 1464, https://doi.org/10.1007/978-3-031-70875-6_3

and their interactions with the surrounding stroma in the normal and neoplastic breast gland. Finally, we will review various *in vitro* and *in vivo* models employed in mammary gland research.

Keywords

Branching morphogenesis · Epithelial remodelling · Stem cells · EMT · Hormonal regulation

Key Points

1. Hormones drive tissue remodelling and branching morphogenesis in the mammary gland.
2. Bi- and unipotent stem cells are present in the mammary gland, giving rise to ductal or alveolar LEP and MEP cells.
3. Advanced research models are essential to study the spatial and temporal dynamics of the breast gland.
4. While studies in mice have advanced our understanding of the mammary gland, there are significant anatomical differences between human and mice.

3.1 Mammary Gland Structure and Composition

The mammary gland, the signature organ of mammals, serves as the nursing organ for newborn mammalian offspring, which, for a varying amount of time for each species, feed solely on milk produced by the glands. Hence, the primary function of the mammary gland is to produce, store, and deliver milk to nourish the young, thus ensuring postnatal survival and reproductive success. The mammary gland is also a source of one of the most common types of cancer, as breast cancer is a global leading cause of death, after gastrointestinal and respiratory cancer (Network 2021).

The development of the female mammary gland is unique, as it occurs in three distinct stages, stretching well into postnatal life. First, a rudimentary ductal tree is formed during embryonic development both in males and females. This ductal tree stays quiescent until puberty, where oestrous hormonal signals in females cause a resurgence in proliferation and the ductal tree undergoes further proliferation and expansion, leading to an enlargement of the glandular tissue and the surrounding stroma (Silberstein 2001). Lastly, and most importantly, the gland reaches its full development and differentiation during pregnancy and lactation, where a new surge of hormonal signals drives the gland's full differential potential, where the branching ductal tree further expands and lactation begins (Biswas et al. 2022). After weaning of the young, the hormonal signals fall, and the gland involutes as cells die and are reduced in numbers via controlled cell death. The senescence and apoptosis of the breast epithelium during involution reduces the gland to a state comparable to what it was before pregnancy. Thanks to tissue stem cells, this cycle is then repeated during each subsequent pregnancy and lactational periods. A minuscule version of this proliferative phase is initiated and aborted during each menstrual cycle (Ramakrishnan et al. 2002). These developmental phases emphasise the spatial and temporal dynamics in the breast gland from puberty to menopause. To study the mechanisms controlling these developmental stages, the correct research models are essential.

3.2 Dynamic Remodelling of the Epithelial Compartment

3.2.1 Hormonal Regulation of Branching Morphogenesis

The mammary gland has a branching phenotype (Biswas et al. 2022), the purpose of which is to produce a large surface area while at the same time limiting total cell volume. The branching phenotype is also found in several other organs in the body, such as the lungs, kidneys, and several glandular organs including the pancreas, apocrine sweat glands, salivary glands, and also in the microvasculature (Hsu and Yamada 2010; Villasenor et al. 2010; Li et al. 2018; Lang et al. 2021). All these organs have the branching mechanism in common during development, and therefore share many of the relevant molecular signalling pathways (Fata et al. 2004; Affolter et al. 2009; Foubert et al. 2010; Goodwin and Nelson 2020; Lang et al. 2021). An interesting aspect of mammary development is the aforementioned delay in development until the onset of puberty and pregnancy, where hypophyseal hormones such as growth hormone (GH), follicular stimulating hormone (FSH), and luteinising hormone (LH) play a crucial role (Sternlicht 2006; Macias and Hinck 2012; Seachrist et al. 2018). GH has been shown to play a pivotal role in both pre-pubescent and adult rats, and is thought to act upstream of IGF-1 signalling (Kleinberg et al. 2000), the lack of which results in a complete absence of ductal development. FSH and LH induce the production of estrogen and progesterone, respectively, in the ovaries. Estrogen and progesterone induce cell proliferation and mucus secretion, respectively, in the uterine epithelium preparing for the implantation of the blastocyst if fertilisation occurs. Additionally, estrogen plays an important role in ductal elongation in the mammary gland, through pathways activated in the estrogen-responsive stromal and epithelial cells within the mammary gland, in part via the induction of paracrine secretion of secondary signalling molecules such as amphiregulin, resulting in increased proliferation of luminal progenitors (Mueller et al. 2002; Wilson et al. 2006; Ciarloni et al. 2007). Progesterone is an important inducer of secondary and tertiary branch formation along with lobuloalveolar development (Brisken et al. 1998) and during pregnancy, prolactin and glucocorticoids cooperate with progesterone to reach the maximal alveolar differentiation (Hannan et al. 2023) (Fig. 3.1). Finally, oxytocin produced in the posterior pituitary upon suckling stimulates milk ejection, by initiating contraction in the myoepithelial cells through increased concentration of intracellular calcium. This further results in alveolar and ductal contractions, thereby assisting in transporting milk from the alveoli to the nipple (Stevenson et al. 2020). Based on this, the regulation of mammary gland branching morphogenesis and function is driven through two main endocrine signalling groups, ovarian (estrogen and progesterone), and pituitary (GH, prolactin, oxytocin, FSH, and LH), demonstrating the temporal control over branching morphogenesis, both during puberty, and subsequently during pregnancy, where estrogen, progesterone and prolactin signalling is highly amplified [reviewed in Hannan et al. (2023)].

3.2.2 Stem and Progenitor Cells in Branching Morphogenesis

The elaborate branching ducts of the human mammary gland culminate in the terminal duct lobular units (TDLUs) (Fig. 3.2a). TDLUs are surrounded by cellular-rich loose connective tissue containing a dense network of capillaries, fibroblasts, and immune cells (Ronnov-Jessen et al. 1996). The epithelial cells sit on a basement membrane that plays an important role in maintaining the correct polarity of cells and forms a rigid anchor for the epithelium through integrins at focal adhesion contacts and hemidesmosomes (Petersen et al. 1992; Gudjonsson et al. 2002a; Lee and Streuli 2014). The human breast epithelium is composed of two main epithelial cell lineages; the luminal epithelial (LEP) and myoepithelial cells (MEP) (Pechoux et al. 1999) (Fig. 3.2b). The LEPs line the lumen of the hollow ducts and acini of the breast gland and in the latter, they are the milk producing component, whereas the MEPs surround the LEPs and serve as the contractile component during suckling. Myoepithelial cells are important regulators of cellular polarity of LEPs and contribute to large extent to the formation of the basement membrane (Gudjonsson et al. 2002a; Shams 2022). A subset of LEPs express estrogen (ER) and progesterone receptors (PR) (Petersen et al. 1987; Clarke 2003). ER-positive cells are believed to be non-proliferative (Duss et al. 2007) but act as sensors for proliferation in adjacent ER-negative cells via growth factor signalling through amphi-

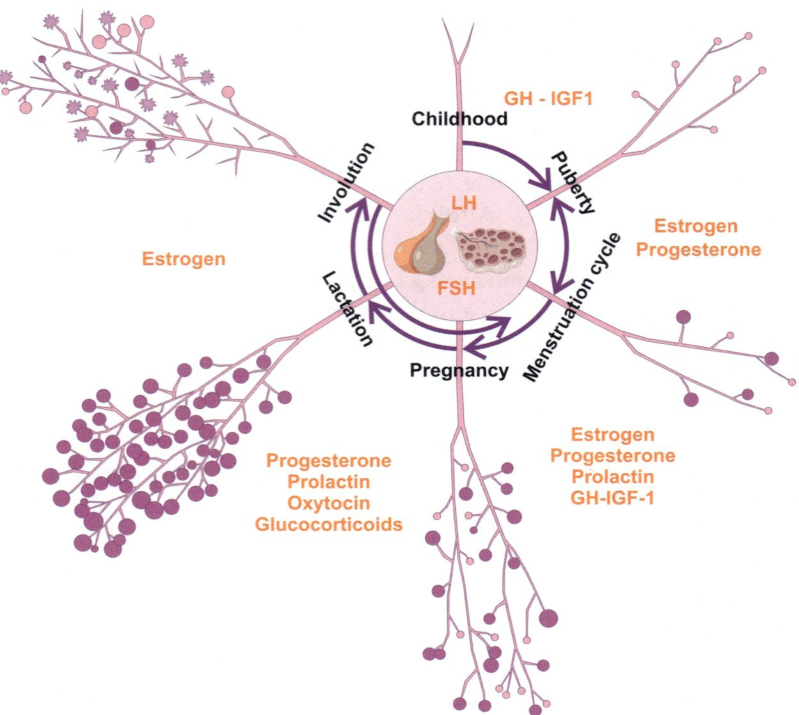

Fig. 3.1 Hormonally induced changes of the mammary gland from childhood to menopause. Morphogenic and functional changes in the mammary gland are regulated by a complex integration of hormonal signals from several organs including hypothalamus/pituitary, ovaries, liver, and adrenal glands. Hormonal stimulation induces branching morphogenesis in the mammary gland at the onset of menarche and to a greater extent if pregnancy occurs. The mammary epithelium reaches full differential potential during lactation, followed by involution when hormonal signals fall. This pattern repeats with each subsequent pregnancy and a miniscule version is initiated and aborted during each menstruation cycle. After menopause, the glandular structure further involutes upon the cessation of ovarian-derived hormonal signalling (not shown). *GH* growth hormone, *LH* luteinising hormone, *FSH* follicular stimulating hormone, *IGF-1* insulin-like growth factor-1 (Created with Biorender)

regulin (LaMarca and Rosen 2007). The origin of LEPs and MEPs has been discussed for decades, but they have been shown to share a common bipotent progenitor that can differentiate into either of the two cell types (Gudjonsson et al. 2002b; Villadsen et al. 2007; Petersen and Polyak 2010; Fu et al. 2020). The existence of stem cells is highly important during development, when the breast gland is growing and differentiating but also during the adult developmental stages of the breast gland such as during pregnancy.

The presence and location of adult stem cells and progenitor cells in the human breast gland have been intensely studied (Gudjonsson et al. 2002b; Clarke et al. 2003; Villadsen et al. 2007; Eirew et al. 2008; Fu et al. 2020). We have previously shown that in the adult breast, cells can be found that are described as suprabasal, i.e. cells that lie *between* the two aforementioned cell lineages, they don't reach the lumen, but are not fully embedded in the MEP cell layer either. These suprabasal epithelial cells harbour stem cell properties and share several of the marker proteins expressed by the two cell lineages. For instance, these suprabasal cells harbour luminal epithelial properties but lack expression of Mucin-1 (MUC1) a marker that identifies fully matured luminal epithelial cells. They also express cytokeratins 18, 19 (LEP), and 14 (MEP) and express TP63, which is an important basal cell marker and has been shown to be important in adult cell progenitor populations (Gudjonsson

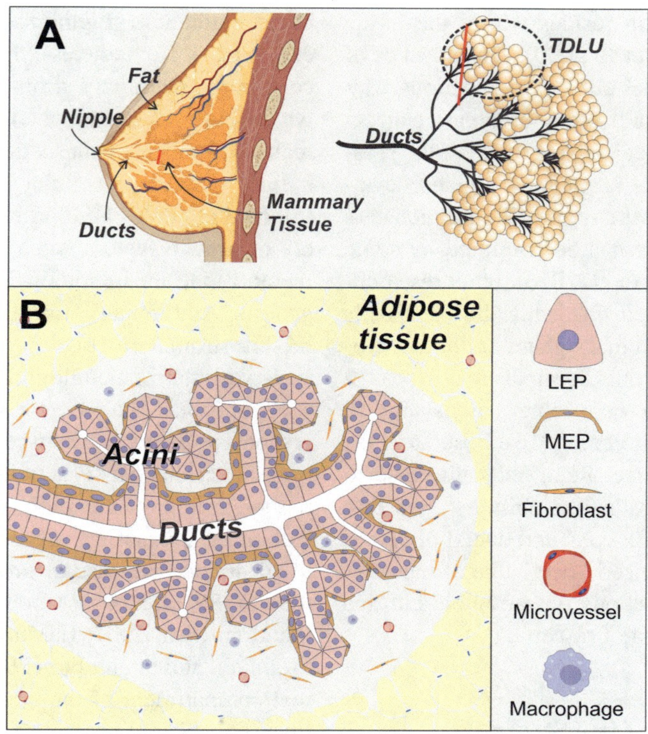

Fig. 3.2 Anatomy of the human female breast. (**a**) The human female breast is comprised of a glandular ductal tree and grape-like lobuloalveolar structures. Originating at the nipple, the mammary ducts extend towards the terminal duct lobular units (TDLUs) which are the functional units of the gland. The breast parenchyma is embedded in fat tissue and collagen-rich stroma. (**b**) The bilayered mammary epithelium is composed of an outer layer of myoepithelial cells (MEP) and an inner layer of luminal epithelial cells (LEP). The mammary acini are embedded in loose, cellular-rich intralobular stroma whereas more collagen-rich, dense interlobular stroma surrounds TDLUs and ducts. (Created with Biorender)

et al. 2002b). Indeed, TP63 is a well-known stem cell marker in other epithelial tissues such as in trachea/bronchi (Arason et al. 2014; Zuo et al. 2015) and in basal layer of the epidermis (Pellegrini et al. 2001). Using biopsies from reduction mammoplasties, we isolated suprabasal cells and demonstrated that these cells were able to give rise to both luminal and myoepithelial cells. A cell line, D492, generated from these subrabasal cells has a unique differentiation potential of being continuously able to generate LEPs and MEPs and furthermore, when cultivated in 3D matrices such as Matrigel, they are capable of forming branching structures reminiscent of TDLU (Gudjonsson et al. 2002b). For the past decade, our research group has used the D492 cell line to gain insight into branching morphogenesis, EMT, and cancer progression (Hilmarsdottir et al. 2015; Ingthorsson et al. 2016; Briem et al. 2019a, b; Morera et al. 2019; Budkova et al. 2020; Steinhaeuser et al. 2020; Sigurdardottir et al. 2021; Sigurdardottir et al. 2022).

Lineage tracing is an important approach to identify progenitor populations within tissues, and while that approach is impossible to utilise in human tissues, it has been successfully used in mouse models of mammary gland development. Jane Visvader's lab has convincingly demonstrated, using sophisticated animal models and lineage tracing, that within the adult mouse mammary gland, cells exist that can clonally expand portions of the mammary tree, both the MEPs and LEPs, supporting the notion that a true bipotential cell population resides within the tissue (Rios et al. 2014; Fu et al. 2020). The presence of these bipotent cells has clinical implications, as it is believed that certain types of breast cancers originate from these cells. Nevertheless, the presence of bipotent cells in mammary gland development and adult tissue remodelling is debated. While their existence has been refuted by some researchers (Wuidart et al. 2016), other researchers have demonstrated that while bipotent cells reside within the mammary gland, unipotent progenitors (giving off only luminal or only basal/myoepithelial cells) contribute extensively to alveologenesis (Davis et al. 2016). Based on this, progenitors are diverse. Stem cells give rise to progenitor cells with distinct ability to generate ductal or alveolar LEP cells and ductal or alveolar MEP cells. Enhanced knowledge of these bi- and unipotent populations is warranted and this topic is an active field of research.

3.2.3 The Role of the Stromal Microenvironment in Normal Breast Physiology

The stromal compartment of the human breast, surrounding the epithelial parenchyma, includes a variety of extracellular matrix proteins and multiple cell types. It has become increasingly recognised that stroma is not merely a structural support for the epithelium but rather plays a dominant role in regulating breast morphogenesis and maintaining homeostasis (Shekhar et al. 2001; Wiseman and Werb 2002; Gudjonsson et al. 2003; Parmar and Cunha 2004; Rauner and Kuperwasser 2021). The adult non-lactating mammary stroma is highly rich of adipocytes. During pregnancy, the adipocytic compartment regresses as the epithelium expands but reappears after weaning. Thus, during the lactation cycle of the breast gland the adipocytic component displays a high degree of plasticity with de- and re-differentiation of the adipocytes (Wang et al. 2018). In the microvessels surrounding the TDLUs, endothelial cells are not merely passive counterparts of the conducting system but rather provide proliferative and niche signals to the breast epithelium (Ingthorsson et al. 2010; Wang et al. 2021). Nevertheless, the most predominant cells in the mammary stroma are the fibroblasts, which play an instrumental role in modulating mammary morphogenesis through paracrine signalling and extracellular matrix production (Sumbal et al. 2021). Fibroblasts produce a variety of growth factors (such as fibroblast growth factors) that are important inducers of morphogenesis. Additionally, fibroblasts can induce, or inhibit stromal remodelling via secretion of a variety of matrix metalloproteinases (MMPs). As such, fibroblasts can secrete MMP2 via estrogen-responsive pathways, as well as promote inhibition of various MMP activities via secretion of tissue inhibitor of metalloproteases (TIMP). This can affect paracrine signalling by regulating MMP-induced release of growth factors such as the EGFR ligands Amphiregulin and EGF (Ciarloni et al. 2007; LaMarca and Rosen 2007; Sternlicht and Sunnarborg 2008). Within the stromal compartment of the human breast, two distinct fibroblast lineages exist, each conveying various differential and regulatory cues on the epithelium (Morsing et al. 2016; Morsing et al. 2020).

3.2.4 Epithelial to Mesenchymal Transition in Breast Morphogenesis

In a dynamic tissue such as the breast gland, a certain degree of plasticity in both stroma and the epithelium is necessary to accomplish the remodelling process. The continuous remodelling seen during each menstruation cycle and more profoundly during pregnancy is made possible due to the plasticity of epithelial cells as they need to invade the surrounding stroma to initiate branching morphogenesis. This epithelial plasticity is seen as a transient change in the epithelium where leading cells lose epithelial properties and gain mesenchymal phenotype that helps them to invade surrounding stroma. This process, known as epithelial-to-mesenchymal transition (EMT), is a developmental process seen during gastrulation, formation of neural crest cells, and in organogenesis (Kim et al. 2017; Francou and Anderson 2020). In its strict definition, EMT means that cells completely lose epithelial phenotype and gain mesenchymal phenotype and properties. However, complete EMT rarely occurs. Instead, a wide spectrum of partial EMT (p-EMT) exists. During branching breast morphogenesis, the leading cells need to undergo p-EMT to be able to invade the surrounding stroma. Cancer cells also use p-EMT to invade the surrounding tissue. The reverse concept, mesenchymal to epithelial transition (MET), brings the tissue back to the epithelial phenotype (Nakaya and Sheng 2013). Both EMT and MET are under control of a number of conserved signalling pathways, including EGF, Wnt, TGFb1, and FGF pathways among many others (Thiery et al. 2009; Singh et al. 2018). These signalling pathways activate several transcription factors (TFs) that are responsible for the phenotypic changes seen in EMT (Stemmler et al. 2019). Moreover, in recent years non-coding RNA (ncRNA), both long noncoding RNA (lncRNA) and microRNA, have been shown to participate in the EMT process (Wright et al. 2010; Hilmarsdottir et al. 2015; Richards et al. 2015). However, while understanding of the role of lncRNA in EMT/MET is limited, several miRNAs have been shown to play a pivotal role in the regulation of EMT. Most importantly, it is firmly established that members of the miR-200 family are powerful regulators of EMT/MET through a feedback loop with ZEB1/2 transcription factors, which control the expression of E-cadherin (Gregory et al. 2008; Park et al. 2008; Hilmarsdottir et al. 2015).

The ErbB family of receptor tyrosine kinases via Epidermal Growth Factor (EGF) signalling pathways have a fundamental role in EMT regulation [reviewed in Hardy et al. (2010)]. In mouse mammary gland, the ErbB/EGF axis regulates EMT in end bud by inducing the expression of Snail1 and Slug that repress expression of E-cadherin and upregulate expression of mesenchymal markers conferring the cap cells with migration properties to invade the surrounding stroma (Hardy et al. 2010). Also, ErbB/EGF pathways induce expression of metalloproteinases such as MMP2, MMP9, and MT1-MMP (Majumder et al. 2019). These enzymes break down the basement membrane and the interstitial collagen allowing the leading cells to migrate into the surrounding stroma.

3.3 From Normal Development to Cancer

3.3.1 Signalling Pathways in Breast Development and Cancer

Cancer evolves when signalling pathways essential for cell proliferation, differentiation, and survival become dysregulated. In the breast, abnormal signalling is driven by overly active hormonal or growth factor receptors or by constitutively active signalling cascades due to gene amplifications or genetic alterations of oncogenes or tumour-suppressor genes. In adult life, remodelling of the breast gland is dependent on the activity of epithelial stem and progenitor cells and accumulating evidence points towards these cells as the cells of origin of many breast cancers (see Sections III and IV for further reading).

The Wnt, Notch, and Hedgehog signalling pathways are evolutionary conserved pathways that regulate differentiation and homeostasis throughout the body. In the developing mammary gland, canonical Wnt signalling mediates placode development and initial morphogenesis, whereas Notch signalling regulates cell renewal and cell fate decisions (Dontu et al. 2004; Boras-Granic and Wysolmerski 2008). Despite having opposing effects on cell fate decisions during development (Acar et al. 2021), evidence suggests that Wnt and Notch pathways may interact and cooperate during breast cancer initiation (Ayyanan et al. 2006). Oncogenic alterations in core Notch genes are well known in hematological malignancies and have also been described in solid tumours, including breast cancer (Wang et al. 2015). Somatic mutations of key regulators of the Wnt pathway are uncommon in breast cancers, (Geyer et al. 2011), and activation of the pathway is rather mediated through overexpression of canonical ligands (Howe and Brown 2004). Hedgehog signalling pathway, which is important for pubertal morphogenesis of the mammary gland, is to a lesser degree than the other two pathways ascribed a role in breast cancer initiation but rather in breast cancer progression and metastasis formation (O'Toole et al. 2011; Riaz et al. 2018).

3.3.2 Tumour Microenvironment

As already described, the normal mammary gland is a highly organised ecosystem where the epithelial compartment is separated from the surrounding cellular-rich stroma by the basement membrane. Nevertheless, reciprocal signalling between the epithelium and stroma is pivotal for formation and homeostasis of the mammary gland. Breast cancer originates predominantly in the epithelial compartment and mainly in the luminal epithelial cells. In fact, myoepithelial cells have been assigned a role as tumour suppressors as continuous layer of myoepithelial cells and unbroken basement membranes are hallmarks of breast cancer in situ (Deugnier et al. 2002; Shams 2022). When the myoepithelial layer gets discontinuous and the basement membrane is breeched, cancer cells can invade the adjacent microenvironment and extravasate to the lymph or blood vessels (Fig. 3.3). When cancer cells encounter the microenvironment/stroma, heterotypic interactions can take place between the cancer cells and adjacent stromal cells creating a tumour microenvironment that may further facilitate cancer progression (Ingthorsson et al. 2022). In the activated stroma, the main stromal cell type, fibroblasts undergo phenotypic changes to become myofibroblasts and direct physical interaction between myofibroblasts and cancer cells further drives the oncogenic process (Ronnov-Jessen et al. 1995). In addition to the myofibroblasts, the tumour microenvironment includes a number of non-tumourigenic cell types, such as immune cells, endothelial cells, pericytes, adipose cells, and neurons. Although previously thought not to contribute to cancer progression, these cells are now acknowledged as active players of the tumoural niche, promoting tumour proliferation through cell–cell contact as well as paracrine signalling (de Visser and Joyce 2023).

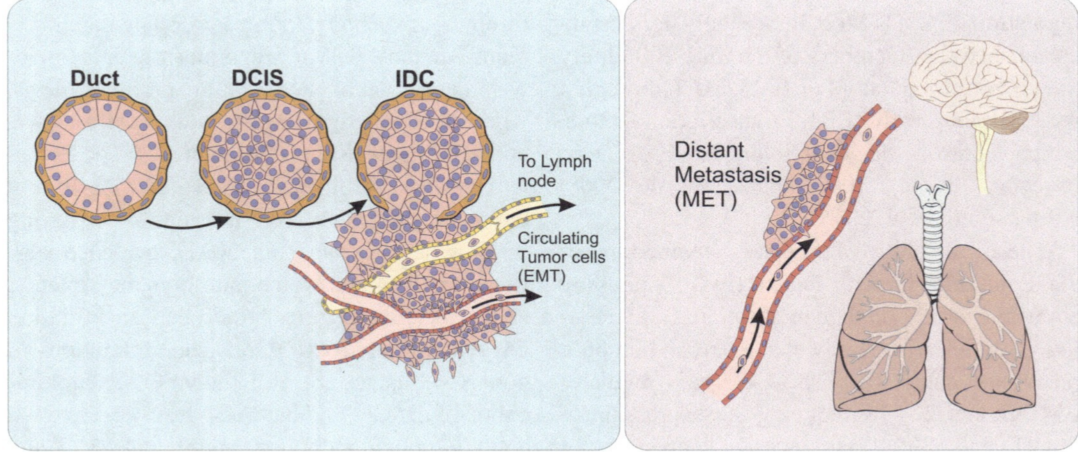

Fig. 3.3 Breast cancer progression and formation of distant metastases. Breast cancer progresses from ductal carcinoma in situ (DCIS) to invasive ductal carcinoma (IDC) when the basement membrane surrounding the epithelial compartment is breached. Epithelial-to-mesenchymal transition (EMT) equips cancer cells with enhanced motility so they can extravasate into and survive the transport through the circulatory system. Cancer cells colonise and form distant metastases through the reverse process, mesenchymal-to-epithelial transition (MET). (Created with Biorender)

3.4 Experimental Models in Breast Biology Research

3.4.1 Advancing from Conventional Monolayer Cell Culture to Three-Dimensional Context

The current materials/model systems to study the dynamic changes during breast gland development are heavily based on rodents, particularly mice and rats, as access to early developmental and pregnant human tissues, due to ethical reasons, are hard to come by. To address this scarcity, mammary gland researchers have developed sophisticated cell culture models that capture certain aspects of mammary gland development *in vitro* (Fig. 3.4). Indeed, cell culture models have been pivotal in advancing our understanding of breast epithelial differentiation and morphogenesis. Many normal mammary epithelial and breast cancer cell lines exist and have been used extensively for dissecting biological processes in normal development and cancer. However, genetic, and phenotypic drifting from the origin is a limiting factor for the biological relevance of cell lines. Nevertheless, continuous, or immortalised cell lines have the advantage of being easily expanded and therefore provide a good source material for long-term studies. Primary cells, isolated from fresh tissue, have the advantage of

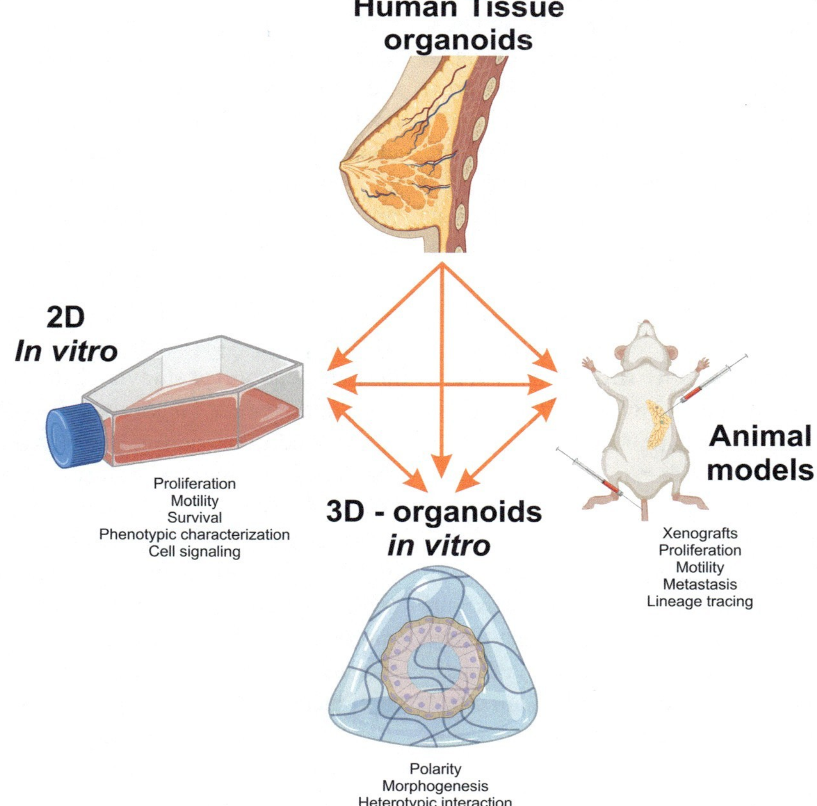

Fig. 3.4 Model systems. Normal and cancerous breast glands are modelled in vitro utilising 2D or 3D cellular systems and in vivo, predominantly employing rodent models. Conventional 2D cell culture models with immortalised cell lines or primary cells from fresh tissue are widely used for characterisation of cellular phenotype and cellular behaviour. Increased complexity with regards to morphogenesis and cell-cell/cell-ECM interaction is obtained by moving into 3D context. For in vivo studies, rodent models have long been the gold standard in mammary gland research, although other models, both mammalian and non-mammalian are also used. (Created with Biorender)

being close in phenotype to their in vivo counterparts, yet limited lifespan complicates long-term studies. Still, culture conditions for the maintenance of primary mammary epithelial cells have been improved and new protocols developed, including for culturing ER+ cells (Fridriksdottir et al. 2015). Using cell sorting technologies, it is possible to separate cells from the donor tissue into its structural components. Access to normal breast tissue from reduction mammoplasties enables cultivation of most cellular components of the breast gland such as epithelial cells, fibroblasts, and endothelial cells (Ronnov-Jessen et al. 1996; Pechoux et al. 1999; Sigurdsson et al. 2006; Fridriksdottir et al. 2015).

From healthy mammary tissue, luminal and myoepithelial cells can be isolated for further analysis *in vitro*. These cells can be manipulated genetically and chemically to simulate changes that occur during crucial developmental processes. Thus, changes to cell migration and invasion behaviour and changes to proliferative rates and metabolic changes can be studied and compared with events seen in malignancies. Additionally, basic heterotypic interactive studies of the different cell populations, be it interaction between the main epithelial components (LEPs and MEPs) or crosstalk between different histological components such as stromal cells (e.g., fibroblasts and endothelial cells) and the epithelial compartment can be simulated in a simplified manner. Additionally, cells can be isolated from tumour explants. Primary cells from malignant lesions are notoriously difficult to culture, owing mainly to the highly specific environment within the tumour, which strongly affects the behaviour of the cells once removed from the correct tissue context. This is also true with regards to cells isolated from healthy tissue and must be kept close in mind when designing experiments in monolayer cultures.

While epithelial structures can be considered in a way to exhibit a two-dimensional architecture, as they are bound to a basement membrane and form flat sheets that can be formed into tubes, they exist within the body which is anything but flat. Beneath the epithelial component is a vast stromal compartment, where correct histoarchitecture is of utmost importance to maintain tissue homeostasis, as previously described in this chapter. The study of this histoarchitectural arrangement and changes within require more sophisticated models in three dimensions.

3.4.2 Recapitulating Breast Tissue Complexity with Organoids

In recent decades, the use of breast organoids for studying breast morphogenesis and cancer has received increasing attention. Owing to advancements in organoid technology, long-term culture of normal human mammary tissue with preserved structural, cellular, and microenvironmental features is now possible (Rosenbluth et al. 2020; Mohan et al. 2021). Furthermore, methods for characterisation of cellular subtypes in organoids, such as single-cell sequencing and cytometry by time of flight (CyTOF) have had a huge impact on the understanding of cellular structures and composition. Human and rodent-derived breast organoid models have been utilised for the study of normal development and function of the mammary gland as well as breast cancer progression. As breast organoids capture the heterogeneity and phenotypic traits of *in vivo* conditions, they are suitable for studying heterotypic interactions in the breast gland, thus partially replacing mouse studies. However, one must keep in mind the donor-to-donor variability of human breast organoids (Kim et al. 2020). Patient-derived breast cancer organoids hold great promise as a tool for the development of patient-specific therapeutic options and therefore offer a realistic approach for the advancement of personalised therapy (Psilopatis et al. 2023). The most common method of simulating the *in vivo* condition in a three-dimensional culture occurs using a variety of hydrogels that contain several of the extracellular building blocks found within the stroma. These gels are highly varied with regards to their ingredients, but most contain collagen I to simulate stromal environment, with additions of Collagen IV and laminins to mimic the basement membrane, and other molecules such as fibronectin and growth factors. Collectively these gels (such as Matrigel) enable sophisticated ways to study homo- and heterotypic interactions of cellular components. Culturing cells in a three-dimensional context allows for crucial cell–cell and cell–extracellular matrix (ECM) interactions and is therefore undoubtedly more biologically relevant than the conventional monolayer cell culture. In fact, mammary gland biologists were forerunners in the development of 3D cell culture methods and these systems have been pivotal for elucidation of regulatory mechanisms of both normal and neoplastic mammary glands (Emerman et al. 1979; Bissell 1981; Streuli et al. 1991; Petersen et al. 1992; Weaver et al. 1995; Weaver et al. 1997). Ranging from simple spheroid cultures to complex co-cultures, 3D cell culture systems remain an integral part of mammary gland and breast cancer research (Sumbal et al. 2020). Interestingly, both fibroblasts and endothelial cells control growth and morphogenesis of breast epithelial cells in 3D culture. Thus, it has been shown that intralobular fibroblasts stimulate TDLU-like formation in co-culture with epithelial progenitor cells whereas interductal fibroblasts support epithelial duct formation (Morsing et al. 2020). Endothelial cells stimulate breast epithelial growth and branching morphogenesis in 3D culture. We have convincingly demonstrated that when endothelial cells are co-cultured with both primary cells and cancer-derived cell lines, they vastly induce proliferation and phenotypic changes. By coculturing endothelial cells in reconstituted basement membrane (rBM) together with the breast epithelial stem cell line D492 we saw both induced branching morphogenesis and EMT (Sigurdsson et al. 2011). In fact, the branching structures generated were akin to TDLUs *in vivo*. Furthermore, the formation of spindle-shaped colonies was seen. These spindle-like structures were phenotypically mesenchymal, indicating a cell population that has completed its EMT program. A cell line generated from these colonies, referred to as D492M is restricted in its mesenchymal state and thus not able to revert to its original epithelial phenotype. Intriguingly, overexpression of miRNA200c and P63 in D492 M-induced MET resulting in restoration of the branching epithelial structures (Ingthorsson et al. 2010; Sigurdsson et al. 2011; Hilmarsdottir et al. 2015).

3.4.3 In Vivo Models: Utilising Rodent Models, Primarily Mice

A lot has been learned about stem cells, the molecular mechanisms of branching morphogenesis, and cancer progression by studying the mouse mammary gland (Borowsky 2011; Fu et al. 2020). As such, studies in mice have advanced our knowledge on mammary development through elegant models including genetic knock-in and knock-out experiments and cellular lineage tracing, where cells can be fluorescently labelled and their progeny maintain the fluorescence, enabling researchers to track their location. Owing to recent advances in lineage-tracing methods based on single-cell sequencing, cell fate trajectories can now be tracked more accurately using unique cellular barcodes [reviewed in Yao et al. (2022)]. Due to the short developmental period of mice, as they live and age fast, they are extremely useful to study cancer initiation. The mouse mammary tumour virus (MMTV) is a retrovirus that can be transmitted through the milk of infected females to suckling offspring, where it inserts into the new host's genome and begins its life cycle (Mertz et al. 2005). During puberty the virus infects the cells of the mammary gland, promoting the formation of epithelial breast tumours. Building on the life cycle of the MMTV, several mouse models have been engineered where a genetic element of choice is placed under the control of MMTV promoter sequences, thereby enabling research of the first steps of oncogenesis. Additionally, mice can be used in xenograft studies where human-derived cells are grafted into immunodeficient mice (NOD/SCID, or NSG mice), for studies of primary tumour formation (by either injecting into the mouse mammary fat pad, or via intraductal injections directly into the mammary ducts (Kittrell et al. 2016), or for studies of metastasis (by injecting into the fat pad, and waiting, or by intravenous injections).

Although mouse models are widely used in mammary gland research, the anatomical differences between mice and men cannot be disregarded. The mouse mammary gland is composed of simple ducts that terminate in end buds and the epithelium is surrounded by fat tissue. Hence, diverse epithelial-stromal interactions exist between the mammary glands of human and mouse. Given these anatomical differences, researchers need to be cautious when extrapolating results from mouse studies to humans. This emphasises that while there are similarities, studies on human-derived material are equally important. To address some of these differences, researchers have attempted to "humanize" the mouse gland via addition of human-derived cells like fibroblasts or immune cells (Kuperwasser et al. 2004), hence producing a mouse model that mimics the human mammary gland slightly more. Several other animal models are used to study breast cancer apart from the mouse, which is by far the least costly. These models are both non-mammalian (like zebrafish) and mammalian (e.g. rats, hamsters, tree-shrews, dogs, cats, pigs, and non-human primates). However, mouse models are by far the most common, as husbandry of other animal species can be prohibitively expensive, due to large size, long life-time, and long generation time [reviewed in Zeng et al. (2020)]. Nevertheless, dogs have proven to be quite useful in breast cancer research, as many dog breeds are heavily inbred, and show high incidence of mammary gland tumour formation (Kwon et al. 2023).

3.5 Conclusion

The female mammary gland is a unique structure as most of its developmental phases occur postnatally at the onset of puberty. The mammary gland is under control of the endocrine system mainly the pituitary gland and ovaries with the hypothalamus being the major control organ, regulating both positive and negative feedback. This hormonal regulation is the driver of tissue remodelling and branching morphogenesis in the mammary gland during each menstruation cycle and most profoundly during pregnancy, lactation, and involution. Hormonal regulation is, however, dependent on heterotypic interactions between the epithelial and stromal compartments. The importance of the basement membrane in maintaining the histoarchitecture in the normal breast is becoming increasingly clear, and loss of its integrity may facilitate tumour progression. Much is already known about the stem cells in the mouse mammary gland thanks to advanced lineage tracing methods *in vivo* and many omics methods such as single-cell sequencing. Although knowledge about stem cells in the human female breast gland has advanced, more comprehensive understanding is needed about how mammary stem cells alter their fate during branching morphogenesis in the menstruation cycle and during pregnancy. The stem cell niche includes systematic (hormones) and local components of the stroma. The exact composition of the stem cell niche and how it regulates stem cells in the breast is still poorly defined. Unravelling spatial and temporal regulation of stem cells in the breast, employing advanced research models, will aid in understanding breast cancer progression and hopefully result in new therapeutic targets.

References

Acar A, Hidalgo-Sastre A, Leverentz MK, Mills CG, Woodcock S, Baron M, Collu GM, Brennan K (2021) Inhibition of Wnt signalling by Notch via two distinct mechanisms. Sci Rep 11(1):9096

Affolter M, Zeller R, Caussinus E (2009) Tissue remodelling through branching morphogenesis. Nat Rev Mol Cell Biol 10(12):831–842

Arason AJ, Jonsdottir HR, Halldorsson S, Benediktsdottir BE, Bergthorsson JT, Ingthorsson S, Baldursson O, Sinha S, Gudjonsson T, Magnusson MK (2014) deltaNp63 has a role in maintaining epithelial integrity in airway epithelium. PLoS One 9(2):e88683

Ayyanan A, Civenni G, Ciarloni L, Morel C, Mueller N, Lefort K, Mandinova A, Raffoul W, Fiche M, Dotto GP, Brisken C (2006) Increased Wnt signaling triggers oncogenic conversion of human breast epithelial cells by a Notch-dependent mechanism. Proc Natl Acad Sci USA 103(10):3799–3804

Bissell MJ (1981) The differentiated state of normal and malignant cells or how to define a "normal" cell in culture. Int Rev Cytol 70:27–100

Biswas SK, Banerjee S, Baker GW, Kuo CY, Chowdhury I (2022) The mammary gland: basic structure and molecular signaling during development. Int J Mol Sci 23(7)

Boras-Granic K, Wysolmerski JJ (2008) Wnt signaling in breast organogenesis. Organogenesis 4(2):116–122

Borowsky AD (2011) Choosing a mouse model: experimental biology in context--the utility and limitations of mouse models of breast cancer. Cold Spring Harb Perspect Biol 3(9):a009670

Briem E, Ingthorsson S, Traustadottir GA, Hilmarsdottir B, Gudjonsson T (2019a) Application of the D492 Cell lines to explore breast morphogenesis, EMT and cancer progression in 3D culture. J Mammary Gland Biol Neoplasia 24(2):139–147

Briem E, Budkova Z, Sigurdardottir AK, Hilmarsdottir B, Kricker J, Timp W, Magnusson MK, Traustadottir GA, Gudjonsson T (2019b) MiR-203a is differentially expressed during branching morphogenesis and EMT in breast progenitor cells and is a repressor of peroxidasin. Mech Dev 155:34–47

Brisken C, Park S, Vass T, Lydon JP, O'Malley BW, Weinberg RA (1998) A paracrine role for the epithelial progesterone receptor in mammary gland development. Proc Natl Acad Sci USA 95(9):5076–5081

Budkova Z, Sigurdardottir AK, Briem E, Bergthorsson JT, Sigurdsson S, Magnusson MK, Traustadottir GA, Gudjonsson T, Hilmarsdottir B (2020) Expression of ncRNAs on the DLK1-DIO3 locus is associated with basal and mesenchymal phenotype in breast epithelial progenitor cells. Front Cell Dev Biol 8:461

Ciarloni L, Mallepell S, Brisken C (2007) Amphiregulin is an essential mediator of estrogen receptor alpha function in mammary gland development. Proc Natl Acad Sci USA 104(13):5455–5460

Clarke RB (2003) Steroid receptors and proliferation in the human breast. Steroids 68(10–13):789–794

Clarke RB, Anderson E, Howell A, Potten CS (2003) Regulation of human breast epithelial stem cells. Cell Prolif 36(Suppl 1):45–58

Davis FM, Lloyd-Lewis B, Harris OB, Kozar S, Winton DJ, Muresan L, Watson CJ (2016) Single-cell lineage tracing in the mammary gland reveals stochastic clonal dispersion of stem/progenitor cell progeny. Nat Commun 7:13053

de Visser KE, Joyce JA (2023) The evolving tumor microenvironment: from cancer initiation to metastatic outgrowth. Cancer Cell 41(3):374–403

Deugnier MA, Teuliere J, Faraldo MM, Thiery JP, Glukhova MA (2002) The importance of being a myoepithelial cell. Breast Cancer Res 4(6):224–230

Dontu G, Jackson KW, McNicholas E, Kawamura MJ, Abdallah WM, Wicha MS (2004) Role of Notch signaling in cell-fate determination of human mammary stem/progenitor cells. Breast Cancer Res 6(6):R605–R615

Duss S, Andre S, Nicoulaz AL, Fiche M, Bonnefoi H, Brisken C, Iggo RD (2007) An oestrogen-dependent model of breast cancer created by transformation of normal human mammary epithelial cells. Breast Cancer Res 9(3):R38

Eirew P, Stingl J, Raouf A, Turashvili G, Aparicio S, Emerman JT, Eaves CJ (2008) A method for quantifying normal human mammary epithelial stem cells with in vivo regenerative ability. Nat Med 14(12):1384–1389

Emerman JT, Burwen SJ, Pitelka DR (1979) Substrate properties influencing ultrastructural differentiation of mammary epithelial cells in culture. Tissue Cell 11(1):109–119

Fata JE, Werb Z, Bissell MJ (2004) Regulation of mammary gland branching morphogenesis by the extracellular matrix and its remodeling enzymes. Breast Cancer Res 6(1):1–11

Foubert E, De Craene B, Berx G (2010) Key signalling nodes in mammary gland development and cancer. The Snail1-Twist1 conspiracy in malignant breast cancer progression. Breast Cancer Res 12(3):206

Francou A, Anderson KV (2020) The epithelial-to-mesenchymal transition (EMT) in development and cancer. Annu Rev Cancer Biol 4:197–220

Fridriksdottir AJ, Kim J, Villadsen R, Klitgaard MC, Hopkinson BM, Petersen OW, Ronnov-Jessen L (2015) Propagation of oestrogen receptor-positive and oestrogen-responsive normal human breast cells in culture. Nat Commun 6:8786

Fu NY, Nolan E, Lindeman GJ, Visvader JE (2020) Stem cells and the differentiation hierarchy in mammary gland development. Physiol Rev 100(2):489–523

Geyer FC, Lacroix-Triki M, Savage K, Arnedos M, Lambros MB, MacKay A, Natrajan R, Reis-Filho JS (2011) beta-Catenin pathway activation in breast cancer is associated with triple-negative phenotype but not with CTNNB1 mutation. Mod Pathol 24(2):209–231

Goodwin K, Nelson CM (2020) Branching morphogenesis. Development 147(10)

Gregory PA, Bert AG, Paterson EL, Barry SC, Tsykin A, Farshid G, Vadas MA, Khew-Goodall Y, Goodall GJ (2008) The miR-200 family and miR-205 regulate epithelial to mesenchymal transition by targeting ZEB1 and SIP1. Nat Cell Biol 10(5):593–601

Gudjonsson T, Ronnov-Jessen L, Villadsen R, Rank F, Bissell MJ, Petersen OW (2002a) Normal and tumor-derived myoepithelial cells differ in their ability to interact with luminal breast epithelial cells for polarity and basement membrane deposition. J Cell Sci 115(Pt 1):39–50

Gudjonsson T, Villadsen R, Nielsen HL, Ronnov-Jessen L, Bissell MJ, Petersen OW (2002b) Isolation, immortalization, and characterization of a human breast epithelial cell line with stem cell properties. Genes Dev 16(6):693–706

Gudjonsson T, Ronnov-Jessen L, Villadsen R, Bissell MJ, Petersen OW (2003) To create the correct microenvironment: three-dimensional heterotypic collagen assays for human breast epithelial morphogenesis and neoplasia. Methods 30(3):247–255

Hannan FM, Elajnaf T, Vandenberg LN, Kennedy SH, Thakker RV (2023) Hormonal regulation of mammary gland development and lactation. Nat Rev Endocrinol 19(1):46–61

Hardy KM, Booth BW, Hendrix MJ, Salomon DS, Strizzi L (2010) ErbB/EGF signaling and EMT in mammary development and breast cancer. J Mammary Gland Biol Neoplasia 15(2):191–199

Hilmarsdottir B, Briem E, Sigurdsson V, Franzdottir SR, Ringner M, Arason AJ, Bergthorsson JT, Magnusson MK, Gudjonsson T (2015) MicroRNA-200c-141 and ΔNp63 are required for breast epithelial differentiation and branching morphogenesis. Dev Biol 403(2):150–161

Howe LR, Brown AM (2004) Wnt signaling and breast cancer. Cancer Biol Ther 3(1):36–41

Hsu JC, Yamada KM (2010) Salivary gland branching morphogenesis--recent progress and future opportunities. Int J Oral Sci 2(3):117–126

Ingthorsson S, Sigurdsson V, Fridriksdottir A Jr, Jonasson JG, Kjartansson J, Magnusson MK, Gudjonsson T (2010) Endothelial cells stimulate growth of normal and cancerous breast epithelial cells in 3D culture. BMC Res Notes 3:184

Ingthorsson S, Andersen K, Hilmarsdottir B, Maelandsmo GM, Magnusson MK, Gudjonsson T (2016) HER2 induced EMT and tumorigenicity in breast epithelial progenitor cells is inhibited by coexpression of EGFR. Oncogene 35(32):4244–4255

Ingthorsson S, Traustadottir GA, Gudjonsson T (2022) Cellular plasticity and heterotypic interactions during breast morphogenesis and cancer initiation. Cancers (Basel) 14(21)

Kim DH, Xing T, Yang Z, Dudek R, Lu Q, Chen YH (2017) Epithelial mesenchymal transition in embryonic development, tissue repair and cancer: a comprehensive overview. J Clin Med 7(1)

Kim J, Koo BK, Knoblich JA (2020) Human organoids: model systems for human biology and medicine. Nat Rev Mol Cell Biol 21(10):571–584

Kittrell F, Valdez K, Elsarraj H, Hong Y, Medina D, Behbod F (2016) Mouse mammary intraductal (MIND) method for transplantation of patient derived primary DCIS cells and cell lines. Bio Protoc 6(5)

Kleinberg DL, Feldman M, Ruan W (2000) IGF-I: an essential factor in terminal end bud formation and ductal morphogenesis. J Mammary Gland Biol Neoplasia 5(1):7–17

Kuperwasser C, Chavarria T, Wu M, Magrane G, Gray JW, Carey L, Richardson A, Weinberg RA (2004) Reconstruction of functionally normal and malignant human breast tissues in mice. Proc Natl Acad Sci USA 101(14):4966–4971

Kwon JY, Moskwa N, Kang W, Fan TM, Lee C (2023) Canine as a comparative and translational model for human mammary tumor. J Breast Cancer 26(1):1–13

LaMarca HL, Rosen JM (2007) Estrogen regulation of mammary gland development and breast cancer: amphiregulin takes center stage. Breast Cancer Res 9(4):304

Lang C, Conrad L, Iber D (2021) Organ-specific branching morphogenesis. Front Cell Dev Biol 9:671402

Lee JL, Streuli CH (2014) Integrins and epithelial cell polarity. J Cell Sci 127(Pt 15):3217–3225

Li S, Zheng X, Nie Y, Chen W, Liu Z, Tao Y, Hu X, Hu Y, Qiao H, Qi Q, Pei Q, Cai D, Yu M, Mou C (2018) Defining key genes regulating morphogenesis of apocrine sweat gland in sheepskin. Front Genet 9:739

Macias H, Hinck L (2012) Mammary gland development. Wiley Interdiscip Rev Dev Biol 1(4):533–557

Majumder A, Ray S, Banerji A (2019) Epidermal growth factor receptor-mediated regulation of matrix metalloproteinase-2 and matrix metalloproteinase-9 in MCF-7 breast cancer cells. Mol Cell Biochem 452(1–2):111–121

Mertz JA, Simper MS, Lozano MM, Payne SM, Dudley JP (2005) Mouse mammary tumor virus encodes a self-regulatory RNA export protein and is a complex retrovirus. J Virol 79(23):14737–14747

Mohan SC, Lee TY, Giuliano AE, Cui X (2021) Current status of breast organoid models. Front Bioeng Biotechnol 9:745943

Morera E, Steinhauser SS, Budkova Z, Ingthorsson S, Kricker J, Krueger A, Traustadottir GA, Gudjonsson T (2019) YKL-40/CHI3L1 facilitates migration and invasion in HER2 overexpressing breast epithelial progenitor cells and generates a niche for capillary-like network formation. In Vitro Cell Dev Biol Anim 55(10):838–853

Morsing M, Klitgaard MC, Jafari A, Villadsen R, Kassem M, Petersen OW, Ronnov-Jessen L (2016) Evidence of two distinct functionally specialized fibroblast lineages in breast stroma. Breast Cancer Res 18(1):108

Morsing M, Kim J, Villadsen R, Goldhammer N, Jafari A, Kassem M, Petersen OW, Ronnov-Jessen L (2020) Fibroblasts direct differentiation of human breast epithelial progenitors. Breast Cancer Res 22(1):102

Mueller SO, Clark JA, Myers PH, Korach KS (2002) Mammary gland development in adult mice requires epithelial and stromal estrogen receptor alpha. Endocrinology 143(6):2357–2365

Nakaya Y, Sheng G (2013) EMT in developmental morphogenesis. Cancer Lett 341(1):9–15

Network GBoDC (2021) Global burden of disease study 2019 (GBD 2019) reference life table

O'Toole SA, Machalek DA, Shearer RF, Millar EK, Nair R, Schofield P, McLeod D, Cooper CL, McNeil CM, McFarland A, Nguyen A, Ormandy CJ, Qiu MR, Rabinovich B, Martelotto LG, Vu D, Hannigan GE, Musgrove EA, Christ D, Sutherland RL, Watkins DN, Swarbrick A (2011) Hedgehog overexpression is associated with stromal interactions and predicts for poor outcome in breast cancer. Cancer Res 71(11):4002–4014

Park SM, Gaur AB, Lengyel E, Peter ME (2008) The miR-200 family determines the epithelial phenotype of cancer cells by targeting the E-cadherin repressors ZEB1 and ZEB2. Genes Dev 22(7):894–907

Parmar H, Cunha GR (2004) Epithelial-stromal interactions in the mouse and human mammary gland in vivo. Endocr Relat Cancer 11(3):437–458

Pechoux C, Gudjonsson T, Ronnov-Jessen L, Bissell MJ, Petersen OW (1999) Human mammary luminal epithelial cells contain progenitors to myoepithelial cells. Dev Biol 206(1):88–99

Pellegrini G, Dellambra E, Golisano O, Martinelli E, Fantozzi I, Bondanza S, Ponzin D, McKeon F, De Luca M (2001) p63 identifies keratinocyte stem cells. Proc Natl Acad Sci USA 98(6):3156–3161

Petersen OW, Polyak K (2010) Stem cells in the human breast. Cold Spring Harb Perspect Biol 2(5):a003160

Petersen OW, Hoyer PE, van Deurs B (1987) Frequency and distribution of estrogen receptor-positive cells in normal, nonlactating human breast tissue. Cancer Res 47(21):5748–5751

Petersen OW, Ronnov-Jessen L, Howlett AR, Bissell MJ (1992) Interaction with basement membrane serves to rapidly distinguish growth and differentiation pattern of normal and malignant human breast epithelial cells. Proc Natl Acad Sci USA 89(19):9064–9068

Psilopatis I, Mantzari A, Vrettou K, Theocharis S (2023) The role of patient-derived organoids in triple-negative breast cancer drug screening. Biomedicines 11(3)

Ramakrishnan R, Khan SA, Badve S (2002) Morphological changes in breast tissue with menstrual cycle. Mod Pathol 15(12):1348–1356

Rauner G, Kuperwasser C (2021) Microenvironmental control of cell fate decisions in mammary gland development and cancer. Dev Cell 56(13):1875–1883

Riaz SK, Khan JS, Shah STA, Wang F, Ye L, Jiang WG, Malik MFA (2018) Involvement of hedgehog pathway in early onset, aggressive molecular subtypes and metastatic potential of breast cancer. Cell Commun Signal 16(1):3

Richards EJ, Zhang G, Li ZP, Permuth-Wey J, Challa S, Li Y, Kong W, Dan S, Bui MM, Coppola D, Mao WM, Sellers TA, Cheng JQ (2015) Long non-coding RNAs (LncRNA) regulated by transforming growth factor (TGF) beta: LncRNA-hit-mediated TGFbeta-induced epithelial to mesenchymal transition in mammary epithelia. J Biol Chem 290(11):6857–6867

Rios AC, Fu NY, Lindeman GJ, Visvader JE (2014) In situ identification of bipotent stem cells in the mammary gland. Nature 506(7488):322–327

Ronnov-Jessen L, Petersen OW, Koteliansky VE, Bissell MJ (1995) The origin of the myofibroblasts in breast cancer. Recapitulation of tumor environment in culture unravels diversity and implicates converted fibroblasts and recruited smooth muscle cells. J Clin Invest 95(2):859–873

Ronnov-Jessen L, Petersen OW, Bissell MJ (1996) Cellular changes involved in conversion of normal to malignant breast: importance of the stromal reaction. Physiol Rev 76(1):69–125

Rosenbluth JM, Schackmann RCJ, Gray GK, Selfors LM, Li CM, Boedicker M, Kuiken HJ, Richardson A, Brock J, Garber J, Dillon D, Sachs N, Clevers H, Brugge JS (2020) Organoid cultures from normal and cancer-prone human breast tissues preserve complex epithelial lineages. Nat Commun 11(1):1711

Seachrist DD, Donaubauer E, Keri RA (2018) Hypothalamic–pituitary–mammary gland (HPM) axis. Encyclopedia of reproduction, 2nd edn. M. K. Skinner, Academic Press

Shams A (2022) Re-evaluation of the myoepithelial cells roles in the breast cancer progression. Cancer Cell Int 22(1):403

Shekhar MP, Werdell J, Santner SJ, Pauley RJ, Tait L (2001) Breast stroma plays a dominant regulatory role in breast epithelial growth and differentiation: implications for tumor development and progression. Cancer Res 61(4):1320–1326

Sigurdardottir AK, Jonasdottir AS, Asbjarnarson A, Helgudottir HR, Gudjonsson T, Traustadottir GA (2021) Peroxidasin enhances basal phenotype and inhibits branching morphogenesis in breast epithelial progenitor cell line D492. J Mammary Gland Biol Neoplasia 26(4):321–338

Sigurdardottir AK, Hilmarsdottir B, Gudjonsson T, Traustadottir GA (2022) Application of 3D culture assays to study breast morphogenesis, epithelial plasticity, and cellular interactions in an epithelial progenitor cell line. Methods Mol Biol 2429:391–403

Sigurdsson V, Fridriksdottir AJ, Kjartansson J, Jonasson JG, Steinarsdottir M, Petersen OW, Ogmundsdottir HM, Gudjonsson T (2006) Human breast microvascular endothelial cells retain phenotypic traits in long-term finite life span culture. In Vitro Cell Dev Biol Anim 42(10):332–340

Sigurdsson V, Hilmarsdottir B, Sigmundsdottir H, Fridriksdottir AJ, Ringner M, Villadsen R, Borg A, Agnarsson BA, Petersen OW, Magnusson MK, Gudjonsson T (2011) Endothelial induced EMT in breast epithelial cells with stem cell properties. PLoS One 6(9):e23833

Silberstein GB (2001) Postnatal mammary gland morphogenesis. Microsc Res Tech 52(2):155–162

Singh M, Yelle N, Venugopal C, Singh SK (2018) EMT: mechanisms and therapeutic implications. Pharmacol Ther 182:80–94

Steinhaeuser SS, Morera E, Budkova Z, Schepsky A, Wang Q, Rolfsson O, Riedel A, Krueger A, Hilmarsdottir B, Maelandsmo GM, Valdimarsdottir B, Sigurdardottir AK, Agnarsson BA, Jonasson JG, Ingthorsson S, Traustadottir GA, Oskarsson T, Gudjonsson T (2020) ECM1 secreted by HER2-overexpressing breast cancer cells promotes formation of a vascular niche accelerating cancer cell migration and invasion. Lab Investig 100(7):928–944

Stemmler MP, Eccles RL, Brabletz S, Brabletz T (2019) Non-redundant functions of EMT transcription factors. Nat Cell Biol 21(1):102–112

Sternlicht MD (2006) Key stages in mammary gland development: the cues that regulate ductal branching morphogenesis. Breast Cancer Res 8(1):201

Sternlicht MD, Sunnarborg SW (2008) The ADAM17-amphiregulin-EGFR axis in mammary development and cancer. J Mammary Gland Biol Neoplasia 13(2):181–194

Stevenson AJ, Vanwalleghem G, Stewart TA, Condon ND, Lloyd-Lewis B, Marino N, Putney JW, Scott EK, Ewing AD, Davis FM (2020) Multiscale imaging of basal cell dynamics in the functionally mature mammary gland. Proc Natl Acad Sci USA 117(43):26822–26832

Streuli CH, Bailey N, Bissell MJ (1991) Control of mammary epithelial differentiation: basement membrane induces tissue-specific gene expression in the absence of cell-cell interaction and morphological polarity. J Cell Biol 115(5):1383–1395

Sumbal J, Budkova Z, Traustadottir GA, Koledova Z (2020) Mammary organoids and 3D cell cultures: old dogs with new tricks. J Mammary Gland Biol Neoplasia 25(4):273–288

Sumbal J, Belisova D, Koledova Z (2021) Fibroblasts: the grey eminence of mammary gland development. Semin Cell Dev Biol 114:134–142

Thiery JP, Acloque H, Huang RY, Nieto MA (2009) Epithelial-mesenchymal transitions in development and disease. Cell 139(5):871–890

Villadsen R, Fridriksdottir AJ, Ronnov-Jessen L, Gudjonsson T, Rank F, LaBarge MA, Bissell MJ, Petersen OW (2007) Evidence for a stem cell hierarchy in the adult human breast. J Cell Biol 177(1):87–101

Villasenor A, Chong DC, Henkemeyer M, Cleaver O (2010) Epithelial dynamics of pancreatic branching morphogenesis. Development 137(24):4295–4305

Wang K, Zhang Q, Li D, Ching K, Zhang C, Zheng X, Ozeck M, Shi S, Li X, Wang H, Rejto P, Christensen J, Olson P (2015) PEST domain mutations in Notch receptors comprise an oncogenic driver segment in triple-negative breast cancer sensitive to a gamma-secretase inhibitor. Clin Cancer Res 21(6):1487–1496

Wang QA, Song A, Chen W, Schwalie PC, Zhang F, Vishvanath L, Jiang L, Ye R, Shao M, Tao C, Gupta RK, Deplancke B, Scherer PE (2018) Reversible De-differentiation of mature white adipocytes into preadipocyte-like precursors during lactation. Cell Metab 28(2):282–288 e283

Wang J, Song W, Yang R, Li C, Wu T, Dong XB, Zhou B, Guo X, Chen J, Liu Z, Yu QC, Li W, Fu J, Zeng YA (2021) Endothelial Wnts control mammary epithelial patterning via fibroblast signaling. Cell Rep 34(13):108897

Weaver VM, Howlett AR, Langton-Webster B, Petersen OW, Bissell MJ (1995) The development of a functionally relevant cell culture model of progressive human breast cancer. Semin Cancer Biol 6(3):175–184

Weaver VM, Petersen OW, Wang F, Larabell CA, Briand P, Damsky C, Bissell MJ (1997) Reversion of the malignant phenotype of human breast cells in three-dimensional culture and in vivo by integrin blocking antibodies. J Cell Biol 137(1):231–245

Wilson CL, Sims AH, Howell A, Miller CJ, Clarke RB (2006) Effects of oestrogen on gene expression in epithelium and stroma of normal human breast tissue. Endocr Relat Cancer 13(2):617–628

Wiseman BS, Werb Z (2002) Stromal effects on mammary gland development and breast cancer. Science 296(5570):1046–1049

Wright JA, Richer JK, Goodall GJ (2010) microRNAs and EMT in mammary cells and breast cancer. J Mammary Gland Biol Neoplasia 15(2):213–223

Wuidart A, Ousset M, Rulands S, Simons BD, Van Keymeulen A, Blanpain C (2016) Quantitative lineage tracing strategies to resolve multipotency in tissue-specific stem cells. Genes Dev 30(11):1261–1277

Yao M, Ren T, Pan Y, Xue X, Li R, Zhang L, Li Y, Huang K (2022) A new generation of lineage tracing dynamically records cell fate choices. Int J Mol Sci 23(9)

Zeng L, Li W, Chen CS (2020) Breast cancer animal models and applications. Zool Res 41(5):477–494

Zuo W, Zhang T, Wu DZ, Guan SP, Liew AA, Yamamoto Y, Wang X, Lim SJ, Vincent M, Lessard M, Crum CP, Xian W, McKeon F (2015) p63(+)Krt5(+) distal airway stem cells are essential for lung regeneration. Nature 517(7536):616–620

Single-Cell Analysis in the Mouse and Human Mammary Gland

4

Catriona Corbishley, Patrick Rainford, Austin Reed, and Walid Khaled

Abstract

The mammary gland is a complex organ, host to a rich array of different cell types. As the only organ to complete its development in adulthood, it delicately balances both cell intrinsic and external signalling from hormones, growth factors and other stimulants. The gland can undergo vast proliferation, restructuring and functional maturation during pregnancy and undo these gross changes to a nearly identical resting state during involution. The adaptive nature of the mammary gland underpins its function but also increases its susceptibility to cancer. While already characterised at a macro scale, understanding the complexities of mammary gland morphogenesis, development and tumorigenesis requires interrogation of cellular and molecular mechanisms. As outlined below, single-cell analysis is a key approach for this, allowing us to unbiasedly explore and characterise the functions and properties of individual cells from the genome to the proteome. Here, we introduce key single-cell analysis methods and give brief introductions to their respective workflows. We then discuss the structure, cell types and development of the mammary gland from birth, puberty and through pregnancy, as well as cancer formation. Additionally, we highlight the benefits and caveats of implementing single-cell methodologies and mouse models for studying critical time points of human development and disease. Finally, we highlight some limitations and future directions of single-cell techniques. This chapter provides a starting point for users hoping to further their understanding of mammary gland development and its link to cancer as explained by single-cell analysis studies.

Keywords

Single-cell analysis · Mammary gland · Mouse models · Development · Cell lineage and hierarchy · Breast cancer · Techniques

Catriona Corbishley, Patrick Rainford and Austin Reed contributed equally to this work and share first authorship.

C. Corbishley
Department of Pharmacology, University of Cambridge, Cambridge, UK

Cambridge Stem Cell Institute, University of Cambridge, Cambridge, UK

Hit Discovery, Discovery Sciences, R&D, AstraZeneca, Cambridge, UK

P. Rainford · A. Reed · W. Khaled (✉)
Department of Pharmacology, University of Cambridge, Cambridge, UK

Wellcome-MRC Cambridge Stem Cell Institute, University of Cambridge, Cambridge, UK
e-mail: wtk22@cam.ac.uk

T. Sørlie, R. B. Clarke (eds.), *A Guide to Breast Cancer Research*, Advances in Experimental Medicine and Biology 1464, https://doi.org/10.1007/978-3-031-70875-6_4

Key Points

- The mammary gland is a unique organ that undergoes dynamic changes during its lifespan orchestrated by changes to its cellular composition. These processes can become dysregulated in disease states such as cancer.
- Mouse and human mammary glands share many similarities, making mice a useful model for studying mammary gland development and breast cancers. Key differences also exist between human and mice which require careful consideration.
- Single-cell technologies allow us to study changes in DNA, RNA, protein and epigenetic state. Each technique requires its own sample preparation, processing methods and analysis and provides complementary insight into different levels of the central dogma.
- Single-cell technology facilitates detailed molecular characterisation of dynamic processes such as development, pregnancy and involution at single-cell resolution to improve biological modelling and understanding.
- Single-cell sequencing has redefined our concept of cell type and revealed the full cellular heterogeneity apparent within the mammary gland and the lineage relationships between them.
- Current single-cell approaches have several caveats and limitations which is important to be aware of when designing experiments. Technological advancements are seeking to address existing limitations and produce new modalities of analysis.

4.1 Single-Cell Sequencing

4.1.1 Introduction

In order to understand the biological processes occurring in the mammary gland, both in healthy and diseased states, we first need to identify and characterise the cells which comprise the mammary gland and the lineage hierarchies from which they are derived. While historically, anatomists examined and researched organs such as the mammary gland by analysing its structure and gross functional properties, research has advanced significantly in its ability to interrogate organs with increasing depth. Following the original discovery of cells by Robert Hooke (1665), the initial foray of biologists into single-cell analyses involved studying the morphology of cells using microscopy. However, over time, technological advances in flow cytometry, imaging and high-throughput sequencing have greatly expanded the scope and depth of single-cell analysis. High-throughput sequencing facilitates the analysis of molecular and functional properties of individual cells in an unbiased fashion, revealing heterogeneity and dynamics that would be missed with traditional bulk analysis methods. The advent of single-cell analysis has therefore revolutionised our knowledge of biology and disease by identifying previously unknown cell types. Single-cell data has characterised the biological processes and mechanisms involved in development, homeostasis and disease states which has unveiled new therapeutic strategies. Finally, it has even redefined what a cell type is and revealed the plastic and amorphous nature of cells both in health and disease. However, single-cell analyses are not without their limitations, and the future direction of new single-cell analysis technologies needs to work towards addressing these challenges. Before diving into the contributions single-cell analyses have made in furthering our understanding of mouse and human mammary gland biology, an overview of the techniques involved is required.

4.1.2 Single-Cell RNA Sequencing

Single-cell RNA sequencing (scRNA-seq) is one of the most widely used sequencing approaches and enables comprehensive analysis of cellular heterogeneity by exploring the entire transcriptome of individual cells. By sampling the mRNA molecules present in each cell, scRNA-seq provides valuable insights into transcriptional activity and cellular diversity within a sample. This section provides an overview of the general workflow involved in scRNA-seq, highlighting the key steps in the process and a basic workflow for generic analysis.

4.1.2.1 Library Preparation and Sequencing

The workflow of scRNA-seq begins with the isolation and preparation of single cells. Cells can be obtained from various sources such as tissues or cell cultures. Techniques like fluorescence-activated cell sorting (FACS) or microfluidic platforms are commonly employed to isolate individual cells of interest and distribute them into separate reaction wells or droplets. Maintaining cell viability and integrity is crucial at this stage to ensure reliable downstream analysis.

Following single-cell isolation, the cells undergo lysis to release their RNA content which is captured, converted to cDNA and stabilised to prevent degradation (Fig. 4.1). Several protocols and commercial kits are available for RNA capture, utilising strategies like oligo-dT priming, random priming, or unique molecular identifiers (UMIs) to tag individual RNA molecules both for identifying sample and cell of origin and distinguishing amplification artefacts. To ensure sufficient quantities of cDNA are available for easy detection and downstream analysis, PCR amplification is commonly employed to increase yield. The resulting library is then ready for high-throughput sequencing using platforms like Illumina.

4.1.2.2 Read Realignment and Quality Control

Sequencing outputs a large list of raw reads indicating the distinct nucleotide sequences detected. These are then computationally aligned to the corresponding reference genome and using the integrated genetic barcodes (identifying cell of origin and/or UMI), these reads are mapped to the corresponding individual cell. This then allows the identification of which genes are being expressed and their relative counts, which after accounting for PCR duplicates are often denoted UMI counts. Quality control is performed based on three main metrics: UMI counts (or equivalent), number of distinct genes detected and percentage of mitochondrial RNA observed in each cell/droplet. Barcodes containing particularly few transcripts or other low-quality outliers are removed, likely representing ambient RNA contamination or damaged cells. The counts are often normalised and transformed into log-counts to account for both sequencing depth variation between cells or samples and standardise the counts distribution which can be skewed by rounds of PCR duplication. Then, computational approaches are often used to identify barcodes likely to represent doublets. Cell barcodes identifying high quality cells are then passed on for downstream analysis.

4.1.2.3 Downstream Analysis

From this stage, the typical workflow can vary greatly depending on the experimental design and initial purpose of the sequencing. In an experiment where sequencing was completed over several batches (perhaps on different days or even collated from different labs) batch correction/integration is often required to account for technical effects common in scRNA-seq. This can be completed via a continually evolving repertoire of integration methods such as scVI or fastMNN (Lopez et al. 2018; Haghverdi et al. 2018). Once accounted for, one of the first steps would usually involve qualitatively exploring the structure of the data through dimension reduction and visualisation. Each gene is considered as a distinct 'dimension' which together describes the activity of a cell. Typically, a subset of genes (approx. 2000–5000 depending on the use case) with the highest individual variance across all cells is then selected, both to reduce computational effort and high-dimensional noise. From this set of highly variable genes, principal component analysis (PCA) is performed to identify the linear combinations of genes which show the highest variability across cells. These principal components hope to capture the major heterogeneity present in the dataset from which cells can be clustered based on similarity into discrete or continuously varying cell types/states.

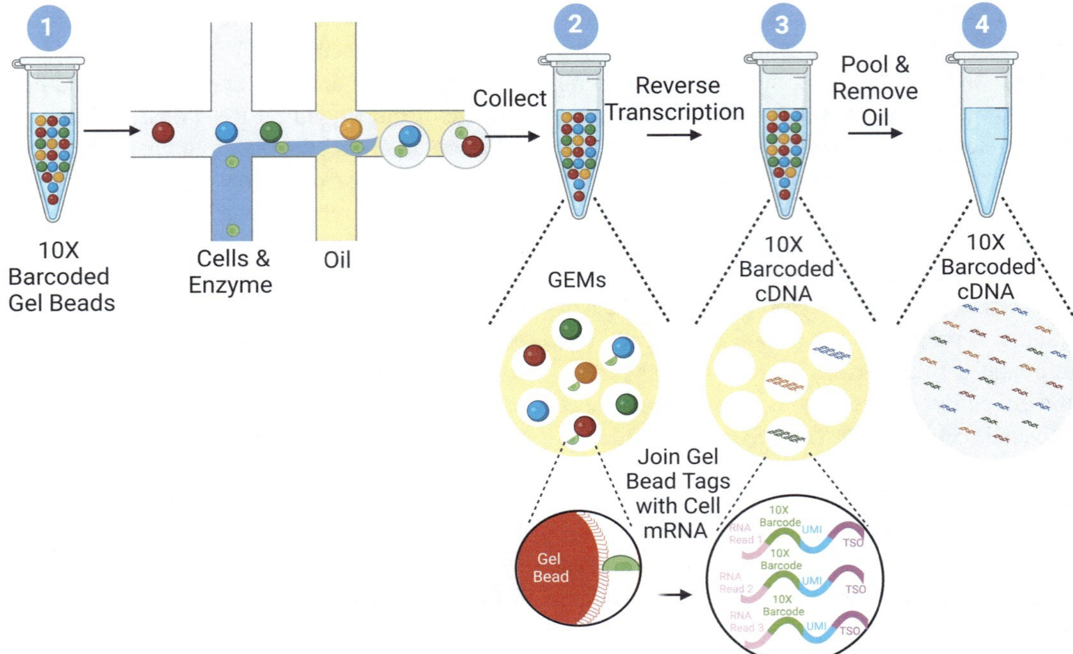

Fig. 4.1 Microfluidics-based single-cell RNA sequencing. Schematic representation of a typical library preparation workflow for microfluidics-based single-cell RNA sequencing. First, hydrogel beads are prepared each containing a unique 10X barcode on its surface (1). Next, isolated cells are delivered using limiting dilution to ensure single cells combine with individual beads and reverse transcriptase enzyme inside partitioning oil to generate a Gel Beads-in-Emulsion, known as GEMs (2). Once captured in GEMs, reverse transcription takes place, converting RNA to unique barcoded cDNA (3). Transcripts originating from the same cell can be identified using the associated 10X barcode, while transcripts can be distinguished from one another using the Unique Molecular Identifier (UMI). Finally, barcoded cDNA can be pooled and oil removed before cDNA is converted to a library for use in high-throughput sequencing platforms (4) (created with BioRender.com)

There is a wealth of literature detailing many different ways to cluster data into cell types. Most commonly the Leiden clustering algorithm is used based on its robustness and high performance in high-dimensional scRNA datasets. Leiden is an unbiased network-based approach which identifies clusters as collections of cells with high connectivity on the data's K-nearest neighbour graph (for more details see: Traag et al. 2019), i.e., identifying groups of cells with high transcriptional similarity. Commonly, a further dimensionality reduction technique such as Uniform Manifold Approximation and Projection (UMAP) is then used on the PCA coordinates to visualise the dataset in a 2D or 3D plot which aims to preserve local structure (i.e. the algorithm attempts to plot similar cells closer to each other). This helps to explore and understand complex datasets more easily, allowing the identifications of trends, groupings or outliers that might not be obvious in the original high-dimensional data. However, the UMAP plot can only give qualitative insights into the data due to its non-linear nature. To quantitatively study transcriptional variation in particular cell types or across test groups, various statistical approaches are used. New methods are continually developing in this field to assess various additional aspects such as cell–cell communication, gene regulatory networks and inferred copy number variation profiles.

4.1.3 CyTOF

In addition to single-cell RNA sequencing (scRNA-seq), another powerful approach that has revolutionised the field of single-cell analysis is Cytometry by Time-of-Flight (CyTOF) (Bandura et al. 2009). CyTOF is a cutting-edge technology that enables the high-resolution analysis of protein expression in individual cells. By assaying protein expression rather than RNA, CyTOF can give better insight into the current behaviour of the cell accounting for the variety of post-translational and post-transcriptional effects which scRNA-seq is blind to. Unfortunately, this comes with a cost, which lies in the number of different proteins able to be quantified in one experiment. The following section will provide an overview of the general workflow involved in CyTOF, highlighting its key steps in implementation and basic analysis.

4.1.3.1 Sample Preparation and Acquisition

The CyTOF workflow begins with the preparation of single-cell suspensions, which can be obtained from various sources, including tissues or cell cultures. Unlike traditional flow cytometry, which relies on fluorescence-based detection, CyTOF employs metal-conjugated antibodies for cell labelling. Each metal is associated with a specific antibody, allowing for the simultaneous measurement of multiple cellular markers with minimal spectral overlap. This feature greatly expands the number of parameters that can be assessed in a single experiment.

Once the cells are appropriately labelled with metal-conjugated antibodies, they are introduced into the CyTOF instrument for acquisition. In CyTOF, cells are atomised into individual droplets, and a high-powered laser is used to vaporise them. As the cells vaporise, the metal ions associated with specific antibodies are released and measured based on their time-of-flight in a mass spectrometer. This process generates highly detailed data on the expression of numerous cell surface and intracellular markers at the single-cell level. Current CyTOF technology allows the quantification of up to 40 distinct metal probes and can perform a very high cell throughput, matching or exceeding that of most scRNA-seq protocols (Iyer et al. 2022).

4.1.3.2 Data Analysis and Interpretation

The data generated by CyTOF is complex and multidimensional, often encompassing dozens of cellular markers for each cell. Similar to RNA sequencing, CyTOF provides a large matrix with protein counts for each of your chosen markers across each individual cell. To make sense of this wealth of information, various computational approaches are employed very similarly to scRNA-seq workflows. The analysis begins with normalisation, batch correction and quality control to account for variations in signal variation over time or between batches and remove dead or damaged cells from downstream analysis. Various packages have been developed to perform these steps such as CATALYST (Crowell et al. 2023, github). Then, matching scRNA-seq data analysis pipelines, unbiased clustering and dimension reduction is completed to annotate cell types and visualise the data. Furthermore, CyTOF data analysis involves the quantification of protein expression levels, allowing for the identification of differentially expressed proteins in specific cell populations. This information can provide insights into functional differences between cell types or reveal key regulatory proteins involved in cellular processes.

4.1.4 ATAC Sequencing

Identifying genes or proteins differentially regulated in individual cells is a great approach to distinguish cellular states or the effects of treatment conditions. However, this often provides little explanation of the underlying mechanisms which drive the change in gene or protein expression which may lie higher up the hierarchy of the central dogma. One aspect of this could lie in epigenetic changes such as changes in chromosomal structure and accessibility. This affects gene expression directly by manipulating the physical accessibility of different regions of the genome to macromolecules involved in transcription. ATAC (Assay for Transposase-Accessible Chromatin) sequencing is commonly used to investigate the accessibility of chromatin regions within individual cells (Buenrostro et al. 2013). It provides insights into the organisation of chromatin and regulatory elements such as promoters and enhancers, which play a crucial role in gene expression. In this section, we will provide an overview of the general workflow involved in ATAC sequencing, highlighting the key steps in the process.

4.1.4.1 Nuclei Isolation and Transposition

The ATAC sequencing workflow begins with the isolation of nuclei from the cells of interest. Cells can be obtained from various sources, such as tissues or cell cultures. The isolated nuclei contain intact chromatin, including both DNA and associated proteins. Next, the isolated nuclei undergo transposition, a process that involves the enzymatic digestion and insertion of sequencing adapters into open chromatin regions.

4.1.4.2 Tagmentation and DNA Amplification

During the transposition step, a transposase enzyme is used to fragment the chromatin and simultaneously add adapters to the open regions. This process, known as tagmentation, tags the accessible DNA regions with the adapters. Following tagmentation, PCR amplification is performed to selectively amplify the tagged DNA fragments, which include the regions of open chromatin. The amplified DNA fragments serve as the input for subsequent sequencing library preparation.

4.1.4.3 Library Preparation, Sequencing and Data Analysis

After DNA amplification, the ATAC sequencing library is prepared. This involves adding sequencing adapters to the amplified DNA fragments, which allows them to be sequenced on high-throughput sequencing platforms such as Illumina. The library preparation step may also incorporate unique molecular identifiers (UMIs) or barcodes to enable the identification of PCR duplicates and to facilitate downstream analysis.

The prepared ATAC sequencing library is subjected to high-throughput sequencing, generating a large number of short DNA sequence reads. These sequence reads represent the accessible chromatin regions in the original cells. The raw sequencing data then undergoes bioinformatic analysis to process and interpret the results. This analysis typically involves read alignment to a reference genome, quality control assessment and identification of accessible regions (Grandi et al. 2022).

4.1.4.4 Downstream Analysis

The downstream analysis of ATAC sequencing data involves exploring the accessibility landscape of the genome within individual cells. This can include identifying regions of open chromatin, analysing chromatin accessibility patterns across different cell types or conditions and investigating regulatory elements such as promoters and enhancers. Advanced computational techniques, including peak calling, clustering and differential accessibility analysis, are applied to gain insights into the functional implications of chromatin accessibility. Generally, this analysis is performed in bulk per test condition; however, newer approaches are being developed to explore chromatin accessibility at a single-cell level in the so-called scATAC sequencing (Cusanovich et al. 2015).

4.1.5 Single-Cell DNA Sequencing

While scRNA-seq has been transformative in our understanding of transcriptional diversity at the single-cell level, single-cell DNA sequencing (scDNA-seq) offers a parallel view into the genomic heterogeneity of individual cells. A further step up the chain to ATAC sequencing, scDNA-seq allows exploration of the mutational landscape of tissue, identifying single nucleotide polymorphisms, copy number variations or even structural variations and rearrangements at a single-cell level. This section will overview the general workflow involved in scDNA-seq, highlighting its key steps and the valuable insights it provides into the genetic landscape of cells.

4.1.5.1 Sample Preparation and Sequencing

The scDNA-seq workflow begins with the isolation and preparation of single cells, similar to scRNA-seq. Single cells can be sourced from various biological samples, including tissues or cell cultures. Techniques such as fluorescence-activated cell sorting (FACS) or microfluidic platforms are commonly used to isolate individual cells, ensuring their viability and integrity throughout the process.

Once single cells are isolated, they undergo a process of DNA extraction, amplification and library preparation. The exact order and protocols used in this stage vary significantly across scDNA-seq methods. Direct Library Preparation (DLP) sequencing uses nanowells for single-cell isolation and lysis. Then the DNA is fragmented and tagged performing minimal PCR for amplification indexing and adaptor incorporation (Zahn et al. 2017). The resulting DNA libraries are ready for high-throughput sequencing using platforms such as Illumina. Each sequenced read represents a segment of the genomic DNA from a single cell.

4.1.5.2 Data Analysis and Interpretation

The data generated by scDNA-seq is complex, with each cell's genomic content represented in the form of sequencing reads. To extract meaningful information, advanced computational techniques are applied to mould the results into a more interpretable form. The first step often involves mapping and aligning the sequencing reads to a reference genome to determine the number of reads for each genomic region with tools such as Bowtie2 (Langmead and Salzberg 2012). This process allows the identification of genomic features, such as copy number variations and mutations.

One of the primary applications of scDNA-seq is the detection of copy number alterations at the single-cell level. By analysing the depth of sequencing coverage across the genome, changes in the copy number can be inferred, including amplifications and deletions, within individual cells using software such as scAbsolute (Schneider et al. 2023). Additionally, scDNA-seq can enable the identification of somatic mutations and genetic heterogeneity within tissues or cell populations. This is completed by comparing population references and the pool of cells sequenced, to identify unique polymorphisms specific to individual cells or subclones. This analysis can provide important insights on clonal evolution and the role of genetic variation in disease progression. However, single-cell somatic mutation analysis is currently limited by the cost of increased sequencing depth for scDNA-seq experiments. Further advancements in the sequencing technology aim to reduce costs and broaden its usability.

4.2 Comparing Mouse and Human Mammary Glands

4.2.1 Mouse Models

Mammary gland development and breast cancer development are highly dynamic and complex events involving cross talk between multiple cell types and stimuli. The frequency and variety of these changes throughout the life of a mammary gland makes it a challenging tissue to study, particularly using a single time point and/or cell-line based models. Human breast donor samples are typically only available at one or very few time points, preventing the study of a continuum of states which fairly reflect the native physiology. To overcome this limitation, experimental animal models from which multiple time points can be studied more easily are widely utilised in mammary gland modelling and are a key research tool for understanding breast cancer biology.

Animal models represent a gold standard preclinical model, encapsulating the complexity of living organisms and more accurately reflecting the native biological state (Boix-Montesinos et al. 2021). Mammalian animals offer a closely related model to study human disease. Rodent models are the most popular mammalian animal models, with rats (*Rattus norvegicus*) and mice (*Mus musculus*) the most widely used rodents. Mice are widely utilised in disease modelling and offer a valuable model for studying processes which are well-conserved between rodents and primate lineages. Practically, mice have many advantages over other larger animals including small size facilitating easier management, handling and cheaper associated costs. Mouse models also generate highly reproducible results within relatively short timeframes owing to their short reproductive cycles and lifespans. However, while there are many similarities between human and mouse mammary glands, there are also several differences. Understanding these similarities and differences is important for ensuring that the design, execution, analyses and conclusions of model experiments are carefully reasoned.

4.2.2 Mouse and Human Mammary Glands

4.2.2.1 Structural Differences

Mammary glands of mice and humans share very similar physiology, structure and function, making mice a useful model for studying breast development and cancer (Cardiff and Wellings 1999; Boix-Montesinos et al. 2021). Single-cell technologies are now allowing us to interrogate the cellular properties underpinning these similarities as well as differences and the lineage relationships of the cells composing the mammary gland. This is not only useful for linking cellular properties with physiological function in different animals, but also allows us to determine the strengths and limitations of mouse models for mammary gland research.

Human and mice mammary glands exist in highly dynamic states and undergo dramatic morphogenetic changes throughout their lifespan. To orchestrate these physiological changes, specific cell lineages and their stem and progenitor functions are required as summarised in Fig. 4.2.

The hierarchy of epithelial cells is notably similar in mouse and human mammary systems. Both systems comprise a heterogeneous cellular

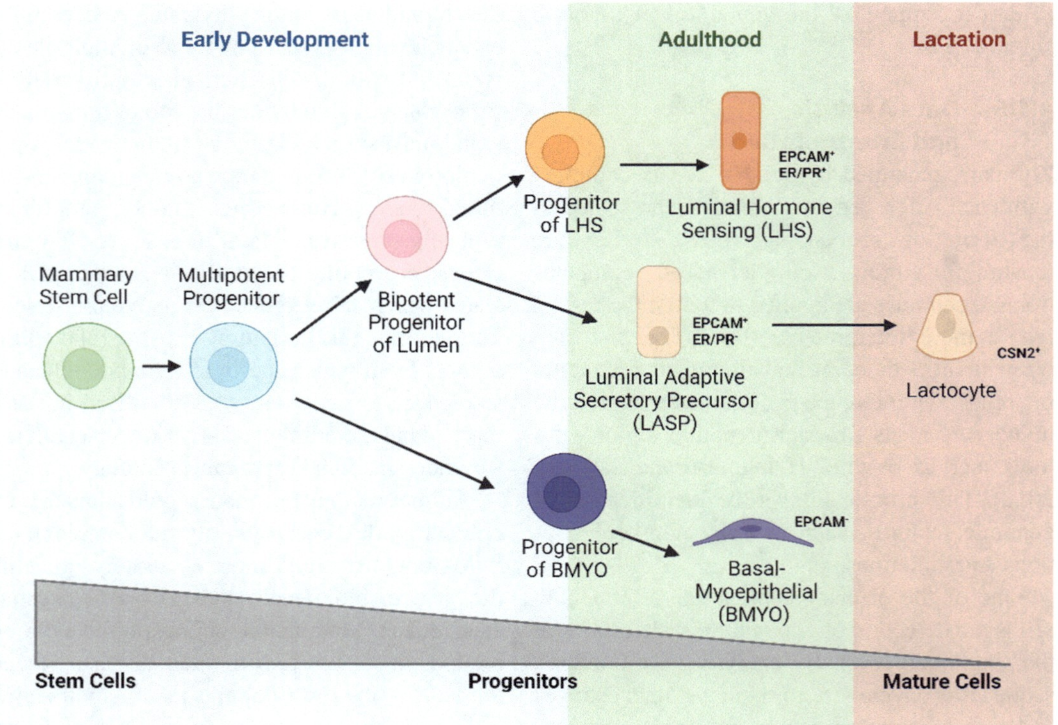

Fig. 4.2 Mammary cell lineage hierarchy schematic. Schematic representation of the current proposed model for mammary gland cell lineage hierarchy, showing progression from a stem cell-like state to a mature cell state (created with BioRender.com)

compartment containing luminal and basal tissue layers which can be further subclassified. The central luminal lactocyte cells are responsible for milk production whilst the basal layer contracts to expel milk along the duct towards the nipple through which milk is released during lactation. Architecturally, adult human and mouse mammary glands are both organised into bi-layered epithelial branching structures which sit within the fat pad along with a lymph node. The human breast is a branching network of ducts that forms 12–20 structures known as lobes. Each of these lobes comprises 20–40 grape-like terminal ductal lobular units (TDLUs), also known as lobules. These lobules are each made up of many alveoli, the functional units of the breast which go on to produce milk in pregnancy. A schematic overview of the human gland is given below in Fig. 4.3. The adult mouse mammary epithelial tree, at rest, is similarly composed of a branching ductal structure that terminates in blunt-ended ductal termini (Paine and Lewis 2017) but does not form TDLUs. Instead, during pregnancy, the ductal structures undergo massive proliferation and branching, ultimately forming milk-producing lobules filled with alveoli (Richert et al. 2000). Single-cell RNA sequencing of mouse mammary glands during different stages of gestation and lactation suggests that this process is driven by hyperproliferation and differentiation of LASP cells into lactocytes (Bach et al. 2017).

Whilst sharing many similarities, key differences exist between mice and human mammary gland systems. For example, the number and distribution of mammary glands differs. Mice have five pairs of mammary glands along the mammary line, while humans have two mammary glands located on the chest. Furthermore, mouse mammary glands have fewer and shorter ductal

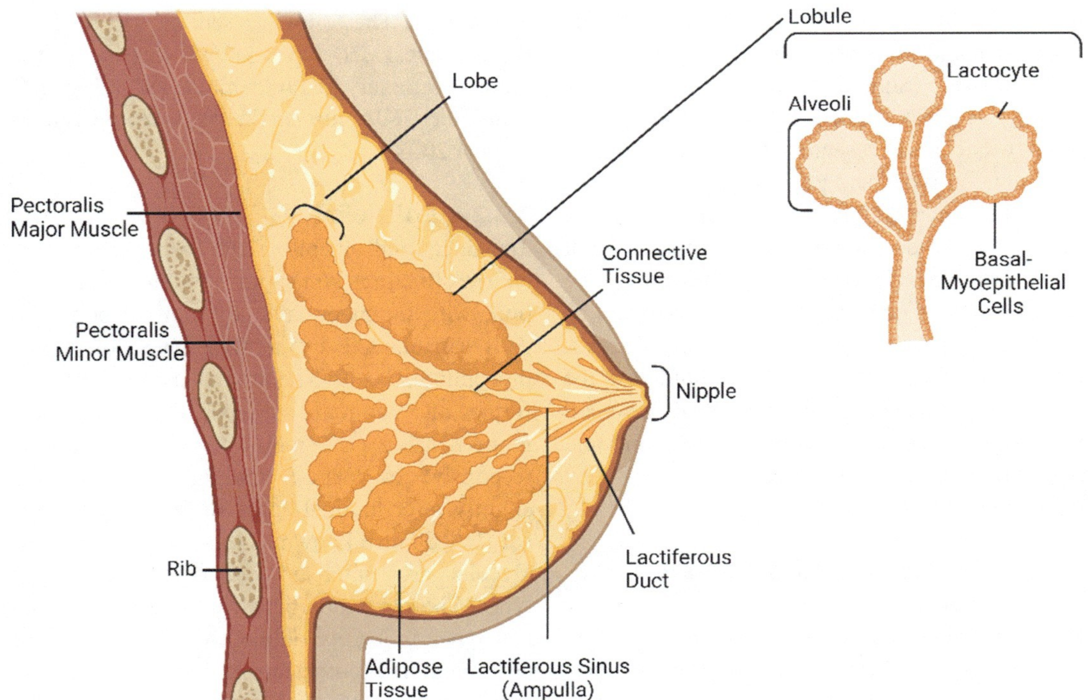

Fig. 4.3 Anatomy of a lactating human mammary gland. The mammary gland is a network of lobules and ducts. Each breast comprises 12–20 lobes, each of which is made up of 20–40 lobules that branch away from the nipple. Each lobule itself is made up of several alveoli, the site of milk synthesis. Alveoli are joined to the nipple via lactiferous ducts which act as a channel for milk during lactation. Adipose tissue, blood vessels and connective tissue fill the space around the ductal tree (created with BioRender.com)

branches with less sophisticated branching patterns whilst human glands exhibit more extensive baseline branching. In addition to structural differences, mice experience a greater demand for milk production compared with humans due to larger litter sizes and shorter reproductive and gestational periods. To accommodate these demands, mice undergo more extensive and dynamic involution and remodelling to a baseline morphology, in contrast to human TDLUs which retain more extensive branching following lactation. In addition to structural differences observed, key cellular differences exist between mice and human mammary glands.

4.2.2.2 Cell Type Differences

The mammary gland is a unique organ that is able to undergo vast structural and functional changes upon hormonal stimulation during pregnancy and then largely reverse these changes returning to a resting state through the processes of involution. Being both the only secretory organ that matures during adulthood under normal homoeostatic conditions and the most common origin for cancer worldwide (Sung et al. 2021), the mammary gland is of great interest in both developmental biology and cancer research. There are a range of different cell types and populations that contribute to the structural integrity and functionality of the breast. Understanding the composition of these cell types is crucial for unravelling the complexities of mammary gland biology and its potential implications in breast-related diseases. Recent advancements in single-cell studies of the human breast have shed light on the diverse cell populations present in the mammary gland and have provided valuable insights into how they compare to mouse cell types.

4.2.2.3 Cell Types of the Mammary Gland

High-throughput scRNA-seq is a commonly used and effective technique for identifying and characterising cell types. Clustering of gene expression data allows an unbiased way to identify populations of cells with similar expression profiles and comparison to previously identified marker genes facilitates the annotation of clusters. However, the resolution of clustering and the variety of cell types captured in a particular experiment can vary, often making the task of annotation a manual labour-intensive stage of analysis. An additional issue, particularly in the breast/mammary gland field, is the inconsistency of cell type nomenclature, with many groups using various synonyms for the same group of cells. The Human Cell Atlas (HCA) is a consorted global effort to address these issues and characterise all cell types within the human body. It hopes to provide an all-encompassing resource of scRNA-seq datasets with standardised cell type labels for all to use. This centralised effort hopes to remove some of the biases related to manual cluster annotations creating a reference of the standard distribution of cellular states and their categorisation. One way in which the HCA is attempting to standardise cell nomenclature is through organised meetings in which experts come together to agree on universal cell type annotations. The following section will describe the canonical cell types known to exist in the human mammary gland (summarised in Fig. 4.4) using the HCA nomenclature agreed upon in August 2023.

4.2.2.4 Epithelial

The ducts and alveoli of the resting breast are hollow structures and appear similar in composition, with an inner layer of luminal epithelial cells surrounded by a thin layer of basal-myoepithelial cells. The luminal cells can be split further into two main subtypes, the luminal hormone sensing (LHS; also known as hormone responsive or mature luminal) cells and the slightly rarer luminal adaptive secretory precursor (LASP; also known as luminal progenitor or alveolar progenitor or secretory luminal) cell types. The separation between these two luminal cell types is largely defined by the presence of oestrogen and progesterone receptors on hormone sensing cells which are absent on LASPs (Sleeman et al. 2007; Mallepell et al. 2006). Within the mouse, several studies have shown that the LASP cell type can differentiate to give

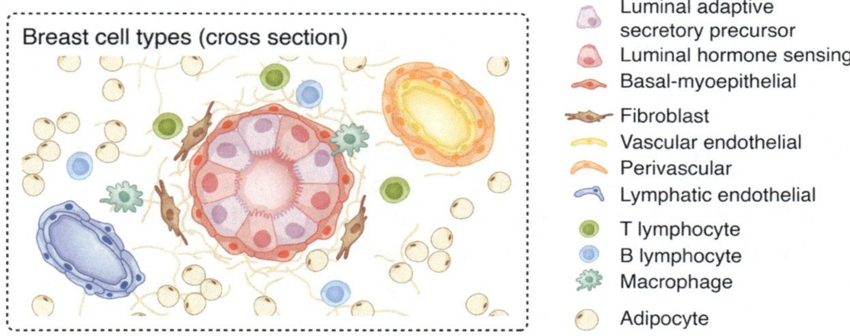

Fig. 4.4 Schematic of the cell types present within the breast. The ducts and alveoli of the human breast are composed of epithelial cells, which are embedded in a microenvironment supported and maintained by stromal cells and further protected by the presence of several immune cells

rise to functional alveolar cells which secrete milk (Bach et al. 2017; Pal et al. 2017). The differentiation of LASPs into functional alveolar cells has also been evidenced in the human mammary gland through single-cell analysis of cells excreted in human milk (Twigger et al. 2022). Additionally, within some strains of mice, a third luminal population has been identified which displays a mix of both LASP and luminal hormone sensing gene markers. These have been labelled hormone sensing progenitors; however, the functional significance of the cells is unknown and no human equivalent has been identified (Bach et al. 2017).

Throughout normal development and lifespan, the ratio of luminal and basal-myoepithelial cells fluxes to change the cellular composition of the mammary gland. During early development, multipotent mammary stem cells are thought to give rise to the early ductal tree and help control cell type compositions. Recently, there has been debate regarding the existence of multipotent mammary stem cells in the adult gland; however, lineage-tracing experiments suggest that each of the three epithelial cell types maintain their own lineages throughout adulthood (Saeki et al. 2021). This suggests that multipotent cell types are lost during earlier stages of development. Alternative single-cell data points away from a unidirectional, hierarchical differentiation trajectory, instead suggesting that mammary basal-myoepithelial cells exist in dynamic non-hierarchical transcriptional states (Gutierrez et al. 2022). Dysregulation and perturbations of the cell lineage ratios have been linked extensively to breast cancer, thus greater understanding of the dynamics of these processes is vital to the field.

4.2.2.5 Stroma

The microenvironment surrounding the mammary gland's epithelial ductal tree consists of an array of stroma which help maintain the structural integrity and natural homeostasis of the breast. The composition of the stromal compartment is largely conserved between mice and humans, although there are some structural differences. Some of the main structural differences include the number and location of glands and the presence of a prominent fat pad in mice, whereas human mammary glands have adipose tissue spread throughout the breast. In both species, the stromal compartment can be classified into four primary categories: fibroblasts, endothelial cells, perivascular cells and adipocytes. Fibroblasts are responsible for producing and maintaining the extracellular matrix, which provides structural support to the gland. Fibroblasts also secrete various extracellular proteins which contribute to the organisation and integrity of the gland during processes such as tissue remodelling and wound healing (Avagliano et al. 2020). Single-cell sequencing studies have highlighted a great diversity in the subtypes of fibroblast cells in both the mouse and human mammary glands

(Bach et al. 2021; Reed et al. 2023), adding to earlier characterisations which distinguish between intralobular and interlobular fibroblasts based on their proximity to the epithelial ducts and lobules (Fleming et al. 2008). In particular, there has been a lot of recent interest regarding cancer-associated fibroblasts, a subpopulation of fibroblast cells which support a pro-tumour microenvironment. It is suggested that these cells could play a role in the formation of cancer through the secretion of protumourigenic factors (Nee et al. 2023). Despite these findings, there is still a significant knowledge gap regarding the functional diversity of fibroblasts in the mammary gland and its relationship to disease. The endothelial cells consist of vascular endothelial and lymphatic endothelial cell types which construct the veins, arteries and lymphatic vessels spread throughout the breast. Related to these cells are the perivascular cells (also known as vascular mural, vascular accessory or pericytes), which play a crucial role in supporting the function of blood vessels by modulating blood flow, vessel permeability and contributing to angiogenesis (Sweeney and Foldes 2018). The final category of stromal cells is adipocytes, or fat cells, which constitute a significant proportion of the breast. Adipocytes contribute to the microenvironment by secreting various adipokines and growth factors that influence the behaviour of neighbouring cells (Church et al. 2012).

4.2.2.6 Immune

There are a variety of immune cells present in and around the mammary gland of both lymphoid and myeloid lineages. The various types and subtypes of immune cells can be defined in many ways. Traditionally, marker proteins have been used with FACS sorting to distinguish functionally distinct cell types. However, they can also be separated by their development origin with some immune cells remaining tissue-resident and originating from early embryonic immune cells while others continually enter the tissue from circulation after maturing elsewhere in the body. The main immune cell types found in the mammary gland are T cells, B cells, plasma cells, natural killer cells, innate lymphoid cells, mast cells, neutrophils, macrophages and dendritic cells. These have now been identified in many scRNA-seq studies; however, due both to differences in protein and RNA correlation and the physical size or fragility of some of these cells, most single-cell studies to date struggle to capture or annotate the full range of immune cells present in the mammary gland (Reed et al. 2023; Kumar et al. 2023). Efforts such as the Immune Cell Atlas are working to address some of these shortcomings (Domínguez Conde et al. 2022).

4.3 Single-Cell Analyses of Mouse Mammary Gland Development

The mammary gland undergoes dynamic changes during its lifespan. The development of the mammary gland can be broadly divided into six different stages: embryonic, pre-pubertal, pubertal, pregnancy, lactation and involution. Each phase of development is tightly regulated via a different mechanism and mammary glands comprise various cell types and cell states to facilitate these changes. Given the poor availability of human mammary gland samples outside of adult resting states or diseased states such as cancer, the majority of single-cell analyses of mammary gland development have been conducted on mouse tissues. For example, Henry et al. used single-cell profiling of mouse models to characterise gene expression signatures and identified cellular heterogeneity across diverse stages of mammary gland maturation and development (Henry et al. 2021).

4.3.1 Embryonic Development

Most of the mammary gland development occur postnatally, during adolescence and adulthood. However, during embryonic development, a rudimental gland is formed which is present at birth. Murine embryonic mammary gland development begins shortly after mid-gestation at embryonic day (E)10.5 and continues until E18.5. At E10.5, development begins with emergence of bilateral ridges known as milk lines which form through thickening of the ectoderm/epidermis and run between the anterior and posterior limb buds. Between E11 and E12 ectodermal cells coalesce into five pairs of mammary placodes, transient lens shaped structures, which form along the milk lines at the site of each future nipple. The placodes then invaginate and become bulb-shaped epithelial buds known as the primary mammary rudiment which are distinct from the surrounding epidermis (Sternlicht et al. 2006). At E13.5 mammary gland development in the female embryos temporarily pauses whilst in male embryos androgen receptor activation in the mesenchyme causes permanent degradation of the mammary buds between E13.5 and 15.5. At E15.5, mammary development in the females resumes and the glands begin to proliferate. The primary rudiment penetrates the mesenchyme layer and invades a preadipocyte cluster which later becomes the mammary fat pad. Limited branching begins around E16 when each sprout forms a lumen which opens at the surface of the skin where epidermal invagination creates the nipple. Thus, a hollow rudimentary ductal tree occupying a small portion of the fat pad is present at birth (Hens and Wysolmerski 2005; Sakakura et al. 1987).

Our understanding of embryonic mammary gland development has been deepened using singe cell analysis. For example, single-cell chromatin data from Chung et al. suggests that by late embryonic development (E18) most cells are already weakly biased towards either a luminal or a basal fate, priming cells to rapidly differentiate into the respective cell types upon microenvironmental stimuli following birth (Chung et al. 2019). Multiple single-cell lineage-tracing and genetic studies suggest bipotent foetal mammary stem cells are present in the embryo, and separate lineage-committed stem/progenitor populations for basal and luminal lineages are maintained in the postnatal gland (Elias et al. 2017; Lilja et al. 2018). Regan & Smalley found these lineage restrictions could be loosened to form multilineage potential upon loss of homeostasis/injury (Regan and Smalley 2020).

4.3.2 Pubertal Development

At birth, the mouse mammary gland consists of a small epithelial rudiment embedded in the stromal tissue. Prior to puberty, the epithelial rudiment is quiescent, and the growth rate of the mammary gland matches overall animal growth. During puberty, the mammary gland undergoes significant changes and develops from a rudimentary tree into a complex branched epithelial ductal tree capable of supporting alveolar and milk production during pregnancy and lactation. With the onset of puberty at approximately 3–4 weeks of age, ovarian and pituitary-derived hormones stimulate accelerated epithelial cell migration and ductal extension, amplification and branching, a process known as branching morphogenesis. From week 4, terminal end buds (TEBs), highly proliferative large club-shaped structures at the tip of growing ducts are seen. TEBs are formed of multiple inner layers of cells known as body cells and a single outer leading layer of cells known as cap cells. TEBs drive the process of ductal elongation and invasion of the surrounding fat pad under the control of oestradiol and the oestrogen receptor. TEBs undergo bifurcation to produce new primary ducts, and secondary side branches form, filling the entire fat pad with a branched ductal tree. Sexual maturity is reached at approximately 5 weeks; however, the mammary glands undergo further growth until puberty is complete at approximately 10–12 weeks of age. At the end of puberty when ducts reach the end of the mammary fat pad, TEBs regress and the body cells and outer cap cells differentiate into the luminal and myoepithelial cells, respectively, that line the mature ducts (Fu et al. 2020). At this point, the mature ductal network which acts as a channel for milk during lactation is fully formed and most of the stroma is invaded. Some space remains within the fat pad to enable additional expansion during oestrus or pregnancy. Mature ducts undergo dynamic changes of branching and regression during each oestrus cycle due to fluctuations in ovarian hormones which drive sprouting of additional tertiary side branches to produce a fuller ductal tree in preparation for potential lactation (Fata et al. 2004).

Oestrus Cycle Pop Out Box

- In mice, the reproductive cycle is commonly known as the oestrus cycle and takes 4–5 days to complete.
- The oestrus cycle consists of proestrus, estrus, metestrus and diestrus stages which cycle until interrupted either by pregnancy, pseudopregnancy or anestrus (a non-breeding period when reproductive organs are quiescent).
- Driven by fluctuations in levels of oestrogen, progesterone and prolactin hormones, the mammary gland undergoes well-characterised morphological changes during each stage of the estrus cycle.
- Ductal branching and proliferation are seen during proestrus and estrus stages whilst regression is seen during metestrus and diestrus phases.
- Estrus stage can be evaluated in a number of ways; however, vaginal cytology is widely accepted as the most accurate method.

4.3.3 Pregnancy/Gestation

Pregnancy triggers significant mammary gland remodelling to produce lactation competent glands capable of feeding the offspring. Pregnancy related morphogenesis is tightly controlled through the complex interplay of multiple factors including oestrogen, progesterone, prolactin and insulin-like growth factor. Gestation related mammary changes can be divided into distinct development stages: ductal growth and expansion, alveologenesis and secretory initiation.

4.3.4 Ductal Growth, Alveologenesis, Secretory Initiation

The early onset of pregnancy related hormones triggers ductal epithelial cells to rapidly proliferate and begin further ductal branching. This ductal branching forms the underlying structure for the mature gland. Next, in preparation for lactation, alveolar structures capable of milk production form in a process known as alveologenesis. Ultimately, this results in specialised grape-shaped structures called alveoli to generate the structures required to support lactation (Brisken 2002). In this process, elevated levels of serum prolactin and progesterone activate the alveolar switch, a genetic program responsible for coordinating changes in mammary epithelial cell proliferation, migration, differentiation and deletion (Oakes et al. 2006). Alveologenesis halts around mid-pregnancy and the secretory initiation phase begins. After this point, maturation of luminal cells within the alveoli forms lactocyte cells capable of milk production.

4.3.5 Lactation

During the lactation stage, the mammary gland produces and secretes milk in a phase known as secretory activation. Secretory activation phase occurs nearing parturition when alveolar tight junctions close, leading to the secretion of milk and lipid proteins into the alveolar lumen in preparation for active milk secretion post-partum (Oakes et al. 2006). Following birth, the removal of the placenta causes progesterone levels to drop which in combination with elevated levels of prolactin, cortisol and insulin stimulates lactation. Stimulation of the nipples and milk removal triggers prolactin and oxytocin release to maintain milk production. In mice, lactation continues for approximately 3 weeks post-partum unless otherwise weaned.

It is important to highlight that most of our understanding of the mammary gland during pregnancy and lactation is based on results from mouse models. This is generally due to obvious ethical and practical limitations of sampling tissue from women during lactation. Recent single-cell studies looking at live cells ejected within the milk of lactating mothers suggest that there may be more differences at the cellular level of lactation than had previously been appreciated. Twigger et al. (2022) found two distinct populations of lactocytes cells both expressing similar but distinct expression profiles to that of the singular alveolar/lactocyte population characterised in the mouse (Bach et al. 2017; Pal et al. 2017). By considering gene signatures this study showed both lactocyte populations were most closely related to the human LASP cell type of the resting breast. This suggests a similar lineage trajectory from LASP to lactocyte operates in the human gland. However, more work needs to be done in this area to understand how the cellular composition of the mouse and human mammary gland relate and what this may mean functionally and for milk composition and production.

4.3.6 Involution

Following a period of lactation, the mammary gland undergoes a multi-step process known as involution to return glands to a near pre-pregnant quiescent state in preparation for future pregnancies (Hennighausen and Robinson 1998). Involution is a complex and tightly controlled extensive tissue remodelling process, triggered by weaning and orchestrated by hormones, proteases and elements of the immune system. During involution, apoptosis of mammary ductal and alveolar cells is observed along with increased immune cell recruitment to the mammary gland. Degradation of stagnant milk and apoptotic cell death also occur prior to repopulation of the mammary gland with fat cells (Nonnecke and Smith 1984; Hurley 1989; Strange et al. 1992; Watson 2006; Strange et al. 1992; Watson 2006).

Involution can be broadly divided into a reversible and irreversible phase (Lund et al. 1996). In mice, the reversible phase occurs during the first 2 days postweaning via locally controlled lysosomal mediated programmed cell death. Following weaning, stagnant milk accumulates within the mammary gland which triggers increased expression of death-inducing signalling molecules (Stein et al. 2007). This causes significant apoptosis of epithelial cells; however, mammary gland morphology largely remains unchanged and lactation can be reinitiated (Strange et al. 1992). After 48 h post weaning, the irreversible phase begins driven by systemic hormonal changes and mitochondrial-mediated apoptosis. During the irreversible phase, milk is cleared, the basement membrane degraded, and alveoli structures collapse. In mice, involution takes approximately 2 weeks to complete during which time the gland regresses back to a nearly pre-pregnant state ready to initiate another cycle of pregnancy, lactation and involution.

Mammary tumour progression often mimics or hijacks involution-associated pathways. For example, one single-cell transcriptomics study identified a novel driver of alveolar lineage differentiation in tumours, with concomitant acquisition of metastasis and offers a putative link between the poor prognosis of breast cancer associated with a short period following childbirth (Valdés-Mora et al. 2021).

4.3.7 Effect of Parity

Pregnancy-induced mammary gland changes have been shown to induce lasting changes which persist beyond involution. For example, one single-cell RNA-sequencing study showed cells in the luminal compartment of parous and nulliparous mice have different transcriptional profiles (Bach et al. 2017). Faster initiation of ductal branching is observed in parous compared with nulliparous mice and one study looking at DNA methylation of various mammary cell types suggests epigenetic changes underpin these differences (dos Santos et al. 2015). Hanasoge Somasundara et al. (2021) used single-cell RNA sequencing to profile epithelial and non-epithelial cells in mammary tissue from nulliparous and parous mice. They showed that pregnancy-induced changes modulate the communication between mammary epithelial and immune cells, offering one link between pregnancy, the immune microenvironment and mammary oncogenesis (Hanasoge Somasundara et al. 2021).

4.3.8 Breast Cancer

Breast cancer is the most commonly diagnosed cancer in the world (Sung et al. 2021). As prognosis is typically better the earlier a cancer is diagnosed and treated, there is a pressing need to develop effective diagnostics and therapeutics targeting early breast cancers. To facilitate this, understanding the cellular origins and mechanisms of breast cancer development and progression is key. However, multiple breast cancer subtypes exist, each hypothesised to arise from a different cell of origin or molecular drivers and in turn each associated with different phenotypes and clinical outcomes. Due to a lack of pre-clinical mouse models which can recapitulate the human breast cancer subtypes, the majority of understanding of breast cancer origin is limited to the triple-negative breast cancer (TNBC) subtype. Nevertheless, these studies provide an interesting insight into how the endogenous dynamism of the developing mammary gland can be repurposed to potentially initiate or drive cancer.

4.3.8.1 Stratification and Modelling of Breast Cancer Subtypes

Breast cancers can be classified both according to traditional histopathological and molecular markers such as gene expression signatures. Traditional markers such as histopathology, grade and stage are widely used to inform clinical prognosis and treatment decisions. For example, the vast majority of breast cancers are mammary ductal carcinomas, meaning they originate from the mammary epithelial tissue. H&E (hematoxylin and eosin) staining can differentiate in-situ carcinomas, which are still demarcated to epithelial structures, from invasive carcinomas which have invaded the surrounding tissue. This may indicate the progression or aggressiveness of a patient's tumour, and therefore may influence the clinical treatment regimen required.

Breast cancers are also commonly stratified using immunohistochemistry (IHC) according to molecular markers such as tumour expression of oestrogen (ER), progesterone (PR) and HER2 receptors. TNBC is negative for ER, PR and HER2 overexpression. The presence/absence of these receptors will influence treatment choice due to differential efficacies of targeted therapeutics such as trastuzumab. Trastuzumab is a monoclonal antibody that targets HER2 receptors and induces immune-mediated internalisation of HER2 receptors. However, more increasingly, sequencing of tumour biopsies is now being used to subcategorise breast cancers to highly specific subcategories.

In addition to subcategorisation based on receptor status, breast cancer research has previously used molecular markers such as DNA, transcriptomics and epigenetic sequencing as a form of classification. A commonly used classification divides breast cancer into five molecular subtypes: luminal A, luminal B, basal-like, HER2-enriched and claudin-low (Koboldt et al. 2012; Prat et al. 2010). While different to receptor-based classification, there are expected relationships between these two systems of classification (Table 4.1).

Additional studies which have integrated both genomic and transcriptomic data have since further subclassified breast cancer into ten molecular subgroups, each associated with different clinical features and prognoses (Dawson et al. 2013). These studies have truly illustrated the ability of interrogative molecular characterisation and sequencing in identifying new subtypes of cell or disease, which therefore improves our understanding of the underlying biology of these processes.

Despite the advantages of subclassification, understanding the origin and mechanism of progression of each subtype remains difficult. This is because developing an appropriate model which

Table 4.1 Receptor overexpression within breast cancer molecular subcategories. Breast cancer can be stratified into different molecular subcategories, each typically with different clinical phenotypes. This is traditionally done by inspecting the tumour expression status of Human Epidermal Growth Factor Receptor 2 (HER2), oestrogen receptors (ER) and progesterone receptors (PR)

Molecular subcategory	Receptor overexpression
Luminal A	HER2–, ER+ and/or PR+
Luminal B	HER2+, ER+ and/or PR+
HER2-enriched	HER2+, ER– and PR–
Basal-like	HER2–, ER– and PR–
Claudin-low	HER2–, ER– and PR–

recapitulates each subtype is challenging and largely depends on epidemiological studies of each subtype revealing modifying factors which greatly increase the risk of each specific subtype. While highly penetrant monogenic risk factors can be relatively easily recreated in mouse models, recapitulating complex polygenic or environmental risk factors can prove much more difficult.

Modelling spontaneous tumours which are typically induced by an accumulation of lower-risk genetic or environmental factors such as age, diet, etc. can be challenging to achieve in an experimental setting. Thus, a common approach to model breast cancer development often involves considering the most penetrant and commonly mutated genes per breast cancer subtype. Epidemiological studies have shown *BRCA1* mutations greatly elevate the risk of breast cancer with a TNBC phenotype, whereas *BRCA2* mutations have a greater disposition towards luminal-like breast cancers than *BRCA1* (Vargas et al. 2010). As a result, these genes are commonly mutated in mouse models to explore the origins of the separate breast cancer subtypes with greater granularity.

4.3.8.2 Cellular Changes Associated with BRCA1, Ageing, Parity and Their Relationship with Breast Cancer

Studying the effects of processes such as ageing and parity has revealed temporary or long-lasting cellular changes which can affect future functioning of the mammary gland and breast cancer tumorigenesis. For example, studying human mammary tissues from *BRCA1* carriers or targeted deletion of *Brca1* in mouse models was used to identify LASPs (also known as luminal progenitors) as the putative cell of origin for TNBC. In these studies, human *BRCA1* carrier mammary gland samples showed expanded LASP populations and the transcriptome of *BRCA1*-deficient basal-like tumours were found to most resemble LASPs (Lim et al. 2009). Furthermore, targeted deletion of *Brca1* in mouse LASPs generated basal-like tumours similar to human TNBC, whereas *Brca1* deletion in basal-myoepithelial cells did not (Molyneux et al. 2010). Identifying LASPs as the putative cell of origin has since facilitated studies which have improved our understanding of the mechanism of early tumorigenesis. For example, time-resolved scRNA-seq of mammary glands from mice with *Brca1/Trp53* perturbed LASPs demonstrated LASP expansion and hormone-independent aberrant differentiation to lactocytes (also known as alveolar cells) (Bach et al. 2021). This process resembles mammary gland remodelling induced by pregnancy and lactation, which is visibly apparent in wholemounts relative to nulliparous wildtype mice (Fig. 4.5). Moreover, within a *BRCA1* deficient background, scRNA-seq data has showed increased chromatin accessibility at alveologenesis genes *Csn2* and *Wap*, genes nor-

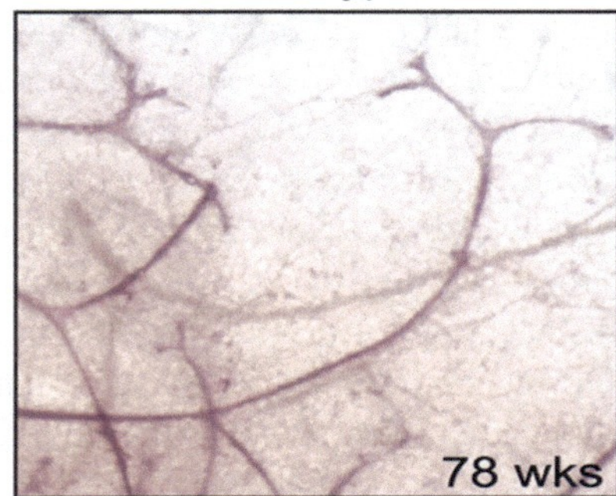

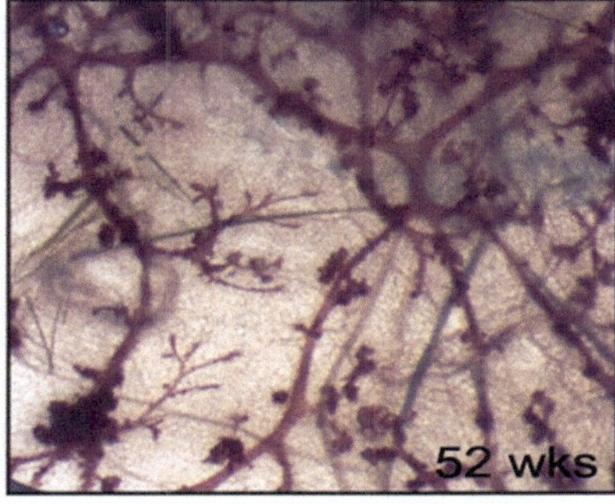

Fig. 4.5 Wholemount imaging of aberrant alveologenesis phenotype. Wholemounts of mammary glands from wildtype and *Blg-Cre*; *Brca1*$^{f/f}$; *Trp53*$^{+/-}$ animals. Mouse age is labelled in the bottom right. Wholemount imaging of the mammary glands shows a marked branching and alveologenesis phenotype in the *Blg-Cre*; *Brca1*$^{f/f}$; *Trp53*$^{+/-}$ mice, independently of pregnancy-induced hormonal signalling

mally only expressed during pregnancy and lactation, and associated expression of *Csn2* (Bach et al. 2021). These findings were further substantiated by CSN2 immunofluorescent staining and imaging. While many further studies are required to understand the cell of origin and mechanisms of early tumorigenesis in different breast cancer subtypes, initial research into *BRCA1*-deficiency-induced TNBC indicated a hijacking of transcriptional programmes apparently endogenous to the cell of origin. Whether hijacking of other mammary gland developmental programmes is also utilised by other breast cancer subtypes is still to be determined; however, the above findings serve as a key reminder as to why a general understanding of mammary gland development is important when studying both health and disease.

In addition, investigating changes in mammary epithelial cells caused by processes such as ageing and parity has unveiled the dynamic nature of these cells and their impact on the breast more generally, even providing links to changing disease risk statuses. Various epidemiological studies have shown that parity has an age-dependent and protective effect against breast cancer generally (MacMahon and Pugh 1970). Looking at the age of pregnancy showed that this protective effect is magnified in younger pregnancies and lessened in older pregnancies. However, when separated by individual breast cancer subtypes, similar studies found that parity instead increases the risk of TNBC specifically (Fortner et al. 2019; Redondo et al. 2012). Several recent studies have utilised omics approaches to characterise the changes imparted on the breast by pregnancy at a cellular level. Of note, increases in some subtypes of natural killer immune cells are reported alongside epigenetic alterations of the LASP compartment priming the gland for further pregnancies (Hanasoge Somasundara et al. 2021; dos Santos et al. 2015). Assuming aberrant differentiation is TNBC specific, these effects combined could provide some explanation behind the varying impact of parity on breast cancer risk. A missing piece in this puzzle remains the impact and cellular changes imposed by ageing on the mammary gland (as well as its interplay with parity). Generally, ageing is known as one of the greatest risk factors in most cancers and is also closely linked to epigenetic dysregulation (Campisi and Yaswen 2009; Yu et al. 2020). In the breast, ageing is associated with various changes, most notably the loss of lineage fidelity in LASP cells, in part thought to also contribute towards increased breast cancer risk (Gray et al. 2022; Shalabi et al. 2021; LaBarge et al. 2016). These findings briefly highlight the importance of understanding the biological impact of key natural processes within the breast to understand the mechanisms driving tumour formation.

4.4 Limitation of Single-Cell Studies

While single-cell analyses have been incredibly useful for elucidating cell types and functions in both healthy and diseased tissue states, there are limitations which require tackling to improve their utility as the field progresses. Ongoing advances to single-cell technologies and novel applications are seeking to address these challenges.

4.4.1 Single-Cell Omic Analyses: An Incomplete Picture

Many single-cell analyses provide only a limited perspective of the inner workings of a cell. While analyses such as scRNA-seq can capture enough information to characterise and identify cell types, understanding functional differences between cell types is much more difficult. Typically, biological function is inferred by looking at differentially expressed genes and prescriptively associating them with biological processes, often using gene ontology (GO) analysis packages such as Goseq (Young et al. 2010). However, there are a few problems with this approach. Firstly, while useful for initially getting a sense of on-going biological processes, reliance on GO enrichment analysis can ultimately prove overly reductionist unless the analyser manually verifies that it is consistent with the biology. For instance, the enrichment of components of a signalling pathway might identify the pathway as a differentially active biological process within a cell. However, it's crucial for the user to manually validate whether the enriched components truly function as drivers of the pathway, such as transcription factors, rather than downstream components which may be affected by other processes. Furthermore, as many genes play roles in multiple biological functions, it is important to verify that GO-enriched functions are consistent with biological expectations. For example, it is unreasonable to infer that if neuronal development gene signatures are flagged in a mammary gland cell that this is inducing neurogenesis. Additionally, depending on where in the central dogma single-cell analysis targets, there may be subsequent downstream factors which negate or alter inferred biological function. For example, we infer from DNA and RNA sequencing that this eventually impacts protein expression and therefore biological function. However, this does not account for additional complicating factors affecting RNA stability such as miRNA and siRNA which may inhibit RNA translation. Additionally, post-translational modifications which affect subsequent protein function or target it for degradation may further invalidate the inferred biological significance of DNA and RNA sequencing. Resultantly, it is important that the inferred biological significance of single-cell analyses such as RNA sequencing is considered with a critical perspective. Ideally, it is often necessary to evaluate findings through subsequent validation experiments which use functional readouts or immunohistochemistry to confirm findings.

4.4.2 Single-Cell Proteomics

Proteomics is a particularly reliable modality of single-cell analyses due to the enhanced stability of proteins relative to mRNA. This means it is less likely to be affected by stress-induced artefacts caused during sample preparation, and additionally, is a better predictor of on-going or short-term future behaviour as a protein is typically more stable and thus has a longer duration of effect. Moreover, the multimodal combination of RNA sequencing and proteomics is particularly valuable as the correlation between mRNA and protein is not always linear due to unobserved factors such as miRNA and siRNA interference, or variations in protein stability and degradation. Finally, unlike the post-transcriptional hurdles faced by mRNA, information on protein post-translation modifications can be captured during proteomics analysis and provide key additional information on protein state and function. However, despite this, proteomics is still a single-cell modality which is more rarely used. This is because single-cell proteomics faces several technical challenges which currently limits, but does not eliminate, its utility. Unlike nucleic acids, proteins cannot be amplified prior to analysis meaning the protein quantities within a single cell to be analysed are exceedingly small. Consequently, sample preparation must have minimal loss of cell content, and furthermore, the technology must be extremely sensitive. Additionally, it is currently very difficult to observe single-cell proteomics in a way that is not restricted to a limited number of markers. Recently, mass-spectrometry based methods of single-cell proteomics have been published which quantify the proteomes of single cells in an unbiased and unlabelled manner (Brunner et al. 2022). However, the throughput is restricted to only approximately 40 cells a day, which is insufficient to capture full cellular heterogeneity or observe rare, stochastic biological processes.

Alternatively, other next-generation sequencing-based strategies utilise protein-binding antibodies labelled with unique oligonucleotide barcodes to improve scalability (as summarised in Fig. 4.6); however, these approaches require targeted analysis. Provided there are suitable antibodies available, the use of barcodes means that many different proteins can be sequenced in combination, all at single-cell resolution. Additionally, popular methods such as CITE-seq (Stoeckius et al. 2017) use this sequencing to combine proteomics with RNA sequencing, providing a more comprehensive characterisation of single cells. However, CITE-seq is currently restricted to extracellular proteins which limits its

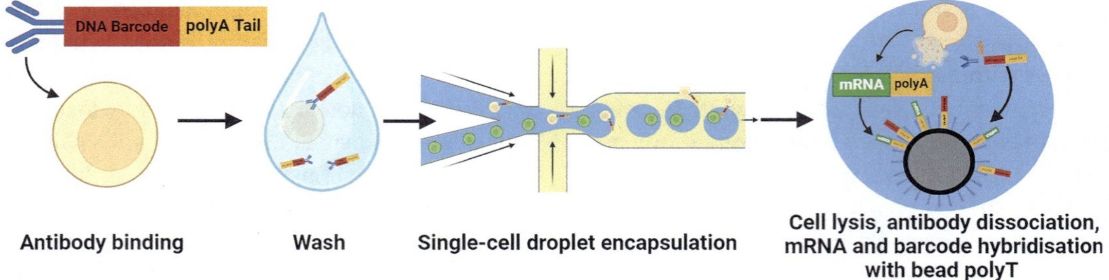

Fig. 4.6 Typical workflow of antibody-barcode single-cell proteomics. Schematic representation of a workflow of an antibody-oligonucleotide barcode-based method of single-cell proteomics, such as CITE-Seq. Cells are labelled with specific protein-binding antibodies, each bound to a unique oligonucleotide antibody, before washing to remove excess unbound antibodies. Microfluidics are utilised to encapsulate cells into individual droplets, along with a bead/microparticle containing polyT tails, due to the immiscibility of water in oil. Cells are lysed to release mRNA while oligonucleotide barcodes are released from antibodies, both of which are pulled down by microparticle polyT tails. Bound sequences are converted to cDNA, amplified and labelled for high-throughput sequencing platforms in a similar manner to Fig. 4.1 (created with BioRender.com)

utility. Furthermore, while barcodes enable the use of many antibodies in combination, the risk of antibody cross-reactivity increases with an expanding panel and thus limits panel size. This issue is particularly exacerbated when the panel of proteins being analysed contains highly homologous proteins, which are typically difficult to differentiate with antibodies without significant cross-reactivity. Overall, while single-cell proteomics has made great advancements recently, no method is currently available which offers sensitivity, high-throughput and unbiased analysis.

4.4.3 Multiomics

The potential disconnection between different modalities of single-cell analysis, caused by potentially unobserved confounding factors such as chromatin accessibility or post-transcriptional/translational modifications, is partially being addressed by multiomics. This is where multiple modalities are analysed in parallel on a single-cell scale, providing a more complete characterisation of a cell state at the time (see Sect. 4.5). However, while specific multiomic technologies may experience their own technical difficulties, multiomics as a whole faces its own share of overarching challenges. Firstly, combining multiple modalities of single-cell analysis requires more complex sample preparation and processing which significantly increases the associated cost. The expense of multiomics may prove prohibitive for many projects, and even when implemented, tends to limit the number of samples which may be analysed. Resultantly, multiomics technology is currently underrepresented, and when used, the smaller samples sizes reduce the resolution of analyses meaning subtle changes may be missed. Furthermore, while improving, integrating differing -omics datasets relatively seamlessly without significant batch effects proves difficult. Development of new methods for dataset integration and batch effect correction are seeking to improve this, but nevertheless, unification of datasets remains challenging. Finally, sequencing single cells with multiple modalities generates vast and complex datasets. Resultantly, the computational demand for analysing and storing these datasets continues to grow, posing an often-overlooked challenge of its own. Optimal strategies for effectively archiving, sharing and maintaining these expansive datasets in the long term is a topic of on-going discussion.

4.4.4 Pseudotime Analysis Limitations

An additional limitation of these analyses is that they only represent a snapshot of the sample, and the biological processes occurring, at the time of sample collection. If using in-vivo samples, the relevant biological processes being observed will effectively stop (or become unreliable to observe) once the mammary glands are extracted. Moreover, until the glands are digested to single cells and then lysed or fixed (analysis-dependent), the signalling and processes within cells will continue to change. Resultantly, stress signalling is a common artefact in RNA sequencing, although less common in proteomics as more time is required to mediate protein level changes. While these methods only represent a snapshot of the cell state, pseudotime analyses attempt to recapitulate dynamic and transitional processes by inferring a trajectory connecting cell types or states. In cases where samples are acquired across different time points, this trajectory can span time intervals, providing insight into temporal changes. However, as current scRNA-seq-based predictions of lineage tracing can only explore evolving or differentiating cells at the time of sequencing on a scale of only hours, the resolution of pseudotime analyses is limited by the size of the time intervals and the sample size collected within each interval. This is because cell states intermediary between the points of interest need observing and characterisation for the analysis to work. If the progression between states is rapid, rare or stochastic, the likelihood of observing this process is rare, and so a greater number of closely distributed samples are required. Given the expense of these analyses, this degree of resolution is difficult to acquire, and resultantly recapitulating cellular temporal changes and biological processes can be difficult.

4.4.5 Cell States and Cellular Taxonomy

Another issue arises in how to rationalise and interpret very high-resolution data interrogating complex biological systems. Some scRNA-seq datasets have now grown to encompass millions of cells each containing read counts for over 20,000 genes. Such large-scale analysis poses not only computational challenges but also conceptual hurdles that need to be addressed. One approach is to subcategorise data and analyses to distinct, entirely functional observations such as changes in signalling pathways which are well defined. However, interpreting data becomes much more subjective when grappling with less well-defined categories such as cell types. Traditionally, a cell type was thought to be an immutable property of a cell determined by morphology, functionality and anatomical location. However, single-cell technologies have since revealed the remarkable heterogeneity of cells. This is an issue, as this can cause divergence and inconsistent cell taxonomy within biological fields. Clustering scRNA-seq data in high-dimensional transcriptional space has revealed marked variation even within defined cell type populations, and moreover, it has revealed that cellular states believed to be discreetly separated can be connected by a continuum of intermediate cells. This has triggered a movement of thinking away from strictly defined cell types to a more amorphous identity as a cell state. However, while more accurately representing biological heterogeneity, this poses a challenge for cell taxonomy and how we comprehend and discuss cells. Cell atlases, generated from large-scale scRNA-sequencing of various mouse and human organs, have generated rich datasets for the scientific community to explore and rationalise their own data through comparison. However, the necessity of defining and annotating cell types through clustering cells with similar transcriptomes naturally reinforces the idea of immutable cell types due to presentation of distinct cell types on two-dimensional embeddings such as UMAPs. Some argue that shifting from cell atlases to cell trees, through integration of lineage data, would better demonstrate the dynamic nature of cell states and make cell identification more consistent throughout the field (Domcke and Shendure 2023). Nevertheless, as cells are characterised in dynamic processes with increasing interrogative depth, how cells are rationalised and annotated in a consistent and comprehensible way is still subject to debate. Currently, forums are being held for those most experienced in single-cell analyses (particularly those generating cell atlases) to facilitate a medium by which the scientific field can arrive at a consensus for cell taxonomy. Efforts like this are vital, as without a functioning and unified system to facilitate data sharing and comparison, the reproducibility crisis already on-going in the scientific community will only be exacerbated.

4.5 Future Directions

4.5.1 Introduction

Single-cell multiomics, the process of sequencing and analysing multiple modalities of the cell state in parallel, is helping to provide a holistic understanding of cellular mechanisms and behaviour at rest or during biological processes. Not only does this provide more comprehensive characterisation of cellular states but helps to offset the challenges of potentially confounding factors (see Sect. 4.4.1) which may have otherwise gone unobserved. Resultantly, conclusions drawn from multiomic single-cell analyses are reinforced with more evidence and thus tend to be more reliable. Currently, multiomics is a rapidly expanding field, with an influx of new methodologies each with their own mechanisms, advantages and disadvantages. This section intends to briefly explore a few techniques chosen to showcase the different modalities being combined in new multiomic approaches and to illustrate the future direction of advancements in single-cell multiomic technologies. Additionally, this section hopes to demonstrate the developments in single-cell analyses which are seeking to address or mitigate the limitations previously described.

4.5.2 Integrating DNA, RNA and Epigenomics

Across many facets of biological research, scRNA-seq has been the most widely implemented single-cell analysis for several reasons. This includes its ability to identify and characterise new cell types, as well as its utility in scrutinising on-going biological processes in naturally occurring phenomena such as differentiation and in response to extrinsic factors such as drug treatment. However, countless phenomena beyond the scope of scRNA-seq may affect the transcriptome, such as chromatin accessibility or chromosomal instability. Resultantly, observations from scRNA-seq may not have the biological effect inferred from the data or may be caused by another upstream phenomenon. Consequently, many multiomic technologies have endeavoured to combine scRNA-seq with scDNA-seq and chromatin accessibility assays to provide a more complete understanding of the processes affecting cellular transcription during dynamic biological processes.

When studying disease states such as cancer, the integration of scDNA-seq with scRNA-seq has proven useful in understanding perturbations in transcription. This is because many cancers, such as triple-negative breast cancer, are known for marked chromosomal instability which can cause aneuploidy or copy number variations (CNVs). Aneuploidy, when somatic cells have inherited an abnormal number of chromosomes due to incorrect chromosomal segregation, can perturb transcription by altering the number of gene copies a cell carries. This affects transcription as overrepresentation or underrepresentation of a gene alters the likelihood of transcription. Similarly, CNVs are caused by duplication or deletions of segments of DNA which can alter transcription of genes found within affected segments. Chromosomal instability has since been linked with multiple facets of cancer, including immune evasion and suppression, metastasis and chemoresistance (Bakhoum and Cantley 2018). Thus, there is clear interest in integrating scDNA-seq with scRNA-seq when studying cancer.

Multiple methods exist for parallel scDNA-seq and scRNA-seq, with many differing in how they separate DNA and RNA in their sample preparation. For example, this can be done physically via complete lysis of the cell and separation of mRNA by poly-T beads. However, Direct Nuclear Tagmentation and RNA-sequencing (DNTR-seq) (Zachariadis et al. 2020) operates via partial lysis of the cell and nuclear separation from the RNA via centrifugation and aspiration. RNA is converted to cDNA, and both are prepared for sequencing via tagmentation. This involves the splitting of DNA into fragments which are then PCR amplified to append sequencing adapters. Both RNA (as cDNA) and genomic DNA are then sequenced and aligned to the reference genome. The counts of RNA allow quantification of gene transcription, while counts of genomic DNA detail sequencing coverage and potential CNVs. This was used to identify CNVs in colon adenocarcinoma cell lines following DNA damaging agents (X-ray or etoposide), which was then used to contextualise gene transcription. They found that the majority of cells demonstrate a linear relationship between gene copy and transcription (i.e. gene doubling ≈ transcription doubling); however, key cancer genes such as MYC experienced strong feedback regulation which meant their transcription was relatively unaffected (Zachariadis et al. 2020). This study highlights the advantages offered by combining scDNA-seq and scRNA-seq. Relying solely on scDNA-seq could lead to the inference of elevated MYC expression, lacking the context provided by scRNA-seq. Conversely, scRNA-seq might suggest the absence of MYC copy number variations. Only through their synergistic use can the full cellular state be observed.

Another important factor when contextualising scRNA-seq data is the epigenetic state of a cell. This is because it can help explain the cause of altered gene transcription, or conversely, help infer the consequences of altered transcription. For example, increased chromatin accessibility may help explain elevated transcription of genes observed in scRNA-seq data, whereas if scRNA-seq data observed increased expression of a transcription factor, observing the accessibility of its binding sites can help predict the transcription factor effect. Resultantly, a useful multiomic strategy is to combine scRNA-seq with chromatin accessibility assays. Depending on the scientific question, this approach can be untargeted or targeted. Untargeted strategies include SNARE-seq2 (Plongthongkum et al. 2021), in which samples are fixed and permeabilised. mRNA is captured using oligo-dT oligos and reverse transcribed to cDNA, while the DNA is tagmented through transposase Tn5. This method is unbiased as Tn5 will tagment any open and accessible chromatin without any specific targeting. Following a series of low cycle PCRs for barcoding and introduction of sequencing adapters, the cDNA and tagmented DNA is sequenced, mapped and analysed. The benefit of this unbiased approach is that all accessible chromatin is sequenced, providing a more complete picture of the cellular epigenome. However, it does not have any ability to investigate what is inducing increased accessibility of certain regions. This is where targeted approaches are required.

Targeted strategies include Paired-Tag (Zhu et al. 2021), which shares a similar mechanism to untargeted approaches but targets tagmentation to areas affected by specific histone modifications. In Paired-Tag, permeabilised nuclei are first incubated with antibodies targeting specific histone modifications such as methylation H3K4me1. This targets transposase Tn5 to areas affected by the targeted histone modifications, which then undergoes the same steps of tagmentation, reverse transcription, etc. By specifically targeting tagmentation to areas affected by specific histone modifications, the differing epigenetic regulation of single cells can be assessed, which in combination with scRNA-seq data can contextualise changes in transcription at single-cell resolution. Additionally, whereas scRNA-seq alone provides a snapshot of the cell state at the instant of cell lysis, epigenetic regulation has a more lasting effect on cell state. Resultantly, this provides information not only on the cell state, but potentially the cell fate also.

Impressively, ambitious methods are now being published which can combine more than two modalities of single-cell sequencing. One example is Single-cell Nucleosome, Methylation and Transcription sequencing (scNMT-seq) (Clark et al. 2018), which is capable of sequencing RNA, as well as assessing chromatin accessibility and the methylation status of DNA. scNMT-seq first involves the physical separation of DNA and RNA, followed by the treatment of DNA with GpC methyltransferases. GpC methyltransferases methylate accessible guanines located prior to a cytosine, which in mammalian cells is much rarer than CpG methylation. GpC methylation therefore detects areas of open and accessible chromatin without altering endogenous methylation. DNA is then submitted for bisulfite sequencing, which determines which nucleotides are methylated. Given the relative rarity of GpC and CpG methylation, bisulfite sequencing therefore determines accessible chromatin as well as assaying endogenous methylation. RNA undergoes SmartSeq2 sequencing as previously described. Overall, scNMT-seq is a data-rich method for assessing transcription and epigenetics with single-cell resolution.

4.5.3 Spatial Omics

Given the limitation of loss of spatial information in traditional single-cell sequencing, which is particularly important when studying solid tissue, there has been great effort to develop single-cell sequencing technologies which retains spatial information. This is important in observing cell-to-cell signalling and dynamic processes such as cell migration and invasion which would otherwise be lost. For example, spatial information was used to observe improved T-cell infiltration and activity in a 4T1 murine breast cancer tumour model following TGFβ blockade (Grauel et al. 2020), illustrating the efficacy and mechanism of potential therapeutics. Spatial-omics is a rapidly developing field which has been most widely utilised for RNA sequencing, but now, is also beginning to encompass multiomic data. Spatial transcriptomics have largely been separated into two classes of methodology: imaging and sequencing. Imaging methods use fluorescent probes to detect or sequence target mRNA in situ, whereas sequencing methods prepare the sample for traditional sequencing methods in a way that retains spatial information.

4.5.4 Imaging Methods

In-situ Hybridisation (ISH), which includes Multiplexed Error-Robust Fluorescence In Situ Hybridisation (MERFISH) (Xia et al. 2019), is one imaging method which utilises fluorescently labelled probes which bind to target mRNA of interest. In MERFISH, a panel of target genes for which expression will be measured is designed, and a probe is designed for each gene which binds the target gene mRNA with high affinity and specificity. The probe is composed of a sequence of binary elements which can either bind or cannot bind a fluorescent probe. The fluorescent probes are added and imaged sequentially, assigning a 1 to a transcript if fluorescent or 0 if not. After many rounds of imaging, each transcript will be decoded a unique binary sequence (e.g. 100111010110) according to the sequence of fluorophore binding, which is then used to assign a transcript identity and its spatial location. Alternatively, in-situ sequencing (ISS) methods such as ExSeq (Alon et al. 2021) function by serially hybridising probes which bind two nucleotides at a time. Each 2-nucleotide probe binds a different fluorophore and is serially imaged, hence sequencing each mRNA transcript two bases at a time. These imaging-based spatial transcriptomic methods are incredibly powerful and data-rich and provide better spatial resolution than sequencing methods. However, these methods often are not yet truly single-cellular, as the spatial resolution may be larger than a cell, and even if not, the area imaged may partially fall outside of a cell's spatial morphology. Additionally, the area to be analysed is still relatively small, and the approach is biased due to the pre-selection of a panel of genes of interest. Nevertheless, the spatial resolution provided is still sufficient to provide interesting insights into cellular spatial relationships.

4.5.5 Sequencing Methods

Array-based technology enables samples to be divided into small subsections each with a unique barcode, which enables the spatial origin of transcripts to be mapped onto the sample following sequencing. For example, High-Definition Spatial Transcriptomics (HDST) (Vickovic et al. 2019) utilised 1.4 million 2 μm wells (each with a unique barcode) to divide and label transcripts within a frozen tissue section into 2 μm regions.

Transcripts are then processed and sequenced as normal; however, the capturing of the barcode allows spatial mapping of the transcripts. This allows much larger tissue samples to be sequenced in an unbiased method. However, this method does have poorer resolution than imaging-based methods.

An alternative and more generalisable method of utilising existing multiomic methodologies in a way that retains spatial information is to dissect out regions of interest (ROI) using technologies such as laser capture microdissection and then uniquely labelling or sequencing each ROI, separately. While enabling the use of existing multiomic technologies, this is relatively low throughput and restricted to a pre-defined ROI. More recently, methods such as Dithiobis(Succinimidyl Propionate) (DSP) (Merritt et al. 2020) have facilitated larger scale spatial RNA and protein sequencing by conjugating antibodies or RNA probes to unique barcodes joined by a photocleavable linker. When UV light is shone on a small region, the linker is cleaved, releasing the barcodes in that region which will then be sequenced. From this, the spatial location of proteins and transcripts can be recapitulated. This has the benefit of an adjustable region of interest with a resolution as small as a single cell; however, it is a biased approach due to the use of specific probes. Additionally, UV exposure can damage the samples and result in artefacts.

4.5.6 Future of Single-Cell Proteomics

Existing methods of single-cell proteomics (respectively) have differing strengths and weaknesses that typically relate to throughput or a restriction on the type or number of proteins which can be studied. While CITE-seq is excellent for sequencing many proteins in combination with RNA-sequencing, currently it is limited to extracellular staining due to high background intracellular staining preventing accurate reads. Nevertheless, efforts are underway to optimise such methods. Intranuclear Cellular Indexing of Transcriptomes and Epitopes Sequencing (incite-SEQ) (Chung et al. 2021) is an adapted form of CITE-seq capable of staining some intranuclear proteins; however, the number of intranuclear proteins that can be targeted is very limited. While further optimisation may improve this, it is unlikely that in the current format, this method will be able to substantially sequence many intracellular proteins without significant background staining. Instead, another useful form of single-cell proteomics is CyTOF, which utilises antibodies conjugated to inorganic metal ions to label both extracellular and intracellular proteins. Ions then undergo high-throughput via time-of-flight mass cytometry. While CyTOF still encounters the hazards of antibody cross-reactivity, which limits panel size to ~40 markers, the approach is still able to characterise and discriminate between cell types provided the markers chosen are appropriate. For example, as part of the Human Cell Atlas, CyTOF was used alongside scRNA-sequencing to identify and characterise the diverse cellular subtypes found within the human mammary gland (Gray et al. 2022). CyTOF was able to recapitulate the cellular diversity identified by scRNA-seq, thus illustrating that even with a panel of only 40 selected markers, this method can provide complementary and unique insights into biological processes.

4.6 Conclusion

Single-cell analyses have revolutionised our understanding of the mammary gland. The high-throughput nature of these technologies has generated vast sums of data interrogating various molecular modalities at single-cell resolution, enabling a new understanding of the cellular heterogeneity within the mammary gland, and facilitating close interrogation of the cellular programmes mediating biological change. Improved throughput has allowed characterisation of the dynamic mechanisms driving pre-pubertal and post-pubertal change, including pregnancy, lactation and involution, providing new insights into the developmental biology of the mammary gland. Additionally, it has been used to characterise the cellular programmes driving function and dysfunction, such as the transcriptional programmes engaged to enable milk protein production, and how this becomes dysregulated during tumorigenesis to facilitate pre-malignant expansion. Nevertheless, despite their utility, careful experimental design is required before implementing single-cell analysis of the mammary gland. For example, while the human and mouse mammary gland have many similarities, there are also some key structural and cellular differences. When using mouse models, it is important to be aware of these differences to ensure that the process being studied is sufficiently recapitulated in mice to provide useful information. Moreover, there are a wide range of single-cell technologies available which are growing at an accelerating rate. Selecting the most appropriate technique requires knowledge of the strengths and limitations of each, as well as awareness during analysis of which conclusions can be made confidently and which require further follow-up functional validation. Overall, given the unique plasticity of the mammary gland through pre- and post-pubertal development, it is important to study the mechanisms regulating and driving these changes which has been facilitated by the multimodal scrutiny of single-cell analyses. As single-cell technology rapidly expands to improve on existing techniques or to provide entirely new methodologies, it is likely that these methods will only grow in relevance as we seek to further understand the mammary gland in both health and disease.

References

Alon S, Goodwin DR, Sinha A, Wassie AT, Chen F, Daugharthy ER, Bando Y, Kajita A, Xue AG, Marrett K, Prior R, Cui Y, Payne AC, Yao CC, Suk HJ, Wang R, Yu CJ, Tillberg P, Reginato P, Pak N et al (2021) Expansion sequencing: Spatially precise in situ transcriptomics in intact biological systems. Science 371

Avagliano A, Fiume G, Pelagalli A, Sanità G, Ruocco MR, Montagnani S, Arcucci A (2020) Metabolic plasticity of melanoma cells and their crosstalk with tumor microenvironment. Front Oncol 10:722

Bach K, Pensa S, Grzelak M, Hadfield J, Adams DJ, Marioni JC, Khaled WT (2017) Differentiation dynamics of mammary epithelial cells revealed by single-cell RNA sequencing. Nat Commun 8(1)

Bach K, Pensa S, Zarocsinceva M, Kania K, Stockis J, Pinaud S, Lazarus KA, Shehata M, Simões BM, Greenhalgh AR, Howell SJ, Clarke RB, Caldas C, Halim TYF, Marioni JC, Khaled WT (2021) Time-resolved single-cell analysis of *Brca1* associated mammary tumourigenesis reveals aberrant differentiation of luminal progenitors. Nat Commun 12:1502

Bakhoum SF, Cantley LC (2018) The multifaceted role of chromosomal instability in cancer and its microenvironment. Cell 174:1347–1360

Bandura DR, Baranov VI, Ornatsky OI, Antonov A, Kinach R, Lou X, Pavlov S, Vorobiev S, Dick JE, Tanner SD (2009) Mass cytometry: technique for real time single cell multitarget immunoassay based on inductively coupled plasma time-of-flight mass spectrometry. Anal Chem 81(16):6813–6822

Boix-Montesinos P, Soriano-Teruel PM, Armiñán A, Orzáez M, Vicent MJ (2021) The past, present, and future of breast cancer models for nanomedicine development. Adv Drug Deliv Rev 173:306–330

Brisken C (2002) Hormonal control of alveolar development and its implications for breast carcinogenesis. J Mammary Gland Biol Neoplasia 7(1)

Brunner AD, Thielert M, Vasilopoulou C, Ammar C, Coscia F, Mund A, Hoerning OB, Bache N, Apalategui A, Lubeck M, Richter S, Fischer DS, Raether O, Park MA, Meier F, Theis FJ, Mann M (2022) Ultra-high sensitivity mass spectrometry quantifies single-cell proteome changes upon perturbation. Mol Syst Biol 18

Buenrostro JD, Giresi PG, Zaba LC, Chang HY, Greenleaf WJ (2013) Transposition of native chromatin for fast and sensitive epigenomic profiling of open chromatin, DNA-binding proteins and nucleosome position. Nat Methods 10(12):1213–1218

Campisi J, Yaswen P (2009) Aging and cancer cell biology. Aging Cell 8(3):221–225

Cardiff RD, Wellings SR (1999) The comparative pathology of human and mouse mammary glands. J Mammary Gland Biol Neoplasia 4(1)

Chung CY, Ma Z, Dravis C, Preissl S, Poirion O, Luna G, Hou X, Giraddi RR, Ren B, Wahl GM (2019) Single-cell chromatin analysis of mammary gland development reveals cell-state transcriptional regulators and lineage relationships. Cell Rep 29(2):495–510

Chung H, Parkhurst CN, Magee EM, Phillips D, Habibi E, Chen F, Yeung BZ, Waldman J, Artis D, Regev A (2021) Joint single-cell measurements of nuclear proteins and RNA in vivo. Nat Methods 18:1204–1212

Church C, Horowitz M, Rodeheffer M (2012) WAT is a functional adipocyte? Adipocyte 1(1):38–45

Clark SJ, Argelaguet R, Kapourani CA, Stubbs TM, Lee HJ, Alda-Catalinas C, Krueger F, Sanguinetti G, Kelsey G, Marioni JC, Stegle O, Reik W (2018) scNMT-seq enables joint profiling of chromatin accessibility DNA methylation and transcription in single cells. Nat Commun 9:781

Crowell H, Zanotelli V, Chevrier S, Robinson M (2023) CATALYST: Cytometry dATa anALYSis Tools. R package version 1.26.0. https://bioconductor.org/packages/CATALYST, https://doi.org/10.18129/B9.bioc.CATALYST

Cusanovich DA, Daza R, Adey A, Pliner HA, Christiansen L, Gunderson KL, Steemers FJ, Trapnell C, Shendure J (2015) Multiplex single cell profiling of chromatin accessibility by combinatorial cellular indexing. Science 348(6237):910–914

Dawson S-J, Rueda OM, Aparicio S, Caldas C (2013) A new genome-driven integrated classification of breast cancer and its implications. EMBO J 32:617–628

Domcke S, Shendure J (2023) A reference cell tree will serve science better than a reference cell atlas. Cell 186:1103–1114

Domínguez Conde C, Xu C, Jarvis LB, Rainbow DB, Wells SB, Gomes T, Howlett SK, Suchanek O, Polanski K, King HW, Mamanova L, Huang N, Szabo PA, Richardson L, Bolt L, Fasouli ES, Mahbubani KT, Prete M, Tuck L, Richoz N et al (2022) Cross-tissue immune cell analysis reveals tissue-specific features in humans. Science 376(6594)

dos Santos CO, Dolzhenko E, Hodges E, Smith AD, Hannon GJ (2015) An epigenetic memory of pregnancy in the mouse mammary gland. Cell Rep 11(7):1102–1109

Elias S, Morgan MA, Bikoff EK, Robertson EJ (2017) Long-lived unipotent Blimp1-positive luminal stem cells drive mammary gland organogenesis throughout adult life. Nat Commun 8(1)

Fata JE, Werb Z, Bissell MJ (2004) Regulation of mammary gland branching morphogenesis by the extracellular matrix and its remodelling enzymes. Breast Cancer Res 6(1):1–11. https://doi.org/10.1186/bcr634

Fleming JM, Long EL, Ginsburg E, Gerscovich D, Meltzer PS, Vonderhaar BK (2008) Interlobular and intralobular mammary stroma: genotype may not reflect phenotype. BMC Cell Biol 9:46

Fortner RT, Sisti J, Chai B, Collins LC, Rosner B, Hankinson SE, Tamimi RM, Eliassen AH (2019) Parity, breastfeeding, and breast cancer risk by hormone receptor status and molecular phenotype: results from the Nurses' Health Studies. Breast Cancer Res 21(1):40

Fu NY, Nolan E, Lindeman GJ, Visvader JE (2020) Stem cells and the differentiation hierarchy in mammary gland development. Physiol Rev 100(2):489–523

Grandi FC, Modi H, Kampman L, Corces MR (2022) Chromatin accessibility profiling by ATAC-seq. Nat Protoc 17:1518–1552

Grauel AL, Nguyen B, Ruddy D, Laszewski T, Schwartz S, Chang J, Chen J, Piquet M, Pelletier M, Yan Z, Kirkpatrick ND, Wu J, deWeck A, Riester M, Hims M, Geyer FC, Wagner J, MacIsaac K, Deeds J, Diwanji R et al (2020) TGFβ-blockade uncovers stromal plasticity in tumors by revealing the existence of a subset of interferon-licensed fibroblasts. Nat Commun 11:6315

Gray GK, Li CMC, Rosenbluth JM, Selfors LM, Girnius N, Lin JR, Schackmann RCJ, Goh WL, Moore K, Shapiro HK, Mei S, D'Andrea K, Nathanson KL, Sorger PK, Santagata S, Regev A, Garber JE, Dillon DA, Brugge JS (2022) A human breast atlas integrating single-cell proteomics and transcriptomics. Dev Cell 57(11):1400–1420

Gutierrez G, Sun P, Han Y, Dai X (2022) Defining mammary basal cell transcriptional states using single-cell RNA-sequencing. Sci Rep 12(1)

Haghverdi L, Lun ATL, Morgan MD, Marioni JC (2018) Batch effects in single-cell RNA-sequencing data are corrected by matching mutual nearest neighbors. Nat Biotechnol 36(5):421–427

Hanasoge Somasundara AV, Moss MA, Feigman MJ, Chen C, Cyrill SL, Ciccone MF, Trousdell MC, Vollbrecht M, Li S, Kendall J, Beyaz S, Wilkinson JE, dos Santos CO (2021) Parity-induced changes to mammary epithelial cells control NKT cell expansion and mammary oncogenesis. Cell Rep 37(10)

Hennighausen L, Robinson GW (1998) Think globally, act locally: the making of a mouse mammary gland. www.genesdev.org

Henry S, Trousdell MC, Cyrill SL, Zhao Y, Feigman MJ, Bouhuis JM, Aylard DA, Siepel A, dos Santos CO (2021) Characterization of gene expression signatures for the identification of cellular heterogeneity in the developing mammary gland. J Mammary Gland Biol Neoplasia 26(1):43–66

Hens JR, Wysolmerski JJ (2005) Molecular mechanisms involved in the formation of the embryonic mammary gland. Breast Cancer Res 7(5):220–224

Hooke R, 1635–1703 (1665) Micrographia, or, some physiological descriptions of minute bodies made by magnifying glasses: with observations and inquiries thereupon. Printed for James Allestry, London, 111667

Hurley WL (1989) Mammary gland function during involution. J Dairy Sci 72(6):1637–1646

Iyer A, Hamers AAJ, Pillai AB (2022) CyTOF® for the masses. Front Immunol 13:815828

Koboldt DC, Fulton RS, McLellan MD, Schmidt H, Kalicki-Veizer J, McMichael JF, Fulton LL, Dooling DJ, Ding L, Mardis ER, Wilson RK, Ally A, Balasundaram M, Butterfield YSN, Carlsen R, Carter C, Chu A, Chuah E, Chun HJE et al (2012) Comprehensive molecular portraits of human breast tumours. Nature 490:61–70

Kumar T, Nee K, Wei R, He S, Nguyen QH, Bai S, Blake K, Pein M, Gong Y, Sei E, Hu M, Casasent AK, Thennavan A, Li J, Tran T, Chen K, Nilges B, Kashikar N, Braubach O, Ben Cheikh B et al (2023) A spatially resolved single-cell genomic atlas of the adult human breast. Nature 620(7972):181–191

LaBarge MA, Mora-Blanco EL, Samson S, Miyano M (2016) Breast cancer beyond the age of mutation. Gerontology 62(4):434–442

Langmead B, Salzberg S (2012) Fast gapped-read alignment with Bowtie 2. Nat Methods 9:357–359

Lilja AM, Rodilla V, Huyghe M, Hannezo E, Landragin C, Renaud O, Leroy O, Rulands S, Simons BD, Fre S (2018) Clonal analysis of Notch1-expressing cells reveals the existence of unipotent stem cells that retain long-term plasticity in the embryonic mammary gland. Nat Cell Biol 20(6):677–687

Lim E, Vaillant F, Wu D, Forrest NC, Pal B, Hart AH, Asselin-Labat ML, Gyorki DE, Ward T, Partanen A, Feleppa F, Huschtscha LI, Thorne HJ, kConFab, Fox SB, Yan M, French JD, Brown MA, Smyth GK, Visvader JE et al (2009) Aberrant luminal progenitors as the candidate target population for basal tumor development in BRCA1 mutation carriers. Nat Med 15:907–913

Lopez R, Regier J, Cole MB, Jordan MI, Yosef N (2018) Deep generative modelling for single-cell transcriptomics. Nat Methods 15(12):1053–1058

Lund LR, Rømer J, Thomasset N, Solberg H, Pyke C, Mina J, Bissell MJ, Danø K, Zena Werb Z (1996) Two distinct phases of apoptosis in mammary gland involution: proteinase-independent and -dependent pathways. Development 112(1):181–193

MacMahon B, Pugh TF (1970) Epidemiology; principles and methods, 1st edn. Little Brown, Boston

Mallepell S, Krust A, Chambon P, Brisken C (2006) Paracrine signaling through the epithelial estrogen receptor alpha is required for proliferation and morphogenesis in the mammary gland. Proc Natl Acad Sci USA 103(7):2196–2201

Merritt CR, Ong GT, Church SE, Barker K, Danaher P, Geiss G, Hoang M, Jung J, Liang Y, McKay-Fleisch J, Nguyen K, Norgaard Z, Sorg K, Sprague I, Warren C, Warren S, Webster PJ, Zhou Z, Zollinger DR, Dunaway DL et al (2020) Multiplex digital spatial profiling of proteins and RNA in fixed tissue. Nat Biotechnol 38:586–599

Molyneux G, Geyer FC, Magnay FA, McCarthy A, Kendrick H, Natrajan R, Mackay A, Grigoriadis A, Tutt A, Ashworth A, Reis-Filho JS, Smalley MJ (2010) BRCA1 basal-like breast cancers originate from luminal epithelial progenitors and not from basal stem cells. Cell Stem Cell 7:403–417

Nee K, Ma D, Nguyen QH et al (2023) Preneoplastic stromal cells promote *BRCA1*-mediated breast tumorigenesis. Nat Genet 55:595–606

Nonnecke BJ, Smith KL (1984) Biochemical and antibacterial properties of bovine mammary secretion during mammary involution and at parturition. J Dairy Sci 67(12):2863–2872

Oakes SR, Hilton HN, Ormandy CJ (2006) Key stages in mammary gland development: The alveolar switch: Coordinating the proliferative cues and cell fate decisions that drive the formation of lobuloalveoli from ductal epithelium. Breast Cancer Res 8(2)

Paine IS, Lewis MT (2017) The terminal end bud: the little engine that could. J Mammary Gland Biol Neoplasia 22:93–108

Pal B, Chen Y, Vaillant F, Jamieson P, Gordon L, Rios AC, Wilcox S, Fu N, Liu KH, Jackling FC, Davis MJ, Lindeman GJ, Smyth GK, Visvader JE (2017) Construction of developmental lineage relationships in the mouse mammary gland by single-cell RNA profiling. Nat Commun 8(1)

Plongthongkum N, Diep D, Chen S, Lake BB, Zhang K (2021) Scalable dual-omics profiling with single-nucleus chromatin accessibility and mRNA expression sequencing 2 (SNARE-seq2). Nat Protoc 16:4992–5029

Prat A, Parker JS, Karginova O, Fan C, Livasy C, Herschkowitz JI, He X, Perou CM (2010) Phenotypic and molecular characterization of the claudin-low intrinsic subtype of breast cancer. Breast Cancer Res 12

Redondo CM, Gago-Domínguez M, Ponte SM, Castelo ME, Jiang X, García AA, Fernández MP, Tomé MA, Fraga M, Gude F, Martínez ME, Garzón VM, Carracedo Á, Castelao JE (2012) Breast feeding, parity and breast cancer subtypes in a Spanish Cohort. PLoS One 7(7)

Reed AD, Pensa S, Steif A, Stenning J, Kunz DJ, He P, Twigger A-J, Kania K, Barrow-McGee R, Goulding I, Gomm JJ, Jones L, Marioni JC, Khaled WT (2023) A human breast cell atlas mapping the homeostatic cellular shifts in the adult breast. BioRxiv. https://doi.org/10.1101/2023.04.21.537845

Regan JL, Smalley MJ (2020) Integrating single-cell RNA-sequencing and functional assays to decipher mammary cell states and lineage hierarchies. NPJ Breast Cancer 6(1)

Richert MM, Schwertfeger KL, Ryder JW, Anderson SM (2000) An atlas of mouse mammary gland development. J Mammary Gland Biol Neoplasia 5:227–241

Saeki K, Chang G, Kanaya N, Wu X, Wang J, Bernal L, Ha D, Neuhausen SL, Chen S (2021) Mammary cell gene expression atlas links epithelial cell remodelling events to breast carcinogenesis. Commun Biol 4(1)

Sakakura T, Kusano I, Kusakabe M, Inaguma Y, Nishizuka Y (1987) Biology of mammary fat pad in fetal mouse: capacity to support development of various fetal epithelia in vivo. Development 100

Schneider MP, Cullen A, Pangonyte J, Skelton J, Major H, Van Oudenhove E, Garcia MJ, Chaves-Urbano B, Piskorz AM, Brenton JD, Macintyre G, Markowetz F (2023) Scabsolute: measuring single-cell ploidy and replication status. BioRxiv. https://doi.org/10.1101/2022.11.14.516440

Shalabi SF, Miyano M, Sayaman RW, Lopez JC, Jokela TA, Todhunter ME, Hinz S, Garbe JC, Stampfer MR, Kessenbrock K, Seewaldt VE, LaBarge MA (2021) Evidence for accelerated aging in mammary epithelia of women carrying germline *BRCA1* or *BRCA2* mutations. Nat Aging 1(9):838–849

Sleeman KE, Kendrick H, Robertson D, Isacke CM, Ashworth A, Smalley MJ (2007) Dissociation of estrogen receptor expression and in vivo stem cell activity in the mammary gland. J Cell Biol 176(1):19–26

Stein T, Salomonis N, Gusterson BA (2007) Mammary gland involution as a multi-step process. J Mammary Gland Biol Neoplasia 12(1):25–35

Sternlicht MD (2006) Key stages in mammary gland development: the cues that regulate ductal branching morphogenesis. Breast Cancer Res 8(1):201

Sternlicht MD, Kouros-Mehr H, Lu P, Werb Z (2006) Hormonal and local control of mammary branching morphogenesis. Differ Res Biol Diver 74(7):365–381. https://doi.org/10.1111/j.1432

Stoeckius M, Hafemeister C, Stephenson W, Houck-Loomis B, Chattopadhyay PK, Swerdlow H, Satija R, Smibert P (2017) Simultaneous epitope and transcriptome measurement in single cells. Nat Methods 14:865–868

Strange R, Li F, Saurer S, Burkhardt A, Friis RR (1992) Apoptotic cell death and tissue remodelling during mouse mammary gland involution. Development 115

Sung H, Ferlay J, Siegel RL, Laversanne M, Soerjomataram I, Jemal A, Bray F (2021) Global Cancer Statistics 2020: GLOBOCAN estimates of incidence and mortality worldwide for 36 cancers in 185 countries. CA Cancer J Clin 71(3):209–249

Sweeney M, Foldes G (2018) It takes two: endothelial-perivascular cell cross-talk in vascular development and disease. Front Cardiovasc Med 5:154

Traag VA, Waltman L, van Eck NJ (2019) From Louvain to Leiden: guaranteeing well-connected communities. Sci Rep 9:5233

Twigger AJ, Engelbrecht LK, Bach K, Schultz-Pernice I, Pensa S, Stenning J, Petricca S, Scheel CH, Khaled WT (2022) Transcriptional changes in the mammary gland during lactation revealed by single cell sequencing of cells from human milk. Nat Commun 13(562)

Valdés-Mora F, Salomon R, Gloss BS, Law AMK, Venhuizen J, Castillo L, Murphy KJ, Magenau A, Papanicolaou M, Rodriguez de la Fuente L, Roden DL, Colino-Sanguino Y, Kikhtyak Z, Farbehi N, Conway JRW, Sikta N, Oakes SR, Cox TR, O'Donoghue SI et al (2021) Single-cell transcriptomics reveals involution mimicry during the specification of the basal breast cancer subtype. Cell Rep 35(2)

Vargas AC, Silva LD, Lakhani SR (2010) The contribution of breast cancer pathology to statistical models to predict mutation risk in *BRCA* carriers. Fam Cancer 9:545–553

Vickovic S, Eraslan G, Salmén F, Klughammer J, Stenbeck L, Schapiro D, Äijö T, Bonneau R, Bergenstråhle L, Navarro JF, Gould J, Griffin GK, Borg Å, Ronaghi M, Frisén J, Lundeberg J, Regev A, Ståhl PL (2019) High-definition spatial transcriptomics for in situ tissue profiling. Nat Methods 16:987–990

Watson CJ (2006) Key stages in mammary gland development—involution: apoptosis and tissue remodelling that convert the mammary gland from milk factory to a quiescent organ. Breast Cancer Res 8:203

Xia C, Fan J, Emanuel G, Hao J, Zhuang X (2019) Spatial transcriptome profiling by MERFISH reveals subcellular RNA compartmentalization and cell cycle-dependent gene expression. Proc Natl Acad Sci USA 116:19490–19499

Young MD, Wakefield MJ, Smyth GK, Oshlack A (2010) Gene ontology analysis for RNA-seq: accounting for selection bias. Genome Biol 11:14

Yu M, Hazelton WD, Luebeck GE, Grady WM (2020) Epigenetic aging: more than just a clock when it comes to cancer. Cancer Res 80(3):367–374

Zachariadis V, Cheng H, Andrews N, Enge M (2020) A highly scalable method for joint whole-genome sequencing and gene-expression profiling of single cells. Mol Cell 80:541–553

Zahn H, Steif A, Laks E, Eirew P, VanInsberghe M, Shah SP, Aparicio S, Hansen CL (2017) Scalable whole-genome single-cell library preparation without preamplification. Nat Methods 14(2):167–173

Zhu C, Zhang Y, Li YE, Lucero J, Behrens MM, Ren B (2021) Joint profiling of histone modifications and transcriptome in single cells from mouse brain. Nat Methods 18:283–292

Part II

Development and Cancer: Model Systems and Approaches

Therese Sørlie and Robert Clarke

This part introduces advanced methodologies and model systems used to study mammary gland development and breast cancer progression. Key advances include the use of cellular barcoding techniques to trace cell lineages and understand cellular hierarchies, as well as various models for studying the progression of ductal carcinoma in situ (DCIS) to invasive ductal carcinoma (IDC). The efficacy of patient-derived xenografts (PDX) in preserving the characteristics of human breast tumors for therapeutic research is highlighted, along with the renewed significance of rat models, particularly with the advent of CRISPR/Cas9 technology, in exploring aspects of breast cancer that are challenging to model in mice.

In Chap. 5, Silvia Fre and her colleague from Institut Curie in Paris, France, describe how lineage tracing methods, through genetic and optical barcodes, have significantly advanced our understanding of cell behavior and hierarchies during normal and tumor development. These techniques enable the integration of lineage information with single-cell profiling, allowing for the identification of markers and pathways that define specific stem cell states and those promoting tumor progression and therapy resistance.

In Chap. 6, Fariba Behbod and her colleague from the University of Missouri, USA, explore how models simulating the transition from ductal carcinoma in situ (DCIS) to invasive ductal carcinoma (IDC) have been developed to understand the molecular and cellular mechanisms underlying this progression. Continuous advancement of these models, including how to incorporate epithelial–stromal interactions, will be crucial for predicting when DCIS lesions remain indolent and when they progress to malignancy.

In Chap. 7, Elisabetta Marangoni from the Curie Institute in Paris, France, proposes that patient-derived xenografts (PDX) are highly effective preclinical models for studying human breast cancer biology and evaluating new treatments. They preserve the phenotypic and molecular characteristics of donor

T. Sørlie
Oslo, Norway

R. Clarke
Manchester, UK

tumors, providing strong predictive value for translating cancer therapeutics into clinical settings. However, limitations include the absence of a human immune system and low take rates for certain breast cancer subtypes.

Finally, in Chap. 8, Yi Li and his colleague from Baylor College of Medicine, Houston, USA, describe how rats, historically significant in breast cancer research, have regained importance with advancements in genetic engineering, particularly the CRISPR/Cas9 technology. Rat models are especially valuable for studying estrogen receptor-positive breast cancer, providing insights that are difficult to achieve with mouse models. This section reviews the evolution of rat models and their application in breast cancer research, emphasizing their potential to address unresolved challenges.

By exploring these advanced model systems and approaches, this part of the book aims to enhance our understanding of mammary gland development and breast cancer, offering insights crucial for developing effective therapeutic strategies.

5 Recording Lineage History with Cellular Barcodes in the Mammary Epithelium and in Breast Cancer

Candice Merle and Silvia Fre

Abstract

Lineage tracing methods have extensively advanced our understanding of physiological cell behaviour *in vivo* and *in situ* and have vastly contributed to decipher the phylogeny and cellular hierarchies during normal and tumour development. In recent years, increasingly complex systems have been developed to track thousands of cells within a given tissue or even entire organisms. Cellular barcoding comprises all techniques designed to genetically label single cells with unique DNA sequences or with a combination of fluorescent proteins, in order to trace their history and lineage production in space and time. We distinguish these two types of cellular barcoding as genetic or optical barcodes. Furthermore, transcribed cellular barcodes can integrate the lineage information with single-cell profiling of each barcoded cell. This enables the potential identification of specific markers or signalling pathways defining distinct stem cell states during development, but also signals promoting tumour growth and metastasis or conferring therapy resistance.

In this chapter, we describe recent advances in cellular barcoding technologies and outline experimental and computational challenges. We discuss the biological questions that can be addressed using single-cell dynamic lineage tracing, with a focus on the study of cellular hierarchies in the mammary epithelium and in breast cancer.

Keywords

Cellular barcoding · Optical barcodes · Genetic barcodes · Single-cell lineage tracing · Mouse genetics

Key Points

- Lineage tracing is an essential tool to study stem cells and cancer biology.
- Different cellular barcoding methods have been developed to perform clonal analyses.
- Transcribed barcodes record both clonal history and cell identity.
- There are current challenges in lineage tracing and cellular barcoding approaches.
- Perspectives: Human lineage tracing will allow the exploration of human cell behaviour *in vivo* and *in situ*, in homeostasis and disease.

C. Merle · S. Fre (✉)
Laboratory of Genetics and Developmental Biology, Institut Curie, INSERM U934, CNRS UMR3215, Paris, France
e-mail: candice.merle@curie.fr; silvia.fre@curie.fr

T. Sørlie, R. B. Clarke (eds.), *A Guide to Breast Cancer Research*, Advances in Experimental Medicine and Biology 1464, https://doi.org/10.1007/978-3-031-70875-6_5

Lineage tracing is currently the gold-standard approach to study cellular hierarchies and cell fate *in vivo*. Indeed, it has become clear that removing stem cells or tumour cells from their physiological environment can dramatically change their characteristics and their behaviour. In the mammary gland, for example, it was found that cell dissociation induces reactivation of multipotency in otherwise unipotent progenitor cells, and the phenotype of dissociated cells in transplantation assays has created confusion regarding the identity and existence of multipotent mammary stem cells. Interestingly, it has been shown that under different stress conditions, such as transplantation, enzymatic digestion, or oncogene expression, cells can undergo lineage conversion, changing their physiological potency and commitment (Van Keymeulen et al. 2011, 2015; Rodilla et al. 2015; Koren et al. 2015; Jardé et al. 2016; Lilja et al. 2018; Wuidart et al. 2018; Rodilla and Fre 2018; Lloyd-Lewis et al. 2019; Centonze et al. 2020). Likewise, tumour cells can modify their invasive traits or their drug resistance when they are dissociated from their original tumour niche (Plaks et al. 2015). These findings may have important consequences in interpreting results generated upon cell dissociation, *in vitro* manipulation, as in studies of clonal evolution in breast cancer using Patient-Derived Xenografts (PDXs) infected *in vitro* with lentiviral barcode libraries (Nguyen et al. 2014; Echeverria et al. 2018; Merino et al. 2019). It is thus important to design methods that allow us to genetically trace the *in vivo* behaviour and fate of cancer cells *in situ*, thus within the physiological tumour microenvironment, comprising stromal and immune cells.

Given the paramount importance of clonal fate mapping studies performed *in vivo* in physiological conditions, we discuss here the new generation of cellular barcoding techniques, which provide an efficient and quantitative strategy to unbiasedly mark individual cells with unique and heritable tags that can be followed *in vivo* in time and space.

5.1 Introduction

Biological systems are composed of millions of cells with unique past and future lineages. Differently from *C. elegans*, where every cell can be traced to its immediate mother to generate the complete cell lineage tree of this multicellular organism (Sulston et al. 1983), more complex animals present more serious challenges and our ability to track the fate of cells within a mouse or a human remains very limited. However, recent years have seen great efforts of developmental biologists, cancer geneticists, and technology developers to find methods to reconstruct cellular ancestries, one of the next great frontiers in biological research. In this chapter, we will present two major types of lineage tracing approaches: the ones based on imaging and tracking fluorescently labelled cells and the ones using genetic DNA barcodes to mark single cells and trace their progeny over time.

A cell's history is written in its genome: every mutation acquired that gets passed on to daughter cells serves as a record. This is why any lineage tracing strategy requires the ability to genetically mark the cell genome. This was initially and successfully achieved by engineering heritable "lineage recorders" thanks to the development of mice expressing an inducible version of the Cre recombinase under the control of cell or tissue specific promoters, combined with the presence of a Cre-responsive reporter gene (Hoess et al. 1986). This technique employs inducible Cre to trigger the permanent expression of a reporter gene in defined cells that can be tracked throughout several generations [reviewed in Liu et al. (2020)]. However, reporter expression can also be triggered by other types of recombinases, such as in the Dre/Rox (Sauer and McDermott 2004), Tet/TetO (Gossen and Bujard 1992), or Flp/FRT (Cox 1983) systems, or even by external stimuli, like a heat shock or a drug.

Cre-mediated clonal analysis, mostly relying on the expression of coloured reporters (lacZ or fluorescent proteins), has seen an explosion of studies in the past 20 years, and it has generated an enormous amount of crucial information on *in vivo* stem cell behaviour in physiological contexts and in tumours. The many methods developed over the past century for tracing cells have been reviewed elsewhere (Kretzschmar and Watt 2012). The most widely used methods for clonal analysis involve the use of fluorescent tags to label the cells to track. However, the use of a single fluorescent reporter is not suitable for the study of a high number of labelled cells, because cells with different cellular origins cannot be distinguished if all derived clones share the same colour. The development of multicolour reporter mice, such as the Brainbow (Livet et al. 2007) and its second-generation version called Confetti (Snippert et al. 2010), improved the ability to perform quantitative clonal analysis through the combinatorial expression of different fluorescent proteins that can genetically label a larger number of cells. However, these models still require complex statistical frameworks to infer the clonal origin of each tracked cell from a defined and unique progenitor.

Fluorescence-based lineage tracing approaches are limited by the number of distinct clones that can be simultaneously followed. In contrast, the very recent development of fate mapping by DNA barcodes, retrospectively achieved by high-throughput sequencing, provides another route to map a cell's history, enabling researchers to theoretically record every single division event in a given tissue. Furthermore, these powerful tools can be combined with other single-cell measurements, such as single-cell RNA or ATAC sequencing.

In this chapter, we will review the two main cell tracing techniques currently used: multicolour tracing using combinations of fluorescent proteins (that we have termed optical barcodes) and fate mapping approaches based on unique nucleic acid sequences (that we refer to as genetic barcodes) (Table 5.1).

Table 5.1 Overview of cellular barcoding studies in mammary gland and in breast cancer

Barcode system	Models	Phenotype analysed	Transcriptomic analysis coupled with lineage information	References
Library	Cell lines MDA-MB-231 and SUM-149	Describe clonal growth patterns	No	Nguyen et al. (2014)
Library	Cell lines 4T1	Identify molecular mechanisms supporting metastasis	No	Wagenblast et al. (2015)
Library	Metastatic PDX	Clonal dynamics in metastasis	No	Echeverria et al. (2018)
Library	TNBC PDX	Clonal distribution before and after treatment	No	Echeverria et al. (2019)
Library	TNBC PDX	Clonal distribution of metastasis and relapsing tumours	No	Merino et al. (2019)
Library	MMTV-rtTA;TetO-neu	Clonal distribution after treatment	No	Walens et al. (2020)
Library	E9.5 embryos	Quantification of pluripotent progenitors	No	Ying and Beronja (2020)
Optical barcodes	Cell line MDA-MB-231	Define clonal distribution coupled with transcriptomic analysis in metastasis	Yes	Berthelet et al. (2021)
Library CellTracker	Cell line MDA-MB-231	Clonal distribution after treatment	No	Patwardhan et al. (2021)
CRISPR-Cas9	Cell lines MDA-MB-231 and AT-3	Identify the origin of secondary metastases	No	Zhang et al. (2021)

5.2 Methods for Cellular Barcoding

5.2.1 Optical Barcodes

Optical barcodes label individual cells by the stable expression of a fluorescent protein that is transmitted to their daughters, allowing researchers to track the derived clones by imaging, without loss of spatial information on the localisation of the traced cells. This also permits the retrieval of fluorescent cells by fluorescence-activated cell sorting (FACS) for cell type quantifications and further molecular analyses (Fig. 5.1a). Methods recording lineages in living animals and tissues and retaining the spatial context (*in situ*) are essential for understanding the physiological growth conditions and *in vivo* cell behaviour.

Optical barcoding is based on the combination of several fluorescent proteins in one cell and was implemented with the development of the LeGO (Lentiviral Gene Ontology) vectors used for RGB (Red-Green-Blue) marking (Weber et al. 2008, 2010). This technique relies on lentiviral vectors encoding a wide spectrum of different fluorescent proteins, creating a diverse palette of colours for each infected cell. This unique colour combination is genetically encoded, hence transmitted to the clonal progeny of single, easily identifiable cells, allowing the efficient *in vivo* tracing of individual clones. Optical barcodes have the prerogative of being detected by microscopy in intact tissues, hence preserving essential information on the spatial distribution of the traced cells within a tissue or tumour. Indeed, reconstructing the relationship between closely related cells can be challenged by the fact that daughter cells may travel far away and be dispersed across a given tissue. This is a particular issue in tissues undergoing extensive remodelling during development, such as branching morphogenesis, or in metastatic tumours. In these cases, successive generations of cells could venture far from their ancestral home, and only spatial lineage tracing with optical barcodes can provide this crucial information. The first LeGO systems based on the combination of RGB fluorescence allowed the detection of up to seven colour combinations (Weber et al. 2011). Recent methods improved the RGB system with the development of new reporters carrying a combination of 6 different colours, allowing to track up to 64 unique clones (Malide et al. 2014; Mohme et al. 2017; Shembrey et al. 2022).

Recent years saw the advent of a new optical barcoding technology featuring the combinatorial use of 4 fluorescent proteins targeted to different subcellular compartments, generating "visual barcodes" (Kaufman et al. 2022). They used blue (BFP), cyan (CFP), green (GFP), and yellow (YFP) fluorescent proteins, each expressed in different cellular locations: in the nucleus, the endoplasmic reticulum, the cytoplasm, in peroxisomes, and throughout the whole cell. The authors of this study combined 4 fluorescent proteins with 3 different localisations, producing 12 visual barcodes that, in combination, can detect up to 60 different clones.

The major concern about these optical barcoding approaches is that currently cells need to be infected by viruses to introduce barcode libraries, implying *in vitro* manipulations. However, optical barcoding techniques offer several advantages: the ability to image, quantify and track the fate of individual cells and the behaviour of their progeny *in vivo* while maintaining the spatial context of each traced cell is crucial. In addition, barcoded fluorescent cells can be sorted by flow cytometry and probed for their plasticity in transplantation assays, 3D organoids, or tissue explant cultures, or they can be assayed with other downstream molecular analyses.

5.2.2 Genetic Barcodes

Genetic barcoding can be used to track millions of cells in parallel, and thus it is an efficient approach for investigating heterogeneous cell populations or rare cell states.

With the term genetic barcodes, we include both known DNA tags that are introduced into cells to create a readable permanent record in the cell genome (stable barcodes) (Fig. 5.1b) (Kebschull and Zador 2018) and more complex techniques that rely on the genome editing tool CRISPR-Cas9 to target traceable mutations to a

A. Optical barcodes

Confetti or Brainbow

Last generation of optical barcode

B. Stable genetic barcodes

Barcode library

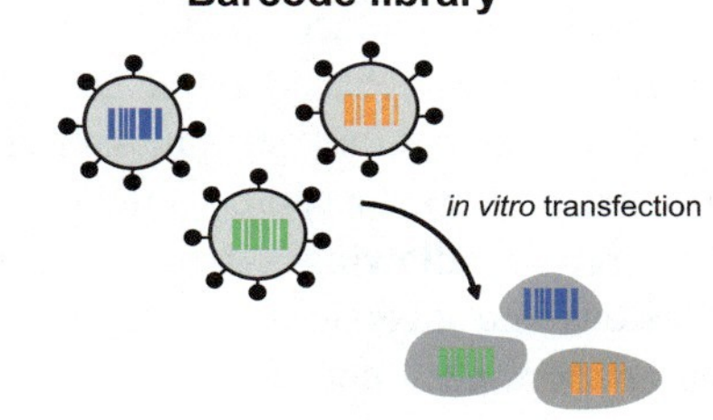

Barcoding based on Cre recombination

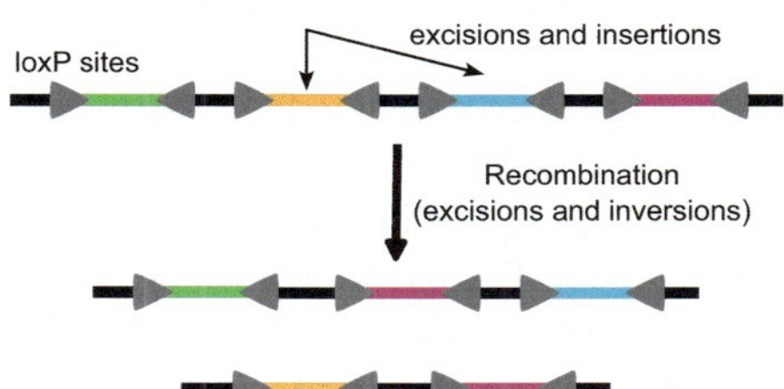

Transposons

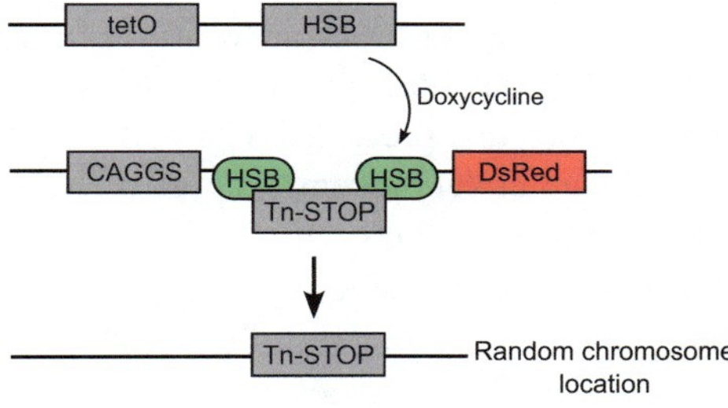

DRAG mice

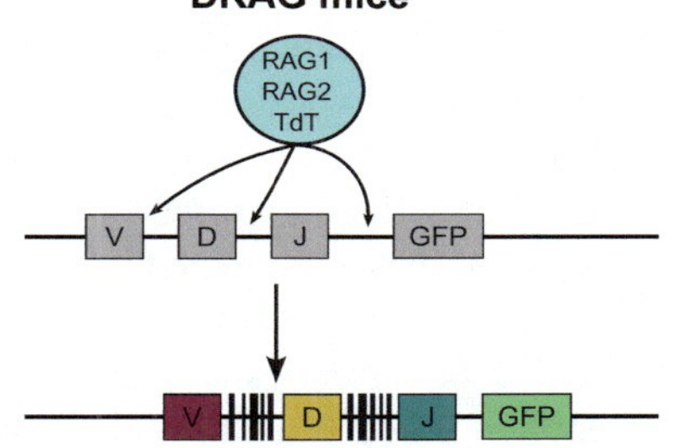

C. Evolving genetic barcodes

CRISPR/Cas9

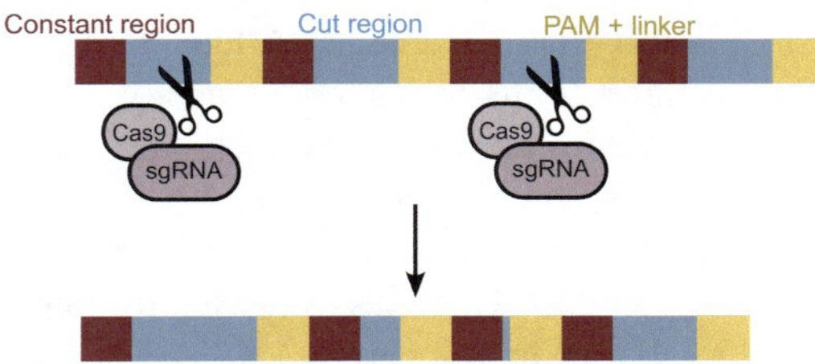

Fig. 5.1 Cellular barcoding systems used for lineage tracing. (**a**) Optical barcodes provide the spatial information of each clone identified through a combination of fluorescent proteins. (**b**) Stable genetic barcodes allow to trace the lineage history of even rare cells from a common ancestor. (**c**) Evolving genetic barcodes, recording cell generations, allow the reconstruction of branching phylogenetic lineage trees for each labelled cell

selected part of the genome (evolving barcodes) (Fig. 5.1c). Due to the error-prone nature of repair of Cas9-induced double-stranded DNA breaks, this technology can record the evolution of barcodes throughout cell generations and thus draw genealogy trees of mapped cells.

5.2.2.1 Stable Barcodes

Barcode Libraries

Historically, genetic barcoding was developed in two major studies performed by Jordan and Lemishka and Walsh and Cepko (Jordan and Lemischka 1990; Walsh and Cepko 1992) in the early 90s, when the authors used retroviral infection to introduce a reference library of known short and very diverse DNA sequences (barcodes) to decipher the clonal history of hematopoietic stem cells and mouse cerebral cortex cells.

Recent years have witnessed the implementation of many different barcode libraries of increasing diversity and complexity. These approaches allow lineage tracing at a different scale than optical barcoding, since barcode libraries typically contain thousands of unique and heritable barcodes, usually encoded in lentiviral or retroviral vectors, each containing a distinct DNA sequence. It is important to stress the fact that cell viral infection is considered biologically neutral, and it allows the clonal outputs of the original transduced cells to be inferred from the barcode content of DNA extracted from their progeny. To distinguish barcoded cells from non-infected cells, barcode libraries typically contain selectable reporters, such as a fluorescent protein or a gene conferring an antibiotic resistance. The barcode sequences are then retrieved by parallel deep DNA sequencing. Many recent libraries, such as Watermelon (Oren et al. 2021), lineage and RNA recovery (LARRY) (Weinreb et al. 2020) CellTagging (Biddy et al. 2018), ClonMapper (Gutierrez et al. 2021), and single-cell profiling and lineage tracing (SPLINTR) (Fennell et al. 2021), have been developed. These allow the detection of transcribed barcodes, which are highly expressed and readily captured within each single-cell transcriptome, enabling the recording of clonal history over time, in parallel with gathering information on the cell identity and differentiation status of the clonal progeny.

Genetic Barcode Technologies Based on Cre-recombination for In Vivo Studies

One of the major disadvantages of genetic barcodes encoded in viral libraries is that they require dissociation of the cells from a given tissue or tumour to be infected *in vitro* and then the infected cells need to be transplanted back into a mouse. For this reason, some original mouse models have been recently generated to allow barcode-based lineage tracing *in vivo* and *in situ*, avoiding *in vitro* cell manipulations. The first mouse model that induces genetic barcoding is the Polylox mouse, based on a DNA cassette composed of several loxP sites in alternating orientations (Polylox), spaced by unique sequences of DNA blocks, allowing a defined combination of excisions and inversions. Upon Cre-mediated recombination, each cell can undergo a specific recombination pattern (Peikon et al. 2014; Pei et al. 2017, 2019, 2020). A more recent version of the Polylox mouse harbours transcribed barcodes (Pei et al. 2020). In hematopoietic cells, this system was shown to be capable of generating on average 740 barcodes per mouse, with 88% of the targeted cells that presented a barcode.

Two studies very recently reported the generation of mice carrying the LoxCode construct (Weber et al. 2023; Biben et al. 2023). Similar to the Polylox system, the LoxCode construct (Weber et al. 2016) carries 14 loxP sites in alternate orientation interspersed with 13 short DNA segments with a unique sequence. Cre-mediated recombination generates an impressively high theoretical barcode diversity, reportedly up to 30×10^9 unique barcodes. Although highly promising in terms of barcode diversity, it should be noted that potential drawbacks of this approach are represented by the length of the barcodes (leading to more complex code sequencing) and the probability of barcode tagging that heavily relies on Cre efficiency.

Transposons

A less widely embraced method is based on the temporally restricted expression of a Hyperactive Sleeping Beauty (HSB) transposase, an enzyme that mediates the genomic mobilisation of a cognate DNA transposon (Tn). The HSB transposase is expressed upon doxycycline administration to mice, triggering the integration of a DNA transposon in a quasi-random position in the genome (Sun et al. 2014). Because the Tn is randomly inserted in the genome, each cell that underwent transposition carries a unique insertion site that represents a permanent tag and is transmitted to the progeny. This technique allows the detection of 5 to 25 clones per 10,000 cells. The transposon-mediated approach for clonal mapping was recently used to identify distinct embryonic waves of multipotent hematopoietic progenitors (Patel et al. 2022). However, the Sleeping Beauty transposase appears to have some bias towards insertions within specific DNA motifs (Vigdal et al. 2002). To overcome this limitation, a new system called TracerSeq was developed, using the Tol2 transposase to mobilise transposons and allowing to combine lineage tracing and transcriptomic analyses (Wagner et al. 2018).

DRAG Barcoding Mice

This approach takes advantage of the V(D)J recombination system that is used by our immune system to produce a high degree of genetic diversity in the repertoire of T cell receptors in lymphoid lineages [reviewed in Bassing et al. (2002)]. V(D)J recombination is initiated by the RAG1 and RAG2 enzymes through the introduction of DNA double-strand breaks between the V (Variable), D (Diversity), and J (Joining) coding segments flanked by Recombination Signal Sequences (RSS). To induce endogenous cellular barcoding of all cellular lineages in an organism in a temporally controlled manner, a DNA cassette was designed, called DRAG (Diversity through RAG), composed of a promoter, a RAG/TdT (Terminal deoxynucleotidyl Transferase) coding sequence surrounded by two loxP sites, a VDJ sequence and a GFP coding sequence. Upon Cre-mediated recombination, the segment between the two loxP sites is inverted, leading to the transient expression of the enzymes RAG1, RAG2, and TdT. As a consequence, RAG-mediated recombination between the V, D, and J segments is induced at the time of Cre induction and in the cells where Cre is expressed, and additional diversity is generated through deletions and insertions mediated by TdT at the junction sites. The VDJ sequence thus generated (barcode) is stable over time, heritable and is also transcribed, allowing to couple transcriptomic and lineage information (Cosgrove et al. 2023). This system was recently reported to efficiently trace cells and derived lineages in the mouse brain, mammary gland, and hematopoietic cells (Urbanus et al. 2023).

Most of the genetic barcodes are coupled with one single fluorescent tag. Therefore, different barcodes cannot be distinguished by flow cytometry, and the cells corresponding to one clone cannot be selected. An approach called COLBERT (Control of Lineages by Barcode-Enabled Recombinant Transcription) was developed to overcome this limitation (Al'Khafaji et al. 2018). Using this technique, a population of cells is tagged with a barcode-gRNA under the control of a specific promoter. Cells are then transfected with a Cas9 cassette and a "Recall" plasmid encoding a lineage barcode of interest, upstream of a gene leading to the expression of a fluorescent protein. The pool of cells containing the defined barcode will express the corresponding fluorescent protein and can be sorted by flow cytometry. This method was used to study drug-resistant clones in a leukaemia cell line using the ClonMapper library (Gutierrez et al. 2021). A similar strategy, CRISPRa Tracing of Clones in Heterogenous cell populations (CaTCH) was developed to sort live cell clones with defined and specific barcode sequences (Umkehrer et al. 2021). Even if these methods are very efficient for selecting the labelled cells of interest, they require an *in vitro* cell manipulation, potentially inducing changes in cell potency and features, as explained above.

5.2.2.2 Evolving Barcodes for Dynamic Lineage Tracing

Compared to stable barcodes that are common to all cells within a clone, evolving barcodes provide another dimension to lineage tracing, namely the temporal or generational component. Indeed, dynamic clonal tracing methods can achieve the reconstruction of branching phylogenetic lineage trees for each labelled cell (Fig. 5.1c).

The advent of the CRISPR-Cas9 technology has allowed the development of methods based on evolving barcodes. Indeed, the error-prone non-homologous end joining (NHEJ) cell machinery used to repair Cas9-induced double-strand breaks, generates a high diversity of unique and heritable barcodes, by introducing insertions or deletions at a targeted locus. The resulting random "edits", the evolving barcodes, permit the identification of distinct copies of the CRISPR target sequence differentially repaired in individual cells. The first CRISPR/Cas9 barcoding system, termed Genome Editing of Synthetic Target Arrays for Lineage Tracing (GESTALT) was applied to the zebrafish *Danio rerio* by injecting the CRISPR/Cas9 editing reagents in single-cell fish embryos, targeting a genomic barcode with 10 sgRNA target sites, absent from the zebrafish genome and predicted to be highly editable (McKenna et al. 2016). Tracing was performed from fertilised eggs to adulthood and showed that a small number of early forming embryonic lineages generates the majority of the cells in a given organ of adult zebrafish, demonstrating clonal dominance. In this study, the GESTALT approach provided the lineage relationships of hundreds of thousands of differentiated cells.

A couple of years later, the single-cell sequencing strategy ScarTrace was developed, also based on the CRISPR-Cas9 system (Alemany et al. 2018). This technique enables the quantification of clonal history and cell types for thousands of cells collected from different organs in zebrafish. ScarTrace labels cells with unique barcodes in a zebrafish embryo. CRISPR/Cas9 technology induces insertions and deletions, called "scars", at different positions in eight tandem copies of a histone-GFP transgene. The authors developed a protocol to allow the detection of scars in the cDNA of labelled cells. Unlike the first GESTALT system, this new method accomplished the goal of obtaining a quantitative analysis of the clonal origin of each cell concomitantly with information on cell identity by single-cell RNA sequencing.

The original GESTALT system was then further modified in several versions, such as scGESTALT, studying single cells in the zebrafish brain (Raj et al. 2018), LINNAEUS (Lineage tracing by Nuclease-Activated Editing of Ubiquitous Sequences) applied to zebrafish (Spanjaard et al. 2018) or the Mouse for Actively Recording Cells (MARC1) system (Kalhor et al. 2018), initially providing only lineage information, and later combined with scRNAseq profiles (Chan et al. 2019), delivering cell fate maps during gastrulation or the first steps of embryo development from a zygote.

Another related method called macsGESTALT (multiplexed, activatable, clonal, and subclonal GESTALT) has been recently developed (Simeonov et al. 2021). With this strategy, each barcode is encoded by a combination of a 10 bp constant region coupled with 250 bp of editable CRISPR target sites. The constant region is used for clonal reconstruction and the evolving region for phylogenetic recordings. Unlike the previous GESTALT models, macsGESTALT requires cell manipulation *in vitro*, since the dox-inducible Cas9 and the gRNAs array are introduced into cells through lentiviral transduction followed by a PiggyBac-transposition to insert the multiplexed barcodes. Despite these limitations, macsGESTALT remains the first approach that was used to retrace phylogenies in a cancer model. This technique was employed to track about 100 clones and reconstruct the dissemination of ~28,000 single cells across multiple metastatic sites in a mouse model of metastatic pancreatic cancer.

The models described above require the generation of mouse embryos for each experimental replicate, and the resulting transgenic mice are not fit for breeding because of the high number of randomly inserted transgenes. In addition, macsGESTALT necessitates *in vitro* cell manipulation, carrying along all the pitfalls linked to cell dissociation that were previously described.

To overcome these limitations, another model of CRISPR-edited barcodes was developed by the team of Camargo. They designed a genetic system where the induction of doxycycline leads to concomitant Cas9 expression and generation of double-strand breaks in a target array (Bowling et al. 2020). The breaks are randomly repaired, forming new DNA sequences called CARLIN (CRISPR Array Repair LINeage tracing) alleles. Sequential pulses of doxycycline can be used to build multi-level, hierarchical cell histories for lineage reconstruction. For this model, barcodes were detected in only 10% of the cells and 12% of CARLIN alleles are generated at high frequency, often leading to reproduction of the same barcode in different cells. This model is able to create up to 44,000 distinct alleles. A filtering step is critical to ensure that a detected allele indeed derives from the traced cells and does not represent a "popular" sequence shared by two different cells of origin. CARLIN alleles are also transcribed, allowing to couple lineage and transcriptomic information. This is also the first inducible mouse model, offering the advantage of controlling the starting time of cellular barcoding. In this model, the deletion and insertions generated by Cas9 are contained in defined genomic loci, minimising the deleterious and uncontrollable effects of non-targeted double-strand breaks in the genome. Moreover, and most importantly, CARLIN mice are kept as stable transgenic mouse lines, and they can therefore be bred to any genetic model of interest and used to study any organ, except for the brain. A second generation, improved version of this system was recently developed, called DARLIN for Cas9-TdT CARLIN (Li et al. 2023). Starting from the CARLIN model, the authors showed that CRISPR/Cas9 editing is more prone to insertions than deletions, leading to some alleles generated at high frequencies. In this second model, they used the terminal deoxynucleotidyl transferase (TdT) that can insert random nucleotides at both overhang and blunt 3′ ends. The coexpression of Cas9 and TdT generates more insertions than deletions compared to Cas9 alone. In the DARLIN mice, 65% of alleles were observed only once compared to 30% of unique barcodes in the CARLIN mouse model. This improved system allowed barcode detection in 60% of profiled single cells. The authors also developed a new sequencing method, called Camellia-seq, to simultaneously measure DNA methylation, chromatin accessibility, gene expression, and lineage information in each individual cell.

5.3 Cellular Barcoding Applied to Mammary Stem Cells and Breast Cancer

5.3.1 Unravelling Embryonic Cell Fate Specification in the Mouse Mammary Gland

The early stages of embryonic mammary gland development and the hierarchy of foetal mammary stem cells (fMaSCs) have been poorly studied until recent years, partly because of the small size and difficulty of detecting early embryonic mammary placodes and buds.

However, recent evidence indicates that, different from the majority of tissues, which are maintained by multipotent stem cells, in the mammary gland only unipotent progenitors sustain tissue homeostasis. Indeed, several lineage-tracing studies found that at birth, the mammary epithelium arises predominantly from basal and luminal progenitors that are unipotent and fully lineage committed. These unexpected findings prompted several groups to investigate the lineage potential of fMaSCs, in order to establish if multipotent mammary stem cells exist in the embryonic gland and to understand when and how lineage specification occurs in this tissue. Indeed, although fMaSCs have multipotent activity upon transplantation, their true developmental potential *in situ* can only be revealed by lineage tracing at clonal density.

In the past decade, technological developments in single-cell analyses (mainly scRNAseq and scATACseq) combined with the use of lineage tracing techniques have provided exciting new insights into embryonic mammary gland development and the origin and potency of fMaSCs. We have undertaken a systematic and technically delicate clonal analysis *in vivo* during embryonic and perinatal mammary gland development, using combinations of multicolour optical barcodes to trace the clonal fate of individual fMaSCs. Indeed, population-based studies do not have the resolution of addressing the important question of whether individual embryonic stem cells exhibit multipotent potential at the clonal level or comprise distinct stem cell subsets already committed towards a specific cell lineage. In addition, it was unclear when cell fate restriction occurs during mammary gland development and what are the responsible mechanisms. We performed lineage tracing analysis using the multicolour Confetti reporter mouse, combined with whole mount immunofluorescence, mathematical modelling of clonal dynamics, molecular profiling, and functional studies in mouse mutants, to comprehend embryonic mammary gland development and lineage specification. We identified the critical developmental times for cell identity acquisition for all mammary lineages and, unexpectedly, found that early embryonic development of the mouse mammary gland relies on the proliferative activity of multipotent MaSCs that progressively differentiate into lineage-restricted unipotent precursors that fuel late embryonic and post-natal growth and branching morphogenesis. Cellular barcoding in this context revealed that the embryonic mammary gland contains exclusively unipotent lineage-committed stem cells starting from embryonic day E15.5, surprisingly early in mammogenesis. In addition, this approach allowed us to define the specific developmental time points for mammary cell fate restriction, both for basal and luminal lineages (at post-natal day P3), but also for luminal ERalfa^{pos} and ERalfa^{neg} cell fate (between P15 and P21, at the onset of puberty). Importantly, lineage tracing was also used to track the fate of mutant cells and revealed that the unipotency of mammary progenitors belies a remarkable degree of plasticity that allows cell-autonomous factors to redirect cell identity and differentiation potential, irrespective of the cellular environment and the degree of commitment of the targeted cells (Lilja et al. 2018). Concomitantly, the lab of Prof Blanpain demonstrated the bipotency and early fate commitment of fMaSCs using the multicolour Confetti optical barcodes coupled to tetracycline-induced cell-specific inducible Cre expression (Wuidart et al. 2018).

In addition, an elegant study used genetic barcoding induced by intra-amniotic injection of lentiviruses packed with a library of known genetic barcodes to tag embryonic epidermal cells at E9.5 (before mammary placode formation). Clonal tracing of barcoded cells showed that mammary glands are derived from bipotent fMaSCs that appear very early in embryogenesis (E9.5). Furthermore, they estimated that the mammary epithelium originates from a relatively small number of ectodermal progenitors (~120) that exhibit an equivalent long-term potential (Ying and Beronja 2020).

Application of cellular barcoding in the context of embryonic mammary gland development has thus provided an in-depth characterisation of the origin, *in vivo* behaviour and fate, differentiation potential, and extensive plasticity of mammary stem cells.

5.3.2 Analysis of Intra-tumoural Cell and Clonal Heterogeneity

The first cellular barcoding study in breast cancer reported the characterisation, through known stable genetic barcodes, of mammary tumours grown and serially transplanted from either human breast cancer cell lines (MDA-MB-231 and SUM-49) or breast cancer PDXs (Nguyen et al. 2014). The unbiased genetic barcoding approach taken in this pioneering study allowed the authors to infer clonal outputs of the original transduced cells in a prospective and quantitative fashion, although a strong limitation to this approach consists in the drawback that cells belonging to each clone could not be isolated and molecularly characterised. By counting the numbers and size of multiple barcoded clones detected in each tumour and correlating them to the number of initially transplanted cells, the authors calculated the frequency of barcoded cells able to generate a detectable tumour clone, which they defined as the "clone-initiating cells" (CICs). This study revealed extensive heterogeneity between tumours in terms of CICs frequency. Through the evaluation of the clonal frequency and heterogeneity in serially transplanted tumours, they found that only a minority of barcodes was conserved between primary and secondary tumours, despite the supposed clonal origin of the tumours. Notwithstanding the limitations of this original study that suffered the lack of single-cell analyses not available at the time, the first fate mapping analysis by genetic barcoding in serial transplants of breast cancer revealed five patterns of clonal growth amongst transplanted tumours: constant, increasing, decreasing, fluctuating, and delayed growth (Nguyen et al. 2014). Similarly, Merino et al. infected a genetic barcode library into PDXs from metastatic TNBC breast cancer, then selected the barcoded cells and transplanted them into the mammary fat pads of immunodeficient mice to concomitantly track the spatio-temporal fate of multiple barcoded clones in primary tumours and their metastases. To assess clonal mosaicism in primary tumours, the authors assessed the number of shared barcodes between different samples of the same PDX that were collected and dissected into pieces of similar size, called biopsies. This experimental setup allowed them to reconstruct the 3D clonal composition and the architecture of the primary tumour. Although each piece of primary tumour contained a unique profile of barcodes, both in terms of sequence and frequency, some barcodes were shared among adjacent tumour pieces, whereas others were homogeneously distributed throughout the tumour. Notwithstanding the extensive heterogeneity observed, the authors could propose a model in which tumour cells within PDXs grow in spatial "patches", partially recapitulating the clonal mosaicism typical of patient tumours (Merino et al. 2019). Both these studies, however, required the use of tumour cells cultured *in vitro*, infected with a lentiviral library and then transplanted in host mice. These experimental manipulations inevitably impact and alter cell behaviour as well as their interaction with the tumour microenvironment. It is thus conceivable that the clonal composition and evolution of tumour clones would also be affected and differ from the original tumours. In this respect, the development of mouse models for cellular barcoding that do not require cell infection with barcode libraries currently represents the best solution for clonal fate mapping *in vivo*. The possibility of tracking human cells in patients using "natural" barcodes (or somatic mutations) will be discussed in the Perspectives section. In addition, the new generation of cellular barcoding techniques described here allows the combination of barcode detection to gather lineage information and transcriptomic analysis of single barcoded cells to reveal cell identity. In the context of primary breast cancer, however, a study applying this combined approach to correlate single-cell transcriptomic analyses with clonal fate mapping is still currently missing.

5.3.3 Identification of Metastasis-Initiating Cells

Cellular barcoding approaches can generate a high diversity of tags, allowing the detection of clones even when they are composed of a small proportion of cells. This feature can also provide a better comprehension of metastatic diseases. If we focus on breast cancer, several studies using cell lines or PDXs and employing different systems for cellular barcoding, reached the important conclusion that clone abundance within a primary tumour does not necessarily correlate with a higher frequency of circulating tumour cells or secondary lesions and metastases (Wagenblast et al. 2015; Echeverria et al. 2018; Merino et al. 2019; Berthelet et al. 2021; Umeki et al. 2022). Indeed, numerous clones have the capacity to seed metastases, but only a few of them are able to proliferate and establish dominant expanding clones at distant sites (Echeverria et al. 2018; Merino et al. 2019). These findings also provided us with the ability of distinguishing clonal features of shedding, seeding and drug resistance. Although several clones can leave the primary tumour and disseminate progeny into blood and lung ("shedders"), only a small proportion will survive and proliferate at distal sites ("seeders") and will eventually establish stable metastases. This study thus established that the proportion of one clone in the primary tumour does not necessarily correlate with its metastatic potential (Merino et al. 2019).

Using optical barcodes in cell lines derived from Triple Negative Breast Cancer (TNBC), Berthelet and colleagues tracked cells from the primary tumours to lung and liver metastases (Berthelet et al. 2021). Corroborating previous studies, they found that the barcode diversity decreased in the metastases compared to the original primary tumours (Wagenblast et al. 2015; Echeverria et al. 2018; Merino et al. 2019; Guo et al. 2022). They found a similar clonal composition between liver and lung metastases, although the proportion of each clone was different between the two distant sites. The observation that lung metastases were mainly polychromatic whereas liver ones typically presented one single colour also suggested an influence of the metastatic niche on the clonal composition and evolution of the metastatic tumour cells. Thanks to the fluorescence of optical barcodes, clones of interest could then be captured and processed for scRNA sequencing. Based on the distinct distribution of some clones in the liver or the lung, this analysis allowed the identification of transcriptomic changes influenced by the metastasis microenvironment and identified specific signatures supporting selective metastatic seeding in each secondary organ.

Furthermore, a recent study used genetic barcodes generated with the CRISPR/cas9 system to analyse differences and similarities between different sites of metastasis. The authors found that the majority of metastases are indeed polyclonal, carrying several different barcodes, irrespective of the metastatic organ. In this study, cellular barcoding allowed the authors to show that secondary metastases could even arise from primary bone metastases (Zhang et al. 2021).

These studies beautifully illustrate how cellular barcoding can be valuable in providing insights into the spatio-temporal diversity of clones in metastatic disease, a fundamental question with significant therapeutic implications.

5.3.4 Prediction of Drug Resistance or Tumour Relapse

Our capacity of predicting which cells can survive and acquire resistance to therapy relies on a deep characterisation of the pathways that govern residual cancer cell survival after treatment and that confer a proliferative advantage to these cells. Such knowledge is essential if we aspire to propose new strategies for targeted therapeutic approaches tailored at preventing tumour relapse. Cellular barcoding provides sufficient resolution to track the clonal fate of cells before and after treatment and, by comparative analysis of the transcriptional landscape of the barcoded cells that survive therapy, to potentially identify the mechanisms conferring drug resistance. Unlike in acute myeloid leukaemia, where these kinds of studies are facilitated by the possibility of obtaining liquid biopsies before and after treatment, for breast cancer, only a few labs have used cellular barcoding to study resistance to therapy. Moreover, these studies relied on barcode libraries transduced *in vitro* into established cell lines or dissociated PDXs that were then transplanted into immunodeficient host mice and lacked a correlated transcriptional analysis of individual barcoded cells. Notwithstanding these limitations, some studies have described the changes in clonal composition observed in relapsing tumours after treatment, using either cell lines or PDX models of TNBC (Merino et al. 2019; Echeverria et al. 2019; Patwardhan et al. 2021). Surprisingly, though, they observed only minor differences before and after treatment, since most clones survived treatment, leading to a similar profile of intra-tumoral heterogeneity between tumours treated with vehicle compared with chemotherapy. Interestingly, these results seem to indicate that all clones in the primary tumour have a similar fitness providing them with the capacity of surviving chemotherapy. By contrast, relapsing tumours that reappear after treatment harbour fewer barcodes than the primary tumours (Echeverria et al. 2019). This important observation suggests that clones able to re-grow after treatment are probably characterised by intrinsic properties supporting their proliferation and expansion.

Another study used cellular barcoding to monitor clonal dynamics during tumour recurrence in a mouse model of primary Her2-driven mammary tumours that were dissociated and infected *in vitro* with a lentiviral barcode library

(Walens et al. 2020). In this model, doxycycline induced the expression of the Her2/neu oncogene, leading to invasive mammary tumours. The withdrawal of doxycycline led to tumour regression, mimicking the effect of anti-Her2 targeted therapy. However, a small proportion of cancer cells survived (equivalent to the clinical definition of "residual tumour") and restarted to divide within relapsing tumours. This study revealed that, in this specific mouse model, clonal complexity decreases in residual tumours compared to primary tumours resulting in the enrichment or selection of a small number of clones. However, when the authors assessed the clonal composition of recurrent tumours, they observed two routes for tumour relapse from dormant residual cells: either only a few clones resume growth, giving rise to reduced clonal diversity, as was the case for the residual cells, or most clones can restart proliferating, leading to recurrent tumours with a clonal distribution comparable to the cell repertoire of the primary tumour. It is noteworthy that the authors complemented the cellular barcoding approach with single-cell RNA sequencing and whole exome sequencing of residual and recurrent cells (Walens et al. 2020).

A few studies also used cellular barcoding to evaluate the clonal composition of primary tumours and to study the clonal dynamics during metastatic spread and in relapsing tumours. However, most of these studies used cancer cell lines and required long *in vitro* manipulations and selections to introduce barcode libraries into the cells. Through the work of several labs, important differences between *in vitro* and *in vivo* experimental conditions were indeed observed, reiterating the sharp and urgent need for *in vivo* and *in situ* cellular barcoding analyses that do not demand *in vitro* cell manipulations (Wagenblast et al. 2015; Walens et al. 2020; Berthelet et al. 2021).

5.4 Limitations and Perspectives of Cellular Barcoding

The high number of different approaches being developed in recent years and discussed in this chapter clearly proves the growing interest in cellular barcoding techniques that can provide sufficient resolution to answer fundamental questions in developmental and cancer biology.

The *in situ* visualisation of homeostatic cell turnover and fate as well as early oncogene-induced changes in cell behaviour have been limited to the static analysis of snapshots of fixed tissues and therefore the dynamic changes in developmental cell state or cancer-triggered cell plasticity remain poorly understood. In perspective, optical barcodes will be uniquely suited for real-time or *in situ* lineage tracing experiments, an emerging approach combining fate mapping with time-lapse multispectral microscopy. Wholemount immunofluorescence at the end of the time-lapse microscopy on fixed samples will provide the missing spatial information on the tracked cells, necessary to reveal how lineage-traced cells maintain or alter their fate, position, or behaviour. Ongoing technological developments combining intravital and time-lapse microscopy with unbiased marking of individual cells using unique, heritable barcodes, will allow the simultaneous attribution of positional clonal fate and cell identity with high spatio-temporal resolution.

Notwithstanding the attractiveness of these strategies, current cellular barcoding approaches still present certain limitations. Although genetic barcodes are superior to optical ones because of their high diversity, all systems developed up to now have witnessed a bias towards certain DNA sequences that are more often generated, what we define as "popular" barcodes. Such barcode redundancy is dangerous because it can lead to wrongful assumptions of monoclonality, even when cells carrying the same barcode derive in reality from different progenitors. Popular barcodes thus need to be identified and removed from clonal quantification and assessment. In addition, point mutations occur frequently during sequencing and PCR amplification (about 1% of base calling, on average), thus it is important to design strategies for distinguishing true barcodes from sequencing errors in systems where a reference library of known barcodes is not available. These potential biases can lead to misinterpretations in the reconstruction of lineage trees or in the assessment of stem cell lineage potential.

Processing of cellular barcoding data requires a deep knowledge of statistics and bioinformatics and the expertise to design probabilistic frameworks. Modelling of clonal information that can be run in simulations is a necessity which can then be tested against the experimental data acquired.

As mentioned above, another limitation of genetic barcoding approaches is the lack of spatial information on the positions of the cells both at the time of barcode induction (to locate the mothers or cells of origin) and at later time points (to follow the daughter cells). Although this drawback can be overcome with optical barcodes, the high barcode diversity will be lost.

5.4.1 Human Lineage Tracing

The introduction of an optical or genetic barcode into a cell requires viral infection *in vitro* or the generation of transgenic model organisms. A big challenge is currently represented by several attempts to develop methods allowing us to track human cells, in their physiological environment, using "natural" somatic mutations or microsatellite instability to retrospectively infer lineages in patients [reviewed in Baron and van Oudenaarden (2019)]. Lineage tracing in humans is based on identifying "natural" barcodes that could fall into the following categories: copy number variants (CNVs), single nucleotides variants (SNVs), single nucleotide polymorphisms (SNPs), retroelement transposons, and microsatellite repeats. In addition, natural barcodes can also be found in mitochondrial DNA (Ludwig et al. 2019).

In 2005, the computer scientist Ehud Shapiro proposed that researchers could use the natural mutations in individual human cells to piece together how they are related (Frumkin et al. 2005). This approach focused on repetitive stretches of DNA spread throughout the genome, called microsatellites.

Lineage tracing studies have been performed in humans using CNVs (Navin et al. 2011; Wang et al. 2014; Casasent et al. 2018), long interspersed nuclear element-1 (LINE-1) retrotransposons (Hwang et al. 2019) and somatic Single Nucleotide Variants (sSNVs) (Xu et al. 2012; Lodato et al. 2015; Leung et al. 2017; Bizzotto et al. 2021). However, such applications in humans remain costly and difficult to apply at the level of the whole organism.

Specifically for breast cancer, a recent elegant study used mutations progressively acquired by breast cancer cells to define clones (Lomakin et al. 2022). The authors developed a workflow, termed Base-Specific *in situ* Sequencing (BaSISS), to spatially localise genetic clones across sections of human tumours. To this end, they first detected different subclones using bulk whole-genome sequencing (WGS) data, then they designed specific probes to detect the different subclones they had identified and finally they used spatial transcriptomics to correlate lineage information and transcriptomic properties. This original study found that clonal territories are correlated with a defined transcriptional phenotype possibly related with specific immune and stromal niches. However, this method suffers from a low sensitivity that is not compatible with the high clonal diversity typically found in human tumours. Also, clonal identification requires an initial step of high-depth WGS that is not always possible. Regardless, this ground-breaking approach revealed the transcriptional characteristics and the spatial localisation of each tumour clone, a remarkable step in human cancer biology.

5.5 Conclusions

There is little doubt that the coming years will see an increasing amount of cellular barcoding studies and the advent of new techniques to perform these kinds of analyses. Here we reviewed the two major current systems for cellular barcoding: optical barcodes allowing spatial visualisation of cell fate and genetic barcoding to follow high numbers of cells and couple lineage history with single-cell molecular analyses.

Ideally, the future will also bring about new methods capable of simultaneously profiling lineage barcodes, the transcriptome, and the epigenome in single cells.

Cellular barcoding methods have not yet been systematically employed for studying the mammary cellular hierarchies, or the plasticity and lineage conversion potential of different mammary cells. Furthermore, most studies on clonal evolution and dynamics in breast cancer involved *in vitro* manipulation and selection, underlining the demand of new studies using *in vivo* generated barcodes as presented above, as well as the implementation of more efficient methods for tracking naturally occurring barcodes in humans.

Glossary

Cellular barcoding a meth od used to track cells and their progeny in space and time with a specific tag.

Optical barcodes defined by a combination of several fluorescent proteins in a single cell.

Genetic barcodes stable and heritable DNA sequences unique to each cell.

Clone all cells marked by the same barcode, reflecting the fact that they arose from a single ancestor.

Popular barcodes barcode DNA sequences or colour combinations that are commonly generated and can be shared by two different cells of origin, creating the merging of different clones that become indistinguishable.

Cellular barcoding at clonal density the targeted labelling of a small number of cells, allowing each unique clone to be easily identified.

References

Al'Khafaji AM, Deatherage D, Brock A (2018) Control of lineage-specific gene expression by functionalized gRNA barcodes. ACS Synth Biol 7:2468–2474. https://doi.org/10.1021/acssynbio.8b00105

Alemany A, Florescu M, Baron CS et al (2018) Whole-organism clone tracing using single-cell sequencing. Nature 556:108–112. https://doi.org/10.1038/nature25969

Baron CS, van Oudenaarden A (2019) Unravelling cellular relationships during development and regeneration using genetic lineage tracing. Nat Rev Mol Cell Biol 20:753–765. https://doi.org/10.1038/s41580-019-0186-3

Bassing CH, Swat W, Alt FW (2002) The mechanism and regulation of chromosomal V(D)J recombination. Cell 109:S45–S55. https://doi.org/10.1016/S0092-8674(02)00675-X

Berthelet J, Wimmer VC, Whitfield HJ et al (2021) The site of breast cancer metastases dictates their clonal composition and reversible transcriptomic profile. Sci Adv 7:eabf4408. https://doi.org/10.1126/sciadv.abf4408

Biben C, Weber TS, Potts KS et al (2023) In vivo clonal tracking reveals evidence of haemangioblast and haematomesoblast contribution to yolk sac haematopoiesis. Nat Commun 14:41. https://doi.org/10.1038/s41467-022-35744-x

Biddy BA, Kong W, Kamimoto K et al (2018) Single-cell mapping of lineage and identity in direct reprogramming. Nature 564:219–224. https://doi.org/10.1038/s41586-018-0744-4

Bizzotto S, Dou Y, Ganz J et al (2021) Landmarks of human embryonic development inscribed in somatic mutations. Science 371:1249–1253. https://doi.org/10.1126/science.abe1544

Bowling S, Sritharan D, Osorio FG et al (2020) An engineered CRISPR-Cas9 mouse line for simultaneous readout of lineage histories and gene expression profiles in single cells. Cell 181:1693–1694. https://doi.org/10.1016/j.cell.2020.06.018

Casasent AK, Schalck A, Gao R et al (2018) Multiclonal invasion in breast tumors identified by topographic single cell sequencing. Cell 172:205–217.e12. https://doi.org/10.1016/j.cell.2017.12.007

Centonze A, Lin S, Tika E et al (2020) Heterotypic cell–cell communication regulates glandular stem cell multipotency. Nature 584:608–613. https://doi.org/10.1038/s41586-020-2632-y

Chan MM, Smith ZD, Grosswendt S et al (2019) Molecular recording of mammalian embryogenesis. Nature 570:77–82. https://doi.org/10.1038/s41586-019-1184-5

Cosgrove J, Lyne A-M, Rodriguez I et al (2023) Metabolically primed multipotent hematopoietic progenitors fuel innate immunity. BioRxiv 2023(01):24.525166. https://doi.org/10.1101/2023.01.24.525166

Cox MM (1983) The FLP protein of the yeast 2-microns plasmid: expression of a eukaryotic genetic recombination system in Escherichia coli. Proc Natl Acad Sci USA 80:4223–4227. https://doi.org/10.1073/pnas.80.14.4223

Echeverria GV, Powell E, Seth S et al (2018) High-resolution clonal mapping of multi-organ metastasis in triple negative breast cancer. Nat Commun 9:5079. https://doi.org/10.1038/s41467-018-07406-4

Echeverria GV, Ge Z, Seth S et al (2019) Resistance to neoadjuvant chemotherapy in triple-negative breast cancer mediated by a reversible drug-tolerant state. Sci Transl Med 11:eaav0936. https://doi.org/10.1126/scitranslmed.aav0936

Fennell KA, Vassiliadis D, Lam EYN et al (2021) Non-genetic determinants of malignant clonal fitness at single-cell resolution. Nature 1–7. https://doi.org/10.1038/s41586-021-04206-7

Frumkin D, Wasserstrom A, Kaplan S et al (2005) Genomic variability within an organism exposes its cell lineage tree. PLoS Comput Biol 1:e50. https://doi.org/10.1371/journal.pcbi.0010050

Gossen M, Bujard H (1992) Tight control of gene expression in mammalian cells by tetracycline-responsive promoters. Proc Natl Acad Sci USA 89:5547–5551. https://doi.org/10.1073/pnas.89.12.5547

Guo Q, Spasic M, Maynard AG et al (2022) Clonal barcoding with qPCR detection enables live cell functional analyses for cancer research. Nat Commun 13:3837. https://doi.org/10.1038/s41467-022-31536-5

Gutierrez C, Al'Khafaji AM, Brenner E et al (2021) Multifunctional barcoding with ClonMapper enables high-resolution study of clonal dynamics during tumor evolution and treatment. Nat Cancer 2:758–772. https://doi.org/10.1038/s43018-021-00222-8

Hoess RH, Wierzbicki A, Abremski K (1986) The role of the loxP spacer region in P1 site-specific recombination. Nucleic Acids Res 14:2287–2300

Hwang B, Lee W, Yum S-Y et al (2019) Lineage tracing using a Cas9-deaminase barcoding system targeting endogenous L1 elements. Nat Commun 10:1234. https://doi.org/10.1038/s41467-019-09203-z

Jardé T, Lloyd-Lewis B, Thomas M et al (2016) Wnt and Neuregulin1/ErbB signalling extends 3D culture of hormone responsive mammary organoids. Nat Commun 7:13207. https://doi.org/10.1038/ncomms13207

Jordan CT, Lemischka IR (1990) Clonal and systemic analysis of long-term hematopoiesis in the mouse. Genes Dev 4:220–232. https://doi.org/10.1101/gad.4.2.220

Kalhor R, Kalhor K, Mejia L et al (2018) Developmental barcoding of whole mouse via homing CRISPR. Science 361:eaat9804. https://doi.org/10.1126/science.aat9804

Kaufman T, Nitzan E, Firestein N et al (2022) Visual barcodes for clonal-multiplexing of live microscopy-based assays. Nat Commun 13:2725. https://doi.org/10.1038/s41467-022-30008-0

Kebschull JM, Zador AM (2018) Cellular barcoding: lineage tracing, screening and beyond. Nat Methods 15:871–879. https://doi.org/10.1038/s41592-018-0185-x

Koren S, Reavie L, Couto JP et al (2015) PIK3CA H1047R induces multipotency and multi-lineage mammary tumours. Nature 525:114–118. https://doi.org/10.1038/nature14669

Kretzschmar K, Watt FM (2012) Lineage tracing. Cell 148:33–45. https://doi.org/10.1016/j.cell.2012.01.002

Leung ML, Davis A, Gao R et al (2017) Single-cell DNA sequencing reveals a late-dissemination model in metastatic colorectal cancer. Genome Res 27:1287–1299. https://doi.org/10.1101/gr.209973.116

Li L, Bowling S, Yu Q et al (2023) A mouse model with high clonal barcode diversity for joint lineage, transcriptomic, and epigenomic profiling in single cells. BioRxiv. https://doi.org/10.1101/2023.01.29.526062

Lilja AM, Rodilla V, Huyghe M et al (2018) Clonal analysis of Notch1-expressing cells reveals the existence of unipotent stem cells that retain long-term plasticity in the embryonic mammary gland. Nat Cell Biol 20:677–687. https://doi.org/10.1038/s41556-018-0108-1

Liu K, Jin H, Zhou B (2020) Genetic lineage tracing with multiple DNA recombinases: a user's guide for conducting more precise cell fate mapping studies. J Biol Chem 295:6413–6424. https://doi.org/10.1074/jbc.REV120.011631

Livet J, Weissman TA, Kang H et al (2007) Transgenic strategies for combinatorial expression of fluorescent proteins in the nervous system. Nature 450:56–62. https://doi.org/10.1038/nature06293

Lloyd-Lewis B, Mourikis P, Fre S (2019) Notch signalling: sensor and instructor of the microenvironment to coordinate cell fate and organ morphogenesis. Curr Opin Cell Biol 61:16–23. https://doi.org/10.1016/j.ceb.2019.06.003

Lodato MA, Woodworth MB, Lee S et al (2015) Somatic mutation in single human neurons tracks developmental and transcriptional history. Science 350:94–98. https://doi.org/10.1126/science.aab1785

Lomakin A, Svedlund J, Strell C et al (2022) Spatial genomics maps the structure, nature and evolution of cancer clones. Nature 1–9. https://doi.org/10.1038/s41586-022-05425-2

Ludwig LS, Lareau CA, Ulirsch JC et al (2019) Lineage tracing in humans enabled by mitochondrial mutations and single cell genomics. Cell 176:1325–1339.e22. https://doi.org/10.1016/j.cell.2019.01.022

Malide D, Métais J-Y, Dunbar CE (2014) In vivo clonal tracking of hematopoietic stem and progenitor cells marked by five fluorescent proteins using confocal and multiphoton microscopy. J Vis Exp JoVE:51669. https://doi.org/10.3791/51669

Merino D, Weber TS, Serrano A et al (2019) Barcoding reveals complex clonal behavior in patient-derived xenografts of metastatic triple negative breast cancer. Nat Commun 10:766. https://doi.org/10.1038/s41467-019-08595-2

McKenna A, Findlay GM, Gagnon JA, Horwitz MS, Schier AF, Shendure J (2016) Whole-organism lineage tracing by combinatorial and cumulative genome editing. Science 353(6298):aaf7907. https://doi.org/10.1126/science.aaf7907. Epub 2016 May 26. PMID: 27229144; PMCID: PMC4967023

Mohme M, Maire CL, Riecken K et al (2017) Optical barcoding for single-clone tracking to study tumor heterogeneity. Mol Ther 25:621–633. https://doi.org/10.1016/j.ymthe.2016.12.014

Navin N, Kendall J, Troge J et al (2011) Tumor evolution inferred by single cell sequencing. Nature 472:90–94. https://doi.org/10.1038/nature09807

Nguyen LV, Cox CL, Eirew P et al (2014) DNA barcoding reveals diverse growth kinetics of human breast tumour subclones in serially passaged xenografts. Nat Commun 5:5871. https://doi.org/10.1038/ncomms6871

Oren Y, Tsabar M, Cuoco MS et al (2021) Cycling cancer persister cells arise from lineages with distinct programs. Nature 596:576–582. https://doi.org/10.1038/s41586-021-03796-6

Patel SH, Christodoulou C, Weinreb C et al (2022) Lifelong multilineage contribution by embryonic-born blood progenitors. Nature 606:747–753. https://doi.org/10.1038/s41586-022-04804-z

Patwardhan GA, Marczyk M, Wali VB et al (2021) Treatment scheduling effects on the evolution of drug resistance in heterogeneous cancer cell populations. NPJ Breast Cancer 7:60. https://doi.org/10.1038/s41523-021-00270-4

Pei W, Feyerabend TB, Rössler J et al (2017) Polylox barcoding reveals haematopoietic stem cell fates realized in vivo. Nature 548:456–460. https://doi.org/10.1038/nature23653

Pei W, Wang X, Rössler J et al (2019) Using Cre-recombinase-driven Polylox barcoding for in vivo fate mapping in mice. Nat Protoc 14:1820–1840. https://doi.org/10.1038/s41596-019-0163-5

Pei W, Shang F, Wang X et al (2020) Resolving fates and single-cell transcriptomes of hematopoietic stem cell clones by PolyloxExpress barcoding. Cell Stem Cell 27:383–395.e8. https://doi.org/10.1016/j.stem.2020.07.018

Peikon ID, Gizatullina DI, Zador AM (2014) In vivo generation of DNA sequence diversity for cellular barcoding. Nucleic Acids Res 42:e127. https://doi.org/10.1093/nar/gku604

Plaks V, Kong N, Werb Z (2015) The cancer stem cell niche: how essential is the niche in regulating stemness of tumor cells? Cell Stem Cell 16:225–238. https://doi.org/10.1016/j.stem.2015.02.015

Raj B, Wagner DE, McKenna A et al (2018) Simultaneous single-cell profiling of lineages and cell types in the vertebrate brain. Nat Biotechnol 36:442–450. https://doi.org/10.1038/nbt.4103

Rodilla V, Fre S (2018) Cellular plasticity of mammary epithelial cells underlies heterogeneity of breast cancer. Biomedicines 6:103. https://doi.org/10.3390/biomedicines6040103

Rodilla V, Dasti A, Huyghe M et al (2015) Luminal progenitors restrict their lineage potential during mammary gland development. PLoS Biol 13:e1002069. https://doi.org/10.1371/journal.pbio.1002069

Sauer B, McDermott J (2004) DNA recombination with a heterospecific Cre homolog identified from comparison of the pac-c1 regions of P1-related phages. Nucleic Acids Res 32:6086–6095. https://doi.org/10.1093/nar/gkh941

Shembrey C, Smith J, Grandin M et al (2022) Longitudinal monitoring of intra-tumoural heterogeneity using optical barcoding of patient-derived colorectal tumour models. Cancers 14:581. https://doi.org/10.3390/cancers14030581

Simeonov KP, Byrns CN, Clark ML et al (2021) Single-cell lineage tracing of metastatic cancer reveals selection of hybrid EMT states. Cancer Cell 39:1150–1162.e9. https://doi.org/10.1016/j.ccell.2021.05.005

Snippert HJ, van der Flier LG, Sato T et al (2010) Intestinal crypt homeostasis results from neutral competition between symmetrically dividing Lgr5 stem cells. Cell 143:134–144. https://doi.org/10.1016/j.cell.2010.09.016

Spanjaard B, Hu B, Mitic N et al (2018) Simultaneous lineage tracing and cell-type identification using CRISPR–Cas9-induced genetic scars. Nat Biotechnol 36:469–473. https://doi.org/10.1038/nbt.4124

Sulston JE, Schierenberg E, White JG, Thomson JN (1983) The embryonic cell lineage of the nematode Caenorhabditis elegans. Dev Biol 100:64–119. https://doi.org/10.1016/0012-1606(83)90201-4

Sun J, Ramos A, Chapman B et al (2014) Clonal dynamics of native haematopoiesis. Nature 514:322–327. https://doi.org/10.1038/nature13824

Umeki Y, Ogawa N, Uegaki Y et al (2022) DNA barcoding and gene expression recording reveal the presence of cancer cells with unique properties during tumor progression. Cell Mol Life Sci 80:17. https://doi.org/10.1007/s00018-022-04640-4

Umkehrer C, Holstein F, Formenti L et al (2021) Isolating live cell clones from barcoded populations using CRISPRa-inducible reporters. Nat Biotechnol 39:174–178. https://doi.org/10.1038/s41587-020-0614-0

Urbanus J, Cosgrove J, Beltman JB et al (2023) DRAG in situ barcoding reveals an increased number of HSPCs contributing to myelopoiesis with age. Nat Commun 14:2184. https://doi.org/10.1038/s41467-023-37167-8

Van Keymeulen A, Rocha AS, Ousset M et al (2011) Distinct stem cells contribute to mammary gland development and maintenance. Nature 479:189–193. https://doi.org/10.1038/nature10573

Van Keymeulen A, Lee MY, Ousset M et al (2015) Reactivation of multipotency by oncogenic PIK3CA induces breast tumour heterogeneity. Nature 525:119–123. https://doi.org/10.1038/nature14665

Vigdal TJ, Kaufman CD, Izsvák Z et al (2002) Common physical properties of DNA affecting target site selection of sleeping beauty and other Tc1/mariner transposable elements. J Mol Biol 323:441–452. https://doi.org/10.1016/S0022-2836(02)00991-9

Wagenblast E, Soto M, Gutiérrez-Ángel S et al (2015) A model of breast cancer heterogeneity reveals vascular mimicry as a driver of metastasis. Nature 520:358–362. https://doi.org/10.1038/nature14403

Wagner DE, Weinreb C, Collins ZM et al (2018) Single-cell mapping of gene expression landscapes and lineage in the zebrafish embryo. Science 360:981–987. https://doi.org/10.1126/science.aar4362

Walens A, Lin J, Damrauer JS et al (2020) Adaptation and selection shape clonal evolution of tumors during residual disease and recurrence. Nat Commun 11:5017. https://doi.org/10.1038/s41467-020-18730-z

Walsh C, Cepko CL (1992) Widespread dispersion of neuronal clones across functional regions of the cerebral cortex. Science 255:434–440. https://doi.org/10.1126/science.1734520

Wang Y, Waters J, Leung ML et al (2014) Clonal evolution in breast cancer revealed by single nucleus genome sequencing. Nature 512:155–160. https://doi.org/10.1038/nature13600

Weber K, Bartsch U, Stocking C, Fehse B (2008) A multicolor panel of novel lentiviral "Gene Ontology" (LeGO) vectors for functional gene analysis. Mol Ther 16:698–706. https://doi.org/10.1038/mt.2008.6

Weber K, Mock U, Petrowitz B et al (2010) Lentiviral gene ontology (LeGO) vectors equipped with novel drug-selectable fluorescent proteins: new building blocks for cell marking and multi-gene analysis. Gene Ther 17:511–520. https://doi.org/10.1038/gt.2009.149

Weber K, Thomaschewski M, Warlich M et al (2011) RGB marking facilitates multicolor clonal cell tracking. Nat Med 17:504–509. https://doi.org/10.1038/nm.2338

Weber TS, Dukes M, Miles DC et al (2016) Site-specific recombinatorics: in situ cellular barcoding with the Cre Lox system. BMC Syst Biol 10:43. https://doi.org/10.1186/s12918-016-0290-3

Weber T, Biben C, Miles D et al (2023) LoxCode in vivo barcoding resolves epiblast clonal fate to fetal organ. BioRxiv. https://doi.org/10.1101/2023.01.02.522501

Weinreb C, Rodriguez-Fraticelli A, Camargo FD, Klein AM (2020) Lineage tracing on transcriptional landscapes links state to fate during differentiation. Science 367:eaaw3381. https://doi.org/10.1126/science.aaw3381

Wuidart A, Sifrim A, Fioramonti M et al (2018) Early lineage segregation of multipotent embryonic mammary gland progenitors. Nat Cell Biol 20:666–676. https://doi.org/10.1038/s41556-018-0095-2

Xu X, Hou Y, Yin X et al (2012) Single-cell exome sequencing reveals single-nucleotide mutation characteristics of a kidney tumor. Cell 148:886–895. https://doi.org/10.1016/j.cell.2012.02.025

Ying Z, Beronja S (2020) Embryonic barcoding of equipotent mammary progenitors functionally identifies breast cancer drivers. Cell Stem Cell 26:403–419.e4. https://doi.org/10.1016/j.stem.2020.01.009

Zhang W, Bado IL, Hu J et al (2021) The bone microenvironment invigorates metastatic seeds for further dissemination. Cell 184:2471–2486.e20. https://doi.org/10.1016/j.cell.2021.03.011

Models for Studying Ductal Carcinoma In Situ Progression

6

Isabella Nair and Fariba Behbod

Abstract

An estimated 55,720 new cases of ductal carcinoma in situ (DCIS) will be diagnosed in 2023 in the USA alone because of the increased use of screening mammography. The treatment goal in DCIS is early detection and treatment with the hope of preventing progression into invasive disease. Previous studies show progression into invasive cancer as well as reduction in mortality from treatment is not as high as previously thought. So, are we overdiagnosing and over-treating DCIS? An understanding of the natural progression of DCIS is paramount to address this. The purpose of this chapter is to describe various models that have been developed to simulate the processes involved in DCIS to invasive ductal carcinoma (IDC) transition. While each model possesses a unique set of strengths and weaknesses, they have collectively contributed to the current understanding of the molecular and cellular mechanisms underlying this transition. Even though much has been learned, continued advancement of the current models to best match the composition of DCIS epithelial and stromal microenvironment including the extracellular matrix (ECM), stromal cell types, and immune microenvironment will be essential. These advances will undoubtedly pave the way toward a full understanding of mechanisms associated with progression and in predicting when a DCIS lesion remains indolent and when triggers tip in the balance toward progression to malignancy.

Keywords

Ductal carcinoma in situ · Invasive ductal carcinoma · Mouse-INtraDuctal (MIND) model · Breast cancer · Animal models · Precancer biology · Nonmalignant breast cancers

Supplementary Information The online version contains supplementary material available at https://doi.org/10.1007/978-3-031-70875-6_6. The videos can be accessed individually by clicking the DOI link in the accompanying figure caption or by scanning this link with the SN More Media App.

I. Nair
Department of General Surgery, University of Missouri - Kansas City, Kansas City, MO, USA
e-mail: isn5g8@mail.umkc.edu

F. Behbod (✉)
Department of Pathology and Laboratory Medicine, MS 3045, The University of Kansas Medical Center, Kansas City, KS, USA
e-mail: fbehbod@kumc.edu

T. Sørlie, R. B. Clarke (eds.), *A Guide to Breast Cancer Research*, Advances in Experimental Medicine and Biology 1464, https://doi.org/10.1007/978-3-031-70875-6_6

Key Points

1. Annual diagnosis of DCIS has drastically increased due to the adoption of screening mammography. DCIS is considered a non-obligate precursor to IDC; the goal of treating DCIS is to prevent invasive progression and/or metastasis.
2. Previous human DCIS models have shown that progressive potential into IDC as well as the reduction in mortality from treating DCIS is not as great as researchers once thought. This raises the question: are we overdiagnosing and over-treating DCIS? To answer this an understanding of the natural progression of DCIS is paramount.
3. Previous animal models have yielded useful data regarding invasive potential but were limited in their ability to replicate the natural progression of DCIS that has been observed in human models.
4. The Mouse INtraDuctal (MIND) model provides the platform to replicate the natural progression of human DCIS in an *in vivo* animal model. The models mimic all histological subtypes of human DCIS, express similar biomarkers, and a fraction progress to IDC.
5. Previous research has identified numerous biomarkers that can reflect the risk of recurrence and prognostic outcomes of breast cancer. Data obtained from the MIND models have identified useful biomarkers for invasive progression. However, there is still much to be learned.
6. Limitations of the MIND model include the inability to address the role of the immune system in influencing invasive progression as the mice used are immunocompromised. The use of immunocompetent mouse mammary precancer progression models described in this review is one way to overcome the immune deficiencies of the MIND models.
7. Computer-assisted bioprinting to create a 3D *in vitro* model of human breast will provide future powerful tools for studying DCIS progression.

6.1 Introduction

The annual diagnosis of ductal carcinoma in situ (DCIS) has increased; this is a result of advanced radiographic technology in combination with the widespread adoption of screening mammography in women's health maintenance (Ozanne et al. 2011). According to 2023 data provided by the American Cancer Society, it is estimated that 297,790 new cases of invasive breast cancer and 55,720 new cases of DCIS will be diagnosed in the USA (Ted 2023). DCIS is defined as a proliferation of neoplastic cells that are confined to the ductal system of the breast. If malignant cells continue to grow and progress beyond the membrane of the ductal system, the diagnosis of invasive ductal carcinoma (IDC) is made. The standard treatment after a diagnosis of DCIS includes a multimodal approach including surgical resection (mastectomy or breast-conserving lumpectomy), radiation therapy and hormone-blocking agents (van Seijen et al. 2019). The goal of early detection and treatment of DCIS is to prevent the progression into IDC. Interestingly though, the risk of natural progression was found to be lower than anticipated based on data from the Surveillance, Epidemiology, and End Results (SEER) registry (Ozanne et al. 2011). In addition, autopsies completed on middle-aged women (age 40–70), with no documented history of breast disease, discovered undiagnosed DCIS lesions in 8.9% (Welch and Black 1997). If the risk of progression to invasive cancer is less than what was initially thought and if women with no known breast disease are found to have undiagnosed DCIS lesions on autopsy, it is reasonable to question, are we overtreating DCIS?

Despite numerous previous studies, the sequela of DCIS progression to invasive disease is still not well understood. The purpose of this chapter is to introduce the readers to the various *in vitro* and *in vivo* models that have been developed in the recent years to study the sequence of events that mediate a transition from DCIS to invasive breast cancer.

6.2 *In vitro* Models

Research across all fields of cancer continues to identify the contribution that the local microenvironment yields in the natural progression of cancer from a pre-malignant lesion to an invasive lesion. Prior research has suggested that signals produced by the microenvironment as well as remodeling of the ECM have the potential to contribute to the progression of DCIS (Zhao et al. 2004; Jedeszko et al. 2009). One challenge has been how to best match the composition of breast stroma and the ECM *in vitro*. Collagen and Matrigel are commonly used to replicate human breast ECM. A number of synthetic hydrogels have also been developed [reviewed in Ma et al. (2018)]. Matrigel is the "gold standard" and contains primarily laminin, type IV collagen, and entactin, as well as proteoglycans and growth factors (Ma et al. 2018). Collagen is also commonly used as it is the most abundant constituent of ECM. One needs to keep in mind that to provide a suitable microenvironment for cancer growth, the ECM should mimic breast stroma with respect to cellular composition, structure, stiffness, and permeability (Ma et al. 2018). Numerous *in vitro* models have been designed to mimic the breast stroma to investigate the contribution of various factors in the microenvironment of breast epithelium on the progression of DCIS to invasive disease. The following are examples of such 3D *in vitro* culture systems.

Yoonseok Choi et al. micro-engineered a 3D *in vitro* assimilation of human DCIS and fibroblasts (Choi et al. 2015). They utilized a human normal mammary epithelial cell line (HMT-3522), a DCIS cell line (MCF10DCIS.COM), and human primary fibroblasts (HMF). Each cell type was labeled separately using a fluorescent dye, RFP labeled mammary epithelial cells, CFP labeled fibroblasts and GFP labeled MCF10DCIS.COM. A microdevice reflective of an extracellular membrane was constructed independently. After sterilization, the microdevice was serially treated until its contents were reflective of the stromal tissue of a mammary duct. The DCIS spheroids were then subsequently introduced into the microdevice (Fig. 6.1a). This ability to create an *in vitro* replication of human microenvironments created a platform where chemotherapeutic agents could be trialed before being used in *in vivo* studies (Fig. 6.1b). This study specifically evaluated paclitaxel, a commonly used chemotherapy agent. The cytotoxic effects were determined by measuring lactate dehydrogenase (LDH). Results showed a statistically significant increase in the amount of cytotoxicity compared to a group of cells that had not been treated with the agent. The effects of the drug were further highlighted when the DCIS spheroids were examined. The treated cell spheroids showed a decreased or unchanged size in comparison to the untreated spheroids which demonstrated continuous proliferation and size enlargement. It was also noted that proliferating DCIS spheroids displaced the adjacent epithelial cells without invading the underlying stroma. These findings suggest that the disease model accurately represents the confined growth of DCIS within the ducts, as observed in clinical cases. Furthermore, the results also highlight the ability to use these models as screening platforms for potential therapeutic agents. Authors of this study plan to continue modifying the contents of the microenvironment to include additional cell types found in human stromal tissue in addition to fibroblasts. They also plan to work on the recipe used to create their microenvironment so that it can continue to evolve during the progression of DCIS to invasive cancer as would be seen in clinical cases. In comparison to the xenografts used in the MIND study; this process eliminates the need for extensive treatment of DCIS samples followed by serial complex intraductal injections that lack the ability to maintain control of the microenvironment.

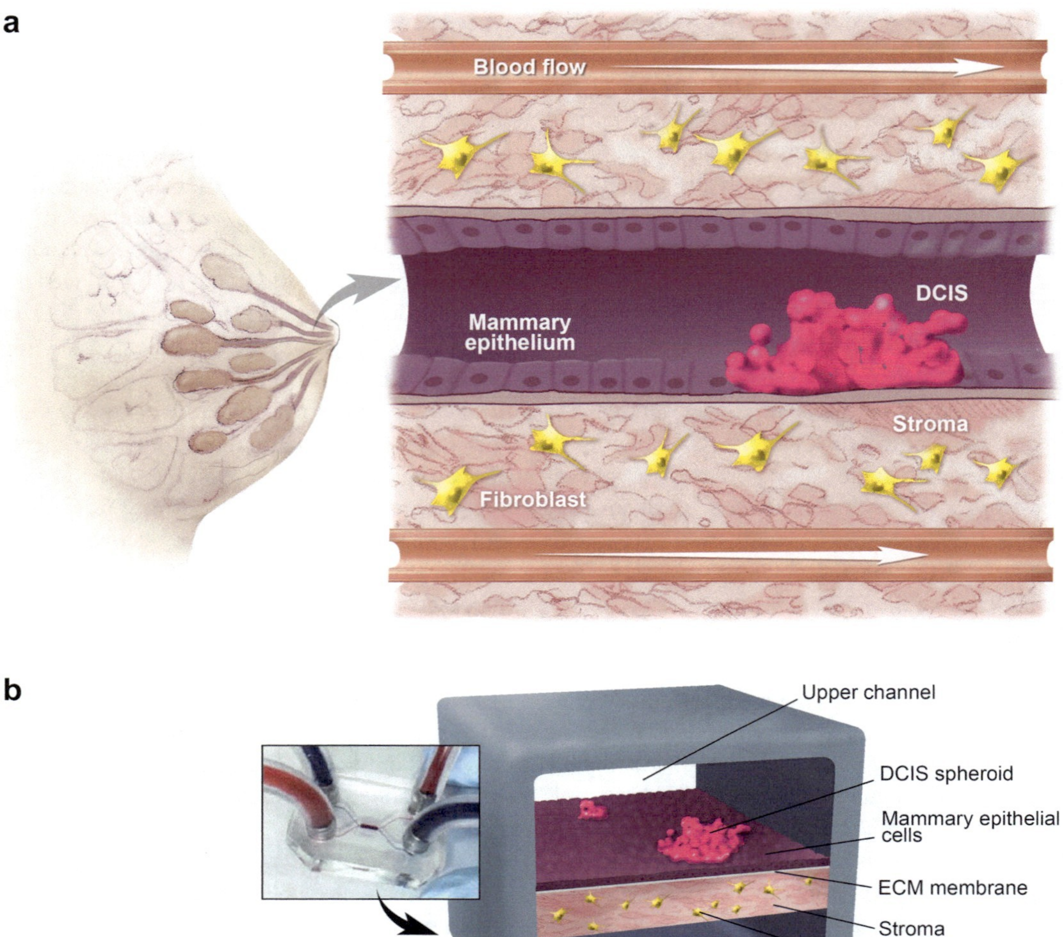

Fig. 6.1 (**a**) Illustration depicting DCIS cancer cells confined within the mammary duct. At this stage, the cells are considered in situ because they have not extended beyond the basement membrane which is surrounded by stromal tissue containing fibroblasts. (**b**) Breast cancer on a chip microdevice recapitulates the microarchitecture of DCIS and surrounding tissues. The upper channel consists of mammary epithelium with embedded DCIS spheroids while the lower chamber mimics the *in vivo* basement membrane with surrounding fibroblast containing stromal tissue [published with permission from The Royal Society of Chemistry; adapted from Choi et al. (2015)]

Mammary Architecture and Microenvironment Engineering (MAME) is another example of a 3D *in vitro* culture system that was developed to study DCIS progression. In this 3D co-culture system, epithelial and stromal cell components, i.e., fibroblasts and myoepithelial cells, are placed in close proximity to the epithelial cells in order to study cell:cell interactions that regulate DCIS to IDC transition. The MAME cocultures consist of multiple layers. Fibroblasts are embedded in the bottom layer mixed with a solution of type I collagen. A layer of reconstituted basement membrane (rBM) is then placed on top of the collagen layer on which DCIS cells and other stromal cell components such as myoepithelial cells are seeded. The medium is then

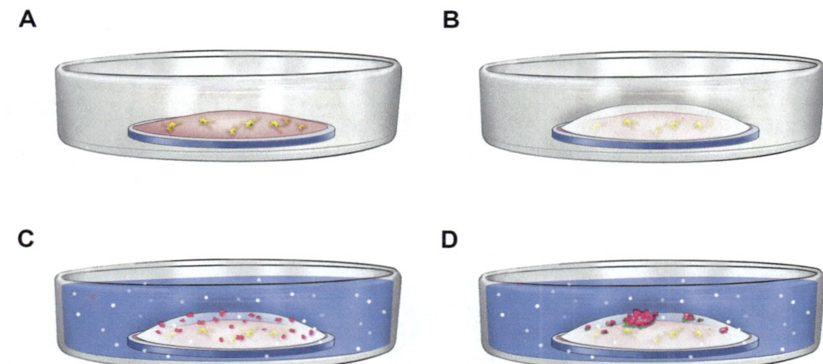

Fig. 6.2 Illustration of MAME cocultures. First layer of the coculture is coated with collagen I consisting of DQ-collagen I and fibroblasts. The second layer consists of DQ-collagen IV which recapitulates a basement membrane. Tumor cells are then added on top and overlaid with culture media. The green dots seen in sub-image D reflect cleavage products of DQ collagen I and IV [published with permission from the Journal of Visual Experiments; adapted from Sameni et al. (2012)]

mixed with 2% rBM which is used to feed the cells (Sameni et al. 2012) (Fig. 6.2). Since DCIS to IDC transition involves degradation of the basement membrane via proteolysis, both Collagen I and IV (present in rBM) become fluorogenic upon hydrolysis. The fluorogenic DQ™ collagen can be used to directly monitor collagenase activity. DQ™ substrates have an excessive number of fluorescent dyes so that the fluorescence signal is quenched. This quenching of the signal is caused by the proximity of the dyes on the intact substrate. The enzyme-driven lysis of collagen results in the separation of the dye molecules from one another and the subsequent increase in fluorescent signals. Additionally, each cellular component, i.e., fibroblasts, epithelial cells, etc., may be labeled separately. For example, the migration of fibroblasts and their incorporation into invasive edges of DCIS may be imaged over time. Fluorescent collagen fragments can also be found in association with invasive DCIS. Furthermore, drugs that target the proteolytic pathways or any other processes that either induce or suppress invasiveness may be evaluated in a temporal manner. By utilizing MAME, the interplay between human breast myoepithelial cells and cancer-associated fibroblasts on DCIS progression was studied. Their studies showed that myoepithelial cells reduced the size of 3D DCIS structures and their ability to degrade extracellular matrix. They went on to show that the tumor-suppressive effects of myoepithelial cells on DCIS were linked to inhibition of urokinase plasminogen activator/urokinase plasminogen activator receptor-mediated proteolysis via plasminogen activator inhibitor 1. Furthermore, myoepithelial cells inhibited the tumor-promoting effects of cancer-associated fibroblasts by attenuating interleukin 6 signaling pathways. The MAME models can be used for live-cell imaging of DCIS invasion over time. Molecules of interest can be downregulated with shRNAs or drugs and their contribution to DCIS invasive progression can be evaluated, imaged, and quantified. In addition, conditioned media from MAME models can be sampled to measure changes in secretion of proteases, cytokines, pH, oxygen tension, etc., during the process of DCIS invasive progression (Sameni et al. 2012, 2017; Osuala et al. 2015).

What most 3D *in vitro* co-culture systems lack is the ability to replicate the normal anatomical lumen seen in breast tissue which has been identified as having an impact on cancer progression (Nelson and Bissell 2006; Verbridge et al. 2013; Bischel et al. 2014, 2015; Duchamp et al. 2019). Bischel et al. proposed an *in vitro* model that recapitulates a native mammary duct model including a physiologically accurate lumen design (Fig. 6.3). A viscous finger pat-

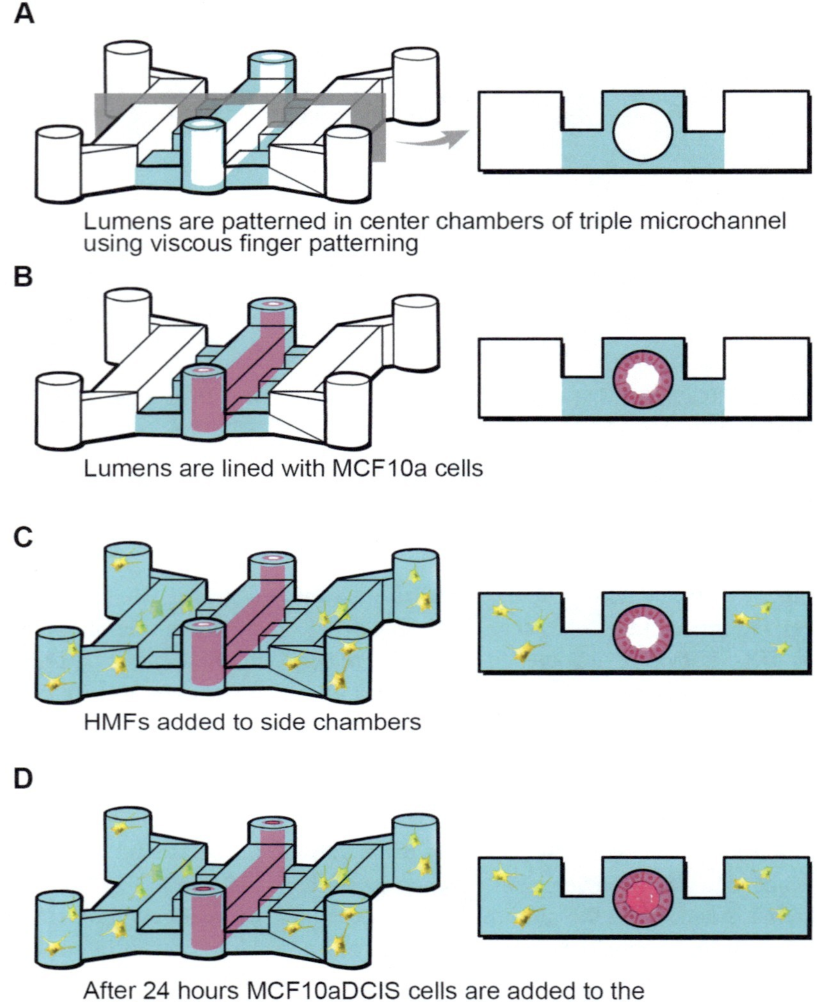

A
Lumens are patterned in center chambers of triple microchannel using viscous finger patterning
B
Lumens are lined with MCF10a cells
C
HMFs added to side chambers
D
After 24 hours MCF10aDCIS cells are added to the MCF10a-lined lumens

Fig. 6.3 Overview of model patterning methods. Viscous finger patterning is used to line the center chamber of a triple microchannel. The lumen is then coated with a matrigel lining followed by the injection of MCF10a cells, which recapitulate the anatomic mammary duct structure. HMF cells are then added to the side chambers. A healthy mammary duct has been mimicked with the above process; DCIS is then modeled by injecting MCF10aDCIS cells into the lumen (published under open access; adapted from Bischel et al. (2015), originally published under CC-BY 4.0)

terning method was used to coat lumen structures with a mixture reflective of an anatomic basement membrane (Bischel et al. 2012; Bischel et al. 2013; Bischel et al. 2015; Duchamp et al. 2019). Lumens were then filled with either healthy epithelial cells or DCIS cells, representing a normal mammary duct and a DCIS-containing mammary duct, respectively. The formation of adherens junctions between the injected cells and the artificial basement membrane was confirmed by staining for E-cadherin; the identification of these connections confirmed that this model has the ability to accurately recapitulate the normal histology of mammary ducts. Despite being an *in vitro* model, the ability to closely replicate an *in vivo* setting allows for the invasive progression that occurs when epithelial cells are co-cultured with fibroblasts to be closely studied. Furthermore, the paracrine signaling that occurred between the DCIS cells and surrounding fibroblasts was observed and validated by multiple endpoints. Invasiveness of the DCIS lesions was manually quantified using bright field images by evaluating the frequency as well as the total area of invasion. Quantification of the lesion was parallel to tumor size and invasive margins used in humans. The degree of collagen modification surrounding invasive lesions was quantified using second-harmonic generation images. Results also showed that cells demonstrating an invasive transition had decreased levels of E-cadherin indicating progression of cells beyond the basement membrane. Bischel et al. have successfully developed a clinically relevant *in vitro* model that recapitulates a native mammary duct model including a physiologically accurate lumen design. This study design has provided the foundation to study the invasive transition of DCIS in response to microenvironmental factors. In addition, this study was able to depict more advanced stages of DCIS in comparison to previous studies by using a high number of DCIS cells. The design of this study can be used to further investigate other environmental factors that have potential to contribute to invasion as well as serve a potential arena to study the effects of potential therapeutic interventions.

Bioprinting technology has become increasingly popular for generating 3D *in vitro* culture systems. One example is a study by Duchamp and colleagues who reported the generation of mammary duct-like structures using bioprinting (Duchamp et al. 2019). When a breast cancer cell line, MCF7, was placed inside these duct-like structures, the generation of in situ lesions followed by their subsequent invasion could be modeled. This bioprinted mammary ductal carcinoma model provided a proof-of-concept demonstrating the value of bioprinting for modeling carcinoma in situ invasive progression. The bioprinting procedure involved first filling of a polydimethylsiloxane (PDMS) mold with a layer of Gelatin-Methacryloyl (GelMA). To generate duct-like structures, an agarose microfiber was placed onto the GelMA layer using a bioprinter, followed by placing another layer of GelMA and photo crosslinking of the entire construct. In the final steps, the agarose microfiber is removed to form the hollow microchannels. The microchannel within the hydrogel can then be seeded with cancer cells (Fig. 6.4). Through the programming of the bioprinter, various mammary ductal structures may be generated. By seeding breast cancer cells inside the mammary duct-like structures, the investigators demonstrated that the cancer cells proliferated, invaded through the matrix, and deposited basement membrane molecules such as collagen. It would be worthwhile to adopt a similar bioprinting system using patient-derived DCIS cells and/or organoids.

Recently, computer-assisted bioprinting technologies have provided a powerful tool for translational research. For example, a 3D bioprinted glioma model was generated in which the brain tissue was bioprinted using mouse macrophage cells and mouse glioma cells with both cell types in a GelMA/gelatin blend bioink (Dai et al. 2016). The glioblastoma cells recruited macrophages which were polarized into tumor-associated macrophages. The model was used to study the efficacy of chemotherapy and immunotherapy on glioblastoma. Similar strategies have been used to generate a 3D cervical cancer tumor model, and a metastatic lung cancer model (Zhao et al. 2014; Meng et al. 2019). Likewise, computer-assisted 3D bioprinting may be designed for studying the transition to DCIS to IDC.

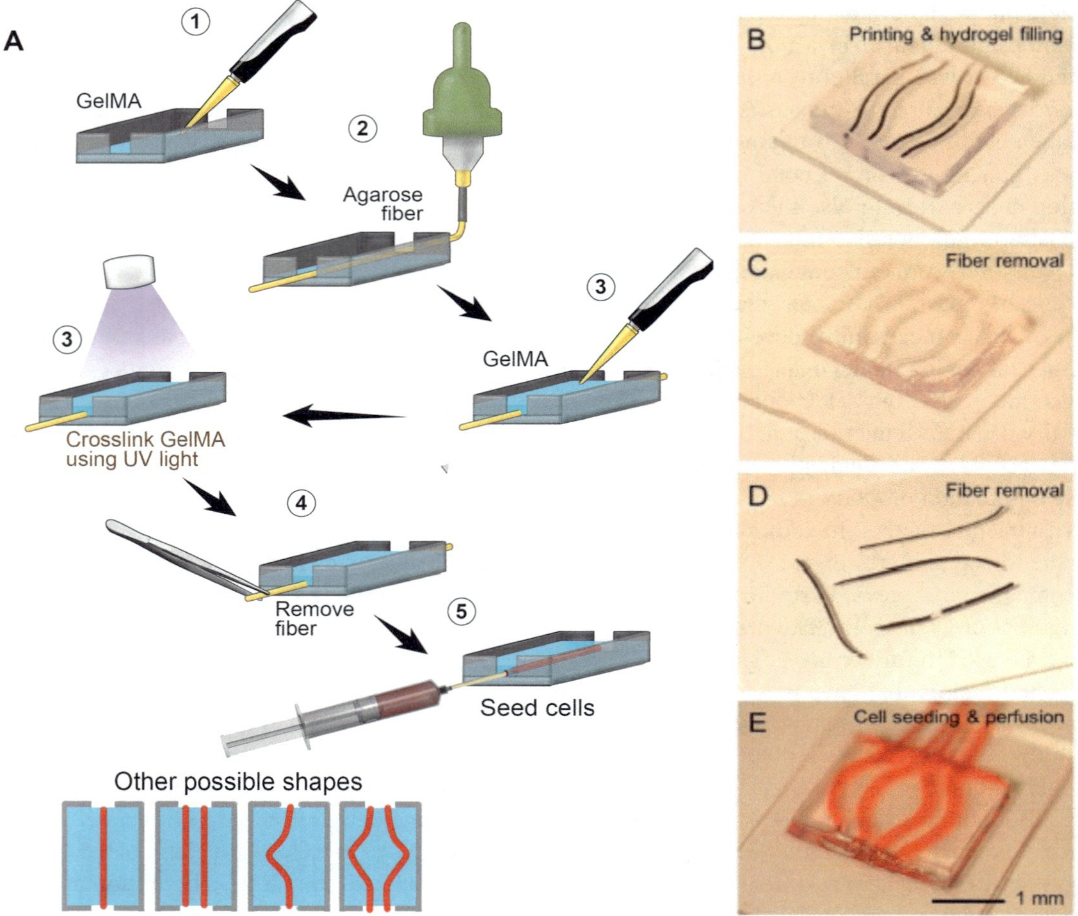

Fig. 6.4 Schematic of sacrificial bioprinting process. First, a thin layer of GelMA is deposited in the mold followed by a layer of microfibers and then a layer of casting GelMA polymer. Photo crosslinking is stimulated with UV light. The microfiber is then removed and followed by the seeding of mammary ductal carcinoma cells into the microchannel. Sub images B-D depict the described process. Image E shows the perfusion of the microchannels [published with permission from John Wiley & Sons; adapted from Duchamp et al. (2019)]

6.3 *In vivo* Models

The first patient-derived xenograft model of DCIS was developed by Espina *et al* by xenotransplantation of freshly procured DCIS organoids and propagated *in vitro* DCIS spheroids from biopsy and surgical specimens. They reported that invasive tumors formed at a rate of ~80% (21/27 cases transplanted) from both freshly procured as well as *in vitro* propagated organoids (Espina et al. 2010; Espina and Liotta 2011).

With the idea that human DCIS initiates inside the ducts, Behbod and colleagues developed the Mouse-INtraDuctal (MIND) model (Fig. 6.5 and Movie 1). MIND involves intraductal injection of DCIS cell lines or patient-derived DCIS epithelial cells into the mammary ducts of immunocompromised mice (Behbod et al. 2009). Similar to the human condition, intraductally injected DCIS epithelial cells initially form *in situ* lesions and in some cases where the DCIS epithelial cells acquire a malignant transformation, the lesions undergo invasive progression as evident by the loss of a continuous myoepithelial cell layer

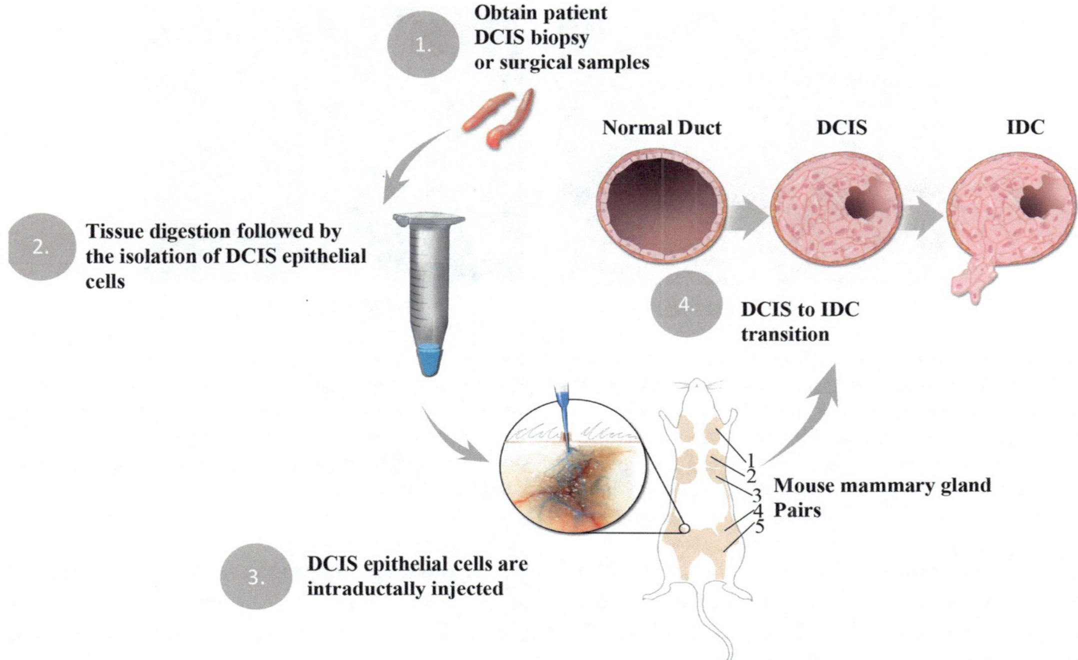

Fig. 6.5 Mouse INtraDuctal (MIND) Model. Model involves obtaining DCIS epithelial cells from human subjects diagnosed with DCIS. The DCIS cells are isolated through tissue processing and then injected into the mammary ducts of immunocompromised mice. The progression of DCIS into invasive ductal carcinoma can be simulated once the cells extend beyond the myoepithelial layer and basement membrane (published under open access; adapted from Hong et al. (2022), originally published under CC-BY 4.0). Method for Intraductal Injection of cancer cells for generating the MIND models (published under open access; originally published in Breast Cancer Research 2009)

(smooth muscle actin positive cell layer) and/or the basement membrane (Behbod et al. 2009; Valdez et al. 2011; Kittrell et al. 2016; Hong et al. 2022) (Fig. 6.6). MIND was initially established using DCIS cell lines, MCF10DCIS (DCIS.COM) and SUM225CWN (SUM225) cell lines and epithelial cells obtained from one case of a patient-derived DCIS tissue (Behbod et al. 2009). The DCIS-like lesions were formed inside the mammary ducts and slowly progressed to invasive lesions by 8–10 weeks (Behbod et al. 2009). DCIS-like lesions formed by the DCIS.COM cell line lacked expression of ER, PR, and HER2, while DCIS-like lesions generated by SUM225 were HER2-positive and lacked expression of ER and PR (Behbod et al. 2009). To generate an ER/PR positive DCIS cell line model, Villanueva and colleagues stably expressed different combinations of human ER/PR including PR (A or B isoforms), ER-α alone, or both ER-α and PR in DCIS.COM cells (Villanueva et al. 2019). DCIS.COM ER/PR positive cells showed E2 responsiveness shown by upregulation of known ER targets, i.e., GREB1. Microarray RNA profiling of ER + PR-B positive DCIS.COM cell lines also showed a luminal signature compared to the parental DCIS.COM cells which showed a basal/HER2 signature. The ER/PR positive DCIS.COM cell line was used in the MIND system and showed responsiveness to hormones (Villanueva et al. 2019).

Following the success of the MIND models in mimicking invasive progression of DCIS cell lines, it was important to also show that the MIND models mimicked the natural progression of patient-derived DCIS epithelial cells *in vivo*. For this purpose, over the course of ~13 years, beginning from 2009, human tissue specimens with radiographic suspicion for DCIS were obtained from radiology and surgical suites from

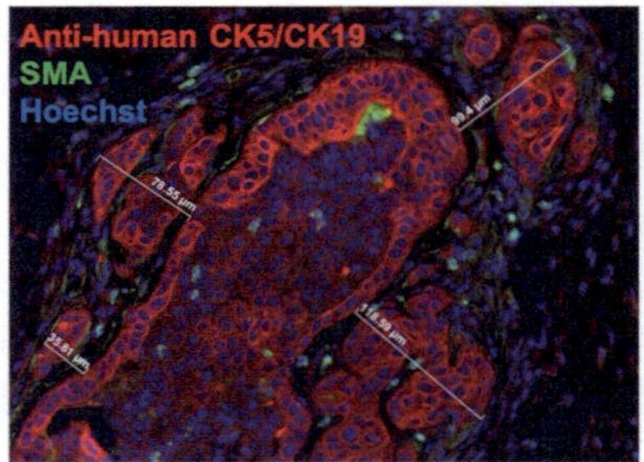

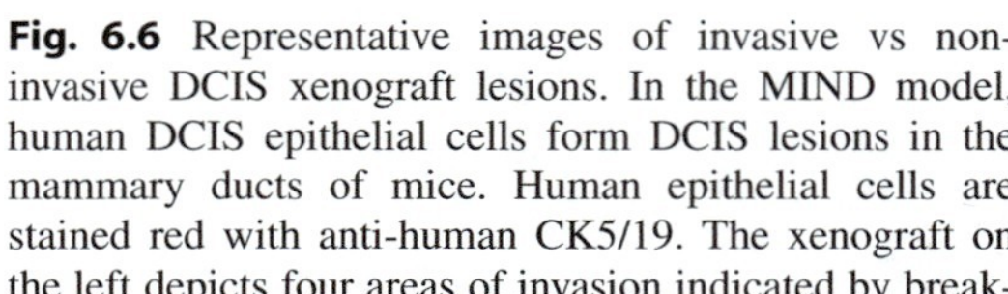

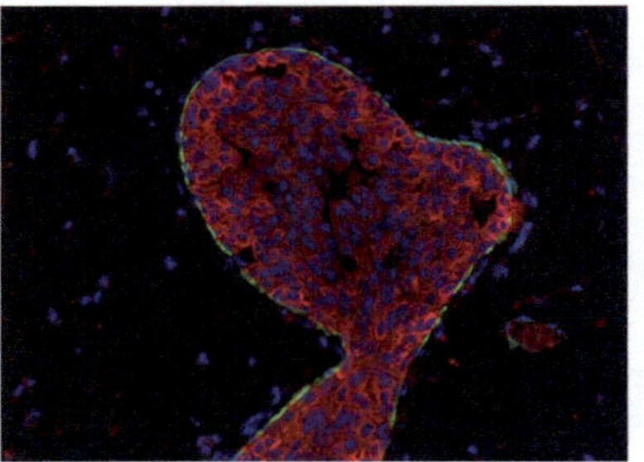

Non-invasive

Fig. 6.6 Representative images of invasive vs non-invasive DCIS xenograft lesions. In the MIND model, human DCIS epithelial cells form DCIS lesions in the mammary ducts of mice. Human epithelial cells are stained red with anti-human CK5/19. The xenograft on the left depicts four areas of invasion indicated by breakdown of SMA and cell invasion beyond the SMA layer. The distance of invasion beyond the SMA is measured by the white lines. In comparison, the xenograft on the right shows an intact SMA boarder, indicating no areas of invasion (original figure published with permission from Farbia Behbod)

several institutions in Kansas City (University of Kansas Medical Center, Truman Hospital and St. Luke's hospital) as well as in Wichita, KS (Heartland Pathology). Following an overnight digestion of the specimens, DCIS epithelial cells were isolated and cryopreserved until a confirmed diagnosis of pure DCIS was obtained. Successful intraductal transplantation of injected DCIS epithelial cells within mouse mammary glands was assessed using IF staining. Anti-smooth actin (SMA) and CK19 were identified; SMA served as a marker of myoepithelial cell layer and perimeter of the xenografted DCIS lesions and CK19 reflected human DCIS epithelial cells. Compromised myoepithelium was reflected by disruption in the SMA border indicating invasive progression of the xenograft (Hong et al. 2022). A total of 37 patient samples were injected using the MIND method; over a median duration of 9 months, 20 samples (54%) injected into 95 xenografts showed in vivo invasive progression while 17 (46%) samples injected into 107 xenografts showed no invasive progression. Within the progressed xenografts, 9 patient samples out of 54 showed a mixed pattern where some of the xenografts progressed and the others remained non-progressed.

For majority of cases, patient DCIS lesions and their corresponding xenografts expressed similar biomarkers, ER, PR, HER2, Ki67, and TP53. Concordance between the biomarkers showed a higher trend for the progressed compared to non-progressed samples. Concordance in biomarker expression for non-progressed versus progressed for ER was 64% versus 89%, PR 47% versus 91%, HER2 82% versus 87%, Ki67 53% versus 60%, and p53 67% versus 83%, respectively. Lack of a 100% concordance between patient DCIS and xenografted DCIS with respect to biomarker expression may be due to intra-tumoral heterogeneity and/or evolution of xenografted DCIS over a 9-month duration of follow-up.

Given the life span limitations of mice, after 12 months the xenografts were harvested with the intention for sequential transplantation into a second generation of mice. Using flow cytometry, the xenograft was separated into human epithelial cells and mouse cells (exclusion of mouse using anti-MHC I/II antibody by magnetic sorting). The resulting human epithelial cells were transplanted into a second generation of mice. IF images demonstrated maintained cribriform histology through both the first transplanted generation and into the second generation. Additionally, our results demonstrated that patient-derived DCIS MIND models mimicked all histologic subtypes of human DCIS including micropapillary, papillary, cribriform, solid, and comedo. Among the clinically relevant biomarkers, only progesterone receptor expression in patient DCIS and extent of *in vivo* growth in xenografts predicted an invasive outcome. Analysis of the frequency of cancer-related pathogenic mutations among the groups showed no significant differences (KW: $P > 0.05$) between the invasive and non-invasive models. There were also no differences in the frequency of high, moderate, or low-severity mutations (KW; $P > 0.05$). These results suggest that genetic changes in the DCIS are not the primary driver for the development of invasive disease.

Hutten and colleagues utilized the MIND models to generate and characterize 115 patient-derived DCIS MIND models. Their studies demonstrated that DCIS high grade, HER2 amplification, expansive 3D growth, and high burden of copy number aberrations were associated with DCIS MIND invasive progression (Hutten et al. 2023).

6.4 Immunocompetent Mouse Mammary Precancer Progression Models

A comprehensive review of transgenic mouse models of DCIS has been previously published (Behbod et al. 2018). In this chapter, we will present three novel mouse models of mammary precancer progression representing three distinct breast cancer subtypes (ER⁺/PR⁺, triple-negative breast cancer [TNBC], and HER2 overexpressing) (Du et al. 2006; Reddy et al. 2010; Haricharan et al. 2013; Bu and Li 2020). The models are generated by intraductal injection of lentiviruses that express either an oncogene or a Cre recombinase (Fig. 6.7).

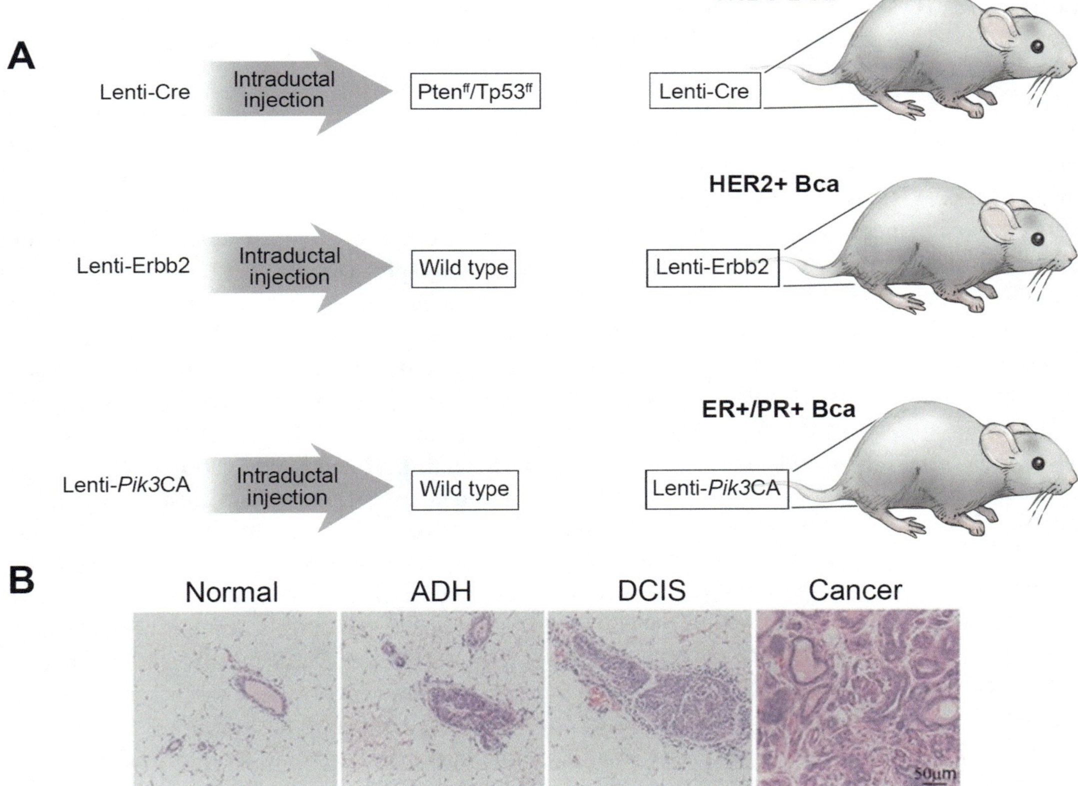

Fig. 6.7 Immunocompetent mouse mammary pre-cancer progression models. (**a**) To generate the TNBC models, $Pten^{ff}/Tp53^{ff}$ mice will be intraductally injected using Lenti-Cre to delete Pten and Tp53 in mammary ductal epithelial cells. Lentiviral vectors that express an oncogene (Lenti-Erbb2 or Lenti-Pik3CA) will be intraductally injected to generate HER2+ and ER+/PR+ breast cancer models, respectively. (**b**) H&E stain of a mouse mammary precancer progression model showing a sequential transition from normal to ADH to DCIS and invasive breast cancer. *Bca* Breast Cancer (original figure published with permission from Dr. Yi Li)

Pik3ca-H1047R model *PIK3CA* is mutated in 40% of luminal human invasive breast cancers and approximately 70% of human breast atypical ductal hyperplasia, with the *H1047R* mutation in the kinase domain being the most frequent (Ang et al. 2014). The fourth mammary glands of mice (i.e., FVB or Balb/C) are intraductally injected with a lentivirus expressing Lenti-Pik3ca-H1047R at a dose of 1.5×10^7 units. Pik3ca-H1047R expression in mammary epithelial cells will result in the formation of atypical ductal hyperplasia (ADH) with a median duration of 4 weeks that advances to DCIS with a median duration of 8 weeks and to IDC with a median duration of 20 weeks. The role of specific gene KO on ADH-DCIS-IDC may be studied by co-expression of a Cre recombinase. For example, intraductal injection of a lentivirus expressing Lenti-Pik3ca-H1047R-P2A-Cre in a transgenic mouse model expressing a gene of interest flanked by LoxP sites will result in overexpression of Pik3CA and simultaneous KO of a gene of interest in the same ductal epithelial cells. Studies in Dr. Li's lab have demonstrated that the invasive tumors in this model are highly differentiated adenocarcinoma with small areas of squamous differentiation (Young et al. 2022). Using the clinical cut-off of 1% as positive, estrogen receptor (Esr1) scored positive in 90% of the invasive tumors, with an average of 35% of tumor cells positive while progesterone receptor (Pgr) was positive in 100% of invasive tumors, with an average of 20% of tumor cells positive.

Lenti-ca-Erbb2 (activated Erbb2) model ERBB2 is amplified and overexpressed in 20–30% of primary human invasive breast cancers and correlates with poor patient outcomes. Transgenic mouse models that overexpress an activated form of rat NEU (activated Erbb2) initiate mammary invasive tumors with a median latency of 120 days (Reddy et al. 2010). Similar to the methods above, the fourth mammary glands of FVB or Balb/C mice are intraductally injected with lentiviruses that express constitutively activated rat *Neu* (*Lenti-ca-Erbb2*). Similar to the method described above, when combined with Cre recombinase (Lenti-ca-Erbb2-P2A-Cre) one will be able to examine the role of specific gene KO in progression of ADH to DCIS to IDC.

TNBC models Both *TP53* and *PTEN* are often inactivated in TNBC. Dr. Yi Li's group has shown that mammary glands with both *Tp53* and *Pten* deleted from TNBC invasive tumors in a median 5 months (Martinez et al. 2022). To generate *Pten*$^{f/f}$/*Tp53*$^{f/f}$ mice, a lenti-Cre lentivirus is injected into the fourth mammary gland of transgenic mice with both *Tp53* and *Pten* flanked by LoxP sites. Similarly, to test the impact of a gene of interest on precancer progression, a transgenic mouse model carrying *Pten/Tp53 and a gene of interest* flanked by LoxP sites may be generated followed by intraductal injection of Lenti-Cre to simultaneously delete *Pten*, Tp53 and the gene of interest in the mammary ductal epithelial cells. This will allow one to examine the role of a gene of interest in the progression of ADH to DCIS to IDC in a TNBC model.

6.5 Conclusion

The annual diagnosis of DCIS continues to uptick because of the widespread adoption of screening mammography. Despite the ever-increasing number of diagnoses per year, statistics do not seem to see the expected correlation of increased mortality. This data has forced researchers to stop and address the question: Are we overdiagnosing and overtreating DCIS? The natural progression of DCIS into IDC and identification of factors that contribute to that progression must first be understood before addressing this question. Numerous models, both *in vitro* and *in vivo,* have been developed to better understand this topic. From these studies, key information has been gleaned. Progression from DCIS into IDC is multifactorial; the microenvironment carcinoma cells and their cross-talks have all been identified as contributing factors and may serve as predictive biomarkers associated with progression. While all of these models have their limitations, they serve as a foundation yielding essential knowledge to a better understanding of this disease and how we as a community of researchers can best support our patients with DCIS diagnoses.

References

Ang DC, Warrick AL, Shilling A, Beadling C, Corless CL, Troxell ML (2014) Frequent phosphatidylinositol-3-kinase mutations in proliferative breast lesions. Mod Pathol 27(5):740–750. https://doi.org/10.1038/modpathol.2013.197

Behbod F, Kittrell FS, LaMarca H, Edwards D, Kerbawy S, Heestand JC, Young E, Mukhopadhyay P, Yeh HW, Allred DC, Hu M, Polyak K, Rosen JM, Medina D (2009) An intraductal human-in-mouse transplantation model mimics the subtypes of ductal carcinoma in situ. Breast Cancer Res 11(5):R66. https://doi.org/10.1186/bcr2358

Behbod F, Gomes AM, Machado HL (2018) Modeling human ductal carcinoma in situ in the mouse. J Mammary Gland Biol Neoplasia 23(4):269–278. https://doi.org/10.1007/s10911-018-9408-0

Bischel LL, Lee SH, Beebe DJ (2012) A practical method for patterning lumens through ecm hydrogels via viscous finger patterning. J Lab Autom 17(2):96–103. https://doi.org/10.1177/2211068211426694

Bischel LL, Young EW, Mader BR, Beebe DJ (2013) Tubeless microfluidic angiogenesis assay with three-dimensional endothelial-lined microvessels. Biomaterials 34(5):1471–1477. https://doi.org/10.1016/j.biomaterials.2012.11.005

Bischel LL, Sung KE, Jimenez-Torres JA, Mader B, Keely PJ, Beebe DJ (2014) The importance of being a lumen. FASEB J 28(11):4583–4590. https://doi.org/10.1096/fj.13-243733

Bischel LL, Beebe DJ, Sung KE (2015) Microfluidic model of ductal carcinoma in situ with 3d, organotypic structure. BMC Cancer 15:12. https://doi.org/10.1186/s12885-015-1007-5

Bu W, Li Y (2020) Intraductal injection of lentivirus vectors for stably introducing genes into rat mammary epithelial cells in vivo. J Mammary Gland Biol Neoplasia 25(4):389–396. https://doi.org/10.1007/s10911-020-09469-w

Choi Y, Hyun E, Seo J, Blundell C, Kim HC, Lee E, Lee SH, Moon A, Moon WK, Huh D (2015) A microengineered pathophysiological model of early-stage breast cancer. Lab Chip 15(16):3350–3357. https://doi.org/10.1039/c5lc00514k

Dai X, Ma C, Lan Q, Xu T (2016) 3d bioprinted glioma stem cells for brain tumor model and applications of drug susceptibility. Biofabrication 8(4):045005. https://doi.org/10.1088/1758-5090/8/4/045005

Du Z, Podsypanina K, Huang S, McGrath A, Toneff MJ, Bogoslovskaia E, Zhang X, Moraes RC, Fluck M, Allred DC, Lewis MT, Varmus HE, Li Y (2006) Introduction of oncogenes into mammary glands in vivo with an avian retroviral vector initiates and promotes carcinogenesis in mouse models. Proc Natl Acad Sci USA 103(46):17396–17401. https://doi.org/10.1073/pnas.0608607103

Duchamp M, Liu T, van Genderen AM, Kappings V, Oklu R, Ellisen LW, Zhang YS (2019) Sacrificial bioprinting of a mammary ductal carcinoma model. Biotechnol J 14(10):e1700703. https://doi.org/10.1002/biot.201700703

Espina V, Liotta LA (2011) What is the malignant nature of human ductal carcinoma in situ? Nat Rev Cancer 11(1):68–75. https://doi.org/10.1038/nrc2950

Espina V, Mariani BD, Gallagher RI, Tran K, Banks S, Wiedemann J, Huryk H, Mueller C, Adamo L, Deng J, Petricoin EF, Pastore L, Zaman S, Menezes G, Mize J, Johal J, Edmiston K, Liotta LA (2010) Malignant precursor cells pre-exist in human breast dcis and require autophagy for survival. PLoS One 5(4):e10240. https://doi.org/10.1371/journal.pone.0010240

Haricharan S, Dong J, Hein S, Reddy JP, Du Z, Toneff M, Holloway K, Hilsenbeck SG, Huang S, Atkinson R, Woodward W, Jindal S, Borges VF, Gutierrez C, Zhang H, Schedin PJ, Osborne CK, Tweardy DJ, Li Y (2013) Mechanism and preclinical prevention of increased breast cancer risk caused by pregnancy. elife 2:e00996. https://doi.org/10.7554/eLife.00996

Hong Y, Limback D, Elsarraj HS, Harper H, Haines H, Hansford H, Ricci M, Kaufman C, Wedlock E, Xu M, Zhang J, May L, Cusick T, Inciardi M, Redick M, Gatewood J, Winblad O, Aripoli A, Huppe A, Balanoff C, Wagner JL, Amin AL, Larson KE, Ricci L, Tawfik O, Razek H, Meierotto RO, Madan R, Godwin AK, Thompson J, Hilsenbeck SG, Futreal A, Thompson A, Hwang ES, Fan F, Behbod F, Grand Challenge PC (2022) Mouse-intraductal (mind): an in vivo model for studying the underlying mechanisms of dcis malignancy. J Pathol 256(2):186–201. https://doi.org/10.1002/path.5820

Hutten SJ, de Bruijn R, Lutz C, Badoux M, Eijkman T, Chao X, Ciwinska M, Sheinman M, Messal H, Herencia-Ropero A, Kristel P, Mulder L, van der Waal R, Sanders J, Almekinders MM, Llop-Guevara A, Davies HR, van Haren MJ, Martin NI, Behbod F, Nik-Zainal S, Serra V, van Rheenen J, Lips EH, Wessels LFA, Grand Challenge PC, Wesseling J, Scheele C, Jonkers J (2023) A living biobank of patient-derived ductal carcinoma in situ mouse-intraductal xenografts identifies risk factors for invasive progression. Cancer Cell 41(5):986–1002 e1009. https://doi.org/10.1016/j.ccell.2023.04.002

Jedeszko C, Victor BC, Podgorski I, Sloane BF (2009) Fibroblast hepatocyte growth factor promotes invasion of human mammary ductal carcinoma in situ. Cancer Res 69(23):9148–9155. https://doi.org/10.1158/0008-5472.CAN-09-1043

Kittrell F, Valdez K, Elsarraj H, Hong Y, Medina D, Behbod F (2016) Mouse mammary intraductal (mind) method for transplantation of patient derived primary dcis cells and cell lines. Bio Protoc 6(5)

Ma Y, Lin M, Huang G, Li Y, Wang S, Bai G, Lu TJ, Xu F (2018) 3d spatiotemporal mechanical microenvironment: A hydrogel-based platform for guiding stem cell fate. Adv Mater 30(49):e1705911. https://doi.org/10.1002/adma.201705911

Martinez JD, Mo Q, Xu Y, Qin L, Li Y, Xu J (2022) Common genomic aberrations in mouse and human breast cancers with concurrent p53 deficiency and activated pten-pi3k-akt pathway. Int J Biol Sci 18(1):229–241. https://doi.org/10.7150/ijbs.65763

Meng F, Meyer CM, Joung D, Vallera DA, McAlpine MC, Panoskaltsis-Mortari A (2019) 3d bioprinted in vitro metastatic models via reconstruction of tumor microenvironments. Adv Mater 31(10):e1806899. https://doi.org/10.1002/adma.201806899

Nelson CM, Bissell MJ (2006) Of extracellular matrix, scaffolds, and signaling: Tissue architecture regulates development, homeostasis, and cancer. Annu Rev Cell Dev Biol 22:287–309. https://doi.org/10.1146/annurev.cellbio.22.010305.104315

Osuala KO, Sameni M, Shah S, Aggarwal N, Simonait ML, Franco OE, Hong Y, Hayward SW, Behbod F, Mattingly RR, Sloane BF (2015) Il-6 signaling between ductal carcinoma in situ cells and carcinoma-associated fibroblasts mediates tumor cell growth and migration. BMC Cancer 15:584. https://doi.org/10.1186/s12885-015-1576-3

Ozanne EM, Shieh Y, Barnes J, Bouzan C, Hwang ES, Esserman LJ (2011) Characterizing the impact of 25 years of dcis treatment. Breast Cancer Res Treat 129(1):165–173. https://doi.org/10.1007/s10549-011-1430-5

Reddy JP, Peddibhotla S, Bu W, Zhao J, Haricharan S, Du YC, Podsypanina K, Rosen JM, Donehower LA, Li Y (2010) Defining the atm-mediated barrier to tumorigenesis in somatic mammary cells following erbb2 activation. Proc Natl Acad Sci USA 107(8):3728–3733. https://doi.org/10.1073/pnas.0910665107

Sameni M, Anbalagan A, Olive MB, Moin K, Mattingly RR, Sloane BF (2012) Mame models for 4d live-cell imaging of tumor: Microenvironment interactions that impact malignant progression. J Vis Exp(60). https://doi.org/10.3791/3661

Sameni M, Cavallo-Medved D, Franco OE, Chalasani A, Ji K, Aggarwal N, Anbalagan A, Chen X, Mattingly RR, Hayward SW, Sloane BF (2017) Pathomimetic avatars reveal divergent roles of microenvironment in invasive transition of ductal carcinoma in situ. Breast Cancer Res 19(1):56. https://doi.org/10.1186/s13058-017-0847-0

Ted, A.C.S.D.A.R.A.M.A.P.B.N.D.B.A.B.E.C.M.F.-B.M.F.N.F., 2023. *Cancer facts and figures 2023*. Available from chrome-extension://efaidnbmnnnibpcajpcglclefindmkaj/https://www.cancer.org/content/dam/cancer-org/research/cancer-facts-and-statistics/annual-cancer-facts-and-figures/2023/2023-cancer-facts-and-figures.pdf

Valdez KE, Fan F, Smith W, Allred DC, Medina D, Behbod F (2011) Human primary ductal carcinoma in situ (dcis) subtype-specific pathology is preserved in a mouse intraductal (mind) xenograft model. J Pathol 225(4):565–573. https://doi.org/10.1002/path.2969

van Seijen M, Lips EH, Thompson AM, Nik-Zainal S, Futreal A, Hwang ES, Verschuur E, Lane J, Jonkers J, Rea DW, Wesseling J, P. team (2019) Ductal carcinoma in situ: To treat or not to treat, that is the question. Br J Cancer 121(4):285–292. https://doi.org/10.1038/s41416-019-0478-6

Verbridge SS, Chakrabarti A, DelNero P, Kwee B, Varner JD, Stroock AD, Fischbach C (2013) Physicochemical regulation of endothelial sprouting in a 3d microfluidic angiogenesis model. J Biomed Mater Res A 101(10):2948–2956. https://doi.org/10.1002/jbm.a.34587

Villanueva H, Grimm SL, Dhamne S, Rajapakshe K, Visbal AP, Davis CM, Ehli EA, Hartig SM, Coarfa C, Edwards DP (2019) Correction to: The emerging roles of steroid hormone receptors in ductal carcinoma in situ (dcis) of the breast. J Mammary Gland Biol Neoplasia 24(1):109–110. https://doi.org/10.1007/s10911-018-9421-3

Welch HG, Black WC (1997) Using autopsy series to estimate the disease “reservoir” for ductal carcinoma in situ of the breast: How much more breast cancer can we find? Ann Intern Med 127(11):1023–1028

Young A, Bu W, Jiang W, Ku A, Kapali J, Dhamne S, Qin L, Hilsenbeck SG, Du YN, Li Y (2022) Targeting the pro-survival protein bcl-2 to prevent breast cancer. Cancer Prev Res (Phila) 15(1):3–10. https://doi.org/10.1158/1940-6207.CAPR-21-0031

Zhao YG, Xiao AZ, Park HI, Newcomer RG, Yan M, Man YG, Heffelfinger SC, Sang QX (2004) Endometase/matrilysin-2 in human breast ductal carcinoma in situ and its inhibition by tissue inhibitors of metalloproteinases-2 and -4: A putative role in the initiation of breast cancer invasion. Cancer Res 64(2):590–598. https://doi.org/10.1158/0008-5472.can-03-1932

Zhao Y, Yao R, Ouyang L, Ding H, Zhang T, Zhang K, Cheng S, Sun W (2014) Three-dimensional printing of hela cells for cervical tumor model in vitro. Biofabrication 6(3):035001. https://doi.org/10.1088/1758-5082/6/3/035001

7 Patient-Derived Xenografts of Breast Cancer

Elisabetta Marangoni

Abstract

Patient-derived xenografts (PDX) of breast cancer, obtained from the engraftment of tumour samples into immunodeficient mice, are the most effective preclinical models for studying the biology of human breast cancer and for the evaluation of new anti-cancer treatments. Notably, breast cancer PDX preserve the phenotypic and molecular characteristics of the donor tumours and reproduce the diversity of breast cancer. This preservation of breast cancer biology involves a number of different aspects, including tumour architecture and morphology, patterns of genomic alterations and gene expression, mutational status, and intra-tumour heterogeneity. For these reasons, these models have a strong predictive value in the translation of cancer therapeutics into clinical settings and can be considered as powerful and clinically relevant research tools for the identification of new treatments, mechanisms of drug resistance, and predictive biomarkers. PDX models have also been successfully used to analyse breast cancer metastasis and persister cancer cells surviving chemotherapy. Limitations of breast cancer PDX include the lack of a human immune system and the low take rate, especially for estrogen receptor (ER) and HER2-positive subtypes.

Keywords

PDX · Breast cancer · Drug response · Predictive biomarker · Drug resistance

Key Points

- PDX models are obtained from the engraftment of patients' tumour fragments directly in immunodeficient mice. These models maintain the histological and molecular features of the donor tumours with high fidelity.
- PDX models have been used to analyse mechanisms driving treatment resistance and to identify new therapeutic targets and predictive biomarkers of treatment response and resistance.
- PDX models of ductal carcinoma in situ (DCIS) and rare subtypes of breast cancers have been developed, allowing the identification of biomarkers for DCIS progression and therapeutic targets for rare histological types of breast cancers.
- The main limitations of breast cancer PDX models are the lack of a human tumour microenvironment, the low take rate, and differences in drug metabolism.

E. Marangoni (✉)
Laboratory of Preclinical Investigation, Translational Research Department, Institut Curie, Paris, France
e-mail: elisabetta.marangoni@curie.fr

T. Sørlie, R. B. Clarke (eds.), *A Guide to Breast Cancer Research*, Advances in Experimental Medicine and Biology 1464, https://doi.org/10.1007/978-3-031-70875-6_7

7.1 Introduction

In the last 70 years, different kinds of preclinical models of cancer have been developed to study the biological behaviour of cancer *in vivo* and to identify new drugs against cancer. Until the beginning of 2000, cell line-derived xenografts models (CDX), obtained from the injection of cancer cell lines cultured *in vitro* in artificial conditions, were the most used preclinical models of cancer. These models are genetically well defined and easy to manipulate; however, they are poorly predictive of treatment response in the clinics due to the genetic and epigenetic alterations accumulated in cell culture and fail to recapitulate both the inter-tumour and intra-tumour heterogeneity of human cancers. These limitations have restricted the use of CDX models for preclinical evaluation of efficacy of anti-cancer drugs (Gillet et al. 2011, 2013). To circumvent these limitations, patient-derived xenografts (PDX) models, obtained from the engraftment of patients' tumour fragments, have been developed. In this chapter, we will address the main characteristics and applications of PDX models in breast cancer research and will discuss their advantages and limitations.

7.2 Historical Considerations and Phenotypic Fidelity of PDX

Even if the PDX models of breast cancer (BC) have been extensively developed in the early 2000s, it should be highlighted that the first serial growth of human tumours in immunodeficient mice was described in 1969 (Rygaard and Povlsen 1969) and the first large series of BC PDX was reported 10 years later (Bailey et al. 1980, 1981). The preservation of histopathological characteristics, chromosome number, and tumour-marker production as well as the low tumour take, a characteristic of BC PDX, were already described in these pioneer manuscripts. Since then, several studies have reported the establishment of different collections of BC PDX. A review was published in 2016 by a consortium of academic institutions developing PDX models of BC, with more than 500 models identified across different countries (Dobrolecki et al. 2016). Success rates of generating stable transplantable PDX models of BC are typically low (around 20%), although variations exist among the different studies. Triple-negative breast cancer (TNBC) have typically a higher take rate as compared to ER-positive and HER2-positive BC (Dobrolecki et al. 2016). Other biological and clinical factors that have been shown to influence the take rate are the tumour stage, the origin of the sample (primary breast tumour or metastatic lesion), and the histological subtype of BC (lobular BCs are more difficult to establish than ductal carcinomas). Interestingly, different groups showed that tumour engraftment is a prognostic indicator of disease outcome for women with newly diagnosed BC (DeRose et al. 2011; du Manoir et al. 2014).

Different immunocompromised mouse models have been used to generate BC PDX, including athymic nude mice, SCID mice, and NSG mice. A detailed description of these strains is described elsewhere (Dobrolecki et al. 2016).

The phenotype and the molecular profile of PDX models and matched patents' tumours have been compared in several studies. Comparative analyses have demonstrated that PDX models are almost indistinguishable from the corresponding patients' tumours, both at the morphological and immunohistochemistry levels (Marangoni et al. 2007; Cottu et al. 2012; DeRose et al. 2013; Kabos et al. 2012; Zhang et al. 2013; Li et al. 2013; Bruna et al. 2016). Concordance between PDX and matched patients' tumour samples was also found at the gene expression level (Reyal et al. 2012; Zhang et al. 2013; DeRose et al. 2013) and at the genomic level, by analysis of copy number alterations (CNA) and mutational profiles (Bergamaschi et al. 2009; Reyal et al. 2012; Zhang et al. 2013; DeRose et al. 2013; Bruna et al. 2016; Li et al. 2013; du Manoir et al. 2014; Savage et al. 2020). Analysis of large series of matched patients' primary tumours and PDX of BC showed strong CNA conservation from primary tumours through early and late-passage PDX (Woo et al. 2021; Bruna et al. 2016). Moreover, only a small fraction of sample pairs showed large CNA discordance, suggesting that clonal selection out of a genomically heterogeneous population is rare. These results indicate that the variations observed in PDX are mainly due to spontaneous intratumoral evolution, rather than murine pressures. At the mutational level, Li et al. found a good correlation of the variant allele frequencies between primary tumours and PDX and identified some unique mutations in the PDX models, but most of them were in genes not expressed (Li et al. 2013). Moreover, in BC PDX comparative allelic frequencies of cancer-associated genes are typically maintained (Zhang et al. 2013; Coussy et al. 2019; Bruna et al. 2016; Gao et al. 2015).

7.3 Prediction of Treatment Response

The failure to translate promising preclinical candidates into clinical advances can be partially explained by the inability of CDX models to accurately predict anticancer activity in clinical trials. As mentioned above, CDX models fail to represent both the intra- and inter-tumour heterogeneity of human cancers, mainly because of the pronounced differences in molecular profiles between cell lines and patients' tumour samples of the same pathology (Honkala et al. 2022; Domcke et al. 2013; Jiang et al. 2016). The diversity across tumour types and the limitations of cell lines to fully capture key aspects of tumour biology led to the development of PDX as preclinical models that can reliably reflect prognostic and treatment outcomes of cancer patients. For breast cancer, two retrospective studies demonstrated that the treatment responses of PDX models are concordant with the responses of the corresponding patients (Marangoni et al. 2007; Zhang et al. 2013). PDX models were also generated from tumour biopsies and surgical samples in the prospective study BEAUTY, where women with high-risk primary breast cancers were treated with neo-adjuvant chemotherapy. Eight PDX models derived from biopsy samples (prior to neoadjuvant chemotherapy) were assessed for *in vivo* paclitaxel response and a complete concordance with patients' response was found (Yu et al. 2017).

Furthermore, a large study screened PDX established for 92 patients with various solid tumours, including ten patients with BC, against the same treatments that were administered clinically and correlated patient outcomes with the responses in corresponding models. This analysis demonstrated that PDXs accurately replicated patients' clinical outcomes, with very high positive and negative predictive values, even when patients received several additional cycles of therapy over time (Izumchenko et al. 2017). Finally, response rates to standard chemotherapies used in BC treatment such as anthracyclines, taxanes, capecitabine, and platinum salts are similar in PDX cohorts and clinical trials (Marangoni et al. 2018; Ter Brugge et al. 2016; Marangoni et al. 2007).

7.4 PDX Models of Ductal Carcinoma In Situ (DCIS) and Rare Forms of Breast Cancer

The progression of DCIS into invasive breast carcinoma is still poorly understood and consensus biomarkers for DCIS progression are lacking, prompting the need for preclinical *in vivo* models that allow longitudinal monitoring of DCIS progression. Development of a PDX model of DCIS was first reported in 1975 by Outzen and Custer who successfully transplanted a dysplastic breast lesion in nude mice (Outzen and Custer 1975). PDX models of DCIS were also reported later by Warnberg et al. who used them to test the *in vivo* effects of a farnesyl transferase inhibitor (Wärnberg et al. 2006).

Hong et al. developed an *in vivo* model, Mouse-INtraDuctal (MIND), in which patient-derived DCIS epithelial cells are injected intraductally and allowed to progress naturally in mice. Similar to human DCIS, the cancer cells formed in situ lesions inside the mouse mammary ducts and mimicked all histologic subtypes (Hong et al. 2022). More recently, Hutten et al. utilised the same injection technique to generate a deeply characterised biobank of 115 PDX models of DCIS (Hutten et al. 2023). Authors identified different factors correlated with high-risk, including HER2 and MYC amplification, high

CNA burden, solid growth pattern, grade 3, high Ki67 level, and distinct 3D growth pattern, whereas a luminal A subtype or columnar growth correlated with low-risk DCIS.

Rare cancers are insufficiently represented in clinical trials. Treatment decisions depend on data extrapolated from related common cancers, which may differ from the rare cancer in question, resulting in failure of the therapy regimens received by the patient. Basket trials (where many tumour types carrying the same molecular aberration are grouped together) have been proposed as one of the alternatives to standard clinical trials. Indeed, rare cancers are thought to arise owing to an initial genetic driver mutation, without the need for as many concurrent mutations as in more common cancers (Barker and Scott 2019).

PDX models are ideal for studying the tumour biology of rare cancers and evaluating drug response, where no other *in vivo* models are likely to exist. For example, a unique PDX model of malignant adenomyoepithelioma of the breast, an extremely rare form of BC with a high frequency of HRAS mutations, allowed to demonstrate significant anti-tumour activity of a MEK inhibitor (Bieche et al. 2021). The same group established different PDX models of metaplastic breast cancer, a rare and heterogeneous group of breast cancers characterised by differentiation of the neoplastic epithelium into squamous and/or mesenchymal elements, including spindle, chondroid, osseous, and rhabdomyoid cells (Coussy et al. 2020a). These tumours are typically enriched for PIK3CA mutations and/or copy number alterations of genes in the RTK-MAPK pathway. A combination of PI3K and MEK inhibitors was found to be highly effective in these PDX.

7.5 Clonal Evolution and Intra-Tumour Heterogeneity in PDX Models

Breast cancers, like other cancers, include multiple clones evolving dynamically in space and time (Aparicio and Caldas 2013). PDX models of BC have emerged as powerful preclinical models able to reproduce intra-tumour heterogeneity (Cassidy et al. 2015). Using single-cell sequencing of BC PDX analysed at different passages, Eirew et al. showed that clonal selection occurs at varying degrees at the first engraftment and through serial propagation of PDX. They showed that similar clonal expansion patterns can emerge in independent grafts of the same patient's tumour, indicating that genomic aberrations can be reproducible determinants of evolutionary trajectories (Eirew et al. 2015). In a different study, Ding et al. found that the mutational profile of a TNBC PDX was closer to the patient's brain metastasis than the primary tumour from which it was derived, suggesting similar evolutionary pressures during progression to metastasis and establishment of a xenograft (Ding et al. 2010). Li et al. analysed by whole genome sequencing a set of 17 matched patients' tumours and PDX showing that for many mutations the variant allele frequencies (VAF) were preserved in the PDX, even in the case of rare mutations (Li et al. 2013). This implies that the original clonal representation can be transplantable, and that the different clones maintain their relative prevalence in equilibrium.

PDX models of HER2-positive BC have been used to explore the role of intra-tumour heterogeneity on the response to different HER2-targeting treatments. Stromal determinants were found to be better predictors of response than tumour epithelial cells, and the authors identified alveolar epithelial and fibroblastic reticular cells as well as lymphatic vessel endothelial hyaluronan receptor 1–positive (Lyve1+) macrophages as putative drivers of therapeutic resistance to HER2-targeting agents (Janiszewska et al. 2021).

7.6 Applications of PDX Models

The potential applications of PDX models are vast and include the preclinical evaluation of new treatments including toxicity, efficacy, and pharmacodynamics studies, the identification of novel combinations of therapy, and optimal treatment schedules. Possible applications also include the molecular analysis of tumour response, the identification of biomarkers indicating drug responder or non-responder, and mechanisms of drug resistance.

7.7 Mechanisms and Driver of Treatment Response and Resistance

PDX models of BC have been used to identify mechanisms of treatment resistance. By the genetic analysis of PDX models established from liver metastases of patients treated by aromatase inhibitors, Li et al. identified alterations of the ER gene (mutations and translocations) that confer resistance to aromatase inhibitors (Li et al. 2013). In another study, PDX models of TNBC were used to identify mechanisms of resistance to DNA-damaging drugs and poly(ADP-ribose) polymerase (PARP) inhibitors. In BRCA1 methylated tumours that re-expressed BRCA1, authors found de novo gene fusions that placed BRCA1 under the transcriptional control of a heterologous promoter, resulting in re-expression of BRCA1 and acquisition of therapy resistance (Ter Brugge et al. 2016). More recently, PDX of TNBC were used to demonstrate that incomplete methylation of BRCA1 is associated with residual BRCA1 gene expression, restoration of a functional homologous recombination repair, and resistance to cisplatin (Menghi et al. 2022; Ter Brugge et al. 2023). Finally, by integrating chromatin conformation capture, RNA-seq, and whole-genome sequencing obtained in a carboplatin-resistant TNBC PDX, Dozmorov et al. highlighted the role of long noncoding RNAs and amplification of ABC transporters and prioritise mitochondrial metabolism and oxidative phosphorylation pathways as the possible mechanisms of carboplatin resistance (Dozmorov et al. 2023).

7.8 Modelling Residual Disease with PDX Models

Tumour recurrence is frequent and associated with poor survival in TNBC patients showing residual disease after neo-adjuvant chemotherapy (NAC). PDX models have been successively employed to model residual disease and tumour recurrence in TNBC. Echeverria et al. used PDX models of TNBC to isolate and analyse residual tumours remaining after treatment with standard chemotherapies and found that chemotherapy resistance can be mediated by a reversible chemotherapy-tolerant state. Gene expression signatures of the residual tumours identified mitochondrial oxidative phosphorylation as a potential dependency in residual tumours, and inhibition of oxidative phosphorylation delayed tumour regrowth in the models (Echeverria et al. 2019). PDX models established from residual tumours in patients treated by NAC have been reported by different groups. Marangoni et al. established a panel of residual disease-derived PDX with cross-resistance to anthracyclines, taxanes, and platins. These models responded to the anti-metabolite capecitabine and predictive biomarkers were identified by transcriptomic and immunohistological analysis in a cohort of 32 TNBC PDX (Marangoni et al. 2018). Yu et al. established PDX models both sensitive and resistant to standard NAC by engrafting pre-chemotherapy biopsies and post-chemotherapy surgical samples. These models exhibited similar biological and drug response characteristics as the patients' primary tumours (Yu et al. 2017).

7.9 PDX for Studies on Stem-Cell and Metastasis

PDX models of BC have also been used to analyse cancer stem cells (CSC) and tumour-initiating cells. Charafe-Jauffret et al. reported that the successful engraftment of BC PDX was correlated with the presence of ALDH1-positive CSCs, which predicted prognosis in patients. The xenografts developed showed a hierarchical cell organisation of BC with the ALDH1-positive CSCs constituting the tumorigenic cell population (Charafe-Jauffret et al. 2013). Analysis of gene expression from those CSCs identified a transcriptional program of 19 genes shared with murine embryonic, hematopoietic, and neural stem cells. In another study, combined FAK and paclitaxel treatment reduced tumour size, Ki67, ex-vivo mammospheres, and ALDH+ expression in PDX models of TNBC (Timbrell et al. 2021). Singh et al. investigated the role of IL-8 in the regulation of CSC activity using PDX and determined the potential benefit of combining CXCR1/2 inhibition with HER2-targeted therapies (Singh et al. 2013). The same group showed that short-term treatment with the anti-estrogens tamoxifen or fulvestrant decreased cell proliferation but increased stem cell activity through JAG1-NOTCH4 receptor activation both in patient-derived samples and PDX of ER-positive BC (Simoes et al. 2015). They also highlighted the importance of STAT3 signalling in CSC-mediated resistance to endocrine therapy and the potential of SFX-01, a stabilised formulation of sulforaphane, for its effects on breast CSC activity that were demonstrated in ER+ PDX (Simoes et al. 2020).

Breast cancer PDX models have also been employed to explore mechanisms and dynamics governing the metastatic dissemination. Using single-cell RNA sequencing of metastatic PDX models, Davis et al. identified a distinct transcriptomic program in micrometastases with oxidative phosphorylation among the top enriched pathways (Davis et al. 2020). Pharmacological inhibition of oxidative phosphorylation attenuated metastatic seeding in the lungs, which demonstrates the functional importance of oxidative phosphorylation in metastasis. Another interesting study addressed the question of clonal dynamics during metastasis using a PDX model established from a metastatic TNBC. Genomic sequencing of the PDX model revealed alterations in the clonal architecture between the primary tumour and the different metastases in the mice. Lung, liver, and brain metastases were enriched for an identical population of high-abundance subclones, demonstrating that primary tumour clones harbor properties enabling them to seed and thrive in multiple organ sites. However, the RNA sequencing revealed that, while the activation status of some pathways was concordant between liver and lung metastases (such as downregulation of EMT, TGF-β signalling, and hypoxia in metastases compared to the primary tumour), some pathways were differentially regulated in the two sites (e.g. cholesterol homeostasis). These results demonstrate that while the clonal and genomic origins of metastases in distinct organs are similar, gene expression programs can be more variable, likely due to the diverse organ microenvironments (Echeverria et al. 2018).

PDX models established from biopsies of BC metastases have been reported by different groups. One example is illustrated in the work of Montaudon et al. who established different PDX from the engraftment of bone metastases biopsies from patients progressing on endocrine treatments and CDK4/6 inhibitors (Montaudon et al. 2020). Transcriptomic analyses reveal enrichment of the G2/M checkpoint and up-regulation of Polo-like kinase 1 (PLK1) in the bone metastases-derived PDX. PLK1 inhibition resulted in tumour shrinkage in CCND1-driven PDX, including different RB-positive PDX with acquired palbociclib resistance (Montaudon et al. 2020).

The lack of clinically relevant models for studying breast cancer metastasis to a human bone microenvironment has stunted the development of effective treatments for this condition. To address this problem, Lefley et al. have developed humanised mouse models with bone implants in which BC PDXs were found to metastasise to the human bone. Breast cancer cells underwent expression changes of IL-1B, IL-1R1, S100A4, CTSK, SPP1, and RANK as they progressed from primary tumours to bone metastasis and inhibiting IL-1B signalling significantly reduced bone metastasis (Lefley et al. 2019).

Another interesting study was published recently by Kabraji and colleagues, who presented the results of a hybrid study with preclinical and clinical evaluation of the activity of trastuzumab deruxtecan (T-DXd) on brain metastases from advanced HER2-positive BC (Kabraji et al. 2023). T-DXd inhibited tumour growth and prolonged survival in orthotopic PDX models of HER2-positive (IHC 3+) and HER2-low (IHC 2+/FISH ratio < 2) BC brain metastases and this was confirmed in a T-DM1–resistant model (Kabraji et al. 2023).

7.10 Identification of Predictive Biomarkers and New Therapeutic Targets

Gene-expression profiling and other genome-wide high-throughput technologies have advanced our understanding of cancer biology, enabling the discovery of biomarkers for the prediction of tumour response to treatment using PDX models (Tentler et al. 2012; Byrne et al. 2017).

Large cohorts of TNBC PDX have been used in "xenotrial" to identify predictive markers of chemotherapy response. In a panel of 55 PDX models, Ter Brugge et al. demonstrate that the HRD status, determined from shallow whole genome sequencing, predicted response to platinum drugs (Ter Brugge et al. 2023). This genomic characterisation of tumours allowed the identification of gene alterations such as ORC1 mutations and XRCC3 deletions that were driving cisplatin response in 2 PDX models. In another study, the same group tested the activity of a TOP1 inhibitor, irinotecan, in 40 PDX of TNBC. The HRD status, determined from a genomic signature, combined with high SLFN11 expression and RB1 loss identified highly sensitive tumours, consistent with the notion that deficiencies in cell cycle checkpoints and DNA repair result in high sensitivity to TOP1 inhibitors. Treatment with the ATR inhibitor VE-822 increased sensitivity to irinotecan in SLFN11-negative PDXs and abolished irinotecan-induced phosphorylation of checkpoint kinase 1 (CHK1) (Coussy et al. 2020b). PDX models of BC have also been used to identify RAD51 foci as marker of PARP inhibitors response in BRCA-mutated and non-mutated BC (Castroviejo-Bermejo et al. 2018; Cruz et al. 2018). The same authors also used PDX models of ER-positive BC to identify high p16 expression and heterozygous RB1 loss as biomarkers for CDK4/6 inhibitor resistance (Palafox et al. 2022). Using both patients' samples and PDX models, Ciscar et al. showed that RANK is a poor prognosis factor and a therapeutic target in ER-negative postmenopausal BC (Ciscar et al. 2023). In ER- breast PDX, RANKL inhibition reduced tumour cell proliferation and stemness, regulated tumour immunity and metabolism, and improved response to chemotherapy.

7.11 Epigenetic and Metabolism

Metabolism and epigenetic reprogramming are two fundamental hallmarks of cancer connected to each other whose importance was not recognised until recently. In some cases, reprogrammed metabolic activities can be exploited to diagnose, monitor, and treat cancer.

Metabolic dysregulation and reprogramming are prominent features in cancer, but they remain poorly characterised in patients' derived BC samples. In a recent study, untargeted metabolomics analysis of patients' tumours and PDX models revealed two major metabolic groups independent of BC histologic subtypes: a "Nucleotide/Carbohydrate-Enriched" group and a "Lipid/Fatty Acid-Enriched" group. Targeting the Nucleotide/Carbohydrate-Enriched PDX with a pyrimidine biosynthesis inhibitor or a glutaminase inhibitor led to therapeutic efficacy (Liao et al. 2022). In another study, concentrations of choline-derived metabolites were measured in PDX established from basal-like and luminal-like BC subtypes (Moestue et al. 2010, 2013). Differences in choline metabolite concentrations observed between these two models in mice correlated well with similar profiles and gene-expression patterns observed in material from patients with ER-positive and PR-positive BC, and triple-negative breast cancer, suggesting that these PDX xenografts are relevant models for studying choline metabolism in these subtypes.

Finally, El Botty et al. performed a global metabolomics analysis of patients' tumours and bone metastasis-derived PDX of patients progressing on endocrine treatments and CDK4/6 inhibitors. They could demonstrate that a fraction of metastatic ER + BC is highly reliant on oxidative phosphorylation (OXPHOS). *In vivo* treatment with a OXPHOS inhibitor strongly inhibited PDX tumour growth and the response was associated with decreased levels of metabolites of the glutathione, glycogen and pentose phosphate pathways in treated tumours (El-Botty et al. 2023).

Recent cancer genome projects highlighted the role of epigenetic alterations in cancer development. Restrictive chromatin states may prevent appropriate induction of tumour suppressor programs or block differentiation. By contrast, permissive or "plastic" states may allow stochastic oncogene activation or non-physiologic cell fate transitions (Flavahan et al. 2017).

Using cell lines and PDX models of TNBC, Marsolier et al. investigated which epigenetic modifiers could regulate expression programs of persister or chemo-resistant cells (Marsolier et al. 2022). They showed that even prior to treatment, the epigenome is already a key player, with a priming of the persister program. By monitoring epigenomes, transcriptomes, and lineages with single-cell resolution, authors found that the repressive histone mark H3K27me3 regulates cell fate at the onset of chemotherapy and that a persister expression program is primed with both H3K4me3 and H3K27me3 in unchallenged cells, H3K27me3 being the lock to its transcriptional activation. They further demonstrated that preventing H3K27me3 demethylation simultaneously to chemotherapy inhibits the transition to a drug-tolerant state, and delays tumour recurrence in vivo (Marsolier et al. 2022).

Another elegant study analysed the phenotypic plasticity in BC endocrine resistance. By using matched culture models and PDX models of endocrine-resistant and sensitive BC, authors showed that changes in transcription factors and enhancer interactions can reorganise the landscape of ERα-bound enhancers, resulting in gene program transitions that promote plasticity and endocrine therapy resistance (Bi et al. 2020).

7.12 Limitations of Breast Cancer PDX Models

PDX models also have different limitations. One of the major limitations is that the human tumour microenvironment (TME) is lost and partially replaced by a murine TME, lacking different components of the immune system, depending on the mice strains. NGS mice lack B and T lymphocytes and NK cells, while nude mice lack only T lymphocytes. For that reason, PDX models cannot be used to test treatments that target the immune system, such as immune checkpoint inhibitors, nor to address the role of the immune system in the response to standard treatments. To overcome this limitation, various strategies have been developed to humanise mice through the engraftment of peripheral blood stem cells or human bone marrow cells. However, some challenges and limitations remain regarding the translational value of these humanised mice, such as HLA class I and II incompatibilities between PDX and human hematopoietic stem and progenitor cells, and the expensive and time-consuming generation of humanised PDX models (Chen et al. 2023).

Other limitations of PDX models include differences in drug metabolism between humans and mice, which result in differences in drug metabolite levels and activities (Martignoni et al. 2006).

Finally, the low take rate, especially for ER-positive and early stage breast cancers, together with the slow growth and long latency period (several months), are other well-known limitations of breast cancer PDX.

7.13 Conclusions

In conclusion, PDX models of BC represent powerful and reliable preclinical models that reproduce with high fidelity the biology of the donor breast tumours. They represent both the inter-tumour and intra-tumour heterogeneity of breast cancers. They can be used to identify mechanisms of drug resistance, test new anti-cancer treatments, identify predictive biomarkers, and model key aspects of cancer progression such as metastasis and tumour recurrence. The lack of immune cells and other stromal components represents the major limitation of PDX models.

References

Aparicio S, Caldas C (2013) The implications of clonal genome evolution for cancer medicine. N Engl J Med 368:842–851

Bailey MJ, Gazet JC, Peckham MJ (1980) Human breast-cancer xenografts in immune-suppressed mice. Br J Cancer 42:524–529

Bailey MJ, Ormerod MG, Imrie SF, Humphreys J, Roberts JD, Gazet JC, Neville AM (1981) Comparative functional histopathology of human breast carcinoma xenografts. Br J Cancer 43:125–134

Barker HE, Scott CL (2019) Preclinical rare cancer research to inform clinical trial design. Nat Rev Cancer 19:481–482

Bergamaschi A, Hjortland GO, Triulzi T, Sorlie T, Johnsen H, Ree AH, Russnes HG, Tronnes S, Maelandsmo GM, Fodstad O, Borresen-Dale AL, Engebraaten O (2009) Molecular profiling and characterization of luminal-like and basal-like in vivo breast cancer xenograft models. Mol Oncol 3:469–482

Bi M, Zhang Z, Jiang YZ, Xue P, Wang H, Lai Z, Fu X, De Angelis C, Gong Y, Gao Z, Ruan J, Jin VX, Marangoni E, Montaudon E, Glass CK, Li W, Huang TH, Shao ZM, Schiff R, Chen L, Liu Z (2020) Enhancer reprogramming driven by high-order assemblies of transcription factors promotes phenotypic plasticity and breast cancer endocrine resistance. Nat Cell Biol 22:701–715

Bieche I, Coussy F, El-Botty R, Vacher S, Chateau-Joubert S, Dahmani A, Montaudon E, Reyes C, Gentien D, Reyal F, Ricci F, Nicolas A, Marchio C, Vincent-Salomon A, Lae M, Marangoni E (2021) HRAS is a therapeutic target in malignant chemo-resistant adenomyoepithelioma of the breast. J Hematol Oncol 14:143

Bruna A, Rueda OM, Greenwood W, Batra AS, Callari M, Batra RN, Pogrebniak K, Sandoval J, Cassidy JW, Tufegdzic-Vidakovic A, Sammut S-J, Jones L, Provenzano E, Baird R, Eirew P, Hadfield J, Eldridge M, McLaren-Douglas A, Barthorpe A, Lightfoot H, O'Connor MJ, Gray J, Cortes J, Baselga J, Marangoni E, Welm AL, Aparicio S, Serra V, Garnett MJ, Caldas C (2016) A biobank of breast cancer explants with preserved intra-tumor heterogeneity to screen anticancer compounds. Cell

Byrne AT, Alferez DG, Amant F, Annibali D, Arribas J, Biankin AV, Bruna A, Budinska E, Caldas C, Chang DK, Clarke RB, Clevers H, Coukos G, Dangles-Marie V, Eckhardt SG, Gonzalez-Suarez E, Hermans E, Hidalgo M, Jarzabek MA, de Jong S, Jonkers J, Kemper K, Lanfrancone L, Maelandsmo GM, Marangoni E, Marine JC, Medico E, Norum JH, Palmer HG, Peeper DS, Pelicci PG, Piris-Gimenez A, Roman-Roman S, Rueda OM, Seoane J, Serra V, Soucek L, Vanhecke D, Villanueva A, Vinolo E, Bertotti A, Trusolino L (2017) Interrogating open issues in cancer precision medicine with patient-derived xenografts. Nat Rev Cancer

Cassidy JW, Caldas C, Bruna A (2015) Maintaining tumor heterogeneity in patient-derived tumor xenografts. Cancer Res 75:2963–2968

Castroviejo-Bermejo M, Cruz C, Llop-Guevara A, Gutiérrez-Enríquez S, Ducy M, Ibrahim YH, Gris-Oliver A, Pellegrino B, Bruna A, Guzmán M, Rodríguez O, Grueso J, Bonache S, Moles-Fernández A, Villacampa G, Viaplana C, Gómez P, Vidal M, Peg V, Serres-Créixams X, Dellaire G, Simard J, Nuciforo P, Rubio IT, Rodrigo D, Carl Barrett J, Caldas C, Baselga J, Saura C, Cortés J, Déas O, Jonkers J, Masson J-Y, Cairo S, Judde J-G, O'Connor MJ, Díez O, Balmaña J, Serra V (2018) A RAD51 assay feasible in routine tumor samples calls PARP inhibitor response beyond BRCA mutation. EMBO Mol Med

Charafe-Jauffret E, Ginestier C, Bertucci F, Cabaud O, Wicinski J, Finetti P, Josselin E, Adelaide J, Nguyen TT, Monville F, Jacquemier J, Thomassin-Piana J, Pinna G, Jalaguier A, Lambaudie E, Houvenaeghel G, Xerri L, Harel-Bellan A, Chaffanet M, Viens P, Birnbaum D (2013) ALDH1-positive cancer stem cells predict engraftment of primary breast tumors and are governed by a common stem cell program. Cancer Res 73:7290–7300

Chen A, Neuwirth I, Herndler-Brandstetter D (2023) Modeling the tumor microenvironment and cancer immunotherapy in next-generation humanized mice. *Cancers (Basel)* 15

Ciscar M, Trinidad EM, Perez-Chacon G, Alsaleem M, Jimenez M, Jimenez-Santos MJ, Perez-Montoyo H, Sanz-Moreno A, Vethencourt A, Toss M, Petit A, Soler-Monso MT, Lopez V, Gomez-Miragaya J, Gomez-Aleza C, Dobrolecki LE, Lewis MT, Bruna A, Mouron S, Quintela-Fandino M, Al-Shahrour F, Martinez-Aranda A, Sierra A, Green AR, Rakha E, Gonzalez-Suarez E (2023) RANK is a poor prognosis marker and a therapeutic target in ER-negative postmenopausal breast cancer. EMBO Mol Med 15:e16715

Cottu P, Marangoni E, Assayag F, de Cremoux P, Vincent-Salomon A, de Ch Guyader L, Plater C, Elbaz N, Karboul JJ, Fontaine S, Chateau-Joubert P, Boudou-Rouquette S, Alran V, Dangles-Marie D, Gentien MF, Poupon, and D. Decaudin. (2012) Modeling of response to endocrine therapy in a panel of human luminal breast cancer xenografts. Breast Cancer Res Treat 133:595–606

Coussy F, de Koning L, Lavigne M, Bernard V, Ouine B, Boulai A, El Botty R, Dahmani A, Montaudon E, Assayag F, Morisset L, Huguet L, Sourd L, Painsec P, Callens C, Chateau-Joubert S, Servely JL, Larcher T, Reyes C, Girard E, Pierron G, Laurent C, Vacher S, Baulande S, Melaabi S, Vincent-Salomon A, Gentien D, Dieras V, Bieche I, Marangoni E (2019) A large collection of integrated genomically characterized patient-derived xenografts highlighting the heterogeneity of triple-negative breast cancer. Int J Cancer 145:1902–1912

Coussy F, El Botty R, Lavigne M, Gu C, Fuhrmann L, Briaux A, de Koning L, Dahmani A, Montaudon E, Morisset L, Huguet L, Sourd L, Painsec P, Chateau-Joubert S, Larcher T, Vacher S, Melaabi S, Salomon AV, Marangoni E, Bieche I (2020a) Combination of PI3K and MEK inhibitors yields durable remission in PDX models of PIK3CA-mutated metaplastic breast cancers. J Hematol Oncol 13:13

Coussy F, El-Botty R, Chateau-Joubert S, Dahmani A, Montaudon E, Leboucher S, Morisset L, Painsec P, Sourd L, Huguet L, Nemati F, Servely JL, Larcher T, Vacher S, Briaux A, Reyes C, La Rosa P, Lucotte G, Popova T, Foidart P, Sounni NE, Noel A, Decaudin D, Fuhrmann L, Salomon A, Reyal F, Mueller C, Ter Brugge P, Jonkers J, Poupon MF, Stern

MH, Bieche I, Pommier Y, Marangoni E (2020b) BRCAness, SLFN11, and RB1 loss predict response to topoisomerase I inhibitors in triple-negative breast cancers. Sci Transl Med 12

Cruz C, Castroviejo-Bermejo M, Gutiérrez-Enríquez S, Llop-Guevara A, Ibrahim YH, Gris-Oliver A, Bonache S, Morancho B, Bruna A, Rueda OM, Lai Z, Polanska UM, Jones GN, Kristel P, de Bustos L, Guzman M, Rodríguez O, Grueso J, Montalban G, Caratú G, Mancuso F, Fasani R, Jiménez J, Howat WJ, Dougherty B, Vivancos A, Nuciforo P, Serres-Créixams X, Rubio IT, Oaknin A, Cadogan E, Barrett JC, Caldas C, Baselga J, Saura C, Cortés J, Arribas J, Jonkers J, Díez O, O'Connor MJ, Balmaña J, Serra V (2018) RAD51 foci as a functional biomarker of homologous recombination repair and PARP inhibitor resistance in germline BRCA-mutated breast cancer. Ann Oncol 29:1203–1210

Davis RT, Blake K, Ma D, Gabra MBI, Hernandez GA, Phung AT, Yang Y, Maurer D, Aeyt Lefebvre H, Alshetaiwi Z, Xiao J, Liu JW, Locasale MA, Digman E, Mjolsness M, Kong ZW, Lawson DA (2020) Transcriptional diversity and bioenergetic shift in human breast cancer metastasis revealed by single-cell RNA sequencing. Nat Cell Biol 22:310–320

DeRose YS, Wang G, Lin YC, Bernard PS, Buys SS, Ebbert MT, Factor R, Matsen C, Milash BA, Nelson E, Neumayer L, Randall RL, Stijleman IJ, Welm BE, Welm AL (2011) Tumor grafts derived from women with breast cancer authentically reflect tumor pathology, growth, metastasis and disease outcomes. Nat Med 17:1514–1520

DeRose YS, Gligorich KM, Wang G, Georgelas A, Bowman P, Courdy SJ, Welm AL, Welm BE (2013) Patient-derived models of human breast cancer: protocols for in vitro and in vivo applications in tumor biology and translational medicine. Curr Protoc Pharmacol, Chapter 14: Unit14 23

Ding L, Ellis MJ, Li S, Larson DE, Chen K, Wallis JW, Harris CC, McLellan MD, Fulton RS, Fulton LL, Abbott RM, Hoog J, Dooling DJ, Koboldt DC, Schmidt H, Kalicki J, Zhang Q, Chen L, Lin L, Wendl MC, McMichael JF, Magrini VJ, Cook L, McGrath SD, Vickery TL, Appelbaum E, Deschryver K, Davies S, Guintoli T, Lin L, Crowder R, Tao Y, Snider JE, Smith SM, Dukes AF, Sanderson GE, Pohl CS, Delehaunty KD, Fronick CC, Pape KA, Reed JS, Robinson JS, Hodges JS, Schierding W, Dees ND, Shen D, Locke DP, Wiechert ME, Eldred JM, Peck JB, Oberkfell BJ, Lolofie JT, Du F, Hawkins AE, O'Laughlin MD, Bernard KE, Cunningham M, Elliott G, Mason MD, Thompson DM Jr, Ivanovich JL, Goodfellow PJ, Perou CM, Weinstock GM, Aft R, Watson M, Ley TJ, Wilson RK, Mardis ER (2010) Genome remodelling in a basal-like breast cancer metastasis and xenograft. Nature 464:999–1005

Dobrolecki LE, Airhart SD, Alferez DG, Aparicio S, Behbod F, Bentires-Alj M, Brisken C, Bult CJ, Cai S, Clarke RB, Dowst H, Ellis MJ, Gonzalez-Suarez E, Iggo RD, Kabos P, Li S, Lindeman GJ, Marangoni E, McCoy A, Meric-Bernstam F, Piwnica-Worms H, Poupon MF, Reis-Filho J, Sartorius CA, Scabia V, Sflomos G, Tu Y, Vaillant F, Visvader JE, Welm A, Wicha MS, Lewis MT (2016) Patient-derived xenograft (PDX) models in basic and translational breast cancer research. Cancer Metastasis Rev 35:547–573

Domcke S, Sinha R, Levine DA, Sander C, Schultz N (2013) Evaluating cell lines as tumour models by comparison of genomic profiles. Nat Commun 4:2126

Dozmorov MG, Marshall MA, Rashid NS, Grible JM, Valentine A, Olex AL, Murthy K, Chakraborty A, Reyna J, Figueroa DS, Hinojosa-Gonzalez L, Lee ED-I, Baur BA, Roy S, Ay F, Harrell JC (2023) Rewiring of the 3D genome during acquisition of carboplatin resistance in a triple-negative breast cancer patient-derived xenograft. Sci Rep 13:5420

du Manoir S, Orsetti B, Bras-Goncalves R, Nguyen TT, Lasorsa L, Boissiere F, Massemin B, Colombo PE, Bibeau F, Jacot W, Theillet C (2014) Breast tumor PDXs are genetically plastic and correspond to a subset of aggressive cancers prone to relapse. Mol Oncol 8:431–443

Echeverria GV, Powell E, Seth S, Ge Z, Carugo A, Bristow C, Peoples M, Robinson F, Qiu H, Shao J, Jeter-Jones SL, Zhang X, Ramamoorthy V, Cai S, Wu W, Draetta G, Moulder SL, Symmans WF, Chang JT, Heffernan TP, Piwnica-Worms H (2018) High-resolution clonal mapping of multi-organ metastasis in triple negative breast cancer. Nat Commun 9:5079

Echeverria GV, Ge Z, Seth S, Zhang X, Jeter-Jones S, Zhou X, Cai S, Tu Y, McCoy A, Peoples M, Sun Y, Qiu H, Chang Q, Bristow C, Carugo A, Shao J, Ma X, Harris A, Mundi P, Lau R, Ramamoorthy V, Wu Y, Alvarez MJ, Califano A, Moulder SL, Symmans WF, Marszalek JR, Heffernan TP, Chang JT, Piwnica-Worms H (2019) Resistance to neoadjuvant chemotherapy in triple-negative breast cancer mediated by a reversible drug-tolerant state. Sci Transl Med 11

Eirew P, Steif A, Khattra J, Ha G, Yap D, Farahani H, Gelmon K, Chia S, Mar C, Wan A, Laks E, Biele J, Shumansky K, Rosner J, McPherson A, Nielsen C, Roth AJ, Lefebvre C, Bashashati A, de Souza C, Siu C, Aniba R, Brimhall J, Oloumi A, Osako T, Bruna A, Sandoval JL, Algara T, Greenwood W, Leung K, Cheng H, Xue H, Wang Y, Lin D, Mungall AJ, Moore R, Zhao Y, Lorette J, Nguyen L, Huntsman D, Eaves CJ, Hansen C, Marra MA, Caldas C, Shah SP, Aparicio S (2015) Dynamics of genomic clones in breast cancer patient xenografts at single-cell resolution. Nature 518:422–426

El-Botty R, Morriset L, Montaudon E, Tariq Z, Schnitzler A, Bacci M, Lorito N, Sourd L, Huguet L, Dahmani A, Painsec P, Derrien H, Vacher S, Masliah-Planchon J, Raynal V, Baulande S, Larcher T, Vincent-Salomon A, Dutertre G, Cottu P, Gentric G, Mechta-Grigoriou F, Hutton S, Driouch K, Bieche I, Morandi A, Marangoni E (2023) Oxidative phosphorylation is a metabolic vulnerability of endocrine therapy and palbociclib resistant metastatic breast cancers. Nat Commun 14(1):4221. Accession Number: 37452026;

PMCID: PMC10349040; https://doi.org/10.1038/s41467-023-40022-5

Flavahan WA, Gaskell E, Bernstein BE (2017) Epigenetic plasticity and the hallmarks of cancer. Science 357

Gao H, Korn JM, Ferretti S, Monahan JE, Wang Y, Singh M, Zhang C, Schnell C, Yang G, Zhang Y, Balbin OA, Barbe S, Cai H, Casey F, Chatterjee S, Chiang DY, Chuai S, Cogan SM, Collins SD, Dammassa E, Ebel N, Embry M, Green J, Kauffmann A, Kowal C, Leary RJ, Lehar J, Liang Y, Loo A, Lorenzana E, Robert McDonald E 3rd, McLaughlin ME, Merkin J, Meyer R, Naylor TL, Patawaran M, Reddy A, Roelli C, Ruddy DA, Salangsang F, Santacroce F, Singh AP, Tang Y, Tinetto W, Tobler S, Velazquez R, Venkatesan K, Von Arx F, Wang HQ, Wang Z, Wiesmann M, Wyss D, Xu F, Bitter H, Atadja P, Lees E, Hofmann F, Li E, Keen N, Cozens R, Jensen MR, Pryer NK, Williams JA, Sellers WR (2015) High-throughput screening using patient-derived tumor xenografts to predict clinical trial drug response. Nat Med

Gillet JP, Calcagno AM, Varma S, Marino M, Green LJ, Vora MI, Patel C, Orina JN, Eliseeva TA, Singal V, Padmanabhan R, Davidson B, Ganapathi R, Sood AK, Rueda BR, Ambudkar SV, Gottesman MM (2011) Redefining the relevance of established cancer cell lines to the study of mechanisms of clinical anti-cancer drug resistance. Proc Natl Acad Sci USA 108:18708–18713

Gillet JP, Varma S, Gottesman MM (2013) The clinical relevance of cancer cell lines. J Natl Cancer Inst 105:452–458

Hong Y, Limback D, Elsarraj HS, Harper H, Haines H, Hansford H, Ricci M, Kaufman C, Wedlock E, Xu M, Zhang J, May L, Cusick T, Inciardi M, Redick M, Gatewood J, Winblad O, Aripoli A, Huppe A, Balanoff C, Wagner JL, Amin AL, Larson KE, Ricci L, Tawfik O, Razek H, Meierotto RO, Madan R, Godwin AK, Thompson J, Hilsenbeck SG, Futreal A, Thompson A, Hwang ES, Fan F, Behbod F, Precision Consortium Grand Challenge (2022) Mouse-INtraDuctal (MIND): An in vivo model for studying the underlying mechanisms of DCIS malignancy. J Pathol 256:186–201

Honkala A, Malhotra SV, Kummar S, Junttila MR (2022) Harnessing the predictive power of preclinical models for oncology drug development. Nat Rev Drug Discov 21:99–114

Hutten SJ, de Bruijn R, Lutz C, Badoux M, Eijkman T, Chao X, Ciwinska M, Sheinman M, Messal H, Herencia-Ropero A, Kristel P, Mulder L, van der Waal R, Sanders J, Almekinders MM, Llop-Guevara A, Davies HR, van Haren MJ, Martin NI, Behbod F, Nik-Zainal S, Serra V, van Rheenen J, Lips EH, Wessels LFA, Precision Consortium Grand Challenge, Wesseling J, Scheele C, Jonkers J (2023) A living biobank of patient-derived ductal carcinoma in situ mouse-intraductal xenografts identifies risk factors for invasive progression. Cancer Cell 41:986–1002 e9

Izumchenko E, Paz K, Ciznadija D, Sloma I, Katz A, Vasquez-Dunddel D, Ben-Zvi I, Stebbing J, McGuire W, Harris W, Maki R, Gaya A, Bedi A, Zacharoulis S, Ravi R, Wexler LH, Hoque MO, Rodriguez-Galindo C, Pass H, Peled N, Davies A, Morris R, Hidalgo M, Sidransky D (2017) Patient-derived xenografts effectively capture responses to oncology therapy in a heterogeneous cohort of patients with solid tumors. Ann Oncol

Janiszewska M, Stein S, Metzger Filho O, Eng J, Kingston NL, Harper NW, Rye IH, Aleckovic M, Trinh A, Murphy KC, Marangoni E, Cristea S, Oakes B, Winer EP, Krop IE, Russnes HG, Spellman PT, Bucher E, Hu Z, Chin K, Gray JW, Michor F, Polyak K (2021) The impact of tumor epithelial and microenvironmental heterogeneity on treatment responses in HER2+ breast cancer. JCI Insight 6

Jiang G, Zhang S, Yazdanparast A, Li M, Pawar AV, Liu Y, Inavolu SM, Cheng L (2016) Comprehensive comparison of molecular portraits between cell lines and tumors in breast cancer. BMC Genomics 17(Suppl 7):525

Kabos P, Finlay-Schultz J, Li C, Kline E, Finlayson C, Wisell J, Manuel CA, Edgerton SM, Harrell JC, Elias A, Sartorius CA (2012) Patient-derived luminal breast cancer xenografts retain hormone receptor heterogeneity and help define unique estrogen-dependent gene signatures. Breast Cancer Res Treat 135:415–432

Kabraji S, Ni J, Sammons S, Li T, Van Swearingen AED, Wang Y, Pereslete A, Hsu L, DiPiro PJ, Lascola C, Moore H, Hughes M, Raghavendra AS, Gule-Monroe M, Murthy RK, Winer EP, Anders CK, Zhao JJ, Lin NU (2023) Preclinical and clinical efficacy of trastuzumab deruxtecan in breast cancer brain metastases. Clin Cancer Res 29:174–182

Lefley D, Howard F, Arshad F, Bradbury S, Brown H, Tulotta C, Eyre R, Alferez D, Wilkinson JM, Holen I, Clarke RB, Ottewell P (2019) Development of clinically relevant in vivo metastasis models using human bone discs and breast cancer patient-derived xenografts. Breast Cancer Res 21:130

Li S, Shen D, Shao J, Crowder R, Liu W, Prat A, He X, Liu S, Hoog J, Lu C, Ding L, Griffith OL, Miller C, Larson D, Fulton RS, Harrison M, Mooney T, McMichael JF, Luo J, Tao Y, Goncalves R, Schlosberg C, Hiken JF, Saied L, Sanchez C, Giuntoli T, Bumb C, Cooper C, Kitchens RT, Lin A, Phommaly C, Davies SR, Zhang J, Kavuri MS, McEachern D, Dong YY, Ma C, Pluard T, Naughton M, Bose R, Suresh R, McDowell R, Michel L, Aft R, Gillanders W, DeSchryver K, Wilson RK, Wang S, Mills GB, Gonzalez-Angulo A, Edwards JR, Maher C, Perou CM, Mardis ER, Ellis MJ (2013) Endocrine-therapy-resistant ESR1 variants revealed by genomic characterization of breast-cancer-derived xenografts. Cell Rep 4:1116–1130

Liao C, Glodowski CR, Fan C, Liu J, Mott KR, Kaushik A, Vu H, Locasale JW, McBrayer SK, DeBerardinis RJ, Perou CM, Zhang Q (2022) Integrated metabolic profiling and transcriptional analysis reveals therapeutic modalities for targeting rapidly proliferating breast cancers. Cancer Res 82:665–680

Marangoni E, Vincent-Salomon A, Auger N, Degeorges A, Assayag F, de Cremoux P, de Plater L, Guyader C,

De Pinieux G, Judde JG, Rebucci M, Tran-Perennou C, Sastre-Garau X, Sigal-Zafrani B, Delattre O, Dieras V, Poupon MF (2007) A new model of patient tumor-derived breast cancer xenografts for preclinical assays. Clin Cancer Res 13:3989–3998

Marangoni E, Laurent C, Coussy F, El-Botty R, Chateau-Joubert S, Servely JL, de Plater L, Assayag F, Dahmani A, Montaudon E, Nemati F, Fleury J, Vacher S, Gentien D, Rapinat A, Foidart P, Sounni NE, Noel A, Vincent-Salomon A, Lae M, Decaudin D, Roman-Roman S, Bieche I, Piccart M, Reyal F (2018) Capecitabine efficacy is correlated with TYMP and RB1 expression in PDX established from triple-negative breast cancers. Clin Cancer Res 24:2605–2615

Marsolier J, Prompsy P, Durand A, Lyne AM, Landragin C, Trouchet A, Bento ST, Eisele A, Foulon S, Baudre L, Grosselin K, Bohec M, Baulande S, Dahmani A, Sourd L, Letouze E, Salomon AV, Marangoni E, Perie L, Vallot C (2022) H3K27me3 conditions chemotolerance in triple-negative breast cancer. Nat Genet 54:459–468

Martignoni M, Groothuis GM, de Kanter R (2006) Species differences between mouse, rat, dog, monkey and human CYP-mediated drug metabolism, inhibition and induction. Expert Opin Drug Metab Toxicol 2:875–894

Menghi F, Banda K, Kumar P, Straub R, Dobrolecki L, Rodriguez IV, Yost SE, Chandok H, Radke MR, Somlo G, Yuan Y, Lewis MT, Swisher EM, Liu ET (2022) Genomic and epigenomic BRCA alterations predict adaptive resistance and response to platinum-based therapy in patients with triple-negative breast and ovarian carcinomas. Sci Transl Med 14:eabn1926

Moestue SA, Borgan E, Huuse EM, Lindholm EM, Sitter B, Borresen-Dale AL, Engebraaten O, Maelandsmo GM, Gribbestad IS (2010) Distinct choline metabolic profiles are associated with differences in gene expression for basal-like and luminal-like breast cancer xenograft models. BMC Cancer 10:433

Moestue SA, Dam CG, Gorad SS, Kristian A, Bofin A, Maelandsmo GM, Engebraten O, Gribbestad IS, Bjorkoy G (2013) Metabolic biomarkers for response to PI3K inhibition in basal-like breast cancer. Breast Cancer Res 15:R16

Montaudon E, Nikitorowicz-Buniak J, Sourd L, Morisset L, El Botty R, Huguet L, Dahmani A, Painsec P, Nemati F, Vacher S, Chemlali W, Masliah-Planchon J, Chateau-Joubert S, Rega C, Leal MF, Simigdala N, Pancholi S, Ribas R, Nicolas A, Meseure D, Vincent-Salomon A, Reyes C, Rapinat A, Gentien D, Larcher T, Bohec M, Baulande S, Bernard V, Decaudin D, Coussy F, Le Romancer M, Dutertre G, Tariq Z, Cottu P, Driouch K, Bieche I, Martin LA, Marangoni E (2020) PLK1 inhibition exhibits strong anti-tumoral activity in CCND1-driven breast cancer metastases with acquired palbociclib resistance. Nat Commun 11:4053

Outzen HC, Custer RP (1975) Growth of human normal and neoplastic mammary tissues in the cleared mammary fat pad of the nude mouse. J Natl Cancer Inst 55:1461–1466

Palafox M, Monserrat L, Bellet M, Villacampa G, Gonzalez-Perez A, Oliveira M, Braso-Maristany F, Ibrahimi N, Kannan S, Mina L, Herrera-Abreu MT, Odena A, Sanchez-Guixe M, Capelan M, Azaro A, Bruna A, Rodriguez O, Guzman M, Grueso J, Viaplana C, Hernandez J, Su F, Lin K, Clarke RB, Caldas C, Arribas J, Michiels S, Garcia-Sanz A, Turner NC, Prat A, Nuciforo P, Dienstmann R, Verma CS, Lopez-Bigas N, Scaltriti M, Arnedos M, Saura C, Serra V (2022) High p16 expression and heterozygous RB1 loss are biomarkers for CDK4/6 inhibitor resistance in ER(+) breast cancer. Nat Commun 13:5258

Reyal F, Guyader C, Decraene C, Lucchesi C, Auger N, Assayag F, De Plater L, Gentien D, Poupon MF, Cottu P, De Cremoux P, Gestraud P, Vincent-Salomon A, Fontaine JJ, Roman-Roman S, Delattre O, Decaudin D, Marangoni E (2012) Molecular profiling of patient-derived breast cancer xenografts. Breast Cancer Res 14:R11

Rygaard J, Povlsen CO (1969) Heterotransplantation of a human malignant tumour to "Nude" mice. Acta Pathol Microbiol Scand 77:758–760

Savage P, Pacis A, Kuasne H, Liu L, Lai D, Wan A, Dankner M, Martinez C, Munoz-Ramos V, Pilon V, Monast A, Zhao H, Souleimanova M, Annis MG, Aguilar-Mahecha A, Lafleur J, Bertos NR, Asselah J, Bouganim N, Petrecca K, Siegel PM, Omeroglu A, Shah SP, Aparicio S, Basik M, Meterissian S, Park M (2020) Chemogenomic profiling of breast cancer patient-derived xenografts reveals targetable vulnerabilities for difficult-to-treat tumors. Commun Biol 3:310

Simoes BM, O'Brien CS, Eyre R, Silva A, Yu L, Sarmiento-Castro A, Alferez DG, Spence K, Santiago-Gomez A, Chemi F, Acar A, Gandhi A, Howell A, Brennan K, Ryden L, Catalano S, Ando S, Gee J, Ucar A, Sims AH, Marangoni E, Farnie G, Landberg G, Howell SJ, Clarke RB (2015) Anti-estrogen resistance in human breast tumors is driven by JAG1-NOTCH4-dependent cancer stem cell activity. Cell Rep 12:1968–1977

Simoes BM, Santiago-Gomez A, Chiodo C, Moreira T, Conole D, Lovell S, Alferez D, Eyre R, Spence K, Sarmiento-Castro A, Kohler B, Morisset L, Lanzino M, Ando S, Marangoni E, Sims AH, Tate EW, Howell SJ, Clarke RB (2020) Targeting STAT3 signaling using stabilised sulforaphane (SFX-01) inhibits endocrine resistant stem-like cells in ER-positive breast cancer. Oncogene 39:4896–4908

Singh JK, Farnie G, Bundred NJ, Simoes BM, Shergill A, Landberg G, Howell SJ, Clarke RB (2013) Targeting CXCR1/2 significantly reduces breast cancer stem cell activity and increases the efficacy of inhibiting HER2 via HER2-dependent and -independent mechanisms. Clin Cancer Res 19:643–656

Tentler JJ, Tan AC, Weekes CD, Jimeno A, Leong S, Pitts TM, Arcaroli JJ, Messersmith WA, Eckhardt SG (2012) Patient-derived tumour xenografts as models for oncology drug development. Nat Rev Clin Oncol 9:338–350

Ter Brugge P, Kristel P, van der Burg E, Boon U, de Maaker M, Lips E, Mulder L, de Ruiter J, Moutinho C, Gevensleben H, Marangoni E, Majewski I, Jozwiak K, Kloosterman W, van Roosmalen M, Duran K, Hogervorst F, Turner N, Esteller M, Cuppen E, Wesseling J, Jonkers J (2016) Mechanisms of therapy resistance in patient-derived Xenograft models of BRCA1-deficient breast cancer. J Natl Cancer Inst 108

Ter Brugge P, Moser SC, Bieche I, Kristel P, Ibadioune S, Eeckhoutte A, de Bruijn R, van der Burg E, Lutz C, Annunziato S, de Ruiter J, Masliah Planchon J, Vacher S, Courtois L, El-Botty R, Dahmani A, Montaudon E, Morisset L, Sourd L, Huguet L, Derrien H, Nemati F, Chateau-Joubert S, Larcher T, Salomon A, Decaudin D, Reyal F, Coussy F, Popova T, Wesseling J, Stern MH, Jonkers J, Marangoni E (2023) Homologous recombination deficiency derived from whole-genome sequencing predicts platinum response in triple-negative breast cancers. Nat Commun 14:1958

Timbrell S, Aglan H, Cramer A, Foden P, Weaver D, Pachter J, Kilgallon A, Clarke RB, Farnie G, Bundred NJ (2021) FAK inhibition alone or in combination with adjuvant therapies reduces cancer stem cell activity. NPJ Breast Cancer 7:65

Wärnberg F, White D, Anderson E, Knox F, Clarke RB, Morris J, Bundred NJ (2006) Effect of a farnesyl transferase inhibitor (R115777) on ductal carcinoma in situ of the breast in a human xenograft model and on breast and ovarian cancer cell growth in vitro and in vivo. Breast Cancer Res 8

Woo XY, Giordano J, Srivastava A, Zhao ZM, Lloyd MW, de Bruijn R, Suh YS, Patidar R, Chen L, Scherer S, Bailey MH, Yang CH, Cortes-Sanchez E, Xi Y, Wang J, Wickramasinghe J, Kossenkov AV, Rebecca VW, Sun H, Mashl RJ, Davies SR, Jeon R, Frech C, Randjelovic J, Rosains J, Galimi F, Bertotti A, Lafferty A, O'Farrell AC, Modave E, Lambrechts D, Ter Brugge P, Serra V, Marangoni E, El Botty R, Kim H, Kim JI, Yang HK, Lee C, Dean DA 2nd, Davis-Dusenbery B, Evrard YA, Doroshow JH, Welm AL, Welm BE, Lewis MT, Fang B, Roth JA, Meric-Bernstam F, Herlyn M, Davies MA, Ding L, Li S, Govindan R, Isella C, Moscow JA, Trusolino L, Byrne AT, Jonkers J, Bult CJ, Medico E, Chuang JH, Pdxnet Consortium, and Opdx Consortium Eur (2021) Conservation of copy number profiles during engraftment and passaging of patient-derived cancer xenografts. Nat Genet 53:86–99

Yu J, Qin B, Moyer AM, Sinnwell JP, Thompson KJ, Copland JA 3rd, Marlow LA, Miller JL, Yin P, Gao B, Minter-Dykhouse K, Tang X, McLaughlin SA, Moreno-Aspitia A, Schweitzer A, Lu Y, Hubbard J, Northfelt DW, Gray RJ, Hunt K, Conners AL, Suman VJ, Kalari KR, Ingle JN, Lou Z, Visscher DW, Weinshilboum R, Boughey JC, Goetz MP, Wang L (2017) Establishing and characterizing patient-derived xenografts using pre-chemotherapy percutaneous biopsy and post-chemotherapy surgical samples from a prospective neoadjuvant breast cancer study. Breast Cancer Res 19:130

Zhang X, Claerhout S, Prat A, Dobrolecki LE, Petrovic I, Lai Q, Landis MD, Wiechmann L, Schiff R, Giuliano M, Wong H, Fuqua SW, Contreras A, Gutierrez C, Huang J, Mao S, Pavlick AC, Froehlich AM, Wu MF, Tsimelzon A, Hilsenbeck SG, Chen ES, Zuloaga P, Shaw CA, Rimawi MF, Perou CM, Mills GB, Chang JC, Lewis MT (2013) A renewable tissue resource of phenotypically stable, biologically and ethnically diverse, patient-derived human breast cancer xenograft models. Cancer Res 73:4885–4897

Rat Models of Breast Cancer

8

Wen Bu and Yi Li

Abstract

As the first mammal to be domesticated for research purposes, rats served as the primary animal model for various branches of biomedical research, including breast cancer studies, up until the late 1990s and early 2000s. During this time, genetic engineering of mice, but not rats, became routine, and mice gradually supplanted rats as the preferred rodent model. But recent advances in creating genetically engineered rat models, especially with the assistance of CRISPR/Cas9 technology, have rekindled the significance of rats as a critical model in exploring various facets of breast cancer research. This is particularly pronounced in the study of the formation and progression of the estrogen receptor-positive subtype, which remains challenging to model in mice. In this chapter, we embark on a historical journey through the evolution of rat models in biomedical research and provide an overview of the general and histological characteristics of rat mammary glands. Next, we critically review major rat models for breast cancer research, including those induced by carcinogens, hormones, radiation, germline transgenes, germline knockouts, and intraductal injection of retrovirus/lentivirus to deliver oncogenic drivers into mature mammary glands. We also discuss the advances in building rat models using somatic genome editing powered by CRISPR/Cas9. This chapter concludes with our forward-looking perspective on future applications of advanced rat models in critical areas of breast cancer research that have continued to challenge the mouse model community.

Keywords

Rat · Mammary gland · Carcinogen · Transgenic model · Knockout model · Viral vector · Intraductal injection · Somatic genome editing

Key Points

- Summary of the evolution of rat models in biomedical research.
- Comparison of the general and histological characteristics of rat mammary glands with those of mice and humans.
- Evaluation of conventional rat models induced by carcinogens, hormones, radiation, germline transgenes, and germline knockouts.
- Description of somatic rat models generated by intraductal injection of retro-

W. Bu · Y. Li (✉)
Lester & Sue Smith Breast Center, Baylor College of Medicine, Houston, TX, USA
e-mail: liyi@bcm.edu

T. Sørlie, R. B. Clarke (eds.), *A Guide to Breast Cancer Research*, Advances in Experimental Medicine and Biology 1464, https://doi.org/10.1007/978-3-031-70875-6_8

virus/lentivirus to deliver oncogenic drivers into mature mammary glands.
- Review of the latest advances in building next-generation precision rat models using somatic genome editing technology.

8.1 Rat Evolution and Domestication

Rats are medium-sized, long-tailed rodents belonging to the *Rattus* genus, while the smaller-sized mice belong to the *Mus* genus. Rats and mice diverged from a common ancestor over 23 million years ago (Adkins et al. 2001). However, they both belong to the *Murinae* sub-family within the *Muridae* family (Hedrich 2020) (Fig. 8.1).

The Norway rat (*Rattus norvegicus,* also knowns as the brown rat) is one of over 60 species in the *Rattus* genus. It was the first mammal

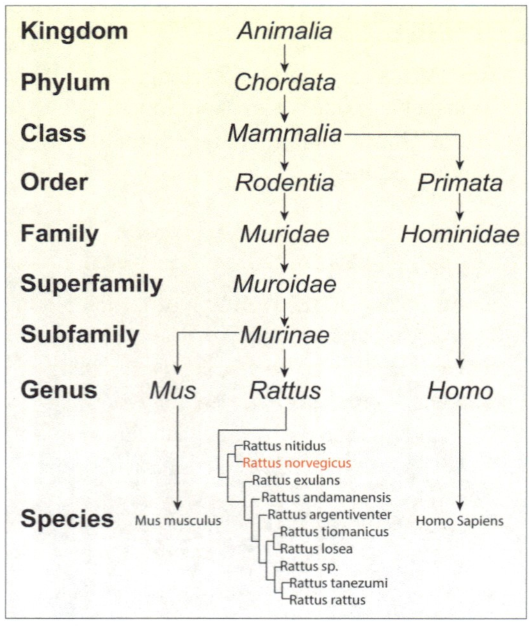

Fig. 8.1 Diagram of the taxonomy tree of Mus, Rattus, and Homo genus that mice, rats, and human belong to, respectively. Selected rat species (Hedrich 2020) are noted

to be domesticated for research purposes. Norway rats likely came into captivity for a rat-baiting sport that was popular in France and England as early as 1800 (Suckow and Baker 2020). The term "Norway rat" may have originated from the belief that they arrived in England from Norway aboard ships in the eighteenth century (Modlinska and Pisula 2020). But the actual origin of this rat species is unclear. It is generally agreed that this species originally came from Asia and spread to Europe and then to the USA (Adkins et al. 2001; Suckow and Baker 2020; Zeng et al. 2018). The earliest known fossils of *R. norvegicus* were discovered in China (Modlinska and Pisula 2020; Muss and Carleton 2005; Wu and Wang 2012).

Fragmented literature suggests that rats were used for fasting and other nutritional studies in Europe prior to 1850, but the earliest documented experiment on the rat was probably an adrenalectomy study in Norway rats by the French scientist J. M. Philipeaux (1856). After 1893, the American neurologist Henry Donaldson at the University of Chicago began using albino rats. In 1905, he became the research director of the Wistar Institute in Philadelphia and brought these rats with him. Together with other scientists there, he initiated efforts to standardize these albino rats for biomedical research, giving rise to Wistar and Wistar-derived rat strains. In 1912, the Wistar Institute began to supply these rat strains commercially. These rats likely contributed significant genetic materials to other currently used rat strains (Modlinska and Pisula 2020; Smith et al. 2019; Suckow and Baker 2020). Common stocks of outbred laboratory rats include Wistar, Sprague Dawley (SD), and Long-Evans (Table 8.1). Inbred strains offer an advantage for studying characteristics/phenotypes (such as coat color) and their genetic controls, and for minimizing variables, thus reducing sample sizes. They are generated by at least 20 sequential generations of brother-sister matings. In 1909, Helen King at Wistar started inbreeding using their albino Norway rats (King 1918). (Mouse inbreeding had begun in 1907 by Clarence Cook Little, then a Harvard undergraduate (Staats 1966)). Common inbred laboratory rat strains include the Brown

Table 8.1 Common laboratory rats

Name	Immune status	Inbred/ outbred	Coat color
Wistar	Competant	Outbred	White
Sprague Dawley	Competant	Outbred	White
Long Evans	Competant	Outbred	White
Brown Norway	Competant	Inbred	Non-agouti brown
Buffalo	Competant	Inbred	White
Copenhagen	Competant	Inbred	White with a brown hood
Fischer	Competant	Inbred	White
Lewis	Competant	Inbred	White
WAG	Competant	Inbred	White
Nude rat	T-cell deficient	Outbred	White or black or black and white
SRG rat	B, T, and NK cell deficient	Inbred	White

Norway, Fischer 344, and Lewis strains (Table 8.1) (Suckow et al. 2006).

8.2 Rats as Models for Biomedical Research

Rats have been used for biomedical research for over 160 years (Smith et al. 2019). They are a leading model for research in behavior/psychology, physiology, pharmacology, and toxicology, and for the study of a wide range of common, genetically complex human diseases. In fact, the rat was the first and most commonly used model species until the late 1990s and early 2000s when routine genetic engineering of mice advanced these smaller rodents as the most commonly used model species in biology (Aitman et al. 2016; Dwinell 2010; Homberg et al. 2017). However, the breakthrough of CRISPR/Cas9 technology has now cleared the technological hurdles for generating transgenic and knockout rats. The utilization of rat models will likely increase substantially in the coming years.

There are multiple advantages to the rat as a model for biomedical research. While the rat and the mouse are approximately 93% identical in nucleotide sequences and 94% in amino acid sequences (Wolfe and Sharp 1993), the genome structure of rats is more similar to the human's than is the mouse genome organization. Rats have 21 pairs of chromosomes, two pairs less than the human's 23 pairs, while mice harbor only 20 pairs. Furthermore, rat chromosomes are metacentric, with their centrosomes located toward the middle of the chromosomes similar to human centrosome arrangements, while mouse chromosomes are telocentric (Larsson et al. 1998). In addition, the genome size of rats is also more similar to humans—2.75 base-pairs in rats and 2.9 billion in humans vs. 2.5 billion in mice (Gibbs et al. 2004). This closer similarity in genome organization and size to human beings may explain some closer physiological and pathophysiological similarities between rats and humans.

The rat's larger brain size and higher cognition relative to mice make rats a better model for neuronal and behavioral studies (Smith et al. 2019; Suckow et al. 2006). The ten-fold larger body size of rats over mice often renders them a better choice for many physiological experiments since physiological measurements and experimental procedures are a lot easier to carry out in rats, including blood pressure measurements and serial blood draws (which are much challenging in the mouse), catheterization, and sophisticated surgical procedures. This advantage combined with the rat being the first and the most commonly used model until the last two decades has resulted in rat physiology being extremely well documented. Consequently, the rat has been a preferred animal model for studying physiological processes of virtually every organ system in humans (Suckow et al. 2006). These experiments have led to the identification of most of the essential amino acids, vitamins, and essential trace elements (Smith et al. 2019; Suckow et al. 2006). Furthermore, many discoveries in endocrinology came from early rat experiments, beginning with the 1856 adrenalectomy study by Philipeaux (1856). Like this study, many of the early studies of endocrinology involved observing the physiological effects of ablating rat endocrine glands, including castration, the removal of thyroid/parathyroid, ovariectomy and ovarian transplantation, and removal of the mammary glands (Smith et al. 2019; Suckow et al. 2006).

Rats have been extensively utilized in pharmacology and toxicology studies due to their larger body size compared to mice, their extensive history of physiological measurements, and their sharing with humans similar pathways for eradicating toxins (Huang et al. 2011). The size advantage allows for easier clinical and repeated sampling of blood, urine, tissues, and other physiological measurements. Almost every drug developed for human treatment has been tested in rats, highlighting their significance in pharmacology and toxicology (Mashimo and Serikawa 2009; Smith et al. 2019). Additionally, the National Cancer Institute (NCI) and National Toxicology Program (NTP) have amassed a vast publicly available dataset from over more than three decades of standardized bioassays of carcinogenicity using rats, encompassing thousands of chemical compounds (Bucher 2002; Zeiger 2017).

Compared to rabbits and pigs, rats are still relatively small, cost-effective, and easy to breed and handle. Due to a short life span (less than 3 years) they are also suitable for aging studies. In addition, the omnivorous feeding patterns of rats position them as a better model for nutrition studies than a strict herbivore, such as the rabbit. Furthermore, the ability to quickly breed rats and select for specific traits, coupled with the extensive history of rat physiological measurements, makes rats an ideal model for studying specific diseases in humans. For example, there exist specific rat lines carrying traits of human cardiovascular diseases, such as GH (genetically hypertensive) rats, SS (salt-sensitive) rats, SHR (spontaneously hypertensive) rats, SHRSP (stroke-prone spontaneously hypertensive) rats, and LH (Lyon hypertensive) rats (Smith et al. 2019). Moreover, rat breeding has also selected lines that are highly prone to developing cancer, stroke, Alzheimer's disease, Parkinson's disease, diabetes, obesity, asthma, etc. In addition, the causative genes for numerous disease phenotypes have been identified in rat models, and these findings have been successfully translated to humans in many instances (Szpirer 2020, 2022). Detailed information on rat strains and rat models of human diseases can be found at the Rat Genome Database (RGD, https://rgd.mcw.edu/) (Wang et al. 2019).

8.3 Rat vs. Mouse Mammary Glands: Compare and Contrast

Rats and mice, as rodents, share many similarities in their mammary glands. However, due to their distinct genera, they also exhibit significant differences. Grossly, both rats and mice have bilaterally and symmetrically located mammary glands along the ventral milk lines, extending from the neck to the perianal area. Interestingly, while mice have five pairs of mammary glands, rats have six (Cardiff et al. 2018). Each mammary gland in mature mice and rats possesses a single lactiferous duct and ostia while women's breast contains multiple.

Prior to adolescence, the mammary glands of both mice and rats consist of a tubular ductal tree that ends in a baseball bat-shape structure called the terminal end bud (TEB). A TEB is comprised of an outer layer of cap cells and multilayered body cells. Body cells are the precursor to luminal cells, while cap cells are the precursor to basal cells (also known as myoepithelial cells) (Sreekumar et al. 2017). At this stage, this ductal tree is primitive, occupying a small area near the nipple. At the onset of puberty, both mice and rats initiate similar estrous cycles lasting 4–5 days, during which surging ovarian hormones cause the resting TEBs to grow and branch out (Figs. 8.2a, b, 8.3a, b), depositing along the way more mature ducts—a single layer of luminal cells and a layer of basal cells—and ending in either terminal ducts (mice and rats) or alveolar buds (rats only). As estrous cycles continue in rats, these alveolar buds further branch and expand into lobules, each of which contains a group of alveoli (also referred to as acini) surrounded by dense intralobular stroma, a connective tissue (Figs. 8.2d, 8.3d). Luminal cells in

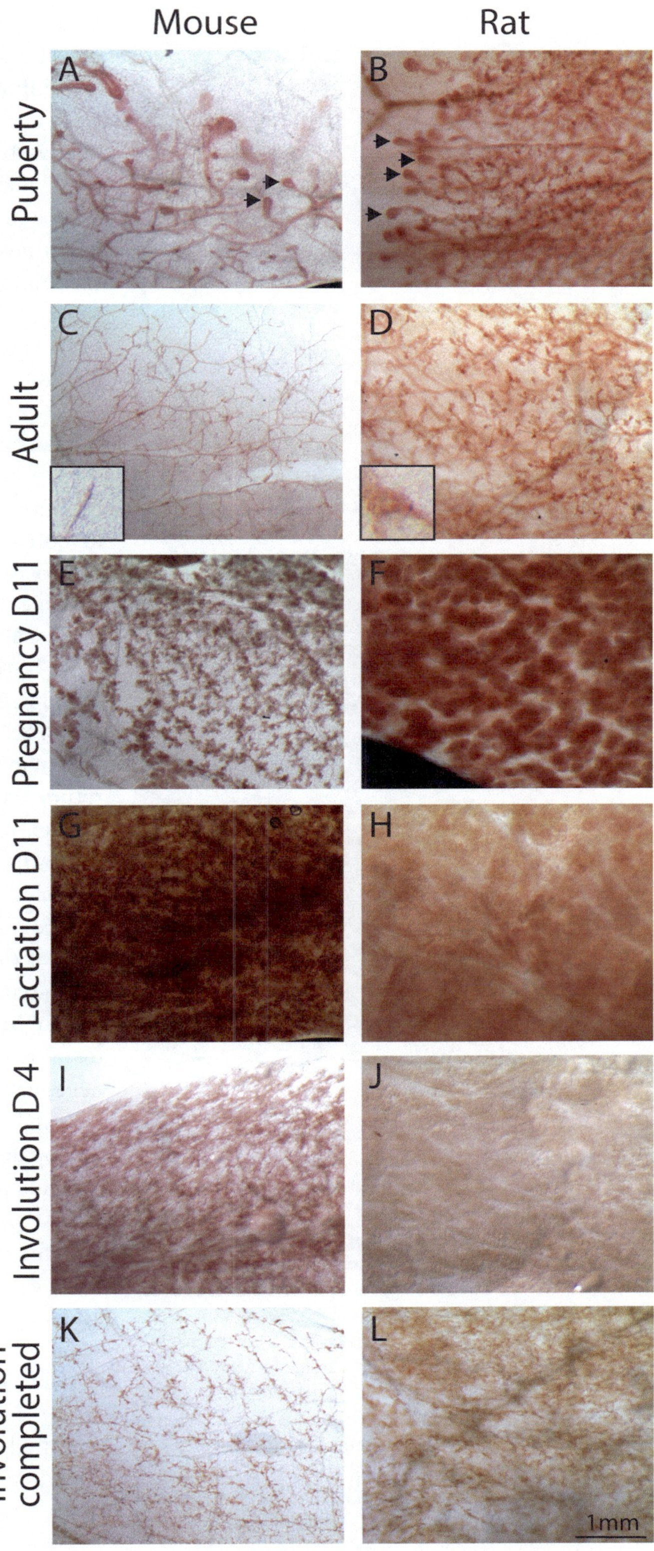

Fig. 8.2 Whole mount neutral red staining of mouse and rat mammary glands at different developmental stages. (**a**) Branching ducts and TEBs in a 36-day-old FVB/n mouse. (**b**) Dense branching ducts and TEBs in a 38-day-old SD rat. (**c**) Duct and ductal termini, but not lobules, in an 86-day-old FVB/n mouse. Inset is a high-magnification view of ducts. (**d**) Alveolar buds and TDLUs in an 80-day-old SD rat. Inset is a high-magnification view of a TDLU. (**e**, **f**) Lobule appearance in a day 11 pregnant FVB/n mouse vs extensive lobular development in a day 11 pregnant SD rat. (**g**, **h**) Dense lobules in an FVB/n mouse and a SD rat at day 11 of lactation. (**i**, **j**) Collapsing lobules in an FVB/n mouse and a SD rat at day 4 of involution. (**k**, **l**) Loss and degeneration of lobules in a fully involuted mammary gland in a retired mouse breeder (8 months old) and a retired rat breeder (5 months old). Of note, the densely stained structures are dilated ducts and degenerated residual lobules

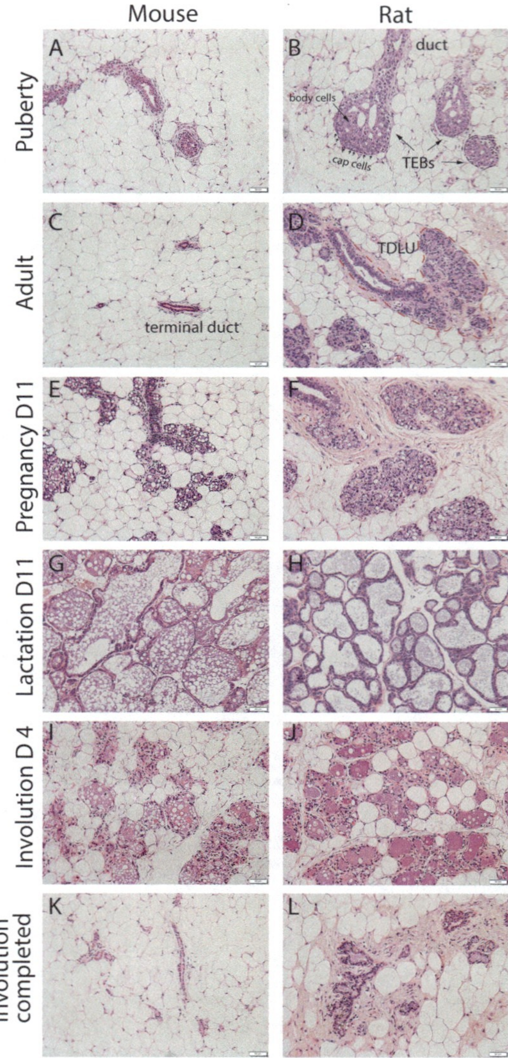

Fig. 8.3 H&E staining of sections of mouse and rat mammary glands at different developmental stages. (**a**) Ducts and a partial TEB in a 36-day-old FVB/n mouse. (**b**) Three TEBs in a 38-day-old SD rat. (**c**) Ducts, but not lobules, in an 86-day-old FVB/n mouse. A potential terminal duct is indicated. (**d**) A typical TDLU showing both a terminal duct and clusters of alveoli (acini), and multiple other lobules in an 80-day-old SD rat. Note the appreciable amounts of connective tissue between alveoli and around the duct as well as dispersed in the fat pad versus the general lack of connective tissue in the mouse. (**e, f**) Lobule appearance in a day 11 pregnant FVB/n mouse vs extensive lobular development in a day 11 pregnant SD rat. Milk droplets in various sizes are seen in the alveolar cells. (**g, h**) Milk secretion causing distension of the alveolar lumen in an FVB/n mouse and a SD rat at day 11 of lactation. (**i, j**) Collapsing lobules in an FVB/n mouse and a SD rat at day 4 of involution. (**k, l**) Loss and degeneration of lobules in a fully involuted mammary gland in a retired mouse breeder (8 months old) and a retired rat breeder (5 months old). Note the abundant amounts of connective tissue in the rat

alveoli are commonly referred to as alveolar cells (or acinar cells). The ductal trees in women are similarly organized (Fig. 8.4), but the ductal trees in mice lack lobules and involve little connective tissue, and the tree branches end in terminal ducts only (Cardiff et al. 2018) (Figs. 8.2c, 8.3c, and 8.4). Consequently, rats may serve as a better model for studying human breast development and cancer, which is generally considered to arise from a terminal duct lobular unit (TDLU), a term referring to a lobule and its associated duct.

In pregnancy, the lobules in both rats and humans enlarge and differentiate to prepare for milk production (Figs. 8.2f, 8.3f). At this stage, the mouse mammary ductal tree also develops alveoli and lobules (Figs. 8.2e, 8.3e). Upon parturition, the alveolar cells in all three species become terminally differentiated and produce milk, causing lumen distension (Figs. 8.2g, h, 8.3g, h). Upon weaning, excess alveolar cells in both mice and rats as well as humans rapidly die (Figs. 8.2i, j, 8.3i, j). In approximately 3 weeks, the mammary glands in both mice and rats return largely to their pre-pregnancy state, and mouse mammary glands lose lobules gained during pregnancy/lactation (Figs. 8.2k, l, 8.3k, l). Interestingly, some of the alveolar cells gained in pregnancy/lactation may linger as progenitor or even stem cells based on transplantation studies in mice (Boulanger et al. 2004). Unlike humans, aged rodents do not experience menopause and the menopause-associated fast degeneration of the ductal tree. However, rodents may be induced to go into artificial menopause by ovariectomy.

Male mice possess only rudimentary glandular tissue, while male rats have more prominent glandular structures that differ morphologically from those of female rats. Male rat mammary glands are characterized by a predominance of lobules of acini and fewer ducts compared to female rat mammary glands (Cardiff et al. 2018). Notably, the ducts in male rats have a stratified epithelium and epithelial cells with abundant and vacuolated cytoplasm, in contrast to the single-layered epithelial cells with sparse cytoplasm lining the intralobular ducts in female rat mammary glands (Cardiff et al. 2018).

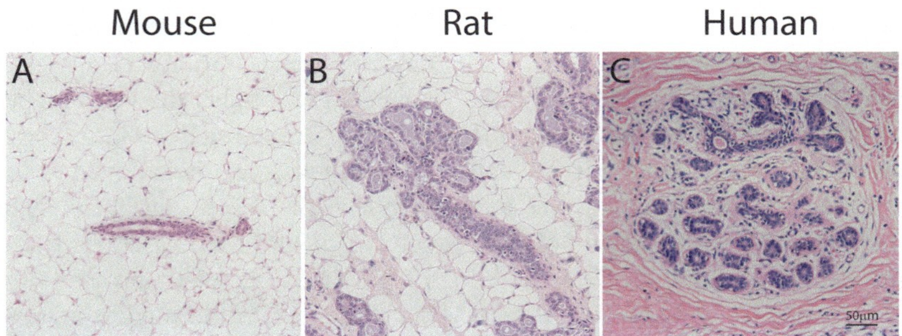

Fig. 8.4 H&E staining of sections of adult mouse, rat, and human mammary glands. (**a**) Ducts, but not lobules, in an 86-day-old FVB/n mouse. (**b**) A typical TDLU showing both a terminal duct and clusters of alveoli (acini), and multiple other lobules in an 80-day-old SD rat. Note the appreciable amounts of connective tissue between alveoli and around the duct as well as dispersed in the fat pad versus the general lack of connective tissue in the mouse. (**c**) A typical TDLU in a woman of unknown age. Note the extensive connective tissue and the relatively minor adipocyte component

8.4 Chemical-, Hormone-, and Radiation-Induced Rat Mammary Tumor Models

Breast cancer is caused by the combination of multiple external and internal risk factors, including chemical carcinogens, radiation, and hormone levels. Rats have been the primary animal model for studying the tumorigenic mechanism of these risk factors on mammary tumors. Tumor models induced by these risk factors are also valuable for evaluating the impact of other risk factors, such as diet and reproduction history, on breast tumorigenesis. Furthermore, these models have also been frequently used for preclinical drug testing.

"One of the most remarkable experiments in cancer research is the induction of cancer which occurs preferentially in the breast of rats following the feeding of carcinogenic hydrocarbons," Charles Huggins wrote in 1961 when reporting his finding of a single feeding of polynuclear hydrocarbons inducing hormone-dependent mammary tumors in rats (Huggins et al. 1961). This groundbreaking finding, along with his discovery of hormone dependence of prostate cancer, led to his Nobel Prize in physiology or medicine in 1966. In this experiment, Huggins showed that a single intragastric injection of 20 mg of DMBA into 50-day-old SD rats resulted in mammary tumors with 100% incidence in just 2 months following treatment (Huggins et al. 1961). Since then, carcinogens have been used extensively in rats to study mammary tumors and their hormone dependence. These carcinogens include 3-methylcholanthrene (MCA), N-ethyl-N-nitrosourea (ENU, otherwise known as N-nitroso-N-ethylurea [NEU]), 1-butyl-1-nitrosourea (BNU), N-methyl-N-nitrosourea (MNU, also known as N-nitroso-N-methylurea [NMU]) and 7,12-dimethylbenz[a]anthracene (DMBA) (Welsch 1985). The two most commonly used are MNU and DMBA for their mammary organotropism, but they are very different chemicals. MNU directly alkylates oxygen and nitrogen atoms in nucleotides to produce DNA adducts (Richardson et al. 1987). The formation of these adducts can lead to improper nucleotide incorporation during DNA replication in highly proliferating cells. MNU primarily induces a G → A transition (Singer and Kuśmierek 1982). On the other hand, DMBA, a lipophilic polycyclic aromatic hydrocarbon, must be metabolized into an active form (diol–epoxides) to bind to DNA to create DNA adducts. This metabolism is accomplished by the cytochrome P450 (CYP) 1 family enzymes. Therefore, gastric-delivered DMBA is metabolized first in the liver by CYP1A enzymes and subsequently in mammary glands by CYP1A and CYP1B isoforms (Lin et al. 2012; Williams and Phillips 2000). Unlike MNU, the bulky DMBA molecule forms large adducts with G and A residues, leading to excision repair and thus point mutations of undefined specificity (Singer and Kuśmierek 1982).

The efficiency of chemically induced tumor formation in rats is highly dependent on the strain, age, and dosage of carcinogen (Russo and Russo 1996; Welsch 1985). Outbred SD and inbred Wistar-Furth (WF), NSD, and Lewis rats are highly susceptible to DMBA. The inbred Fischer 344 and August Copenhagen Irish (ACI) rats are moderate (Isaacs 1986), while the inbred Copenhagen line is highly resistant to DMBA (Isaacs 1986). Similar strain differences exist when MNU is administered (Isaacs 1986). MNU can be delivered into sensitive strains via intravenous, subcutaneous, or intraperitoneal routes. The gastric route is not needed since MNU does not need to be metabolized in liver. A single dose of MNU at 25 or 50 mg/kg body weight causes tumors with a latency and incidence similar to those observed with DMBA treatment (Russo and Russo 1996). The reasons for strain differences in sensitivity are not well understood (Wood et al. 2002), but a single autosomal genetic allele has been implicated (Isaacs 1986).

Rats reach sexual maturity at approximately 6 weeks of age (Sengupta 2013). During puberty and early adolescence, the rat mammary gland is most susceptible to carcinogen-induced tumorigenesis (Medina 2007). For example, when DMBA (100 mg/kg) was administered intragastrically into SD rats at different ages and monitored for 22 weeks, the four groups treated at young ages (30, 40, 46, and 55 days) all developed tumors with a high incidence (93, 89, 100, and 97%, respectively) and multiplicity (3.4, 3.9, 5.6, and 3.6, respectively), but either or both measurements decreased substantially in the three older groups (70, 140, and 180 days), with the oldest group showing the lowest incidence and multiplicity (54% and 1.4) (Russo et al. 1979). In another experiment, MNU was injected intravenously into SD in two doses (5 mg/100 g body weight/injection, 1 week apart) beginning at the age of 35, 50, 80, 140, or 200 days. When evaluated at 6 months after the initial injection, incidence rates of 100% and 94% were observed in the day 35 and 50 groups, respectively, but the incidence dropped to 59% in the day 80 group, 30% in the day 140 group, and only 22% in the day 200 group (Grubbs et al. 1983b). The two younger groups also showed a higher tumor multiplicity (Grubbs et al. 1983b). The high sensitivity at a young age is believed to be due to high numbers of TEBs and their fast-proliferating cells (Ip 1996; Medina 2007; Russo and Russo 1996). TEBs are maximum at 4–8 weeks of age but disappear in the mature mammary gland at 10–12 weeks of age (Medina 2007). Besides age, tumor incidence rates and the number of tumors per rat also correlate with the dose of the carcinogens administered until a plateau is reached (Huggins et al. 1961; McCormick et al. 1981). In addition, additional treatments following the initial dose of carcinogen accelerate tumor development, and these subsequent treatments have been suggested to cause secondary and collaborative genetic events (Isaacs 1985).

Carcinogen-treated rats first develop intraductal proliferations (alveolar hyperplasia and ductal hyperplasia), which then progress to ductal carcinoma in situ (DCIS) and finally invasive carcinomas. Tumors induced by MNU and DMBA can present different histological forms, as thoroughly examined by Jose Russo & Irma Russo (Russo and Russo 2000). DMBA-induced tumors are mostly papillary and papillary cystic adenocarcinomas and fibroadenomas (which are benign and are characterized by a proliferative connective tissue admixed with normal appearing mammary epithelia of ductal or lobular structures) (Medina 2007). MNU-induced tumors are primarily adenocarcinoma or adenomyoepithelioma (Gil Del Alcazar et al. 2022; Medina 2007). Of note, even some large lesions in these rats are still confined within the duct (therefore DCIS) and surrounded by a basal layer and collagen-rich stroma (Gil Del Alcazar et al. 2022). Also, tumors in these models generally expand with a pushing margin and lack leading strands of tumor cells infiltrating the surrounding stroma (Medina 2007). Distant metastases to lung, bone, or other organs are generally rare (Medina 2007) although in rats treated at a peripubertal age (but not 50 days of age) with MNU, metastases to visceral organs were detected in small proportions (Thompson et al. 1992).

The overwhelming majority of the tumors induced by DMBA or MNU produce estrogen receptor (ER) and progesterone receptor (PR), and they depend on estrogen for continued growth since ovariectomy can block growth of 85–90% of these tumors, as reviewed by Clifford Welsch (1985). Estrogen is critical also for the initiation of these types of tumors since ovariectomy prior to carcinogen treatment can diminish tumor formation (Welsch 1985). Besides, the estrus phase at the time of carcinogen injection affects tumor induction by carcinogens, with the estrus and proestrus phases being more susceptible than diestrus (Lindsey et al. 1981; Ratko and Beattie 1985).

Pregnancy affects human breast cancer risk—while a first pregnancy before the age of 22 decreases the lifetime risk of breast cancer by as much as 50%, a first pregnancy delayed to after 35 increases lifetime breast cancer risk by as much as 40% (Albrektsen et al. 2005; MacMahon et al. 1970), and a pregnancy at any age leads to a short term rise of breast cancer risk (Schedin 2006). Parity status in rats has a substantial impact on sensitivity of the mammary gland to tumor induction by DMBA and MNU (Medina 2007). Mating within a few weeks following carcinogen treatment stimulates mammary tumor development (Dao et al. 1960; Dao and Sunderland 1959; Grubbs et al. 1983a), likely due to pregnancy stimulation of premalignant cell expansion and progression to cancer (Haricharan et al. 2013; Haricharan and Li 2014). Our work in mouse models suggests that this may be due to STAT5, which is normally activated during pregnancy and lactation, abetting precancerous cells in dismantling the apoptosis anticancer barrier that would otherwise slow tumorigenesis (Haricharan et al. 2013). Tumors developed during pregnancy accelerate growth until weaning, when these tumors will usually regress (Ip 1996; Welsch 1985). On the other hand, pregnancy prior to carcinogen administration suppresses tumor development (Ip 1996; Welsch 1985). Protection also occurs if rats were pretreated for 3 weeks with estradiol + progesterone at levels that yield circulating hormone levels similar to those occurring during mid-pregnancy (Medina 2007). The underlying mechanism has been suggested to be pregnancy and pregnancy hormones-induced loss of TEBs and stem cells, reduction of cell proliferation, differentiation of mammary cells, alterations of mammary cell fate, epigenetic and chromatic remodeling, and stromal remodeling, based on work in both rats and mice, as reviewed by several groups (Medina 2005, 2007; Meier-Abt and Bentires-Alj 2014; Russo and Russo 2011; Siwko et al. 2008b).

Tumors induced by both DMBA and MNU do not show any aneuploidy, but specific cancer-driving genetic changes caused by DMBA vs. MNU are quite different. More than 80% of MNU-induced mammary tumors were reported to carry activating *Hras* mutations (primarily codon 12 G->A transition) (Sukumar et al. 1983; Zarbl et al. 1985). Later, Samuelson et al. (2009) confirmed this finding. But when analyzing 71 DMBA-induced mammary tumors, they could not detect hot spot mutations in any *Ras* gene member (*Hras*, *Kras*, and *Nras*) (Samuelson et al. 2009). However, other groups reported mutations in a different hot spot codon of HRAS (codon 61) in low proportions of tumors (~20%) (El-Sohemy and Archer 2000; Kito et al. 1996). Despite these discrepancies, it is evident that DMBA-induced mammary tumors do not involve *Ras* mutations as frequent as MNU-induced tumors, and even when they do, the mutations are different; therefore, these two carcinogens induce mammary tumors through inflicting different types of genetic alterations. Of note, whole genome sequencing of 31 MNU tumors identified additional mutations in several other genes including *Foxa1*, *Brca2*, *Pik3ca*, and *Tp53* (Gil Del Alcazar et al. 2022).

It is not entirely clear why mammary glands in rats are so much more sensitive to DMBA and MNU than other tissues. (This selectivity does not apply in the mouse—DMBA-treated mice develop leukemias and tumors in the skin, lung, stomach, and ovary at significant rates (~25%) often leading to early euthanasia (Medina 2007)). However, three possible explanations are worth noting: (1) Cell proliferation is certainly a factor as discussed above regarding age vs. carcinogen sensitivity, but the gastrointestinal tract and skin, which also go through cycles of rapid proliferation followed by cell shedding, only infrequently present tumors in these carcinogen-treated rats. Perhaps the organotropism of these carcinogens in rats arises from these rapidly expanding mammary cells at puberty in these sensitive rat lines being especially prone to DNA damage and mutations caused by these carcinogens, and/or being less able to repair DNA damage. (Colon cancer is induced in rodents most commonly with the colon-organotrophic 1,2-dimethylhydrazine (DMH) and azoxymethane (AOM) (Rosenberg et al. 2009), while skin cancer is commonly induced by a single topical application of a sub-carcinogenic dose of DMBA followed by repeated applications of a pro-inflammatory phorbol ester, such as 12-O-tetra decanoylphorbol-13-acetate (TPA) (Neagu et al. 2016). MNU can also induce skin tumors if applied topically (Graffi et al. 1967)). (2) Although capable of transforming multiple epithelial tissues to cancer, carcinogen-induced mutated Ras may transform rodent mammary cells more swiftly than the epithelial cells in other organs, and possibly without the need for secondary mutations or other assisting changes, leading to mammary tumor appearance and euthanasia before appearance of gross tumors in other organs—we found that mutated Ras can induce mammary tumors in rats or mice in only a few weeks (Bu and Li 2020, 2024), and Connie Eaves and colleagues reported high sensitivity of human breast epithelial cells to Ras transformation (Nguyen et al. 2015). (3) DMBA does not often involve Ras mutations, but three other factors may contribute to its mammary organotropism. DMBA is a neuroendocrine disruptor leading to increased secretion of estrogen and prolactin, which are themselves breast cancer risk factors (Kerdelhue et al. 2016). Furthermore, high levels of CYP1B in mammary glands facilitate metabolizing DMBA to the final active form. In addition, the lipophilic nature of DMBA might lead to higher levels of accumulation in the adipocyte-rich mammary gland than in other epithelial tissues, therefore inflicting more severe DNA damage than in non-mammary glands. However, these factors apply in mice too; yet, mice do not exhibit high organotropism to DMBA.

Besides carcinogens, radiation has also been found to induce mammary tumors readily. Ionizing radiation, such as X-rays, γ-rays, and neutrons, can damage DNA and initiate tumorigenesis. The mammary gland is one of the tissues with the highest sensitivity of radiation carcinogenesis (Russo and Russo 1996), although radiation in general is less potent than carcinogens in causing mammary tumors (Shellabarger 1972). When applied to susceptible rat strains, such as SD rats, at around 9 weeks of age when sexual maturity has been reached and TEB numbers have already expanded, sublethal doses (either single or fractionated) of radiation, such as X-rays or neutrons, lead to palpable tumors in approximately 5–12 months. Many tumors induced by radiation are primarily benign papillomas and fibroadenomas, while the incidence of carcinomas is much lower than those induced by chemical agents. Most radiation-induced epithelial tumors are hormone receptor-positive and depend on ovaries for continued growth, similar to carcinogen-induced tumors (Russo and Russo 1996). Radiation-induced tumors do not typically carry *Hras* mutations (Imaoka et al. 2007, 2009).

Besides being required for formation and growth of carcinogen-induced tumors in rats, estrogen at high levels can also induce mammary tumors in rats. After continuous administration of exogenous estrogen to achieve blood estrogen levels similar to those experienced by women during the periovulatory phase of the menstrual cycle or during pregnancy, tumors appear with a relatively long latency (Shull et al. 2018). Both 17β-estradiol (E2, the primary form of estrogen made during women's reproductive years) and synthetic estrogens, such as diethylstilbestrol (DES), have been used for this purpose (Shull et al. 2018). They are administered with repeated intravenous injections or chronic release via subcutaneous interscapular pellet or silastic tubing implantation. The optimal age to start hormone treatment is 8–9 weeks. This is about 2–3 weeks after the optimal age for carcinogen treatment. The A-strain Copenhagen Irish (ACI) strain of rats is particularly susceptible to tumor induction by estrogen while SD is resistant, unlike the strain preference observed in carcinogen models. Estrogen treatment leads to diffuse lobuloalveolar hyperplasia rapidly (within 1 week), followed by focal atypical epithelial hyperplasia (~10 weeks), and then palpable tumors with a median latency of ~18 weeks (Shull et al. 2018). These palpable tumors include both ductal carcinoma in situ (DCIS) and invasive carcinomas (Shull et al. 2018). Estrogen-induced tumors produce ER and PR, and they depend on this exogenous estrogen for continued growth—tumors completely regress if E2 implants are removed or if rats are treated with tamoxifen (Harvell et al. 2000; Shull et al. 2018). Exogenous estrogen-initiated mammary tumorigenesis requires intact ovarian functions and progesterone since E2 fails to induce tumors in ovariectomized rats or in intact rats treated with the progesterone receptor antagonist mifepristone (Shull et al. 2018). Interestingly, 70–80% of estrogen-induced tumors exhibit chromosomal aneuploidy, a common feature of human breast cancer (Harvell et al. 2000; Li et al. 2002; Shull et al. 2018), unlike the mostly diploid tumor cells seen in carcinogen-induced mammary tumors. The underlying molecular mechanisms are unclear, but persistent high levels of estrogen may lead to accumulations of excess adducts and cause overexpression of aurora kinase A (AURKA), and oxidative stress (Shull et al. 2018), both of which are implicated in DNA damage and genomic instability.

Carcinogen, radiation, and hormone-induced tumor models provide powerful tools for studying tumorigenesis and progression driven by external and internal risk factors. They are also valuable for evaluating preventive measures and therapeutic drugs (Alečković et al. 2022; Bhat et al. 2001; Tinsley et al. 2023). However, these models have noticeable limitations, which include: (1) Genetic mutations in these models are either not frequently observed in human breast tumors (e.g., *HRAS*) or are unclear, and carcinogen and radiation models lack the chromosomal aneuploidy commonly seen in human breast cancer. (2) Carcinogens and irradiation may not be among the major risk factors in women—for instance, neither DMBA nor MNU has been implicated in the etiology of human breast cancer. (3) Atypical lesions, the earliest breast change known to confer an increased risk of breast cancer, are diagnosed typically in a breast that is already fully developed, although clonal expansions of breast cells with a driver mutation could emerge at a prepubertal stage (Nishimura et al. 2023). While the pubertal age at which rats are most susceptible to chemical inducers suggests adolescent girls at this age may be particularly susceptible to potential harm from certain environmental carcinogens, these carcinogen models build on an abnormally developed ductal tree, decreasing their value for modeling early breast cancer formation and testing new chemoprevention treatments. (4) The overwhelming majority of the tumors in MNU and DMBA-induced tumors do not invade the basement membrane. These in situ ductal carcinomas do not spread to distant organs, largely precluding these models from studies of late stages of breast cancer progression. (5) These tumors are predominantly hormone receptor-positive, precluding their use for modeling other breast cancer sub-types. When considered together, these limitations, particularly the unpredictable and clinically irrelevant genetic alterations, hinder the broader use of these models for studying molecular mechanisms driving breast tumorigenesis and for testing targeted therapies.

8.5 Germline Transgenic and Knockout Rat Models of Breast Cancer

To overcome the limitations of chemical-, hormone-, and radiation-induced tumor models, it is crucial to create tumor models that carry specific oncogenic drivers. This can be accomplished by introducing these genetic drivers into mammary epithelial cells through genetic engineering methods, such as transgenic expression of oncogenes or knockout of tumor suppressor genes. The technology for developing transgenic animal models was first reported in mice in 1981 (Brinster et al. 1981; Gordon and Ruddle 1981) but was not established in rats until a decade later (Hammer et al. 1990; Mullins et al. 1990). Similar to generating a mouse transgenic model, transgenic rats are made by introducing a transgenic construct into fertilized rat oocytes through pronuclear microinjection. The successfully injected eggs are then implanted through microsurgery into the oviduct of a pseudo-pregnant surrogate mother. The resulting pups are screened for the presence of the transgene by genotyping methods such as PCR. The transgene-positive rats are then bred to confirm stable expression and to establish a founder line (Mullins et al. 2002).

However, this process is much more technically challenging and much less efficient in rats than in mice. For example, the generation of transgenic rats requires a continuous infusion of FSH (follicle-stimulating hormone) for superovulation, contrasting with the single injection needed for producing transgenic mice (Mullins et al. 2002). Furthermore, the success rates for producing rat founders are much lower than those for producing mouse founders (Mullins et al. 2002). For instance, in the creation of an *HRAS* transgenic rat line, 1145 embryos underwent pronuclear injection, but only one founder with long-term transgene transmission was established (Asamoto et al. 2000). This low success rate may be attributed to the physical characteristics of rat embryos, which with their less elastic and spongier texture are more susceptible to damage during injection. Furthermore, oviduct transfers in rats tend to be less successful, leading to fewer successful pregnancies and generally smaller litter sizes. Moreover, some of the initial transgenic offspring exhibited mosaicism, suggesting that the transgene integration into the host genome did not occur until after at least one round of cell division (Charreau et al. 1996). On the other hand, the mouse transgenic technologies rapidly became routine. Transgenic models allowed studying specific oncogenic drivers in breast tumorigenesis and therapeutic implications, and they rapidly displaced carcinogen and radiation rat models as the preferred models to study breast cancer. Nevertheless, several transgenic rat mammary tumor models have been reported including those transgenic for human *ERBB2* (i.e., *HER2*), rat *Neu* (a constitutively activated version of *Erbb2*), human *TGFα*, and human *HRAS* (Table 8.2). These models are briefly discussed below:

In 1999, Davies et al. reported the first two transgenic rat models of breast cancer—transgenic *ERBB2* (WT) and *TGFα* (WT) (which encodes a key ligand for members of the ERB family of receptor tyrosine kinases) under the control of the Molony mammary tumor virus (MMTV) long terminal repeats (Davies et al. 1999). Transgenic mRNA expression was detectable only upon pregnancy, and after multiple cycles of pregnancy and lactation, benign lesions appeared including lobular and ductal hyperplasia, fibroadenomas, cystic dilations, and papillary adenomas. A small subset of the rats eventually developed ductal carcinoma in situ and invasive carcinoma, but no metastasis was detected. The ER status was not documented in these models.

In 2002, Watson et al. described a different rat transgenic line expressing cDNA encoding a mutated and constitutively activated version of ERBB2 (also designed as NEU), driven by the MMTV promoter. This line exhibited a different mammary tumorigenic impact (Watson et al. 2002) compared to rats transgenic for human *ERBB2* (wild-type) reported by Davies et al.

Table 8.2 Germline transgenic and knockout rat mammary tumor models

Gene name	Method	References
ERBB2	Transgenic	Davies et al. (1999)
TGFB1	Transgenic	Davies et al. (1999)
Neu	Transgenic	Watson et al. (2002)
Hras	Transgenic	Asamoto et al. (2000), Tsuda et al. (2001)
P53	ES cells knockout	Tong et al. (2010), Yan et al. (2012)
Brca1	Carcinogen-based germline mutatation	Zan et al. (2003)
Brca2	Carcinogen-based germline mutatation	Zan et al. (2003)
Brca1	CRISPR/Cas9-based L63X mutation	Nakamura et al. (2022)
Nf1	CRISPR/Cas9-based indel	Dischinger et al. (2018)

(1999). Specifically, transgenic *Neu* females did not develop mammary tumors, but transgenic males did. This observation led Watson et al. to treat these females with androgen, which led to mammary tumors. The resulting tumors were positive for the androgen receptor (AR), but negative for both estrogen and progesterone receptors (Watson et al. 2002). These data are a bit surprising since mice transgenic for *Neu* developed tumors with high penetrance and a short latency (Ursini-Siegel et al. 2007).

HRAS has also been engineered as a transgene into rats. The HRAS128 rat line carries three copies of the WT human *HRAS* gene and its own promoter region (Asamoto et al. 2000). These rats were not studied for tumor development on their own, but they were found to exhibit high susceptibility to mammary tumorigenesis induced by MNU (Asamoto et al. 2000; Tsuda et al. 2001). Histological analyses of these tumors revealed solid tubular or papillary tubular adenocarcinomas. The ER status and the occurrence of metastasis were not reported. In addition, transgenic rats lines carrying 3–7 copies of wild-type rat *Hras* or *Kras* under the control of rat *Hras* promoter have been reported to exhibit no substantial impact on mammary glands when compared to non-transgenic littermates (Thompson et al. 2002). Unexpectedly, they were found to have a decreased sensitivity to MNU-induced tumorigenesis compared to non-transgenic littermates (Thompson et al. 2002).

Tumor suppressor genes need to be studied in knockout animals. The establishment of mouse embryonic stem (ES) cell lines in 1981 by Martin Evans and Gail Martin (Evans and Kaufman 1981; Martin 1981) led to the creation of knockout mice by Mario R. Capecchi, Martin Evans, and Oliver Smithies in 1989 (Koller et al. 1989; Kuehn et al. 1987; Mansour et al. 1990). After that, creating knockout mice quickly became routine, and now virtually all known cancer-significant genes have been knocked out in mice. However, rat ES cells weren't available until 2008 (Buehr et al. 2008; Li et al. 2008). In 2010, Tong et al. reported the successful deletion of *Tp53* in rat ES cells by homologous recombination and the birth of the first ES cell-based knockout rat (Tong et al. 2010) (Of note, a year earlier, Geurts et al. reported the successful use of injection of mRNA encoding zinc-finger nucleases into the one-cell stage of rat embryos to disrupt endogenous genes (Geurts et al. 2009), which led to the creation of several knockout rat lines later on (Huang et al. 2012; Rumi et al. 2014)). Even after this initial success, adapting the mouse knockout technology to rats has been challenging due to difficulties in maintaining rat ES cell pluripotency using mouse ES cell culture conditions although recent advances in culture conditions and pluripotency manipulation have eased this roadblock (Buehr et al. 2008; Chenouard et al. 2021; Jacob et al. 2010). Two additional factors contributed to the challenges of engineering knockout rats—the inefficient incorporation of genetically modified ES cells into developing rat embryos leading to fewer chimeric offspring compared to the relatively high efficiency in mice, and the low chances of germline transmission from chimeric offspring. As a result, only a small number of rat lines from ES knockouts have been reported, and only a few of them have been characterized for mammary tumorigenesis (Table 8.2). For example, *Tp53* heterozygote knockout rats generated by this method developed mammary tumors (with a frequency of 20%) and other tumors in a pattern similar to Li-Fraumeni patients (Tong et al. 2010; Yan et al. 2012), while *Tp53* knockout mice rarely developed epithelial tumors before they succumbed to lymphomas and sarcomas.

Prior to the application of these genetic engineering tools, two hereditary breast cancer genes had been deactivated in rats by a more primitive method. *Brca1* and *Brca2* knockout rat models were created through chemical mutagenesis—male outbred SD rats were treated with a split dose of ENU (2 × 60 mg/kg) to induce mutations in sperm (Zan et al. 2003). These rats were then bred with wild-type female SD rats to produce F1 pups, which were screened for the presence of mutant alleles of *Brca1* and *Brca2* using Agouti yeast cDNA/gDNA truncation assays (Zan et al. 2003). This was a labor-extensive and inefficient approach that potentially introduced mutations in other alleles too. Notwithstanding, the resulting *Brca1+/−* rats were viable, whereas *Brca1−/−*

rats died during embryogenesis (Zan et al. 2003), similar to what was observed in mice (Dine and Deng 2013). On the other hand, both *Brca2+/−* and *Brca2−/−* rats were viable, although *Brca2−/−* rats were notably smaller and were infertile compared to Brca2+/− and wild-type littermates. Unlike human *BRCA1/2* carriers who have a lifetime risk of up to 80% for breast cancer, neither *Brca1+/−* nor *Brca2+/−* rats developed mammary tumors, a trait they shared with mouse carriers (Evers and Jonkers 2006). Furthermore, *Brca1+/−* and *Brca2+/−* rats did not even show increased mammary tumor multiplicity compared to their wild-type littermates after treatment with ENU (Zan et al. 2003). However, these *Brca2−/−* rats exhibited underdeveloped mammary glands, and later in life they succumbed to a variety of tumors, among which osteosarcoma was the most common type (Zan et al. 2003).

With the arrival of CRISPR-Cas9 technology, many knockout rat lines have been produced using methods that bypassed the need for ES cells. CRISPR-Cas9-mediated direct genome editing of rat zygotes also resulted in multiple knockout rat models relevant to breast cancer research. For example, the *Nf1* knockout rat line was generated by injecting two single-guide RNAs (sgRNAs) and Cas9 mRNA into the fertilized eggs from SD rats (Dischinger et al. 2018). These eggs were then implanted into pseudopregnant foster mothers. Out of the 19 pups born, 18 carried insertion and deletion (indel) mutations. Remarkably, all 11 female rats from this generation (G0) developed multiple mammary tumors at the relatively young age of 6–8 weeks, presenting a 100% penetrance rate. These tumors displayed a mixed variety of histological types, including acinar, solid, ductular, and cystic, and they stained positive for ER and PR.

A *Brca1* CRISPR knockout rat line was generated using a method similar to that employed for generating the *Nf1* knockout line, except that a short stretch of oligodeoxynucleotides serving as a homology-directed repair (HDR) donor was co-injected along with the sgRNA and Cas9 mRNA to achieve a precise genetic alteration (Nakamura et al. 2022). The resulting nonsense point mutation at codon 63 (Leucine), which is a founder mutation in patients, led to the birth of Brca1L63X rats. Rats homozygous for this truncation mutant died embryonically. Heterozygous Brca1L63X rats develop normally with no mammary tumors. Following MNU treatment, they did not even develop more tumors than their wild-type littermates, similar to *Brca1+/−* rats generated by ENU mutagenesis. Interestingly, however, Brca1L63X/+ rats, but not their wild-type littermates, exhibited dose-dependent mammary carcinogenesis in response to ionizing radiation, suggesting that *BRCA1* carriers in the human population may be at increased risk to radiation. The resulting tumors showed no evidence of somatic mutations of the wild-type allele, unlike tumors in human carriers, and produced low levels of estrogen receptor α staining (Nakamura et al. 2022).

8.6 Somatic Rat Mammary Tumor Models by Retrovirus/Lentivirus-Mediated Oncogene Delivery

While having played a critical role in understanding cancer biology, transgenic models of mice or rats both suffer a few critical drawbacks. Transgenic expression before the mammary gland is fully developed may impair mammary stem cells, mammary cell differentiation and homeostasis, and normal mammary gland development, thus subsequently impacting tumorigenesis. Expression of a transgenic oncogene in the entire mammary epithelia fails to mimic the evolution of sporadic breast cancers in humans. To overcome these spatiotemporal drawbacks of transgenic rodent models in general and to bypass the technical difficulty in engineering transgenic rats, an alternative approach has been employed to introduce oncogenic drivers in rats to model breast cancer. This approach involves the somatic delivery of an oncogene or other relevant genetic materials into mammary epithelial cells in situ in fully developed mammary glands. This is accomplished through the intraductal injection of a viral vector. Controlling the viral dosage allows for infection and therefore oncogene expression in tiny fractions of the mammary cell population. Each rat mammary gland consists of a ductal tree lined by epithelial cells, all converging into a single opening at the tip of the nipple. This structure allows easy access for viral vectors, which can be delivered into the lumen of the ductal tree via intraductal injection. The "up-the-teat" injection technique is the most commonly used for this purpose. Michael Gould at the University of Wisconsin initially reported this approach to mammary tumor induction in 1991 (Wang et al. 1991a, b).

Several types of viral vectors may be used for the intraductal delivery of genetic material, including vectors derived from retrovirus (Thompson et al. 1998; Wang et al. 1991a, b; Woditschka et al. 2006), lentivirus (Bu and Li 2020, 2024), adenovirus (a double-stranded DNA virus), and adenovirus-associated virus (a single-stranded DNA virus; AAV) (Bu and Li 2024). All of these vectors are engineered to be "gutless" so that they express no viral genes to avoid immune rejection. Retrovirus and lentivirus vectors integrate permanently into the host genome, thus stably introducing the genes of interest into the mammary epithelial cells. While retrovirus requires cell proliferation for efficient genomic integration, lentivirus integrates into the genome of any cell it encounters, whether proliferating or quiescent. Adenoviral and AAV vectors infect both proliferating and quiescent cells, but they do not integrate into the genome of infected cells, and they get diluted out after a few cycles of cell proliferation. Therefore, genes cloned into these vectors are expressed for a short window of time. This feature can be advantageous when the gene of interest needs to be expressed for only a short amount of time, such as the Cre recombinase gene, which is used to delete floxed tumor suppressor genes. Due to the architecture of the mammary gland, where the luminal epithelium is largely insulated from the underlying basal layer by various cell–cell junctions between luminal cells, viruses delivered into the ductal lumen primarily infect primarily luminal epithelial cells (Bu and Li 2024), the counterpart of which is the primary cell of origin for human breast cancer.

The luminal epithelial layer consists of distinct cell subtypes, including luminal stem cells, progenitor cells, and several groups of differentiated cells. To selectively infect specific cell subsets within this population, the TVA technology can be utilized. This approach allows avian leukosis virus-derived RCAS vectors or pseudotyped lentiviral vectors to infect only specific cells expressing TVA (tumor virus A), the receptor for RCAS. We have adapted this technology to mice for studying breast cancer origin in different subsets of mammary cells, by making transgenic mice expressing *Tva* using several cell type/differentiation-selective promoters including MMTV, WAP, cytokeratin 6a, and the Wnt-responding synthetic promoter TOP (Bu and Li 2024). We plan to make *Tva* transgenic rats in the near future.

Compared to traditional transgenic rat models, where the gene of interest is introduced at the stage of fertilized eggs through microinjection, the intraductal virus injection method offers several advantages:

1. Viral intraductal injection eliminates the time-consuming process of creating a transgenic rat line for each gene of interest. Therefore, many genetic alterations can be tested swiftly.
2. Infection and thus oncogenic activation occurs in a small number of cells in otherwise completely normal mammary epithelia, closely mimicking the evolution of sporadic human breast cancer, which accounts for over 90% of all breast cancer cases.
3. Viral intraductal injection circumvents potential disruptions to early mammary gland formation caused by the premature and mammary gland-wide expression of a potential oncogenic driver engineered into the germline (although this shortcoming of conventional transgenic models can be mitigated by inducible transgenic expression).
4. Viral intraductal injection allows for the introduction of a gene of interest at any desired time after puberty including different stages of reproduction. This temporal control is important for studying the impact of genes

of interest specifically at distinct stages of adult mammary development.

5. One viral vector can be used to introduce multiple genes of interest.
6. Multiple viral vectors can be co-injected to study genetic collaboration. Co-injected cells will be enriched over time if the two genetic events collaborate in driving cancer formation.
7. Viral vectors can be injected into existing lines of genetically engineered models to study genetic interactions between a virus-mediated gene and a previously well-characterized transgenic or knockout gene.
8. Viral vectors can be injected into existing lines of rodent models whose stromal cells are modified by genetic engineering or other means to investigate the impact of stromal cells on cancer evolution initiated by virus-mediated activation of oncogenic drivers.
9. Viral vectors can be injected into any strain of rodents, eliminating the need to breed from one strain into another, a common time-consuming task in using genetically engineered germline models.
10. When combined with the TVA technology, this viral method can introduce the gene of interest into a specific cell population. This modification can help study the cell origin of tumorigenesis and conduct cell lineage-tracing assays in the mammary glands.

Somatic rat mammary tumor models via virus vector-mediated oncogene delivery were initially reported using retroviral vectors (Wang et al. 1991a, b). Since retrovirus infects primarily proliferating cells, Michael Gould's lab treated rats with the mammary mitogen perphenazine (an antipsychotic drug that increases serum prolactin levels) before they injected the retroviral vector pJR carrying an activated form of *Hras* or *Neu* (Wang et al. 1991a, b). Among the pJR-*Hras* injected rats, palpable tumors were detected within 5 weeks. The resulting tumors exhibited a wide range of histopathologies ranging from well differentiated to anaplastic morphologies (Wang et al. 1991b). Among the pJR-*Neu* injected rats, carcinomas started to appear in 3 weeks. The resulting tumors are cribriform-comedocarcinomas. Importantly, progression from hyperplasia to carcinoma in situ and further to infiltrating carcinoma was also observed in this model, as in carcinogen models. Furthermore, approximately 50% of the tumors are hormone-dependent and can be prevented or slowed by tamoxifen treatment (Wang et al. 1991a). This contrasts with ER being generally absent in *Neu* transgenic rat or mouse tumors. In humans, approximately 50% of HER2-positive tumors are also ER+ and benefit from endocrine therapy.

To overcome the cell proliferation limitation of retroviral vectors and any concern about mitogen pre-treatment disturbing the homeostasis seen in a resting mammary gland, we have taken lentiviral vectors for oncogene delivery in mice (Bu et al. 2009; Siwko et al. 2008a) and adapted them for delivery into rat mammary glands (Bu and Li 2020, 2024). This approach allows us to target any luminal cells, regardless of their proliferation status, and eliminates the need for mammary mitogen pre-treatment. By performing an intraductal injection of the lentiviral vector FUCGW carrying the mutated oncogene *HrasQ61L* into SD rats (8-week-old; 7×10^7 IUs/gland) (Fig. 8.5), we induced tumors with a median onset time of only 25 days (Bu and Li 2020). These tumors were classified as adenocarcinomas and were strongly positive for both ER and PR (Fig. 8.5). Furthermore, these tumors were hormone-dependent, as demonstrated by tumor shrinkage following ovariectomy (Fig. 8.5) (Bu and Li 2020). These findings are in dramatic contrast to tumors induced by the same *HasQ61L* lentivirus delivered intraductally into mice. The resulting tumors in mice are metaplastic carcinomas with heavy squamous differentiation and no hormone receptors (Bu et al. 2023; Bu and Li 2024). It is yet to be determined whether this tumor difference in rats vs. mice is due to certain unique properties of rat luminal epithelial cells or to the rat mammary microenvironment.

Besides *Hras*, intraductal injection of a lentivirus vector carrying *Braf* (Fig. 8.6) or a mutated *Pik3ca* (Bu and Li 2020) also induced hormone receptor-positive tumors in rats. We are testing

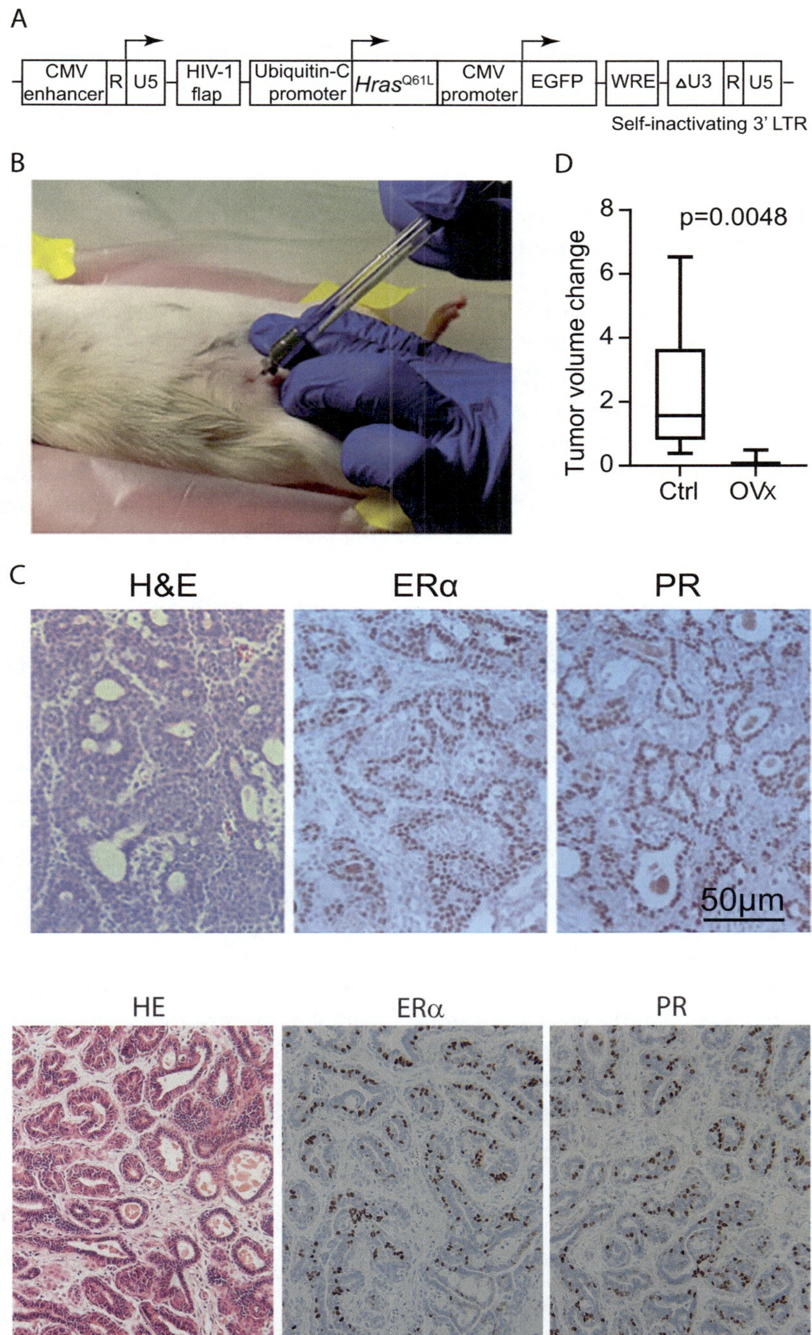

Fig. 8.5 ER$^+$ rat mammary tumors generated by intraductal injection of lentivirus vector carrying HrasQ61L. (**a**) Diagram of the lentiviral vector carrying HrasQ61L (Bu and Li 2020). (**b**) A picture showing a Hamilton syringe fitted with a blunt needle being inserted into the nipple opening. (**c**) Tumor size changes at 2 weeks following ovariectomy. (**d**) H&E and immunohistochemical images of estrogen receptor α (ERα) and progesterone receptor (PR) in tumors

Fig. 8.6 ER$^+$ rat mammary tumors generated by intraductal injection of lentivirus vector carrying *Braf*^{V600E}. H&E and immunohistochemical staining for estrogen receptor α (ERα) and progesterone receptor (PR)

other oncogenic drivers to determine whether they also cause ER+ tumors in rats. Nevertheless, these rat models provide a valuable tool for studying ER+ breast cancer in an immunocompetent setting, which has been difficult in mice since few of them develop ER+ tumors.

This intraductal virus-based somatic gene delivery method provides a robust and convenient way to create clinically relevant rodent models of breast cancer (Bu and Li 2024). However, there are also some drawbacks and limitations that should be considered when using this method in both rats and mice:

1. Each animal needs to be injected intraductally with virus, and up-the-teat injection requires extensive training before reproducible injection can be achieved. In contrast, experimental animals from genetically engineered lines can be easily produced from standard breeding of previously created and characterized stocks of animals.
2. The gene of interest in the virus vector is under the control of exogenous promoters (e.g., viral LTR or a housekeeping gene). Therefore, these virus-delivered genes lack the physiological transcriptional control inherent in their native loci.
3. Retroviruses and lentiviruses largely integrate randomly into the genome of the infected cells, leading to unpredictable copy numbers and position effects on expression of the gene of interest. Therefore, oncogene expression levels may vary among the individual infected cells. High expressers are likely to be more competitive and are therefore selected for in tumor evolution.
4. The random integration of lentivirus/retrovirus into the host genome may disrupt the expression of the host genes at the integration site, potentially complicating the interpretation of the results from these experiments, although this is a highly unlikely event since the overwhelming majority of the genome does not encode and there are two alleles of most genes except for those on sex chromosomes.
5. Epitope tags and markers such as HA, FLAG, green fluorescent protein (GFP), and luciferase are often included in these viral vectors for virus titer determination and for detection of the infected cells. However, these tags and markers could trigger a host immune reaction, confounding the tumor immune microenvironment.

These concerns potentially dampen the value of these models in mimicking human breast cancer and should be considered in virus construction and data interpretation. For example, oncogene drivers should be of a rat origin if their human or mouse orthologs are substantially different in amino acid sequences. When studying tumor microenvironment, every effort should be made to avoid the use of tags and markers that may provoke an immune response to these ectopic epitopes unrelated to tumorigenesis in patients.

8.7 Somatic Gene-Editing-Based Rat Mammary Tumor Models

The CRISPR-Cas9 technology enables the direct modification of endogenous genes precisely at their native loci, providing a more accurate representation of gene function and regulation in physiological conditions (Anzalone et al. 2020; Bu et al. 2023; Bu and Li 2024; Kaltenbacher et al. 2022; Katti et al. 2022). This technology could overcome major limitations of producing cancer models using virus-mediated delivery of oncogenes. Multiple mouse tumor models have been created by somatic indel-editing of tumor suppressor genes. This process is mediated by sgRNA-directed, Cas9-catalyzed double-strand breaks at specific genomic sites, followed by error-prone non-homologous end joining repair (NHEJ), leading to insertions and deletions, and consequently, loss of function (Anzalone et al. 2020). To harness these technical advances for modeling breast cancer in rats, we injected intraductally an AAV vector carrying sgRNA against *Nf1*, *Tp53*, or both in rats transgenic for *Cas9* (Fig. 8.7). Indel editing of *Tp53* led to tumor development in a few months, but indel editing of *Nf1* or both *Tp53* and Nf1 led to tumors in only a few weeks. The resulting tumors in all three groups are adenocarcinomas and express ER and PR (Fig. 8.7). At least in the case of *Nf1* and *Tp53/Nf1* indel editing, the tumors are dependent on ovarian hormones (the *Tp53* group of tumors is being tested). Compared to the germline

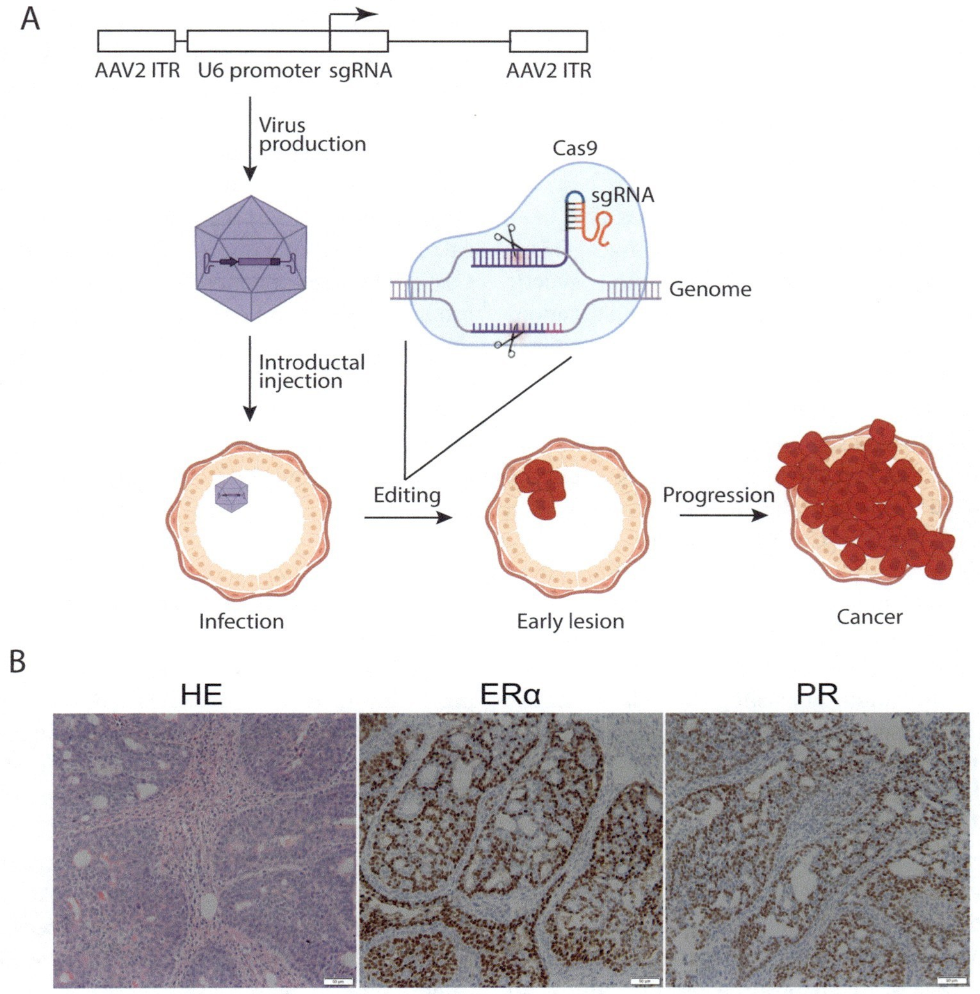

Fig. 8.7 ER⁺ rat mammary tumors generated by somatic editing of the *Nf1* gene. (**a**) Diagram of the process of somatic editing-induced tumorigenesis in rats. (**b**) H&E staining and immunohistochemical staining for estrogen receptor α (ERα) and progesterone receptor (PR) in tumors

knockout rat models, this somatic genome editing method provides several benefits:

1. Time and Cost Efficiency: Generating germline knockout rat lines is a labor-intensive process that can take a few years, while somatic editing requires only constructing an AAV vector carrying sgRNAs, producing viruses, confirming their targeting efficacy and specificity (in vitro and/or in vivo), and performing intraductal injection into a group of *Cas9*-transgenic rats.
2. Clinical Relevance: Germline knockout, especially if both alleles are disrupted, may impair embryogenesis and organ development, producing models that may not mimic the great majority of human breast cancers, which are sporadic. Somatic genome editing takes place at any adult age with temporal control, thereby offering models that may better mimic sporadic human breast cancers.
3. Multiplexing Capability: Producing compound mutant rodent lines usually involves breeding multiple lines together, a time-

consuming process. Simultaneous editing of multiple genes is easily achievable with somatic genome editing, as demonstrated by our concurrent somatic editing of both *Nf1* and *Tp53*.

The CRISPR-Cas9 technology has also been used to engineer precise point mutations. This is important since most cancer-causing genetic alterations in humans involve point mutations that disable tumor suppressor genes or activate proto-oncogenes. Introducing missense mutations into proto-oncogenes can be achieved using various Cas9-based methods (Anzalone et al. 2020): (1) The deaminase-mediated base-editing approach introduces transition mutations using a nuclease-deficient Cas9 fused with either a cytidine or adenine deaminase. However, this method often results in bystander mutations and lacks the capability to perform all possible base changes (Annunziato et al. 2020; Zafra et al. 2018). (2) The prime editor, consisting of a Cas9 nickase fused with a reverse transcriptase and a pegRNA, can theoretically introduce any point mutation and has been successfully used to introduce the S45F mutation into β-catenin and induce liver tumors in mice (Liu et al. 2021). However, its high-pressure injection method is currently not practical for many organs. (3) The incorporation of homology-directed repair (HDR) into vectors carrying sgRNA enables the introduction of all 12 types of point mutations (Anzalone et al. 2020). This HDR-mediated precise editing is now widely used in cell cultures (Anzalone et al. 2020; Dou et al. 2023; Katti et al. 2022). However, its application in cancer modeling has been less successful. For instance, Platt and colleagues designed an editing vector for both indel-editing of *Tp53* and *Lkb1* tumor suppressor genes as well as the creation of a missense mutation in the *Kras* locus in the respiratory epithelium to model lung cancer (Platt et al. 2014). While the resulting tumors showed high levels of indel mutations in *Tp53* and *Lkb1*, the *KrasG12D* missense mutation was practically undetectable (Platt et al. 2014). This finding is contrary to the well-documented strong cooperative effect between KrasG12D and loss of function of P53 or LKB1 in mouse lung tumorigenesis models (Ji et al. 2007), suggesting that their HDR-based *Kras* editing may not be highly successful. Another group used a similar vector targeting these three genes to create lung cancer mouse models, but the efficiency of *Kras* editing remained a concern (Winters et al. 2017). To overcome these technical challenges, we have refined the CRISPR/Cas9/HDR-based method for somatic editing of proto-oncogenes in vivo and achieved high flexibility and efficiency (Bu et al. 2023). Using this improved approach, we successfully generated several mouse models of breast cancer (Bu et al. 2023). Now we have also successfully adapted this updated vector for introducing somatic point mutations in rats including *Esr1* and *Pik3ca*.

8.8 Future Development

Technological advances in rat genetic engineering, viral-mediated oncogene delivery, and somatic genome editing are unlocking significant potential for rapidly creating rat models of breast cancer and enhancing their resemblance to the initiation and evolution of human breast cancer. These rat models could help answer many critical questions that remain unresolved. A major strength is the clinically relevant ER+ breast cancer models—a feat that has not been achieved using mouse models. Despite constituting about 70% of all human breast cancers, ER+ breast cancer is poorly represented in current animal models, especially in terms of genetic alterations, hormone-dependence, metastasis, tumor microenvironment, and immunological changes. The lack of such models has hampered our understanding of the development and progression of ER+ breast cancer, thereby hindering the identification of new preventative measures and treatments.

Addressing this research gap involves establishing rat mammary tumor models that carry common oncogenic genetic alterations found in clinical ER+ breast cancer specimens. Somatic genome-editing techniques can be deployed swiftly and accurately for this purpose. Systemic profiling of these rat ER+ tumor models at DNA, epigenome, RNA, protein, metabolic, and immunological levels will shed light on the mechanisms underlying ER+ breast cancer development and progression, guiding the identification of new preventative and therapeutic strategies.

Human ER+ breast cancers typically show low immune cell infiltration and resistance to immune checkpoint treatment. These new rat models may offer an opportunity to investigate why these tumors are devoid of immune cells and how they can be converted into immune "hot" so that they can be treated effectively with immune checkpoint therapy. More importantly, since patient ER+ tumors are treated with surgical resection and then adjuvant endocrine therapy to kill and suppress tumor cells that have disseminated, these rat models offer an excellent opportunity to investigate clinically relevant questions including how ER+ tumor cells survive in distant organs and escape treatment.

Human ER+ breast cancer primarily metastasizes to the bones (Kennecke et al. 2010; Smid et al. 2008), but there are no germline or somatic mouse models of ER+ breast cancer that spontaneously metastasize to bone. All our knowledge regarding ER+ breast cancer bone metastasis has been gleaned from xenografted models, which lack the immune component that is now known to be critical in cancer progression and treatment. These rat ER+ models may offer a rare opening to study how ER+ tumors survive in bones and develop resistance to therapy and whether they can be converted into immune hot for immune checkpoint treatment. Initial characterization of these rat models indicates that some of their tumors indeed disseminate to bones.

Rats may also be valuable for studying other subtypes of breast cancer. Lobular breast cancer comprises approximately 15% of human breast cancer cases and expresses ER. Patients with lobular tumors are treated with endocrine therapy (Oesterreich et al. 2022). Deactivation of E-cadherin is a key feature of these tumors. However, tumors in mice harboring knockout of *Cdh1* (which encodes E-cadherin) do not fully mimic human lobular tumors, especially in lacking estrogen dependence (Annunziato et al. 2016; Doornebal et al. 2013). Since rat mammary glands mimic human breasts more closely than mouse mammary tissues, it will be interesting to test whether *Cdh1* knockout in rat mammary cells leads to lobular tumors that better mimic human lobular breast cancer. In the same vein, rat models of HER2+ and triple-negative breast cancer (TNBC) may also provide valuable insights, particular in metastasis and therapy. HER2 breast cancer and TNBC exhibit metastases more often in visceral organs including liver, lung, and brain (Dent et al. 2009; Gerratana et al. 2015). Comparing these rat models among themselves and with mouse models may help understand organotropic spread of these subtypes of breast cancer.

In conclusion, the breakthroughs in rat mammary tumor modeling techniques are offering unprecedented opportunities to advance our understanding of human breast cancer and have paved the way for investigating new preventative and therapeutic strategies. Progress in this field in the coming years, especially concerning ER+ breast cancer metastasis, is expected to be rapid and exciting.

Acknowledgments The authors thank Drs. Chandandeep Nagi and Carolina Gutierrez for assistance in pathological confirmation of rat tumors and Drs. Jeffrey Rosen and Gary Chamness for critical reading of this manuscript.

References

Adkins RM, Gelke EL, Rowe D, Honeycutt RL (2001) Molecular phylogeny and divergence time estimates for major rodent groups: evidence from multiple genes. Mol Biol Evol 18:777–791

Aitman T, Dhillon P, Geurts AM (2016) A RATional choice for translational research? Dis Model Mech 9:1069–1072

Albrektsen G, Heuch I, Hansen S, Kvale G (2005) Breast cancer risk by age at birth, time since birth and time intervals between births: exploring interaction effects. Br J Cancer 92:167–175

Alečković M, Cristea S, Gil Del Alcazar CR, Yan P, Ding L, Krop ED, Harper NW, Rojas Jimenez E, Lu D, Gulvady AC et al (2022) Breast cancer prevention by short-term inhibition of TGFβ signaling. Nat Commun 13:7558

Annunziato S, Kas SM, Nethe M, Yucel H, Del Bravo J, Pritchard C, Bin Ali R, van Gerwen B, Siteur B, Drenth AP et al (2016) Modeling invasive lobular breast carcinoma by CRISPR/Cas9-mediated somatic genome editing of the mammary gland. Genes Dev 30:1470–1480

Annunziato S, Lutz C, Henneman L, Bhin J, Wong K, Siteur B, van Gerwen B, de Korte-Grimmerink R, Zafra MP, Schatoff EM et al (2020) In situ CRISPR-Cas9 base editing for the development of genetically engineered mouse models of breast cancer. EMBO J 39:e102169

Anzalone AV, Koblan LW, Liu DR (2020) Genome editing with CRISPR-Cas nucleases, base editors, transposases and prime editors. Nat Biotechnol 38:824–844

Asamoto M, Ochiya T, Toriyama-Baba H, Ota T, Sekiya T, Terada M, Tsuda H (2000) Transgenic rats carrying human c-Ha-ras proto-oncogenes are highly susceptible to N-methyl-N-nitrosourea mammary carcinogenesis. Carcinogenesis 21:243–249

Bhat KP, Lantvit D, Christov K, Mehta RG, Moon RC, Pezzuto JM (2001) Estrogenic and antiestrogenic properties of resveratrol in mammary tumor models. Cancer Res 61:7456–7463

Boulanger CA, Wagner KU, Smith GH (2004) Parity-induced mouse mammary epithelial cells are pluripotent, self-renewing and sensitive to TGF-beta1 expression. Oncogene 24:552–560

Brinster RL, Chen HY, Trumbauer M, Senear AW, Warren R, Palmiter RD (1981) Somatic expression of herpes thymidine kinase in mice following injection of a fusion gene into eggs. Cell 27:223–231

Bu W, Li Y (2020) Intraductal injection of lentivirus vectors for stably introducing genes into rat mammary epithelial cells in vivo. J Mammary Gland Biol Neoplasia 25:389–396

Bu W, Li Y (2024) Advances in immunocompetent mouse and rat models. Cold Spring Harb Perspect Med 14(3):a041328

Bu W, Xin L, Toneff M, Li L, Li Y (2009) Lentivirus vectors for stably introducing genes into mammary epithelial cells in vivo. J Mammary Gland Biol Neoplasia 14:401–404

Bu W, Creighton CJ, Heavener KS, Gutierrez C, Dou Y, Ku AT, Zhang Y, Jiang W, Urrutia J, Jiang W et al (2023) Efficient cancer modeling through CRISPR-Cas9/HDR-based somatic precision gene editing in mice. Sci Adv 9:eade0059

Bucher JR (2002) The National Toxicology Program rodent bioassay: designs, interpretations, and scientific contributions. Ann N Y Acad Sci 982:198–207

Buehr M, Meek S, Blair K, Yang J, Ure J, Silva J, McLay R, Hall J, Ying QL, Smith A (2008) Capture of authentic embryonic stem cells from rat blastocysts. Cell 135:1287–1298

Cardiff RD, Jindal S, Treuting PM, Going JJ, Gusterson B, Thompson HJ (2018) Mammary gland. In: Treuting P, Dintzis S, Montine KS (eds) Comparative anatomy and histology. Elsevier, pp 487–509

Charreau B, Tesson L, Soulillou JP, Pourcel C, Anegon I (1996) Transgenesis in rats: technical aspects and models. Transgenic Res 5:223–234

Chenouard V, Remy S, Tesson L, Menoret S, Ouisse LH, Cherifi Y, Anegon I (2021) Advances in genome editing and application to the generation of genetically modified rat models. Front Genet 12:615491

Dao TL, Sunderland H (1959) Mammary carcinogenesis by 3-methylcholanthrene. I. Hormonal aspects in tumor induction and growth. J Natl Cancer Inst 23:567–585

Dao TL, Bock FG, Greiner MJ (1960) Mammary carcinogenesis by 3-methylcholanthrene. II. Inhibitory effect of pregnancy and lactation on tumor induction. J Natl Cancer Inst 25:991–1003

Davies BR, Platt-Higgins AM, Schmidt G, Rudland PS (1999) Development of hyperplasias, preneoplasias, and mammary tumors in MMTV-c-erbB-2 and MMTV-TGFalpha transgenic rats. Am J Pathol 155:303–314

Dent R, Hanna WM, Trudeau M, Rawlinson E, Sun P, Narod SA (2009) Pattern of metastatic spread in triple-negative breast cancer. Breast Cancer Res Treat 115:423–428

Dine J, Deng CX (2013) Mouse models of BRCA1 and their application to breast cancer research. Cancer Metastasis Rev 32:25–37

Dischinger PS, Tovar EA, Essenburg CJ, Madaj ZB, Gardner EE, Callaghan ME, Turner AN, Challa AK, Kempston T, Eagleson B et al (2018) NF1 deficiency correlates with estrogen receptor signaling and diminished survival in breast cancer. NPJ Breast Cancer 4:29

Doornebal CW, Klarenbeek S, Braumuller TM, Klijn CN, Ciampricotti M, Hau CS, Hollmann MW, Jonkers J, de Visser KE (2013) A preclinical mouse model of invasive lobular breast cancer metastasis. Cancer Res 73:353–363

Dou Y, Katsnelson L, Gritsenko MA, Hu Y, Reva B, Hong R, Wang YT, Kolodziejczak I, Lu RJ, Tsai CF et al (2023) Proteogenomic insights suggest druggable pathways in endometrial carcinoma. Cancer Cell 41:1586–1605.e1515

Dwinell MR (2010) Online tools for understanding rat physiology. Brief Bioinform 11:431–439

El-Sohemy A, Archer MC (2000) Inhibition of N-methyl-N-nitrosourea- and 7,12-dimethylbenz[a] anthracene-induced rat mammary tumorigenesis by dietary cholesterol is independent of Ha-Ras mutations. Carcinogenesis 21:827–831

Evans MJ, Kaufman MH (1981) Establishment in culture of pluripotential cells from mouse embryos. Nature 292:154–156

Evers B, Jonkers J (2006) Mouse models of BRCA1 and BRCA2 deficiency: past lessons, current understanding and future prospects. Oncogene 25:5885–5897

Gerratana L, Fanotto V, Bonotto M, Bolzonello S, Minisini AM, Fasola G, Puglisi F (2015) Pattern of metastasis and outcome in patients with breast cancer. Clin Exp Metastasis 32:125–133

Geurts AM, Cost GJ, Freyvert Y, Zeitler B, Miller JC, Choi VM, Jenkins SS, Wood A, Cui X, Meng X et al (2009) Knockout rats via embryo microinjection of zinc-finger nucleases. Science 325:433

Gibbs RA, Worley KC, Okwuonu G, Lewis L, Hawes A, Gill R, Holt RA, Adams MD, Amanatides PG, Barnstead M et al (2004) Genome sequence of the

Brown Norway rat yields insights into mammalian evolution. Nature 428:493–521

Gil Del Alcazar CR, Trinh A, Aleckovic M, Rojas Jimenez E, Harper NW, Oliphant MUJ, Xie S, Krop ED, Lulseged B, Murphy KC et al (2022) Insights into immune escape during tumor evolution and response to immunotherapy using a rat model of breast cancer. Cancer Immunol Res 10:680–697

Gordon JW, Ruddle FH (1981) Integration and stable germ line transmission of genes injected into mouse pronuclei. Science 214:1244–1246

Graffi A, Hoffmann A, Schütt M (1967) Nmethyl-N-nitrosourea as a strong topical carcinogen when painted on skin of rodents. Nature 214:611

Grubbs CJ, Hill DL, McDonough KC, Peckham JC (1983a) N-nitroso-N-methylurea-induced mammary carcinogenesis: effect of pregnancy on preneoplastic cells. J Natl Cancer Inst 71:625–628

Grubbs CJ, Peckham JC, Cato KD (1983b) Mammary carcinogenesis in rats in relation to age at time of N-nitroso-N-methylurea administration. J Natl Cancer Inst 70:209–212

Hammer RE, Maika SD, Richardson JA, Tang JP, Taurog JD (1990) Spontaneous inflammatory disease in transgenic rats expressing HLA-B27 and human beta 2m: an animal model of HLA-B27-associated human disorders. Cell 63:1099–1112

Haricharan S, Li Y (2014) STAT signaling in mammary gland differentiation, cell survival and tumorigenesis. Mol Cell Endocrinol 382:560–569

Haricharan S, Dong J, Hein S, Reddy JP, Du Z, Toneff M, Holloway K, Hilsenbeck SG, Huang S, Atkinson R et al (2013) Mechanism and preclinical prevention of increased breast cancer risk caused by pregnancy. eLife 2:e00996

Harvell DM, Strecker TE, Tochacek M, Xie B, Pennington KL, McComb RD, Roy SK, Shull JD (2000) Rat strain-specific actions of 17beta-estradiol in the mammary gland: correlation between estrogen-induced lobuloalveolar hyperplasia and susceptibility to estrogen-induced mammary cancers. Proc Natl Acad Sci USA 97:2779–2784

Hedrich HJ (2020) Taxonomy and stocks and strains. In: Suckow MA, Hankenson FC, Wilson RP, Foley PL (eds) The laboratory rat. Elsevier, pp 47–76

Homberg JR, Wöhr M, Alenina N (2017) Comeback of the rat in biomedical research. ACS Chem Neurosci 8:900–903

Huang G, Ashton C, Kumbhani DS, Ying QL (2011) Genetic manipulations in the rat: progress and prospects. Curr Opin Nephrol Hypertens 20:391–399

Huang L, Be X, Tchaparian EH, Colletti AE, Roberts J, Langley M, Ling Y, Wong BK, Jin L (2012) Deletion of Abcg2 has differential effects on excretion and pharmacokinetics of probe substrates in rats. J Pharmacol Exp Ther 343:316–324

Huggins C, Grand LC, Brillantes FP (1961) Mammary cancer induced by a single feeding of polymucular hydrocarbons, and its suppression. Nature 189:204–207

Imaoka T, Nishimura M, Kakinuma S, Hatano Y, Ohmachi Y, Yoshinaga S, Kawano A, Maekawa A, Shimada Y (2007) High relative biologic effectiveness of carbon ion radiation on induction of rat mammary carcinoma and its lack of H-ras and Tp53 mutations. Int J Radiat Oncol Biol Phys 69:194–203

Imaoka T, Nishimura M, Iizuka D, Daino K, Takabatake T, Okamoto M, Kakinuma S, Shimada Y (2009) Radiation-induced mammary carcinogenesis in rodent models: what's different from chemical carcinogenesis? J Radiat Res 50:281–293

Ip C (1996) Mammary tumorigenesis and chemoprevention studies in carcinogen-treated rats. J Mammary Gland Biol Neoplasia 1:37–47

Isaacs JT (1985) Determination of the number of events required for mammary carcinogenesis in the Sprague-Dawley female rat. Cancer Res 45:4827–4832

Isaacs JT (1986) Genetic control of resistance to chemically induced mammary adenocarcinogenesis in the rat. Cancer Res 46:3958–3963

Jacob HJ, Lazar J, Dwinell MR, Moreno C, Geurts AM (2010) Gene targeting in the rat: advances and opportunities. Trends Genet 26:510–518

Ji H, Ramsey MR, Hayes DN, Fan C, McNamara K, Kozlowski P, Torrice C, Wu MC, Shimamura T, Perera SA et al (2007) LKB1 modulates lung cancer differentiation and metastasis. Nature 448:807–810

Kaltenbacher T, Löprich J, Maresch R, Weber J, Müller S, Oellinger R, Groß N, Griger J, de Andrade KN, Avramopoulos P et al (2022) CRISPR somatic genome engineering and cancer modeling in the mouse pancreas and liver. Nat Protoc 17:1142–1188

Katti A, Diaz BJ, Caragine CM, Sanjana NE, Dow LE (2022) CRISPR in cancer biology and therapy. Nat Rev Cancer 22:259–279

Kennecke H, Yerushalmi R, Woods R, Cheang MC, Voduc D, Speers CH, Nielsen TO, Gelmon K (2010) Metastatic behavior of breast cancer subtypes. J Clin Oncol 28:3271–3277

Kerdelhue B, Forest C, Coumoul X (2016) Dimethyl-Benz(a)anthracene: a mammary carcinogen and a neuroendocrine disruptor. Biochim Open 3:49–55

King HD (1918) Studies on inbreeding. I. The effects in inbreeding on the growth and variability in the body weight of the albino rat. J Exp Zool 26:1–54

Kito K, Kihana T, Sugita A, Murao S, Akehi S, Sato M, Tachibana M, Kimura S, Ueda N (1996) Incidence of p53 and Ha-ras gene mutations in chemically induced rat mammary carcinomas. Mol Carcinog 17:78–83

Koller BH, Hagemann LJ, Doetschman T, Hagaman JR, Huang S, Williams PJ, First NL, Maeda N, Smithies O (1989) Germ-line transmission of a planned alteration made in a hypoxanthine phosphoribosyltransferase gene by homologous recombination in embryonic stem cells. Proc Natl Acad Sci USA 86:8927–8931

Kuehn MR, Bradley A, Robertson EJ, Evans MJ (1987) A potential animal model for Lesch-Nyhan syndrome through introduction of HPRT mutations into mice. Nature 326:295–298

Larsson M, Asp E, Johansson LXC, Röhme D, Levan G (1998) Sublocalizing the centromeric region in linkage groups from three metacentric rat chromosomes by FISH. Mamm Genome 9:479–481

Li JJ, Papa D, Davis MF, Weroha SJ, Aldaz CM, El-Bayoumy K, Ballenger J, Tawfik O, Li SA (2002) Ploidy differences between hormone- and chemical carcinogen-induced rat mammary neoplasms: comparison to invasive human ductal breast cancer. Mol Carcinog 33:56–65

Li P, Tong C, Mehrian-Shai R, Jia L, Wu N, Yan Y, Maxson RE, Schulze EN, Song H, Hsieh CL et al (2008) Germline competent embryonic stem cells derived from rat blastocysts. Cell 135:1299–1310

Lin Y, Yao Y, Liu S, Wang L, Moorthy B, Xiong D, Cheng T, Ding X, Gu J (2012) Role of mammary epithelial and stromal P450 enzymes in the clearance and metabolic activation of 7,12-dimethylbenz(a)anthracene in mice. Toxicol Lett 212:97–105

Lindsey WF, Das Gupta TK, Beattie CW (1981) Influence of the estrous cycle during carcinogen exposure on nitrosomethylurea-induced rat mammary carcinoma. Cancer Res 41:3857–3862

Liu P, Liang SQ, Zheng C, Mintzer E, Zhao YG, Ponnienselvan K, Mir A, Sontheimer EJ, Gao G, Flotte TR et al (2021) Improved prime editors enable pathogenic allele correction and cancer modelling in adult mice. Nat Commun 12:2121

MacMahon B, Cole P, Lin TM, Lowe CR, Mirra AP, Ravnihar B, Salber EJ, Valaoras VG, Yuasa S (1970) Age at first birth and breast cancer risk. Bull World Health Organ 43:209–221

Mansour SL, Thomas KR, Deng CX, Capecchi MR (1990) Introduction of a lacZ reporter gene into the mouse int-2 locus by homologous recombination. Proc Natl Acad Sci USA 87:7688–7692

Martin GR (1981) Isolation of a pluripotent cell line from early mouse embryos cultured in medium conditioned by teratocarcinoma stem cells. Proc Natl Acad Sci USA 78:7634–7638

Mashimo T, Serikawa T (2009) Rat resources in biomedical research. Curr Pharm Biotechnol 10:214–220

McCormick DL, Adamowski CB, Fiks A, Moon RC (1981) Lifetime dose-response relationships for mammary tumor induction by a single administration of N-methyl-N-nitrosourea. Cancer Res 41:1690–1694

Medina D (2005) Mammary developmental fate and breast cancer risk. Endocr Relat Cancer 12:483–495

Medina D (2007) Chemical carcinogenesis of rat and mouse mammary glands. Breast Dis 28:63–68

Meier-Abt F, Bentires-Alj M (2014) How pregnancy at early age protects against breast cancer. Trends Mol Med 20:143–153

Modlinska K, Pisula W (2020) The Norway rat, from an obnoxious pest to a laboratory pet. eLife 9:e50651

Mullins JJ, Peters J, Ganten D (1990) Fulminant hypertension in transgenic rats harbouring the mouse Ren-2 gene. Nature 344:541–544

Mullins LJ, Brooker G, Mullins JJ (2002) Transgenesis in the rat. Methods Mol Biol 180:255–270

Muss GG, Carleton MD (2005) Superfamily Muroidea. In: Wilson DE, Reeder DM (eds) Mammal species of the world: a taxonomic and geographic reference. The Johns Hopkins University Press

Nakamura Y, Kubota J, Nishimura Y, Nagata K, Nishimura M, Daino K, Ishikawa A, Kaneko T, Mashimo T, Kokubo T et al (2022) Brca1(L63X) (/+) rat is a novel model of human BRCA1 deficiency displaying susceptibility to radiation-induced mammary cancer. Cancer Sci 113:3362–3375

Neagu M, Caruntu C, Constantin C, Boda D, Zurac S, Spandidos DA, Tsatsakis AM (2016) Chemically induced skin carcinogenesis: updates in experimental models (review). Oncol Rep 35:2516–2528

Nguyen LV, Pellacani D, Lefort S, Kannan N, Osako T, Makarem M, Cox CL, Kennedy W, Beer P, Carles A et al (2015) Barcoding reveals complex clonal dynamics of de novo transformed human mammary cells. Nature 528:267–271

Nishimura T, Kakiuchi N, Yoshida K, Sakurai T, Kataoka TR, Kondoh E, Chigusa Y, Kawai M, Sawada M, Inoue T et al (2023) Evolutionary histories of breast cancer and related clones. Nature 620:607–614

Oesterreich S, Nasrazadani A, Zou J, Carleton N, Onger T, Wright MD, Li Y, Demanelis K, Ramaswamy B, Tseng G et al (2022) Clinicopathological features and outcomes comparing patients with invasive ductal and lobular breast cancer. J Natl Cancer Inst 114:1511–1522

Philipeaux J (1856) Note sur le extirpation des capsules surrenales chez les rats albinos (Mus ratus). C R Acad Sci 43:904–906

Platt RJ, Chen S, Zhou Y, Yim MJ, Swiech L, Kempton HR, Dahlman JE, Parnas O, Eisenhaure TM, Jovanovic M et al (2014) CRISPR-Cas9 knockin mice for genome editing and cancer modeling. Cell 159:440–455

Ratko TA, Beattie CW (1985) Estrous cycle modification of rat mammary tumor induction by a single dose of N-methyl-N-nitrosourea. Cancer Res 45:3042–3047

Richardson KK, Richardson FC, Crosby RM, Swenberg JA, Skopek TR (1987) DNA base changes and alkylation following in vivo exposure of Escherichia coli to N-methyl-N-nitrosourea or N-ethyl-N-nitrosourea. Proc Natl Acad Sci USA 84:344–348

Rosenberg DW, Giardina C, Tanaka T (2009) Mouse models for the study of colon carcinogenesis. Carcinogenesis 30:183–196

Rumi MA, Dhakal P, Kubota K, Chakraborty D, Lei T, Larson MA, Wolfe MW, Roby KF, Vivian JL, Soares MJ (2014) Generation of Esr1-knockout rats using zinc finger nuclease-mediated genome editing. Endocrinology 155:1991–1999

Russo J, Russo IH (1996) Experimentally induced mammary tumors in rats. Breast Cancer Res Treat 39:7–20

Russo J, Russo IH (2000) Atlas and histologic classification of tumors of the rat mammary gland. J Mammary Gland Biol Neoplasia 5:187–200

Russo IH, Russo J (2011) Pregnancy-induced changes in breast cancer risk. J Mammary Gland Biol Neoplasia 16:221–233

Russo J, Wilgus G, Russo IH (1979) Susceptibility of the mammary gland to carcinogenesis: I Differentiation of the mammary gland as determinant of tumor incidence and type of lesion. Am J Pathol 96:721–736

Samuelson E, Nilsson J, Walentinsson A, Szpirer C, Behboudi A (2009) Absence of Ras mutations in rat DMBA-induced mammary tumors. Mol Carcinog 48:150–155

Schedin P (2006) Pregnancy-associated breast cancer and metastasis. Nat Rev Cancer 6:281–291

Sengupta P (2013) The laboratory rat: relating its age with human's. Int J Prev Med 4:624–630

Shellabarger CJ (1972) Mammary neoplastic response of Lewis and Sprague-Dawley female rats to 7,12-dimethylbenz(a)anthracene or x-ray. Cancer Res 32:883–885

Shull JD, Dennison KL, Chack AC, Trentham-Dietz A (2018) Rat models of 17β-estradiol-induced mammary cancer reveal novel insights into breast cancer etiology and prevention. Physiol Genomics 50:215–234

Singer B, Kuśmierek JT (1982) Chemical mutagenesis. Annu Rev Biochem 51:655–693

Siwko SK, Bu W, Gutierrez C, Lewis B, Jechlinger M, Schaffhausen B, Li Y (2008a) Lentivirus-mediated oncogene introduction into mammary cells in vivo induces tumors. Neoplasia 10:653–662

Siwko SK, Dong J, Lewis MT, Liu H, Hilsenbeck SG, Li Y (2008b) Evidence that an early pregnancy causes a persistent decrease in the number of functional mammary epithelial stem cells--implications for pregnancy-induced protection against breast cancer. Stem Cells 26:3205–3209

Smid M, Wang Y, Zhang Y, Sieuwerts AM, Yu J, Klijn JG, Foekens JA, Martens JW (2008) Subtypes of breast cancer show preferential site of relapse. Cancer Res 68:3108–3114

Smith JR, Bolton ER, Dwinell MR (2019) The rat: a model used in biomedical research. Methods Mol Biol 2018:1–41

Sreekumar A, Toneff MJ, Toh E, Roarty K, Creighton CJ, Belka GK, Lee DK, Xu J, Chodosh LA, Richards JS et al (2017) WNT-mediated regulation of FOXO1 constitutes a critical axis maintaining pubertal mammary stem cell homeostasis. Dev Cell 43:436–448

Staats J (1966) The laboratory mouse. In: Greeen EL (ed) Biology of the laboratory mouse. McGraw-Hill, New York, pp 1–9

Suckow MA, Baker HJ (2020) Historical foundations. In: Suckow MA, Hankenson FC, Wilson RP, Foley PL (eds) The laboratory rat. Elsevier, pp 3–46

Suckow MA, Weisbroth SH, Franklin CL (2006) The laboratory rat. Elsevier Science, San Diego

Sukumar S, Notario V, Martin-Zanca D, Barbacid M (1983) Induction of mammary carcinomas in rats by nitroso-methylurea involves malignant activation of H-ras-1 locus by single point mutations. Nature 306:658–661

Szpirer C (2020) Rat models of human diseases and related phenotypes: a systematic inventory of the causative genes. J Biomed Sci 27:84

Szpirer C (2022) Rat models of human diseases and related phenotypes: a novel inventory of causative genes. Mamm Genome 33:88–90

Thompson HJ, Adlakha H, Singh M (1992) Effect of carcinogen dose and age at administration on induction of mammary carcinogenesis by 1-methyl-1-nitrosourea. Carcinogenesis 13:1535–1539

Thompson TA, Kim K, Gould MN (1998) Harvey ras results in a higher frequency of mammary carcinomas than Kirsten ras after direct retroviral transfer into the rat mammary gland. Cancer Res 58:5097–5104

Thompson TA, Haag JD, Lindstrom MJ, Griep AE, Lohse JK, Gould MN (2002) Decreased susceptibility to NMU-induced mammary carcinogenesis in transgenic rats carrying multiple copies of a rat ras gene driven by the rat Harvey ras promoter. Oncogene 21:2797–2804

Tinsley HN, Mathew B, Chen X, Maxuitenko YY, Li N, Lowe WM, Whitt JD, Zhang W, Gary BD, Keeton AB et al (2023) Novel non-cyclooxygenase inhibitory derivative of Sulindac inhibits breast cancer cell growth in vitro and reduces mammary tumorigenesis in rats. Cancers 15

Tong C, Li P, Wu NL, Yan Y, Ying QL (2010) Production of p53 gene knockout rats by homologous recombination in embryonic stem cells. Nature 467:211–213

Tsuda H, Asamoto M, Ochiya T, Toriyama-Baba H, Naito A, Ota T, Sekiya T, Terada M (2001) High susceptibility of transgenic rats carrying the human c-Ha-ras proto-oncogene to chemically-induced mammary carcinogenesis. Mutat Res 477:173–182

Ursini-Siegel J, Schade B, Cardiff RD, Muller WJ (2007) Insights from transgenic mouse models of ERBB2-induced breast cancer. Nat Rev Cancer 7:389–397

Wang B, Kennan WS, Yasukawa-Barnes J, Lindstrom MJ, Gould MN (1991a) Frequent induction of mammary carcinomas following neu oncogene transfer into in situ mammary epithelial cells of susceptible and resistant rat strains. Cancer Res 51:5649–5654

Wang BC, Kennan WS, Yasukawa-Barnes J, Lindstrom MJ, Gould MN (1991b) Carcinoma induction following direct in situ transfer of v-Ha-ras into rat mammary epithelial cells using replication-defective retrovirus vectors. Cancer Res 51:2642–2648

Wang SJ, Laulederkind SJF, Zhao Y, Hayman GT, Smith JR, Tutaj M, Thota J, Tutaj MA, Hoffman MJ, Bolton ER et al (2019) Integrated curation and data mining for disease and phenotype models at the rat genome database. Database 2019

Watson PA, Kim K, Chen KS, Gould MN (2002) Androgen-dependent mammary carcinogenesis in rats transgenic for the Neu proto-oncogene. Cancer Cell 2:67–79

Welsch CW (1985) Host factors affecting the growth of carcinogen-induced rat mammary carcinomas: a review and tribute to Charles Brenton Huggins. Cancer Res 45:3415–3443

Williams JA, Phillips DH (2000) Mammary expression of xenobiotic metabolizing enzymes and their potential role in breast cancer. Cancer Res 60:4667–4677

Winters IP, Chiou SH, Paulk NK, McFarland CD, Lalgudi PV, Ma RK, Lisowski L, Connolly AJ, Petrov DA, Kay MA et al (2017) Multiplexed in vivo homology-directed repair and tumor barcoding enables parallel quantification of Kras variant oncogenicity. Nat Commun 8:2053

Woditschka S, Haag JD, Waller JL, Monson DM, Hitt AA, Brose HL, Hu R, Zheng Y, Watson PA, Kim K et al (2006) Neu-induced retroviral rat mammary carcinogenesis: a novel chemoprevention model for both hormonally responsive and nonresponsive mammary carcinomas. Cancer Res 66:6884–6891

Wolfe KH, Sharp PM (1993) Mammalian gene evolution: nucleotide sequence divergence between mouse and rat. J Mol Evol 37:441–456

Wood GA, Korkola JE, Archer MC (2002) Tissue-specific resistance to cancer development in the rat: phenotypes of tumor-modifier genes. Carcinogenesis 23:1–9

Wu X, Wang Y (2012) Fossil materials and migrations of Mus musculus and Rattus norvegicus. Res China's Front Archaeol 1:1–9

Yan HX, Wu HP, Ashton C, Tong C, Ying QL (2012) Rats deficient for p53 are susceptible to spontaneous and carcinogen-induced tumorigenesis. Carcinogenesis 33:2001–2005

Zafra MP, Schatoff EM, Katti A, Foronda M, Breinig M, Schweitzer AY, Simon A, Han T, Goswami S, Montgomery E et al (2018) Optimized base editors enable efficient editing in cells, organoids and mice. Nat Biotechnol 36:888–893

Zan Y, Haag JD, Chen KS, Shepel LA, Wigington D, Wang YR, Hu R, Lopez-Guajardo CC, Brose HL, Porter KI et al (2003) Production of knockout rats using ENU mutagenesis and a yeast-based screening assay. Nat Biotechnol 21:645–651

Zarbl H, Sukumar S, Arthur AV, Martin-Zanca D, Barbacid M (1985) Direct mutagenesis of Ha-ras-1 oncogenes by N-nitroso-N-methylurea during initiation of mammary carcinogenesis in rats. Nature 315:382–385

Zeiger E (2017) Reflections on a career and on the history of genetic toxicity testing in the National Toxicology Program. Mutat Res Rev Mutat Res 773:282–292

Zeng L, Ming C, Li Y, Su LY, Su YH, Otecko NO, Dalecky A, Donnellan S, Aplin K, Liu XH et al (2018) Out of southern East Asia of the Brown rat revealed by large-scale genome sequencing. Mol Biol Evol 35:149–158

Part III

Development and Cancer: Cells of Origin and Heterogeneity

Therese Sørlie and Robert Clarke

Breast cancer's heterogeneity stems from the intrinsic properties of breast epithelial precursor cells and the influence of the microenvironment. Key areas of focus include the identification of cells of origin, the regulatory mechanisms governing cell fate, and the implications for cancer classification.

In Chap. 9, Jane Visvader and her colleague from the University of Melbourne, Australia, explain how both intrinsic and extrinsic mechanisms contribute to the profound heterogeneity observed in breast cancer. The intrinsic characteristics of breast epithelial precursor cells, or "cells of origin," influence tumor phenotype and susceptibility to mutagenesis upon exposure to oncogenic stimuli. Molecular profiling has revealed strong concordance between the gene expression profiles of breast cancer subtypes and specific cell types within normal breast epithelium. Mouse models and patient-derived breast tissues are critical for delineating the normal mammary stem cell hierarchy and identifying targets of neoplastic transformation. Additionally, the microenvironment of premalignant cells can influence tumor initiation, offering potential targets for cancer prevention.

In Chap. 10, Alexandra Van Keymeulen from Université Libre de Bruxelles, Belgium, describes how cell fate regulation in breast development occurs predominantly postnatally and involves the microenvironment, transcription factors, and master regulators. These factors are essential for determining basal and luminal cell identities and their fate choices, such as differentiating into ER-positive or ER-negative cells. Oncogene expression can induce reprogramming and change the fate of mammary epithelial cells before tumor appearance, playing a crucial role in tumorigenesis. Understanding these regulatory mechanisms provides insights into how cell fate decisions contribute to breast cancer development.

In Chap. 11, Richard Iggo and his colleague from the University of Bordeaux, France, explain how the classification of breast cancer through cell

---

T. Sørlie · R. Clarke
Oslo, Norway

Manchester, UK

identity is based on the structure of the mammary epithelium, which consists of an inner luminal layer with ER-positive hormone-sensing cells and ER-negative alveolar/secretory cells, and an outer basal layer with myoepithelial/stem cells. The Intrinsic classification system categorizes hormone-sensing tumors into luminal A/B and HER2-E/molecular apocrine/LAR classes, and alveolar/secretory tumors into the basal-like class. The human tendency to develop hormone-sensing cell tumors, possibly due to specific genetic events during adolescence, further highlights the need for precise classification systems.

By exploring the origins, regulatory mechanisms, and classification of breast cancer, this part of the book aims to enhance our understanding of the disease's heterogeneity and inform the development of targeted therapies.

9 Cells-of-Origin of Breast Cancer and Intertumoral Heterogeneity

Rachel Joyce and Jane E. Visvader

Abstract

Both intrinsic and extrinsic mechanisms underpin the profound intertumoral heterogeneity in breast cancer. Increasing evidence suggests that the intrinsic characteristics of breast epithelial precursor cells may influence tumour phenotype. These "cells-of-origin" of cancer preside in normal breast tissue and are uniquely susceptible to mutagenesis upon exposure to distinct oncogenic stimuli. Notably, molecular profiling studies have revealed strong concordance between the gene expression profiles of breast cancer subtypes and discrete cell types within the normal breast epithelium. Further characterisation of cells-of-origin of breast cancer requires comprehensive delineation of the normal mammary stem cell hierarchy. To this end, mouse models have provided valuable tools for exploring stem and progenitor cell function and identifying potential targets of neoplastic transformation via in vivo lineage-tracing studies. Nonetheless, the murine mammary differentiation hierarchy does not fully recapitulate human biology, and complementary studies using patient-direct breast tissue are critical. There is also accumulating evidence that extrinsic factors such as the microenvironment of premalignant cells can influence tumour initiation, highlighting opportunities for targeting cancer cells-of-origin via deconvolution of the premalignant epithelial niche. Pertinently, the identification of premalignant clones and targetable molecular perturbations responsible for driving their oncogenic transformation has critical implications for disease management and prevention.

Keywords

Breast cancer · Cells-of-origin of cancer · Mammary gland development · *BRCA1* · *BRCA2*

Key Points

1. The relative tumour-forming potential of distinct mammary epithelial cell types is highly context-specific.
2. The lineage-specificity of premalignant cells can directly influence their susceptibility to certain oncogenic events, and their intrinsic molecular characteristics may be conserved through the journey of oncogenic transformation.

R. Joyce · J. E. Visvader (✉)
Cancer Biology and Stem Cells Division, The Walter and Eliza Hall Institute of Medical Research, Parkville, VIC, Wurundjeri Country, Melbourne, Australia

Department of Medical Biology, The University of Melbourne, Parkville, VIC, Wurundjeri Country, Melbourne, Australia
e-mail: visvader@wehi.edu.au

T. Sørlie, R. B. Clarke (eds.), *A Guide to Breast Cancer Research*, Advances in Experimental Medicine and Biology 1464, https://doi.org/10.1007/978-3-031-70875-6_9

3. Hormone receptor-negative luminal progenitor cells have emerged as important targets in *BRCA1*-mutant hereditary breast cancer.
4. Extrinsic factors can influence precursor cells to drive intertumoral heterogeneity in breast cancer.
5. Interrogating putative cells-of-origin of heritable breast cancers may reveal clinically actionable cellular perturbations responsible for driving tumour development and inform targeted anticancer therapy design.

9.1 Introduction

Breast cancer remains the most commonly diagnosed cancer globally and is responsible for a high proportion of cancer-associated mortalities; approximately one woman is estimated to die each minute from the disease (Sung et al. 2021). As molecular profiling technologies paint increasingly resolved pictures of breast cancer genomic, transcriptomic and proteomic landscapes, remarkable heterogeneity has become evident at both the single cell and spatial levels. Understanding the fundamental stem and progenitor cell biology underlying normal mammary gland development can provide significant insights into breast tumour aetiology and offer critical opportunities for the identification of novel therapeutic strategies for breast cancer treatment and prevention. This chapter will explore the cell-of-origin model of intertumoral heterogeneity as it relates to breast cancer development and its application to identifying novel strategies for anticancer therapies, with a focus on *BRCA*-mutant hereditary breast cancers.

9.2 Intertumoral Heterogeneity in Breast Cancer

In the early 2000s, transcriptional profiling of breast tumours and downstream hierarchical clustering using intrinsic gene expression resolved four principle molecular subtypes of breast cancer: basal-like, ERBB2 overexpressing/HER2-enriched, luminal A, luminal B (Perou et al. 2000; Sørlie et al. 2001, 2003), and this was subsequently extended to a larger dataset (Koboldt et al. 2012). In 2007, an additional subgroup was defined, the claudin-low subgroup (Herschkowitz et al. 2007), which may also be reflective of a distinct cellular state (Fougner et al. 2020). Normal-like tumours have also been described but show significant contamination with normal breast tissue and thus remain poorly understood. Histopathological characteristics and immunophenotyping on the basis of KI67, HER2 and estrogen receptor (ER) and progesterone receptor (PR) expression are often used as intrinsic markers to stratify patient breast tumours into clinical subtypes: HER2-enriched tumours express HER2 through focal amplification or increased transcription, have a high proliferative index and are frequently ER/PR-negative; luminal cancers express ER/PR, although the luminal B subtype has a high proliferative index while luminal A tumours express the highest levels of hormone receptors (HRs) and a low proliferative index; basal-like breast tumours have a high proliferative index and are ER/PR/HER2-negative; claudin-low tumours also tend to lack ER/PR/HER2 expression and express mesenchymal characteristics, as well as low levels of adhesion and proliferation proteins (Prat et al. 2010; Harbeck et al. 2019). This immunophenotypic and histopathological approach to breast tumour subtyping enables clinicians to coordinate a more tailored strategy for treatment and decision-making throughout the course of disease (reviewed in Harbeck et al. 2019; Nolan et al. 2023). In recent years, transcriptomic profiling assays for rapid and refined clinical breast cancer subtyping have emerged, including the Prosigna assay, which has shown promise for providing improved prognostic patient data in retrospective trials (Parker et al. 2009), and is now being prospectively trialled in the OPTIMA study (ISRCTN42400492).

A proteomic approach to breast cancer classification has also been made possible due to advances in high-resolution mass spectrometry technologies and computational tools (Mann et al. 2013). Several studies have now shown that proteomic profiling and downstream unsupervised hierarchical clustering can be reliably used to stratify breast cancers into subtypes which are generally reflective of those identified via molecular profiling (Tyanova et al. 2016; Johansson et al. 2019; Asleh et al. 2022). These analyses have been particularly helpful in uncovering heterogeneity amongst basal-like breast cancers, which are relatively homogeneous at the mRNA level (Sørlie et al. 2003), including identification of "immune-hot" and "immune cold" basal-like subtypes (Johansson et al. 2019; Asleh et al. 2022). Molecular profiling of patient tumours at the single-cell level has uncovered an unprecedented degree of intratumoral heterogeneity in breast cancers, including the presence of multiple intrinsic molecular subtypes within a single tumour (Chung et al. 2017; Wu et al. 2021). Notably, the influence of these smaller cellular subsets on overall breast tumour behaviour and their clinical relevance in disease remain uncertain. The integration of single-cell sequencing, spatial transcriptomics and immunophenotyping has enabled spatial mapping of tumour neighbourhoods and suggested that nine unique "ecotypes" of breast cancer are associated with distinct clinical outcomes (Wu et al. 2021).

Historically, two central models have been put forth to explain the biological mechanisms underlying intertumoral heterogeneity observed amongst cancers: the genetic mutation and the cell-of-origin hypotheses. The genetic mutation model predicts that the phenotype of a tumour is dependent on the type of oncogenic mutation that occurs in a given cell. Alternatively, the cell-of-origin of cancer model predicts that tumour phenotype is a direct reflection of the intrinsic nature of the precursor cell that is initially exposed to an oncogenic insult (Visvader 2011). Stem and lineage-restricted progenitor cells within the differentiation hierarchy are prime candidates for malignant transformation owing to their proliferative potential and self-renewal capacity. Indeed, the lifetime risk of cancer has been linked to the total number of stem cell divisions that maintain tissue homeostasis over an average lifespan (Tomasetti et al. 2017). Of note, even though the initial driver mutation may occur in a stem cell, transformation may only be manifest once the stem cell has differentiated to a committed progenitor cell, exemplified by chronic myeloid leukaemia (Lytle et al. 2018). In the case of breast cancer, long-term protection conferred by a single early pregnancy and increased incidence associated with irradiation in teenagers underscore the contribution of long-lived breast stem cells to oncogenesis (Pike et al. 1981; Land and McGregor 1979). Remarkably, recent phylogenetic analyses of early evolutionary events in breast tissue indicated that mutations can be acquired in early puberty (Nishimura et al. 2023). It is also possible for differentiated cells to serve as cancer cells-of-origin due to cellular plasticity within the stem cell hierarchy, where context-specific dedifferentiation may lead to the acquisition of self-renewal properties (Schwitalla et al. 2013; Tetteh et al. 2015; Sutherland and Visvader 2015). The lineage-specificity of premalignant cells has been shown to directly influence their susceptibility to certain oncogenic events in mouse models (reviewed in Visvader 2011; Balani et al. 2017), and elucidation of the molecular mechanisms underpinning oncogenic transformation of precursor cells has proven especially valuable for hereditary breast cancer (see below). In addition to influencing primary tumour development, cells-of-origin of cancer have been implicated in promoting tumour relapse: recent studies on leukaemias have revealed the existence of premalignant haematopoietic stem cells, which evade chemotherapy and persist during remission (Shlush et al. 2014; Corces-Zimmerman et al. 2014). Thus, the identification and characterisation of mammary epithelial subsets that serve as putative cancer cells-of-origin can provide valuable biological insights into breast cancer development and relapse and may inform design of effective cancer treatment and prevention strategies.

Although the cell-of-origin can profoundly impact tumour subtype, genotype also has a deterministic role. For example, targeting *Rb1* and/or *Trp53* mutations to mammary progenitor cells in transgenic mouse models supports a role for genetic lesions in directly influencing tumour phenotype (Jiang et al. 2010). Moreover, targeting different mutations to luminal progenitor

(LP) cells using BLG-cre also demonstrated that genetic drivers are key determinants of tumour phenotype (Melchor et al. 2014). Substantial evidence has accumulated over the past two decades indicating that the genetic mutation and cell-of-origin models of intertumoral heterogeneity are not mutually exclusive but cooperate with one another, in concert with microenvironmental factors, to yield diverse tumour phenotypes (Itzkowitz and Yio 2004; Tlsty and Coussens 2006; Schwitalla et al. 2013).

9.3 The Mammary Stem Cell Hierarchy as a Framework for Identifying Cells-of-Origin of Cancer

Human breast tissue comprises a branched ductal epithelial system that extends inward from the nipple into the surrounding fat pad, where it interacts with various subsets of fibroblasts, immune cells, endothelial cells and adipocytes. Luminal cells constitute the inner layer of the ductal tree while myoepithelial cells form the outer (basal) epithelial layer. The ductal tree terminates in terminal ductal lobular units (TDLUs), with each TDLU consisting of a small cluster of lobules emanating from a terminal duct (Wellings et al. 1975). During pregnancy, these units undergo differentiation to produce and secrete milk in preparation for lactation. Although mice lack TDLUs, mouse mammary glands contain alveolar cells which terminally differentiate during pregnancy to likely perform an analogous function. Notably, there is evidence that TDLUs, rather than ductal regions, serve as the major sites of breast cancer initiation (Wellings 1980; Russo et al. 1982). The extensive regeneration and remodelling that the mammary gland undergoes during puberty, pregnancy and involution is orchestrated through the mammary stem cell (MaSC) hierarchy, a simplified model of which may be described as follows: the MaSC sits at the top of the hierarchy and differentiates into increasingly lineage-restricted intermediates, including HR-positive (HR^+) ductal LPs; HR-negative (HR^-) alveolar LPs; basal/myoepithelial progenitors; and differentiated ductal, alveolar and myoepithelial cells (Visvader 2009). Although there are substantial parallels between the differentiation hierarchies in mice and humans, distinct cell populations can be resolved using the same or similar cell surface markers (Fu et al. 2020). In humans, EPCAM and CD49f readily fractionate the mammary epithelium into $EPCAM^+CD49f^-$ mature luminal, $EPCAM^+CD49f^+$ LP, $EPCAM^-CD49f^+$ basal/myoepithelial (enriched for MaSCs) and $EPCAM^-CD49f^-$ stromal cells (Lim et al. 2009), whereas in mice, EpCAM and CD49f only distinguish the basal and luminal compartments such that $EpCAM^{hi}CD49f^+$ defines luminal cells and $EpCAM^{med}CD49f^{hi}$ defines basal cells (Shehata et al. 2012). The markers CD24 and CD29 are also commonly used to differentiate the mouse luminal and basal mammary populations; luminal cells are $CD24^+CD29^{lo}$ whereas basal cells are $CD24^+CD29^{hi}$ (Shackleton et al. 2006). CD14 can be used to further fractionate the mouse luminal compartment into $CD14^+$ progenitors and $CD14^-$ mature luminal cells, while Sca1 expression enriches for HR^+ LPs (Asselin-Labat et al. 2011; Shehata et al. 2012). Definitive markers for HR^+ and HR^- LP cells in human tissue are yet to be defined. Nevertheless, the HR^+ progenitor subset differs in proportions between these two species: in human tissue the LP population comprises an average of approximately 25% of HR^+ cells (albeit large interpatient variation) whereas a much smaller fraction (approximately 5%) of HR^+ progenitors can be discerned in the mouse mammary gland (Asselin-Labat et al. 2007; Shehata et al. 2012).

Despite the identification and prospective isolation of distinct mammary epithelial subsets that constitute stem and progenitor cell-enriched fractions in mice and in humans, the precise structure of the different cellular compartments and their relationship to one another have not yet been fully elucidated. Lineage-tracing and transplantation studies suggest that rare multipotent MaSCs exist in the postnatal mammary gland and give rise to lineage-restricted progenitors that differentiate into the mature cells of the gland (Fu et al. 2020). However, other lineage-tracing studies suggest that multipotent MaSCs only exist in the embryo and posit that lineage-restricted progenitors perform all functions within the postnatal mammary gland (Lloyd-Lewis et al. 2017; Fu et al. 2020). The ability of a single cell from the basal compartment to regenerate an entire ductal epithelial tree in vivo may reflect the presence of facultative stem cells, that is, cells that can assume a stem cell state under specific conditions (Shackleton et al. 2006). While the types of lineage-tracing approaches performed in mice are not amenable to humans, mitochondrial mutational profiling coupled with single-cell genomics can be used as an alternative method to track cell fate in vitro and infer clonal relationships (Ludwig et al. 2019). Studies on X chromosome inactivation patterning in breast tissue (Tsai et al. 1996) and more recent mitochondrial-genomic analyses of formalin-fixed, paraffin-embedded primary patient breast tissue samples, coupled with histological analysis, support the existence of multipotent MaSCs in the human breast (Cereser et al. 2018).

The LP compartment of the stem cell hierarchy appears to be especially complex. Lineage tracing of luminal cells in various mouse models has demonstrated that they are sustained by unipotent LP cells (e.g. van Keymeulen et al. 2011; Davis et al. 2016). Long-term lineage tracing studies spanning at least 1 year demonstrate that luminal cells may also derive from long-lived bipotent stem cells (Rios et al. 2019). Compelling evidence from murine lineage tracing experiments suggests that the ER^+ and ER^- luminal cell lineages are independently maintained in the postnatal mammary gland by unipotent ER^+ and ER^- LP cells (Wang et al. 2017; van Keymeulen et al. 2017; Lilja et al. 2018). Moreover, lineage tracing studies based on Elf5, a definitive marker of LP cells (Rios et al. 2014), have indicated the exclusive labelling of ER^- progeny (data not shown). Nevertheless, mouse models of ER^- luminal cell-driven mammary tumorigenesis have shown that both ER^+ and ER^- tumours may arise from an ER^- cell, suggesting flux between the two subsets in a pathogenic setting (Melchor et al. 2014). In human breast, the LP population comprises both ER^+ and ER^- cells (Clarke et al. 2005; Eirew et al. 2008; Lim et al. 2009), but it remains to be determined whether these progenitors are exclusively unipotent.

Accumulating evidence suggests that cellular identities within the stem cell hierarchy can transition in a multidirectional manner upon exposure to distinct oncogenic insults and extrinsic factors, such as from the niche or cells within the wider microenvironment. This type of cellular plasticity has been described in stem cell hierarchies for kidney, lung and intestinal tract (Tetteh et al. 2015). In the case of breast cancer, potential dedifferentiation has been described in a number of different mouse models, discussed in Sect. 9.4. It therefore seems likely that various pathogenic scenarios can modulate the differentiation trajectory of mammary epithelial cells in a context-specific manner.

Elucidation of robust cell surface markers for the fractionation of human breast epithelial subsets has enabled deep molecular profiling of cellular compartments within the stem cell hierarchy. Notably, comparison of gene expression signatures derived from normal epithelial cell subsets exhibits strong concordance with the molecular signatures of the principal breast cancer subtypes (Fig. 9.1): claudin-low breast tumours are strikingly similar to MaSCs while basal-like, HER2-enriched and luminal breast tumours harbour increasingly differentiated molecular profiles akin to normal LP (basal-like) and more differentiated luminal cells (HER2-enriched, luminal A and luminal B) (Lim et al. 2009; Prat and Perou 2011). Fetal MaSC-enriched populations in mouse appear to be unique and show similarity to both basal-like and $HER2^+$ tumours (Spike et al. 2012). Cumulatively, these data indicate that distinct cells-of-origin along the MaSC hierarchy may underpin intertumoral heterogeneity in breast cancer.

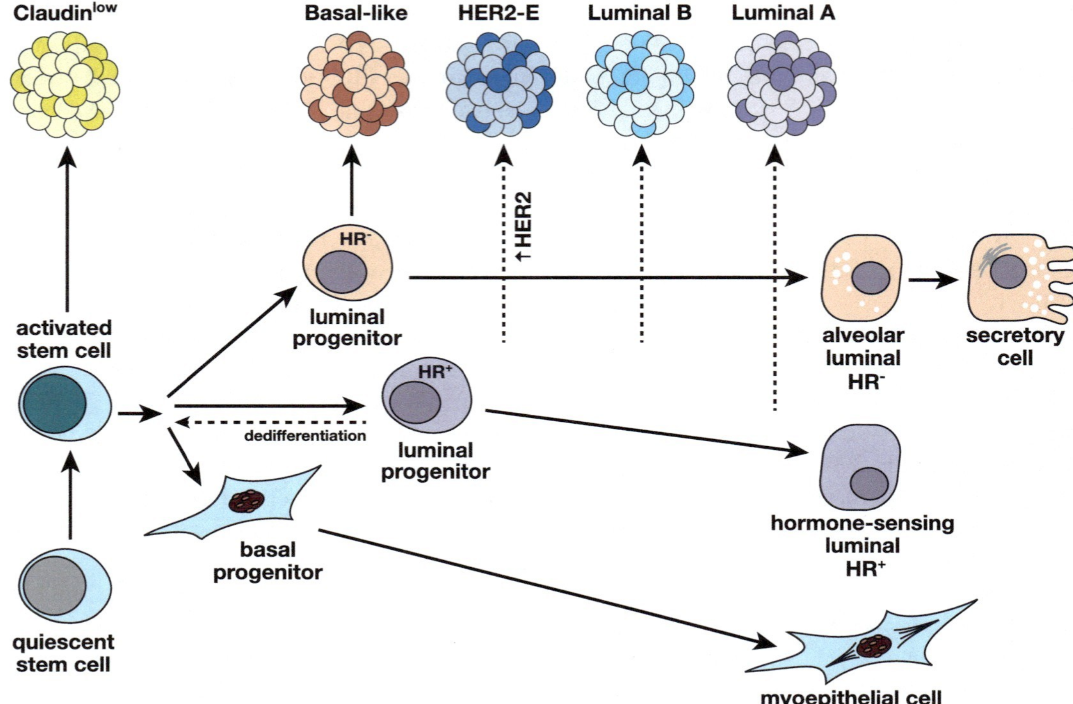

Fig. 9.1 The MaSC hierarchy and breast cancer cells-of-origin. Schematic depicting relationships between the normal breast stem cell hierarchy and the intrinsic breast cancer subtypes. Both activated and quiescent stem cells comprise the MaSC compartment; MaSCs differentiate into LP cells, which may be HR$^+$ or HR$^-$, and basal progenitors; HR$^+$ LP cells generate mature hormone-sensing luminal cells, and HR$^-$ LP cells give rise to HR$^-$ alveolar luminal cells. Secretory cells arise from HR$^-$ alveolar epithelium in late pregnancy. Vertical arrows denote the putative cells-of-origin of cancer for each tumour subtype based on conservation of their transcriptional signatures. Under pathogenic conditions, LP cells may undergo dedifferentiation (depicted by dotted line) and acquire basal/myoepithelial cell properties. HR, hormone receptor

9.4 Experimental Techniques for Identifying Breast Cancer Cells-of-Origin

Several experimental strategies are currently used to identify potential cancer cells-of-origin and their vulnerabilities, which may be exploited to improve patient outcomes (Visvader 2011). One such approach involves ex vivo transduction of primary patient lineage-specific cell subsets and downstream transplantation assays to assess the tumour-forming capacity of modulated cells. Normal patient tissue biopsies can be fractionated into distinct cell subsets using fluorescence-activated cell sorting (FACS), then transduced with lentiviral constructs containing one or more oncogenes linked to a fluorescent tag; these oncogene-activated cell populations can be transplanted into immunocompromised mice, which are then monitored for tumour development. The harvesting of tumours allows the subsequent characterisation of fluorescent-labelled progeny. In the context of familial cancers, primary tissue samples donated by informed and consenting patients harbouring germline mutations in tumour suppressor genes such as *BRCA1/2*, *PALB2* or *ATM* may be fractionated into cell subsets by FACS and subjected to transcriptomic and proteomic profiling as well as ex vivo functional assays in order to identify perturbations unique to these populations that render them susceptible to transformation.

Utilising primary patient specimens for these types of studies can be rewarding but challenging, due to limited quantities of available biological material and high levels of intrinsic patient variation. Genetically engineered mouse models have served as robust models of tumorigenesis and disease but are reliant on the identification of lineage-specific promoters to study the cell subsets of interest. Mice that express lineage-specific promoter-driven cre-recombinase can direct the expression of oncogenes or loss of tumour suppressor genes, to a specific population of cells and drive distinct pathways of tumour development. For example, targeted loss of *Brca1* and *Trp53* using *Blg* (expressed in luminal mammary epithelium) and *Krt14* (expressed in basal mammary epithelium) promoter-driven cre-recombinase results in the formation of high-grade invasive ductal carcinomas and adenomyoepitheliomas, respectively (Molyneux et al. 2010). Targeted mutations in mammary luminal cells or restricted LPs in mouse models affecting key drivers such as *Pi3K*, *Trp53* and *Pten* frequently give rise to basal-like tumours (Koren et al. 2015; van Keymeulen et al. 2015; Wang et al. 2016, 2019; Tao et al. 2017), underscoring inherent plasticity and the dedifferentiation of LPs to basal-like cells. Stem cells have also been implicated in mouse models of breast cancer. For example, mouse mammary tumour virus (MMTV)-driven Wnt-1 overexpression in the mammary epithelium results in dramatic expansion of the basal/MaSC but not the luminal compartment in preneoplastic tissue from transgenic mice (Shackleton et al. 2006). Moreover, expansion of functional stem cells occurs in the *Trp53*-null mouse model of breast cancer (Zhang et al. 2008).

Clonal in vivo lineage tracing of modulated cell subsets provides a method by which the identity of a cancer cell-of-origin can be definitively proven. This technique incorporates an inducible cre-recombinase system, such as creER^{T2}, which enables dose-dependent expression of cre-recombinase in response to tamoxifen treatment in a restricted proportion of cells, which may then be tracked at the single-cell level using a fluorescent tag (Barker et al. 2009). Interestingly, in vivo lineage-tracing studies have revealed that upon targeting the polyoma middle T-antigen (PyMT) or ERBB2 overexpression to the luminal epithelium, oncogene-activated luminal cells can dedifferentiate into basal-like cells, with the resultant hyperplastic regions and tumours containing cells of both lineages (Hein et al. 2016). In another manifestation of plasticity, lineage tracing in mouse "Confetti" models in which *Pten* and *Trp53* were inactivated in basal or luminal mammary epithelial cells revealed frequent acquisition of mesenchymal features in a small subset of cells within each tumour clone (Rios et al. 2019). Together, these studies point to an inherent plasticity within the mammary epithelium during carcinogenesis, which likely contributes to breast cancer heterogeneity.

Importantly, there are potential limitations and caveats associated with mouse models that must be considered when extrapolating to human breast stem and progenitor cell dynamics. There are clear morphological differences in the mammary epithelial tree structure between the two species, including the presence of TDLUs in human breast only, and distinctions between their respective differentiation hierarchies. Mice, unlike humans, do not undergo menopause although ageing and menopause have been shown to influence the transcriptomic profiles of subsets within the MaSC hierarchy of mice and humans (Li et al. 2020; Shalabi et al. 2021), with some evidence from common marmosets revealing parallel changes in progenitor clonogenicity (Wu et al. 2016). As mouse models may not always accurately recapitulate key features of human stem and progenitor cell biology, complementary studies on patient-derived breast tissue, where possible, is vital to confirming their clinical relevance in specific contexts.

9.5 Interrogating Precursor Cells to Identify Targeted Strategies for the Prevention of *BRCA*-Mutant Breast Cancer

Hereditary breast and ovarian cancer (HBOC) syndrome refers to the inheritance of germline mutations in genes that predispose to breast and ovarian tumorigenesis, resulting in a significantly elevated lifetime cancer risk. Intriguingly, these genes predominantly encode proteins which function in common pathways of genome maintenance and repair (Nielsen et al. 2016). Mutations in *BRCA1* and *BRCA2* are estimated to account for one-quarter of the HBOC cases (Kast et al. 2016), and are among the most closely studied of HBOC susceptibility genes, leading to the development of numerous genetically engineered mouse models of *BRCA*-deficient mammary tumorigenesis (Evers and Jonkers 2006). Although germline mutations affect all cells of the body, *BRCA* mutation carriers have a strong propensity to develop breast and/or ovarian cancers. Indeed, interrogation of mammary epithelial cells, mammary fibroblasts and skin fibroblasts from preneoplastic *BRCA1* mutation carriers and noncarriers revealed increased genomic instability in mammary epithelial cells alone, suggesting these cells are particularly susceptible to neoplastic transformation upon *BRCA1* haploinsufficiency (Sedic et al. 2015). A multitude of oncogenic *BRCA* variants have been reported, the bulk of which (approximately 80%) are classified as frameshift and nonsense mutations that are either known or predicted to result in a truncated and dysfunctional BRCA protein (Landrum et al. 2017). A smaller percentage of oncogenic missense mutations in *BRCA1* and *BRCA2* have also been described (Landrum et al. 2017). Recent analyses of hundreds of informative pedigrees with either pathogenic missense variants or truncating variants in *BRCA1* or *BRCA2* have revealed a decreased estimated breast cancer risk for *BRCA1* mutation carriers harbouring pathogenic missense versus truncating variants, while a trend of decreased risk was observed for *BRCA2* mutation carriers when considering patients 50 years or older (Li et al. 2022).

The *BRCA1* gene was first described using positional cloning methods in 1994 (Miki et al. 1994). In the decades since, significant progress has been made in developing our understanding of *BRCA1*-mutant breast cancer aetiology and disease. Early observations of the histological and immunophenotypes of *BRCA1*-mutant and sporadic breast cancers revealed that *BRCA1* mutation carriers develop poorly differentiated, HR^- breast tumours (Lynch et al. 1998; Verhoog et al. 1998). Approximately 10 years after characterisation of the *BRCA1* gene, the intrinsic molecular subtypes of breast cancer were uncovered, and *BRCA1*-mutant breast cancers were characterised as transcriptionally "basal-like" (Sørlie et al. 2003). Owing to the poorly differentiated phenotype of *BRCA1*-mutant breast cancers and expression of basal cytokeratins, it was proposed that these cancers arose from MaSCs, leading to studies on BRCA1-mediated MaSC function and maintenance (Liu et al. 2008; Vassilopoulos et al. 2008). Unexpectedly, analysis of preneoplastic breast tissue from *BRCA1* mutation carriers revealed an expanded and aberrant LP subset that possessed transcriptional profiles strikingly similar to those of basal-like breast cancers, particularly *BRCA1*-mutant tumours (Lim et al. 2009). These findings indicated that LPs are a key cancer-initiating population in BRCA1 mutation carriers. It is notable that interrogation of patient-derived preneoplastic mammary organoids, isolated from germline *BRCA1* mutation carriers and noncarriers, has revealed an enrichment of LP cells in organoids from *BRCA1*-deficient patients (Rosenbluth et al. 2020).

Importantly, engineered mouse models of BRCA1-deficient breast cancer have demonstrated that targeting *Brca1* loss to the luminal, but not basal compartment, leads to the formation of mammary tumours that phenocopy human disease (Molyneux et al. 2010). In addition, transcriptomic profiling of premalignant *Brca1*-deficient LP cells in mouse models revealed aberrant expression of basal and alveolar differentiation genes in these cells (Wang et al. 2019; Bach et al. 2021). Thus, LP cells are more susceptible to *Brca1*-deficient tumorigenesis and may be reprogrammed to acquire certain basal-like characteristics upon transformation.

Further fractionation of the human LP population in preneoplastic tissue from *BRCA1* mutation versus noncarriers by flow cytometry has demonstrated expansion of a $RANK^+$ LP subset, which displayed increased colony forming activity ex vivo, increased levels of DNA damage and a transcriptional signature closely aligned with that of basal-like breast cancers (Nolan et al. 2016). Although RANK$^+$ LP cells are HR$^-$, they are responsive to circulating progesterone via paracrine RANK ligand (RANKL) signalling: RANKL is secreted by neighbouring PR$^+$ cells in response to progesterone, which potentiates a paracrine, pro-proliferative signal to RANK$^+$ progenitors. Profiling studies of wildtype versus *BRCA1*-mutant mammary epithelial cell lines have suggested that BRCA1 deficiency may promote autocrine RANKL/RANK signalling to promote proliferation (Cuyàs et al. 2017). Nonetheless, serum progesterone levels are increased in *BRCA* mutation carriers (Widschwendter et al. 2013), and elevated PR signalling has been reported in breast tissue from *BRCA1* mutation carriers as well as mouse models of *Brca1*-deficiency (Poole et al. 2006; King et al. 2004). Hence, dysregulation of hormonal signalling may occur as one of the earliest events in *BRCA1* mutation carriers during the precancerous phase. In complementary work, Sau and colleagues identified aberrant levels of noncanonical NF-κB activity in the luminal epithelium of *BRCA1* mutation carriers and identified DNA damage-induced NF-κB signalling as a key mediator of hormone-independent clonogenicity in a mouse model of BRCA1 deficiency (Sau et al. 2016). Taken together, a subset of aberrant LP cells in *BRCA1*-mutant tissue exhibits hyperactivation of RANK and NF-κB signalling, as well as defective DNA repair mechanisms, culminating in a population that is highly susceptible to neoplastic transformation (Fig. 9.2).

Notably, in preclinical studies, RANKL inhibition using the decoy receptor osteoprotegerin (OPG) effectively delayed mammary tumorigenesis in the MMTV-cre-driven mouse model of Brca1-deficient breast cancer (Nolan et al. 2016). Further, the occurrence of preneoplastic lesions was markedly attenuated upon treatment with OPG or the recombinant RANKL antagonist RANK-Fc (Sigl et al. 2016; Nolan et al. 2016). The potential therapeutic benefit of RANKL inhibition in *BRCA1* mutation carriers has culminated in the establishment of the BRCA-P study (CTR 2017-002505-35) – a randomized, double-blind placebo-controlled international phase 3 clinical trial that aims to determine the efficacy of denosumab as a chemo-preventative agent for women harbouring a *BRCA1* germline mutation (Fig. 9.2).

BRCA2 mutation carriers are prone to developing breast cancers with variable molecular profiles including both HR$^+$ and HR$^-$ disease (Sørlie et al. 2003; Stevens et al. 2013). In contrast to *BRCA1* mutation carriers, preneoplastic mammary epithelium of *BRCA2*$^{mut/+}$ patients does not harbour an expanded RANK$^+$ LP population (Nolan et al. 2016). Recent work, however, has implicated aberrant LPs as the likely "cells-of-origin" of cancer in *BRCA2* mutation carriers, including an ERBB3^{lo} progenitor subset. These cells are expanded in pathologically normal breast tissue from premenopausal *BRCA2* mutation carriers and exhibit hyperactive mTORC1 signalling and disrupted proteostasis (Joyce et al. 2024). Increased mTORC1 signalling appears to be a conserved feature of preneoplastic *BRCA2*-deficient LP cells in mice and patient-derived luminal cell lines (Joyce et al. 2024; Shalabi et al. 2021). Further, somatic copy number variations, potentially reflecting an intrinsic susceptibility to DNA damage, have been reported in primary *BRCA2*$^{mut/+}$ LPs but not basal cells (Karaayvaz-Yildirim et al. 2020). Intriguingly, single ERBB3^{lo} LPs were shown to give rise to colonies containing both ER$^+$ and ER$^-$ cells ex vivo, suggesting that these progenitors may be precursors for either ER$^+$ or ER$^-$ disease (Joyce et al. 2024). Notably, short-term treatment with the mTORC1 inhibitor everolimus significantly delayed mammary tumour development in a preclinical mouse model, providing functional evidence for the mTORC1 pathway serving as a driver in *BRCA2*-deficient breast oncogenesis (Joyce et al. 2024) (Fig. 9.2).

In the mammary gland, the microenvironment of premalignant *BRCA1*-mutant epithelium has emerged as a potential novel therapeutic target for chemoprevention. Precancer-associated fibroblasts, or "pre-CAFs" were identified in preneoplastic breast tissue of *BRCA1* mutation carriers, and functional assays using *Brca1*- and *Trp53*-deficient murine mammary epithelial

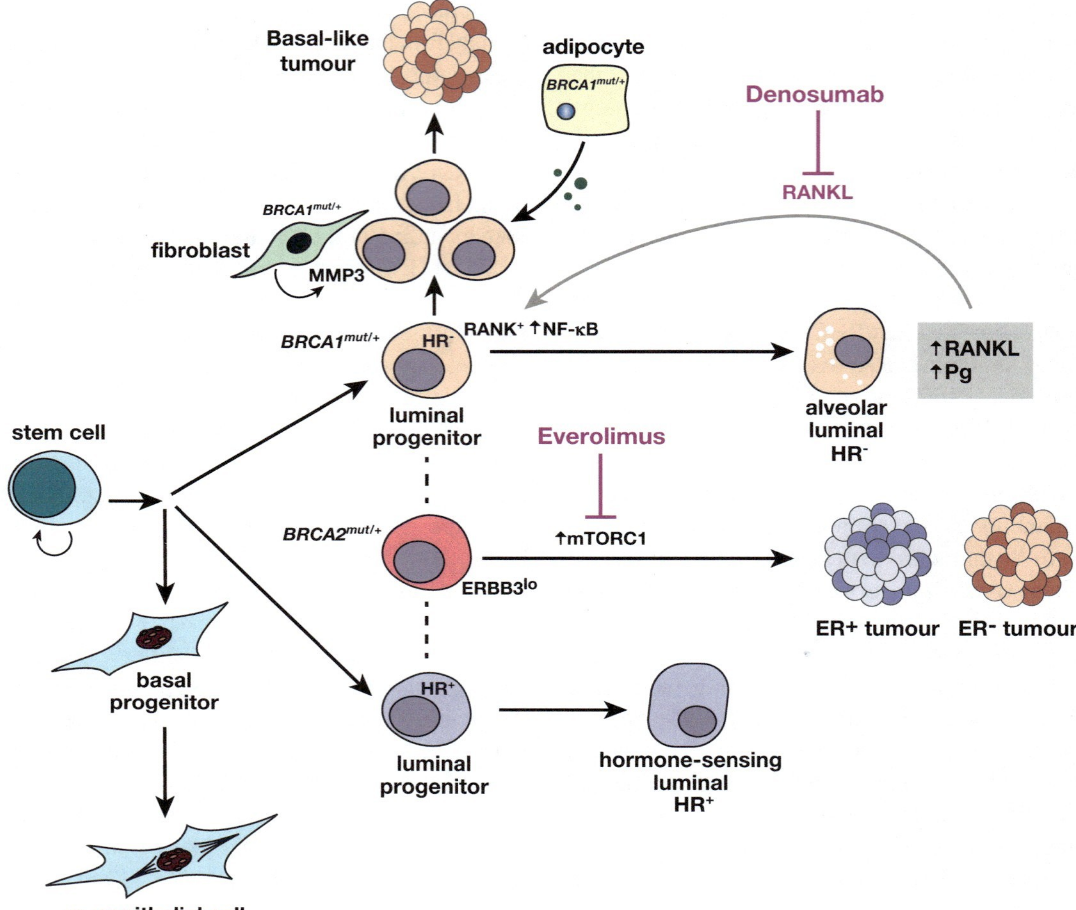

Fig. 9.2 LPs serve as putative breast cancer cells-of-origin in germline *BRCA* mutation carriers. Schematic model of oncogenesis in *BRCA* mutation carriers. In premenopausal *BRCA1* mutation carriers, expansion of RANK$^+$ LPs, enriched for HR$^-$ cells, occurs in premalignant tissue. These cells can receive proliferative signals from progesterone (Pg) via the secretion of RANKL from mature hormone-sensing cells. RANKL can bind and activate the RANK receptor on the aberrant LP subset. This results in the activation of pro-proliferative pathways such as NF-κB, which also occurs in response to DNA damage accumulated through defective DNA repair machinery. RANK signalling also initiates the DNA damage response and can trigger the proliferation of RANK$^+$ cells. Extrinsic influences can impact breast epithelial cell growth, including *BRCA1*$^{mut/+}$ fibroblasts that may be primed for the synthesis of metalloprotease MMP3 or *BRCA1*$^{mut/+}$ adipocytes through as yet undefined secreted factors that likely alter metabolism. For *BRCA2* mutation carriers, aberrant ERBB3^{lo} LPs with disrupted proteostasis and increased mTORC1 signalling expand in pathologically normal, premenopausal breast tissue, giving rise to ER$^+$ or ER$^-$ tumours. Potential breast cancer prevention strategies include blockade of the RANKL (denosumab) and mTORC1 (everolimus) pathways in *BRCA1* and *BRCA2* mutation carriers, respectively. HR, hormone receptor, ER, oestrogen receptor

cells suggested that these cells can promote *Brca1*-deficient tumour initiation in vivo (Nee et al. 2023). Moreover, *BRCA1*-deficient pericytes in preneoplastic tissue were shown to be enriched for nerve growth factor (NGF) and to exert a proliferative effect on mammary basal cells, which express the NGF receptor (Nee et al. 2023). The breast adipose microenvironment was also recently implicated in promoting DNA damage in the breast epithelium of *BRCA* mutation carriers, providing evidence for a relationship between increased weight and breast cancer risk in these patients (Bhardwaj et al. 2023). Thus, close interrogation of the niches in which cells-of-origin of cancer reside and their influence on oncogenesis may provide unique opportunities for the identification of chemoprevention targets.

9.6 Concluding Remarks

Foundational studies of normal mammary epithelial cell biology and breast tumour precursor cells have driven significant progress towards identifying targeted breast cancer prevention options for *BRCA1* mutation carriers. Whether deciphering the aetiology of breast cancer in germline *BRCA2* mutation carriers and patients carrying additional HBOC gene variants can lead to much-needed targets for cancer treatment and prevention strategies remains to be seen. As multiomics single-cell and spatial technologies continue to develop, their integration will lead to the further unravelling of mechanisms by which breast tumour precursor cells are influenced by their microenvironment and reveal novel avenues for therapeutic intervention. Further characterisation of the extrinsic and intrinsic factors which cooperate to drive cellular transformation of distinct cancer cells-of-origin may provide an opportunity to design targeted chemoprevention strategies for patients with HBOC, conceptualise improved cancer screening strategies for earlier detection and identify methods to combat tumours which have relapsed after initial treatment. Pertinently, progress towards these ends will require a refined understanding of the breast stem cell hierarchy on the basis of functional characterisation, in addition to the molecular descriptors offered by single-cell profiling approaches.

Acknowledgements We thank P. Maltezos for assistance with figure illustrations. RJ is supported by a Peeneeyt Thanampool (Strong Women) Aunty Joan Vickery and Aunty Angela Clarke Indigenous Post-doctoral Fellowship. JEV is supported by NHMRC Fellowship/Investigator Grant #1037230 and #1102742.

References

Asleh K, Negri GL, Spencer SE, Miko SC, Hughes CS, Wang XQ, Gao D et al (2022) Proteomic analysis of archival breast cancer clinical specimens identifies biological subtypes with distinct survival outcomes. Nat Commun 13(1):896. https://doi.org/10.1038/s41467-022-28524-0

Asselin-Labat M-L, Sutherland KD, Barker H, Thomas R, Shackleton M, Forrest NC, Hartley L et al (2007) Gata-3 is an essential regulator of mammary-gland morphogenesis and luminal-cell differentiation. Nat Cell Biol 9(2):201–209. https://doi.org/10.1038/ncb1530

Asselin-Labat M-L, Sutherland KD, Vaillant F, Gyorki DE, Di W, Holroyd S, Breslin K et al (2011) Gata-3 negatively regulates the tumor-initiating capacity of mammary luminal progenitor cells and targets the putative tumor suppressor Caspase-14. Mol Cell Biol 31(22):4609–4622. https://doi.org/10.1128/mcb.05766-11

Bach K, Pensa S, Zarocsinceva M, Kania K, Stockis J, Pinaud S, Lazarus KA et al (2021) Time-resolved single-cell analysis of Brca1 associated mammary tumourigenesis reveals aberrant differentiation of luminal progenitors. Nat Commun 12(1):1502. https://doi.org/10.1038/s41467-021-21783-3

Balani S, Nguyen LV, Eaves CJ (2017) Modeling the process of human tumorigenesis. Nat Commun 8(1):15422. https://doi.org/10.1038/ncomms15422

Barker N, Ridgway RA, van Es JH, van de Wetering M, Begthel H, van den Born M, Danenberg E, Clarke AR, Sansom OJ, Clevers H (2009) Crypt stem cells as the cells-of-origin of intestinal cancer. Nature 457(7229):608–611. https://doi.org/10.1038/nature07602

Bhardwaj P, Iyengar NM, Zahid H, Carter KM, Byun DJ, Choi MH, Sun Q et al (2023) Obesity promotes breast epithelium DNA damage in women carrying a germline mutation in BRCA1 or BRCA2. Sci Transl Med 15(684):eade1857. https://doi.org/10.1126/scitranslmed.ade1857

Cereser B, Jansen M, Austin E, Elia G, McFarlane T, van Deurzen CHM, Sieuwerts AM et al (2018) Analysis of clonal expansions through the normal and premalignant human breast epithelium reveals the presence of luminal stem cells. J Pathol 244(1):61–70. https://doi.org/10.1002/path.4989

Chung W, Eum HH, Lee H-O, Lee K-M, Lee H-B, Kim K-T, Ryu HS et al (2017) Single-cell RNA-Seq enables comprehensive tumour and immune cell profiling in primary breast cancer. Nat Commun 8(1):15081. https://doi.org/10.1038/ncomms15081

Clarke RB, Spence K, Anderson E, Howell A, Okano H, Potten CS (2005) A putative human breast stem cell population is enriched for steroid receptor-positive cells. Dev Biol 277(2):443–456. https://doi.org/10.1016/j.ydbio.2004.07.044

Corces-Zimmerman MR, Hong W-J, Weissman IL, Medeiros BC, Majeti R (2014) Preleukemic mutations in human acute myeloid leukemia affect epigenetic regulators and persist in remission. Proc Natl Acad Sci 111(7):2548–2553. https://doi.org/10.1073/pnas.1324297111

Cuyàs E, Corominas-Faja B, María MM-S, Martin-Castillo B, Lupu R, Brunet J, Bosch-Barrera J, Menendez JA (2017) BRCA1 Haploinsufficiency cell-autonomously activates RANKL expression and generates Denosumab-responsive breast cancer-initiating cells. Oncotarget 8(21):35019–35032. https://doi.org/10.18632/oncotarget.16558

Davis FM, Lloyd-Lewis B, Harris OB, Kozar S, Winton DJ, Muresan L, Watson CJ (2016) Single-cell lineage tracing in the mammary gland reveals stochastic clonal dispersion of stem/progenitor cell progeny. Nat Commun 7(1):13053. https://doi.org/10.1038/ncomms13053

Eirew P, Stingl J, Raouf A, Turashvili G, Aparicio S, Emerman JT, Eaves CJ (2008) A method for quantifying normal human mammary epithelial stem cells with in vivo regenerative ability. Nat Med 14(12):1384–1389. https://doi.org/10.1038/nm.1791

Evers B, Jonkers J (2006) Mouse models of BRCA1 and BRCA2 deficiency: past lessons, current understanding and future prospects. Oncogene 25(43):5885–5897. https://doi.org/10.1038/sj.onc.1209871

Fougner C, Bergholtz H, Norum JH, Sørlie T (2020) Re-definition of Claudin-low as a breast cancer phenotype. Nat Commun 11(1):1787. https://doi.org/10.1038/s41467-020-15574-5

Fu NY, Nolan E, Lindeman GJ, Visvader JE (2020) Stem cells and the differentiation hierarchy in mammary gland development. Physiol Rev 100(2):489–523. https://doi.org/10.1152/physrev.00040.2018

Harbeck N, Penault-Llorca F, Cortes J, Gnant M, Houssami N, Poortmans P, Ruddy K, Tsang J, Cardoso F (2019) Breast cancer. Nat Rev Dis Prim 5(1):66. https://doi.org/10.1038/s41572-019-0111-2

Hein SM, Haricharan S, Johnston AN, Toneff MJ, Reddy JP, Dong J, Bu W, Li Y (2016) Luminal epithelial cells within the mammary gland can produce basal cells upon oncogenic stress. Oncogene 35(11):1461–1467. https://doi.org/10.1038/onc.2015.206

Herschkowitz JI, Simin K, Weigman VJ, Mikaelian I, Usary J, Zhiyuan H, Rasmussen KE et al (2007) Identification of conserved gene expression features between murine mammary carcinoma models and human breast tumors. Genome Biol 8(5):R76. https://doi.org/10.1186/gb-2007-8-5-r76

Itzkowitz SH, Yio X (2004) Inflammation and cancer IV. Colorectal cancer in inflammatory bowel disease: the role of inflammation. Am J Physiol Gastrointest Liver Physiol 287(1):G7–G17. https://doi.org/10.1152/ajpgi.00079.2004

Jiang Z, Deng T, Jones R, Li H, Herschkowitz JI, Liu JC, Weigman VJ et al (2010) Rb deletion in mouse mammary progenitors induces luminal-B or basal-like/EMT tumor subtypes depending on P53 status. J Clin Invest 120(9):3296–3309. https://doi.org/10.1172/jci41490

Johansson HJ, Socciarelli F, Vacanti NM, Haugen MH, Zhu Y, Siavelis I, Fernandez-Woodbridge A et al (2019) Breast cancer quantitative proteome and proteogenomic landscape. Nat Commun 10(1):1600. https://doi.org/10.1038/s41467-019-09018-y

Joyce R, Pascual R, Heitink L, Capaldo BD, Vaillant F, Christie M, Tsai M et al (2024) Identification of aberrant luminal progenitors and MTORC1 as a potential breast cancer prevention target in BRCA2 mutation carriers. Nat Cell Biol 26(1):138–152. https://doi.org/10.1038/s41556-023-01315-5

Karaayvaz-Yildirim M, Silberman RE, Langenbucher A, Saladi SV, Ross KN, Zarcaro E, Desmond A et al (2020) Aneuploidy and a deregulated DNA damage response suggest haploinsufficiency in breast tissues of BRCA2 mutation carriers. Sci Adv 6(5):eaay2611. https://doi.org/10.1126/sciadv.aay2611

Kast K, Rhiem K, Wappenschmidt B, Hahnen E, Hauke J, Bluemcke B, Zarghooni V et al (2016) Prevalence of BRCA1/2 germline mutations in 21 401 families with breast and ovarian cancer. J Med Genet 53(7):465. https://doi.org/10.1136/jmedgenet-2015-103672

Keymeulen V, Van A, Rocha AS, Ousset M, Beck B, Bouvencourt G, Rock J, Sharma N, Dekoninck S, Blanpain C (2011) Distinct stem cells contribute to mammary gland development and maintenance. Nature 479(7372):189–193. https://doi.org/10.1038/nature10573

Keymeulen V, Van A, Lee MY, Ousset M, Brohée S, Rorive S, Giraddi RR, Wuidart A et al (2015) Reactivation of multipotency by oncogenic PIK3CA induces breast tumour heterogeneity. Nature 525(7567):119–123. https://doi.org/10.1038/nature14665

Keymeulen V, Van A, Fioramonti M, Centonze A, Bouvencourt G, Achouri Y, Blanpain C (2017) Lineage-restricted mammary stem cells sustain the development, homeostasis, and regeneration of the estrogen receptor positive lineage. Cell Rep 20(7):1525–1532. https://doi.org/10.1016/j.celrep.2017.07.066

King TA, Gemignani ML, Li W, Giri DD, Panageas KS, Bogomolniy F, Arroyo C et al (2004) Increased progesterone receptor expression in benign epithelium of BRCA1-related breast cancers. Cancer Res 64(15):5051–5053. https://doi.org/10.1158/0008-5472.can-04-1283

Koboldt DC, Fulton RS, McLellan MD, Schmidt H, Kalicki-Veizer J, McMichael JF, Fulton LL et al (2012) Comprehensive molecular portraits of human breast tumours. Nature 490(7418):61–70. https://doi.org/10.1038/nature11412

Koren S, Reavie L, Couto JP, De Silva D, Stadler MB, Roloff T, Britschgi A et al (2015) PIK3CAH1047R induces multipotency and multi-lineage mammary tumours. Nature 525(7567):114–118. https://doi.org/10.1038/nature14669

Land CE, McGregor DH (1979) Breast cancer incidence among atomic bomb survivors: implications for radiobiologic risk at low doses. JNCI J Natl Cancer Inst. https://doi.org/10.1093/jnci/62.1.17

Landrum MJ, Lee JM, Benson M, Brown GR, Chao C, Chitipiralla S, Baoshan G et al (2017) ClinVar: improving access to variant interpretations and supporting evidence. Nucleic Acids Res 46(D1):D1062–D1067. https://doi.org/10.1093/nar/gkx1153

Li CM-C, Shapiro H, Tsiobikas C, Selfors LM, Chen H, Rosenbluth J, Moore K et al (2020) Aging-associated alterations in mammary epithelia and stroma revealed by single-cell RNA sequencing. Cell Rep 33(13):108566. https://doi.org/10.1016/j.celrep.2020.108566

Li H, Engel C, de la Hoya M, Peterlongo P, Yannoukakos D, Livraghi L, Radice P et al (2022) Risks of breast and ovarian cancer for women harboring pathogenic missense variants in BRCA1 and BRCA2 compared with those harboring protein truncating variants. Genet Med 24(1):119–129. https://doi.org/10.1016/j.gim.2021.08.016

Lilja AM, Rodilla V, Huyghe M, Hannezo E, Landragin C, Renaud O, Leroy O, Rulands S, Simons BD, Fre S (2018) Clonal analysis of Notch1-expressing cells reveals the existence of unipotent stem cells that retain long-term plasticity in the embryonic mammary gland. Nat Cell Biol 20(6):677–687. https://doi.org/10.1038/s41556-018-0108-1

Lim E, Vaillant F, Di W, Forrest NC, Pal B, Hart AH, Asselin-Labat M-L et al (2009) Aberrant luminal progenitors as the candidate target population for basal tumor development in BRCA1 mutation carriers. Nat Med 15(8):907–913. https://doi.org/10.1038/nm.2000

Liu S, Ginestier C, Charafe-Jauffret E, Foco H, Kleer CG, Merajver SD, Dontu G, Wicha MS (2008) BRCA1 regulates human mammary stem/progenitor cell fate. Proc Natl Acad Sci 105(5):1680–1685. https://doi.org/10.1073/pnas.0711613105

Lloyd-Lewis B, Harris OB, Watson CJ, Davis FM (2017) Mammary stem cells: premise, properties, and perspectives. Trends Cell Biol 27(8):556–567. https://doi.org/10.1016/j.tcb.2017.04.001

Ludwig LS, Lareau CA, Ulirsch JC, Christian E, Muus C, Li LH, Pelka K et al (2019) Lineage tracing in humans enabled by mitochondrial mutations and single-cell genomics. Cell 176(6):1325–1339.e22. https://doi.org/10.1016/j.cell.2019.01.022

Lynch BJ, Holden JA, Buys SS, Neuhausen SL, Gaffney DK (1998) Pathobiologic characteristics of hereditary breast cancer. Hum Pathol 29(10):1140–1144. https://doi.org/10.1016/s0046-8177(98)90427-0

Lytle NK, Barber AG, Reya T (2018) Stem cell fate in cancer growth, progression and therapy resistance. Nat Rev Cancer 18(11):669–680. https://doi.org/10.1038/s41568-018-0056-x

Mann M, Kulak NA, Nagaraj N, Cox J (2013) The coming age of complete, accurate, and ubiquitous proteomes. Mol Cell 49(4):583–590. https://doi.org/10.1016/j.molcel.2013.01.029

Melchor L, Molyneux G, Mackay A, Magnay F-A, Atienza M, Kendrick H, Nava-Rodrigues D et al (2014) Identification of cellular and genetic drivers of breast cancer heterogeneity in genetically engineered mouse tumour models. J Pathol 233(2):124–137. https://doi.org/10.1002/path.4345

Miki Y, Swensen J, Donna Shattuck-Eidens P, Futreal A, Harshman K, Tavtigian S, Liu Q et al (1994) A strong candidate for the breast and ovarian cancer susceptibility gene BRCA1. Science 266(5182):66–71. https://doi.org/10.1126/science.7545954

Molyneux G, Geyer FC, Magnay F-A, McCarthy A, Kendrick H, Natrajan R, MacKay A et al (2010) BRCA1 basal-like breast cancers originate from luminal epithelial progenitors and not from basal stem cells. Cell Stem Cell 7(3):403–417. https://doi.org/10.1016/j.stem.2010.07.010

Nee K, Ma D, Nguyen QH, Pein M, Pervolarakis N, Insua-Rodríguez J, Gong Y et al (2023) Preneoplastic stromal cells promote BRCA1-mediated breast tumorigenesis. Nat Genet 55(4):595–606. https://doi.org/10.1038/s41588-023-01298-x

Nielsen FC, van Overeem Hansen T, Sørensen CS (2016) Hereditary breast and ovarian cancer: new genes in confined pathways. Nat Rev Cancer 16(9):599–612. https://doi.org/10.1038/nrc.2016.72

Nishimura T, Kakiuchi N, Yoshida K, Sakurai T, Tatsuki R, Kataoka EK, Chigusa Y et al (2023) Evolutionary histories of breast cancer and related clones. Nature 620(7974):607–614. https://doi.org/10.1038/s41586-023-06333-9

Nolan E, Vaillant F, Branstetter D, Pal B, Giner G, Whitehead L, Lok SW et al (2016) RANK ligand as a potential target for breast cancer prevention in BRCA1-mutation carriers. Nat Med 22(8):933–939. https://doi.org/10.1038/nm.4118

Nolan E, Lindeman GJ, Visvader JE (2023) Deciphering breast cancer: from biology to the clinic. Cell 186(8):1708–1728. https://doi.org/10.1016/j.cell.2023.01.040

Parker JS, Mullins M, Cheang MCU, Leung S, Voduc D, Vickery T, Davies S et al (2009) Supervised risk predictor of breast cancer based on intrinsic subtypes. J Clin Oncol 27(8):1160–1167. https://doi.org/10.1200/jco.2008.18.1370

Perou CM, Sørlie T, Eisen MB, van de Rijn M, Jeffrey SS, Rees CA, Pollack JR et al (2000) Molecular portraits of human breast tumours. Nature 406(6797):747–752. https://doi.org/10.1038/35021093

Pike MC, Henderson BE, Casagrande JT, Rosario I, Gray GE (1981) Oral contraceptive use and early abortion as risk factors for breast cancer in young women. Br J Cancer 43(1):72–76. https://doi.org/10.1038/bjc.1981.10

Poole AJ, Li Y, Kim Y, Lin S-CJ, Lee W-H, Lee EY-HP (2006) Prevention of Brca1-mediated mammary tumorigenesis in mice by a progesterone antagonist. Science 314(5804):1467–1470. https://doi.org/10.1126/science.1130471

Prat A, Perou CM (2011) Deconstructing the molecular portraits of breast cancer. Mol Oncol 5(1):5–23. https://doi.org/10.1016/j.molonc.2010.11.003

Prat A, Parker JS, Karginova O, Fan C, Livasy C, Herschkowitz JI, He X, Perou CM (2010) Phenotypic and molecular characterization of the Claudin-low intrinsic subtype of breast cancer. Breast Cancer Res 12(5):R68. https://doi.org/10.1186/bcr2635

Rios AC, Nai Yang F, Lindeman GJ, Visvader JE (2014) In situ identification of bipotent stem cells in the mammary gland. Nature 506(7488):322–327. https://doi.org/10.1038/nature12948

Rios AC, Capaldo BD, Vaillant F, Pal B, van Ineveld R, Dawson CA, Chen Y et al (2019) Intraclonal plasticity in mammary tumors revealed through large-scale single-cell resolution 3D imaging. Cancer Cell 35(4):618–632.e6. https://doi.org/10.1016/j.ccell.2019.02.010

Rosenbluth JM, Ron CJ, Schackmann GK, Gray LM, Selfors CM-C, Li MB, Kuiken HJ et al (2020) Organoid cultures from normal and cancer-prone human breast tissues preserve complex epithelial lineages. Nat Commun 11(1):1711. https://doi.org/10.1038/s41467-020-15548-7

Russo J, Tay LK, Russo IH (1982) Differentiation of the mammary gland and susceptibility to carcinogenesis. Breast Cancer Res Treat 2(1):5–73. https://doi.org/10.1007/bf01805718

Sau A, Lau R, Cabrita MA, Nolan E, Crooks PA, Visvader JE, Christine Pratt MA (2016) Persistent activation of NF-KB in BRCA1-deficient mammary progenitors drives aberrant proliferation and accumulation of DNA damage. Cell Stem Cell 19(1):52–65. https://doi.org/10.1016/j.stem.2016.05.003

Schwitalla S, Fingerle AA, Cammareri P, Nebelsiek T, Göktuna SI, Ziegler PK, Canli O et al (2013) Intestinal tumorigenesis initiated by dedifferentiation and acquisition of stem-cell-like properties. Cell 152(1–2):25–38. https://doi.org/10.1016/j.cell.2012.12.012

Sedic M, Skibinski A, Brown N, Gallardo M, Mulligan P, Martinez P, Keller PJ et al (2015) Haploinsufficiency for BRCA1 leads to cell-type-specific genomic instability and premature senescence. Nat Commun 6(1):7505. https://doi.org/10.1038/ncomms8505

Shackleton M, Vaillant F, Simpson KJ, Stingl J, Smyth GK, Asselin-Labat M-L, Li W, Lindeman GJ, Visvader JE (2006) Generation of a functional mammary gland from a single stem cell. Nature 439(7072):84–88. https://doi.org/10.1038/nature04372

Shalabi SF, Miyano M, Sayaman RW, Lopez JC, Jokela TA, Todhunter ME, Hinz S et al (2021) Evidence for accelerated aging in mammary epithelia of women carrying germline BRCA1 or BRCA2 mutations. Nat Aging 1(9):838–849. https://doi.org/10.1038/s43587-021-00104-9

Shehata M, Teschendorff A, Sharp G, Nikola Novcic I, Russell A, Avril S, Prater M et al (2012) Phenotypic and functional characterisation of the luminal cell hierarchy of the mammary gland. Breast Cancer Res 14(5):R134. https://doi.org/10.1186/bcr3334

Shlush LI, Zandi S, Mitchell A, Chen WC, Brandwein JM, Gupta V, Kennedy JA et al (2014) Identification of pre-leukaemic haematopoietic stem cells in acute leukaemia. Nature 506(7488):328–333. https://doi.org/10.1038/nature13038

Sigl V, Owusu-Boaitey K, Joshi PA, Kavirayani A, Wirnsberger G, Novatchkova M, Kozieradzki I et al (2016) RANKL/RANK control Brca1 mutation-driven mammary tumors. Cell Res 26(7):761–774. https://doi.org/10.1038/cr.2016.69

Sørlie T, Perou CM, Tibshirani R, Aas T, Geisler S, Johnsen H, Hastie T et al (2001) Gene expression patterns of breast carcinomas distinguish tumor subclasses with clinical implications. Proc Natl Acad Sci 98(19):10869–10874. https://doi.org/10.1073/pnas.191367098

Sørlie T, Tibshirani R, Parker J, Trevor Hastie JS, Marron AN, Deng S et al (2003) Repeated observation of breast tumor subtypes in independent gene expression data sets. Proc Natl Acad Sci 100(14):8418–8423. https://doi.org/10.1073/pnas.0932692100

Spike BT, Engle DD, Lin JC, Cheung SK, La J, Wahl GM (2012) A mammary stem cell population identified and characterized in late embryogenesis reveals similarities to human breast cancer. Cell Stem Cell 10(2):183–197. https://doi.org/10.1016/j.stem.2011.12.018

Stevens KN, Vachon CM, Couch FJ (2013) Genetic susceptibility to triple-negative breast cancer. Cancer Res 73(7):2025–2030. https://doi.org/10.1158/0008-5472.can-12-1699

Sung H, Ferlay J, Siegel RL, Laversanne M, Soerjomataram I, Jemal A, Bray F (2021) Global cancer statistics 2020: GLOBOCAN estimates of incidence and mortality worldwide for 36 cancers in 185 countries. CA Cancer J Clin 71(3):209–249. https://doi.org/10.3322/caac.21660

Sutherland KD, Visvader JE (2015) Cellular mechanisms underlying intertumoral heterogeneity. Trends Cancer 1(1):15–23. https://doi.org/10.1016/j.trecan.2015.07.003

Tao L, Xiang D, Xie Y, Bronson RT, Li Z (2017) Induced P53 loss in mouse luminal cells causes clonal expansion and development of mammary tumours. Nat Commun 8(1):14431. https://doi.org/10.1038/ncomms14431

Tetteh PW, Farin HF, Clevers H (2015) Plasticity within stem cell hierarchies in mammalian epithelia. Trends Cell Biol 25(2):100–108. https://doi.org/10.1016/j.tcb.2014.09.003

Tlsty TD, Coussens LM (2006) Tumor stroma and regulation of cancer development. Annu Rev Pathol 1(1):119–150. https://doi.org/10.1146/annurev.pathol.1.110304.100224

Tomasetti C, Li L, Vogelstein B (2017) Stem cell divisions, somatic mutations, cancer etiology, and cancer prevention. Science 355(6331):1330–1334. https://doi.org/10.1126/science.aaf9011

Tsai YC, Lu Y, Nichols PW, Zlotnikov G, Jones PA, Smith HS (1996) Contiguous patches of Normal human mammary epithelium derived from a single stem cell: implications for breast carcinogenesis. Cancer Res 56(2):402–404

Tyanova S, Albrechtsen R, Kronqvist P, Cox J, Mann M, Geiger T (2016) Proteomic maps of breast cancer subtypes. Nat Commun 7(1):10259. https://doi.org/10.1038/ncomms10259

Vassilopoulos A, Wang R-H, Petrovas C, Ambrozak D, Koup R, Deng C-X (2008) Identification and characterization of cancer initiating cells from BRCA1 related mammary tumors using markers for normal mammary stem cells. Int J Biol Sci 4(3):133–142. https://doi.org/10.7150/ijbs.4.133

Verhoog LC, Brekelmans CTM, Seynaeve C, van den Bosch LMC, Dahmen G, van Geel AN, Tilanus-Linthorst MMA et al (1998) Survival and tumour characteristics of breast-cancer patients with germline mutations of BRCA1. Lancet 351(9099):316–321. https://doi.org/10.1016/s0140-6736(97)07065-7

Visvader JE (2009) Keeping abreast of the mammary epithelial hierarchy and breast tumorigenesis. Genes Dev 23(22):2563–2577. https://doi.org/10.1101/gad.1849509

Visvader JE (2011) Cells of origin in cancer. Nature 469(7330):314–322. https://doi.org/10.1038/nature09781

Wang S, Liu JC, Kim D, Datti A, Zacksenhaus E (2016) Targeted Pten deletion plus P53-R270H mutation in mouse mammary epithelium induces aggressive Claudin-low and basal-like breast cancer. Breast Cancer Res 18(1):9. https://doi.org/10.1186/s13058-015-0668-y

Wang C, Christin JR, Oktay MH, Guo W (2017) Lineage-biased stem cells maintain estrogen-receptor-positive and -negative mouse mammary luminal lineages. Cell Rep 18(12):2825–2835. https://doi.org/10.1016/j.celrep.2017.02.071

Wang H, Xiang D, Liu B, He A, Randle HJ, Zhang KX, Dongre A et al (2019) Inadequate DNA damage repair promotes mammary transdifferentiation, leading to BRCA1 breast cancer. Cell 178(1):135–151.e19. https://doi.org/10.1016/j.cell.2019.06.002

Wellings SR (1980) A hypothesis of the origin of human breast cancer from the terminal ductal lobular unit. Pathol Res Pract 166(4):515–535. https://doi.org/10.1016/s0344-0338(80)80248-2

Wellings SR, Jensen HM, Marcum RG (1975) An atlas of subgross pathology of the human breast with special reference to possible precancerous lesions. J Natl Cancer Inst 55(2):231–273

Widschwendter M, Rosenthal AN, Philpott S, Rizzuto I, Fraser L, Hayward J, Intermaggio MP et al (2013) The sex hormone system in carriers of BRCA1/2 mutations: a case-control study. Lancet Oncol 14(12):1226–1232. https://doi.org/10.1016/s1470-2045(13)70448-0

Wu A, Dong Q, Gao H, Shi Y, Chen Y, Zhang F, Bandyopadhyay A et al (2016) Characterization of mammary epithelial stem/progenitor cells and their changes with aging in common marmosets. Sci Rep 6(1):32190. https://doi.org/10.1038/srep32190

Wu SZ, Al-Eryani G, Roden DL, Junankar S, Harvey K, Andersson A, Thennavan A et al (2021) A single-cell and spatially resolved atlas of human breast cancers. Nat Genet 53(9):1334–1347. https://doi.org/10.1038/s41588-021-00911-1

Zhang M, Behbod F, Atkinson RL, Landis MD, Kittrell F, Edwards D, Medina D et al (2008) Identification of tumor-initiating cells in a P53-null mouse model of breast cancer. Cancer Res 68(12):4674–4682. https://doi.org/10.1158/0008-5472.can-07-6353

10 Mechanisms of Regulation of Cell Fate in Breast Development and Cancer

Alexandra Van Keymeulen

Abstract

This chapter focuses on the mechanisms of regulation of cell fate in breast development, occurring mainly after birth, as well as in breast cancer. First, we will review how the microenvironment of the breast, as well as external cues, plays a crucial role in mammary gland cell specification and will describe how it has been shown to reprogram non-mammary cells into mammary epithelial cells. Then we will focus on the transcription factors and master regulators which have been established to be determinant for basal (BC) and luminal cell (LC) identity, and will describe the experiments of ectopic expression or loss of function of these transcription factors which demonstrated that they were crucial for cell fate. We will also discuss how master regulators are involved in the fate choice of LCs between estrogen receptor (ER)-positive cells and ER− cells, which will give rise to alveolar cells upon pregnancy and lactation. We will describe how oncogene expression induces reprogramming and change of fate of mammary epithelial cells before tumor appearance, which could be an essential step in tumorigenesis. Finally, we will describe the involvement of master regulators of mammary epithelial cells in breast cancer.

Keywords

Cell fate · Mammary gland · Master regulators · Change of fate · Breast cancer · Cell reprogramming

Key Points

- The microenvironment of the breast and external cues are crucial for mammary gland cell specification.
- Luminal and basal cell identities are defined by master regulators.
- Oncogene expression induces reprogramming and change of fate of mammary epithelial cells.
- Master regulators of mammary epithelial cells are involved in breast cancer.

10.1 Introduction

As described in the previous chapters, the mammary epithelial cells assemble into a bilayered ductal network of LCs surrounded by BCs, also called myoepithelial cells, during late embryogenesis (Watson and Khaled 2008). Additional heterogeneity within LCs is observed after birth,

A. Van Keymeulen (✉)
Laboratory of Stem Cells and Cancer (LSCC), Université Libre de Bruxelles (ULB), Brussels, Belgium
e-mail: Alexandra.van.keymeulen@ulb.be

T. Sørlie, R. B. Clarke (eds.), *A Guide to Breast Cancer Research*, Advances in Experimental Medicine and Biology 1464, https://doi.org/10.1007/978-3-031-70875-6_10

when around half of the LCs start expressing hormonal receptors like ER and progesterone receptor (PR) (Petersen et al. 1987).

Lineage-tracing and clonal analysis experiments have shown, as extensively discussed in Chap. 5, that BCs are multipotent during embryonic development, giving rise to BCs and LCs, but that after birth, during puberty, in adulthood and throughout pregnancy cycles, BCs, ER− LCs and ER+ LCs are lineage-restricted and self-sustained lineages (Van Keymeulen et al. 2011; Wuidart et al. 2016, 2018; Van Keymeulen et al. 2017; Rodilla et al. 2015; Lloyd-Lewis et al. 2018; Tao et al. 2014).

How multipotent embryonic cells restrict their potential and commit to one of the different lineages is a fascinating question. Also, how oncogenes reprogram committed cells and induce a change of fate or reinduce multipotency and how master regulators of cell fate are involved in tumorigenesis are important questions for which we are starting to accumulate answers.

In this chapter, we will focus on the known mechanisms regulating the cell fate in breast development. In particular, we will focus on the role of the microenvironment and external cues to specify mammary gland cells. We will describe the known transcription factors acting as master regulators of each cell lineage in the mammary gland, responsible for the switch from multipotency to unipotency and the commitment to one-cell lineage. We will then see how oncogenes can induce cell reprogramming and change of fate and will discuss how master regulators of mammary epithelial cells are involved in breast cancer.

10.2 Role of Microenvironment and External Cues in Mammary Gland Cell Specification

The microenvironment is comprised of adjacent cells of different types, like immune cells, mesenchymal cells and epithelial cells, as well as the extracellular matrix (ECM) mainly composed of collagen, fibronectin and laminin molecules. The microenvironment also comprises soluble hormones and molecules secreted by surrounding cells.

The influence of the microenvironment on the mouse mammary gland development and its implication in cell specification were demonstrated by the work of Gilbert H. Smith et al. Their work was based on transplantation experiments similar to those described in the 1950s in which mammary epithelial cells were transplanted into mammary fat pads of prepubescent female mice in which the endogenous epithelium is surgically removed (cleared fat pad) and were able to recapitulate an entire functional mammary outgrowth regardless of age or parity status of the transplanted cells (Deome et al. 1959). They performed a series of transplantation experiments in immunocompromised mice in which they mixed non-mammary cells, labelled with *LacZ* expression, along with non-labelled mammary epithelial cells into a cleared mammary fat pad. Neural stem cells and their progeny were able to adopt the function of the mammary epithelial cells (Booth et al. 2008). Similarly, adult testicular cells isolated from seminiferous tubules and mesoderm-derived bone marrow cells were able to adopt mammary epithelial properties and differentiate into functional mammary epithelial cells (Boulanger et al. 2007, 2012). Mouse and human cancer cells were also able to be redirected to a normal mammary epithelial cell fate when transplanted along with normal mouse mammary epithelial cells, suppressing their tumorigenic phenotype (Booth et al. 2011; Bussard et al. 2010). Even embryonic stem cells, which form teratomas when transplanted alone, were redirected to a mammary cell fate when transplanted into a cleared mammary fat pad along with normal mammary epithelial cells (Boulanger et al. 2013). These experiments demonstrated that the components of the microenvironment are the ultimate determinants of cell function, regardless of the original nature of the cells transplanted. In these experiments, none of these cells was able to form mammary outgrowth in the absence of mammary epithelial cells, suggesting a crucial contribution of surrounding mammary epithelial cells in the cell fate redirection of non-mammary cells. The group of Gilbert

H. Smith was later able to demonstrate that acellular mammary ECM derived from adult female nulliparous mice was sufficient to direct the differentiation of transplanted testicular-derived cells and embryonic stem cells, in absence of mammary epithelial cells, to form mammary outgrowth in vivo, while ECM derived from other sources did not allow a mammary epithelial cell fate to occur upon transplantation into cleared mammary fat pads (Bruno et al. 2017). These results demonstrated that the non-cellular mammary ECM contains critical factors of the mammary microenvironment which, in conjunction with the mammary fat pad, are sufficient to reprogram non-mammary cells to a mammary epithelial cell fate.

The mammary ECM components responsible for the cell fate determination are likely to be a complex mix of many features, like stiffness, collagen organization, and relative proportions between components and soluble factors rather than one single component. Several components of the mammary ECM have been identified as important for proper mammary gland development and specification. For example, *β1 integrin* ablation was shown to lead to a delay in mammary gland growth, and altered lobuloalveolar development and ductal branching pattern, and be required for mammary epithelial cell differentiation and alveolar development, suggesting that *β1 integrin* is critical for alveolar morphogenesis, for the maintenance of its differentiated function as well as for segregation of the BC/LC lineages (Naylor et al. 2005; Taddei et al. 2008). Similarly, *α3* and *α6 integrin* subunit deletion in LCs resulted in decreased progenitor capacity, retarded alveolar formation, and precocious involution (Romagnoli et al. 2020), and *α2 integrin* knockout mice showed a defect in mammary gland branching morphogenesis (Chen et al. 2002). Laminin-111, composed of *laminin α1, β1, and γ1* chains, has been shown to regulate mammary progenitor self-renewal and establish LC apical–basal polarity (LaBarge et al. 2009; Gudjonsson et al. 2002; Weir et al. 2006). Also, the loss of *laminin α5* in LCs resulted in reduced number and differentiation of ER+ LCs, as well as impaired *Wnt4*-mediated crosstalk between ER+ LCs and BCs (Englund et al. 2021). The collagen receptor *DDR1* has also been shown to have a role in alveologenesis, as *DDR1*-null females showed a failure of alveoli formation in the mammary gland, resulting in the absence of lactation (Vogel et al. 2001). These examples illustrate the importance of the components of the acellular ECM in directing the differentiation fate of mammary epithelial cells.

The stiffness of the ECM also has implications on cell properties and ductal morphogenesis, thereby regulating cell fate. Inappropriate expression of metalloproteinases or inhibitors of metalloproteinases, which regulate the remodeling of the ECM, can lead to aberrant mammary gland phenotypes with branching defects (Fata et al. 2004). Modulation of stiffness in 2D and 3D systems demonstrated that stiffness, on its own, impacts cell shape and tissue morphogenesis (Paszek et al. 2005).

As expected, cellular components of the microenvironment contribute as well to the cell fate of the mammary epithelial cells, through paracrine signaling. In particular, macrophage cells fluctuate during mammary gland development and estrous cycles (Hodson et al. 2013) and play an essential role in mammary ductal morphogenesis, as their depletion results in dramatic reduction of pubertal ductal outgrowth (Gouon-Evans et al. 2000). Macrophages are also required for mammary repopulating ability upon transplantation experiments of mammary stem cell (MaSC)-enriched population (Gyorki et al. 2009). Paracrine signaling involving *Notch* ligand *Delta 1* and *Wnt* between the macrophages and the epithelial cells is involved in this process (Chakrabarti et al. 2018). Macrophages have also been shown to affect differentiation of mammary epithelial cells by influencing estrogen signaling in epithelial cells (Brady et al. 2017). Eosinophils, mast cells, and T-cells can also impact mammary morphogenesis when depleted (Gouon-Evans et al. 2000; Lilla and Werb 2010; Plaks et al. 2015). Other cell types of the mammary microenvironment have been shown to have a role in mammary gland development. For example, ablation of mammary adipocytes has shown that adipocytes are essential for the formation of the ductal network during puberty and to maintain the alveolar structures during adulthood (Landskroner-Eiger et al. 2010; Couldrey et al. 2002). Stromal fibroblasts also influence mammary epithelial cell morphogenesis (Kuperwasser et al. 2004; Medina 2004).

The term MaSCs refers to cells that are able to reconstitute a complete mammary gland in vivo upon transplantation into a cleared mammary fat pad. Alternatively, they are referred to as mammary repopulating units (MRUs). MaSC-enriched population refers to the Fluorescence Activated Cell Sorting (FACS)-sorted population that has been shown to be enriched in MaSCs, which is $CD31^{-}CD45^{-}TER119^{-}(Lin^{-})$ $CD29^{hi}CD24^{+}$. Alternatively, they have been enriched based on $CD31^{-}CD45^{-}TER119^{-}CD140a^{-}(Lin^{-})$ $CD24^{hi}CD49f^{hi}$ cell surface markers. These cells are comprised within the BC compartment and express basal markers. Transplantation of single cells has demonstrated that these MaSCs can be bipotent upon transplantation, giving rise to both the luminal and the basal/myoepithelial lineages and generating functional lobuloalveolar units during pregnancy (Shackleton et al. 2006; Stingl et al. 2006).

The surrounding epithelial cells have a crucial impact on cell fate. Indeed, *K14*-expressing BCs, which have been shown to be unipotent and to only give rise to BCs in vivo by *K14*-reverse tetracycline-controlled transactivator (*rtTA*)-based lineage tracing, were able to give rise to both luminal and basal lineages upon transplantation, when sorted and transplanted alone. However, when the *K14rtTA*-lineage-traced cells were transplanted along with LCs at a physiological ratio, the traced BCs only gave rise to BCs in the outgrowth, suggesting that the presence of LCs restricts the differentiation potential of BCs (Van Keymeulen et al. 2011). The influence of LCs on BC fate was further demonstrated using LC ablation combined with lineage tracing of BCs. These experiments showed, both in vivo and in organoids, that LC ablation leads to reactivation of BC multipotency, traced BCs give rise to both LCs and BCs upon LC ablation. Paracrine signaling was shown to mediate these effects. In particular, tumor necrosis factor (*TNF*), which is secreted by LCs, is involved in the restriction of multipotency of BCs under physiological conditions (Centonze et al. 2020). All these experiments demonstrate that LC presence impacts BC fate by controlling their unipotency/multipotency features.

As described for macrophage and LC effects on mammary gland cell fate, the effects of the surrounding cells are mediated by paracrine signaling molecules. Many paracrine signaling pathways are required for proper mammary gland development. For example, hedgehog signaling also plays a critical role in ductal development (Moraes et al. 2007; Lewis et al. 1999). Besides the numerous paracrine signaling molecules that have been shown to act on mammary gland development and differentiation (not detailed here), hormones, and in particular estrogen, progesterone, and prolactin, have been known for many years to be central in the control of mammary ductal morphogenesis and mammary cell fate decisions (reviewed in Sternlicht et al. (2006)). These hormone cues act on ER+ LCs, which relay the signals to the other cells by paracrine signaling (Brisken et al. 1998; Clarke et al. 1997). Their effect is relayed by transcription factors or master regulators, which determine or maintain the cell identity of each cell type. In the next section, we will focus on the transcription factors associated with cell fate decisions and identities, which are master regulators of mammary epithelial cells.

10.3 Transcription Factors Acting as Master Regulators of Cell Fate in the Mammary Gland

10.3.1 Master Regulators of Luminal Cell Fate

Notch

Four homologs of *Notch* are present in mammals (*Notch1–Notch4*), which interact with five ligands (*Delta-like 1, Delta-like 3, Delta-like 4, Jagged 1, and Jagged 2*) (Qi et al. 1999; Li et al. 1998; Six et al. 2003). They are cell-surface receptors with a single transmembrane domain. Upon ligand binding, *Notch* receptors are cleaved by *presenilin*, which results in the release of the active intracellular form of *Notch*, which translocates to the nucleus and acts as a transcription factor, interacting with partners, to effect transcription (Kadesch 2000).

Activation of *Notch* is crucial to promote commitment to the luminal rather than BC lineage. This has been shown in vivo using a short-term culture system for genetic manipulation followed by in vivo transplantation studies. Introduction of a retrovirus encoding the ligand-independent constitutively active form of the *Notch1* receptor, the *Notch1* intracellular domain (NICD1) (Schroeter et al. 1998) in MaSCs, followed by transplantation, led to nodules composed exclusively of LCs, which were blocked in their ability to undergo differentiation upon pregnancy (Bouras et al. 2008). In vivo inactivation of *Notch* signaling using two distinct approaches, one targeting a downstream partner, and one targeting an enzyme essential for the activity of *Notch* receptors, showed that inactivation of *Notch* leads to expression of basal markers in LCs in pregnancy (Buono et al. 2006). Similarly, genetic deletion of the central mediator *CBF1/RBP-JK* deletion in mammary cells resulted in cells expressing *p63* and which did not contribute to the luminal compartment (Yalcin-Ozuysal et al. 2010). More recently, gain of function experiments *Notch1* combined with lineage tracing demonstrated that *Notch1* forced expression in embryonic multipotent stem cells locks the fate of these cells to ER− LC only. Moreover, forced expression of *Notch1* in differentiated BCs during puberty resulted in a switch in cell fate, as BCs progressively switched their identity to ER− LC within 3 weeks (Lilja et al. 2018), demonstrating that *Notch* activation cell autonomously dictates LC fate specification. Interestingly, in vivo experiments of LC ablation showed that *Notch* signaling is reactivated in unipotent myoepithelial cells when they are reprogrammed into multipotent progenitors to give rise to LCs (Centonze et al. 2020).

In human cells, experiments in 2D culture of isolated human mammary epithelial cells similarly concluded that *NOTCH3* is critical for the differentiation of progenitors into the luminal lineage (Raouf et al. 2008). It was also shown in human cultures that *Notch* signaling downmodulates *p63* expression and that *p63* and *Notch* have antagonistic functions in the control of the basal or luminal identity of mammary epithelial cells (Yalcin-Ozuysal et al. 2010).

Gata3, ERα, and Foxa1

Gata3, *ERα*, and *Foxa1* are coexpressed in ER+ LCs and in luminal tumors, suggesting a modulatory loop maintaining the luminal phenotype. Many studies put together have led to the conclusion that these three transcription factors are key to orchestrating the luminal lineage specification and data are accumulating to suggest a positive feedback loop between these three transcription factors.

Loss of function of *ERα* in mammary epithelial cells results in severely impaired ductal elongation and side branching and prevents terminal end bud formation, shows no development beyond a rudimentary ductal system (Feng et al. 2007; Mallepell et al. 2006), and is clearly a major actor in cell fate control of the mammary gland, relaying the estrogenic cues.

Foxa1 is a key determinant of *ER* function, as almost all *ER*–chromatin interactions and gene expression changes depend on the presence of *Foxa1* (Hurtado et al. 2011). Loss of function of *Foxa1* also causes a defect in ductal elongation and a loss of terminal end bud formation. Loss of *Foxa1* is associated with a loss of *ER* expression, but the expression of *Gata3* is maintained (Bernardo et al. 2010).

Loss of function of *Gata3* in mice mammary gland demonstrated an essential role for *Gata3* in pubertal development, with defect in ductal invasion and terminal end bud formation. Loss of *Gata3* did not result in a transdifferentiation into BCs, as cells retained luminal characters, but with reduced levels of luminal differentiation markers and absence of *ERα*. Chromatin immunoprecipitation of primary mammary epithelial cultures shows that *Gata3* binds to *Foxa1*. These experiments demonstrated that *Gata3* maintains the luminal epithelial differentiation in the adult mammary gland and regulates the transcriptional activity of *ERα* through *Foxa1* (Kouros-Mehr et al. 2006; Asselin-Labat et al. 2007). Overexpression of *Foxa1* and *Gata3* in ER− cells can render them estrogen-responsive to some extent, demonstrating their link with *ER* (Kong et al. 2011). Further experiments of chromatin sequencing demonstrated that *Gata3* acts upstream of *Foxa1* and mediates *ER* binding by shaping enhancer accessibility (Theodorou et al. 2013).

The transcription factor *FoxM1* has also been shown to be a critical regulator of LC fate, through a direct transcriptional repression of *Gata3*. Transgenic mice models were used to show that loss of *FoxM1* results in an increase of differentiated LCs, while increased expression of *FoxM1* led to a decrease in luminal differentiation. In vivo chromatin immunoprecipitation demonstrated that *FoxM1* is able to bind and repress transcription of *Gata3* (Carr et al. 2012).

Tet2 is an epigenetic eraser whose activity is to demethylate DNA. This enzyme has been shown to interact with the transcription factor *Foxp1* to form a complex mediating the demethylation of *ER*, *Gata3*, and *Foxa1*, thereby clearly playing a pivotal role in regulating the luminal lineage commitment (Kim et al. 2020).

In summary, while disrupting the *Gata3* and *Foxa1*, *ER* network does not lead to change of fate toward BCs, as observed when deleting *Notch* signaling, this network has been shown to be crucial for determining the ER+ LC fate.

Runx1

Runx1 is expressed in BCs and in ER+ LCs, but not in milk-producing cells. Deletion of *Runx1* expression in mammary epithelial cells demonstrated that it has a crucial role in controlling the ER+ LCs. Loss of *Runx1* in mammary epithelial cells resulted in a profound reduction in the ER+ LC population. *Runx1* controls their fate by repressing the key transcription factor for alveolar cells *Elf5* and by upregulating the transcription factor *Foxa1* (van Bragt et al. 2014).

10.3.2 Master Regulators of ER−/Alveolar Fate in LCs

Elf5

Elf5 is a key transcription factor that determines luminal alveolar differentiation. Loss of one functional allele of *Elf5* led to the developmental arrest of the mammary gland upon pregnancy, and this effect was cell-autonomous, as transplanted *Elf5* heterozygous cells failed to develop upon pregnancy in wild-type (WT) fat pads of immunodeficient mice (Zhou et al. 2005). Its role in mediating prolactin lobuloalveolar differentiation has first been shown in mice experiments in which reexpression of *Elf5* in prolactin receptor (*Prlr*) nullizygous mammary epithelium restored the lobuloalveolar development and milk production, demonstrating that *Elf5* is capable of substituting for prolactin signaling (Harris et al. 2006). The demonstration that *Elf5* specifies alveolar cells, inducing differentiation during alveolar morphogenesis, was done using *Elf5* knockout and overexpression experiments in mice models. *Elf5* knockout experiments prevented the formation of the secretory epithelium during pregnancy, demonstrating its essential role in alveolar development, and *Elf5* overexpression in virgin mice resulted in alveolar differentiation and milk secretion, demonstrating that *Elf5* is sufficient to specify alveolar cells (Oakes et al. 2008). Interestingly, *Elf5* loss leads to hyperactivation of the *Notch* signaling pathway, which was shown to block differentiation upon pregnancy (Chakrabarti et al. 2012; Bouras et al. 2008).

Stat5

Similar to *Elf5*, absence of *Stat5* in the mammary gland did not affect the ductal tree development but prevented alveolar differentiation upon pregnancy and is activated by prolactin (Miyoshi et al. 2001; Liu et al. 1997). Deletion at different time points using conditional knockout mice showed that *Stat5* is essential not only for pregnancy-induced cell expansion and alveolar differentiation but also for cell survival and cell differentiation maintenance at later time points during pregnancy (Cui et al. 2004). Reexpression of transgenic *Stat5a* in knockout mice was able to rescue alveologenesis, demonstrating that *Stat5* is necessary and sufficient for the establishment of alveolar differentiation (Yamaji et al. 2009). Cross-regulations of *Stat5* and *Elf5* have been shown and suggested that *Stat5* acts upstream of *Elf5* in the gene hierarchy (Yamaji et al. 2009; Oakes et al. 2008).

Runx2

Conditional *Runx2* knockout mice and exogenous *Runx2* expression in mammary gland cells also demonstrated that *Runx2* is a regulator of cell fate in mammary epithelial cells, especially during pregnancy. *Runx2* deletion in the mammary epithelial cells resulted in impaired ductal outgrowth during puberty and disrupted progenitor cell differentiation in pregnancy, leading to a shift toward a more alveolar-committed population with a more differentiated phenotype, while *Runx2* overexpression impaired alveolar differentiation of a mammary epithelial cell line (Owens et al. 2014).

Sox9

Ectopic expression of *Sox9*, together with *Slug*, was first shown to be sufficient to reprogram mature LCs into MaSCs, while *Sox9* expression alone reprogrammed mature LCs into luminal progenitor cells (Guo et al. 2012). *Sox9* deletion, combined with lineage tracing, demonstrated that *Sox9* is essential for luminal lineage commitment and proliferation, as *Sox9*-deleted LCs were lost over time and incapable of contributing to mammary gland development (Malhotra et al. 2014). Establishment of prenatal mammary cell lines from mouse deleted for *Sox9* further showed that *Sox9* is required for embryonic progenitor cells to give rise to luminal progenitor cells that are able to form alveoli (Kogata et al. 2018). Knockout mice for *Sox9* in the mammary gland showed normal ductal tree development in nulliparous mice but showed an alveologenesis defect upon pregnancy, confirming that *Sox9* is an important determinant of alveolar progenitor activity (Christin et al. 2020).

10.3.3 Master Regulators of Basal Cell Fate

p63

It has been shown that *p63* is a critical determinant of BC fate in the mammary gland. Early evidence was shown using isolated primary human breast epithelial cultures. Downmodulation of *p63* by short hairpin (Sh)RNA in BCs resulted in the decreased expression of basal markers and increased expression of luminal markers, suggesting that *p63* is required to maintain the basal versus luminal identity in human mammary epithelial cells. In contrast, ectopic expression of *p63* in LCs was sufficient to induce several hallmarks of the basal phenotype. In vivo, constitutive expression of *p63* in mammary epithelial cells impaired gland reconstitution upon grafting and inhibited the LC fate. Moreover, *Notch* signaling downregulated *p63* expression and mimicked *p63* depletion, while the expression of *p63* partially counteracted the effects of *Notch*, demonstrating antagonistic regulations of *p63* and *Notch* in controlling mammary gland epithelial cell fates (Yalcin-Ozuysal et al. 2010). Experiments combining sustained *p63* expression and lineage tracing further demonstrated in vivo that *p63* expression in embryonic multipotent progenitors promoted BC fate and that its expression in adult LCs was sufficient to reprogram them into BCs (Wuidart et al. 2018).

Wnt/β-Catenin

Many studies have shown that the *Wnt/β-catenin* axis is crucial for stem cell renewal and identity. While it is not possible to describe them all, we will focus on few representative studies which clearly illustrate the involvement of the *Wnt/β-catenin* axis in cell fate. MaSC population is expanded upon ectopic *Wnt* expression in vivo, and an increase in the number of cells lacking expression of differentiation markers is observed, supporting a role as differentiation inhibitor and in stem cell renewal (Liu et al. 2004). Deletion of the *Wnt* signaling receptor *Lrp5* in mammary epithelial cells in vivo led to a delay in ductal development during puberty, and *Lrp5* knockout mammary cells were unable to reconstitute ductal trees through limiting dilution transplant, supporting a role for *Wnt* in stem cell properties (Lindvall et al. 2006). Similarly, deletion of one allele of *Lrp6* reduced the ductal development in mammary gland (Lindvall et al. 2009). On the contrary, constitutive activation of the *Wnt/β-catenin* signaling in BCs, using stabilized N-terminally truncated *β-catenin* under the *K5* promoter, lead to precocious lateral bud formation, increased proliferation, and premature differentiation upon pregnancy (Teulière et al. 2005). Another study demonstrated that stem cells sensitized to *Wnt* signals have a competitive advantage in mammary gland reconstitution assays. In this study, they used inactivated *Axin2* mutant, which encodes a ligand-dependent negative-feedback regulator of the *Wnt* pathway, which dampens the signaling cell autonomously. The mutant results in an elevation of the *Wnt* signaling strength upon ligand activation. By performing competitive repopulation experiments with WT cells, MaSCs from the *Axin2* mutant had a marked increase in the ability to repopulate the fat pad and regenerate a functional mammary gland (Zeng and Nusse 2010). The transcription factor *LBH* was shown to be a direct target gene of the *Wnt/β-catenin* signaling pathway (Rieger et al. 2010) and was also shown to be central in the regulation of basal and stem cell fate. *LBH* conditional knockout mice in the mammary gland showed a pronounced delay in expansion during puberty and pregnancy and an increase in luminal differentiation at the expense of basal differentiation. *LBH* was shown to have a pivotal role in inducing the *p63* transcription factor to promote basal MaSC fate and to repress luminal differentiation genes, including *Esr1* (Lindley et al. 2015).

Slug, Ovol2, and Zeb1

Several masters of epithelial–mesenchymal transition (EMT) regulation are also involved in basal/MaSC identity. *Slug*, a member of the SNAIL family of transcriptional repressors, has also been involved in the regulation of cell fate and stem cell maintenance in the mammary gland. *Slug* is expressed by BCs. Experiments in which *Slug* is knocked down resulted in increased expression of luminal genes, hyperplasia of LCs, and aberrant expression of luminal markers in the BC layer of the mammary gland, indicating that the function of *Slug* is to repress luminal gene transcription program and luminal differentiation, to maintain BC identity (Nassour et al. 2012; Phillips et al. 2014). Interestingly, experiments using *Slug* transient expression in sorted primary murine mammary epithelial cells have shown that *Slug* transient expression in luminal progenitor cells was able to convert them into MaSC, while *Slug* transient expression in differentiated LCs failed to induce organoid-forming cells and therefore did not result in conversion into MaSC. However, transient expression of *Sox9* along with *Slug* induced the formation of organoids from differentiated LCs, suggesting that these two transcription factors cooperated, *Sox9* converted differentiated LCs into luminal progenitor cells and *Slug* converted luminal progenitor cells into MaSC (Guo et al. 2012). *Slug* seems to have a role in maintaining stem cell properties as well, as when *Slug*-deficient mammary epithelial cells are transplanted as single-cell suspensions, they failed to reconstitute a ductal network (Phillips et al. 2014).

Ovol2, a member of the Ovo family of zing finger transcription factor, was shown to protect the epithelial identity of mammary cells by repressing major well-known EMT inducers, using conditional knockout and lineage-tracing approaches in vivo. Deletion of *Ovol2* inhibited mammary ductal morphogenesis, depleted MaSC population, and lead to EMT of mammary epithelial cells (Watanabe et al. 2014).

Zeb1, one of the well-known EMT inducers, was also shown to promote BC fate and their self-renewal capacity. Indeed, *Zeb1* deletion in mammary epithelial cells in vivo resulted in a decrease in basal/luminal ratio, a defect in ductal branching morphogenesis, and an increase in proliferation (Han et al. 2022).

Taz

The hippo transducer *Taz* was identified in a screen of transcription factors that were able to induce lineage switching of mammary epithelial cells. In this screen, transcription factors were expressed in LCs to identify candidates able to induce a basal phenotype. *Taz* was shown to induce basal characteristics when expressed in LCs, and *Taz* depletion in BCs led to luminal differentiation, demonstrating a role for *Yap* in the determination of lineage identity in the mammary gland (Skibinski et al. 2014).

Numb and Numbl

The two homologs *Numb* and *Numbl*, which have previously been associated with asymmetric division (Zhong et al. 1996), also have an impact on cell fate in the mammary gland upon conditional deletion in vivo. *Numb* homologs are expressed in BCs and peak up during pregnancy. Their loss results in an expansion of LCs and a decrease in BCs, in EMT, and in a failure in alveolar forma-

The epigenetic mechanisms regulating mammary cell identity are still poorly understood, but one study clearly demonstrated their importance. Indeed, deletion of *Pygo2*, a histone methylation reader and potential writer through interaction with histone-modifying enzymes, in mammary cells, led to a decrease in basal/MaSC and luminal progenitor populations, and the MaSC showed a luminal differentiation bias. These observations suggested that the loss of the epigenetic regulator *Pygo2* was shifting the BC identity toward a more luminal identity. Mechanistically, *Pygo2* was shown to positively regulate the basal-promoting *Wnt/βcatenin* signaling and suppress the luminal-promoting *Notch* signaling (Gu et al. 2013).

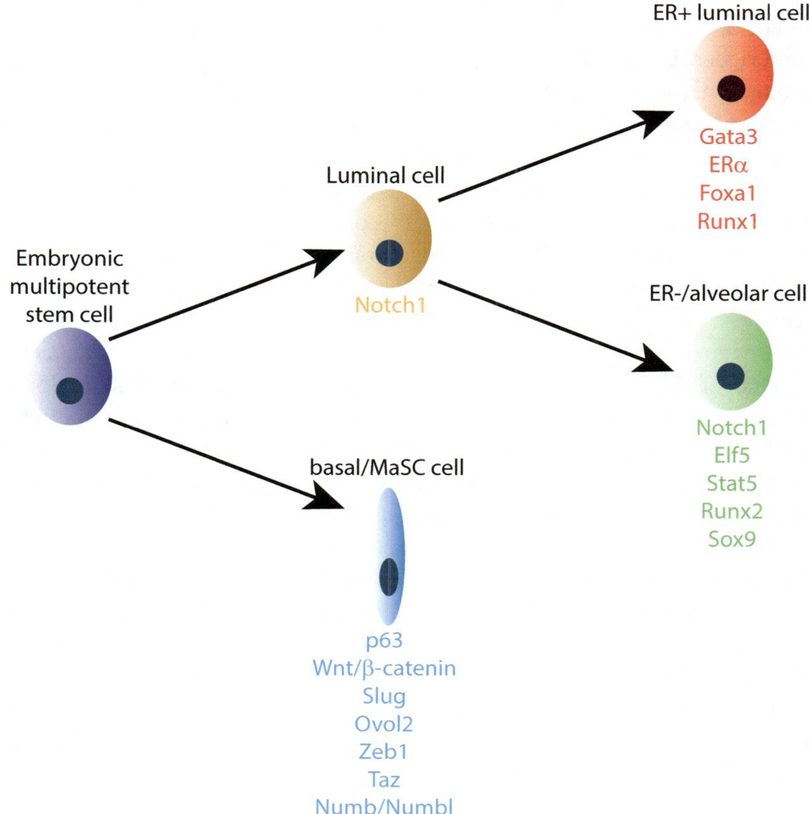

Fig. 10.1 Summary of master regulators involved in cell fate in the mammary gland. Lineage-tracing experiments have demonstrated that embryonic multipotent stem cells give rise to LCs and BCs. After birth, these two cell lineages are self-maintained. Later on, before the onset of puberty, ER+ and ER− LCs become self-maintained as well. The different cell types are depicted in this figure. Arrows point to the cell types arising from the previous cell type. For each cell type after birth, the master regulators involved in their cell specification are listed

tion and lactation, demonstrating their involvement in basal fate, epithelial identity maintenance, and lactation (Zhang et al. 2016a).

Figure 10.1 summarizes the transcription factors which have been associated with a role as master regulators of cell fate in the mammary gland.

10.4 Oncogene-Induced Change of Fate in the Mammary Gland

Historically, it has been often presumed that differentiated cells are determined during development and become irreversibly committed to their fate. However, reactivation of multipotency, cell fate change, and lineage infidelity has been associated with tumor onset and is thought to be an important driver of cancer progression in various types of cancers (Van Keymeulen et al. 2015; Koren et al. 2015; Youssef et al. 2012; Christin et al. 2020; Ge et al. 2017; Malinova et al. 2021; Davies et al. 2021; Walter et al. 2019; Le Magnen et al. 2018). This reprogramming, preceding tumor appearance, could be an essential step in tumorigenesis on which we could act to stop tumorigenesis. The ability of cancer cells to switch phenotypes has also emerged as a mode of targeted therapy evasion in various cancers (reviewed in Boumahdi and de Sauvage (2020)). Understanding the molecular basis of this plasticity could therefore contribute to new therapeutic strategies, which could lead to better clinical response when combined with existing anticancer treatments.

One of the most common oncogenic mutations in breast cancer, *Pik3ca*^{H1047R}, has been shown, upon expression in mice models, to reactivate multipotency in mammary gland epithelial cells. Indeed, expression of the *Pik3ca* mutant, specifically in LCs, combined with lineage tracing, gives rise to basal-like cells before progressing into aggressive basal-like invasive tumors. Similarly, expression of the *Pik3ca* mutant, specifically in BCs, gives rise to luminal-like cells before giving rise to less aggressive luminal-like tumors. These results also demonstrated that expression of basal or luminal markers is not an indicator of the origin of mammary cancers. Expression profile analysis of these cells demonstrated a profound oncogene-induced reprogramming of these newly formed cells into multipotent cells. This change of fate occurs months before tumor appearance and is likely setting the stage for future intratumoral heterogeneity (Van Keymeulen et al. 2015; Koren et al. 2015).

It has been shown, more than 10 years ago, that *BRCA1* mutation carriers show an expanded luminal progenitor population in the mammary gland, reflecting therefore a defect in progenitor cell lineage commitment before tumor appearance in these patients. Moreover, molecular analysis of disease-free breast tissues from *BRCA1* carriers revealed that the transcriptional repressor *Slug* is aberrantly expressed in these tissues and that its expression suppresses luminal differentiation (Lim et al. 2009; Proia et al. 2011). More recently, single-cell analysis from mice models with loss of *Brca1* and *p53* in LCs demonstrated that the loss of *Brca1* induces an aberrant alveolar differentiation preceding tumorigenesis, evolving into tumor cells with basal/mesenchymal transdifferentiation, giving rise eventually to basal-like breast cancers (Bach et al. 2017; Wang et al. 2019).

Other oncogenic stress hits also induce a change of fate in mammary epithelial cells. Introduction of a retroviral vector expressing either *PyMT*, an oncoprotein commonly used to induce mammary gland tumors (Fluck and Schaffhausen 2009), or *ErbB2*, an oncogene amplified in around 15% of human breast cancers according to Cancer Research UK and the American Cancer Society, into LCs in vivo leads to the generation of basal-like cells from the targeted LCs (Hein et al. 2016). Also, expression of the *Etv6-Ntrk3* oncogene in ER− luminal progenitor cells gives rise to basal-like cells before the development of mammary tumors with basal differentiation (Tao et al. 2015). More recently, a mouse model in which *p53* and *Rb* tumor suppressor genes are inactivated showed an increase of *Sox9* expression in LCs, which is correlated with luminal-to-basal plasticity, preceding tumor appearance (Christin et al. 2020).

Deletion or knock down of *Ptpn22* and *Mll3* promotes *PIK3CA*-driven tumorigenesis and causes the expansion of a stem cell-like population, whose identity remains to be fully characterized, with higher stem cell activity, as measured by its organoid-forming ability (Zhang et al. 2016b).

Sh screen targeting tumor suppressor genes experiments in human breast epithelial mammospheres established that ablation of *LATS 1* and *2*, actors of the *Hippo* pathway, promotes the luminal phenotype and increases the number of bipotent and luminal progenitors, through a direct interaction between the *Hippo* and the *ER* signaling (Britschgi et al. 2017).

Altogether, these studies suggest that change of fate and reprogramming are likely to be a common and important early mechanism in tumorigenesis, driven by many cancer drivers.

Besides these early changes of fate, preceding tumorigenesis, the EMT is known to play an essential role in cancer metastasis. EMT transcription factors like *Slug*, *Snail*, and *Zeb1* are usually activated during cancer progression to promote metastasis. Many studies have shown, using overexpression or downregulation of EMT transcription factors, that perturbing this process affects stem cell capacities of the cancer cells, their migration, and their contribution to metastasis (Mani et al. 2008; Guo et al. 2012; Yang et al. 2004). The generation of a mouse model with an endogenous *Snail1* reporter showed that endogenous *Snail1* expression was restricted to primary tumors that ultimately disseminate, providing evidence linking EMT transcription factors to metastasis without perturbing the process by overexpression or downregulation of genes (Tran et al. 2014). Later on, a study using intravital microscopy showed that the motile tumor cells had undergone EMT, while the epithelial tumor cells where not migrating, and that when mesenchymal tumor cells arrived at secondary sites they converted back to an epithelial state, demonstrating that EMT supports migration (Beerling et al. 2016). Similar to other cancer types, tumors arising from the mammary gland display the existence of multiple subpopulations with different EMT stages, from epithelial to completely mesenchymal states, passing through intermediate hybrid states, and these states displayed differences in cellular plasticity, invasiveness, and metastatic potential (Pastushenko et al. 2018).

These studies illustrated that change of fate and lineage plasticity are observed not only before tumor appearance and upon oncogenic stress, but also once the tumor is formed (in the case of EMT). The importance of EMT in invasiveness and metastatic potential has been demonstrated. The role of lineage plasticity preceding tumor appearance is likely to be an important mechanism in tumorigenesis as well.

10.5 Implication of Master Regulators of Cell Fate in Breast Cancer

As discussed in the previous section, the loss of the tumor suppressor *Brca1* leads to the expansion of a cell population with an aberrant alveolar differentiation, despite all animals being nulliparous. Transposase-accessible chromatin sequencing in mouse models with loss of *Brca1* and *p53* in LCs showed significant enrichment for key transcription factors that drive alveolar differentiation, including *Cebpd*, *Elf5*, *Nfkb1*, and *Sox10*, suggesting that luminal progenitors in the *Brca1*/*p53* mouse model are poised to differentiate toward the alveolar fate (Bach et al. 2017). This model shows that master regulators of alveolar fate are involved in the reprogramming of LCs upon *Brca1* loss, which precedes tumor appearance and could constitute the first detectable event in early tumorigenesis. This is of particular interest in the development of new diagnostic or therapeutic strategies to prevent breast cancer in *Brca1* carrier patients.

Aberrant expression of the master regulator can also lead to tumorigenesis.

Constitutive *Notch* signaling in LCs leads to hyperplasia and tumorigenesis in vivo (Bouras et al. 2008). In mouse models of breast cancer, *Notch4* and *Notch1* can induce tumorigenesis

(Diévart et al. 1999; Gallahan and Callahan 1997). In humans, the expression of the *Notch* inhibitor *Numb* is lost in 50% of breast carcinomas (Pece et al. 2004), and increased NICD accumulation is detected in a range of breast cancer cell lines and primary samples (Stylianou et al. 2006). The *Notch* signaling pathway has been targeted for therapeutic use by several strategies (summarized in Edwards and Brennan (2021)).

Gata3 expression level was identified as one of the best predictors of breast cancer survival and is associated with well-differentiated tumors (Jenssen et al. 2002). A potential role as tumor suppressor has also been suggested, as mutations in *Gata3* have been reported in human breast tumors (Usary et al. 2004). Overexpression of *FoxM1*, which represses *Gata3*, is associated with poor outcome in breast cancer, and its expression is elevated in mammary tumors (Bektas et al. 2008). The use of the *MMTV-PyMT* mouse model of breast cancer clearly indicated that *Gata3* is a crucial regulator of tumor differentiation and that its lack of expression underlies the early stages of breast cancer progression. Indeed, tumor progression, which is correlated with loss of luminal differentiation genes, was correlated with the loss of *Gata3* expression, and restoration of *Gata3* expression in late carcinoma was sufficient to induce luminal differentiation (Kouros-Mehr et al. 2008).

Mutations in *Esr1* are associated with resistance to endocrine therapies and tumor relapse (Jeffreys et al. 2020). *Foxa1* expression level correlates with a favorable outcome in breast cancer (Badve et al. 2007). Mutations within the *Foxa1* gene have been found, as well as amplification of the *Foxa1* locus, though not frequently (TCGA 2012).

Runx1 point mutations, frame-shift mutations, and deletions have been associated with breast cancer (TCGA 2012), and mutations have been shown to lead *Runx1* to loss of function (van Bragt et al. 2014). Similarly, *Elf5* has been shown to be lost in breast cancer, suggesting a potential tumor-suppressive role, and was shown to act as a suppressor of EMT and metastasis in breast cancer cells (Chakrabarti et al. 2012; Zhou et al. 1998; Ma et al. 2003).

Sox9 expression is significantly upregulated in basal-like breast cancer molecular subtypes, and higher expression is associated with a shorter relapse-free survival in patients with this cancer subtype. A functional role of *Sox9* in tumorigenesis has been illustrated in a mouse model in which *Sox9* deletion inhibits the progression of benign lesions to invasive tumors (Christin et al. 2020).

Activation of *Wnt* signaling is common in human breast cancers (Lin et al. 2000; Ugolini et al. 2001; Klopocki et al. 2004). Similarly, accumulation of *β-catenin* has been detected in a majority of human breast cancers and particularly in the basal subtype (Nakopoulou et al. 2006; Khramtsov et al. 2010; Geyer et al. 2011). The transcription factor *LBH* is also abnormally overexpressed in the basal subtype of breast cancer (Lamb et al. 2013; Rieger et al. 2010). The functional role of the *Wnt* signaling pathway in tumorigenesis has been demonstrated as deletion of *Lrp5* supressed *Wnt1*-induced tumorigenesis in mice (Lindvall et al. 2006).

Slug is frequently overexpressed in basal-like breast cancer, and high *Slug* expression is correlated with higher metastatic potential and higher tumor grade (Liu et al. 2013).

In summary, most of the transcription factors involved in regulating cell fate in the mammary gland have been shown to be involved in breast cancer.

10.6 Conclusions

While many transcription factors regulating the lineage identity have been identified and are involved in breast cancer, how they interact with each other is still not always clear. The understanding of the molecular actors influencing lineage identity and dynamics in the normal mammary gland will undoubtedly contribute to a better understanding of breast tumor heterogeneity.

References

Asselin-Labat ML, Sutherland KD, Barker H, Thomas R, Shackleton M, Forrest NC, Hartley L, Robb L, Grosveld FG, van der Wees J, Lindeman GJ, Visvader JE (2007) Gata-3 is an essential regulator of mammary-gland morphogenesis and luminal-cell differentiation. Nat Cell Biol 9:201–209

Bach K, Pensa S, Grzelak M, Hadfield J, Adams DJ, Marioni JC, Khaled WT (2017) Differentiation dynamics of mammary epithelial cells revealed by single-cell RNA sequencing. Nat Commun 8:2128

Badve S, Turbin D, Thorat MA, Morimiya A, Nielsen TO, Perou CM, Dunn S, Huntsman DG, Nakshatri H (2007) FOXA1 expression in breast cancer--correlation with luminal subtype A and survival. Clin Cancer Res 13:4415–4421

Beerling E, Seinstra D, de Wit E, Kester L, van der Velden D, Maynard C, Schäfer R, van Diest P, Voest E, van Oudenaarden A, Vrisekoop N, van Rheenen J (2016) Plasticity between epithelial and mesenchymal states unlinks EMT from metastasis-enhancing stem cell capacity. Cell Rep 14:2281–2288

Bektas N, Haaf A, Veeck J, Wild PJ, Lüscher-Firzlaff J, Hartmann A, Knüchel R, Dahl E (2008) Tight correlation between expression of the Forkhead transcription factor FOXM1 and HER2 in human breast cancer. BMC Cancer 8:42

Bernardo GM, Lozada KL, Miedler JD, Harburg G, Hewitt SC, Mosley JD, Godwin AK, Korach KS, Visvader JE, Kaestner KH, Abdul-Karim FW, Montano MM, Keri RA (2010) FOXA1 is an essential determinant of ERalpha expression and mammary ductal morphogenesis. Development 137:2045–2054

Booth BW, Mack DL, Androutsellis-Theotokis A, McKay RD, Boulanger CA, Smith GH (2008) The mammary microenvironment alters the differentiation repertoire of neural stem cells. Proc Natl Acad Sci USA 105:14891–14896

Booth BW, Boulanger CA, Anderson LH, Smith GH (2011) The normal mammary microenvironment suppresses the tumorigenic phenotype of mouse mammary tumor virus-neu-transformed mammary tumor cells. Oncogene 30:679–689

Boulanger CA, Mack DL, Booth BW, Smith GH (2007) Interaction with the mammary microenvironment redirects spermatogenic cell fate in vivo. Proc Natl Acad Sci USA 104:3871–3876

Boulanger CA, Bruno RD, Rosu-Myles M, Smith GH (2012) The mouse mammary microenvironment redirects mesoderm-derived bone marrow cells to a mammary epithelial progenitor cell fate. Stem Cells Dev 21:948–954

Boulanger CA, Bruno RD, Mack DL, Gonzales M, Castro NP, Salomon DS, Smith GH (2013) Embryonic stem cells are redirected to non-tumorigenic epithelial cell fate by interaction with the mammary microenvironment. PLoS One 8:e62019

Boumahdi S, de Sauvage FJ (2020) The great escape: tumour cell plasticity in resistance to targeted therapy. Nat Rev Drug Discov 19:39–56

Bouras T, Pal B, Vaillant F, Harburg G, Asselin-Labat ML, Oakes SR, Lindeman GJ, Visvader JE (2008) Notch signaling regulates mammary stem cell function and luminal cell-fate commitment. Cell Stem Cell 3:429–441

Brady NJ, Farrar MA, Schwertfeger KL (2017) STAT5 deletion in macrophages alters ductal elongation and branching during mammary gland development. Dev Biol 428:232–244

Brisken C, Park S, Vass T, Lydon JP, O'Malley BW, Weinberg RA (1998) A paracrine role for the epithelial progesterone receptor in mammary gland development. Proc Natl Acad Sci USA 95:5076–5081

Britschgi A, Duss S, Kim S, Couto JP, Brinkhaus H, Koren S, De Silva D, Mertz KD, Kaup D, Varga Z, Voshol H, Vissieres A, Leroy C, Roloff T, Stadler MB, Scheel CH, Miraglia LJ, Orth AP, Bonamy GM, Reddy VA, Bentires-Alj M (2017) The Hippo kinases LATS1 and 2 control human breast cell fate via crosstalk with ERα. Nature 541:541–545

Bruno RD, Fleming JM, George AL, Boulanger CA, Schedin P, Smith GH (2017) Mammary extracellular matrix directs differentiation of testicular and embryonic stem cells to form functional mammary glands in vivo. Sci Rep 7:40196

Buono KD, Robinson GW, Martin C, Shi S, Stanley P, Tanigaki K, Honjo T, Hennighausen L (2006) The canonical Notch/RBP-J signaling pathway controls the balance of cell lineages in mammary epithelium during pregnancy. Dev Biol 293:565–580

Bussard KM, Boulanger CA, Booth BW, Bruno RD, Smith GH (2010) Reprogramming human cancer cells in the mouse mammary gland. Cancer Res 70:6336–6343

Carr JR, Kiefer MM, Park HJ, Li J, Wang Z, Fontanarosa J, DeWaal D, Kopanja D, Benevolenskaya EV, Guzman G, Raychaudhuri P (2012) FoxM1 regulates mammary luminal cell fate. Cell Rep 1:715–729

Centonze A, Lin S, Tika E, Sifrim A, Fioramonti M, Malfait M, Song Y, Wuidart A, Van Herck J, Dannau A, Bouvencourt G, Dubois C, Dedoncker N, Sahay A, de Maertelaer V, Siebel CW, Van Keymeulen A, Voet T, Blanpain C (2020) Heterotypic cell-cell communication regulates glandular stem cell multipotency. Nature 584:608–613

Chakrabarti R, Hwang J, Andres Blanco M, Wei Y, Lukačišin M, Romano RA, Smalley K, Liu S, Yang Q, Ibrahim T, Mercatali L, Amadori D, Haffty BG, Sinha S, Kang Y (2012) Elf5 inhibits the epithelial-mesenchymal transition in mammary gland development and breast cancer metastasis by transcriptionally repressing Snail2. Nat Cell Biol 14:1212–1222

Chakrabarti R, Celià-Terrassa T, Kumar S, Hang X, Wei Y, Choudhury A, Hwang J, Peng J, Nixon B, Grady JJ, DeCoste C, Gao J, van Es JH, Li MO, Aifantis I, Clevers H, Kang Y (2018) Notch ligand Dll1 mediates cross-talk between mammary stem cells and the macrophageal niche. Science 360

Chen J, Diacovo TG, Grenache DG, Santoro SA, Zutter MM (2002) The alpha(2) integrin subunit-deficient mouse: a multifaceted phenotype including defects of branching morphogenesis and hemostasis. Am J Pathol 161:337–344

Christin JR, Wang C, Chung CY, Liu Y, Dravis C, Tang W, Oktay MH, Wahl GM, Guo W (2020) Stem cell determinant SOX9 promotes lineage plasticity and progression in basal-like breast cancer. Cell Rep 31:107742

Clarke RB, Howell A, Potten CS, Anderson E (1997) Dissociation between steroid receptor expression and cell proliferation in the human breast. Cancer Res 57:4987–4991

Couldrey C, Moitra J, Vinson C, Anver M, Nagashima K, Green J (2002) Adipose tissue: a vital in vivo role in mammary gland development but not differentiation. Dev Dyn 223:459–468

Cui Y, Riedlinger G, Miyoshi K, Tang W, Li C, Deng CX, Robinson GW, Hennighausen L (2004) Inactivation of Stat5 in mouse mammary epithelium during pregnancy reveals distinct functions in cell proliferation, survival, and differentiation. Mol Cell Biol 24:8037–8047

Davies A, Nouruzi S, Ganguli D, Namekawa T, Thaper D, Linder S, Karaoğlanoğlu F, Omur ME, Kim S, Kobelev M, Kumar S, Sivak O, Bostock C, Bishop J, Hoogstraat M, Talal A, Stelloo S, van der Poel H, Bergman AM, Ahmed M, Fazli L, Huang H, Tilley W, Goodrich D, Feng FY, Gleave M, He HH, Hach F, Zwart W, Beltran H, Selth L, Zoubeidi A (2021) An androgen receptor switch underlies lineage infidelity in treatment-resistant prostate cancer. Nat Cell Biol 23:1023–1034

Deome KB, Faulkin LJ Jr, Bern HA, Blair PB (1959) Development of mammary tumors from hyperplastic alveolar nodules transplanted into gland-free mammary fat pads of female C3H mice. Cancer Res 19:515–520

Diévart A, Beaulieu N, Jolicoeur P (1999) Involvement of Notch1 in the development of mouse mammary tumors. Oncogene 18:5973–5981

Edwards A, Brennan K (2021) Notch signalling in breast development and cancer. Front Cell Dev Biol 9:692173

Englund JI, Ritchie A, Blaas L, Cojoc H, Pentinmikko N, Döhla J, Iqbal S, Patarroyo M, Katajisto P (2021) Laminin alpha 5 regulates mammary gland remodeling through luminal cell differentiation and Wnt4-mediated epithelial crosstalk. Development 148

Fata JE, Werb Z, Bissell MJ (2004) Regulation of mammary gland branching morphogenesis by the extracellular matrix and its remodeling enzymes. Breast Cancer Res 6:1–11

Feng Y, Manka D, Wagner KU, Khan SA (2007) Estrogen receptor-alpha expression in the mammary epithelium is required for ductal and alveolar morphogenesis in mice. Proc Natl Acad Sci USA 104:14718–14723

Fluck MM, Schaffhausen BS (2009) Lessons in signaling and tumorigenesis from polyomavirus middle T antigen. Microbiol Mol Biol Rev 73:542–563

Gallahan D, Callahan R (1997) The mouse mammary tumor associated gene INT3 is a unique member of the NOTCH gene family (NOTCH4). Oncogene 14:1883–1890

Ge Y, Gomez NC, Adam RC, Nikolova M, Yang H, Verma A, Lu CP, Polak L, Yuan S, Elemento O, Fuchs E (2017) Stem cell lineage infidelity drives wound repair and cancer. Cell 169:636–650.e14

Geyer FC, Lacroix-Triki M, Savage K, Arnedos M, Lambros MB, MacKay A, Natrajan R, Reis-Filho JS (2011) β-Catenin pathway activation in breast cancer is associated with triple-negative phenotype but not with CTNNB1 mutation. Mod Pathol 24:209–231

Gouon-Evans V, Rothenberg ME, Pollard JW (2000) Postnatal mammary gland development requires macrophages and eosinophils. Development 127:2269–2282

Gu B, Watanabe K, Sun P, Fallahi M, Dai X (2013) Chromatin effector Pygo2 mediates Wnt-notch crosstalk to suppress luminal/alveolar potential of mammary stem and basal cells. Cell Stem Cell 13:48–61

Gudjonsson T, Rønnov-Jessen L, Villadsen R, Rank F, Bissell MJ, Petersen OW (2002) Normal and tumor-derived myoepithelial cells differ in their ability to interact with luminal breast epithelial cells for polarity and basement membrane deposition. J Cell Sci 115:39–50

Guo W, Keckesova Z, Donaher JL, Shibue T, Tischler V, Reinhardt F, Itzkovitz S, Noske A, Zürrer-Härdi U, Bell G, Tam WL, Mani SA, van Oudenaarden A, Weinberg RA (2012) Slug and Sox9 cooperatively determine the mammary stem cell state. Cell 148:1015–1028

Gyorki DE, Asselin-Labat ML, van Rooijen N, Lindeman GJ, Visvader JE (2009) Resident macrophages influence stem cell activity in the mammary gland. Breast Cancer Res 11:R62

Han Y, Villarreal-Ponce A, Gutierrez G Jr, Nguyen Q, Sun P, Wu T, Sui B, Berx G, Brabletz T, Kessenbrock K, Zeng YA, Watanabe K, Dai X (2022) Coordinate control of basal epithelial cell fate and stem cell maintenance by core EMT transcription factor Zeb1. Cell Rep 38:110240

Harris J, Stanford PM, Sutherland K, Oakes SR, Naylor MJ, Robertson FG, Blazek KD, Kazlauskas M, Hilton HN, Wittlin S, Alexander WS, Lindeman GJ, Visvader JE, Ormandy CJ (2006) Socs2 and elf5 mediate prolactin-induced mammary gland development. Mol Endocrinol 20:1177–1187

Hein SM, Haricharan S, Johnston AN, Toneff MJ, Reddy JP, Dong J, Bu W, Li Y (2016) Luminal epithelial cells within the mammary gland can produce basal cells upon oncogenic stress. Oncogene 35:1461–1467

Hodson LJ, Chua AC, Evdokiou A, Robertson SA, Ingman WV (2013) Macrophage phenotype in the mammary gland fluctuates over the course of the estrous cycle and is regulated by ovarian steroid hormones. Biol Reprod 89:65

Hurtado A, Holmes KA, Ross-Innes CS, Schmidt D, Carroll JS (2011) FOXA1 is a key determinant of estrogen receptor function and endocrine response. Nat Genet 43:27–33

Jeffreys SA, Powter B, Balakrishnar B, Mok K, Soon P, Franken A, Neubauer H, de Souza P, Becker TM (2020) Endocrine resistance in breast cancer: the role of estrogen receptor stability. Cells 9

Jenssen TK, Kuo WP, Stokke T, Hovig E (2002) Associations between gene expressions in breast cancer and patient survival. Hum Genet 111:411–420

Kadesch T (2000) Notch signaling: a dance of proteins changing partners. Exp Cell Res 260:1–8

Khramtsov AI, Khramtsova GF, Tretiakova M, Huo D, Olopade OI, Goss KH (2010) Wnt/beta-catenin pathway activation is enriched in basal-like breast cancers and predicts poor outcome. Am J Pathol 176:2911–2920

Kim MR, Wu MJ, Zhang Y, Yang JY, Chang CJ (2020) TET2 directs mammary luminal cell differentiation and endocrine response. Nat Commun 11:4642

Klopocki E, Kristiansen G, Wild PJ, Klaman I, Castanos-Velez E, Singer G, Stöhr R, Simon R, Sauter G, Leibiger H, Essers L, Weber B, Hermann K, Rosenthal A, Hartmann A, Dahl E (2004) Loss of SFRP1 is associated with breast cancer progression and poor prognosis in early stage tumors. Int J Oncol 25:641–649

Kogata N, Bland P, Tsang M, Oliemuller E, Lowe A, Howard BA (2018) Sox9 regulates cell state and activity of embryonic mouse mammary progenitor cells. Commun Biol 1:228

Kong SL, Li G, Loh SL, Sung WK, Liu ET (2011) Cellular reprogramming by the conjoint action of ERα, FOXA1, and GATA3 to a ligand-inducible growth state. Mol Syst Biol 7:526

Koren S, Reavie L, Couto JP, De Silva D, Stadler MB, Roloff T, Britschgi A, Eichlisberger T, Kohler H, Aina O, Cardiff RD, Bentires-Alj M (2015) PIK3CA(H1047R) induces multipotency and multi-lineage mammary tumours. Nature 525:114–118

Kouros-Mehr H, Slorach EM, Sternlicht MD, Werb Z (2006) GATA-3 maintains the differentiation of the luminal cell fate in the mammary gland. Cell 127:1041–1055

Kouros-Mehr H, Bechis SK, Slorach EM, Littlepage LE, Egeblad M, Ewald AJ, Pai SY, Ho IC, Werb Z (2008) GATA-3 links tumor differentiation and dissemination in a luminal breast cancer model. Cancer Cell 13:141–152

Kuperwasser C, Chavarria T, Wu M, Magrane G, Gray JW, Carey L, Richardson A, Weinberg RA (2004) Reconstruction of functionally normal and malignant human breast tissues in mice. Proc Natl Acad Sci USA 101:4966–4971

LaBarge MA, Nelson CM, Villadsen R, Fridriksdottir A, Ruth JR, Stampfer MR, Petersen OW, Bissell MJ (2009) Human mammary progenitor cell fate decisions are products of interactions with combinatorial microenvironments. Integr Biol (Camb) 1:70–79

Lamb R, Ablett MP, Spence K, Landberg G, Sims AH, Clarke RB (2013) Wnt pathway activity in breast cancer sub-types and stem-like cells. PLoS One 8:e67811

Landskroner-Eiger S, Park J, Israel D, Pollard JW, Scherer PE (2010) Morphogenesis of the developing mammary gland: stage-dependent impact of adipocytes. Dev Biol 344:968–978

Le Magnen C, Shen MM, Abate-Shen C (2018) Lineage plasticity in cancer progression and treatment. Annu Rev Cancer Biol 2:271–289

Lewis MT, Ross S, Strickland PA, Sugnet CW, Jimenez E, Scott MP, Daniel CW (1999) Defects in mouse mammary gland development caused by conditional haploinsufficiency of Patched-1. Development 126:5181–5193

Li L, Milner LA, Deng Y, Iwata M, Banta A, Graf L, Marcovina S, Friedman C, Trask BJ, Hood L, Torok-Storb B (1998) The human homolog of rat Jagged1 expressed by marrow stroma inhibits differentiation of 32D cells through interaction with Notch1. Immunity 8:43–55

Lilja AM, Rodilla V, Huyghe M, Hannezo E, Landragin C, Renaud O, Leroy O, Rulands S, Simons BD, Fre S (2018) Clonal analysis of Notch1-expressing cells reveals the existence of unipotent stem cells that retain long-term plasticity in the embryonic mammary gland. Nat Cell Biol 20:677–687

Lilla JN, Werb Z (2010) Mast cells contribute to the stromal microenvironment in mammary gland branching morphogenesis. Dev Biol 337:124–133

Lim E, Vaillant F, Wu D, Forrest NC, Pal B, Hart AH, Asselin-Labat ML, Gyorki DE, Ward T, Partanen A, Feleppa F, Huschtscha LI, Thorne HJ, Fox SB, Yan M, French JD, Brown MA, Smyth GK, Visvader JE, Lindeman GJ (2009) Aberrant luminal progenitors as the candidate target population for basal tumor development in BRCA1 mutation carriers. Nat Med 15:907–913

Lin SY, Xia W, Wang JC, Kwong KY, Spohn B, Wen Y, Pestell RG, Hung MC (2000) Beta-catenin, a novel prognostic marker for breast cancer: its roles in cyclin D1 expression and cancer progression. Proc Natl Acad Sci USA 97:4262–4266

Lindley LE, Curtis KM, Sanchez-Mejias A, Rieger ME, Robbins DJ, Briegel KJ (2015) The WNT-controlled transcriptional regulator LBH is required for mammary stem cell expansion and maintenance of the basal lineage. Development 142:893–904

Lindvall C, Evans NC, Zylstra CR, Li Y, Alexander CM, Williams BO (2006) The Wnt signaling receptor Lrp5 is required for mammary ductal stem cell activity and Wnt1-induced tumorigenesis. J Biol Chem 281:35081–35087

Lindvall C, Zylstra CR, Evans N, West RA, Dykema K, Furge KA, Williams BO (2009) The Wnt co-receptor Lrp6 is required for normal mouse mammary gland development. PLoS One 4:e5813

Liu X, Robinson GW, Wagner KU, Garrett L, Wynshaw-Boris A, Hennighausen L (1997) Stat5a is mandatory for adult mammary gland development and lactogenesis. Genes Dev 11:179–186

Liu BY, McDermott SP, Khwaja SS, Alexander CM (2004) The transforming activity of Wnt effectors correlates with their ability to induce the accumulation of mammary progenitor cells. Proc Natl Acad Sci USA 101:4158–4163

Liu T, Zhang X, Shang M, Zhang Y, Xia B, Niu M, Liu Y, Pang D (2013) Dysregulated expression of Slug, vimentin, and E-cadherin correlates with poor clinical outcome in patients with basal-like breast cancer. J Surg Oncol 107:188–194

Lloyd-Lewis B, Davis FM, Harris OB, Hitchcock JR, Watson CJ (2018) Neutral lineage tracing of proliferative embryonic and adult mammary stem/progenitor cells. Development 145

Ma XJ, Salunga R, Tuggle JT, Gaudet J, Enright E, McQuary P, Payette T, Pistone M, Stecker K, Zhang BM, Zhou YX, Varnholt H, Smith B, Gadd M, Chatfield E, Kessler J, Baer TM, Erlander MG, Sgroi DC (2003) Gene expression profiles of human breast cancer progression. Proc Natl Acad Sci USA 100:5974–5979

Malhotra GK, Zhao X, Edwards E, Kopp JL, Naramura M, Sander M, Band H, Band V (2014) The role of Sox9 in mouse mammary gland development and maintenance of mammary stem and luminal progenitor cells. BMC Dev Biol 14:47

Malinova A, Veghini L, Real FX, Corbo V (2021) Cell lineage infidelity in PDAC progression and therapy resistance. Front Cell Dev Biol 9:795251

Mallepell S, Krust A, Chambon P, Brisken C (2006) Paracrine signaling through the epithelial estrogen receptor alpha is required for proliferation and morphogenesis in the mammary gland. Proc Natl Acad Sci USA 103:2196–2201

Mani SA, Guo W, Liao MJ, Eaton EN, Ayyanan A, Zhou AY, Brooks M, Reinhard F, Zhang CC, Shipitsin M, Campbell LL, Polyak K, Brisken C, Yang J, Weinberg RA (2008) The epithelial-mesenchymal transition generates cells with properties of stem cells. Cell 133:704–715

Medina D (2004) Stromal fibroblasts influence human mammary epithelial cell morphogenesis. Proc Natl Acad Sci USA 101:4723–4724

Miyoshi K, Shillingford JM, Smith GH, Grimm SL, Wagner KU, Oka T, Rosen JM, Robinson GW, Hennighausen L (2001) Signal transducer and activator of transcription (stat) 5 controls the proliferation and differentiation of mammary alveolar epithelium. J Cell Biol 155:531–542

Moraes RC, Zhang X, Harrington N, Fung JY, Wu MF, Hilsenbeck SG, Allred DC, Lewis MT (2007) Constitutive activation of smoothened (SMO) in mammary glands of transgenic mice leads to increased proliferation, altered differentiation and ductal dysplasia. Development 134:1231–1242

Nakopoulou L, Mylona E, Papadaki I, Kavantzas N, Giannopoulou I, Markaki S, Keramopoulos A (2006) Study of phospho-beta-catenin subcellular distribution in invasive breast carcinomas in relation to their phenotype and the clinical outcome. Mod Pathol 19:556–563

Nassour M, Idoux-Gillet Y, Selmi A, Côme C, Faraldo ML, Deugnier MA, Savagner P (2012) Slug controls stem/progenitor cell growth dynamics during mammary gland morphogenesis. PLoS One 7:e53498

Naylor MJ, Li N, Cheung J, Lowe ET, Lambert E, Marlow R, Wang P, Schatzmann F, Wintermantel T, Schüetz G, Clarke AR, Mueller U, Hynes NE, Streuli CH (2005) Ablation of beta1 integrin in mammary epithelium reveals a key role for integrin in glandular morphogenesis and differentiation. J Cell Biol 171:717–728

Oakes SR, Naylor MJ, Asselin-Labat ML, Blazek KD, Gardiner-Garden M, Hilton HN, Kazlauskas M, Pritchard MA, Chodosh LA, Pfeffer PL, Lindeman GJ, Visvader JE, Ormandy CJ (2008) The Ets transcription factor Elf5 specifies mammary alveolar cell fate. Genes Dev 22:581–586

Owens TW, Rogers RL, Best S, Ledger A, Mooney AM, Ferguson A, Shore P, Swarbrick A, Ormandy CJ, Simpson PT, Carroll JS, Visvader J, Naylor MJ (2014) Runx2 is a novel regulator of mammary epithelial cell fate in development and breast cancer. Cancer Res 74:5277–5286

Pastushenko I, Brisebarre A, Sifrim A, Fioramonti M, Revenco T, Boumahdi S, Van Keymeulen A, Brown D, Moers V, Lemaire S, De Clercq S, Minguijón E, Balsat C, Sokolow Y, Dubois C, De Cock F, Scozzaro S, Sopena F, Lanas A, D'Haene N, Salmon I, Marine JC, Voet T, Sotiropoulou PA, Blanpain C (2018) Identification of the tumour transition states occurring during EMT. Nature 556:463–468

Paszek MJ, Zahir N, Johnson KR, Lakins JN, Rozenberg GI, Gefen A, Reinhart-King CA, Margulies SS, Dembo M, Boettiger D, Hammer DA, Weaver VM (2005) Tensional homeostasis and the malignant phenotype. Cancer Cell 8:241–254

Pece S, Serresi M, Santolini E, Capra M, Hulleman E, Galimberti V, Zurrida S, Maisonneuve P, Viale G, Di Fiore PP (2004) Loss of negative regulation by Numb over Notch is relevant to human breast carcinogenesis. J Cell Biol 167:215–221

Petersen OW, Høyer PE, van Deurs B (1987) Frequency and distribution of estrogen receptor-positive cells in normal, nonlactating human breast tissue. Cancer Res 47:5748–5751

Phillips S, Prat A, Sedic M, Proia T, Wronski A, Mazumdar S, Skibinski A, Shirley SH, Perou CM, Gill G, Gupta PB, Kuperwasser C (2014) Cell-state transitions regulated by SLUG are critical for tissue regeneration and tumor initiation. Stem Cell Rep 2:633–647

Plaks V, Boldajipour B, Linnemann JR, Nguyen NH, Kersten K, Wolf Y, Casbon AJ, Kong N, van den Bijgaart RJ, Sheppard D, Melton AC, Krummel MF, Werb Z (2015) Adaptive immune regulation of mammary postnatal organogenesis. Dev Cell 34:493–504

Proia TA, Keller PJ, Gupta PB, Klebba I, Jones AD, Sedic M, Gilmore H, Tung N, Naber SP, Schnitt S, Lander ES, Kuperwasser C (2011) Genetic predisposition directs breast cancer phenotype by dictating progenitor cell fate. Cell Stem Cell 8:149–163

Qi H, Rand MD, Wu X, Sestan N, Wang W, Rakic P, Xu T, Artavanis-Tsakonas S (1999) Processing of the notch ligand delta by the metalloprotease Kuzbanian. Science 283:91–94

Raouf A, Zhao Y, K. To, Stingl J, Delaney A, Barbara M, Iscove N, Jones S, McKinney S, Emerman J, Aparicio S, Marra M, Eaves C (2008) Transcriptome analysis of the normal human mammary cell commitment and differentiation process. Cell Stem Cell 3:109–118

Rieger ME, Sims AH, Coats ER, Clarke RB, Briegel KJ (2010) The embryonic transcription cofactor LBH is a direct target of the Wnt signaling pathway in epithelial development and in aggressive basal subtype breast cancers. Mol Cell Biol 30:4267–4279

Rodilla V, Dasti A, Huyghe M, Lafkas D, Laurent C, Reyal F, Fre S (2015) Luminal progenitors restrict their lineage potential during mammary gland development. PLoS Biol 13:e1002069

Romagnoli M, Bresson L, Di-Cicco A, Pérez-Lanzón M, Legoix P, Baulande S, de la Grange P, De Arcangelis A, Georges-Labouesse E, Sonnenberg A, Deugnier MA, Glukhova MA, Faraldo MM (2020) Laminin-binding integrins are essential for the maintenance of functional mammary secretory epithelium in lactation. Development 147

Schroeter EH, Kisslinger JA, Kopan R (1998) Notch-1 signalling requires ligand-induced proteolytic release of intracellular domain. Nature 393:382–386

Shackleton M, Vaillant F, Simpson KJ, Stingl J, Smyth GK, Asselin-Labat ML, Wu L, Lindeman GJ, Visvader JE (2006) Generation of a functional mammary gland from a single stem cell. Nature 439:84–88

Six E, Ndiaye D, Laabi Y, Brou C, Gupta-Rossi N, Israel A, Logeat F (2003) The Notch ligand Delta1 is sequentially cleaved by an ADAM protease and gamma-secretase. Proc Natl Acad Sci USA 100:7638–7643

Skibinski A, Breindel JL, Prat A, Galván P, Smith E, Rolfs A, Gupta PB, LaBaer J, Kuperwasser C (2014) The Hippo transducer TAZ interacts with the SWI/SNF complex to regulate breast epithelial lineage commitment. Cell Rep 6:1059–1072

Sternlicht MD, Kouros-Mehr H, Lu P, Werb Z (2006) Hormonal and local control of mammary branching morphogenesis. Differentiation 74:365–381

Stingl J, Eirew P, Ricketson I, Shackleton M, Vaillant F, Choi D, Li HI, Eaves CJ (2006) Purification and unique properties of mammary epithelial stem cells. Nature 439:993–997

Stylianou S, Clarke RB, Brennan K (2006) Aberrant activation of notch signaling in human breast cancer. Cancer Res 66:1517–1525

Taddei I, Deugnier MA, Faraldo MM, Petit V, Bouvard D, Medina D, Fässler R, Thiery JP, Glukhova MA (2008) Beta1 integrin deletion from the basal compartment of the mammary epithelium affects stem cells. Nat Cell Biol 10:716–722

Tao L, van Bragt MP, Laudadio E, Li Z (2014) Lineage tracing of mammary epithelial cells using cell-type-specific cre-expressing adenoviruses. Stem Cell Rep 2:770–779

Tao L, van Bragt MP, Li Z (2015) A long-lived luminal subpopulation enriched with alveolar progenitors serves as cellular origin of heterogeneous mammary tumors. Stem Cell Rep 5:60–74

TCGA (2012) Comprehensive molecular portraits of human breast tumours. Nature 490:61–70

Teulière J, Faraldo MM, Deugnier MA, Shtutman M, Ben-Ze'ev A, Thiery JP, Glukhova MA (2005) Targeted activation of beta-catenin signaling in basal mammary epithelial cells affects mammary development and leads to hyperplasia. Development 132:267–277

Theodorou V, Stark R, Menon S, Carroll JS (2013) GATA3 acts upstream of FOXA1 in mediating ESR1 binding by shaping enhancer accessibility. Genome Res 23:12–22

Tran HD, Luitel K, Kim M, Zhang K, Longmore GD, Tran DD (2014) Transient SNAIL1 expression is necessary for metastatic competence in breast cancer. Cancer Res 74:6330–6340

Ugolini F, Charafe-Jauffret E, Bardou VJ, Geneix J, Adélaïde J, Labat-Moleur F, Penault-Llorca F, Longy M, Jacquemier J, Birnbaum D, Pébusque MJ (2001) WNT pathway and mammary carcinogenesis: loss of expression of candidate tumor suppressor gene SFRP1 in most invasive carcinomas except of the medullary type. Oncogene 20:5810–5817

Usary J, Llaca V, Karaca G, Presswala S, Karaca M, He X, Langerød A, Kåresen R, Oh DS, Dressler LG, Lønning PE, Strausberg RL, Chanock S, Børresen-Dale AL, Perou CM (2004) Mutation of GATA3 in human breast tumors. Oncogene 23:7669–7678

van Bragt MP, Hu X, Xie Y, Li Z (2014) RUNX1, a transcription factor mutated in breast cancer, controls the fate of ER-positive mammary luminal cells. Elife 3:e03881

Van Keymeulen A, Rocha AS, Ousset M, Beck B, Bouvencourt G, Rock J, Sharma N, Dekoninck S, Blanpain C (2011) Distinct stem cells contribute to mammary gland development and maintenance. Nature 479:189–193

Van Keymeulen A, Lee MY, Ousset M, Brohée S, Rorive S, Giraddi RR, Wuidart A, Bouvencourt G, Dubois C, Salmon I, Sotiriou C, Phillips WA, Blanpain C (2015) Reactivation of multipotency by oncogenic PIK3CA induces breast tumour heterogeneity. Nature 525:119–123

Van Keymeulen A, Fioramonti M, Centonze A, Bouvencourt G, Achouri Y, Blanpain C (2017) Lineage-restricted mammary stem cells sustain the development, homeostasis, and regeneration of the estrogen receptor positive lineage. Cell Rep 20:1525–1532

Vogel WF, Aszódi A, Alves F, Pawson T (2001) Discoidin domain receptor 1 tyrosine kinase has an essential role in mammary gland development. Mol Cell Biol 21:2906–2917

Walter DM, Yates TJ, Ruiz-Torres M, Kim-Kiselak C, Gudiel AA, Deshpande C, Wang WZ, Cicchini M, Stokes KL, Tobias JW, Buza E, Feldser DM (2019) RB constrains lineage fidelity and multiple stages of tumour progression and metastasis. Nature 569:423–427

Wang H, Xiang D, Liu B, He A, Randle HJ, Zhang KX, Dongre A, Sachs N, Clark AP, Tao L, Chen Q, Botchkarev VV Jr, Xie Y, Dai N, Clevers H, Li Z, Livingston DM (2019) Inadequate DNA damage repair promotes mammary transdifferentiation, leading to BRCA1 breast cancer. Cell 178:135–151.e19

Watanabe K, Villarreal-Ponce A, Sun P, Salmans ML, Fallahi M, Andersen B, Dai X (2014) Mammary morphogenesis and regeneration require the inhibition of EMT at terminal end buds by Ovol2 transcriptional repressor. Dev Cell 29:59–74

Watson CJ, Khaled WT (2008) Mammary development in the embryo and adult: a journey of morphogenesis and commitment. Development 135:995–1003

Weir ML, Oppizzi ML, Henry MD, Onishi A, Campbell KP, Bissell MJ, Muschler JL (2006) Dystroglycan loss disrupts polarity and beta-casein induction in mammary epithelial cells by perturbing laminin anchoring. J Cell Sci 119:4047–4058

Wuidart A, Ousset M, Rulands S, Simons BD, Van Keymeulen A, Blanpain C (2016) Quantitative lineage tracing strategies to resolve multipotency in tissue-specific stem cells. Genes Dev 30:1261–1277

Wuidart A, Sifrim A, Fioramonti M, Matsumura S, Brisebarre A, Brown D, Centonze A, Dannau A, Dubois C, Van Keymeulen A, Voet T, Blanpain C (2018) Early lineage segregation of multipotent embryonic mammary gland progenitors. Nat Cell Biol 20:666–676

Yalcin-Ozuysal O, Fiche M, Guitierrez M, Wagner KU, Raffoul W, Brisken C (2010) Antagonistic roles of Notch and p63 in controlling mammary epithelial cell fates. Cell Death Differ 17:1600–1612

Yamaji D, Na R, Feuermann Y, Pechhold S, Chen W, Robinson GW, Hennighausen L (2009) Development of mammary luminal progenitor cells is controlled by the transcription factor STAT5A. Genes Dev 23:2382–2387

Yang J, Mani SA, Donaher JL, Ramaswamy S, Itzykson RA, Come C, Savagner P, Gitelman I, Richardson A, Weinberg RA (2004) Twist, a master regulator of morphogenesis, plays an essential role in tumor metastasis. Cell 117:927–939

Youssef KK, Lapouge G, Bouvrée K, Rorive S, Brohée S, Appelstein O, Larsimont JC, Sukumaran V, Van de Sande B, Pucci D, Dekoninck S, Berthe JV, Aerts S, Salmon I, del Marmol V, Blanpain C (2012) Adult interfollicular tumour-initiating cells are reprogrammed into an embryonic hair follicle progenitor-like fate during basal cell carcinoma initiation. Nat Cell Biol 14:1282–1294

Zeng YA, Nusse R (2010) Wnt proteins are self-renewal factors for mammary stem cells and promote their long-term expansion in culture. Cell Stem Cell 6:568–577

Zhang Y, Li F, Song Y, Sheng X, Ren F, Xiong K, Chen L, Zhang H, Liu D, Lengner CJ, Xue L, Yu Z (2016a) Numb and Numbl act to determine mammary myoepithelial cell fate, maintain epithelial identity, and support lactogenesis. FASEB J 30:3474–3488

Zhang Z, Christin JR, Wang C, Ge K, Oktay MH, Guo W (2016b) Mammary-stem-cell-based somatic mouse models reveal breast cancer drivers causing cell fate dysregulation. Cell Rep 16:3146–3156

Zhong W, Feder JN, Jiang MM, Jan LY, Jan YN (1996) Asymmetric localization of a mammalian numb homolog during mouse cortical neurogenesis. Neuron 17:43–53

Zhou J, Ng AY, Tymms MJ, Jermiin LS, Seth AK, Thomas RS, Kola I (1998) A novel transcription factor, ELF5, belongs to the ELF subfamily of ETS genes and maps to human chromosome 11p13-15, a region subject to LOH and rearrangement in human carcinoma cell lines. Oncogene 17:2719–2732

Zhou J, Chehab R, Tkalcevic J, Naylor MJ, Harris J, Wilson TJ, Tsao S, Tellis I, Zavarsek S, Xu D, Lapinskas EJ, Visvader J, Lindeman GJ, Thomas R, Ormandy CJ, Hertzog PJ, Kola I, Pritchard MA (2005) Elf5 is essential for early embryogenesis and mammary gland development during pregnancy and lactation. EMBO J 24:635–644

11 Classification of Breast Cancer Through the Perspective of Cell Identity Models

Richard Iggo and Gaetan MacGrogan

Abstract

The mammary epithelium has an inner luminal layer that contains estrogen receptor (ER)-positive hormone-sensing cells and ER-negative alveolar/secretory cells, and an outer basal layer that contains myoepithelial/stem cells. Most human tumours resemble either hormone-sensing cells or alveolar/secretory cells. The most widely used molecular classification, the Intrinsic classification, assigns hormone-sensing tumours to Luminal A/B and human epidermal growth factor 2-enriched (HER2E)/molecular apocrine (MA)/luminal androgen receptor (LAR)-positive classes, and alveolar/secretory tumours to the Basal-like class. Molecular classification is most useful when tumours have classic invasive carcinoma of no special type (NST) histology. It is less useful for special histological types of breast cancer, such as metaplastic breast cancer and adenoid cystic cancer, which are better described with standard pathology terms. Compared to mice, humans show a strong bias towards making tumours that resemble mammary hormone-sensing cells. This could be caused by the formation in adolescence of der(1;16), a translocation through the centromeres of chromosomes 1 and 16, which only occurs in humans and could trap the cells in the hormone-sensing state.

Keywords

Breast cancer cell of origin · Mammary lineage · Triple-negative breast cancer · Basal-like breast cancer · HER2-enriched breast cancer · Molecular apocrine breast cancer · Luminal AR breast cancer · der(1;16) translocation

Key Points

1. The luminal layer in mammary ducts and lobules contains estrogen receptor (ER)-positive hormone-sensing cells that convert hormonal signals into paracrine growth factor signals, and ER-negative alveolar/secretory cells that expand greatly during lactation to produce milk.
2. Most human tumours resemble hormone-sensing cells. Tumours derived from hormone-sensing cells are classified as Luminal A/B if they retain ER expression. If they lose ER expression they are classified as HER2-enriched/molecular apocrine/luminal androgen receptor (LAR)-positive (HER2E/MA/LAR).

R. Iggo (✉) · G. MacGrogan
INSERM, Bergonie Cancer Institute, University of Bordeaux, Bordeaux, France
e-mail: Richard.Iggo@u-bordeaux.fr; G.MacGrogan@bordeaux.unicancer.fr

T. Sørlie, R. B. Clarke (eds.), *A Guide to Breast Cancer Research*, Advances in Experimental Medicine and Biology 1464, https://doi.org/10.1007/978-3-031-70875-6_11

3. HER2E, MA and LAR tumours have the same RNA profile. Most have *ERBB2* gene amplification, about 11% have activating mutations in *ERBB2*, and the rest are assumed to have activating mutations elsewhere in the HER2 signalling pathway.
4. Human tumours that resemble ER-negative alveolar/secretory cells are called basal-like tumours, but they probably arise from cells in the luminal layer.
5. Mice frequently develop tumours with mixed phenotypes, including myoepithelial and squamous components, either because they arise in the basal/myoepithelial layer or because mouse tumours established in luminal cells rapidly drift towards a basal/myoepithelial phenotype.
6. The difference between the tumour spectrum in mice and humans could be explained by the presence of a der(1;16) translocation, which is only seen in humans. The translocation arises because humans have massively expanded α-satellite arrays in the centromeres of chromosomes 1 and 16.

11.1 Introduction

It has now been over 20 years since the first transcriptomic classification of breast cancer was proposed. During that time, enormous progress has been made in understanding the mammary lineage and the molecular defects in breast cancer. As we brace ourselves for the onslaught of single-cell sequencing data, this is a good time to ask what the first 20 years of breast cancer classification have given us. With the benefit of hindsight, we can see that all of the classifications based on pooled RNA have converged on the same classification. Single-cell data will revolutionise our understanding of stromal cells, but, notwithstanding some new nomenclature, the good news is it seems likely that it will also converge on the same mammary lineage model and tumour cell types.

11.1.1 Classification of Breast Cancer

There are four main molecular classifications of breast cancer. The first, and de facto standard, is the Intrinsic classification, also called the PAM50 classification (Perou et al. 2000). The genius of the authors who developed it was to recognise that by testing two samples from the same tumour and analysing only genes that did not change, they could eliminate trivial differences in the content of normal cells. This is because the cells that do not change between samples are the tumour cells, the cells intrinsic to the tumour. The classification is based on hierarchical clustering of the most variable genes in the dataset. The most variable genes depend on the exact mix of tumours being analysed, so there were small inconsistencies in the classification of individual tumours in some of the early publications. To get around this, the authors fixed the genes used for the clustering, giving birth to the PAM50 gene set, which is used to this day in commercially available clinical tests like Prosigna (Parker et al. 2009). The Intrinsic classification has five classes: Luminal A, Luminal B, Basal-like, HER2-enriched (HER2E) and Normal-like. A recurring theme in breast cancer classification is that the names given to tumour groups are not what they seem, but the names are now firmly entrenched so we should avoid being misled by the names and focus on understanding the biological entities behind the names.

There is disagreement about the significance of the Normal-like class. As the name implies, the expression profile is similar to that of normal tissue. Some maintain that this is a true tumour type, meaning there exist tumour cells so similar to normal cells that they have the same expression profile, while others argue that it is simply an artefact of normal tissue contamination. There are good reasons to think that the latter explanation is correct, as the authors pointed out in the original publication (Perou et al. 2000). One is that Normal-like tumours come back as other classes after xenografting or metastasis (Reyal et al. 2012; Charafe-Jauffret et al. 2013; Aftimos et al. 2021). It is fashionable to ascribe such differences to plasticity, but a far simpler explanation is that the initial assignment was overshadowed by normal tissue contamination. Many scientists underestimate the extent of normal tissue contamination. In the EORTC 10994 phase III study on p53 mutations, for example, we excluded samples containing less than 20% tumour cells (Bonnefoi et al. 2011). Despite taking two samples from most patients, we lost one-fifth of the patients because neither biopsy met the 20% cut-off for tumour cell content. Most of the samples were taken using then-current imaging techniques to help position the needle in the tumour mass, which was itself at least 2 cm in size, so there is no suggestion that the tumours were so tiny as to be easy to miss, or that the biopsies were taken carelessly. Instead, it is simply a fact that tumour cells are often a small minority of the cells in a clinical sample. This should be borne in mind when analysing pooled datasets like TCGA and METABRIC. Hierarchical clustering is a good first test when analysing a new breast cancer dataset: if there is a good mix of ER-positive and ER-negative tumours, and they do not fall into three large groups, there is probably too much normal tissue for meaningful analysis.

The Luminal A and Luminal B classes are the classic ER-positive tumours that make up about 70%–80% of human breast tumours. Luminal A cells have minimally rearranged genomes and a transcriptome that resembles normal ER-positive hormone-sensing cells. Luminal B cells are still recognisably ER-positive hormone-sensing cells, but they have rearranged genomes with multiple amplicons, frequently accompanied by loss of p53 function. While it is easy to see the differences between Luminal A and B at the extremes, it is much more difficult to decide in the middle of the distribution. This is because the distinction is based on proliferation. Proliferation matters because it is one of the best predictors of prognosis. Many groups have developed prognostic signatures, each based on slightly different criteria. Mauro Delorenzi's group compared the signatures and found that the prognostic value lay almost entirely in the proliferation genes; the remaining genes reflected the way the signatures were developed but added little or no prognostic value (Wirapati et al. 2008). Traditionally, pathologists have used Ki-67 staining to score proliferation, but in practice it takes considerable effort to do this well (Dowsett et al. 2011). The logic behind using gene signatures is that by examining multiple genes there is less risk of outliers producing false results. As expected, proliferation is the key determinant of prognosis not just in breast cancer but in almost all tumours, at least in the short term (other factors, like dormancy and immune response, come into play at later time points). Proliferation is the end point that integrates signals from multiple convergent oncogenic pathways. As such, it does not have a bimodal distribution that neatly separates high- from low-proliferation tumours. Instead, it has a unimodal distribution. This has several consequences. First, pathologists classify most tumours as grade 2. At first glance, one might think they were sitting on the fence, dodging difficult decisions. In fact, they are absolutely right to put most tumours in grade 2, because that is where the peak of the distribution lies. The second consequence is that it is dangerous to put a cut-off through the peak of a distribution, because tiny technical variations that affect signal strength in the assay will change the classification of huge numbers of samples. This is the second reason why some tumours moved between classes in the early publications on Intrinsic classification: it is inevitable and in no way justifies the rather uncharitable criticism that was levelled at the classification at the time (Weigelt et al. 2010). To try to address this issue, the PAM50 gene set is heavily biased towards proliferation genes, but this cannot eliminate the fundamental difficulty of placing a cut-off through the peak of a distribution. An alternative is to report prognostic results on a continuous scale, as is done with OncotypeDx, a signature that focuses exclusively on prognosis (Cronin et al. 2007). Unfortunately, oncologists must give either treatment A or treatment B. They do not have the option of giving, say, 20% of treatment A and 80% of treatment B when a tumour has a score at the 80th centile of the proliferation score—so a continuous score is not as useful as one might imagine.

The third group in the Intrinsic classification is now called the HER2E class. "Enriched" was added to the name after we pointed out that many *ERBB2*-amplified tumours have a Luminal B profile, and many tumours with a HER2E profile do not have *ERBB2* amplification (Farmer et al. 2005). To address this issue, and the difficulty of drawing a line between luminal A and B, we suggested that breast tumours should be classified into only three transcriptomic groups: luminal, molecular apocrine (MA) and basal-like—the "LAB" classification (Farmer et al. 2005; Iggo 2018). These are the three large groups seen when clustering datasets that are not heavily contaminated with normal tissue. With the benefit of hindsight, it is now obvious that the HER2E and MA groups are identical. People approaching the problem from the perspective of triple-negative breast cancer (TNBC) (ER-negative, PR-negative, HER2 amplification-negative breast cancer) gave these tumours a third name, luminal androgen receptor (LAR)-positive (Lehmann et al. 2011). In fact, all three names refer to the same biological entity. The name MA was chosen to highlight a potential role for androgens in this androgen receptor (AR)-positive, ER-negative group. There is a well-established pathological breast cancer subtype called apocrine carcinoma. In our original study, one of the clinical pathologists pointed out that some of the tumours had apocrine features but did not meet the full criteria for apocrine carcinoma. Hence, we chose the term MA to avoid confusion. Apocrine glands are the evolutionary ancestors of mammary glands (Oftedal 2002). They are androgen-driven scent glands that are restricted in humans to the axillae and perineum. Women over the age of 25 often have cystic lesions called apocrine metaplasia, where the luminal epithelial cells are AR-positive and ER-negative (Wells and El-Ayat 2007). This phenotype is assumed to be caused by reversion of mammary epithelial cells to their ancestral fate. Since these cells are supposed to be androgen-driven, it was reasonable to suggest that androgen might have replaced estrogen as the key regulator of growth in MA tumours. Subsequent clinical trials with anti-androgens have produced occasional dramatic responses but the majority of patients do not respond (Gucalp et al. 2013; Traina et al. 2018; Bonnefoi et al. 2016; Grellety et al. 2018). We recently showed that MA tumours fall into two groups, one with high expression of androgen receptor target genes (MA^{hi} tumours), and that it is only these MA^{hi} tumours that respond to treatment with anti-androgens (NCT03383679). We have also established a patient-derived xenograft from an MA^{hi} tumour and shown that its growth is dependent on androgens (unpublished data). Hence, we are now sure that androgen-driven MA breast tumours really do exist. In contrast, it has been known for decades that androgens inhibit the growth of ER-positive tumours (Loeser 1939; Adair and Herrmann 1946). MA tumour cells are hormone-sensing cells that have lost ER expression. For androgen to stimulate rather than inhibit proliferation, we postulate that the spectrum of enhancers accessible to AR, and the mix of coactivators and corepressors bound to AR, have changed. This mirrors a possible model for the switch from repression to activation of proliferation by ER in normal and tumour tissue (Clarke et al. 1997). Understanding the pathogenesis of HER2E/MA/LAR tumours is a research question that fascinates biologists. Despite the initial confusion over the name, it is likely that activation of the HER2 pathway is a key element in their formation. Transcriptomes capture RNA phenotype not DNA genotype: the HER2E/MA/LAR class is distinguished by a specific RNA phenotype. *ERBB2* amplification is a DNA genotype; it is the commonest way to activate the HER2 pathway, but point mutations in *ERBB2* can have the same effect: they are present in about 11% of the HER2E/MA tumours that lack *ERBB2* amplification (Jiang et al. 2019), and 27–28% of pleomorphic lobular tumours, most of which should probably be classified as HER2E/MA (Riedlinger et al. 2021; Bergeron et al. 2021). One possibility is that pathological activation of the HER2 pathway leads to plasticity that makes it easier for cells to switch from a mammary to an apocrine fate (pathologists refer to changes in cell fate as metaplasia). Cells that have amplified *ERBB2* but not (yet) changed fate have a Luminal B phenotype. Other genes that are overexpressed (*FGFR4*) or mutated (*TBX3*, *PIK3CA*, *TP53*) in these tumours probably also facilitate the switch. The Luminal B and HER2E/MA classes are tumours of hormone-sensing cells with unstable genomes (commonly caused by loss of p53), so much of their gene expression profile is the same. This similarity explains why it can sometimes be difficult to classify them, which again led to some rather unfair criticism of the early studies on the Intrinsic classification. It would not be surprising if there were intermediate states, where part, but not all, of the differentiation programme had switched to the new state. Drifting back and forth between HER2E/MA and Luminal B phenotypes may even be a common event; this is certainly what we see in our own studies on MA patient-derived xenografts, which, by definition, start ER-negative in the patient, but show ER expression in a low percentage of cells at some xenograft passages (Richard et al. 2016). In summary, HER2E, MA and LAR refer to tumours with the same phenotype, for which the different names have a historical explanation rather than describing fundamental biological differences.

The Basal-like class in the Intrinsic classification is the one that stood out in the original publication (Perou et al. 2000). Contrary to what is often said, Basal-like tumours have a homogeneous expression profile that produces the tightest cluster of any group in heatmaps of breast cancer gene expression data. One unintended but far-reaching consequence of the success of the Intrinsic classification has been ambiguity over the meaning of the term "basal". The name derives from the fact that the tumours express keratins 5 and 17, keratins found in the basal layers of the skin (Taylor-Papadimitriou et al. 1989). Keratins are widely used as markers by pathologists because they are abundant, stable, structural proteins that give strong signals in immunohistochemistry and show striking differences in expression between Luminal and Basal-like tumours. Hence, naming the ER-negative group after the keratins they express was a reasonable choice because it translates directly to clinical practice: to a first approximation, Luminal tumours express keratins 8/18 whereas Basal-like tumours express keratins 5/17. There are two issues that cause confusion. Anatomically, the inner layer in a bilayer duct is called luminal because the cells are in contact with the lumen; the outer layer is called basal because it wraps around the basal pole of the luminal cells. It follows that a cell given the name basal (or Basal-like) should logically lie in the outer layer of the duct. Keratins 5/17 are indeed expressed mainly by cells in the basal layer in the extra-lobular ducts in humans, but they are frequently expressed by luminal cells in terminal duct lobular units (TDLUs) (Gusterson 2009; Santagata et al. 2014), and they are strongly expressed by the epithelial cells in non-atypical ductal hyperplasia, a benign intraepithelial proliferative lesion of the TDLU (Otterbach et al. 2000). Since most human tumours arise from the luminal cells in the TDLUs, human Basal-like tumours probably express keratin 5/17 because they arose in luminal cells that expressed those keratins, not because they arose from cells in the outer layer of the ducts. In deference to the inventors of the Intrinsic classification we thus apply the term "Basal-like" to tumours that are probably derived from luminal cells. This would be a harmless anachronism, like calling E-cadherin-mutant tumours lobular, were it not for the fact that mouse biologists have embraced the term "basal" to describe anything in the outer layer of the ducts, most of which are myoepithelial cells. This leads to endless confusion, particularly when mouse biologists report luminal-to-basal plasticity. Standard sorting protocols barely distinguish between myoepithelial and stem cells, and interconversion of the cells occurs so easily that ambiguity is often desirable. When mouse biologists say a Luminal tumour has converted to a basal phenotype, most famously after inducing mutant PIK3CA expression in luminal cells (Koren et al. 2015; Van Keymeulen et al. 2015), it is not clear whether they really mean the tumour now resembles a mouse stem cell-like tumour or a human Basal-like tumour. The former implies regression to an earlier stage in the lineage, the latter a sideways move from a hormone-sensing phenotype to an alveolar/secretory progenitor phenotype (the terms are explored in more detail below). Both are interesting, but the latter is far more interesting to those studying human breast biology because it implies a switch between the two commonest forms of human breast cancer. Regression to a myoepithelial or stem cell-like phenotype in a mouse is arguably less interesting to those investigating human breast cancer.

The second widely used molecular classification is the TNBCtype classification (Lehmann et al. 2011, 2016). It subdivides triple-negative tumours into four groups. Unlike the Intrinsic classification, the TNBCtype classification was not created by looking for constant features in paired biopsies, so it had no inbuilt ability to correct for normal tissue contamination. Initially it contained six groups, but it subsequently emerged that two were caused by contamination with stromal cells (Lehmann et al. 2011, 2016). One of the remaining groups is the LAR group, which has the same transcriptomic phenotype as the HER2E/MA group mentioned above. The reason HER2E/MA tumours found their way into the TNBCtype classification is due to the difference between RNA phenotype and DNA genotype: the DNA genotype is HER2-negative, meaning *ERBB2* is not amplified, but the RNA phenotype is HER2E/MA, probably because the HER2 pathway is activated, either by *ERBB2* point mutations or by mutations elsewhere in the pathway (Jiang et al. 2019). For clinicians whose decision-making revolves around ER, PR and HER2, the existence of tumours with a HER2-positive phenotype but a HER2-negative genotype is a source of great confusion. This rapidly became clear in a widely cited follow-up paper by the Burstein group on LAR tumours, that perplexingly discovered that ER is one of the best markers for LAR tumours (Burstein et al. 2015). This can only mean that the authors included ER-positive tumours in a study on TNBC. The name LAR is confusing because it implies that AR uniquely identifies this group, but almost all anatomically luminal cells express AR, including classic Luminal A/B ER-positive tumours. Hence, it is important to resist the temptation to classify tumours as LAR simply because they express AR; AR expression only identifies LAR tumours when ER is absent, and the absence of ER can be difficult to establish in practice, as shown by the Burstein study (Burstein et al. 2015). Clinicians are stuck with the concept of TNBC as a class of tumours, but it is a poor starting point for a classification because it mixes things biologists would never knowingly combine (mammary hormone-sensing cells, alveolar/secretory cells, myoepithelial cells and stem cells). The remaining groups in the TNBCtype classification are Basal-like 1 (BL1), Basal-like 2 (BL2) and Mesenchymal (M). BL1 has higher expression of proliferation genes, and BL2 has higher expression of myoepithelial genes. The most interesting explanation for the difference would be that BL2 tumours are derived from mammary stem cells that generate progeny with both luminal and myoepithelial characteristics, but a simpler explanation is that the BL2 group is contaminated with normal mammary tissue, which has a low proliferation rate and contains myoepithelial cells. Finally, the M tumours express epithelial-to-mesenchymal transition (EMT) genes that are assumed to reflect a more stem-like state. Burstein et al. (2015) proposed a slightly different version of the TNBCtype classification, in which the LAR and M classes are the same but the basal-like group is split into immune-activated (BLIA) and immune-suppressed (BLIS) classes, which have high and low immune cell infiltration, respectively. This evolved into a closely-related classification developed by the Jiang group, which uses the terms LAR, BLIS, Mesenchymal (MES, equivalent to M) and Immunomodulatory (IM, equivalent to BLIA) (Jiang et al. 2019; Zhao et al. 2020). They stratified treatment based on this classification and obtained exciting results with combined immune checkpoint and taxane therapy in the IM group (53% partial responders in heavily pretreated patients) (Jiang et al. 2021). The Mesenchymal group (M or MES) in the TNBCtype, Burstein and Jiang classifications is probably the same as the Claudin-low group identified by Perou as an adjunct to the Intrinsic classification (Prat et al. 2010; Herschkowitz et al. 2007). Claudin is a component of tight junctions, the glue used by luminal cells to make water-tight (in this case, milk-tight) tubes. It is lost when cells undergo EMT. If claudin-low status is not scored, most claudin-low tumours fall into the basal-like class

(Thennavan et al. 2021), leading to debate about whether claudin-low should be considered as a class in its own right, or just a refinement within the existing Intrinsic classes (Fougner et al. 2020). In pathological terms, most claudin-low tumours probably correspond to metaplastic tumours (Thennavan et al. 2021). While it makes sense to use molecular classifications to find differences between morphologically similar tumours (essentially, invasive carcinoma of no special type (NST)), it is more questionable to try to supplant well-defined special histological types that pathologists can identify with high confidence (such as metaplastic, tubular, adenoid cystic, squamous, sebaceous and mucinous tumours) and force them to share a molecular class. Biologists can try to guess the cell type from the expression profile (Thennavan et al. 2021), but pathologists can tell at a glance what is going on in these tumours.

The last commonly cited classification, the IntClust classification, is based on combining gene expression data with DNA copy number data (chromosomal gains, losses and amplicons), although the resulting clusters are primarily distinguished by their copy number profiles (Curtis et al. 2012). The basic premise is that oncogenes cooperate, so a tumour with amplification of one gene should co-amplify its preferred partner (or delete it, for tumour suppressor genes). DNA cleavage at ER binding sites near the cooperating genes, with imprecise repair leading to translocations, was recently proposed as a mechanism for co-amplification of cooperating oncogenes in ER-positive tumours (Lee et al. 2023). This should be rich ground for experimental validation, for example, by engineering the corresponding chromosomal abnormalities with CRISPR technology. As expected, all of the breast cancer classes in the Intrinsic classification can be found in the IntClust groups, with strong enrichment in specific IntClust groups. IntClust 4 has an almost flat copy number plot and enrichment for Normal-like tumours, hinting that the samples contained too little tumour tissue for meaningful analysis (the authors dispute this). IntClust 5 has *ERBB2* amplification and strong enrichment for HER2-E tumours. IntClust 10 has a sawtooth copy number profile (Hicks et al. 2006), indicative of defective double-strand break repair, and strong enrichment for Basal-like tumours. The remaining IntClust groups contain mainly Luminal A and B tumours, together with the classic genomic abnormalities seen in those tumours (essentially, different combinations of 1q, 8q and 16p gains together with amplicons containing CCND1 and FGFR1). The study stands out for the multiplicity of platforms and the sophistication of the bioinformatic approaches used, but if you are planning to reanalyse the data you should note that the study contains multiple batches that require correction before pooling to avoid strong batch effects.

In summary, we now have multiple breast cancer classifications that all converge on the classes identified in the Intrinsic gene classification, which has become the de facto standard against which new molecular classifications are judged. The key weakness of all of these studies is that normal tissue dilutes the signal from the tumour cells because the RNA was pooled before analysis. New techniques that analyse single cells will solve this problem, particularly spatial transcriptomic techniques that link expression to individual pathologically verified cells in the same histological section. Not surprisingly, the cell types emerging from single-cell studies are the same as the ones identified in pooled data, albeit sometimes with different names, so the main contribution of single-cell technology is to highlight the diversity of stromal cells in tumours (for example, macrophage and lymphocyte subsets, and cancer-associated fibroblasts) (Wu et al. 2021; Kumar et al. 2023; Jackson et al. 2020; Gray et al. 2022; Chung et al. 2017; Murrow et al. 2022; Pal et al. 2021; Bach et al. 2017; Nee et al. 2023; Nguyen et al. 2018). In studies with pooled RNA, these cells are a barrier to classification; in single-cell studies they are a rich source of new insights into tumour biology.

11.1.2 Mapping Tumours to the Mammary Lineage

The standard model for the mammary lineage showing the mapping to tumours is shown in Fig. 11.1. It has been known for decades that

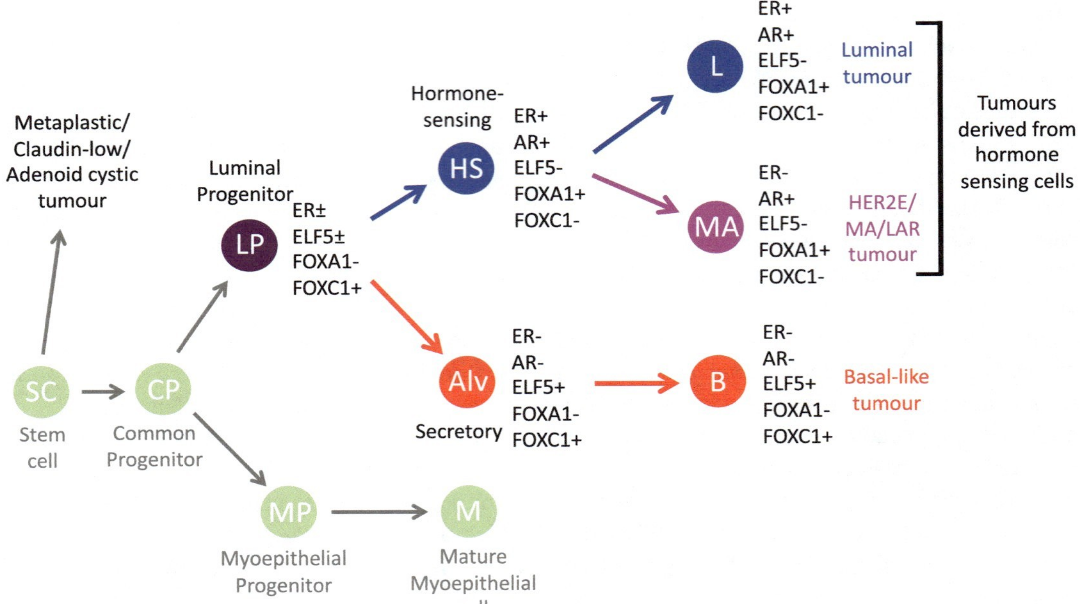

Fig. 11.1 Mammary lineage mapping tumours to cell types. This scheme is slightly modified from the original Lim model (Lim et al. 2009) to take into account the ER-negative, ELF5-positive status of basal-like tumours. *HS*, hormone-sensing cell; *Alv*, alveolar/secretory cell

murine mammary ductal trees can be reconstructed from single cells that can self-renew (Kordon and Smith 1998; DeOme et al. 1959), so we can be sure that mammary stem cells exist. Mammary ducts have an inner luminal layer and an outer myoepithelial layer. The luminal cells are divided into ER-positive and ER-negative populations, where the ER-positive cells are called hormone-sensing cells because their role is to convert systemic hormonal signals into local paracrine growth factor signals. Most human breast cancers are ER-positive and express genes that mark them as being hormone-sensing cells, so understanding the biology of these cells is important to both biologists and clinicians. The ER-negative luminal cells are harder to pin down. In pregnancy and lactation, they expand in number to produce milk, mainly in alveoli at the ends of ducts, but ER-negative cells in the ducts can also produce milk proteins (Smith et al. 1984). ER-negative luminal cells are thus alveolar/secretory cells, although in non-pregnant, non-lactating glands a better term would perhaps be alveolar/secretory progenitors rather than actual milk-secreting cells. The alveolar/secretory cells undergo regular cycles of proliferation, and the myoepithelial cells undergo characteristic morphological changes, such as vacuolisation, during the luteal phase of the menstrual/oestrus cycle (Ramakrishnan et al. 2002; Asselin-Labat et al. 2010; Joshi et al. 2010), in response to progesterone-induced secretion of RANKL and Wnt4 by the hormone-sensing cells (Beleut et al. 2010; Brisken et al. 1998; Rajaram et al. 2015). Conventional lineages assume that stem cells and mature cells are non-proliferating, and connect them with progenitors, which is where the bulk of cell division takes place. These concepts were developed in the haematopoietic system, where it is indeed tremendously difficult to make stem cells or mature cells divide, but there are no hard and fast rules in biology. Conventionally, the mammary lineage is shown with stem cells giving rise to common progenitors, then myoepithelial and luminal progenitors and finally mature myoepithelial and luminal hormone-sensing and alveolar/secretory cells. This simple view does not include changes occurring after lactation. The alveolar/secretory population is massively expanded during lactation, after which the vast majority of the alveolar/secretory cells are eliminated upon weaning. A special population of cells called parity-induced (PI) cells was identified after lactation; it is of intense interest to scientists trying to understand the protective effect of lactation on breast cancer risk in TNBC and *BRCA1*/*BRCA2* mutation carriers (Stordal 2023). Unexpectedly, PI cells exist before pregnancy so they are not strictly a consequence of lactation, despite the name (Booth et al. 2007). Single-cell studies would rather point to them being just ER-negative luminal cells that are slightly more differentiated (i.e., express slightly more milk proteins) than other ER-negative luminal cells (Bach et al. 2017). In normal homeostasis, murine lineage-tracing studies have shown that myoepithelial/basal stem cells maintain the myoepithelial lineage; ER-positive luminal stem cells maintain the hormone-sensing cell lineage, and ER-negative luminal stem cells maintain the alveolar/secretory lineage, where the term "stem cell" is used in the restricted sense that the cell can self-renew, not that it can regenerate a ductal tree containing the full spectrum of cell types in the mammary gland (Van Keymeulen et al. 2011, 2017; Wang et al. 2017). In pathological situations, in particular when luminal cells are missing, myoepithelial/basal cells can convert to luminal cells to fill the gap. They do so in response to local signals, more exactly the loss of TNFα signals from luminal cells that would otherwise inhibit the conversion of myoepithelial/basal cells to luminal cells (Centonze et al. 2020). This makes the point that cells simply respond to local signals; if a signal is always present, we will wrongly conclude that the target cell has a fixed phenotype. To describe differentiation of myoepithelial/basal stem cells to luminal cells as a pathological event stretches the definition of pathology; it is a normal event in circumstances rarely seen in normal homeostasis. The extent to which cells can move around in the lineage is far greater than was originally thought, but this is perhaps not surprising for such a simple lineage. In particular, every myoepithelial cell can convert to a stem cell when the circumstances demand it (Prater et al. 2014). This partly explains why mouse biologists find it so convenient to use the term basal, which encompasses stem cells and myoepithelial cells. It is well established, from grafting and lineage-tracing studies, that basal cells can convert to luminal cells, but it is much harder for luminal cells to convert to myoepithelial/basal cells. External signals are converted to gene expression programmes by transcription factors. Based on the TNFα result, one can surmise that the TNFα signal prevents the activation of the luminal transcriptional programme in myoepithelial/basal cells. Conversion of normal luminal cells into myoepithelial/basal cells was not seen in the classic grafting studies, but it can definitely occur if one short-circuits the signalling step by pulsing mature luminal cells directly with the relevant transcription factors (Sox9 to engage the luminal progenitor programme, then Slug to engage the stem cell programme (Guo et al. 2012). Since it is so easy to move back and forth within the lineage, it should come as no surprise that tumour cells can also change their identity, a phenomenon known as plasticity. In fact, the surprise is not that plasticity occurs, but that the phenotype of human tumours is so stable. Hence, the question we should be asking is not why murine luminal tumours readily convert to a myoepithelial/basal phenotype, but why ER-positive human luminal tumours stay ER-positive for decades, despite the cells being genetically unstable and free to mutationally activate signalling pathways at will. A possible explanation is that human tumour cells are locked into particular states, and for hormone-sensing cells we suspect that the lock is a der(1;16) translocation (see below).

The gene expression profiles at specific points in the lineage were originally defined by analysing cells purified by flow cytometry. For a detailed description of the current situation, see Chap. 9 by Jane Visvader. Flow cytometry uses mainly cell surface proteins to define cell identity. This is unfortunate because cell surface proteins are a consequence not the cause of cell identity. Many studies used EPCAM or CD24 to enrich for epithelial cells, and CD49f/CD29, better known as integrin α6/β1, to enrich for stem cells, the logic being that the integrins would anchor the stem cells in the stem cell niche. In mouse studies, there are two main mammary cell clusters, usually referred to simply as luminal and basal cells, where the former has higher EPCAM expression and the latter has higher integrin expression (Shackleton et al. 2006; Stingl et al. 2006). Most cells in the basal population are myoepithelial cells; only a few are overtly stem cells, in the sense that they lack expression of myoepithelial differentiation markers like the oxytocin receptor, but all myoepithelial cells can convert to stem cells after culture so the distinction is seemingly one of degree (Prater et al. 2014). Flow cytometry of human mammary cells for EPCAM and CD49f (integrin α6) revealed the presence of three mammary cell clusters (Lim et al. 2009): EPCAM single positives were mature luminal cells, CD49f single positives were myoepithelial cells, and double positives were shown by culture and grafting to be luminal progenitors (Lim et al. 2009). The double positives are by far the most interesting for understanding human breast cancer because there is a strong overlap between their gene expression profile and that of Basal-like tumours (Lim et al. 2009). As the name suggests, luminal progenitors have the potential to form both luminal lineages (hormone-sensing cells and alveolar/secretory cells). They express the master regulators for both pathways, ER and ELF5, which are thought to cross-inhibit one another until the cells choose their fate. This leads to a simple and elegant model, where the progenitors become hormone-sensing cells when ER wins, and alveolar/secretory cells when ELF5 wins (Kalyuga et al. 2012) (Fig. 11.2). Expression of ELF5 but not ER is one of the key reasons to think Basal-like tumours belong to the alveolar/secretory lineage.

In summary, human luminal A/B and HER2E/MA/LAR tumours resemble hormone-sensing cells; basal-like tumours resemble luminal progenitors that have committed to the alveolar/secretory lineage, and claudin-low tumours are commonly special pathological types like metaplastic tumours, which resemble mammary stem cells.

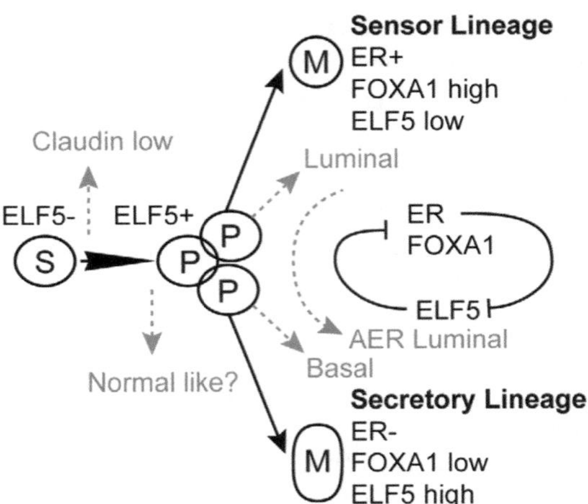

Fig. 11.2 ELF5 and ER compete in luminal progenitors (Kalyuga et al. 2012). *S*, stem cell; *P*, luminal progenitor; *M*, mature cell. (Ref Kalyuga et al. (2012), originally published under CC-BY)

11.1.3 Cell Identity and Cell of Origin

When a cell executes a genetic programme, it makes selective use of the information stored in its genome. Only a small part of that information is encoded directly in protein sequence; the vast majority lies in the sequence of enhancers. The keys to unlocking the information are the transcription factors that bind to those enhancers. The transcription factors at the core of the gene expression clusters in human breast cancer include many discovered by developmental biologists studying mammary gland development (Slepicka et al. 2021). The transcription factors that position mammary glands on the milk line include TBX3, MSX2 and GATA3 (Davenport et al. 2003; Kouros-Mehr et al. 2006; Satokata et al. 2000), which lie at the core of the Luminal gene cluster in heatmaps of human Luminal breast cancer (Perou et al. 2000). TBX3 has impeccable credentials in this respect, since it is not only required for mammary gland development in mice (Davenport et al. 2003), but also responsible for ulnar mammary syndrome, in which affected individuals fail to develop mammary glands (Bamshad et al. 1997). The transcription factors at the core of the Basal-like cluster likewise include several with established roles in development (ELF5, EN1, VGLL1,

FOXC1, SOX10 and BCL11A); ELF5 is the master regulator of lactation and essential for mammary gland development (Oakes et al. 2008; Zhou et al. 2005). When considering how to use this information to define cell identity and cell of origin, it is important to bear in mind that all cells in the mammary lineage have mammary identity, regardless of their position in the lineage. In other words, mammary identity applies equally to stem cells, myoepithelial cells, hormone-sensing cells and milk-secreting cells. It is a property that is established early in development and maintained throughout life. This means it persists in the absence of transcription factors, like ER, which we think of as playing a central role in regulating mammary gene expression, since they are not expressed in stem cells or secretory cells. When genome-wide chromatin immunoprecipitation techniques (ChIP-on-Chip and ChIP-seq) were used to study the location of ER, FOXA1 and GATA3, the most prominent transcription factors in the Luminal tumour cluster, it quickly became apparent that they have overlapping peaks (Kong et al. 2011). Subsequent work has amply confirmed that these transcription factors bind to the same enhancers in mammary epithelial cells (Farcas et al. 2021). In part, this is because those enhancers are more accessible in mammary epithelial cells, so any transcription factor in a mammary epithelial cell is more likely to bind to them, but it is hard not to be impressed by the degree of overlap of the ER, FOXA1 and GATA3 peaks. As more high-quality ChIP-seq datasets become available, the list of factors binding to these sites is sure to grow. For example, it now includes AR (Hickey et al. 2021) and AP-2β (Mustafa, Iggo and Tilley, unpublished data). It is reasonable to conclude that these sites are super-enhancers marked during development that define mammary identity and persist throughout life. This raises many interesting questions, not least how enhancer occupancy changes during differentiation (Holliday et al. 2018). For example, is there a core set of factors that keeps the chromatin accessible at all times? Traditionally, this is the role of polycomb proteins. At particular stages in the lineage, the activity of the super-enhancers is controlled by signalling proteins, the best examples of which are, of course, ER and PR, which act in hormone-sensing cells. Progression through the lineage is regulated by external signals that presumably also converge on these super-enhancers. Notch proteins are possible candidates for this role; they are cell surface receptors that are cleaved on ligand binding to release transcription factors that determine cell fate. Notch1 is particularly interesting because it sends luminal progenitors to the alveolar/secretory (Basal-like) lineage (Rodilla et al. 2015). The two most reciprocally expressed transcription factors in Luminal and Basal-like tumours are FOXA1 and FOXC1 (Fig. 11.3). Both bind to the same sequence motifs. The former is a pioneer factor for ER, where it plays a crucial role in enabling ER to transactivate its target genes (Lupien et al. 2008). This raises the interesting possibilities that FOXC1 could be a pioneer for the transcription factors specific to secretory cells, or that it blocks the binding of FOXA1 to ER-regulated enhancers in alveolar/secretory cells. FOXC2 is an EMT inducer (Mani et al. 2007), whose DNA binding domain is almost identical to that of FOXC1 and whose role seems to overlap with that of FOXC1 in breast cancer (Taube et al. 2010). The two are redundant in chondrogenesis in mice, where Foxc1 is a direct transcriptional target of Sox9 (Almubarak et al. 2021). Human SOX9 is expressed by mammary stem cells and luminal progenitors (Domenici et al. 2019), so it could explain FOXC1 expression in those cells. Sadly, it is easy to speculate but hard to conclude on the complex interactions at mammary super-enhancers because there is currently so little ChIP-seq data available for the lesser-studied transcription factors. Single-cell ATAC-seq combined with RNA-seq has been used to identify motifs in open chromatin in defined mammary cell types (Pervolarakis et al. 2020), but motif analysis does not identify which member within a transcription factor family is bound to a site (Castro-Mondragon et al. 2022) so we still need more ChIP-seq data.

The proteins most commonly used by pathologists to classify breast cancer are ER, PR, HER2 and keratins. The primary role of keratins is to provide physical strength to cells. Keratin genes

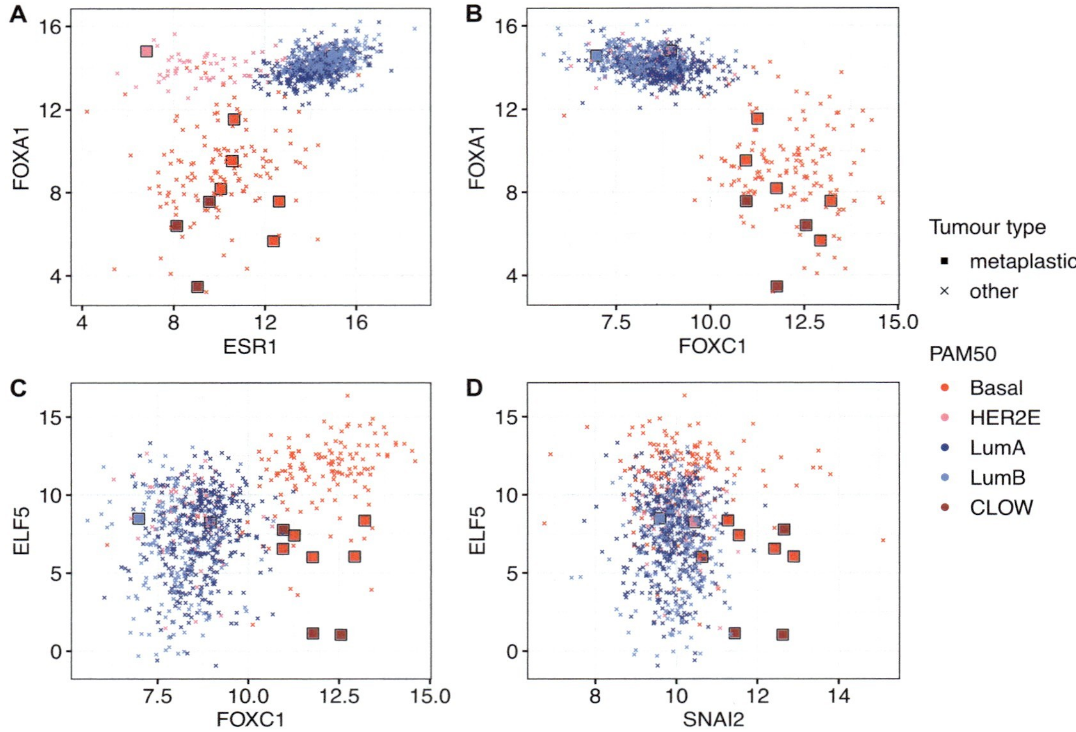

Fig. 11.3 Gene expression plots. (**a**) *ESR1* vs *FOXA1*. These genes conveniently split the major subtypes of human breast cancer. Tumours of hormone-sensing cells are *FOXA1*-positive: those that are *ESR1*-positive are classified as luminal A/B; those that are *ESR1*-negative are classified as HER2E/MA/LAR. The double negatives are Basal-like or Metaplastic. (**b**) *FOXA1* and *FOXC1* show reciprocal expression. Note that *FOXA1* and *FOXC1* do not separate Basal-like from Metaplastic. (**c**, **d**) *ELF5* is high in Basal-like and low in Metaplastic. *SNAI2* is high in most metaplastic and low in most Basal-like. Plotted from TCGA data that was RUVIII-normalised by Molania et al. (2023). The PAM50 assignments and centrally reviewed histology were taken from Thennavan et al. (2021). CLOW, claudin-low

have been duplicated endlessly during evolution, allowing subtle differences in enhancer sequences to emerge, which result in expression of specific keratin genes in particular cells. Pathologists exploit these differences when they use keratins to classify tumour cells, but keratins are normally thought of as being a consequence of cell type, not the cause. In other words, a cell is not a hormone-sensing cell because it expresses keratin 8/18; it expresses keratin 8/18 because it is a hormone-sensing cell. The real genes defining cell identity are the transcription factors that regulate the expression of thousands of genes, not just keratins. Hence, it would be logical to define tumour cell identity with transcription factors rather than keratins. It is quite easy to classify breast tumours in this way with RNA data, as we have shown in the LAB classification (Iggo 2018). In that study we used pools of transcription factors to create robust metagenes that define hormone-sensing (Luminal plus HER2-E/MA) and alveolar/secretory (Basal-like) cells. Translating this to routine pathology requires good antibodies; it works well for ER and PR precisely because so much effort has been put into making good antibodies against those proteins. That said, immunohistochemistry for ER sometimes gives the wrong answer, at least when judged by the more stringent test of gene expression, as shown famously in the TNBC paper by Burstein and colleagues mentioned above (Burstein et al. 2015). Aside from technical problems with antigen preservation and retrieval, the obvious reason for this is that the level of ER protein is itself tightly regulated; in particular, ER degradation is an inherent part of the transcription cycle, so less ER protein may mean more ER activity (Reid et al. 2002, 2003; Metivier et al. 2003). We would argue that FOXA1 (Seachrist et al. 2021) is a better marker for hormone-sensing cells than ER itself (Fig. 11.3), particularly in primary cultures in vitro, where ER expression is rapidly lost (Fridriksdottir et al. 2015). The counterpart of FOXA1 in Basal-like tumours is FOXC1, whose expression is strongly reciprocal to that of FOXA1 in gene expression studies (Fig. 11.3). Use of FOXC1 for immunohistochemistry (IHC) was delayed by a lack of good antibodies, but it is now increasingly used as a marker for Basal-like tumours (reviewed by Han et al. (2017)). Anti-FOXC1 antibodies stain Basal-like tumour cells and the preneoplastic cells in microglandular adenosis (one of the presumed precursors to Basal-like breast cancer), but they also stain most Metaplastic tumours, so one cannot simply conclude from FOXC1 staining that a tumour is Basal-like (Thennavan et al. 2021). Based on gene expression, *SNAI2* and *ELF5* look like they would be a better choice than FOXC1 because they show reciprocal expression in Metaplastic and Basal-like tumours (Fig. 11.3). When one stains real human tissue, it quickly becomes apparent that there is still much to be learnt. In a normal duct or lobule, we expect to see a small number of ER-positive, PR-positive, FOXA1-positive hormone-sensing cells surrounded by a much larger population of ER-negative, PR-negative, FOXC1-positive alveolar/secretory cells. Figure 11.4a shows almost exactly this phenotype: the hormone-sensing cells are indeed ER-positive, PR-positive, FOXA1-positive, and the remaining luminal cells are FOXC1-positive, but many of those FOXC1-positive cells are also ER-positive, meaning they must be luminal progenitors, rather than alveolar/secretory cells, at least when viewed from the perspective of the standard lineage model. Interestingly, this sample also has areas of columnar cell hyperplasia, a preneoplastic condition in which all cells have a perfect hormone-sensing-cell phenotype (Fig. 11.4b). The analysis of human breast tissue is further complicated by hormonal stimulation during the menstrual cycle, which leads to gross changes like vacuolisation of the myoepithelial cells during the luteal phase, as shown in Fig. 11.4c. In that sample, based on the standard model, we would expect to see ER-positive, PR-positive, FOXA1-positive hormone-sensing cells orchestrating the response of the surrounding ER-negative luminal cells through release of RANKL (in response to progesterone), but instead we see mainly ER-positive, FOXC1-positive luminal cells, and almost no cells with a classic hormone-sensing cell phenotype. Note also in this case the presence of large numbers of keratin 5 positive cells in the luminal layer. The only other transcription factors in the LAB metagenes that are commonly used in clinical practice are SOX10, GATA3 and AR. SOX10 is used as a marker for Basal-like tumours. GATA3 and AR are markers for hormone-sensing cells; hence, they are expressed by Luminal and HER2E/MA tumours, with lower GATA3 and higher AR expression in the HER2E/MA group (Bonnefoi et al. 2019). As noted above, high AR does not define the LAR group; in our opinion, to remove hormone-sensing cells from the TNBC group it would be safer to look for FOXA1 (Lehmann-Che et al. 2013), or the ratio of FOXA1 to FOXC1. At first glance, it seems logical to stain for AR when selecting patients for treatment with drugs that target AR. Unfortunately, AR is the target of both the androgen *antagonists* used in clinical trials for HER2E/MA tumours and the androgen *agonists* (selective AR modulators, or SARMs) used in clinical trials for luminal tumours, so using AR staining alone to assign treatment is perilous.We recently showed that MA tumours can be divided into two groups (MA^{lo} and MA^{hi}) on the basis of AR target gene

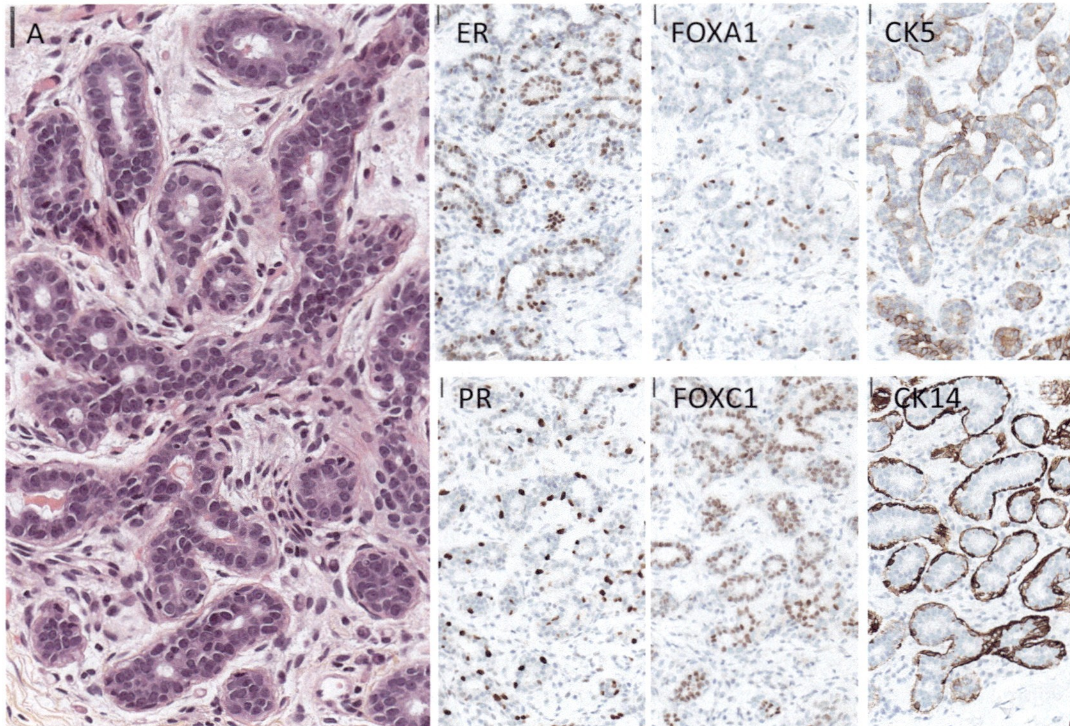

Fig. 11.4 Mammary histology and IHC. (**a**) Normal lobule from a perimenopausal woman. The FOXA1-positive, PR-positive hormone-sensing cells are greatly outnumbered by FOXC1-positive cells. By the pigeonhole principle, most of the latter are ER-positive. In the standard model, they would be classified as luminal progenitors. Occasional luminal cells are keratin 5-positive (CK5). The myoepithelial/basal cells are keratin 14-positive (CK14). (**b**) Columnar cell hyperplasia from the same sample as was used for panel (**a**). All of the cells have a classic hormone-sensing cell phenotype. They are likely to contain the der(1;16) translocation, although a causal relationship has not been proven. (**c**) Normal lobule from a premenopausal woman. The presence of large vacuoles in the myoepithelial cells means the sample was taken during the luteal phase of the menstrual cycle. At this stage, estrogen stimulates ER to transactivate PR expression, and progesterone stimulates PR to transactivate Wnt4 and RANKL expression, which in turn stimulate the myoepithelial/basal cells and alveolar/secretory luminal cells, respectively. Given their role in stimulating the other cells through release of paracrine growth factors, there are strangely few PR-positive, FOXA1-positive hormone-sensing cells. Many luminal cells are keratin 5-positive (CK5). The myoepithelial/basal cells are keratin 14-positive (CK14)

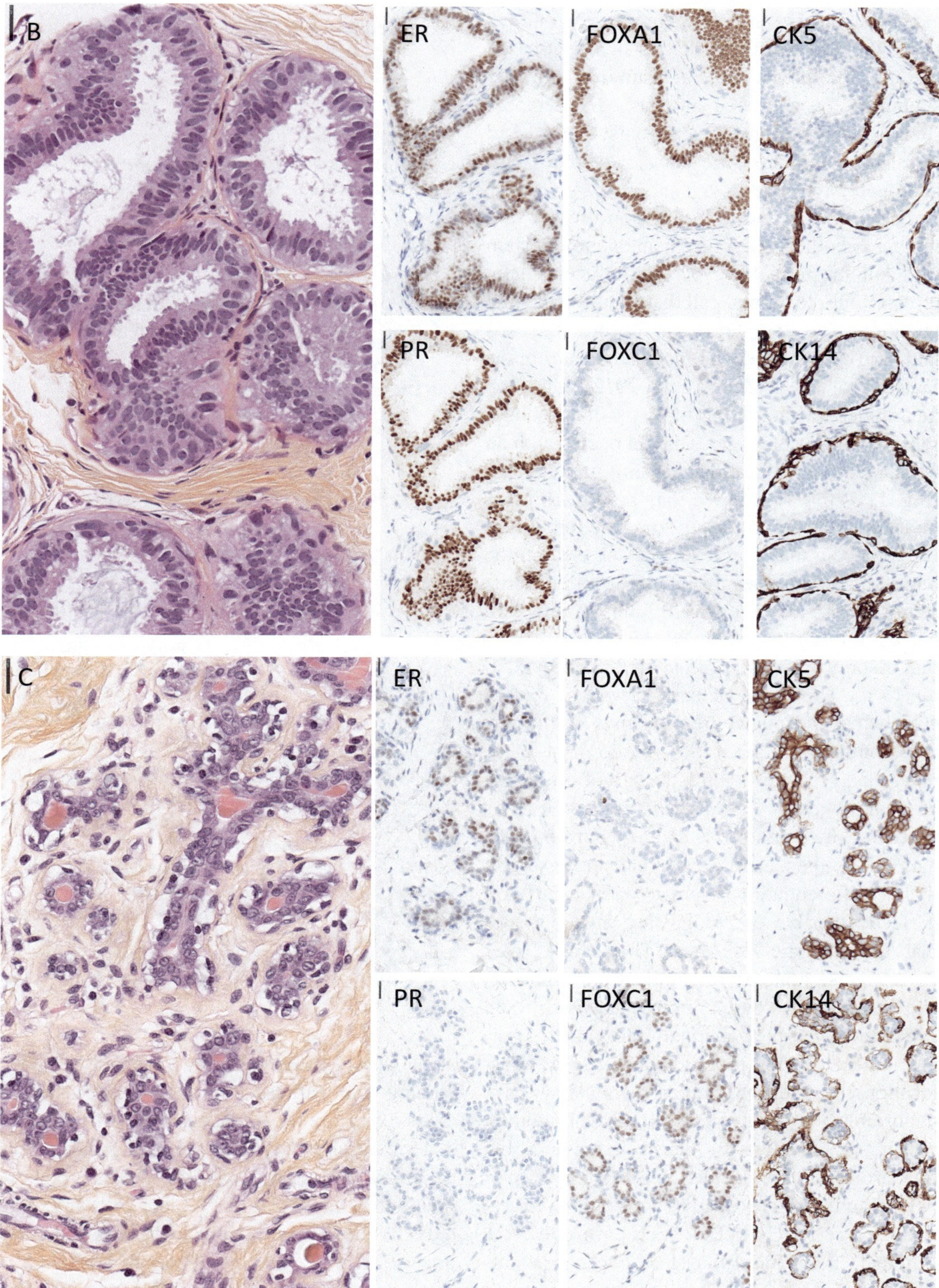

Fig. 11.4 (continued)

expression. This means we now have a rational framework in which to select androgen-based therapy for breast cancer: Luminal tumours should receive androgen agonists; MA^{hi} tumours should receive androgen antagonists; MA^{lo} and Basal-like tumours are not candidates for androgen-based thereapy.

Every cell acquiring a mutation present in a tumour is both a cell of origin and a tumour stem cell, but the term "cell of origin" is normally reserved for the normal cell that acquired the first mutation. The complexity of the problem was laid bare by the molecular clock studies from the Sanger group (Nik-Zainal et al. 2012). Since the mutational trajectory for tumours of hormone-sensing cells in the Sanger model begins with an unbalanced translocation causing trisomy 1q (Fig. 11.5) that is acquired long before any other mutations, the cell of origin for these tumours is likely to be a mammary stem cell. Based on the mouse lineage studies this could be either a true stem cell or a more restricted luminal stem cell. Nishimura recently extended this work to show that trisomy 1q is acquired in adolescence, leading to the expansion of large clones of mutant cells when the ductal tree expands at puberty (Nishimura et al. 2023). So why do most mammary gland biologists think the cell of origin is a luminal progenitor? For human tumours, it is the spectrum of tumours that women develop, and particularly the paucity of tumours with myoepithelial differentiation. Human pathologists are perfectly capable of recognising myoepitheliomas, they just rarely see them. They can also easily recognise tumours with mixed myoepithelial and luminal histology, famously adenoid cystic carcinomas, but they are again rare (albeit fascinating because they contain a MYB-NFIB translocation). In addition, human pathologists have no trouble diagnosing metaplastic carcinomas, which they equate with stem cell tumours, but they are again rare. Instead, the vast majority of human tumours are invasive carcinomas of no special type (IDC NST), which have either the Luminal or the Basal-like gene expression profiles described above. There is broad agreement that ER-positive tumours resemble hormone-sensing cells, but there is room for disagreement about Basal-like tumours, with some people contending that expression of keratins 5 and 17 means they are analogous to cells in the basal layer in the skin (by which they really mean stem cells). As discussed above, the alternative interpretation is that Basal-like tumour cells are luminal cells that have committed to the milk-secreting lineage. The second interpretation would mean that most human tumours resemble luminal cells, in the anatomical sense, and they could therefore theoretically all arise from a luminal progenitor.

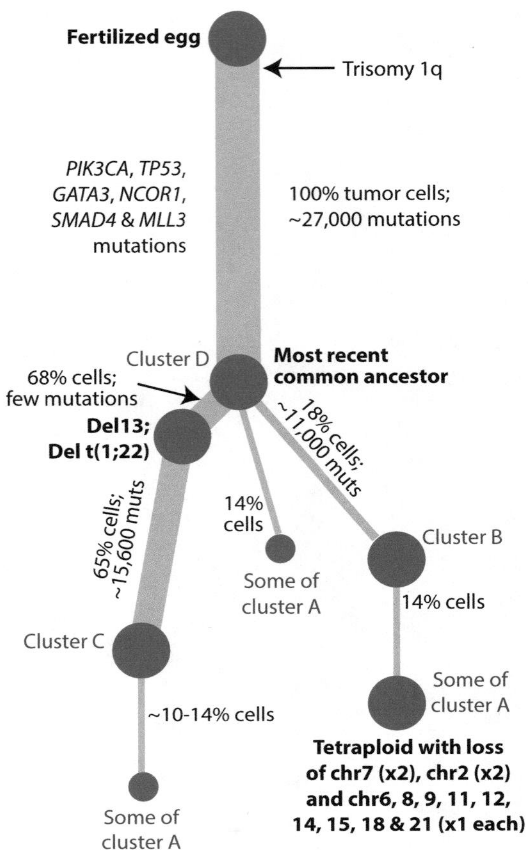

Fig. 11.5 The molecular clock. Analysis of passenger mutations allows bioinformaticians to infer the time when specific mutations and chromosomal rearrangements occur (Nik-Zainal et al. 2012). In the tumour shown, trisomy 1q was the first abnormality detected. Subsequent work by the Nishimura group has confirmed that this event occurs commonly in childhood and adolescence, long before any overtly malignant cells are visible to pathologists (Nishimura et al. 2023). (Ref Nik-Zainal et al. (2012), originally published under CC-BY)

The gene expression profile of Basal-like tumours resembles that of luminal progenitors, including in particular ELF5, the master regulator of lactation. Since the main argument for assigning basal identity to Basal-like tumours is based on keratin expression, it is worth asking whether keratins 5 and 17 really do define basal cells in the human breast. As alluded to above, Gusterson and Ince (Gusterson 2009; Santagata et al. 2014) did exactly that and found that keratins 5 and 17 are expressed by many luminal cells in the TDLUs (Fig. 11.4a, c). Since human tumours are conventionally thought to be derived from the TDLUs rather than the ducts, expression of keratins 5 and 17 is perfectly compatible with an origin from luminal progenitors. Taken together with the similarity of the Basal-like expression profile to that of luminal progenitors, formation of Luminal and Basal-like human tumours from luminal progenitors is the most parsimonious explanation. The classic argument for tumours to arise in stem cells is that multiple mutations are required (Armitage and Doll 1954), which takes such a long time that only stem cells live long enough to acquire all of the mutations. Hence it was a major breakthrough when mouse biologists showed that the ER-positive hormone-sensing cell lineage was maintained, at least in normal homeostatic conditions, by long-lived ER-positive luminal stem cells (Van Keymeulen et al. 2011, 2017; Wang et al. 2017). This was the key missing element in the argument that the cell of origin of ER-positive human breast tumours could be a luminal progenitor or an ER-positive stem cell derived from it.

The reason mouse biologists think mouse mammary gland tumours arise from luminal progenitors is that oncogenic mutations triggered by promoters active in luminal progenitors are particularly good at making mammary gland tumours, some of which show striking similarities to human breast cancers. The problem they encounter is that their promoters always show at least weak activity elsewhere in the lineage, so it becomes a statistical argument. Unlike humans, mice frequently make myoepithelial tumours, and those tumours often have mixed histology that includes myoepithelial and glandular or squamous components (adenomyoepitheliomas and adenosquamous tumours). The simplest explanation for the presence of mixed histology is that the cell of origin is a mammary stem cell. Mixed tumours could arise in a luminal progenitor that dedifferentiated to a common progenitor or stem cell, then redifferentiated to create the luminal and myoepithelial components seen in the tumour, but that is not the most parsimonious explanation. When PIK3CA-H1047R oncogene expression was targeted to luminal cells, mice initially made tumours with a luminal phenotype but with time the cells drifted to a basal phenotype (Koren et al. 2015; Van Keymeulen et al. 2015). Basal in this case means higher integrin $\alpha6/\beta1$ and lower EPCAM expression. This indicates that cells with a basal/myoepithelial phenotype have a selective advantage in mice, meaning cells that do make the change quickly overgrow the hard-earned luminal tumour cells, defeating the best efforts of mouse biologists to model human luminal tumours. Other models for basal-like human breast cancer use promoters targeted to secretory cells, albeit with the caveat that they still show some activity at other steps in the lineage. It makes sense to model ER-negative BRCA1-mutant human breast cancer in this way, and the resulting mouse tumours do indeed resemble their human counterparts, at least histologically (Xu et al. 1999a).

11.1.4 Is There a Signature Translocation in ER-Positive Breast Cancer?

The holy grail for mouse biologists is to make ER-positive models. One of the most popular is MMTV-PyMT, which starts well, with ER-positive hyperplasia, but the tumour cells gradually lose ER expression as the tumours progress (reviewed by Attalla et al. (2021)). Other transgenic models reported to give ER-positive tumours include MMTV-Ccnd1 (reviewed by Dabydeen and Furth (2014)). Szabova et al. recently described an ER-positive model made by inhibiting pocket proteins (Rb, p107and p130) with an SV40 T-antigen fragment (Szabova et al.

2022). Interestingly, the tumours did not amplify *CCND1*, one of the commonest changes in human ER-positive breast cancer. *CCND1* is an ER target gene with two roles: classically, cyclin D1 activates CDK4 to inhibit pocket proteins (most famously Rb), but for breast cancer biologists it is also a transcriptional coactivator for ER (Zwijsen et al. 1997). By focusing on the transcriptional effect on ER, which triggers a positive feedback loop that was assumed to lock in ER-positive identity, we may have overlooked the significance of inhibition of pocket proteins, which silence transcription of the *ESR1* gene itself. The Szabova model looks promising, but it does not explain the failure of the vast majority of mouse models to make ER-positive tumours with relevant histology (meaning histology a human pathologist would call invasive carcinoma of NST, not squamous, adenosquamous or adenomyoepithelioma histology). To put the problem in perspective, if mice were a good model system, we would be struggling to find mouse models that are ER-*negative*, not celebrating the creation of occasional models that are ER-*positive*. The formation of mixed tumours containing myoepithelial components and the progressive loss of ER expression in most mouse models, along with the wholesale drift to a basal phenotype in the beautifully engineered luminal *PIK3CA* models described above, indicates that mouse cells naturally converge on a basal, ER-negative phenotype, where basal in this case means stem/myoepithelial, not Basal-like. To understand what is wrong, it helps to turn the problem around, and ask whether there might be something human-specific that locks in the luminal differentiation of most human breast tumours, preventing their regression to stem/myoepithelial phenotypes. In other words, maybe there is nothing wrong with mice, and the fault lies entirely with humans. There is indeed a human-specific feature of human luminal and HER2E/MA tumours, and it is the trisomy 1q alluded to above (Fig. 11.5). The main effect of trisomy 1q is to increase the copy number of the entire long arm of chromosome 1. Evolution has shuffled the genes on chromosome 1 in the time separating mice from humans, so there is not the slightest chance that trisomy 1q in a mouse could mimic trisomy 1q in a human, not to mention the fact that all mouse chromosomes are acrocentric, so loss of 1p on mouse chromosome 1 is essentially meaningless.

Trisomy 1q is seen in virtually all Luminal and HER2E/MA breast tumours, but the additional copy of 1q is frequently part of a derivative chromosome, abbreviated as der(1;16), resulting from an unbalanced translocation that contains the long arm of chromosome 1 and the short arm of chromosome 16 (Nishimura et al. 2023). The translocation breakpoint lies in the α-satellite repeats in the centromeres of both chromosomes. This occurs because there is a vast expansion of the α-satellite repeats in human centromeres 1 and 16. The repeats must be methylated to prevent recombination. If the DNA methyltransferase *DNMT3B* is mutated in the germline, patients develop the ICF syndrome (ICF for immunoglobulin, chromosome and facial abnormalities), where the chromosomal abnormality is agglutination of centromeres, leading to formation of der(1;16) (Fig. 11.6). It is not known whether the patients are predisposed to breast cancer because they do not live long enough to find out. Rather than containing a single copy of der(1;16), luminal breast cancer cells contain an unstable mixture of derivative chromosomes, including der(1;16) and iso1q. These abnormalities are not unique to breast cancer, occurring, for example, in 40% of multiple

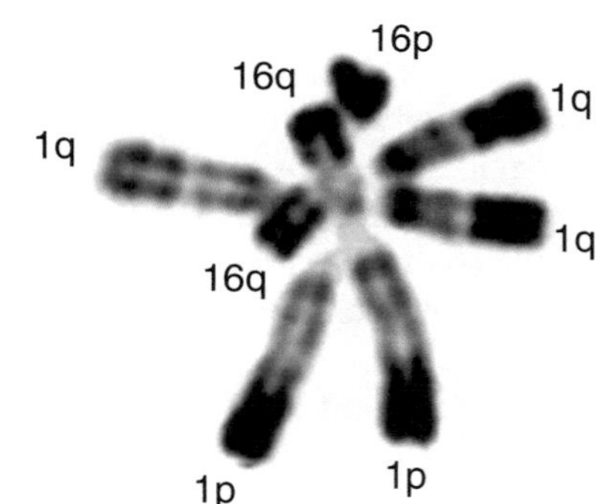

Fig. 11.6 ICF syndrome. Patients with *DNMT3B* mutations are unable to prevent recombination between the α-satellites at the centromeres of chromosomes 1 and 16 (Xu et al. 1999b). Failure to protect these α-satellites is a possible explanation for the formation of the der(1;16) translocation. (Originally published in Ref. Xu et al. (1999b))

myelomas, and they have been known for decades. Indeed, they were among the first genetic abnormalities to be described in tumours (Cruciger et al. 1976; Kovacs 1978; Rowley 1978). It is possible that they are a consequence rather than the cause of Luminal tumour formation, but if there were a signature translocation for Luminal breast cancer, it would look like this. As noted by Nik-Zainal et al. (2012) and confirmed by Nishimura et al. (2023), it is the first mutation recorded with the molecular clock. This means it is present for decades in otherwise normal cells. The great difficulty in studying it is that it does not create a fusion protein because it occurs in non-coding DNA. It slightly increases the copy number of 1q, potentially implicating a very large number of genes, of which many will be sensitive to gene dosage. Alternatively, loss of the entire short arm of chr1 would be an easy way to delete a tumour suppressor gene near the centromere on 1p. NOTCH2 is the first gene in healthy DNA after the pericentromeric repeats on 1p. All four NOTCH genes play interesting roles in asymmetric cell division and lineage decisions (NOTCH1 in the sensory/secretory choice (Rodilla et al. 2015), NOTCH2 at duct branchpoints (Sale et al. 2013), NOTCH3 in the basal/luminal choice (Lafkas et al. 2013) and NOTCH4 in mammary stem cells (Harrison et al. 2010; Gallahan and Callahan 1987)) but it is not clear from these studies how loss of NOTCH2 might alter ER status. In the past it was not possible to create translocations at will, but CRISPR technology makes this potentially an easy task. Rather than providing a direct mitogenic drive to the cell, we suspect that der(1;16) subtly biases the lineage to produce more hormone-sensing cells, then traps the cells in that state. This would explain why women faithfully maintain the ER-positive status of their tumours for decades. Testing this, at least in vitro, will require human cellular models that can recapitulate the lineage. This is currently rather unattractive because it means engineering translocations in short-lived primary human mammary stem cells and testing them before they lose the ability to make ducts, for example, in floating collagen gels (Linnemann et al. 2015), or after injection into mouse ducts (Verbeke et al. 2014) or in humanised mammary fat pads (Kuperwasser et al. 2004). Beyond our focus on molecular subtypes and cells of origin, a real-world inference from this model is that women who develop breast cancer really are completely blameless: their only mistake is to be human, with badly designed centromeres on chromosomes 1 and 16. It also hints at possible new avenues of research for epidemiologists who could usefully look for avoidable environmental exposure of children and adolescents to DNA methylation inhibitors.

11.2 Conclusion

Multiple approaches have converged on a standard model for the mammary lineage and breast cancer molecular classification. Most human tumours resemble either hormone-sensing cells or alveolar/secretory cells. The most widely used molecular classification assigns hormone-sensing tumours to Luminal A/B and HER2E/MA/LAR classes, and alveolar/secretory tumours to the Basal-like class. One problem with the techniques used to create the first generation of molecular classifications was that RNA from contaminating normal cells was pooled with RNA from tumour cells. Single-cell sequencing, particularly when coupled with spatial information, will quietly make this problem fade into history. Notwithstanding the cell types in single-cell studies being given new names, there is fundamentally good agreement between the traditional classification and the emerging classifications based on single cells. Compared to mice, humans show a strong bias towards making tumours that resemble mammary hormone-sensing cells. This could be caused by the formation in adolescence of der(1;16), a translocation through the centromeres of chromosomes 1 and 16, which only occurs in humans.

References

Adair FE, Herrmann JB (1946) The use of testosterone propionate in the treatment of advanced carcinoma of the breast. Ann Surg 123:1023–1035

Aftimos P et al (2021) Genomic and transcriptomic analyses of breast cancer primaries and matched metastases in AURORA, the breast international group (BIG) molecular screening initiative. Cancer Discov 11:2796–2811

Almubarak A et al (2021) Loss of Foxc1 and Foxc2 function in chondroprogenitor cells disrupts endochondral ossification. J Biol Chem 297:101020

Armitage P, Doll R (1954) The age distribution of cancer and a multi-stage theory of carcinogenesis. Br J Cancer 8:1–12

Asselin-Labat ML et al (2010) Control of mammary stem cell function by steroid hormone signalling. Nature 465:798–802

Attalla S, Taifour T, Bui T, Muller W (2021) Insights from transgenic mouse models of PyMT-induced breast cancer: recapitulating human breast cancer progression in vivo. Oncogene 40:475–491

Bach K et al (2017) Differentiation dynamics of mammary epithelial cells revealed by single-cell RNA sequencing. Nat Commun 8:2128

Bamshad M et al (1997) Mutations in human TBX3 alter limb, apocrine and genital development in ulnar-mammary syndrome. Nat Genet 16:311–315

Beleut M et al (2010) Two distinct mechanisms underlie progesterone-induced proliferation in the mammary gland. Proc Natl Acad Sci USA 107:2989–2994

Bergeron A et al (2021) Triple-negative breast lobular carcinoma: a luminal androgen receptor carcinoma with specific ESRRA mutations. Mod Pathol 34(7):1282–1296

Bonnefoi H et al (2011) TP53 status for prediction of sensitivity to taxane versus non-taxane neoadjuvant chemotherapy in breast cancer (EORTC 10994/BIG 1-00): a randomised phase 3 trial. Lancet Oncol 12:527–539

Bonnefoi H et al (2016) A phase II trial of abiraterone acetate plus prednisone in patients with triple-negative androgen receptor positive locally advanced or metastatic breast cancer (UCBG 12-1). Ann Oncol 27:812–818

Bonnefoi H et al (2019) Molecular apocrine tumours in EORTC 10994/BIG 1-00 phase III study: pathological response after neoadjuvant chemotherapy and clinical outcomes. Br J Cancer 120:913–921

Booth BW, Boulanger CA, Smith GH (2007) Alveolar progenitor cells develop in mouse mammary glands independent of pregnancy and lactation. J Cell Physiol 212:729–736

Brisken C et al (1998) A paracrine role for the epithelial progesterone receptor in mammary gland development. Proc Natl Acad Sci USA 95:5076–5081

Burstein MD et al (2015) Comprehensive genomic analysis identifies novel subtypes and targets of triple-negative breast cancer. Clin Cancer Res 21:1688–1698

Castro-Mondragon JA et al (2022) JASPAR 2022: the 9th release of the open-access database of transcription factor binding profiles. Nucleic Acids Res 50:D165–D173

Centonze A et al (2020) Heterotypic cell-cell communication regulates glandular stem cell multipotency. Nature 584:608–613

Charafe-Jauffret E et al (2013) ALDH1-positive cancer stem cells predict engraftment of primary breast tumors and are governed by a common stem cell program. Cancer Res 73:7290–7300

Chung W et al (2017) Single-cell RNA-seq enables comprehensive tumour and immune cell profiling in primary breast cancer. Nat Commun 8:15081

Clarke RB, Howell A, Potten CS, Anderson E (1997) Dissociation between steroid receptor expression and cell proliferation in the human breast. Cancer Res 57:4987–4991

Cronin M et al (2007) Analytical validation of the oncotype DX genomic diagnostic test for recurrence prognosis and therapeutic response prediction in node-negative, estrogen receptor-positive breast cancer. Clin Chem 53:1084–1091

Cruciger QV, Pathak S, Cailleau R (1976) Human breast carcinomas: marker chromosomes involving 1q in seven cases. Cytogenet Cell Genet 17:231–235

Curtis C et al (2012) The genomic and transcriptomic architecture of 2,000 breast tumours reveals novel subgroups. Nature 486:346–352

Dabydeen SA, Furth PA (2014) Genetically engineered ERα-positive breast cancer mouse models. Endocr Relat Cancer 21:R195–R208

Davenport TG, Jerome-Majewska LA, Papaioannou VE (2003) Mammary gland, limb and yolk sac defects in mice lacking Tbx3, the gene mutated in human ulnar mammary syndrome. Development 130:2263–2273

DeOme KB, Faulkin LJ Jr, Bern HA, Blair PB (1959) Development of mammary tumors from hyperplastic alveolar nodules transplanted into gland-free mammary fat pads of female C3H mice. Cancer Res 19:515

Domenici G et al (2019) A Sox2-Sox9 signalling axis maintains human breast luminal progenitor and breast cancer stem cells. Oncogene 38:3151–3169

Dowsett M et al (2011) Assessment of Ki67 in breast cancer: recommendations from the international Ki67 in breast cancer working group. J Natl Cancer Inst 103:1656–1664

Farcas AM, Nagarajan S, Cosulich S, Carroll JS (2021) Genome-wide estrogen receptor activity in breast cancer. Endocrinology 162

Farmer P et al (2005) Identification of molecular apocrine breast tumours by microarray analysis. Oncogene 24:4660–4671

Fougner C, Bergholtz H, Norum JH, Sorlie T (2020) Re-definition of claudin-low as a breast cancer phenotype. Nat Commun 11:1787

Fridriksdottir AJ et al (2015) Propagation of oestrogen receptor-positive and oestrogen-responsive normal human breast cells in culture. Nat Commun 6:8786

Gallahan D, Callahan R (1987) Mammary tumorigenesis in feral mice: identification of a new int locus in mouse mammary tumor virus (Czech II)-induced mammary tumors. J Virol 61:66–74

Gray GK et al (2022) A human breast atlas integrating single-cell proteomics and transcriptomics. Dev Cell 57:1400–1420 e1407

Grellety T, MacGrogan G, Chakiba C, Kind M, Bonnefoi H (2018) Long-term complete response of an androgen receptor–positive triple-negative metastatic breast cancer to abiraterone acetate. JCO Precis Oncol. https://doi.org/10.1200/PO.17.00223

Gucalp A et al (2013) Phase II trial of bicalutamide in patients with androgen receptor-positive, estrogen receptor-negative metastatic breast cancer. Clin Cancer Res 19:5505–5512

Guo W, Keckesova Z, Donaher JL, Shibue T, Tischler V, Reinhardt F, Itzkovitz S, Noske A, Zürrer-Härdi U, Bell G, Tam WL, Mani SA, van Oudenaarden A, Weinberg RA (2012) Slug and Sox9 cooperatively determine the mammary stem cell state. Cell 148(5):1015–1028

Gusterson B (2009) Do 'basal-like' breast cancers really exist? Nat Rev Cancer 9:128–134

Han B et al (2017) FOXC1: an emerging marker and therapeutic target for cancer. Oncogene 36:3957–3963

Harrison H et al (2010) Regulation of breast cancer stem cell activity by signaling through the Notch4 receptor. Cancer Res 70:709–718

Herschkowitz JI et al (2007) Identification of conserved gene expression features between murine mammary carcinoma models and human breast tumors. Genome Biol 8:R76

Hickey TE et al (2021) The androgen receptor is a tumor suppressor in estrogen receptor-positive breast cancer. Nat Med 27:310–320

Hicks J et al (2006) Novel patterns of genome rearrangement and their association with survival in breast cancer. Genome Res 16:1465–1479

Holliday H, Baker LA, Junankar SR, Clark SJ, Swarbrick A (2018) Epigenomics of mammary gland development. Breast Cancer Res 20:100

Iggo R (2018) Classification of breast tumours into molecular apocrine, luminal and basal groups based on an explicit biological model. bioRxiv. https://doi.org/10.1101/270975

Jackson HW et al (2020) The single-cell pathology landscape of breast cancer. Nature 578:615–620

Jiang YZ et al (2019) Genomic and transcriptomic landscape of triple-negative breast cancers: subtypes and treatment strategies. Cancer Cell 35:428–440.e425

Jiang YZ et al (2021) Molecular subtyping and genomic profiling expand precision medicine in refractory metastatic triple-negative breast cancer: the FUTURE trial. Cell Res 31:178–186

Joshi PA et al (2010) Progesterone induces adult mammary stem cell expansion. Nature 465:803–807

Kalyuga M et al (2012) ELF5 suppresses estrogen sensitivity and underpins the acquisition of antiestrogen resistance in luminal breast cancer. PLoS Biol 10:e1001461

Kong SL, Li G, Loh SL, Sung WK, Liu ET (2011) Cellular reprogramming by the conjoint action of ERα, FOXA1, and GATA3 to a ligand-inducible growth state. Mol Syst Biol 7:526

Kordon EC, Smith GH (1998) An entire functional mammary gland may comprise the progeny from a single cell. Development 125:1921–1930

Koren S et al (2015) PIK3CA(H1047R) induces multipotency and multi-lineage mammary tumours. Nature 525:114–118

Kouros-Mehr H, Slorach EM, Sternlicht MD, Werb Z (2006) GATA-3 maintains the differentiation of the luminal cell fate in the mammary gland. Cell 127:1041–1055

Kovacs G (1978) Abnormalities of chromosome no. 1 in human solid malignant tumours. Int J Cancer 21:688–694

Kumar T et al (2023) A spatially resolved single-cell genomic atlas of the adult human breast. Nature 620:181–191

Kuperwasser C et al (2004) Reconstruction of functionally normal and malignant human breast tissues in mice. Proc Natl Acad Sci USA 101:4966–4971

Lafkas D et al (2013) Notch3 marks clonogenic mammary luminal progenitor cells in vivo. J Cell Biol 203:47–56

Lee JJ et al (2023) ERα-associated translocations underlie oncogene amplifications in breast cancer. Nature 618:1024–1032

Lehmann BD et al (2011) Identification of human triple-negative breast cancer subtypes and preclinical models for selection of targeted therapies. J Clin Invest 121:2750–2767

Lehmann BD et al (2016) Refinement of triple-negative breast cancer molecular subtypes: implications for neoadjuvant chemotherapy selection. PLoS One 11:e0157368

Lehmann-Che J et al (2013) Molecular apocrine breast cancers are aggressive estrogen receptor negative tumors overexpressing either HER2 or GCDFP15. Breast Cancer Res 15:R37

Lim E et al (2009) Aberrant luminal progenitors as the candidate target population for basal tumor development in BRCA1 mutation carriers. Nat Med 15:907–913

Linnemann JR et al (2015) Quantification of regenerative potential in primary human mammary epithelial cells. Development 142:3239–3251

Loeser AA (1939) Male hormones in the treatment of cancer of the breast. UICC 4:375

Lupien M et al (2008) FoxA1 translates epigenetic signatures into enhancer-driven lineage-specific transcription. Cell 132:958–970

Mani SA et al (2007) Mesenchyme Forkhead 1 (FOXC2) plays a key role in metastasis and is associated with aggressive basal-like breast cancers. Proc Natl Acad Sci USA 104:10069–10074

Metivier R et al (2003) Estrogen receptor-alpha directs ordered, cyclical, and combinatorial recruitment of cofactors on a natural target promoter. Cell 115:751–763

Molania R et al (2023) Removing unwanted variation from large-scale RNA sequencing data with PRPS. Nat Biotechnol 41:82–95

Murrow LM et al (2022) Mapping hormone-regulated cell-cell interaction networks in the human breast at single-cell resolution. Cell Syst 13:644–664.e648

Nee K et al (2023) Preneoplastic stromal cells promote BRCA1-mediated breast tumorigenesis. Nat Genet 55:595–606

Nguyen QH et al (2018) Profiling human breast epithelial cells using single cell RNA sequencing identifies cell diversity. Nat Commun 9:2028

Nik-Zainal S et al (2012) The life history of 21 breast cancers. Cell 149:994–1007

Nishimura T et al (2023) Evolutionary histories of breast cancer and related clones. Nature 620:607–614

Oakes SR et al (2008) The Ets transcription factor Elf5 specifies mammary alveolar cell fate. Genes Dev 22:581–586

Oftedal OT (2002) The mammary gland and its origin during synapsid evolution. J Mammary Gland Biol Neoplasia 7:225–252

Otterbach F et al (2000) Cytokeratin 5/6 immunohistochemistry assists the differential diagnosis of atypical proliferations of the breast. Histopathology 37:232–240

Pal B et al (2021) A single-cell RNA expression atlas of normal, preneoplastic and tumorigenic states in the human breast. EMBO J 40:e107333

Parker JS et al (2009) Supervised risk predictor of breast cancer based on intrinsic subtypes. J Clin Oncol 27:1160–1167

Perou CM et al (2000) Molecular portraits of human breast tumours. Nature 406:747–752

Pervolarakis N et al (2020) Integrated single-cell transcriptomics and chromatin accessibility analysis reveals regulators of mammary epithelial cell identity. Cell Rep 33:108273

Prat A et al (2010) Phenotypic and molecular characterization of the claudin-low intrinsic subtype of breast cancer. Breast Cancer Res 12:R68

Prater MD et al (2014) Mammary stem cells have myoepithelial cell properties. Nat Cell Biol 16:942–950

Rajaram RD et al (2015) Progesterone and Wnt4 control mammary stem cells via myoepithelial crosstalk. EMBO J 34:641–652

Ramakrishnan R, Khan SA, Badve S (2002) Morphological changes in breast tissue with menstrual cycle. Mod Pathol 15:1348–1356

Reid G, Denger S, Kos M, Gannon F (2002) Human estrogen receptor-alpha: regulation by synthesis, modification and degradation. Cell Mol Life Sci 59:821–831

Reid G et al (2003) Cyclic, proteasome-mediated turnover of unliganded and liganded ERalpha on responsive promoters is an integral feature of estrogen signaling. Mol Cell 11:695–707

Reyal F et al (2012) Molecular profiling of patient-derived breast cancer xenografts. Breast Cancer Res 14:R11

Richard E et al (2016) The mammary ducts create a favourable microenvironment for xenografting of luminal and molecular apocrine breast tumours. J Pathol 240:256–261

Riedlinger GM, Joshi S, Hirshfield KM, Barnard N, Ganesan S (2021) Targetable alterations in invasive pleomorphic lobular carcinoma of the breast. Breast Cancer Res 23:7

Rodilla V et al (2015) Luminal progenitors restrict their lineage potential during mammary gland development. PLoS Biol 13:e1002069

Rowley JD (1978) Abnormalities of chromosome No. 1: significance in malignant transformation. Virchows Arch B Cell Pathol 29:139–144

Sale S, Lafkas D, Artavanis-Tsakonas S (2013) Notch2 genetic fate mapping reveals two previously unrecognized mammary epithelial lineages. Nat Cell Biol 15:451–460

Santagata S et al (2014) Taxonomy of breast cancer based on normal cell phenotype predicts outcome. J Clin Invest 124:859–870

Satokata I et al (2000) Msx2 deficiency in mice causes pleiotropic defects in bone growth and ectodermal organ formation. Nat Genet 24:391–395

Seachrist DD, Anstine LJ, Keri RA (2021) FOXA1: a pioneer of nuclear receptor action in breast cancer. Cancers (Basel) 13

Shackleton M et al (2006) Generation of a functional mammary gland from a single stem cell. Nature 439:84–88

Slepicka PF, Somasundara AVH, Dos Santos CO (2021) The molecular basis of mammary gland development and epithelial differentiation. Semin Cell Dev Biol 114:93–112

Smith GH, Vonderhaar BK, Graham DE, Medina D (1984) Expression of pregnancy-specific genes in preneoplastic mouse mammary tissues from virgin mice. Cancer Res 44:3426–3437

Stingl J et al (2006) Purification and unique properties of mammary epithelial stem cells. Nature 439:993–997

Stordal B (2023) Breastfeeding reduces the risk of breast cancer: a call for action in high-income countries with low rates of breastfeeding. Cancer Med 12:4616–4625

Szabova L et al (2022) Loss of Brca1 and Trp53 in adult mouse mammary ductal epithelium results in development of hormone receptor-positive or hormone receptor-negative tumors, depending on inactivation of Rb family proteins. Breast Cancer Res 24:75

Taube JH et al (2010) Core epithelial-to-mesenchymal transition interactome gene-expression signature is associated with claudin-low and metaplastic breast cancer subtypes. Proc Natl Acad Sci USA 107:15449–15454

Taylor-Papadimitriou J et al (1989) Keratin expression in human mammary epithelial cells cultured from normal and malignant tissue: relation to in vivo phenotypes and influence of medium. J Cell Sci 94(Pt 3):403–413

Thennavan A et al (2021) Molecular analysis of TCGA breast cancer histologic types. Cell Genom 1:100067

Traina TA et al (2018) Enzalutamide for the treatment of androgen receptor-expressing triple-negative breast cancer. J Clin Oncol 36:884–890

Van Keymeulen A et al (2011) Distinct stem cells contribute to mammary gland development and maintenance. Nature 479:189–193

Van Keymeulen A et al (2015) Reactivation of multipotency by oncogenic PIK3CA induces breast tumour heterogeneity. Nature 525:119–123

Van Keymeulen A et al (2017) Lineage-restricted mammary stem cells sustain the development, homeostasis, and regeneration of the estrogen receptor positive lineage. Cell Rep 20:1525–1532

Verbeke S et al (2014) Humanization of the mouse mammary gland by replacement of the luminal layer with genetically-engineered preneoplastic human cells. Breast Cancer Res 16:504

Wang C, Christin JR, Oktay MH, Guo W (2017) Lineage-biased stem cells maintain estrogen-receptor-positive and -negative mouse mammary luminal lineages. Cell Rep 18:2825–2835

Weigelt B et al (2010) Breast cancer molecular profiling with single sample predictors: a retrospective analysis. Lancet Oncol 11:339–349

Wells CA, El-Ayat GA (2007) Non-operative breast pathology: apocrine lesions. J Clin Pathol 60:1313–1320

Wirapati P et al (2008) Meta-analysis of gene expression profiles in breast cancer: toward a unified understanding of breast cancer subtyping and prognosis signatures. Breast Cancer Res 10:R65

Wu SZ et al (2021) A single-cell and spatially resolved atlas of human breast cancers. Nat Genet 53:1334–1347

Xu X et al (1999a) Conditional mutation of Brca1 in mammary epithelial cells results in blunted ductal morphogenesis and tumour formation. Nat Genet 22:37–43

Xu GL et al (1999b) Chromosome instability and immunodeficiency syndrome caused by mutations in a DNA methyltransferase gene. Nature 402:187–191

Zhao S et al (2020) Molecular subtyping of triple-negative breast cancers by immunohistochemistry: molecular basis and clinical relevance. Oncologist 25:e1481–e1491

Zhou J et al (2005) Elf5 is essential for early embryogenesis and mammary gland development during pregnancy and lactation. EMBO J 24:635–644

Zwijsen RM et al (1997) CDK-independent activation of estrogen receptor by cyclin D1. Cell 88:405–415

Part IV
Cellular and Molecular Basis

Therese Sørlie and Robert Clarke

Breast cancer's complexity is driven by a multitude of cellular and molecular factors that influence its development, progression, and response to treatment. This part explores the role of the microenvironment, the molecular underpinnings of tumor heterogeneity, and the specific mechanisms involved in different breast cancer subtypes, offering insights that are crucial for advancing therapeutic strategies.

In Chap. 12, Louise Jones and her colleagues from Barts Cancer Institute, London, UK, explain how ductal carcinoma in situ (DCIS), a precursor to invasive breast cancer, presents a challenge in distinguishing lesions that will progress from those that will remain indolent. While molecular analyses of the carcinoma cells have not consistently revealed differences between progressive and non-progressive lesions, the tumor microenvironment has emerged as a critical factor in tumor progression. Changes in the DCIS microenvironment, including the transformation of myoepithelial cells and the peri-ductal stromal environment, play a significant role in disease progression. Myoepithelial cells, which typically have tumor-suppressor functions, can acquire tumor-promoter properties in DCIS. The transformation of fibroblasts into cancer-associated fibroblasts (CAFs) and alterations in the extracellular matrix (ECM) also contribute to disease dynamics. Detailed studies on the interplay between DCIS epithelial cells and their microenvironment are essential for better predicting disease behavior.

In Chap. 13, Fresia Pareja and her colleague from Memorial Sloan Kettering Cancer Center, USA, describe how breast cancer's heterogeneity encompasses diverse molecular, histological, and clinical variations. The disease's molecular landscape is complex from its earliest stages, with distinct receptor statuses and clinical subtypes influencing therapeutic decisions. Hereditary breast cancer, driven by different susceptibility genes, further

T. Sørlie
Oslo, Norway

R. Clarke
Manchester, UK

complicates this landscape. Each breast cancer subtype has unique metabolic demands and immune microenvironments, and special histologic subtypes exhibit specific genotypic–phenotypic correlations that inform diagnosis and treatment. Understanding the molecular basis of breast cancer heterogeneity is crucial for developing targeted therapies and improving patient outcomes.

Finally, in Chap. 14 Valerie Brunton and her colleague at the University of Edinburgh, Scotland, propose that E-cadherin, a central component of adherens junctions, is vital for epithelial tissue integrity. Its loss is a defining feature of invasive lobular carcinoma (ILC), leading to a distinctive discohesive growth pattern. Despite being common, ILC has been under-researched, with limited clinical trials focused on this subtype. Loss of E-cadherin in ILC results in hyperactivation of growth factor receptors, anoikis resistance, and synthetic lethality with ROS1 inhibition. These molecular changes present potential clinical vulnerabilities that could be targeted to improve treatment outcomes for ILC patients, who currently have limited tailored therapeutic options.

By exploring the microenvironment, molecular heterogeneity, and specific mechanisms of different breast cancer subtypes, this part of the book aims to deepen our understanding of the cellular and molecular basis of breast cancer, with the ultimate aim of better informing future therapeutic strategies.

The Microenvironment in DCIS and Its Role in Disease Progression

12

Mohammad Reza Roozitalab, Niki Prekete, Michael Allen, Richard P. Grose, and J. Louise Jones

Abstract

Ductal carcinoma in situ (DCIS) accounts for ~20% of all breast cancer diagnoses but whilst known to be a precursor of invasive breast cancer (IBC), evidence suggests only one in six patients will ever progress. A key challenge is to distinguish between those lesions that will progress and those that will remain indolent. Molecular analyses of neoplastic epithelial cells have not identified consistent differences between lesions that progressed and those that did not, and this has focused attention on the tumour microenvironment (ME).

The DCIS ME is unique, complex and dynamic. Myoepithelial cells form the wall of the ductal-lobular tree and exhibit broad tumour suppressor functions. However, in DCIS they acquire phenotypic changes that bestow them with tumour promoter properties, an important evolution since they act as the primary barrier for invasion. Changes in the peri-ductal stromal environment also arise in DCIS, including transformation of fibroblasts into cancer-associated fibroblasts (CAFs). CAFs orchestrate other changes in the stroma, including the physical structure of the extracellular matrix (ECM) through altered protein synthesis, as well as release of a plethora of factors including proteases, cytokines and chemokines that remodel the ECM. CAFs can also modulate the immune ME as well as impact on tumour cell signalling pathways. The heterogeneity of CAFs, including recognition of anti-tumourigenic populations, is becoming evident, as well as heterogeneity of immune cells and the interplay between these and the adipocyte and vascular compartments. Knowledge of the impact of these changes is more advanced in IBC but evidence is starting to accumulate for a role in DCIS. Detailed in vitro, in vivo and tissue studies focusing on the interplay between DCIS epithelial cells and the ME should help to define features that can better predict DCIS behaviour.

Keywords

DCIS · Microenvironment · Myoepithelial cell · CAF · Extracellular matrix · Immune cells · Adipocytes

M. R. Roozitalab · N. Prekete · M. Allen · R. P. Grose · J. Louise Jones (✉)
Centre for Tumour Biology, Barts Cancer Institute, John Vane Science Centre, Charterhouse Square, Queen Mary University of London, London, UK
e-mail: m.r.roozitalab@qmul.ac.uk; n.prekete@qmul.ac.uk; m.allen@qmul.ac.uk; r.p.grose@qmul.ac.uk; l.j.jones@qmul.ac.uk

T. Sørlie, R. B. Clarke (eds.), *A Guide to Breast Cancer Research*, Advances in Experimental Medicine and Biology 1464, https://doi.org/10.1007/978-3-031-70875-6_12

Key Points

- There is a need to distinguish between DCIS that progresses and that which remains indolent so treatment can be stratified. The neoplastic epithelial cells of DCIS show no consistent difference to their invasive counterpart, so attention has focused on changes in the microenvironment (ME).
- Myoepithelial cells are a unique component of the DCIS ME. They regulate normal breast duct homeostasis and act as tumour suppressors but acquire tumour-promoter function during DCIS evolution.
- Fibroblasts are key regulators of the stromal ME. In the periductal environment, fibroblasts secrete multiple factors that shape the physical and biological nature of the stroma and influence both myoepithelial and tumour cell function.
- The immune infiltrate can be both pro- and anti-tumourigenic. The composition and function of the immune population is influenced by the stromal ME and neoplastic cells. Results of studies on the impact of the immune ME in DCIS are contradictory, contributed to by a lack of consistency in analysis.
- Adipose tissue is considered an endocrine organ in its own right. Body fat composition has long been associated with breast cancer risk. More recently, changes seen in breast adipose tissue, such as the presence of 'crown-like structures', are starting to indicate how adipose tissue may influence epithelial cell behaviour.
- Every element of the ME interacts. This adds significant complexity to defining the key orchestrators that could be targeted. In almost every aspect, less is known about the DCIS ME compared to IBC, and the challenge is there to be addressed.

12.1 Introduction

Ductal carcinoma in situ (DCIS) is a non-obligate precursor of invasive breast cancer (IBC). It is characterized by a neoplastic proliferation of epithelial cells inside the breast ducts, sometimes extending into lobules, a process known as 'cancerisation', but confined within the ductal-lobular tree by an intact myoepithelial–basement membrane (BM) barrier (Adriance et al. 2005). Earlier stages of the disease, including atypical ductal hyperplasia, where ducts show some but not all the features of DCIS, are also recognized, and confer an increased risk of development of IBC (Ellis 2010). Transition to invasive disease is recognized as penetration of the myoepithelial–BM layer, migration of neoplastic cells into the surrounding stroma and eventual loss of the myoepithelial population (Fig. 12.1).

With the advent of breast screening programmes, DCIS now represents around 20% of all new breast cancer diagnoses (Kerlikowske 2010; Bleyer and Welch 2012; Cancer Research UK 2020). As with IBC, DCIS is a highly heterogeneous disease, which manifests histologically as differences in tumour grade, tumour architecture and disease extent.

Tumour grading is largely based on cytonuclear features of the DCIS with low-grade DCIS being composed of small regular cells, often showing a cribriform or micropapillary architecture. High-grade DCIS is composed of large, pleomorphic cells with frequent mitotic figures, often having a solid architecture and associated necrosis, whilst intermediate-grade DCIS shows nuclear features intermediate between low- and high-grade DCIS. The Van Nuys classification system combines nuclear grade and necrosis, yielding three subgroups of DCIS—non-high-grade without necrosis, non-high-grade with necrosis and high-grade with or without necrosis (Silverstein et al. 1995). Both classification systems show an association between higher-grade disease and local recurrence and disease-free survival (Silverstein et al. 1995; Pinder 2010; Schuh et al. 2015). In most series, ~15–20% of cases are low-grade, 20–40% intermediate grade and ~ 50% are high-grade (Sørum et al. 2010;

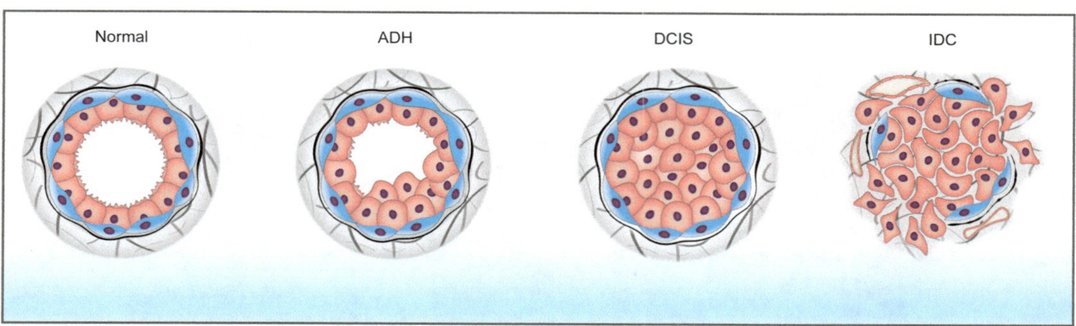

Fig. 12.1 Progressive changes in the human breast duct with development of malignancy. The normal breast duct comprises an inner luminal layer of epithelial cells surrounded by a layer of spindle-shaped myoepithelial cells, which lie in contact with the basement membrane (BM). Ductal carcinoma in situ (DCIS) is characterised by proliferation of neoplastic epithelial cells within the duct with the myoepithelial–BM barrier separating the malignant cells from the interstitial stroma. Earlier stages of atypical ductal hyperplasia (ADH) can be seen, where epithelial cells have some but not all the features of DCIS, such as retaining areas of luminal cell polarity. With disease progression to invasive ductal carcinoma (IDC), neoplastic epithelial cells penetrate the myoepithelial–BM layer, which becomes compromised, and invade the surrounding stroma

Weigel et al. 2015; Van Luijt et al. 2016). However, the potential predictive value of grade is hampered by both poor reproducibility in grading (Ellis et al. 2006) and the presence of more than one grade in almost half of the lesions (Allred et al. 2008).

Standard of care for patients diagnosed with DCIS is surgical excision ± radiotherapy ± endocrine therapy for women with oestrogen receptor (ER)-positive disease, with the rationale of preventing development of IBC. However, numerous studies indicate that only around one in six patients with DCIS would ever progress to invasive disease during their lifetime (Collins et al. 2005; Saunders et al. 2005; Falk et al. 2011; Maxwell et al. 2022); thus, treating all lesions as potentially invasive is significant overtreatment for many women, as recognized in a formal evaluation of the breast screening programme (Independent UK Panel on Breast Cancer Screening 2012). To address this, a number of 'active surveillance' trials have been launched, to avoid surgery in women deemed at low risk of progression (Elshof et al. 2015; Francis et al. 2015; Hwang et al. 2019). These are largely based on DCIS grade and restricted to women with low- or intermediate-grade disease; however, in an audit of women with apparently low-risk disease, nearly 25% had occult invasion on their surgical excision (Pilewskie et al. 2016; Chevez de Paz Villanueva et al. 2017), suggesting that more robust mechanisms of stratification are required.

A number of studies have aimed to identify biomarkers or signatures that could predict which DCIS lesions are most at risk of progression, largely focused on genomic characterization of the neoplastic epithelial cell population. These have shown no consistent changes in invasive disease compared to DCIS, with both disease stages exhibiting similar profiles of copy number aberrations (CNAs), point mutations and epigenetic alterations (Hernandez et al. 2012; Kim et al. 2015; Casasent et al. 2018; Pareja et al. 2020), suggesting DCIS is as molecularly advanced as IBC. This was further supported in a recent large study comparing DCIS with their invasive recurrence: this showed that 75% of invasive recurrences displayed high concordance of driver mutations and chromosomal amplifications with their precursor DCIS (Casasent et al. 2022; Lips et al. 2022), confirming that molecular evolution occurs at a pre-invasive stage and that other factors must be involved in progression to invasion. Other studies have addressed whether changes in transcriptional profiles are associated with DCIS progression (Ma et al. 2003; Lee et al. 2012; Knudsen et al. 2012; Doebar et al. 2017; Rebbeck

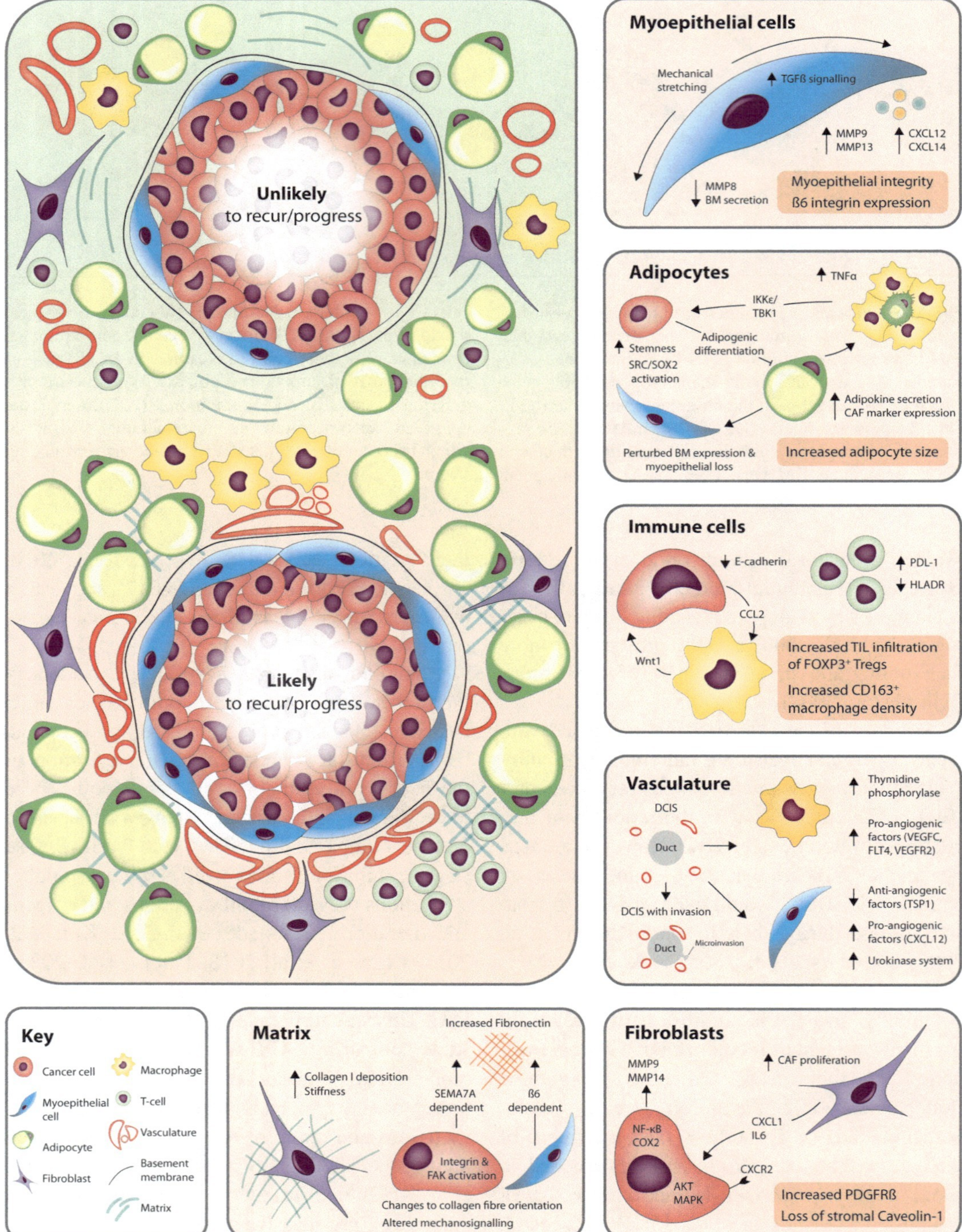

Fig. 12.2 Contribution of the DCIS microenvironment in mediating progression. There is a complex interplay between multiple factors in the breast microenvironment that impact on the behaviour of DCIS, making it unlikely or more likely to progress. Mechanical stretching of the *myoepithelium* in DCIS drives up-regulation of integrin β6, which leads to release of MMP9 and MMP13 through activation of TGFβ signalling. Other changes in DCIS

et al. 2022), and whilst differences have been identified, there are a few consistent changes associated with progression. One exception is in the identification of an epithelial–mesenchymal transition (EMT) expression profile associated with invasion: in a detailed analysis of >2000 regions from 145 patients at different disease stages, Rebbeck et al. identified two EMTs—one in early-stage DCIS, the other where IBC is established (Rebbeck et al. 2022). Interestingly, however, they also identify a change in the gene expression profile, suggesting loss of the myoepithelial cell population, and up-regulation of genes involved in extracellular matrix (ECM) organization with disease progression, emphasizing the role of changes in the microenvironment (ME) with progression.

This has led to a focus on the ME to understand its potential role in influencing disease progression. DCIS has a complex and unique ME (Fig. 12.2) comprising myoepithelial cells, fibroblasts, the ECM, vasculature, immune infiltrate and adipocytes (Gibson et al. 2023a). This chapter will summarize the existing knowledge on the role of each of these components in influencing the behaviour of DCIS and highlight the questions that still remain. Whilst components of the ME are considered separately, they are inextricably linked, with complex cross-talk between different elements, which will be considered: this has implications not only for understanding key points of intervention to prevent progression but also in considering appropriate experimental models to address the significant clinical problem of safely stratifying the management of the increasing number of patients diagnosed with DCIS.

It will be evident that in many areas, the data relating to DCIS is far less advanced than that for IBC. There are a number of possible reasons for this: DCIS is less common than invasive cancer and in itself is not a life-threatening disease so perhaps there is less focus on it; DCIS tissue is more difficult to sample than IBC—it is diffuse and there is a need to ensure occult invasion is not missed; time to progression can span years so

Fig. 12.2 (continued) include altered cytokine and chemokine expression and down-regulation of tumour-suppressor MMP8. *Adipocytes* show increased adipokine secretion, promoting stem-like characteristics of cancer cells through activation of the SRC/SOX2 pathways. They also modulate myoepithelial and macrophage activity, which in turn impact on neoplastic epithelial behaviour, e.g., through IKKε/TBK1-dependent signalling. The *immune cell* infiltrate can generate an immunosuppressive stroma, characterised by increased FOXP3+ TILs, and respective high and low expression of PDL-1 and HLADR, which may promote DCIS progression. Tumour cell–macrophage can drive increased Wnt-1 secretion and cancer cell loss of E-cadherin. *Fibroblasts* become activated to CAFs, which, through release of CXCL1 and IL-6, can drive the activation of AKT/MAPK pathways in the DCIS cells. They also activate tumour cell NF-κB and COX-2 with up-regulation of MMP9 and MMP14. Two *vascular patterns* are observed in DCIS: diffuse stromal and periductal, the latter of which has been associated with a co-existent invasive component. DCIS-associated myoepithelial cells switch from an anti-angiogenic to pro-angiogenic phenotype, emphasising how multiple elements of the microenvironment interact to influence disease behaviour. Changes in *matrix* composition and organisation are seen in DCIS with increased collagen I deposition and changes in fibre orientation that have been related to progression. Increased periductal fibronectin may be mediated in a SEMA7A-dependent or β6-dependent manner. The altered matrix drives changes in downstream mechano-signalling, particularly through integrin and FAK activation in DCIS cells. Features of the tumour microenvironment which may indicate the likelihood of DCIS progression and invasive recurrence are highlighted in associated boxes. Abbreviations: *AKT*, Protein kinase B; *BM*, basement membrane; *CAF*, cancer-associated fibroblasts; *COX2*, Cyclooxygenase-2; CXCL1, (C-X-C motif) chemokine ligand-1; *DCIS*, ductal carcinoma in situ; *FAK*, Focal Adhesion Kinase; *FOXP3*, Forkhead box protein P3; *HLA-DR*, Human Leukocyte Antigen-DR isotype (class II); *IL-6*, Interleukin-6; *MAPK*, Mitogen-activated protein kinase; *MMP*, Matrix Metalloproteinase; *NF-κB*, Nuclear factor-kappa B; *PDGFRβ*, platelet-derived growth factor receptor beta; *PDL-1*, Programmed death ligand-1; *SEMA7A* Semaphorin 7A; SOX2, SRY-box 2; SRC, *proto-oncogene tyrosine protein kinase Src; TIL*, Semaphorin 7A; *SOX2*, SRY-box 2; *SRC*, proto-oncogene tyrosine protein kinase Src; tumour-infiltrating lymphocyte; *TNFα*, tumour necrosis factor α; *VEGF*, vascular endothelial growth factor. Reproduced from Gibson et al. (2023a)

appropriate sample cohorts to study can be challenging; and there are fewer models of DCIS compared to IBC. Against this, we forward the following perspective: most IBCs derive from DCIS though it is clear much DCIS does not progress. If we are to harness the promise of breast screening there is a need to distinguish between those individuals with indolent disease and those that may progress, for whom surgical excision could be life-saving.

12.2 Myoepithelial Cells

Myoepithelial cells are a unique component of the DCIS ME: they are a hybrid cell type with epithelial characteristics, reflected in their expression of cytokeratins (CK) such as CK5 and CK14 and desmosomal proteins, as well as intermediate filament proteins such as vimentin and contractile proteins including α-smooth muscle actin (SMA), more typically associated with mesenchymal cells (Franke et al. 1980; Adriance et al. 2005). Normal myoepithelial cells produce and adhere to the basement membrane (BM). They induce luminal epithelial cell polarity through production of laminin-1 (Gudjonsson et al. 2002) and through expression of specific isoforms of desmosomal proteins (Runswick et al. 2001). Normal myoepithelial cells are widely regarded as having a tumour-suppressor phenotype: they secrete high levels of angiogenic inhibitors, including thrombospondin and tissue inhibitor of metalloproteinase 1 (TIMP1), as well as other proteinase inhibitors such as maspin (Barsky and Karlin 2005), and down-regulate a series of invasion-promoting stromal-derived proteases (Jones et al. 2003). Through their expression of integrin α6β4, which is incorporated into hemidesmosomes, they act as 'rivets' to the BM, contributing to the physical barrier of the duct wall (Bergstraesser et al. 1995). The absence of myoepithelial cells is largely regarded as pathognomonic of invasive disease (Yu et al. 1997; Bofin et al. 2004).

However, it is evident that myoepithelial cells change their phenotype during DCIS evolution. One consistent change is de novo expression of the integrin αvβ6 (Allen et al. 2014). Integrin αvβ6 is not expressed by normal myoepithelial cells but is up-regulated on myoepithelial cells in ~60% of pure DCIS and is almost universally expressed (>90%) in DCIS with a co-existent invasive component. Furthermore, expression of αvβ6 promotes tumour cell invasion through Transforming Growth Factor (TGF)-β-dependent up-regulation of matrix metalloproteinase-(MMP)9 (Allen et al. 2014). Myoepithelial cells in DCIS show altered expression of other MMPs: mechanical stretch generated in myoepithelial cells as ducts become expanded by proliferating neoplastic cells induces both β6 integrin and MMP13 expression (Hayward et al. 2022), and MMP13 promotes myoepithelial-led invasion of luminal cells in 3D in vitro models (Gibson et al. 2023b). Normal myoepithelial cells are a major source of the tumour suppressor MMP8 (Gutiérrez-Fernández et al. 2008), and its loss in DCIS-associated myoepithelial cells leads to destabilization of the myoepithelial barrier, with enhanced invasion and depletion of hemidesmosome structures (Sarper et al. 2017).

Indeed, comprehensive molecular analysis of the DCIS ME has revealed that more numerous and distinct alterations arise in myoepithelial cells than other cell types in DCIS compared to their normal cellular counterparts, including overexpression of C–X–C motif chemokine ligand 12 (CXCL12) and CXCL14—both of which play a role as mediators of monocyte/macrophage homing (Allinen et al. 2004; Kryczek et al. 2007; Sánchez-Martín et al. 2011). DCIS-associated myoepithelial cells also exhibit altered synthesis of ECM proteins (Hayward et al. 2022).

Whilst this body of work points towards destabilization and compromise of the myoepithelial layer pre-disposing to disease progression, a recent study using multiplexed ion beam imaging by time of flight (MIBI-TOF) to define cellular and structural characteristics of normal, DCIS and IBC tissue described a somewhat counterintuitive observation (Risom et al. 2022). Their random forest classifier to predict DCIS progression was heavily weighted towards myoepithelial characteristics; however, they found that an intact myoepithelium with high expression of E-cadherin was associated with non-progressor DCIS lesions, whist those that subsequently progressed had low E-cadherin expression and a thinner less continuous myoepithelial layer, the latter being associated with a higher stromal immune cell infiltrate (Risom et al. 2022). They suggested that this exposure of the intraductal neoplastic cells to the immune system may afford future protection. An association between myoepithelial cell loss and immune cell infiltration has previously been reported (Man and Sang 2004); however, this showed localized disruption of myoepithelial cells to be associated with alterations in the overlying neoplastic epithelial cells, with localized loss of ER and a higher frequency of loss of heterozygosity: they proposed that this local disruption of myoepithelium pre-disposed to development of invasion (Man and Sang 2004; Man 2007). It is currently difficult to reconcile these contradictory findings, and also to reconcile the observations of Risom et al. (2022) with classic histopathological features of neoplastic epithelial cells extending through a breach in the myoepithelial–BM barrier as pathognomonic of invasive disease: at some stage, by definition, invasive progression is characterized by disruption and loss of the myoepithelial cell layer.

It is possible that the findings of Risom et al. (2022) represent a particular stage in disease evolution—perhaps early-stage exposure of DCIS cells to the immune system generates a longer-term anti-tumour response, whereas those cells retained by an intact myoepithelial cell layer develop a more aggressive invasive phenotype and are not challenged by the immune system when they penetrate the myoepithelial barrier.

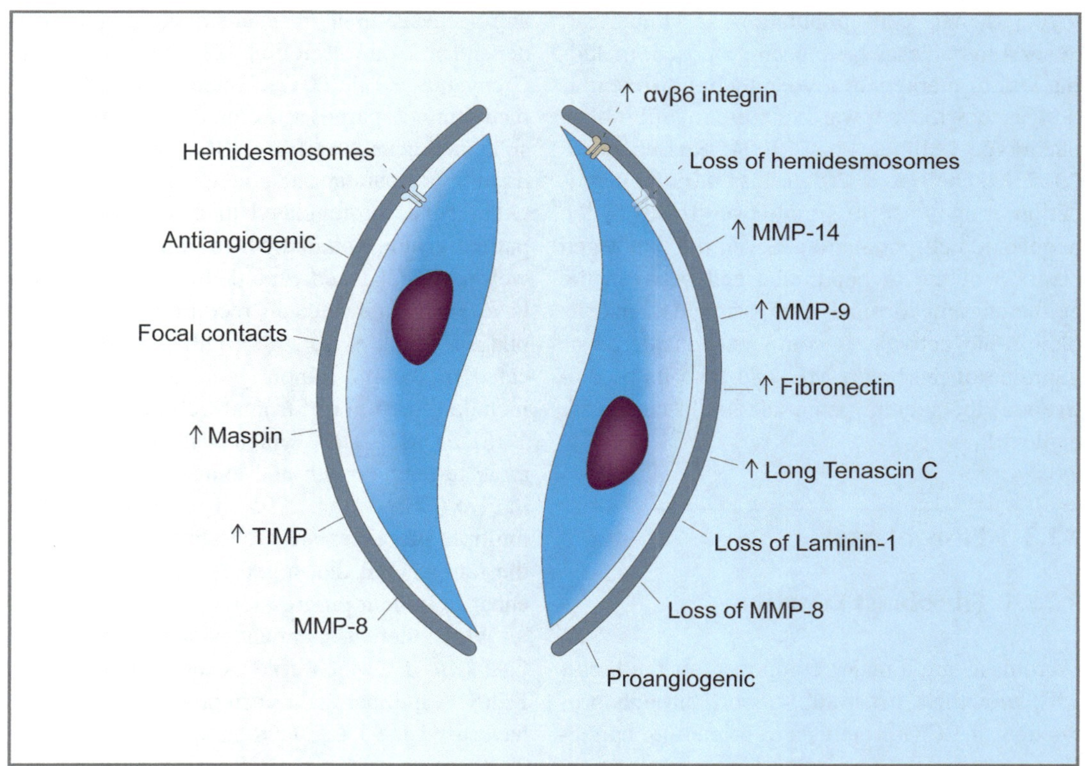

Fig. 12.3 Characteristics of normal and DCIS-associated myoepithelial cells. In normal breast glands, myoepithelial cells exhibit a broad tumour suppressor phenotype, mediating stable adhesion to the basement membrane via hemidesmosomes and focal contacts. They are anti-angiogenic and secrete a range of tumour-suppressor proteases such as Matrix Metalloproteinase (MMP)8 and maspin, and protease inhibitors such as Tissue Inhibitor of Metalloproteinases (TIMP)1. In DCIS ducts, myoepithelial cells show loss of hemidesmosome formation and MMP8 and switch to a pro-angiogenic phenotype. They change their expression of extracellular matrix proteins and show enhanced expression of a series of MMPs, all of which contribute to a pro-tumourigenic environment

Such hypotheses are difficult to address, particularly in the absence of longitudinal tissue sampling of untreated disease, but they are an important consideration in understanding DCIS biology and the eventual development of robust risk signatures.

What is clear is that myoepithelial cells switch their phenotype from tumour suppressor to tumour promoter at some point during DCIS evolution (Fig. 12.3). It is unclear what controls this phenotypic change, whether it is controlled by the neoplastic cells or a physical response to changes in the ME. Identifying the molecular changes associated with this myoepithelial functional switch could help predict DCIS lesions that have a higher likelihood of progression, and may also lead to strategies to inhibit development of invasive disease. Similarly, understanding the factors that lead to the ultimate loss of the myoepithelial cell population is important. Several hypotheses have been proposed, including loss of markers of myoepithelial differentiation, as they move towards a more myofibroblast phenotype (Allinen et al. 2004; Russell et al. 2015; Mitchell et al. 2020), loss through degradation or apoptosis or simple overgrowth by the neoplastic cell population. Given the privileged position of the myoepithelial cell between the epithelial and stromal compartments, and its pleiotropic activity, it could be considered as guardian of the breast ME, and both its predictive and therapeutic potential should be further explored.

12.3 Fibroblasts

12.3.1 Fibroblast Function

Fibroblasts are a major component of the breast ME, providing structural support through production of ECM proteins and promoting epithelial growth and differentiation during development (Lühr et al. 2012; Inman et al. 2015). Whilst relatively quiescent in normal breast, they become activated during development and pregnancy, releasing a range of factors, including proteases such as MMP3, that remodel the breast environment and lead to branching morphogenesis (Wiseman et al. 2003).

Whilst normal fibroblasts have been reported to maintain epithelial homeostasis and suppress proliferation, so inhibiting tumour formation (Bhowmick et al. 2004; Trimboli et al. 2009), cancer-associated fibroblasts (CAFs), widely identified on the basis of their expression of α-SMA, have consistently been shown to promote tumour cell proliferation, invasion and angiogenesis. Indeed, inclusion of CAFs in 3D heterotypic cultures of luminal and myoepithelial cells leads to disruption of normal glandular morphology, indicating their impact on breast tissue structure and phenotype (Holliday et al. 2009). In one study, fibroblasts were isolated from primary human breast carcinoma tissue and incorporated into subcutaneous Matrigel plug assays in mice. In this setting, they were shown to promote angiogenesis in a mechanism at least in part dependent on secretion of adrenomedullin (Benyahia et al. 2017). Interestingly, adrenomedullin was part of a stroma-derived prognostic signature generated from IBC tissues that predicted poor patient outcome (Finak et al. 2008). Other genes up-regulated in this poor-outcome patient group included MMP1 and MMP11, as well as CXCL1 and Endothelin-1 (ET-1) which have been implicated in recruitment of macrophages (Finak et al. 2008). Other factors implicated in the pro-tumourigenic effect of CAFs include secretion of Stromal Cell-derived Factor 1 (SDF1)/CXCL12, which was shown to promote tumour growth and enhance angiogenesis in vivo (Orimo et al. 2005). Thus, it appears that multiple processes are orchestrated by CAFs in the tumour ME that together create a milieu to enhance tumour progression.

Whilst there is abundant evidence for a role of CAFs in IBC, their role is less established in DCIS. A number of in-vitro or xenograft studies have used the DCIS.COM model (Miller et al. 2000) to recapitulate DCIS lesions. In 3D co-culture models in matrigel (Hu et al. 2009) and in microfluidic systems (Sung et al. 2011), addition of fibroblasts led to acquisition of an invasive phenotype by DCIS.COM cells, associated with up-regulation of MMP9 and MMP14 (Hu et al.

2009). In polyoma middle T-virus models of breast cancer, over-expression of CXCL1 in fibroblasts led to enhanced tumour progression from pre-invasive lesions (Bernard et al. 2018). Furthermore, generation of TGFβ-signalling deficient fibroblasts through knock-down of TGFβReceptor2, led to elevated levels of CXCL1 levels in fibroblasts, and these TGFβ-deficient fibroblasts promoted progression of in situ to invasive lesions, with CXCL1 leading to activation of Nuclear factor-kappa B (NFkB), p42/44 Mitogen-Activated protein kinase (MAPK), Protein kinase B (AKT) and Signal transducer and activator of transcription (STAT)3 signalling (Bernard et al. 2018).

12.3.2 Fibroblast Subtypes

These studies support a role for CAFs in promoting tumour progression; however, recent single-cell RNA-sequencing analysis has demonstrated the heterogeneity of fibroblast phenotype in breast and other cancers (Elyada et al. 2019; Sebastian et al. 2020). Thus, CAFs have been divided into three main populations: myofibroblastic CAFs (myCAFs), inflammatory CAFs (iCAFs) and antigen-presenting CAFs (apCAFs) (Fig. 12.4). In general, myCAFs respond to TGFβ, whilst iCAFs express inflammatory mediators such as Interleukin (IL-6) (Öhlund et al. 2017), and apCAFs are characterized by expression of Major Histocompatibility Complex (MHC)II and CD74 (Elyada et al. 2019). Further complexity is demonstrated in analysis of CAF populations from human breast cancer samples, in which four CAF subsets were identified, termed as CAF-S1–CAF-S4, based on differential expression of six markers (Costa et al. 2018). CAF-S1 and CAF-S4 both express high levels of αSMA and could be classed as myCAF, being particularly enriched in the stroma of triple-negative breast cancer. Through functional analysis, they demonstrate that CAF-S1 promotes migration of T-lymphocytes and also

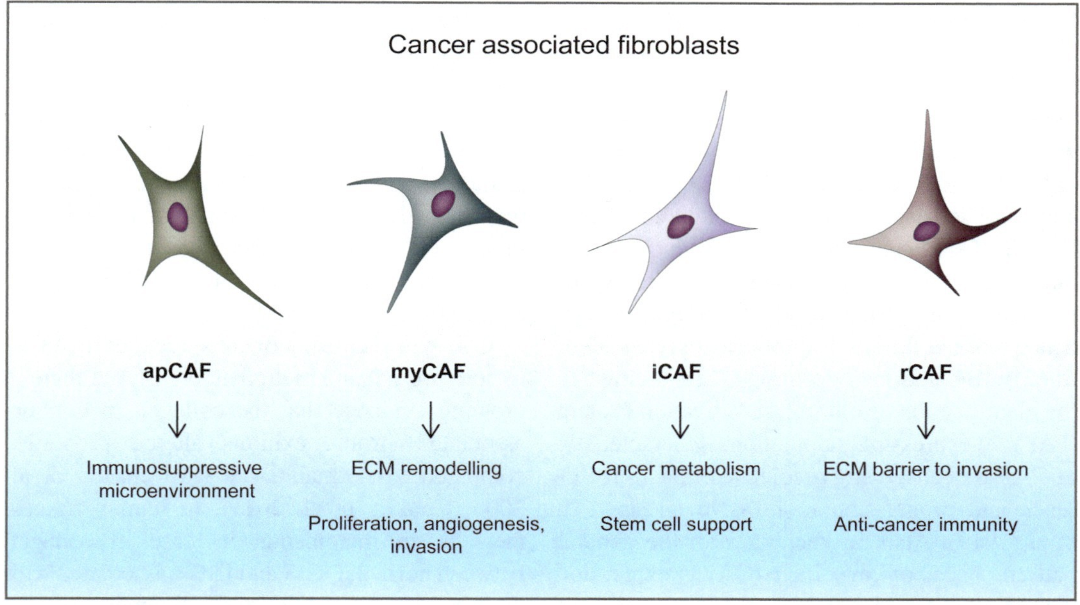

Fig. 12.4 Summary of CAF subtypes and their key roles. At least four distinct subtypes of CAF have been identified with both pro- and anti-tumourigenic properties. The apCAFs have been shown to generate an immunosuppressive tumour microenvironment, whilst classic myCAFs exhibit tumour-promoting effects through ECM remodelling and promotion of tumour cell proliferation and invasion and angiogenesis. The iCAFs, marked by high expression of CXCL12, modulate the tumour metabolic environment and promote cancer stem cell enrichment. In contrast, rCAFs are thought to generate an ECM barrier to cancer cell invasion and promote anti-cancer immunity. Abbreviations: *apCAFs*, antigen-presenting CAFs; *iCAFs*, inflammatory CAFs; *myCAFs*, myofibroblastic CAFs; *rCAFs*, cancer-restraining CAFs

promotes their differentiation into CD25 + Forkhead box protein P3 (FOXP3)+ T-regulatory cells, contributing to an immunosuppressive ME (Costa et al. 2018). Whereas the majority of work favours a pro-tumourigenic function for CAFs, the presence of CAFs acting in an anti-tumour role has been reported (Rhim et al. 2014). Such 'cancer-restraining' CAFs (rCAFs) are thought to form a barrier to tumour cell invasion through modulation of the ECM (Chen et al. 2021). In particular, fibroblasts expressing meflin have been flagged as anti-tumorigenic, since meflin suppresses the activity of lysyl oxidase (LOX) proteins, which are responsible for cross-linking collagen and promoting tumourigenesis (Mizutani et al. 2019) (Fig. 12.4).

Such detailed characterization of the fibroblast phenotype in DCIS is currently lacking, though there is evidence that fibroblasts are altered in DCIS, that there is heterogeneity in fibroblasts in the DCIS peri-ductal space (Chauhan et al. 2003) and that such variation may contribute to disease progression (Osuala et al. 2015; Strell et al. 2019). In one study, Jagged/Notch 2 signalling was found to give rise to a Platelet Derived Growth Factor Receptor (PDGFR)α^{low}/PDGFRβ^{high} fibroblast phenotype, the expression of which in the periductal stroma was associated with increased risk for recurrence in DCIS (Strell et al. 2019). Indirect evidence of a role for iCAFs is provided through co-culture of DCIS.COM cells and CAFs, which abrogated tumour cell migration following knock-down of fibroblast IL-6 (Osuala et al. 2015). Further evidence that the different fibroblast subtypes identified in IBC may evolve during DCIS is shown in the identification of Fibroblast Activation Protein (FAP)^{high} expressing populations, characteristic of CAF-S1 cells, being predictive of DCIS recurrence and progression to invasive disease (Yu et al. 2019). Also, in keeping with the general pattern of loss of caveolin 1 (CAV1) expression in CAFs associated with IBC, reduction or loss of CAV1 has been reported in DCIS, with loss increasing the cumulative incidence of progression to invasive disease by 27-fold (Witkiewicz et al. 2009).

Owing to the use of different technologies and different fibroblast markers, often with only a single marker in an individual study, it is difficult to directly map the fibroblast profile of DCIS lesions onto those identified in IBC. Detailed profiling, including markers for rCAFs, could help determine whether a fibroblast 'phenotypic switch' during DCIS evolution may contribute to progression.

12.4 ECM and Remodelling

12.4.1 ECM Production

Just as the fibroblast phenotype differs in malignant tissue compared to normal, as the major source of the ECM, it is not surprising that the components and function of the ECM itself differ in malignant tissue. The core matrisome consists of ~300 matrix macromolecules comprising collagens, proteoglycans such as hyaluronin and versican, and the complex glycoproteins including laminins, fibronectins and tenascins (Naba et al. 2016). The relative abundance and composition of the matrix varies across tissues in health and disease. The expression of alternative spliced variants (Rekad et al. 2022) and post-translational modification by different enzymes, including proteases and oxidases (Winkler et al. 2020), results in a highly variable and dynamic extracellular environment that can impact on multiple cellular functions (Mouw et al. 2014; Winkler et al. 2020).

Collagen I is the major constituent of the ECM in both normal and malignant breast, but there is growing evidence that the collagen in tumour-associated stroma exhibits altered properties compared to normal tissue (Provenzano et al. 2006; Conklin et al. 2011). In human tissues, there is an incremental increase in collagen between normal, DCIS and IBCs, associated with progressive thickening and alignment of the fibres (Acerbi et al. 2015). Another study described a change in the organization of collagen fibres in a subset of DCIS tissues, with fibres arranged perpendicular to the duct periphery being associated with more aggressive features, including presence of necrosis, Her2 positivity and lack of ER (Conklin et al. 2018). Collagen alignment did not predict disease recurrence in this series of DCIS; however, only 18 of 227 patients developed an ipsilateral recurrence, which likely means the study was under-powered. Further evidence that collagen alignment might impact on DCIS progression comes from a comparison of pure DCIS versus DCIS with co-existent invasion (Toss et al. 2019). This found that collagen arranged perpendicular to the DCIS duct, high collagen density and low fibre dispersity were more frequently seen in DCIS with invasion, and were also associated with shorter local-recurrence-free interval for both high- and non-high-grade disease (Toss et al. 2019). The importance of this perpendicular arrangement of collagen was also demonstrated in mouse models of mammary carcinoma (Provenzano et al. 2008). In apparent contrast to this, Sprague et al. (2021) found greater collagen fibre width and density to associate with a lower disease recurrence in DCIS, with no relationship to fibre angle. It seems clear that collagen characteristics at the DCIS duct periphery can influence behaviour, but further work is needed on larger sample cohorts to develop robust signatures to predict progression.

Other modifications of collagen may also impact on tumour cell behaviour: increased expression of collagen XII, which binds to collagen I fibrils and regulates their organization, has been shown to be a strong predictor of progression-free survival in early-stage breast cancer (Papanicolaou et al. 2022), though its potential role in DCIS progression is unexplored. Collagen properties can also be altered though cross-linking of fibres, largely mediated through LOX enzymes (Vallet and Ricard-Blum 2019). Direct evidence for a tumour-promoting role of LOX was demonstrated by promotion of growth and invasion of pre-malignant MCF10AT mammary epithelial cells when injected into mammary fat pads populated by fibroblasts overexpressing LOX (Levental et al. 2009). A role for LOX, and particularly LOX-like 2 enzymes, has been consistently implicated in mediating aggressive behaviour in IBC (Kirschmann et al. 2002; Ahn et al. 2013), though whether it plays a role in the DCIS ME is unclear.

As well as structural changes, the tumour-associated ECM environment displays a different composition to normal tissues. One protein consistently up-regulated in many solid tumours is tenascin-C (Orend and Chiquet-Ehrismann 2006). Tenascin-C is a hexameric glycoprotein that exists as multiple molecular isoforms generated though alternative splicing (Midwood et al. 2016). Its synthesis is highly regulated, being expressed at low levels in normal adult tissue but increased in both wound healing and cancer (Chiquet-Ehrismann et al. 2014). In normal tissue, tenascin-C primarily exists in its truncated form whereas in cancer-associated stroma, larger splice variants are expressed, sometimes in a tumour-specific pattern (Carnemolla et al. 1999). This has important implications since splicing introduces functional motifs into the mature protein that impact on function (Midwood et al. 2016). In breast, two specific splice variants, one containing exon 14 (TN14), the other containing both exons 14 and 16 (TN 14/16), have been detected in the stroma of IBCs and a subset of DCIS tissues (Adams et al. 2002). In vitro, these isoforms promote tumour cell proliferation and invasion (Hancox et al. 2009). Whether tumour-specific tenascin-C variants in the DCIS peri-ductal stroma can promote progression to invasion is not established, nor whether it has predictive value. However, its multifaceted impact on tumour cell behaviour, as well as its ability to modify other components of the ECM, such as binding to fibronectin (FN) (Huang et al. 2001), and modulation of mechanical properties of the ECM (Miroshnikova et al. 2016) make it worthy of further study.

Fibronectin (FN) has also been shown to be consistently up-regulated in the stroma of IBCs (Koukoulis et al. 1993; Balanis et al. 2013) and is also increased in the peri-ductal stroma of DCIS (Hayward et al. 2022). Interestingly, in 3D culture models of breast acinar development, addition of FN results in filling of the acinar lumen and increased acinar size (Williams et al. 2008). It is evident, however, that the structural organization and not just the deposition of FN influences its impact on epithelial cell behaviour, since disruption of fibril formation rather than depletion of FN per se in an MCF10A normal mammary gland model led to the acquisition of a DCIS phenotype (Magdaleno et al. 2021). Thus, FN may be involved in the development of DCIS as well as potentially influencing progression.

12.4.2 Remodelling of the ECM

As well as changes in the composition of tumour-associated matrix, it also undergoes remodelling, which induces a range of structural changes that influence cell signalling, matrix stiffness, release of growth factors and generation of novel bioactive matrix epitopes that can all impact on tumour behaviour (Egeblad et al. 2010; Winkler et al. 2020). A number of protease families play a role in this matrix remodelling including MMPs, disintegrin and metalloproteinases (ADAMS), disintegrin and metalloproteinases with thrombospondin motifs (ADAMTS), and serine, threonine and cysteine proteases (Page-McCaw et al. 2007; Lu et al. 2011; Bonnans et al. 2014). Of these, MMPs have received particular interest given their therapeutic potential; however, early clinical trials were disappointing (Overall and Dean 2006) and enthusiasm waned. However, it is now apparent that MMPs and ECM proteolysis can generate both anti-tumourigenic effects (Lopez-Otin et al. 2009) as well as the more widely recognized pro-tumourigenic effects (Lu et al. 2011). MMP8 has been shown to exert anti-tumour effects in both breast (Gutiérrez-Fernández et al. 2008) and oral (Åström et al. 2017) carcinoma, as well as in DCIS (Sarper et al. 2017). A novel invasion-suppressor role for the procollagen N-proteinase ADAMTS3, which primarily cleaves the propeptide of fibrillar collagen to allow assembly of mature collagen fibrils (Bekhouche and Colige 2015), has recently been described. In addition to its primary function, it has been shown to degrade FN, and loss of ADAMTS3 in myoepithelial cells resulted in stability of FN and enhancement of tumour invasion (Gibson et al. 2023c). Thus, it is clear that for therapeutic efficacy, detailed understanding of the role of proteases is needed with the ability to generate very specific inhibitors.

In the context of DCIS, the inhibitory effect of MMP8 is countered by expression of a number of other MMPs. Membrane-type 1 (MT1)-MMP is up-regulated in both DCIS and IBC (Jones et al. 1999; Bisson et al. 2003) and has been shown to play a role in tumour cell migration and invasion (Sabeh et al. 2004). In MCF10DCIS.com cells, knock-down of MT1-MMP inhibited invasion in 3D collagen I gels and, in an intraductal xenograft model, knock-down prevented development of invasive tumours (Lodillinsky et al. 2016). Furthermore, MT1-MMP was shown to be up-regulated in these cells on contact with collagen I in a p63-dependent manner (Lodillinsky et al. 2016). In contrast, MT1-MMP-dependent migration is inhibited by interaction with a domain in collagen IV (Pasco et al. 2000), highlighting the complex interplay between tumour cells and matrix components. Other proteases have also been implicated in promoting transition of DCIS to invasion: collagenase 3 (MMP13) is up-regulated in the stroma around areas of DCIS microinvasion (Nielsen et al. 2001) and in DCIS-associated myoepithelial cells (Hayward et al. 2022; Gibson et al. 2023b), and has been shown to promote breast cancer cell invasion (Wang et al. 2012; Sung et al. 2020; Hayward et al. 2022; Gibson et al. 2023b). Stromelysin 3 (MMP11), MMP-2 and TIMP1 have also been shown to be more highly expressed in the stromal environment of DCIS with microinvasion compared to pure DCIS (González et al. 2010), though the functional impact is less clear. Whilst it appears that changes in protease expression may be required for DCIS progression to invasion, what is less clear is the functional redundancy between proteases, which is essential to design appropriate therapeutic strategies. Their predictive value is also not yet established, since the majority of studies have been relatively small and lacking patient outcome.

12.5 The Immune ME

12.5.1 Tumour-Infiltrating Lymphocytes

A role for the immune system across a wide range of solid cancers is well established, and the ability of a tumour to manipulate the immune system is considered a hallmark of cancer (Hanahan and Weinberg 2011). Tumour-infiltrating lymphocytes (TILs) have been shown to relate to breast cancer behaviour, with high density of TILs being associated with a good prognosis (Stanton and Diss 2016; Denkert et al. 2018), and predictive of response to chemotherapy (Denkert et al. 2010) or immunotherapy (Byrne et al. 2020). The relationship of TILs to the behaviour of DCIS is more variable, which may in part be a result of differences in methods of TIL quantification between studies. In a series of almost 1500 cases of DCIS, levels of TILs were analysed using the guidelines established for IBC (Hendry et al. 2017) for their association with recurrent ipsilateral breast events (IBEs), either in situ or invasive disease (Pruneri et al. 2017). No association was found between periductal stromal TILS and recurrence when classed either as continuous variables or as percentage categories. However, a relationship between TIL infiltration and DCIS intrinsic subtype was noted, with high levels of TILS (defined as >50% of periductal stromal area) being more frequent in HER2-positive and TN DCIS compared to luminal-type DCIS (Pruneri et al. 2017). In the SweDCIS randomized radiotherapy trial, where TILS were classified as ≤5% or >5%, 61.9% of 711 DCIS samples had low TIL counts, and those DCIS patients with a high TIL count had a significant increase in IBE at 5 years post-breast conservative surgery. High TILS remained an independent poor prognostic marker for HER2-negative DCIS following multivariate analysis (Schiza et al. 2022). The importance of method of assessment was emphasized by Toss et al. (2018), who compared seven different methods across two DCIS cohorts and found the strongest association to shorter recurrence-free survival with density of 'touching' TILS—defined as lymphocytes in contact with the DCIS duct BM or one lymphocyte diameter away (Toss et al. 2018). The prognostic power of periductal TILs became progressively weaker with increased distance from the duct BM (Toss et al. 2018). They proposed that this interaction between TILs and BM may lead to damage and remodelling of the BM to facilitate invasion (Toss et al. 2018). To some extent, this supports the hypothesis of Man (2007), who correlated immune cell infiltrate with discontinuity of myoepithelial cells and altered features of overlying neoplastic cells. Similarly, digital spatial analysis using deep learning approaches suggested that colocalization of immune cells with the duct rather than total TIL extent may be more important in eliciting an immune response (Narayanan et al. 2021). However, even where there appears to be a similar approach to quantitation, there remains discordance in findings. Badve et al. (2022) found no association between touching lymphocytes and patient outcome in a large DCIS cohort, but found that circumferential TILs were associated with a good prognosis. This itself differs from other studies that report an association between circumferential TILs and a more aggressive DCIS phenotype (Knopfelmacher et al. 2015) and worse prognosis (Thike et al. 2020).

In addition to variation in quantification approaches, the impact on DCIS behaviour is likely to be influenced by the precise immune cell profile present. In general, an anti-tumour response is mediated through CD8+ T-cells with a humoral anti-tumour response mediated by CD20+ B-cells (Nelson 2010), whilst an immunosuppressive response is mediated by CD4+ FOXP3 + T-regulatory cells (Emens 2012; Cruz-Merino et al. 2013). In keeping with this, high FOXP3+ cell counts, together with high stromal TILs and programmed cell death ligand 1 (PD-L1) positivity have been associated with ipsilateral recurrence in DCIS, though interestingly, only Programmed death ligand 1 (PD-L1) was associated with invasive recurrence (Toss et al. 2020). Similarly, in a study comparing pure DCIS to DCIS with co-existent invasion, FOXP3+ TILs were significantly increased in DCIS with invasion, and high FOXP3+ TILs with presence of PD-L1+ immune cells were associated with invasive recurrence in pure DCIS, though numbers are small, with only six patients having an invasive recurrence (Kim et al. 2020).

The data suggest that TILs play a role in modulating DCIS behaviour. However, it seems likely that a combination of TIL phenotype and spatial distribution applied to DCIS cohorts with sufficient frequency of recurrence events will be necessary to establish an algorithm for assessing risk.

12.5.2 Macrophages

Macrophages are a heterogeneous group of cells that play multifunctional roles in the tumour ME. The diversity of their function is dependent on their origin, their tissue of residence and the specific environmental cues they encounter (DeNardo and Rufell 2019). They have long been recognized as having both pro- and anti-tumoural functions (Balkwill et al. 2005; Netea et al. 2017; Propper and Balkwill 2022). Tumour-associated macrophages (TAMs), initially described in relation to the binary M1/M2 paradigm, play an important role in breast cancer (Mantovani et al. 2002; Cassetta et al. 2019). High density of stromal macrophages in breast cancer tissues has been associated with reduced relapse-free and overall survival (Leek et al. 1996; Hao et al. 2012; Yang et al. 2018).

TAM recruitment and phenotype are regulated through autocrine inflammatory circuits as well as cytokine/chemokine-mediated reciprocal interaction with tumours and other cell types. CXCL10, which binds to the interferon γ (IFNγ)-inducible ligand CXCR3, commonly expressed on monocytes, is secreted by both fibroblasts and cancer cells and has been shown to play an important role in the recruitment of monocytes/macrophages (Taub et al. 1993; Yang et al. 2006). In keeping with this, CXCL10 expression has been shown to be significantly higher in IBC compared to DCIS (Ejaeidi et al. 2015). CCL2 is an even more potent chemoattractant that is associated with accumulation of macrophages and modulation of TAM function in breast cancer (Matsushima et al. 1989; Kitamura et al. 2015). Immunohistochemical analyses in primary human breast cancer specimens have shown a significant association between CCL2 expression and CD68^{+} TAM accumulation, with one study demonstrating poorer relapse-free survival in patients with combined high CCL2 and vascular endothelial growth factor (VEGF) tissue expression (Ueno et al. 2000; Saji et al. 2001).

There is accumulating evidence, predominantly, though not exclusively, from mouse models, that macrophages might play a key role in the transition of pre-invasive disease to invasion. In an early study, Lee et al. (1997) reported an association between macrophage infiltrate and the presence of periductal angiogenesis, which has been implicated in promoting DCIS progression. In a Mouse mammary tumour virus-polyoma middle tumour-antigen (MMTV-PyMT) model of breast cancer, genetic deletion of colony stimulating factor 1 (*CSF1*), and thereby macrophages, slowed malignant progression and inhibited formation of metastasis (Lin et al. 2001). Gain of function of *CSF1*, restricted to the mammary gland, restored the TAM phenotype and resulted in tumour progression. Interestingly, lack of TAMs did not impact early tumour development but affected tumour progression more: TAMs specifically appeared to lead to tumour cell invasion through the BM into the stroma (Lin et al. 2001), drawing strong parallels with a potential role in DCIS progression. Further evidence for a role in the progression of pre-invasive lesions is shown in a transplantable p53-null mouse mammary epithelium model, which develops pre-malignant lesions with variable malignant potential (Carron et al. 2017). This showed that macrophages were preferentially recruited to lesions with enhanced progression to invasive disease, and that these macrophages were differentiated towards a tumour-promoting phenotype. The MMTV-Her2 mouse model also generates a series of pre-invasive lesions with variable capacity to progress (Linde et al. 2018); infiltration of macrophages into ducts with features of intramammary epithelial neoplasia—considered a model of human DCIS—was associated with progression to invasive disease, whilst elimination of macrophages from the lesions using CSF1 receptor blocking antibody prevented disease progression. The potential relevance of this to human disease was supported by tissue studies showing significantly more intraductal macrophages in DCIS ducts compared to normal breast ducts (Linde et al. 2018).

Several studies have associated macrophage density with enhanced angiogenesis in breast cancer tissue (Mantovani et al. 1993; Lewis et al. 1995; Lee et al. 1997; Leek and Harris 2002). TAM-derived Vascular Endothelial Growth Factor (VEGF) is a potent chemoattractant for macrophages but has also been implicated in regulating the angiogenic switch and behaviour of perivascular TAMs. Restoration of VEGF-A expression in premalignant mammary lesions of *CSF1*-depleted PyMT models restores macrophage infiltration and disease progression through onset of the angiogenic switch (Lin et al. 2007). Within tumours, it has been demonstrated that cancer cells induce TGFβ-dependent up-regulation of Chemokine receptor (CXCR)4 in monocyte-derived macrophages, which are subsequently recruited towards blood vessels by perivascular fibroblast-derived CXCL12. Following Tie2-dependent attachment to endothelial cells, TAM-secreted VEGF enhances angiogenesis and vascular permeability to permit intravasation of cancer cells (Harney et al. 2015; Arwert et al. 2018).

TAMs also influence other aspects of the tumour ME: they are major suppressors of the immune ME, directly suppressing T-cell function through release of IL-10 stimulated by tumour-cell derived IL-4, IL-13 and TGFβ (Ruffell et al. 2014; Smith et al. 2018). They also suppress T-cell function through expression of PD-L1 (Kuang et al. 2009; Gordon et al. 2017). Further interplay between different elements of the ME is evident, with fibrotic stroma being able to modify the TAM phenotype: CAFs release pro-inflammatory cytokines such as IL-6, Chemokine Ligand (CCL)2, Granulocyte-Macrophage Colony Stimulating Factor (GM-CSF), which can regulate the recruitment, differentiation and activation of TMAs (Wu et al. 2011; Kalluri 2016), locking macrophages into an immunosuppressive state (Mace et al. 2013).

12.5.2.1 TAM Phenotypes

Traditionally, the divergent pro- and anti-tumoural effects of macrophages have been captured in the binary M1/M2 polarization classification, with M1 macrophages being 'classically' activated and M2 macrophages being 'alternatively' activated (Sica and Mantovani 2012; Mills et al. 2000). With growing understanding of the complexity of macrophages, the newer term 'M1-like' has come to define proinflammatory macrophage subsets activated by tumour necrosis factor α (TNFα) and and Interferon (IFN)γ, and characterized by high levels of inducible nitric oxide synthetase (iNOS) or MHCII (Mantovani et al. 2002). The anti-inflammatory, pro-tumoural M2 TAMs are described as expressing high levels of arginase 1, CD163, CD204 or CD206 (Mantovani et al. 2002) and release anti-inflammatory factors such as TGFβ, IL-10 and IL-4 with low levels of pro-inflammatory IL-12, IL-23, IL-1 and chemokines including CXCL10 and CCL5 (Arango Duque and Descoteaux 2014; Mantovani et al. 2004; Briukhovetska et al. 2021).

Recent developments in bulk tissue sequencing, multiplex immunofluorescence and single-cell (sc) RNA sequencing have further emphasized the complexity of TAM phenotypes in cancer, with between five and nine TAM subtypes now identified across a range of cancers (reviewed in Cassetta and Pollard 2023). Using bulk RNA sequencing, Cassetta et al. (2019) revealed significant differences between resident macrophages and TAMs isolated from breast cancer and reduction mammoplasty. Regardless of tissue of origin, macrophages showed no enrichment for M2-associated genes

Table 12.1 Designated macrophage subtypes and key function and gene signatures as described by Ma et al. (2022)

Designation	Key function	Key genes	Breast cancer
IFN-TAMs	Promote proliferation Promote immunosuppression	*CCL2, IFIT1, IFITM1, ISG1*	Y
LA-TAMs	Promote EMT ECM degradation Immunosuppression	*ACPS, APOE, FABP5, SPP1, TREM2*	Y
Angio-TAMs	Promote angiogenesis ECM proteolysis Promote EMT	*AREG, CD163, CEBPB, FN1, SERPINB2, TIMP-1*	Y
Inflam-TAMs	Recruit and regulate immune cells TNF signalling	*CCL3L1, CCL4L2, CXCL1, IL1B, IL6*	N
Reg-TAMs	T-cell suppression Antigen presentation pathway	*CD274*	Y
Prolif-TAMs	High cell proliferation Proinflammatory	*CDK1, HMGN2, MK167, STMN1, TOP2A*	N
Classical TAMS	Inhibit antigen presentation TGFβ and TNF signalling	*CCR2, FCN1, FOS, IL1B, LY6C1, LY6C2*	Y

Seven key macrophage subtypes have been designated on the basis of single-cell (sc) RENA sequencing, scATAC sequencing and cellular indexing of transcriptomes and epitopes by sequencing (CITE-seq). The table indicates the key pathways active in these TAM populations, key genes expressed and whether they have been described in breast cancer

TAM, tissue-associated macrophage; *IFN-TAMs*, interferon-primed TAMs; *LA-TAMs*, lipid-associated TAMS; *Angio-TAMs*, pro-angiogenic TAMs; *Inflam-TAMs*, inflammatory cytokine-enriched TAMs; *Reg-TAMs*, immune regulatory TAMs; Prolif-TAMs, proliferating TAMs

such as *Arg1*, nor did they display differential expression in CD163—a so-called mouse TAM marker. The lack of conformation to traditionally accepted TAM phenotypes was corroborated by Azizi et al. (2018), who used scRNAseq to profile 45,000 immune cells from breast cancer to account for macrophage heterogeneity. In 2021, two large-scale RNAseq analyses aimed to harmonize TAM characteristics from multiple studies (Cheng et al. 2021; Mulder et al. 2021), and recently Ma et al. (2022) proposed a unified classification for TAM subtypes identifying seven distinct TAM subtypes with different effects on the tumour ME (Ma et al. 2022), summarized in Table 12.1. Many of these TAM subtypes have been identified in breast cancer, but it is important to note that none of these studies include analysis of DCIS, so the evolution of macrophage phenotype and its potential role in disease progression remains unresolved. Furthermore, there remains a lack of clear understanding of the spatial biology of different macrophage phenotypes in both DCIS and invasive biology. This is an exciting and rapidly evolving field of research that could help reveal clinically relevant prognostic tools as well as potential novel therapeutic targets (Matusiak et al. 2023).

12.6 Adipocytes

The breast comprises a variable proportion of adipose tissue showing some, but not absolute, correlation with BMI (Iyengar et al. 2019), and higher levels of body fat are associated with an increased risk of post-menopausal breast cancer (Reeves et al. 2007) and poorer outcome in both pre- and post-menopausal women (Dignam et al. 2003). As well as increased adipocyte area in the breast, increased adiposity is associated with increased diameter of individual adipocytes and development of crown-like structures (CLSs), representing a chronic inflammatory response, with macrophages encircling the damaged adipocytes (Sebastiani et al. 2016). Whilst the number of CLSs in benign breast biopsies has previously been shown to be associated with the development of IBC (Vaysse et al. 2017; Carter et al. 2018), no association with CLS and DCIS recurrence has been described to date. However, in a nested case-control study of patients with pure DCIS who did or did not go on to develop an ipsilateral recurrence, both adipocyte diameter and adipocyte area were associated with a significantly increased risk of recurrence (Almekinders et al. 2021). In fact, with each 10-υm increase in adipocyte diameter (at the 75th percentile) there was an increased OR for recurrence of 25% (Almekinders et al. 2021). The number of CLSs showed no association with recurrence (Almekinders et al. 2021). Nonetheless, the potential impact of adipose-related inflammation is suggested by exposure of benign MCF10A cells to macrophage-conditioned media, which led to the acquisition of malignant features (Wilcz-Villega et al. 2020), highlighting the ability of an inflammatory environment to impact epithelial cell function.

Adipose tissue is considered an endocrine organ since it releases a range of growth factors, cytokines, adipokines and proteases that can act on adjacent cells and the ME (Kersgaw and Flier 2004; Walter et al. 2009). It generates a pro-inflammatory environment secreting cytokines, including TNFα, IL-6 and IL-10 as well as factors such as adiponectin and leptin (Trayhurn 2005). In particular, leptin has been shown to have a cancer-promoting role in breast cancer (Andò et al. 2019). Adipose tissue can thus impact surrounding cell structures, and interestingly, in the context of DCIS, human adipose stem cells have been shown to modulate the behaviour of breast myoepithelial cells (Delort et al. 2021). With the caveat that just a single myoepithelial cell line was used, a co-culture model of adipocyte stem cells led to reduced myoepithelial cell viability as well as enhanced expression of leptin and of FN, both of which have been implicated in promoting tumour cell invasion (Andò et al. 2019; Hayward et al. 2022). Obesity has also been shown to reduce the number of myoepithelial cells in mouse models (Chamberlain et al. 2017), which together suggests that the adipose ME could destabilize the myoepithelial duct wall barrier and so facilitate invasive progression. These functional studies, and the work of Almekinders et al. (2021) are compelling, but further validation is essential—using in vitro, in vivo and human tissue studies—to establish the impact and the mechanism of the adipose ME on DCIS progression.

12.7 Blood Vessels and Angiogenesis

Angiogenesis is essential for tumour growth (Weidner et al. 1991) and is considered as one of the hallmarks of cancer (Hanahan and Weinberg 2011). Since blood vessels are restricted to the extra-ductal environment, as DCIS ducts expand, they create a hypoxic environment and reflecting this, DCIS has been associated with enhanced angiogenesis (Guidi et al. 1994; Engels et al. 1997). Two patterns of angiogenesis have been described in DCIS: a diffuse stromal vascularity and a dense rim of periductal vessels encircling the DCIS duct (Guidi et al. 1994; Lee et al. 1997). The periductal vascular density in DCIS has been associated with both in situ and invasive recurrence (Teo et al. 2003). Furthermore, the vessels appear to exhibit an altered phenotype to normal vessels, in particular showing loss of von Willebrand factor (Teo et al. 2003). In addition, expression of thymidine phosphorylase, which is involved in remodelling vasculature, has been shown to be associated with periductal angiogenesis but not diffuse angiogenesis in DCIS (Engels et al. 1997). Interestingly, in a study of pure DCIS versus DCIS with co-existent invasion, higher levels of expression of the pro-angiogenic factors VEGF-C, its receptor Flt-4 and VEGFR2 was found in pure DCIS (Wulfing et al. 2005). This is perhaps not surprising, since the DCIS duct will be particularly hypoxic; once tumour cells escape from the duct, they have greater proximity to vessels compared to the avascular intraductal environment.

As is clear from the preceding discussion, multiple components of the ME can regulate angiogenesis. In DCIS, myoepithelial cells have a distinct role, switching from an anti-angiogenic (Barsky and Karlin 2005) to a pro-angiogenic (Allinen et al. 2004; Nguyen-Ngoc et al. 2012) phenotype. This is mediated in part through up-regulation of plasminogen activator inhibitor-I (PAI-I) (Hildenbrand and Arens 2004), a known pro-angiogenic factor (Isogai et al. 2001). In contrast to this, Bluff et al. (2009) described increased microvessel density in IBC compared to DCIS (Bluff et al. 2009). Thus, while some studies suggest periductal angiogenesis is associated with recurrence (Teo et al. 2003), this is not universal, and the value of angiogenesis as a predictive marker of progression remains uncertain.

12.8 Conclusions

There is a real need to predict which DCIS lesions will progress and which will remain indolent. Since genomic and transcriptomic studies of DCIS epithelial cells have not identified consistent differences to IBC cells, attention has turned to the potential role of the ME. The ME is complex: it comprises multiple components that are dynamic, plastic and interactive. To date, the limiting factors in studies of DCIS progression are lack of power, due to relatively low 'event' rates (either as recurrent DCIS or IBC), restricted marker analysis, when it is clear that many of these components interact, and an inability to analyse both the temporal and spatial evolution of the disease. These are the major challenges. Technological advances—single-cell sequencing, spatial transcriptomics, proteomics, multimodal analysis and AI—will help address these challenges. To leverage this, it is essential that appropriate sample cohorts are assembled for analysis, with linkage to relevant and sophisticated model systems to truly dissect the key modulators of DCIS progression.

References

Acerbi I, Cassereau L, Dean I et al (2015) Human breast cancer invasion and aggression correlates with ECM stiffening and immune cell infiltration. Integr Biol (Camb) 7(10):1120–1134

Adams M, Jones JL, Walker RA et al (2002) Changes in tenascin-C isoform expression in invasive and pre-invasive breast disease. Cancer Res 62:3289

Adriance MC, Inman JL, Petersen OW, Bissell MJ (2005) Myoepithelial cells: good fences make good neighbors. Breast Cancer Res 7(5):190–197

Ahn SG, Dong SM, Oshima A et al (2013) LOXL2 expression is associated with invasiveness and negatively influences survival in breast cancer patients. Breast Cancer Res Treat 141(1):89–99

Allen MD, Thomas GJ, Clark S et al (2014) Altered microenvironment promotes progression of preinvasive breast cancer: myoepithelial expression of alphavbeta6 integrin in DCIS identifies high-risk patients and predicts recurrence. Clin Cancer Res 20(2):344–357

Allinen M, Beroukhim R, Cai L et al (2004) Molecular characterization of the tumor microenvironment in breast cancer. Cancer Cell 6(1):17–32

Allred DC, Yun W, Sufeng M et al (2008) Ductal carcinoma in situ and the emergence of diversity during breast cancer evolution. Clin Cancer Res 14(2):370–378

Almekinders MMM, Scaapveld M, Thijssen B et al (2021) Breast adipocyte size associates with ipsilateral invasive breast cancer risk after ductal carcinoma in situ. NPJ Breast Cancer 7(31)

Andò S, Gelsomino L, Panza S et al (2019) Obesity, leptin and breast cancer: epidemiological evidence and proposed mechanisms. Cancers (Basel) 11(1):62

Arango Duque G, Descoteaux A (2014) Macrophage cytokines: involvement in immunity and infectious diseases. Front Immunol 5:491

Arwert EN, Harney AS, Entenberg D et al (2018) A unidirectional transition from migratory to perivascular macrophage is required for tumor cell intravasation. Cell Rep 23(5):1239–1248

Åström P, Juurikka K, Hadler-Olsen ES et al (2017) The interplay of matrix metalloproteinase-8, transforming growth factor-beta1 and vascular endothelial growth factor-C cooperatively contributes to the aggressiveness of oral tongue squamous cell carcinoma. Br J Cancer 117(7):1007–1016

Azizi E, Carr AJ, Plitas G et al (2018) Single-cell map of diverse immune phenotypes in the breast tumor microenvironment. Cell 174(5):1293–1308 e36

Badve SS, Sanghee C, Lu X et al (2022) Tumor infiltrating lymphocytes in multi-National Cohorts of ductal carcinoma in situ (DCIS) of breast. Cancers (Basel) 14(16):3916

Balanis N, Wendt MK, Schiemann BJ et al (2013) Epithelial to mesenchymal transition promotes breast cancer progression via a fibronectin-dependent STAT3 signaling pathway. J Biol Chem 288:17954–17967

Balkwill F, Charles KA, Mantovani A (2005) Smoldering and polarized inflammation in the initiation and promotion of malignant disease. Cancer Cell 7(3):211–217

Barsky SH, Karlin NJ (2005) Myoepithelial cells: autocrine and paracrine suppressors of breast cancer progression. J Mammary Gland Biol Neoplasia 10(3):249–260

Bekhouche M, Colige A (2015) The procollagen N-proteinases ADAMTS2, 3 and 14 in pathophysiology. Matrix Biol 44-46:46–53

Benyahia Z, Dussault N, Cayol M et al (2017) Stromal fibroblasts present in breast carcinomas promote tumor growth and angiogenesis through adrenomedullin secretion. Oncotarget 8(9):15744–15762

Bergstraesser LM, Srinivasan G, Jones JC et al (1995) Expression of hemidesmosomes and component proteins is lost by invasive breast cancer cells. Am J Pathol 147(6):1823–1839

Bernard S, Myers M, Fang WB et al (2018) CXCL1 derived from mammary fibroblasts promotes progression of mammary lesions to invasive carcinoma through CXCR2 dependent mechanisms. J Mammary Gland Biol Neoplasia 23(4):249–267

Bhowmick NA, Chytil A, Plieth D et al (2004) TGF-beta signaling in fibroblasts modulates the oncogenic potential of adjacent epithelia. Science 303(5659):848–851

Bisson C, Blacher S, Polette M et al (2003) Restricted expression of membrane type 1-matrix metalloproteinase by myofibroblasts adjacent to human breast cancer cells. Int J Cancer 105:7–13

Bleyer A, Welch HG (2012) Effect of three decades of screening mammography on breast-cancer incidence. N Engl J Med 367(21):1998–2005

Bluff JE, Menakuru SR, Cross SS et al (2009) Angiogenesis is associated with the onset of hyperplasia in human ductal breast disease. Br J Cancer 101(4):666–672

Bofin AM, Lydersen S, Hagmar BM (2004) Cytological criteria for the diagnosis of intraductal hyperplasia, ductal carcinoma in situ, and invasive carcinoma of the breast. Diagn Cytopathol 31(4):207–215

Bonnans C, Chou J, Werb Z (2014) Remodelling the extracellular matrix in development and disease. Nat Rev Mol Cell Biol 15:786–801

Briukhovetska D, Dorr J, Endres S et al (2021) Interleukins in cancer: from biology to therapy. Nat Rev Cancer 21(8):481–499

Byrne A, Savas P, Sant S et al (2020) Tissue-resident memory T cells in breast cancer control and immunotherapy responses. Nat Rev Clin Oncol 17(6):341–348

Cancer Research UK (2020). https://www.cancerresearchuk.org/health-professional/cancer-statistics/statistics-by-cancer-type/breast-cancer/incidence-in-situ

Carnemolla B, Castellani P, Ponassi M et al (1999) Identification of a glioblastoma-associated tenascin-C isoform by a high affinity recombinant antibody. Am J Pathol 154(5):1345–1352

Carron EC, Homra S, Rosenberg J et al (2017) Macrophages promote the progression of premalignant mammary lesions to invasive cancer. Oncotarget 8(31):50731–50746

Carter JM, Hoskin TL, Pena MA et al (2018) Macrophagic "crown-like structures" are associated with an increased risk of breast cancer in benign breast disease. Cancer Prev Res (Philos) 11(2):113–119

Casasent AK, Schalck A, Gao R et al (2018) Multiclonal invasion in breast tumors identified by topographic single cell sequencing. Cell 172(1–2):205–217

Casasent AK, Almekinders MM, Mulder C et al (2022) Learning to distinguish progressive and non-progressive ductal carcinoma in situ. Nat Rev Cancer 22(12):663–678

Cassetta L, Pollard JW (2023) A timeline of tumour-associated macrophage biology. Nat Rev Cancer 23(4):238–257

Cassetta L, Fragkogianni S, Sims AH et al (2019) Human tumor-associated macrophage and monocyte transcriptional landscapes reveal cancer-specific reprogramming, biomarkers, and therapeutic targets. Cancer Cell 35(4):588–602.e10

Chamberlain T, D'Amato JV, Arendt LM et al (2017) Obesity reversibly depletes the basal cell population and enhances mammary epithelial cell estrogen receptor alpha expression and progenitor activity. Breast Cancer Res 19(1):128

Chauhan H, Abraham A, Phillips JR et al (2003) There is more than one kind of myofibroblast: analysis of CD34 expression in benign, in situ, and invasive breast lesions. J Clin Pathol 56(4):271–276

Chen Y, McAndrews KM, Kalluri R (2021) Clinical and therapeutic relevance of cancer-associated fibroblasts. Nat Rev Clin Oncol 18(12):792–804

Cheng S, Li Z, Gao R et al (2021) A pan-cancer single - cell transcriptional atlas of tumor infiltrating myeloid cells. Cell 184(3):792–809

Chevez de Paz Villanueva C, Bonev V, Senthil M et al (2017) Factors associated with underestimation of invasive cancer in patients with ductal carcinoma in-situ: precautions for active surveillance et al. JAMA Surg 152:117–114

Chiquet-Ehrismann R, Orend G, Chiquet M et al (2014) Tenascins in stem cell niches. Matrix Biol 37:112–123

Collins LC, Tamimi RM, Baer HJ et al (2005) Outcome of patients with ductal carcinoma in situ untreated after diagnostic biopsy: results from the Nurses' Health Study. Cancer 103(9):1778–1784

Conklin MW, Eickhoff JC, Riching KM et al (2011) Aligned collagen is a prognostic signature for survival in human breast carcinoma. Am J Pathol 178(3):1221–1232

Conklin MW, Gangnon RE, Sprague BL et al (2018) Collagen alignment as a predictor of recurrence after ductal carcinoma in situ. Cancer Epidemiol Biomarkers Prev 27(2):138–145

Costa A, Kieffer Y, Scholer-Dahirel A et al (2018) Fibroblast heterogeneity and immunosuppressive environment in human breast cancer. Cancer Cell 33(3):463–79.e10

Cruz-Merino LD, Barco-sánchez A, Carrasco FH et al (2013) New insights into the role of the immune microenvironment in breast carcinoma. Clin Dev Immunol 2013:785317

Delort L, Cholet J, Decombat C et al (2021) The adipose microenvironment dysregulates the mammary myoepithelial cells and could participate to the progression of breast cancer front cell. Dev Biol 8:571948

DeNardo DG, Rufell D (2019) Macrophages as regulators of tumour immunity and immunotherapy. Nat Rev Immunol 19:369–382

Denkert C, Loibl S, Noske A et al (2010) Tumor-associated lymphocytes as an independent predictor of response to neoadjuvant chemotherapy in breast cancer. J Clin Oncol 28(1):105–113

Denkert C, von Minckwitz G, Darb-Esfahani S et al (2018) Tumour-infiltrating lymphocytes and prognosis in different subtypes of breast cancer: a pooled analysis of 3771 patients treated with neoadjuvant therapy. Lancet Oncol 19(1):40–50

Dignam JJ, Wieand K, Johnson KA et al (2003) Obesity, tamoxifen use, and outcomes in women with estrogen receptor-positive early-stage breast cancer. J Natl Cancer Inst 95(19):1467–1476

Doebar SC, Sieuwerts AM, de Weers V et al (2017) Gene expression differences between ductal carcinoma in situ with and without progression to invasive breast cancer. Am J Pathol 187(7):1648–1655

Egeblad M, Rasch MG, Weaver VM (2010) Dynamic interplay between the collagen scaffold and tumor evolution. Curr Opin Cell Biol 22:697–706

Ejaeidi AA, Craft BS, Puneky LV et al (2015) Hormone receptor-independent CXCL10 production is associated with the regulation of cellular factors linked to breast cancer progression and metastasis. Exp Mol Pathol 99(1):163–172

Ellis IO (2010) Intraductal proliferative lesions of the breast: morphology, associated risk and molecular biology. Mod Pathol 23(Suppl 2):S1–S7

Ellis IO, Coleman D, Wells C et al (2006) Impact of a national external quality assessment scheme for breast pathology in the UK. J Clin Pathol 59(2):138–145

Elshof LE, Tryfonidis K, Slaets L et al (2015) Feasibility of a prospective, randomised, open-label, international multicentre, phase III, non-inferiority trial to assess the safety of active surveillance for low risk ductal carcinoma in situ - the LORD study. Eur J Cancer 51(12):1497–1510

Elyada E, Bolisatty M, Laise P et al (2019) Cross-species single-cell analysis of pancreatic ductal adenocarcinoma reveals antigen-presenting cancer-associated fibroblasts. Cancer Discov 9(8):1102–1123

Emens LA (2012) Breast cancer immunobiology driving immunotherapy: vaccines and immune checkpoint blockade. Expert Rev Anticancer Ther 12(12):1597–1611

Engels K, Fox SB, Whitehouse RM et al (1997) Distinct angiogenic patterns are associated with high-grade in situ ductal carcinomas of the breast. J Pathol 181:207–212

Falk RS, Hofvind S, Skaane P, Haldorsen T (2011) Second events following ductal carcinoma in situ of the breast: a register-based cohort study. Breast Cancer Res Treat 129(3):929–938

Finak G, Bertos N, Pepin F et al (2008) Stromal gene expression predicts clinical outcome in breast cancer. Nat Med 14(5):518–527

Francis A, Thomas J, Fallowfield L et al (2015) Addressing overtreatment of screen detected DCIS; the LORIS trial. Eur J Cancer 51(16):2296–2303

Franke WW, Schmid E, Freudenstain C et al (1980) Intermediate-sized filaments of the prekeratin type in myoepithelial cells. J Cell Biol 84(3):633–654

Gibson SV, Roozitalab RM, Allen MD et al (2023a) Everybody needs good neighbours: the progressive DCIS microenvironment. Trends Cancer 9(4):326–338

Gibson SV, Tomas Bort E, Rodriguez-Fernandez L et al (2023b) TGFβ-mediated MMP13 secretion drives myoepithelial cell dependent breast cancer progression. NPJ Breast Cancer 9(1):9

Gibson SV, Madzharova E, Tan AC et al (2023c) ADAMTS3 restricts cancer invasion in models of early breast cancer progression through enhanced fibronectin degradation. Matrix Biol 121:74–89

González LO, González-Reyes S, Junquera S et al (2010) Expression of metalloproteinases and their inhibitors by tumor and stromal cells in ductal carcinoma in situ of the breast and their relationship with microinvasive events. J Cancer Res Clin Oncol 136(9):1313–1321

Gordon SR, Maute RL, Dulken BW et al (2017) PD-1 expression by tumour-associated macrophages inhibits phagocytosis and tumour immunity. Nature 545(7655):495–499

Gudjonsson T, Rønnov-Jessen L, Villadsen R et al (2002) Normal and tumor-derived myoepithelial cells differ in their ability to interact with luminal breast epithelial cells for polarity and basement membrane deposition. J Cell Sci 115(Pt 1):39–50

Guidi AJ, Fischer L, Harris JR et al (1994) Microvessel density and distribution in ductal carcinoma in situ of the breast. J Natl Cancer Inst 86:614–619

Gutiérrez-Fernández A, Fueyo A, Folgueras AR et al (2008) Matrix metalloproteinase-8 functions as a metastasis suppressor through modulation of tumor cell adhesion and invasion. Cancer Res 68(8):2755–2763

Hanahan D, Weinberg RA (2011) Hallmarks of cancer: the next generation. Cell 144(5):646–674

Hancox RA, Allen MD, Holliday DL et al (2009) Tumour-associated tenascin-C isoforms promote breast cancer cell invasion and growth by matrix metalloproteinase-dependent and independent mechanisms. Breast Cancer Res 11(2):R24

Hao N-B, Lü MH, Fan Y-H et al (2012) Macrophages in tumor microenvironments and the progression of tumors. Clin Dev Immunol 2012:948098

Harney AS, Arwert EN, Entenberg D et al (2015) Real-time imaging reveals local, transient vascular permeability, and tumor cell intravasation stimulated by TIE2hi macrophage-derived VEGFA. Cancer Discov 5(9):932–943

Hayward MK, Allen MD, Gomm JJ et al (2022) Mechanostimulation of breast myoepithelial cells induces functional changes associated with DCIS progression to invasion. NPJ Breast Cancer 8(1):109

Hendry S, Salgado R, Gevaert T et al (2017) Assessing tumor-infiltrating lymphocytes in solid tumors: a practical review for pathologists and proposal for a standardized method from the international immunooncology biomarkers working group: part 1: assessing the host immune response, TILs in invasive breast carcinoma and ductal carcinoma in situ, metastatic tumor deposits and areas for further research. Adv Anat Pathol 24(5):235–251

Hernandez L, Wilkerson PM, Lambros MB et al (2012) Genomic and mutational profiling of ductal carcinomas in situ and matched adjacent invasive breast cancers reveals intra-tumour genetic heterogeneity and clonal selection. J Pathol 227(1):42–52

Hildenbrand R, Arens N (2004) Protein and mRNA expression of uPAR and PAI-1 in myoepithelial cells of early breast cancer lesions and normal breast tissue. Br J Cancer 91(3):564–571

Holliday DL, Brouilette KT, Markert A et al (2009) Novel multicellular organotypic models of normal and malignant breast: tools for dissecting the role of the microenvironment in breast cancer progression. Breast Cancer Res 11(1):R3

Hu M, Peluffo G, Chen H, Polyak K (2009) Role of COX-2 in epithelial–stromal cell interactions and progression of ductal carcinoma in situ of the breast. Proc Natl Acad Sci USA 106(9):3372–3377

Huang W, Chiquet-Ehrismann R, Moyano JV et al (2001) Interference of tenascin-C with syndecan-4 binding to fibronectin blocks cell adhesion and stimulates tumor cell proliferation. Cancer Res 61(23):8586–8594

Hwang ES, Hyslop T, Lynch T et al (2019) The COMET (Comparison of Operative versus Monitoring and Endocrine Therapy) trial: a phase III randomised controlled clinical trial for low-risk ductal carcinoma in situ (DCIS). BMJ Open 9(3):e026797

Independent UK Panel on Breast Cancer Screening (2012) The benefits and harms of breast cancer screening: an independent review. Lancet 380(9855):1778–1786

Inman JL, Robertson C, Mott JD, Bissell MJ (2015) Mammary gland development: cell fate specification, stem cells and the microenvironment. Development 142(6):1028–1042

Isogai C, Laug WE, Shimada H et al (2001) Plasminogen activator inhibitor-1 promotes angiogenesis by stimulating endothelial cell migration toward fibronectin. Cancer Res 61(14):5587–5594

Iyengar NM, Arthur R, Manson JE et al (2019) Association of Body fat and Risk of breast cancer in postmenopausal women with normal body mass index: a secondary analysis of a randomized clinical trial and observational study. JAMA Oncol 5(2):155–163

Jones JL, Glynn P, Walker RA (1999) Expression of MMP-2 and MMP-9, their inhibitors, and the activator MT1-MMP in primary breast carcinomas. J Pathol 189:161–168

Jones JL, Shaw JA, Pringle JH, Walker RA (2003) Primary breast myoepithelial cells exert an invasion-suppressor effect on breast cancer cells via paracrine down-regulation of MMP expression in fibroblasts and tumour cells. J Pathol 201(4):562–572

Kalluri R (2016) The biology and function of fibroblasts in cancer. Nat Rev Cancer 16(9):582–598

Kerlikowske K (2010) Epidemiology of ductal carcinoma in situ. J Natl Cancer Inst Monogr 2010(41):139–141

Kersgaw EE, Flier JS (2004) Adipose tissue as an endocrine organ. J Clin Endocrinol Metab 89(6):2548–2556

Kim SY, Jung SH, Kim MS et al (2015) Genomic differences between pure ductal carcinoma in situ and synchronous ductal carcinoma in situ with invasive breast cancer. Oncotarget 6(10):7597–7607

Kim M, Chung YR, Kim HJ et al (2020) Immune microenvironment in ductal carcinoma in situ: a comparison with invasive carcinoma of the breast. Breast Cancer Res 22(1):32

Kirschmann D, Seftor EA, Fong SFT et al (2002) A molecular role for lysyl oxidase in breast cancer invasion. Cancer Res 62(15):4478–4483

Kitamura T, Qian BZ, Soong D et al (2015) CCL2-induced chemokine cascade promotes breast cancer metastasis by enhancing retention of metastasis associated macrophages. J Exp Med 212(7):1043–1059

Knopfelmacher A, Fox J, Lo Y et al (2015) Correlation of histopathologic features of ductal carcinoma in situ of the breast with the oncotype DX DCIS score. Mod Pathol 28(9):1167–1173

Knudsen ES, Ertel A, Davicioni E et al (2012) Progression of ductal carcinoma in situ to invasive breast cancer is associated with gene expression programs of EMT and myoepithelial. Breast Cancer Res Treat 133(3):1009–1024

Koukoulis GK, Howeedy AA, Korhonene I et al (1993) Distribution of tenascin, cellular fibronectins and integrins in the normal, hyperplastic and neoplastic breast. J Submicrosc Cytol Pathol 25(2):285–295

Kryczek I, Wei S, Keller E et al (2007) Stroma-derived factor (SDF-1/CXCL12) and human tumor pathogenesis. Am J Physiol Cell Physiol 292(3):C987–C995

Kuang DM, Zhao Q, Peng C et al (2009) Activated monocytes in peritumoral stroma of hepatocellular carcinoma foster immune privilege and disease progression through PD-L1. J Exp Med 206(6):1327–1337

Lee AH, Happerfield LC, Bobrow LG, Millis RR (1997) Angiogenesis and inflammation in ductal carcinoma in situ of the breast. J Pathol 181(2):200–206

Lee S, Stewart S, Nagtegaal I et al (2012) Differentially expressed genes regulating the progression of ductal carcinoma in situ to invasive breast cancer. Cancer Res 72(17):4574–4586

Leek RD, Harris AL (2002) Tumor-associated macrophages in breast cancer. J Mammary Gland Biol Neoplasia 7:177–189

Leek RD, Lewis CE, Whitehouse R et al (1996) Association of macrophage infiltration with angio-

genesis and prognosis in invasive breast carcinoma. Cancer Res 56:4625–4629
Levental KR, Yu H, Kass L et al (2009) Matrix crosslinking forces tumor progression by enhancing integrin signaling. Cell 139(5):891–906
Lewis CE, Leek R, Harris A, McGee JO (1995) Cytokine regulation in breast cancer: the role of tumor-associated macrophages. J Leukoc Biol 57:747–751
Lin EY, Nguyen AV, Russell RG, Pollard JW (2001) Colony-stimulating factor 1 promotes progression of mammary tumors to malignancy. J Exp Med 193(6):727–740
Lin EY, Li JF, Bricard G et al (2007) Vascular endothelial growth factor restores delayed tumor progression in tumors depleted of macrophages. Mol Oncol 1(3):288–302
Linde N, Casanova-Acebes M, Sosa MS et al (2018) Macrophages orchestrate breast cancer early dissemination and metastasis. Nat Commun 9(1):21
Lips EH, Kumar T, Megalios A et al (2022) Genomic analysis defines clonal relationships of ductal carcinoma in situ and recurrent invasive breast cancer. Nat Genet 54(6):850–860
Lodillinsky C, Infante E, Guichard A et al (2016) p63/MT1MMP axis is required for in situ to invasive transition in basal-like breast cancer. Oncogene 35(3):344–357
Lopez-Otin C, Palavalli LH, Samuels Y (2009) Protective roles of matrix metalloproteinases: from mouse models to human cancer. Cell Cycle 8:3657–3662
Lu P, Takai K, Weaver VM, Werb Z (2011) Extracellular matrix degradation and remodeling in development and disease. Cold Spring Harb Perspect Biol 3:a005058
Lühr I, Friedl A, Overath T et al (2012) Mammary fibroblasts regulate morphogenesis of normal and tumorigenic breast epithelial cells by mechanical and paracrine signals. Cancer Lett 325(2):175–188
Ma XJ, Salunga R, Tuggle JT et al (2003) Gene expression profiles of human breast cancer progression. Proc Natl Acad Sci USA 100(10):5974–5979
Ma RY, Black A, Qian BZ (2022) Macrophage diversity in cancer revisited in the era of single-cell omics. Trends Immunol 43(7):546–563
Mace TA, Ameen Z, Collins A et al (2013) Pancreatic cancer-associated stellate cells promote differentiation of myeloid-derived suppressor cells in a STAT3-dependent manner. Cancer Res 73(10):3007–3018
Magdaleno C, House T, Pawar JS et al (2021) Fibronectin assembly regulates lumen formation in breast acini. J Cell Biochem 122(5):524–537
Man YG (2007) Focal degeneration of aged or injured myoepithelial cells and the resultant auto-immunoreactions are trigger factors for breast tumor invasion. Med Hypotheses 269(6):1340–1357
Man YG, Sang QX (2004) The significance of focal myoepithelial cell layer disruptions in human breast tumor invasion: a paradigm shift from the "protease-centered" hypothesis. Exp Cell Res 301(2):103–118
Mantovani A, Bottazzi B, Colotta F et al (1993) The origin and function of tumor-associated macrophages. Immunol Today 13:265–270
Mantovani A, Sozzani S, Locati M et al (2002) Macrophage polarization: tumor-associated macrophages as a paradigm for polarized M2 mononuclear phagocytes. Trends Immunol 23(11):549–555
Mantovani A, Sica A, Sozzani S et al (2004) The chemokine system in diverse forms of macrophage activation and polarization. Trends Immunol 25(12):677–686
Matsushima K, Larsen CG, DuBois GC, Oppenheim JJ (1989) Purification and characterization of a novel monocyte chemotactic and activating factor produced by a human myelomonocytic cell line. J Exp Med 169(4):1485–1490
Matusiak M, Hickey J, Luca B et al (2023) A spatial map of human macrophage niches reveals context-dependent macrophage functions in colon and breast cancer. Res Sq 2023 [Not peer reviewed]
Maxwell AJ, Hilton B, Clements K et al (2022) Unresected screen-detected ductal carcinoma in situ: outcomes of 311 women in the forget-me-not 2 study. Breast 61:145–155
Midwood KS, Chiquet M, Tucker RP, Orend G (2016) Tenascin-C at a glance. J Cell Sci 129(23):4321–4327
Miller FR, Santner SJ, Tait L, Dawson PJ (2000) MCF10DCIS.com xenograft model of human comedo ductal carcinoma in situ. J Natl Cancer Inst 92(14):1185–1186
Mills CD, Kincaid K, Alt JM et al (2000) M-1/M2 macrophages and the Th1/Th2 paradigm. J Immunol 164(12):6166–6173
Miroshnikova YA, Mouw JK, Barnes JM et al (2016) Tissue mechanics promote IDH1-dependent HIF1α-tenascin C feedback to regulate glioblastoma aggression. Nat Cell Biol 18(12):1336–1345
Mitchell E, Jindal S, Chan T et al (2020) Loss of myoepithelial calponin-1 characterizes high-risk ductal carcinoma in situ cases, which are further stratified by T cell composition. Mol Carcinog 59(7):701–712
Mizutani Y, Kobayashi H, Iida T et al (2019) Meflin-positive cancer-associated fibroblasts inhibit pancreatic carcinogenesis. Cancer Res 79(20):5367–5381
Mouw JK, Ou G, Weaver VM (2014) Extracellular matrix assembly: a multiscale deconstruction. Nat Rev Mol Cell Biol 15(12):771–785
Mulder K, Patel AA, Kong WT et al (2021) Cross-tissue single-cell landscape of human monocytes and macrophages in health and disease. Immunity 54(8):1883–1900
Naba A, Clauser KR, Ding H et al (2016) The extracellular matrix: tools and insights for the "omics" era. Matrix Biol 49:10–24
Narayanan PL, Raza SEA, Hall AH et al (2021) Unmasking the immune microecology of ductal carcinoma in situ with deep learning. NPJ Breast Cancer 7(1):19
Nelson BH (2010) CD20+ B cells: the other tumor-infiltrating lymphocytes. J Immunol 185(9):4977–4982

Netea MG, Balkwill F, Chonchol M et al (2017) A guiding map for inflammation. Nat Immunol 18(8):826–831

Nguyen-Ngoc KV, Cheung KJ, Brenot A et al (2012) ECM microenvironment regulates collective migration and local dissemination in normal and malignant mammary epithelium. Proc Natl Acad Sci USA 109(39):E2595–E2604

Nielsen BS, Rank F, López JM et al (2001) Collagenase-3 expression in breast myofibroblasts as a molecular marker of transition of ductal carcinoma in situ lesions to invasive ductal carcinomas. Cancer Res 61(19):7091–7100

Öhlund D, Handly-Santana A, Biffu G et al (2017) Distinct populations of inflammatory fibroblasts and myofibroblasts in pancreatic cancer. J Exp Med 214(3):579–596

Orend G, Chiquet-Ehrismann R (2006) Tenascin-C induced signaling in cancer. Cancer Lett 244(2): 143–163

Orimo A, Gupta PB, Sgroi DC et al (2005) Stromal fibroblasts present in invasive human breast carcinomas promote tumor growth and angiogenesis through elevated SDF-1/CXCL12 secretion. Cell 121(3):335–348

Osuala KO, Sameni M, Shah S et al (2015) Il-6 signaling between ductal carcinoma in situ cells and carcinoma-associated fibroblasts mediates tumor cell growth and migration. BMC Cancer 15:584

Overall CM, Dean RA (2006) Degradomics: systems biology of the protease web. Pleiotropic roles of MMPs in cancer. Cancer Metastasis Rev 25:69–75

Page-McCaw A, Ewald AJ, Werb Z (2007) Matrix metalloproteinases and the regulation of tissue remodelling. Nat Rev Mol Cell Biol 8(3):221–233

Papanicolaou M, Parker AL, Yam M et al (2022) Temporal profiling of the breast tumour microenvironment reveals collagen XII as a driver of metastasis. Nat Commun 13(1):4587

Pareja F, Brown DN, Lee JY et al (2020) Whole-exome sequencing analysis of the progression from non-low-grade ductal carcinoma in situ to invasive ductal carcinoma. Clin Cancer Res 26(14):3682–3693

Pasco S, Han J, Gillery P et al (2000) A specific sequence of the noncollagenous domain of the alpha3 (IV) chain of type IV collagen inhibits expression and activation of matrix metalloproteinases by tumor cells. Cancer Res 60(2):467–473

Pilewskie M, Stempel M, Rosenfeld H et al (2016) Do LORIS trial eligibility criteria identify a ductal carcinoma in situ patient population at low risk of upgrade to invasive carcinoma? Ann Surg Oncol 23(11):3487–3493

Pinder SE (2010) Ductal carcinoma in situ (DCIS): pathological features, differential diagnosis, prognostic factors and specimen evaluation. Mod Pathol 23(Suppl 2):S8–S13

Propper DJ, Balkwill FR (2022) Harnessing cytokines and chemokines for cancer therapy. Nat Rev Clin Oncol 19:237–253

Provenzano PP, Eliceiri KW, Campbell JM et al (2006) Collagen reorganization at the tumor-stromal interface facilitates local invasion. BMC Med 4:38

Provenzano PP, Inman DR, Eliceiri KW et al (2008) Collagen density promotes mammary tumor initiation and progression. BMC Med 6:11

Pruneri G, Lazzeronu M, Bagnardi V et al (2017) The prevalence and clinical relevance of tumor-infiltrating lymphocytes (TILs) in ductal carcinoma in situ of the breast. Ann Oncol 28(2):321–328

Rebbeck CA, Xian J, Bornelov S et al (2022) Gene expression signatures of individual ductal carcinoma in situ lesions identify processes and biomarkers associated with progression towards invasive ductal carcinoma. Nat Commun 13:3399

Reeves GK, Pirie K, Beral V et al (2007) Cancer incidence and mortality in relation to body mass index in the million women study: cohort study. BMJ 335(7630):1134

Rekad Z, Izzi V, Lamba R et al (2022) The alternative matrisome: alternative splicing of ECM proteins in development, homeostasis and tumor progression. Matrix Biol 111:26–52

Rhim AD, Oberstein PE, Thomas DH et al (2014) Stromal elements act to restrain, rather than support, pancreatic ductal adenocarcinoma. Cancer Cell 25(6):735–747

Risom T, Glass DR, Averbukh I et al (2022) Transition to invasive breast cancer is associated with progressive changes in the structure and composition of tumor stroma. Cell 185(2):299–310.e18

Ruffell B, Chang-Strachan D, Chan V et al (2014) Macrophage IL-10 blocks $CD8^+$ T cell-dependent responses to chemotherapy by suppressing IL-12 expression in intratumoral dendritic cells. Cancer Cell 26(5):623–637

Runswick SK, O'Hare MJ, Jones L et al (2001) Desmosomal adhesion regulates epithelial morphogenesis and cell positioning. Nat Cell Biol 3(9):823–830

Russell TD, Jindal S, Agunbiade S et al (2015) Myoepithelial cell differentiation markers in ductal carcinoma in situ progression. Am J Pathol 185(11):3076–3089

Sabeh F, Ota I, Holmbeck K et al (2004) Tumor cell traffic through the extracellular matrix is controlled by the membrane anchored collagenase MT1-MMP. J Cell Biol 167:769–781

Saji H, Koike M, Yamori T et al (2001) Significant correlation of monocyte chemoattractant protein-1 expression with neovascularization and progression of breast carcinoma. Cancer 92(5):1085–1091

Sánchez-Martín L, Estecha A, Samaniego R et al (2011) The chemokine CXCL12 regulates monocyte-macrophage differentiation and RUNX3 expression. Blood 117(1):88–97

Sarper M, Allen MD, Gomm J et al (2017) Loss of MMP-8 in ductal carcinoma in situ (DCIS)-associated myoepithelial cells contributes to tumour promotion through altered adhesive and proteolytic function. Breast Cancer Res 19(1):33

Saunders ME, Schuyler PA, Dupont WD, Page DL (2005) The natural history of low-grade ductal carcinoma in situ of the breast in women treated by biopsy only revealed over 30 years of long-term follow-up. Cancer 103(12):2481–2484

Schiza A, Thurfiell V, Tukkberg AS et al (2022) Tumour-infiltrating lymphocytes add prognostic information for patients with low-risk DCIS: findings from the SweDCIS randomised radiotherapy trial. Eur J Cancer 168:128–137

Schuh F, Biazús JV, Resetkova E et al (2015) Histopathological grading of breast ductal carcinoma in situ: validation of a web-based survey through intra-observer reproducibility analysis. Diagn Pathol 10:93

Sebastian A, Hun NR, Martin KA et al (2020) Single-cell transcriptomic analysis of tumor-derived fibroblasts and normal tissue-resident fibroblasts reveals fibroblast heterogeneity in breast cancer. Cancers (Basel) 12(5):1307

Sebastiani F, Cortesi L, Sant M et al (2016) Increased incidence of breast cancer in postmenopausal women with high body mass index at the Modena screening program. J Breast Cancer 19(3):283–291

Sica A, Mantovani A (2012) Macrophage plasticity and polarization: in vivo veritas. J Clin Invest 122:787–795

Silverstein MJ, Poller DN, Waisman JR et al (1995) Prognostic classification of breast ductal carcinoma-in-situ. Lancet 345(8958):1154–1157

Smith LK, Boukhaled GM, Condotta SA et al (2018) Interleukin-10 directly inhibits CD8+ T cell function by enhancing N-glycan branching to decrease antigen sensitivity. Immunity 48(2):299–312

Sørum R, Hofvind S, Skaane P, Haldorsen T (2010) Trends in incidence of ductal carcinoma in situ: the effect of a population-based screening programme. Breast 19:499–505

Sprague BL, Vacek PM, Mulrow SE et al (2021) Collagen organization in relation to ductal carcinoma in situ pathology and outcomes. Cancer Epidemiol Biomarkers Prev 30(1):80–88

Stanton SE, Diss ML (2016) Clinical significance of tumor-infiltrating lymphocytes in breast cancer. J Immunother Cancer 4:59

Strell C, Paulsson J, Jin S-B et al (2019) Impact of epithelial-stromal interactions on Peritumoral fibroblasts in ductal carcinoma in situ. J Natl Cancer Inst 111(9):983–995

Sung KE, Yang N, Pehlke C et al (2011) Transition to invasion in breast cancer: a microfluidic in vitro model enables examination of spatial and temporal effects. Integr Biol (Camb) 3(4):439–450

Sung NJ, Kim NH, Surh YJ, Park SA et al (2020) Gremlin-1 promotes metastasis of breast cancer cells by activating STA3-MMP13 signaling pathway. Int J Mol Sci 21(23):9227

Taub DD, Lloyd AR, Conlon K et al (1993) Recombinant human interferon-inducible protein 10 is a chemoattractant for human monocytes and T lymphocytes and promotes T cell adhesion to endothelial cells. J Exp Med 177(6):1809–1814

Teo NB, Shoker BS, Jarvis C et al (2003) Angiogenesis and invasive recurrence in ductal carcinoma in situ of the breast. Eur J Cancer 39:38–44

Thike AA, Chen X, Koh VCY et al (2020) Higher densities of tumour-infiltrating lymphocytes and CD4+ T cells predict recurrence and progression of ductal carcinoma in situ of the breast. Histopathology 76(6):852–864

Toss MS, Miligy M, Al-Kawaz A et al (2018) Prognostic significance of tumor-infiltrating lymphocytes in ductal carcinoma in situ of the breast. Mod Pathol 31(8):1226–1236

Toss MS, Miligy IM, Gorringe KL et al (2019) Geometric characteristics of collagen have independent prognostic significance in breast ductal carcinoma in situ: an image analysis study. Mod Pathol 32(10): 1473–1485

Toss MS, Abidi A, Lesche D et al (2020) The prognostic significance of immune microenvironment in breast ductal carcinoma in situ. Br J Cancer 122(10):1496–1506

Trayhurn P (2005) Adipose tissue in obesity - an inflammatory issue. Endocrinology 146(3):1003–1005

Trimboli AJ, Cantemir-Stone CZ, Li F et al (2009) Pten in stromal fibroblasts suppresses mammary epithelial tumours. Nature 461(7267):1084–1091

Ueno T, Toi M, Saji H et al (2000) Significance of macrophage chemoattractant protein-1 in macrophage recruitment, angiogenesis, and survival in human breast cancer. Clin Cancer Res 6(8):3282–3289

Vallet SD, Ricard-Blum S (2019) Lysyl oxidases: from enzyme activity to extracellular cross-links. Essays Biochem 63(3):349–364

Van Luijt PA, Heijnsdijk EAM, Fracheboud J et al (2016) The distribution of ductal carcinoma in situ (DCIS) grade in 4232 women and its impact on overdiagnosis in breast cancer screening. Breast Cancer Res 18(1):47

Vaysse C, Lømo J, Garred O et al (2017) Inflammation of mammary adipose tissue occurs in overweight and obese patients exhibiting early-stage breast cancer. NPJ Breast Cancer 3:19

Walter M, Liang S, Ghosh S et al (2009) Interleukin 6 secreted from adipose stromal cells promotes migration and invasion of breast cancer cells. Oncogene 28(30):2745–2755

Wang L, Wang X, Liang Y et al (2012) S100A4 promotes invasion and angiogenesis in breast cancer MDA-MD-231 cells by upregulating matrix metalloproteinase-13. Acta Biochim Pol 59(4):593–598

Weidner N, Semple JP, Welch WR, Folkman J (1991) Tumor angiogenesis amd metastasis – correlation in invasive breast carcinoma. New Engl J Med 324(1):1–8

Weigel S, Hense HW, Heidrich J (2015) Digital mammography screening: does age influence the detection rates of low-, intermediate-, and high-grade ductal carcinoma in situ? Radiology 2015:150322

Wilcz-Villega E, Carter E, Ironside A et al (2020) Macrophages induce malignant traits in mammary epithelium via IKKε/TBK1 kinases and the serine biosynthesis pathway. EMBO Mol Med 12(2):e10491

Williams CM, Engler AJ, Sloane RD et al (2008) Fibronectin expression modulates mammary epithelial cell proliferation during acinar differentiation. Cancer Res 68(9):3185–3192

Winkler J, Abisoye-Ogunniyan A, Metclaf KJ, Werb Z (2020) Concepts of extracellular matrix remodelling in tumour progression and metastasis. Nat Commun 11:5120

Wiseman BS, Sternlicht MD, Lund LR et al (2003) Site-specific inductive and inhibitory activities of MMP-2 and MMP-3 orchestrate mammary gland branching morphogenesis. J Cell Biol 162(6):1123–1133

Witkiewicz AK, Dasgupta A, Nguyen KH et al (2009) Stromal caveolin-1 levels predict early DCIS progression to invasive cancer. Cancer Biol Ther 8(11):1071–1079

Wu MH, Hong H-C, Hong T-M et al (2011) Targeting galectin-1 in carcinoma-associated fibroblasts inhibits oral squamous cell carcinoma metastasis by down-regulating MCP-1/CCL2 expression. Clin Cancer Res 17(6):1306–1316

Wulfing P, Kersting C, Buerger H et al (2005) Expression patterns of angiogenic and lymphangiogenic factors in ductal breast carcinoma in situ. Br J Cancer 92(9):1720–1728

Yang X, Chu Y, Wang Y et al (2006) Targeted in vivo expression of IFN-gamma-inducible protein 10 induces specific antitumor activity. J Leukoc Biol 80(6):1434–1444

Yang M, Zhenhua L, Ren M et al (2018) Stromal infiltration of tumor-associated macrophages conferring poor prognosis of patients with basal-like breast carcinoma J. Cancer 9(13):2308–2316

Yu GH, Sethi S, Cajulis RS et al (1997) Benign pairs. A useful discriminating feature in fine needle aspirates of the breast. Acta Cytol 41(3):721–726

Yu LN, Liu Z, Tian Y et al (2019) FAP-a and GOLPH3 are hallmarks of dcis progression to invasive breast cancer. Front Oncol 9:1424

Molecular Basis of Breast Tumor Heterogeneity

13

Esra Dikoglu and Fresia Pareja

Abstract

Breast cancer (BC) is a profoundly heterogenous disease, with diverse molecular, histological, and clinical variations. The intricate molecular landscape of BC is evident even at early stages, illustrated by the complexity of the evolution from precursor lesions to invasive carcinoma. The key for therapeutic decision-making is the dynamic assessment of BC receptor status and clinical subtyping. Hereditary BC adds an additional layer of complexity to the disease, given that different cancer susceptibility genes contribute to distinct phenotypes and genomic features. Furthermore, the various BC subtypes display distinct metabolic demands and immune microenvironments. Finally, genotypic–phenotypic correlations in special histologic subtypes of BC inform diagnostic and therapeutic approaches, highlighting the significance of thoroughly comprehending BC heterogeneity.

Keywords

Breast cancer · Intratumor heterogeneity · Tumor evolution · Tumor microenvironment · Breast cancer subtypes

Key Points

1. Ductal carcinoma in situ and lobular carcinoma in situ are non-obligate precursors of invasive breast cancer (BC), displaying marked intralesional heterogeneity and sharing molecular similarities with the invasive carcinomas that arise from them.
2. The clinical subtypes of BC are vastly heterogeneous. Beyond the ER+, HER2+, and triple-negative subgroups, additional subtypes have emerged, such as HER2-low BC, which presents novel therapeutic opportunities, with, for example, the use of anti-HER2 antibody drug conjugates.
3. Hereditary BC exhibits profound phenotypic and genomic heterogeneity, exemplified by variations in the histologic subtypes, in ER/HER2 status, and in the presence of genomic scars associated with homologous recombination deficiency.
4. The tumor microenvironment varies across the clinical and histologic subtypes of BC and is associated with particular clinicopathologic and molecular features.
5. BC includes over 20 special histologic subtypes, a subset of which features

E. Dikoglu · F. Pareja (✉)
Department of Pathology and Laboratory Medicine, Memorial Sloan Kettering Cancer Center, New York, NY, USA
e-mail: parejaf@mskcc.org

T. Sørlie, R. B. Clarke (eds.), *A Guide to Breast Cancer Research*, Advances in Experimental Medicine and Biology 1464, https://doi.org/10.1007/978-3-031-70875-6_13

pathognomonic genetic alterations, and constitutes genotypic–phenotypic correlations. These specific genetic alterations hold diagnostic and therapeutic significance.

13.1 Introduction

Breast cancer (BC) is a complex and multifaceted disease characterized by profound phenotypic, molecular, and biological diversity, driven in part by genetic and epigenetic alterations, and influenced by microenvironmental and metabolic factors (Ross and Pareja 2021; Rakha and Pareja 2021; Reina-Campos et al. 2017; Dias et al. 2019).

The advent of advanced molecular techniques has revolutionized our understanding of BC heterogeneity (Chang et al. 2013; Cancer Genome Atlas Network 2012). Temporal heterogeneity, for instance, is evident in the progression from in situ to invasive carcinoma, in the evolutionary trajectories of invasive BCs over time, in the emergence of metastatic disease, as well as in the disease evolution in response to therapy (Middha et al. 2017; Metaxas et al. 2023). Spatial heterogeneity has been unveiled by multiregion sequencing of the same tumor, uncovering subclonal diversification (Yates et al. 2015). Furthermore, the various BC histological subtypes, each characterized by unique phenotypes, molecular profiles, treatment sensitivities, and outcomes, exemplify intertumoral heterogeneity (Fumagalli and Barberis 2021; Turashvili and Brogi 2017).

In this chapter, we will address BC heterogeneity from the molecular pathology perspective. We will explore the heterogeneity during the genesis of BC arising from precursor lesions, cover the diverse clinical subtypes and special histologic subtypes of BC with their molecular correlates, examine the diversity of hereditary BC, and review the metabolic and immune features contributing to BC heterogeneity.

13.2 Heterogeneity in the Progression from In Situ Carcinoma to Invasive BC

Throughout an individual's lifespan, breast tissue acquires genetic alterations with each cell division, and changes due to menstrual cycles, pregnancy, and menopause contribute to the acquisition of these genetic alterations (Nishimura et al. 2023; Cereser et al. 2023). Notably, benign breast tissue exhibits C>T and T>C substitutions, most of them located in introns. These substitutions preferentially affect *NOTCH2* and *RUNX1* in the epithelium and stroma, respectively (Cereser et al. 2023).

The proposed evolutionary models of progression from in situ carcinoma to invasive BC include the independent evolution model, by which in situ and invasive carcinoma are unrelated and follow a parallel evolution, the evolutionary bottleneck model, proposing that a single cell gives rise to various clones, followed by selection of a single clone giving rise to invasive carcinoma, and the multiclonal invasion model positing that evolution occurs at the in situ carcinoma stage, followed by the generation of various clones that migrate and invade together, evolving to invasive carcinoma (Cowell et al. 2013). Invasive BC exhibits similarities at the morphologic, proteomic, and genomic levels with ductal carcinoma in situ (DCIS), a non-obligate precursor (Trinh et al. 2021; Casasent et al. 2017; van Seijen et al. 2019). Clonal decomposition and phylogenetic analyses of synchronously diagnosed lesions revealed that the mechanisms of progression from DCIS to invasive BC are diverse, and that clonal selection might play roles in approximately 30% of the cases (Pareja et al. 2020a). Notably, DCIS exhibiting progression to invasive BC following a clonal selection pattern was found to display higher levels of intratumoral genetic heterogeneity (ITGH) than DCIS where no clonal selection was observed (Pareja et al. 2020a), suggesting that molecular predictors of progression to invasive BC might benefit from inclusion of ITGH assessment.

Lobular carcinoma in situ (LCIS) is a preinvasive breast lesion with genetic similarities to invasive lobular carcinoma (ILC) (Lee et al. 2019), the second most common histologic subtype of BC (Lee et al. 2019; Li et al. 2003). LCIS frequently harbors mutations in *CDH1*, the hallmark genetic alteration of ILC, as well as other alterations known to be enriched in ILC, such as those affecting *PIK3CA*, *TBX3*, and *FOXA1* (Lee et al. 2019). LCIS and ILC can be clonally related, supporting the roles of LCIS as a nonobligate precursor of the latter (Lee et al. 2019). LCIS lesions exhibit genetic heterogeneity (Lee et al. 2019), and interestingly were found to display a shift from aging mutational signatures to the apolipoprotein B mRNA editing enzyme catalytic polypeptide-like (APOBEC) mutational processes during progression to ILC (Lee et al. 2019). Interestingly, compared to classic LCIS, LCIS variants, such as florid and pleomorphic LCIS, were found to show an enrichment in *ERBB2* and *ERBB3* mutations (Harrison et al. 2020; Chen et al. 2009), highlighting the genetic heterogeneity present in these early breast lesions.

13.3 Clinical Subtypes and Receptor Status Heterogeneity in BC

Accurate BC classification and subtyping are crucial for guiding clinical management. Routine histopathologic evaluation of a BC includes the assessment of the biomarker receptors estrogen receptor (ER) and progesterone receptor (PR) by immunohistochemistry (IHC), as well as HER2 by IHC and/or in situ hybridization (ISH), following the American Society of Clinical Oncology/College of American Pathologists (ASCO/CAP) guidelines (Allison et al. 2020; Wolff et al. 2018).

As per the ASCO/CAP guidelines, ER positivity is defined as >1% nuclear staining, and BCs displaying ER expression between 1% and 10% are classified as ER-low (Allison et al. 2020). ER-low BCs are associated with younger age, larger tumor size, higher histological grade, higher rate of lymph node metastasis and higher rate of HER2 positivity, compared to cases with ER expression >10% (Fei et al. 2021; Poon et al. 2020; Yoon et al. 2022; Luo et al. 2022; Yu et al. 2021). ER-low/HER2− BC displays similar molecular features to triple-negative breast cancer (TNBC, i.e., lacking ER and PR expression and lacking HER2 amplification), as well as similar responses to neoadjuvant chemotherapy (NAC) and outcomes (Fujii et al. 2017; Paakkola et al. 2021; Villegas et al. 2021; Dieci et al. 2021; Schrodi et al. 2021; Voorwerk et al. 2023).

BCs displaying HER2 expression of 1+ or 2+ by IHC without HER2 gene amplification constitute the newly recognized HER2-low group of BCs. Identification of these cases holds significant therapeutic implications, given that HER2-low BC patients might benefit from anti-HER2 antibody drug conjugates (ADCs), such as trastuzumab deruxtecan (Modi et al. 2022). A higher *TP53* mutational rate has been observed in metastatic ER+/HER2-low BC compared to HER2-null (HER2 IHC 0) cases (Tarantino et al. 2023). In addition, HER2-low BCs exhibit higher *ERBB2* copy number counts, whereas HER2-null BCs harbor a higher rate of *ERBB2* hemideletions (Tarantino et al. 2023). Nonetheless, the genomic landscape of HER2-low and HER2-null BCs does not appear to be significantly different (Tarantino et al. 2023; Marra et al. 2022).

A subset of TNBCs expresses androgen receptor (AR), and approximately 15% of TNBCs harbor mutations affecting *AR* and *AR* target genes (Lehmann et al. 2011). Interestingly, a subgroup of TNBC, observed predominantly in African American women, is characterized by *AR* splice variants and by a higher rate of AR expression (Asemota et al. 2023).

It is crucial to be cognizant of the fact that receptor status in BC is dynamic and may evolve during treatment and/or tumor progression (Lindström et al. 2012; Dieci et al. 2013; Li et al. 2021). Hence, evaluation of receptor status at multiple time points and consideration of spatiotemporal changes are essential for assessing BC heterogeneity and detecting receptor status conversion (Schrijver et al. 2018). Changes in receptor status following NAC have been reported in approximately 16%–30% of cases, with switches in ER or PR being more common than changes in HER2 status (De La Cruz et al. 2018; Xian et al. 2017; Yoshida et al. 2017; Lluch et al. 2019). Moreover, changes in ER, PR, or HER2 status occur in approximately 30% of the cases during progression (Aurilio et al. 2014). Differences were observed depending on the metastatic site, with an increased rate of ER discordance between the metastatic outgrowth and the primary tumor observed in the central nervous system, bone, and liver metastases (Schrijver et al. 2018; Curigliano et al. 2011; Aurilio et al. 2013).

Notably, a subset of HER2-low BCs exhibit changes in HER2 expression over time, including switches between HER2-null and HER2-low status at relapse, disease progression, or following NAC (Tarantino et al. 2023; Miglietta et al. 2022), underscoring the importance of HER2 status reassessment after NAC (Zhu et al. 2023). In addition, conversion from HER2+ to HER2-low status has been observed in approximately 7% of cases following NAC, and this change has been associated with a worse outcome (Zhu et al. 2023).

13.4 The Diversity of Hereditary BC

Approximately 10%–30% of BC cases are related to hereditary factors (Möller et al. 2016), and 5%–10% of BCs are associated with a germline pathogenic variant or likely pathogenic variant in a cancer predisposition gene (Gage et al. 2012; Prat et al. 2005; Apostolou and Fostira 2013). *BRCA1, BRCA2, CHEK2, PTEN, TP53, ATM, STK11/LKB1, CDH1, NBS1, RAD50, RAD51, BARD1, BRIP1, and PALB2* are BC susceptibility genes of high or moderate penetrance that contribute to the spectrum of hereditary BC (van der Groep et al. 2011; Dorling et al. 2021; Nones et al. 2019; Angeli et al. 2020). There is profound heterogeneity observed in hereditary BC. For instance, BCs associated with germline (g) g*BRCA1* alterations are predominantly invasive ductal carcinomas of no special type (IDC-NST) and TNBC (Reis-Filho and Pusztai 2011; Turner and Reis-Filho 2006; Chen et al. 2018), whereas BCs associated with g*BRCA2* mutations are linked with both ductal and lobular histologic subtypes and are mostly ER+ (Dossus and Benusiglio 2015; Tutt et al. 2021). Akin to g*BRCA2* BCs, BCs associated with g*PALB2* inactivation are ER+. Notably, g*PALB2* and g*BRCA2* alterations are associated with hereditary BC predisposition in males, with *BRCA2* being the most frequently affected susceptibility gene in male BC, contributing to up to 14% of the cases (Couch et al. 1996; Yang et al. 2020). g*BRCA1*, g*BRCA2*, and g*PALB2* BCs are characterized by an array of genomic scars associated with homologous recombination deficiency (HRD; Table 13.1), such as dominant single-base substitution (SBS) mutational signature 3, large-scale transitions (LSTs), and an enrichment in deletions with microhomology, among others (Davies et al. 2017).

BRCA1/2 inactivation disrupts homologous recombination (HR), leading to genomic instability, which can be leveraged therapeutically by platinum agents and PARP inhibitors (PARPi) (Liu et al. 2020; Qu et al. 2023). PARPi induce synthetic lethality in cells homozygous for *BRCA* mutations (Hutchinson 2010) and are employed

Table 13.1 Hereditary predisposition genes associated with breast cancer subtypes and their clinicopathologic and homologous recombination deficiency features

Gene	Clinicopathologic characteristics	Genomic features of HRD
BRCA1	TNBC, high TILs	Yes
BRCA2	ER+ BC, male BC association	Yes
PALB2	ER+ BC, male BC association	Yes
BARD1	TNBC	Yes
RAD51C/D	TNBC	Yes
RAD51B	ER+ BC	Yes
ATM	ER+ BC, low TILs	No
CHEK2	ER+ BC, low TILs, male BC association	No

Abbreviations: *BC*, breast cancer; *ER*, estrogen receptor; *ER+*, ER positive; *HRD*, homologous recombination deficiency; *TILs*, tumor-infiltrating lymphocytes; *TNBC*, triple-negative breast cancer

for the management of metastatic BC occurring in individuals with g*BRCA* mutations (Hutchinson 2010). In preclinical models, *T53BP1* loss results in resistance to PARPi in the setting of *BRCA1* mutations (Jaspers et al. 2013). The combination of *BRCA1* mutations and *TP53P1* loss, however, is synthetic lethal with inhibitors of DNA polymerase or helicase Polθ (Ryan et al. 2023; Zatreanu et al. 2021), illustrating how adaptive response to one therapy leads to vulnerability to another one.

BCs associated with germline alterations in other DNA repair genes, such as *ATM*, *ATR*, *CHEK1*, *CHEK2*, *NBS1*, or *FANC*, show different phenotypes (Lord and Ashworth 2016; Vogel et al. 2024; Heeke et al. 2020). In contrast to BC associated with inactivation of BRCA1/2, the canonical HRD genes, *gATM* and *gCHEK2* BCs lack genomic features of HRD, and display additional distinctive features (Mandelker et al. 2019; Weigelt et al. 2018) (Table 13.1). For instance, *ATM*-associated BCs are predominantly ER+ and display minimal immune infiltrate (Weigelt et al. 2018) (Table 13.1). Notably, g*ATM* variants and somatic *TP53* mutations are mutually exclusive, suggesting an epistatic relationship between these genes (Weigelt et al. 2018). Akin to g*ATM* BCs, g*CHEK2* BCs were found to be mostly ER+ (Smid et al. 2023; Schwartz et al. 2024) (Table 13.1), and BCs with bi-allelic *CHEK2* inactivation were found not to harbor somatic *TP53* mutations (Smid et al. 2023). Given their lack of HRD genomic features, g*ATM* and g*CHECK2* BCs might not benefit from PARPi therapy (Mandelker et al. 2019; Weigelt et al. 2018; Smid et al. 2023; Schwartz et al. 2024; Tung et al. 2020). These patients, however, might be sensitive to DNA damage response (DDR)-focused therapies (Vogel et al. 2024; Bodily et al. 2020; Moon et al. 2023), and inhibition of DDR pathways with the ataxia telangiectasia and Rad3-related (ATR) protein kinase inhibitors, the DNA-dependent protein kinase (DNA-PK) inhibitors, the human tyrosine kinase Wee1 (WEE1) inhibitors, and the checkpoint kinase 1/2 (CHK1/2) inhibitors has shown promising results (Vogel et al. 2024; Topatana et al. 2020). Pathogenic germline mutations in the *RAD51* paralog genes *RAD51B*, *RAD51C*, and *RAD51D* are associated with BCs displaying HRD features. While gRAD51B BCs are predominantly ER+, gRAD51C and gRAD51D are triple-negative (Dorling et al. 2021; Setton et al. 2021; Sun et al. 2017) (Table 13.1).

Significant associations between germline alterations in *CDH1*, *TP53*, and BC characteristics have also been reported. g*CDH1* mutations are associated with early-onset bilateral ILCs (Dossus and Benusiglio 2015) (Table 13.1), and BCs with g*TP53* mutations frequently harbor amplification of *HER2* (Wilson et al. 2010). Genes associated with multiple cancer syndromes that encompass BC include *PTEN* (Cowden syndrome), *TP53* (Li-Fraumeni), *STK11/LKB1* (Peutz-Jeghers), *ATM* (Louis-Bar Syndrome), *NBS1* (Nijmegen breakage syndrome), and *NF1* (neurofibromatosis type 1) (Dorling et al. 2021; Varley 2003; Prokopcova et al. 2007), and additional genes are emerging.

13.5 Diversity in BC Metabolism and Immune Milieu

BC displays vast heterogeneity at the metabolic level. Compared to BCs of other clinical subtypes, TNBC has an increased demand for nicotinamide, 1-ribosyl-nicotinamide, and NAD+ (Voorwerk et al. 2023; Willmann et al. 2016; Navas and Carnero 2021). Furthermore, compared with cancer cells from primary BCs, metastatic BC cells show changes in the metabolism of glucose, fumarate, malate, and succinyl-carnitine, fatty acids, and amino acids (Tarragó-Celada and Cascante 2021; Abdul Kader et al. 2022).

The immune tumor microenvironment (TME) of BC displays marked heterogeneity (Wang et al. 2023; Yu et al. 2023), and assessment of biomarkers, such as PD-L1 expression, DNA mismatch repair (MMR), is useful in the selection of BC patients that can benefit from immunotherapy (Yu et al. 2023). TNBCs exhibit the greatest extent of tumor-infiltrating lymphocytes (TILs), among all BC clinical subtypes (Braunstein and Riaz 2020; Valenza et al. 2023;

Ortiz and Andrechek 2023), whereas ER+ BCs show low TIL levels (Valenza et al. 2023; Ortiz and Andrechek 2023). Recent genomic and transcriptomic studies have found a differential composition of the immune features of ILCs compared to IDC-NSTs (Mouabbi et al. 2023; Tille et al. 2020; Desmedt et al. 2016, 2018). PD-L1 seems to be lower in ILC versus IDC-NST in primary treatment-naïve tumors (Van Baelen et al. 2022). Furthermore, within the ILC group, *ERBB3* mutations are associated with lower TIL extent, whereas *TP53*, *ARID1A*, and *BRCA2* mutations tend be associated with a higher extent of TILs (Desmedt et al. 2018). High TILs are linked to superior clinical outcomes and response to NAC in patients with TNBC and HER2+ BC (Savas et al. 2016; Russo et al. 2019; Salgado et al. 2015). Notably, higher TIL levels in TNBC pre-NAC biopsies correlate with higher rates of pathologic complete response (pCR) and superior outcomes (Issa-Nummer et al. 2013; Yamaguchi et al. 2012). Microsatellite instability occurs in approximately 0.5%–1.7% of BCs (Middha et al. 2017; Bonneville et al. 2017; Willis et al. 2019) and is caused by promoter hypermethylation or inactivating genetic alterations in the MMR genes (Metaxas et al. 2023; Klouch et al. 2022). In addition, specific *MLH1* polymorphisms lead to *MLH1* down-regulation and expression loss, correlating with a high risk of BC onset (Malik et al. 2020). A subset of BCs developing in individuals with Lynch syndrome is etiologically linked to MMR and is mostly ER+/HER2− (Schwartz et al. 2022a).

TMB is a tissue-agnostic biomarker that predicts benefit from immunotherapy; however, data on its role in BC are limited (Barroso-Sousa et al. 2023). Notably, high tumor mutational burden (TMB) in BC is associated with an enrichment in genetic alterations playing roles in resistance to endocrine therapy and cyclin-dependent kinase 4 and 6 (CDK4/6) inhibitors, such as those affecting the phosphatidylinositol 3-kinase/protein kinase B (PI3K-AKT) and receptor Tyrosine Kinase-Ras-Extracellular signal-regulated kinase (RTK-RAS) pathways (Ke et al. 2022; Davis et al. 2023). TMB in BC varies across different BC subtypes. For instance, ER− BCs have a higher TMB than ER+ cases (Xu et al. 2019), and the prevalence of hypermutated tumors is higher among metastatic ILCs compared to metastatic IDC-NSTs (Barroso-Sousa et al. 2020; Sokol et al. 2019). Apolipoprotein B mRNA editing enzyme, catalytic polypeptide (APOBEC) mutagenesis, a key mutational process in BC, has been found to be associated with high TMB (Barroso-Sousa et al. 2023; Sokol et al. 2019). Importantly, patients with ER+ BC showing a dominant APOBEC signature were found to have inferior outcomes to endocrine therapy plus CDK4/6i (Sammons et al. 2022).

13.6 Morphologic Spectrum of BC and Genotypic–Phenotypic Correlations

IDC-NST is the most common histologic subtype of BC, making up approximately 60%–80% of all BC cases (Ellis et al. 1992). However, there are over 20 histologic subtypes of BC, across the ER+ and ER− subgroups, distinguished by unique phenotypes, molecular features, and clinical behaviors (Rakha and Pareja 2021; WHO Classification of Tumors 2019; Pareja et al. 2021). Notably, a subset of these BC subtypes is characterized by pathognomonic genetic alterations (Ross and Pareja 2021; Rakha and Pareja 2021; Pareja et al. 2021). Recognizing these special BC subtypes and understanding their molecular features are crucial for the comprehension of BC heterogeneity and for laying the foundation for the development of novel diagnostic tools and the identification of innovative therapeutic targets.

13.6.1 ER-Positive Special Histologic Subtypes of Breast Cancer

The hallmark genetic alteration of common forms of ER+ BC is concurrent 1q gains and 16q losses (Pareja et al. 2021). In addition, compared to TNBC, ER+ BCs show an enrichment in *PIK3CA* mutations and a lower frequency of *TP53* mutations (Pareja et al. 2021). Although most of the ER+ special histologic BC subtypes are not characterized by a pathognomonic genetic alteration, many of them exhibit an array of genetic features that set them apart from common forms of ER+ BC (Ross and Pareja 2021; WHO Classification of Tumors 2019).

For instance, tubular BCs have a high frequency of *PIK3CA* mutations (Pareja et al. 2021); mucinous BCs lack concurrent 1q gains and 16q losses and show a lower rate of *PIK3CA* and *TP53* mutations compared to ER+ IDC-NST (Pareja et al. 2019; Nguyen et al. 2019). Furthermore, while neuroendocrine tumors molecularly resemble mucinous carcinomas, they are enriched in genetic alterations in chromatin remodeling genes (Pareja et al. 2022; Pareja and D'Alfonso 2020). ILC, on the other hand, is a distinct entity with a hallmark genetic alteration, and a unique molecular profile (WHO Classification of Tumors 2019).

13.6.1.1 Invasive Lobular Carcinoma

ILC is the most common special histologic subtype of BC and shows distinctive features. In comparison to IDC-NSTs, ILCs are more frequently multicentric and bilateral (Choi et al. 2012), and more frequently display metastasis to sites such as ovaries, bone, leptomeninges, digestive tract, orbital tissue, and skin (Arpino et al. 2004; Harris et al. 1984). ILC is characterized by deficiency of E-cadherin, a critical component of the epithelial adhesion complex that results from bi-allelic inactivation of *CDH1* (Ciriello et al. 2015; Caldeira et al. 2006) (Fig. 13.1a). E-cadherin deficiency leads to cellular discohesion that characterizes ILC histologically (WHO Classification of Tumors 2019) (Fig. 13.1a).

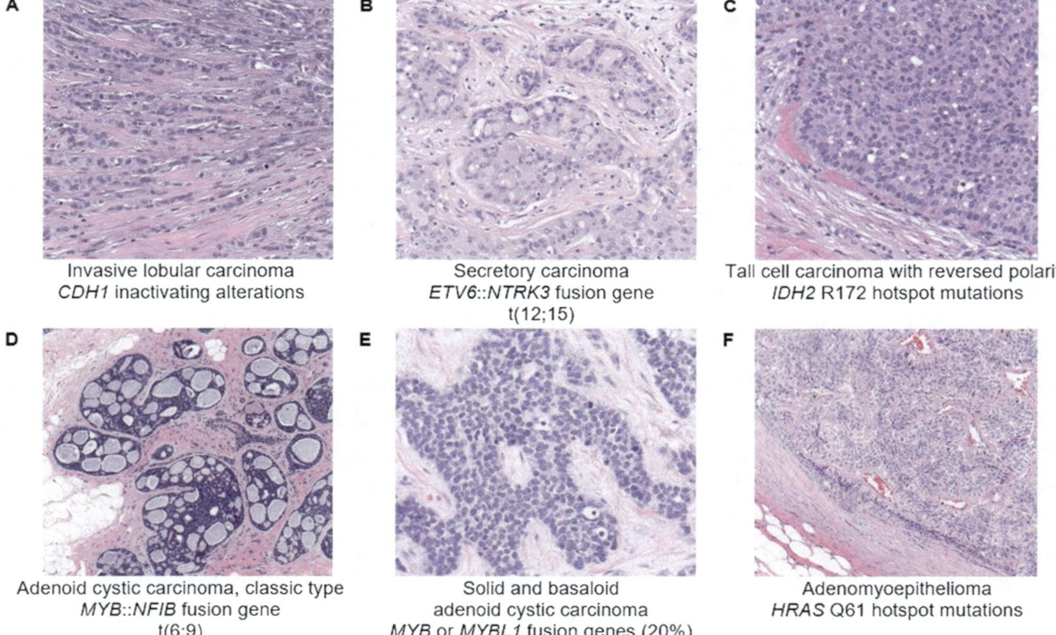

Fig. 13.1 Disease-defining genetic alterations in special histologic subtypes of breast cancer. (**a**–**f**) Representative hematoxylin-and-eosin (H&E) micrographs of special histologic subtypes of breast cancer and their corresponding pathognomonic genetic alterations including (**a**) invasive lobular carcinoma with *CDH1* inactivating genetic alterations; (**b**) secretory carcinoma with *ETV6::NTRK3* fusion gene, t(12;15); (**c**) tall cell carcinoma with reversed polarity with *IDH2* R172 hotspot mutations; (**d**) adenoid cystic carcinoma, classic type with *MYB::NFIB* fusion gene, t(6;9); (**e**) solid and basaloid adenoid cystic carcinoma with 20% of the cases harbor *MYB* or *MYBL1* fusion genes; (**f**) adenomyoepithelioma with *HRAS* Q61 hotspot mutations

CDH1 inactivation in ILC most commonly stems from inactivating mutations associated with loss of heterozygosity (LOH) but can also be due to *CDH1* homozygous deletions or *CDH1* epigenetic silencing via promoter methylation (Desmedt et al. 2016; Ciriello et al. 2015; Pareja et al. 2020b; McCart Reed et al. 2021). A detailed discussion on E-cadherin-mediated cell–cell adhesion and ILC is presented in this chapter.

Importantly, up to 20% of ILCs may lack *CDH1*-inactivating genetic alterations (de Groot et al. 2018). A subset of these cases harbors genetic alterations affecting other crucial cell–cell adhesion proteins that interact with E-cadherin, such as alpha-catenin (*CTNNA1*) and AXIN2, suggesting that ILC constitutes a convergent phenotype (de Groot et al. 2018; Dopeso et al. 2024; Derakhshan et al. 2022). In addition to *CDH1* genetic alterations, ILCs display a distinctive molecular landscape, characterized by an enrichment of genetic alterations in the PI3K pathway, such as *PIK3CA* and *PTEN*, mutations in receptor tyrosine kinases, such as *ERBB2* and *ERBB3*, genetic alterations in transcription factors such as *FOXA1*, *RUNX1*, *TBX3* and *FGFR2*, *ESR1*, and copy number alterations in 1q, 8q, 11q13, and 16q (Desmedt et al. 2016; Ciriello et al. 2015; Pareja et al. 2020b; McCart Reed et al. 2021; Razavi et al. 2018; Privitera et al. 2021).

In addition to classic ILC, several ILC histologic variants are recognized, including pleomorphic, solid, alveolar, and tubulo-lobular ILC, among others (WHO Classification of Tumors 2019), that frequently show a higher histologic grade and greater aggressiveness (Orvieto et al. 2008). At the molecular level, ILC variants differ from classic ILC. For instance, compared to classic ILC, pleomorphic ILCs are more frequently ER− and HER2+ (Simpson et al. 2008), and harbor a greater number of copy number alterations and a higher rate of *TP53*, *ERBB2*, *ERBB3*, *IRS2* and *IGFR1* mutations (Liu et al. 2018; Riedlinger et al. 2021; Batra et al. 2023). Moreover, pleomorphic ILCs exhibit higher scores on gene profiling assays, such as MammaPrint and OncotypeDx (McCart Reed et al. 2021), and are associated with a more aggressive behavior (Liu et al. 2018; Riedlinger et al. 2021; Batra et al. 2023; Shamir et al. 2020; Rosa-Rosa et al. 2019).

Compared to primary tumors, metastatic ILCs display a higher TMB and a greater frequency of genetic alterations in *ESR1*, *FAT1*, *RFWD2*, *NF1*, *AKT1*, *MAP 3K1*, *CCND1*, *CCNE1*, and *IGF1R*, among others (Sokol et al. 2019; Pareja et al. 2020b; Richard et al. 2020; Desmedt et al. 2019). Phylogenetic analyses of paired primary and metastatic ILC samples revealed deletions in *FGFR2*, *PTEN*, and *NCOR1*, and gains/amplifications in *AKT2*, *ZNF217*, *CCND1*, and *EGFR* restricted to the metastasis, supporting their role during progression (Fimereli et al. 2022). Metastatic ILCs show show an enrichment in APOBEC mutational signatures that could contribute to resistance to endocrine therapy (Roberts and Gordenin 2014).

Importantly, loss of E-cadherin results in vulnerabilities in cancer cells (Van Baelen et al. 2022). For instance, synthetic lethality between *ROS1* inhibition and E-cadherin deficiency has been demonstrated (Van Baelen et al. 2022), illustrated by the in vivo anti-tumor effects of *ROS1* inhibitors, such as crizotinib and entrectinib on E-cadherin-deficient BC cells (Bajrami et al. 2018). The effectiveness of ROS1 inhibitors is currently being investigated in ILC (Agostinetto et al. 2022). In addition, preliminary results of prospective trials (SUMMIT-NCT01953926, MutHER trial, part 2-NCT03289039) indicate that targeting HER2 mutations using second-generation HER2 tyrosine kinase inhibitors in combination with endocrine treatment might be more beneficial in ILC than in IDC-NST (Van Baelen et al. 2022).

13.6.2 Triple-Negative Special Histologic Subtypes of BC

TNBCs constitute approximately 10%–20% of BCs, and in addition to common forms of BC, such as IDC-NST, encompass a spectrum of special histologic subtypes, including low-grade and high-grade BCs (Pareja et al. 2016). Common forms of TNBC are characterized by aggressive histopathologic features, larger tumor size, and lymph node positivity, as well as resistance to chemotherapy and poor outcomes (Foulkes et al. 2010). In addition, these BCs are characterized by a high prevalence of *BRCA1* and *BRCA2* mutations (Dwane et al. 2021), HRD (Jiang et al. 2019), high TMB, high levels of genomic instability, and a higher frequency of *NTRK* fusions (Tierno et al. 2023; Bianchini et al. 2022; Song et al. 2024). Common forms of TNBC frequently harbor *TP53* mutations and show an enrichment in genetic alterations affecting *RB1*, *PTEN*, *KMT2C MYC*, and *CCNE1/CDK4*, among others (Cancer Genome Atlas Network 2012; Jiang et al. 2019; Tierno et al. 2023; Dillon et al. 2016; Zheng et al. 2016; Zhang et al. 2020; Banerji et al. 2012; Derakhshan and Reis-Filho 2022). Novel therapeutic strategies for common forms of TNBC are emerging. For instance, a recurrent *MAGI3-AKT3* fusion, which activates the AKT kinase, was identified in TNBC, suggesting that AKT small-molecule inhibitors might be a rational therapeutic strategy to be tested in fusion-positive TNBC patients (Banerji et al. 2012). In addition, TROP2, the target of the novel ADC sacituzumab govitecan, is overexpressed in TNBC (Yao et al. 2023; Hoppe et al. 2022), and this ADC has been FDA-approved for the treatment of metastatic TNBC (de Nonneville et al. 2022). Furthermore, newer ADCs for TNBC are emerging (Nagayama et al. 2020; Dri et al. 2024).

Special histologic subtypes of TNBC include low- and high-grade entities (Schwartz et al. 2023; Weisman et al. 2016). High-grade TNBC special types display complex genomes and despite lacking a pathognomonic genetic alteration, display distinctive genomic features, for instance, apocrine carcinomas exhibit an enrichment in PI3K pathway genetic alterations, such as *PIK3CA* and *PIK3R1* mutations, as well as *NF1* mutations (Schwartz et al. 2023; Weisman et al. 2016). Metaplastic BC shows an enrichment in genetic alterations in the PI3K/AKT/mTOR and canonical Wnt pathways, as well as *TERT* promoter mutations and amplification (Ng et al. 2017; Piscuoglio et al. 2017). On the other hand, low-grade forms of TNBC include various entities with unique phenotypes, histologically resembling their salivary gland counterparts, characterized by quiet genomes and frequently harboring a pathognomonic or disease-defining genetic alteration (WHO Classification of Tumors 2019; Pareja et al. 2016).

13.6.2.1 Secretory Carcinoma

Secretory carcinoma is an exceedingly rare TNBC subtype, with usually favorable clinical outcomes (WHO Classification of Tumors 2019; Pareja et al. 2021). These tumors are composed of cells with vacuolated cytoplasm and abundant intracellular and extracellular secretions and display microcystic, solid, and/or tubular architectures (WHO Classification of Tumors 2019) (Fig. 13.1b). Secretory carcinomas have simple genomes with few copy number alterations and few mutations in cancer genes (Pareja et al. 2021, 2016; Krings et al. 2017). Similarly to the mammary analogue secretory carcinomas of the salivary gland, their counterparts in the salivary gland, secretory carcinomas of the breast are characterized by the translocation t(12;15) resulting in the *ETV6::NTRK3* fusion gene (Tognon et al. 2002; Skálová et al. 2010) (Fig. 13.1b), which can be detected by ISH, next-generation sequencing (NGS) or IHC using pan-TRK antibodies (Harrison et al. 2019; Hechtman et al. 2017). Selective tropomyosin receptor kinase (TRK) inhibitors, such as larotrectinib and entrectinib, have been FDA-approved for the management of solid tumors harboring *NTRK* gene fusions, irrespective of their anatomic location (Amatu et al. 2016; Drilon et al. 2018). Although treatment with TRK inhibitors has shown outstanding responses in patients with recurrent/metastatic breast secretory carcinomas (Drilon et al. 2017, 2018; Laetsch et al. 2018; Shukla et al. 2017), acquired resistance may occur. Repotrectinib and selitrectinib, second-generation TRK inhibitors, can overcome this resistance (Hagopian and Nagasaka 2023), and repotrectinib has been FDA-approved for tumors with NTRK fusions showing progression following prior treatment with TRK inhibitors (Chen et al. 2023).

13.6.2.2 Tall Cell Carcinoma with Reversed Polarity

Tall cell carcinomas with reversed polarity (TCCRPs) are exceptionally rare TNBCs that exhibit histologic features similar to those of tall cell variant of papillary thyroid carcinomas. They display a solid, papillary, and follicular architecture with tall columnar cells demonstrating reversed polarization (apically located nuclei), as well as nuclear clearing and grooves, and intranuclear inclusions (Fig. 13.1c), akin to papillary thyroid carcinoma (Pareja et al. 2021; Masood et al. 2012). TCCRPs are characterized by recurrent *IDH2* R172 hotspot mutations (Fig. 13.1c) like striated duct adenoma, their salivary gland counterparts (Rooper et al. 2023). In addition, genetic alterations affecting the PI3K pathway coexist with *IDH2* mutations in TCCRPs (Chiang et al. 2016; Zhong et al. 2019; Bhargava et al. 2017). In cases lacking *IDH2* R172 mutations, loss-of-function mutations in *TET2* have been reported (Chiang et al. 2016). *IDH2* R172 hotspot mutations can be detected by IHC assays using mutation-specific antibodies or by NGS, aiding in the diagnosis of this rare and challenging tumor (Pareja et al. 2020c, 2021; Alsadoun et al. 2018).

13.6.2.3 Breast Adenoid Cystic Carcinoma

Breast adenoid cystic carcinomas (AdCCs), extremely rare TNBCs, are biphasic epithelial–myoepithelial tumors histologically resembling AdCCs arising in other organs (Marchiò et al. 2010). The classic form of AdCC displays various architectures, including cribriform, tubular ,and trabecular growth patterns (WHO Classification of Tumors 2019) (Fig. 13.1d). Similar to AdCCs arising in other organ systems, most breast classic AdCCs harbor the *MYB::NFIB* gene fusion (Fig. 13.1d) and are characterized by a low mutation rate (D'Alfonso et al. 2014; Persson et al. 2009; Lin et al. 2023). Interestingly, breast classic AdCCs that lack the *MYB::NFIB* fusion gene harbor alternative genetic alterations in the *MYB* pathway, including *MYBL1* fusions or *MYB* amplification (Kim et al. 2018). *MYB*/*MYBL1* fusion genes can be detected using ISH or NGS, and MYB protein overexpression, which characterizes AdCCs, can be detected by IHC (Pareja et al. 2021). Most classic breast AdCCs are indolent, nonetheless recurrences and distant metastases have been reported in a subset of cases (Derakhshan and Reis-Filho 2022; D'Alfonso et al. 2014; Fusco et al. 2016; Sołek et al. 2020) and are associated with an enrichment in genetic alterations in *NOTCH*, *KDM6A*, *CREBBP*, and *SMARCA2* (Ho et al. 2019).

Solid and basaloid adenoid cystic carcinoma (SB-AdCC) is an aggressive and rare TNBC subtype that displays a solid-basaloid architecture (Fig. 13.1e), and, compared to classic AdCC, exhibits a higher histologic grade, and more frequent nodal and distant metastases (WHO Classification of Tumors 2019). SB-AdCCs also differ from classic AdCCs at the genetic level, as only approximately 20% of the cases harbor *MYB* or *MYBL1* fusion genes (Schwartz et al. 2022b) (Fig. 13.1e). In addition, SB-AdCCs show recurrent alterations in *NOTCH* genes, *CREBBP*, and chromatin remodeling genes, such as *KMT2C* and *KMT2D* (Ho et al. 2019; Schwartz et al. 2022b; Masse et al. 2020; Shamir et al. 2023).

There has been limited advancement in targeting of the *MYB–NFIB* fusion gene (Humtsoe et al. 2022). Potential treatment strategies, however, might involve IGF1R/AKT targeting to suppress the activity of this fusion gene, considering that AKT-dependent IGF1R signaling affects the regulation of the *MYB–NFIB* fusion gene (Andersson et al. 2017, 2019). Furthermore, *BUB1* codes for a kinase regulated by MYB, whose inhibition induces synthetic lethality, suggesting potential therapeutic significance in *MYB* fusion-positive AdCCs (Cicirò et al. 2024). CB-103, an oral pan-Notch inhibitor, which reduces the transcriptional activity of the Notch pathway, known to play a role in AdCC (Edwards and Brennan 2021; Raheem et al. 2023), is currently under investigation for the management of *NOTCH*-mutant AdCC in the advanced clinical setting. Promisingly, it has shown disease stabilization in a phase I AdCC study (Hanna et al. 2023; Lehal et al. 2020; Braune et al. 2024).

13.6.2.4 Breast Adenomyoepitheliomas

Adenomyoepitheliomas (AMEs) of the breast are rare epithelial–myoepithelial neoplasms that encompass ER+ and ER− tumors (WHO Classification of Tumors 2019; Nadelman et al. 2006), and benign, atypical and malignant lesions (WHO Classification of Tumors 2019) (Fig. 13.1f). The molecular profiles of ER+ and ER− AMEs are different. While ER+ AMEs show recurrent genetic alterations in the PI3K pathway, such as *PIK3CA* or *AKT1* mutations, ER− AMEs harbor recurrent *HRAS* Q61 hotspot mutations (Fig. 13.1f) that often co-occur with PI3K pathway genetic alterations (Geyer et al. 2018). *HRAS* Q61 mutations can be detected by NGS or IHC with mutation-specific antibodies (Pareja et al. 2020d). Notably, *HRAS* G13 and G12 hotspot mutations have also been reported in malignant AMEs (Baum et al. 2019). Preclinical studies using patient-derived xenografts (PDXs) derived from *HRAS*-mutant AMEs revealed that inhibiting the Ras/RAF/MEK/ERK signaling pathway with the MEK inhibitor trametinib resulted in profound anti-tumor effects. These findings indicate the potential of *HRAS* mutations as a therapeutic target in these tumors (Bièche et al. 2021).

Expression of *KRAS* Q61K depends on the nearby G60G silent substitution to eliminate a cryptic splice donor site (Fackenthal 2023), and *KRAS* Q61K mutant cases in The Cancer Genome Atlas (TCGA) analysis were found to harbor the *KRAS* G60G silent mutation (Kobayashi et al. 2022). A mutation-specific oligonucleotide (MSO) affects *KRAS* splicing, preventing the *KRAS* (Q61K) protein accumulation. This MSO was also found to disrupt splicing of *NRAS* and *HRAS* Q61 mutations and reduce cell viability (Kobayashi et al. 2022), suggesting that these splicing vulnerabilities could be a therapeutic option for *RAS* Q61-mutated AMEs. Furthermore, the combination of trametinib and *IGFR1* inhibitors has shown efficacy in *RAS* Q61-mutant rhabdomyosarcoma preclinical models (Hebron et al. 2023; Garcia et al. 2022), suggesting this as a potential therapeutic approach to explore in *RAS*-mutant AMEs.

13.7 Conclusions and Future Directions

BC displays profound heterogeneity, which is evident even in in situ carcinoma, its precursor. Accurate BC subtyping is essential for guiding therapeutic decision-making. For instance, challenges arise due to the evolving and heterogeneous nature of BC receptor status, exemplified by the recognition of ER-low and HER2-low subgroups, underscoring the importance of the dynamic assessment of biomarkers throughout the disease course.

Histologic subtyping and recognition of special histologic subtypes of BC is paramount for the understanding of BC heterogeneity and for guiding management. The morphologic spectrum of BC, inclusive of the special histologic subtypes, reflects the underlying molecular diversity of this disease. The development of novel diagnostic tools and the implementation of targeted therapies directed at disease-defining genetic alterations, such as TRK inhibitors for *ETV6-NTRK3* fusion gene in secretory carcinomas, highlight the significance of identifying these special BC subtypes in the era of precision medicine. BC immune and metabolic features further contribute to the heterogeneity of BC, with profound implications for treatment eligibility and response, and highlight the need for personalized therapeutic approaches targeting tumor-specific metabolic and immune pathways.

Hereditary BC adds additional complexity to this disease. The genetic landscape and phenotypic features of hereditary BC are diverse and vary according to the cancer susceptibility gene affected, impacting tumor behavior and responses to therapy. Understanding the molecular landscape of hereditary BC can inform targeted therapies, such as the use of PARPi, and underscore the requirement of tailored therapeutic strategies according to genetic predisposition.

Overall, BC heterogeneity presents challenges and opportunities for personalized diagnosis and therapeutics. Emerging strategies and technologies are providing valuable insights into BC diversity. For instance, concurrent tissue based- and liquid biopsy based-genomic profiling of BC has shown to enable the identification of a greater number of patients with targetable variants compared to tissue profiling alone (Iams et al. 2024), including an improved detection of mutations possibly associated with therapeutic resistance, such as *RB1* alterations following CDK4/6 inhibitors, as well as *BRCA1/2* reversion mutations following PARPi (Iams et al. 2024; Sivakumar et al. 2022). Furthermore, artificial intelligence (AI) is transforming pathology by unraveling the BC diversity at an unprecedented pace. AI-based algorithms using digital pathology slides as input have been shown to allow automated cancer detection, classification, biomarker assessment, and prediction of genetic alterations in BC (Steiner et al. 2018; Litjens et al. 2018; Caldonazzi et al. 2023; Lazard et al. 2022; Liu et al. 2023). For example, AI can predict HRD from digital pathology slides with high accuracy (Lazard et al. 2022). These advancements in AI and in other emerging technologies hold promise to further unravel the diversity of BC and allow the refinement of personalized approaches to patient care, ultimately improving outcomes for patients with BC.

References

Abdul Kader S, Dib S, Achkar IW, Thareja G, Suhre K, Rafii A et al (2022) Defining the landscape of metabolic dysregulations in cancer metastasis. Clin Exp Metastasis 39(2):345–362. https://doi.org/10.1007/s10585-021-10140-9

Agostinetto E, Nader-Marta G, Paesmans M, Ameye L, Veys I, Buisseret L et al (2022) ROSALINE: a phase II, neoadjuvant study targeting ROS1 in combination with endocrine therapy in invasive lobular carcinoma of the breast. Future Oncol 18(22):2383–2392. https://doi.org/10.2217/fon-2022-0358

Allison KH, Hammond MEH, Dowsett M, McKernin SE, Carey LA, Fitzgibbons PL et al (2020) Estrogen and progesterone receptor testing in breast cancer: ASCO/CAP guideline update. J Clin Oncol 38(12):1346–1366. https://doi.org/10.1200/jco.19.02309

Alsadoun N, MacGrogan G, Truntzer C, Lacroix-Triki M, Bedgedjian I, Koeb MH et al (2018) Solid papillary carcinoma with reverse polarity of the breast harbors specific morphologic, immunohistochemical and molecular profile in comparison with other benign or malignant papillary lesions of the breast: a comparative study of 9 additional cases. Mod Pathol 31(9):1367–1380. https://doi.org/10.1038/s41379-018-0047-1

Amatu A, Sartore-Bianchi A, Siena S (2016) NTRK gene fusions as novel targets of cancer therapy across multiple tumour types. ESMO Open 1(2):e000023. https://doi.org/10.1136/esmoopen-2015-000023

Andersson MK, Afshari MK, Andrén Y, Wick MJ, Stenman G (2017) Targeting the oncogenic transcriptional regulator MYB in adenoid cystic carcinoma by inhibition of IGF1R/AKT signaling. J Natl Cancer Inst 109(9). https://doi.org/10.1093/jnci/djx017

Andersson MK, Åman P, Stenman G (2019) IGF2/IGF1R signaling as a therapeutic target in MYB-positive adenoid cystic carcinomas and other fusion gene-driven tumors. Cells 8(8):913

Angeli D, Salvi S, Tedaldi G (2020) Genetic predisposition to breast and ovarian cancers: how many and which genes to test? Int J Mol Sci 21(3). https://doi.org/10.3390/ijms21031128

Apostolou P, Fostira F (2013) Hereditary breast cancer: the era of new susceptibility genes. Biomed Res Int 2013:747318. https://doi.org/10.1155/2013/747318

Arpino G, Bardou VJ, Clark GM, Elledge RM (2004) Infiltrating lobular carcinoma of the breast: tumor characteristics and clinical outcome. Breast Cancer Res 6(3):1–8

Asemota S, Effah W, Young KL, Holt J, Cripe L, Ponnusamy S et al (2023) Identification of a targetable JAK-STAT enriched androgen receptor and androgen receptor splice variant positive triple-negative breast cancer subtype. Cell Rep 42(12):113461. https://doi.org/10.1016/j.celrep.2023.113461

Aurilio G, Monfardini L, Rizzo S, Sciandivasci A, Preda L, Bagnardi V et al (2013) Discordant hormone receptor and human epidermal growth factor receptor 2 status in bone metastases compared to primary breast cancer. Acta Oncol 52(8):1649–1656

Aurilio G, Disalvatore D, Pruneri G, Bagnardi V, Viale G, Curigliano G et al (2014) A meta-analysis of oestrogen receptor, progesterone receptor and human epidermal growth factor receptor 2 discordance between primary breast cancer and metastases. Eur J Cancer 50(2):277–289. https://doi.org/10.1016/j.ejca.2013.10.004

Bajrami I, Marlow R, van de Ven M, Brough R, Pemberton HN, Frankum J et al (2018) E-cadherin/ROS1 inhibitor synthetic lethality in breast cancer. Cancer Discov 8(4):498–515. https://doi.org/10.1158/2159-8290.CD-17-0603

Banerji S, Cibulskis K, Rangel-Escareno C, Brown KK, Carter SL, Frederick AM et al (2012) Sequence analysis of mutations and translocations across breast cancer subtypes. Nature 486(7403):405–409. https://doi.org/10.1038/nature11154

Barroso-Sousa R, Jain E, Cohen O, Kim D, Buendia-Buendia J, Winer E et al (2020) Prevalence and mutational determinants of high tumor mutation burden in breast cancer. Ann Oncol 31(3):387–394

Barroso-Sousa R, Pacífico JP, Sammons S, Tolaney SM (2023) Tumor mutational burden in breast cancer: current evidence, challenges, and opportunities. Cancers (Basel) 15(15). https://doi.org/10.3390/cancers15153997

Batra H, Mouabbi JA, Ding Q, Sahin AA, Raso MG (2023) Lobular carcinoma of the breast: a comprehensive review with translational insights. Cancers 15(22):5491

Baum JE, Sung KJ, Tran H, Song W, Ginter PS (2019) Mammary epithelial-myoepithelial carcinoma: report of a case with HRAS and PIK3CA mutations by next-generation sequencing. Int J Surg Pathol 27(4): 441–445. https://doi.org/10.1177/1066896918821182

Bhargava R, Florea AV, Pelmus M, Jones MW, Bonaventura M, Wald A et al (2017) Breast tumor resembling tall cell variant of papillary thyroid carcinoma: a solid papillary neoplasm with characteristic immunohistochemical profile and few recurrent mutations. Am J Clin Pathol 147(4):399–410. https://doi.org/10.1093/ajcp/aqx016

Bianchini G, De Angelis C, Licata L, Gianni L (2022) Treatment landscape of triple-negative breast cancer—expanded options, evolving needs. Nat Rev Clin Oncol 19(2):91–113. https://doi.org/10.1038/s41571-021-00565-2

Bièche I, Coussy F, El-Botty R, Vacher S, Château-Joubert S, Dahmani A et al (2021) HRAS is a therapeutic target in malignant chemo-resistant adenomyoepithelioma of the breast. J Hematol Oncol 14(1):143. https://doi.org/10.1186/s13045-021-01158-3

Bodily WR, Shirts BH, Walsh T, Gulsuner S, King M-C, Parker A et al (2020) Effects of germline and somatic events in candidate BRCA-like genes on breast-tumor signatures. PLoS One 15(9):e0239197

Bonneville R, Krook MA, Kautto EA, Miya J, Wing MR, Chen HZ et al (2017) Landscape of microsatellite instability across 39 cancer types. JCO Precis Oncol 2017. https://doi.org/10.1200/po.17.00073

Braune E-B, Geist F, Tang X, Kalari K, Boughey J, Wang L et al (2024) Identification of a Notch transcriptomic signature for breast cancer. Breast Cancer Res 26(1):4. https://doi.org/10.1186/s13058-023-01757-7

Braunstein LZ, Riaz N (2020) Microenvironmental heterogeneity among triple-negative breast cancer subtypes and the promise of precision medicine. J Natl Cancer Inst 112(7):661–662. https://doi.org/10.1093/jnci/djz209

Caldeira JR, Prando EC, Quevedo FC, Neto FA, Rainho CA, Rogatto SR (2006) CDH1 promoter hypermethylation and E-cadherin protein expression in infiltrating breast cancer. BMC Cancer 6:48. https://doi.org/10.1186/1471-2407-6-48

Caldonazzi N, Rizzo PC, Eccher A, Girolami I, Fanelli GN, Naccarato AG et al (2023) Value of artificial intelligence in evaluating lymph node metastases. Cancers (Basel) 15(9). https://doi.org/10.3390/cancers15092491

Cancer Genome Atlas Network (2012) Comprehensive molecular portraits of human breast tumours. Nature 490(7418):61–70. https://doi.org/10.1038/nature11412

Casasent AK, Edgerton M, Navin NE (2017) Genome evolution in ductal carcinoma in situ: invasion of the clones. J Pathol 241(2):208–218. https://doi.org/10.1002/path.4840

Cereser B, Yiu A, Tabassum N, Del Bel BL, Zagorac S, Ancheta KRZ et al (2023) The mutational landscape of the adult healthy parous and nulliparous human breast. Nat Commun 14(1):5136. https://doi.org/10.1038/s41467-023-40608-z

Chang K, Creighton CJ, Davis C, Donehower L, Drummond J, Wheeler D et al (2013) The cancer genome atlas pan-cancer analysis project. Nat Genet 45(10):1113–1120. https://doi.org/10.1038/ng.2764

Chen YY, Hwang ES, Roy R, DeVries S, Anderson J, Wa C et al (2009) Genetic and phenotypic characteristics of pleomorphic lobular carcinoma in situ of the breast. Am J Surg Pathol 33(11):1683–1694. https://doi.org/10.1097/PAS.0b013e3181b18a89

Chen H, Wu J, Zhang Z, Tang Y, Li X, Liu S et al (2018) Association between BRCA status and triple-negative breast cancer: a meta-analysis. Front Pharmacol 9:909

Chen MF, Yang SR, Shia J, Girshman J, Punn S, Wilhelm C et al (2023) Response to Repotrectinib after development of NTRK resistance mutations on first- and second-generation TRK inhibitors. JCO Precis Oncol 7:e2200697. https://doi.org/10.1200/po.22.00697

Chiang S, Weigelt B, Wen HC, Pareja F, Raghavendra A, Martelotto LG et al (2016) IDH2 mutations define a unique subtype of breast cancer with altered nuclear polarity. Cancer Res 76(24):7118–7129. https://doi.org/10.1158/0008-5472.Can-16-0298

Choi Y, Kim EJ, Seol H, Lee HE, Jang MJ, Kim SM et al (2012) The hormone receptor, human epidermal growth factor receptor 2, and molecular subtype status of individual tumor foci in multifocal/multicentric invasive ductal carcinoma of breast. Hum Pathol 43(1):48–55

Cicirò Y, Ragusa D, Nevado PT, Lattanzio R, Sala G, DesRochers T et al (2024) The mitotic checkpoint kinase BUB1 is a direct and actionable target of MYB in adenoid cystic carcinoma. FEBS Lett 598(2):252–265. https://doi.org/10.1002/1873-3468.14786

Ciriello G, Gatza ML, Beck AH, Wilkerson MD, Rhie SK, Pastore A et al (2015) Comprehensive molecular portraits of invasive lobular breast cancer. Cell 163(2):506–519. https://doi.org/10.1016/j.cell.2015.09.033

Couch FJ, Farid LM, DeShano ML, Tavtigian SV, Calzone K, Campeau L et al (1996) BRCA2 germline mutations in male breast cancer cases and breast cancer families. Nat Genet 13(1):123–125. https://doi.org/10.1038/ng0596-123

Cowell CF, Weigelt B, Sakr RA, Ng CK, Hicks J, King TA et al (2013) Progression from ductal carcinoma in situ to invasive breast cancer: revisited. Mol Oncol 7(5):859–869. https://doi.org/10.1016/j.molonc.2013.07.005

Curigliano G, Bagnardi V, Viale G, Fumagalli L, Rotmensz N, Aurilio G et al (2011) Should liver metastases of breast cancer be biopsied to improve treatment choice? Ann Oncol 22(10):2227–2233

D'Alfonso TM, Mosquera JM, MacDonald TY, Padilla J, Liu YF, Rubin MA et al (2014) MYB-NFIB gene fusion in adenoid cystic carcinoma of the breast with special focus paid to the solid variant with basaloid features. Hum Pathol 45(11):2270–2280. https://doi.org/10.1016/j.humpath.2014.07.013

Davies H, Glodzik D, Morganella S, Yates LR, Staaf J, Zou X et al (2017) HRDetect is a predictor of BRCA1 and BRCA2 deficiency based on mutational signatures. Nat Med 23(4):517–525. https://doi.org/10.1038/nm.4292

Davis AA, Luo J, Zheng T, Dai C, Dong X, Tan L et al (2023) Genomic complexity predicts resistance to endocrine therapy and CDK4/6 inhibition in hormone receptor-positive (HR+)/HER2-negative metastatic breast cancer. Clin Cancer Res 29(9):1719–1729. https://doi.org/10.1158/1078-0432.Ccr-22-2177

de Groot JS, Ratze MA, van Amersfoort M, Eisemann T, Vlug EJ, Niklaas MT et al (2018) αE-catenin is a candidate tumor suppressor for the development of E-cadherin-expressing lobular-type breast cancer. J Pathol 245(4):456–467. https://doi.org/10.1002/path.5099

De La Cruz LM, Harhay MO, Zhang P, Ugras S (2018) Impact of neoadjuvant chemotherapy on breast cancer subtype: does subtype change and, if so, how? : IHC profile and neoadjuvant chemotherapy. Ann Surg Oncol 25(12):3535–3540. https://doi.org/10.1245/s10434-018-6608-1

de Nonneville A, Goncalves A, Mamessier E, Bertucci F (2022) Sacituzumab govitecan in triple-negative breast cancer. Ann Transl Med 10(11):647. https://doi.org/10.21037/atm-22-813

Derakhshan F, Reis-Filho JS (2022) Pathogenesis of triple-negative breast cancer. Annu Rev Pathol 17:181–204. https://doi.org/10.1146/annurev-pathol-042420-093238

Derakhshan F, Dopeso H, Paula ADC, Selenica P, Marra A, da Silva EM et al (2022) Abstract PD14-03: genetic and epigenetic basis of invasive lobular carcinomas lacking CDH1-alterations. Cancer Res 82(4_Supplement):PD14-03-PD14-03. https://doi.org/10.1158/1538-7445.Sabcs21-pd14-03

Desmedt C, Zoppoli G, Gundem G, Pruneri G, Larsimont D, Fornili M et al (2016) Genomic characterization of primary invasive lobular breast cancer. J Clin Oncol 34(16):1872–1881. https://doi.org/10.1200/JCO.2015.64.0334

Desmedt C, Salgado R, Fornili M, Pruneri G, Van den Eynden G, Zoppoli G et al (2018) Immune infiltration in invasive lobular breast cancer. J Natl Cancer Inst 110(7):768–776. https://doi.org/10.1093/jnci/djx268

Desmedt C, Pingitore J, Rothé F, Marchio C, Clatot F, Rouas G et al (2019) ESR1 mutations in metastatic lobular breast cancer patients. NPJ Breast Cancer 5(1):9

Dias AS, Almeida CR, Helguero LA, Duarte IF (2019) Metabolic crosstalk in the breast cancer microenvironment. Eur J Cancer 121:154–171. https://doi.org/10.1016/j.ejca.2019.09.002

Dieci MV, Barbieri E, Piacentini F, Ficarra G, Bettelli S, Dominici M et al (2013) Discordance in receptor status between primary and recurrent breast cancer has a prognostic impact: a single-institution analysis. Ann Oncol 24(1):101–108. https://doi.org/10.1093/annonc/mds248

Dieci MV, Griguolo G, Bottosso M, Tsvetkova V, Giorgi CA, Vernaci G et al (2021) Impact of estrogen receptor levels on outcome in non-metastatic triple negative breast cancer patients treated with neoadjuvant/adjuvant chemotherapy. NPJ Breast Cancer 7(1):101

Dillon J, Mockus S, Ananda G, Spotlow V, Wells W, Tsongalis GJ et al (2016) Somatic gene mutation analysis of triple negative breast cancers. Breast 29:202–207

Dopeso H, Gazzo AM, Derakhshan F, Brown DN, Selenica P, Jalali S et al (2024) Genomic and epigenomic basis of breast invasive lobular carcinomas lacking CDH1 genetic alterations. NPJ Precis Oncol 8(1):33. https://doi.org/10.1038/s41698-024-00508-x

Dorling L, Carvalho S, Allen J, González-Neira A, Luccarini C, Wahlström C et al (2021) Breast cancer risk genes - association analysis in more than 113,000 women. N Engl J Med 384(5):428–439. https://doi.org/10.1056/NEJMoa1913948

Dossus L, Benusiglio PR (2015) Lobular breast cancer: incidence and genetic and non-genetic risk factors. Breast Cancer Res 17:37. https://doi.org/10.1186/s13058-015-0546-7

Dri A, Arpino G, Bianchini G, Curigliano G, Danesi R, De Laurentiis M et al (2024) Breaking barriers in triple negative breast cancer (TNBC) - unleashing the power of antibody-drug conjugates (ADCs). Cancer Treat Rev 123:102672. https://doi.org/10.1016/j.ctrv.2023.102672

Drilon A, Siena S, Ou SI, Patel M, Ahn MJ, Lee J et al (2017) Safety and antitumor activity of the multitargeted pan-TRK, ROS1, and ALK inhibitor Entrectinib: combined results from two phase I trials (ALKA-372-001 and STARTRK-1). Cancer Discov 7(4):400–409. https://doi.org/10.1158/2159-8290.Cd-16-1237

Drilon A, Laetsch TW, Kummar S, DuBois SG, Lassen UN, Demetri GD et al (2018) Efficacy of larotrectinib in TRK fusion-positive cancers in adults and children. N Engl J Med 378(8):731–739. https://doi.org/10.1056/NEJMoa1714448

Dwane L, Behan FM, Gonçalves E, Lightfoot H, Yang W, van der Meer D et al (2021) Project score database: a resource for investigating cancer cell dependencies and prioritizing therapeutic targets. Nucleic Acids Res 49(D1):D1365–D1d72. https://doi.org/10.1093/nar/gkaa882

Edwards A, Brennan K (2021) Notch signalling in breast development and cancer. Front Cell Dev Biol 9:692173. https://doi.org/10.3389/fcell.2021.692173

Ellis IO, Galea M, Broughton N, Locker A, Blamey RW, Elston CW (1992) Pathological prognostic factors in breast cancer. II. Histological type. Relationship with survival in a large study with long-term follow-up. Histopathology 20(6):479–489. https://doi.org/10.1111/j.1365-2559.1992.tb01032.x

Fackenthal JD (2023) Alternative mRNA splicing and promising therapies in cancer. Biomolecules 13(3). https://doi.org/10.3390/biom13030561

Fei F, Siegal GP, Wei S (2021) Characterization of estrogen receptor-low-positive breast cancer. Breast Cancer Res Treat 188(1):225–235. https://doi.org/10.1007/s10549-021-06148-0

Fimereli D, Venet D, Rediti M, Boeckx B, Maetens M, Majjaj S et al (2022) Timing evolution of lobular breast cancer through phylogenetic analysis. EBioMedicine 82:104169. https://doi.org/10.1016/j.ebiom.2022.104169

Foulkes WD, Smith IE, Reis-Filho JS (2010) Triple-negative breast cancer. N Engl J Med 363(20):1938–1948. https://doi.org/10.1056/NEJMra1001389

Fujii T, Kogawa T, Dong W, Sahin AA, Moulder S, Litton JK et al (2017) Revisiting the definition of estrogen receptor positivity in HER2-negative primary breast cancer. Ann Oncol 28(10):2420–2428. https://doi.org/10.1093/annonc/mdx397

Fumagalli C, Barberis M (2021) Breast cancer heterogeneity. Diagnostics (Basel) 11(9). https://doi.org/10.3390/diagnostics11091555

Fusco N, Geyer FC, De Filippo MR, Martelotto LG, Ng CK, Piscuoglio S et al (2016) Genetic events in the progression of adenoid cystic carcinoma of the breast to high-grade triple-negative breast cancer. Mod Pathol 29(11):1292–1305. https://doi.org/10.1038/modpathol.2016.134

Gage M, Wattendorf D, Henry L (2012) Translational advances regarding hereditary breast cancer syndromes. J Surg Oncol 105(5):444–451

Garcia N, Del Pozo V, Yohe ME, Goodwin CM, Shackleford TJ, Wang L et al (2022) Vertical inhibition of the RAF–MEK–ERK Cascade induces myogenic differentiation, apoptosis, and tumor regression in H/NRASQ61X mutant rhabdomyosarcoma. Mol Cancer Ther 21(1):170–183

Geyer FC, Li A, Papanastasiou AD, Smith A, Selenica P, Burke KA et al (2018) Recurrent hotspot mutations in HRAS Q61 and PI3K-AKT pathway genes as drivers of breast adenomyoepitheliomas. Nat Commun 9(1):1816. https://doi.org/10.1038/s41467-018-04128-5

Hagopian G, Nagasaka M (2023) Oncogenic fusions: targeting NTRK. Crit Rev Oncol Hematol 194:104234. https://doi.org/10.1016/j.critrevonc.2023.104234

Hanna GJ, Stathis A, Lopez-Miranda E, Racca F, Quon D, Leyvraz S et al (2023) A phase I study of the pan-Notch inhibitor CB-103 for patients with advanced adenoid cystic carcinoma and other tumors. Cancer Res Commun 3(9):1853–1861. https://doi.org/10.1158/2767-9764.Crc-23-0333

Harris M, Howell A, Chrissohou M, Swindell R, Hudson M, Sellwood R (1984) A comparison of the metastatic pattern of infiltrating lobular carcinoma and infiltrating duct carcinoma of the breast. Br J Cancer 50(1):23–30

Harrison BT, Fowler E, Krings G, Chen YY, Bean GR, Vincent-Salomon A et al (2019) Pan-TRK immunohistochemistry: a useful diagnostic adjunct for secretory carcinoma of the breast. Am J Surg Pathol 43(12):1693–1700. https://doi.org/10.1097/PAS.0000000000001366

Harrison BT, Nakhlis F, Dillon DA, Soong TR, Garcia EP, Schnitt SJ et al (2020) Genomic profiling of pleomorphic and florid lobular carcinoma in situ reveals highly recurrent ERBB2 and ERRB3 alterations. Mod Pathol 33(7):1287–1297

Hebron KE, Wan X, Roth JS, Liewehr DJ, Sealover NE, Frye WJ et al (2023) The combination of trametinib and ganitumab is effective in RAS-mutated PAX-fusion negative rhabdomyosarcoma models. Clin Cancer Res 29(2):472–487

Hechtman JF, Benayed R, Hyman DM, Drilon A, Zehir A, Frosina D et al (2017) Pan-Trk immunohistochemistry is an efficient and reliable screen for the detection of NTRK fusions. Am J Surg Pathol 41(11):1547–1551. https://doi.org/10.1097/pas.0000000000000911

Heeke AL, Xiu J, Elliott A, Korn WM, Lynce F, Pohlmann PR et al (2020) Actionable co-alterations in breast tumors with pathogenic mutations in the homologous recombination DNA damage repair pathway. Breast Cancer Res Treat 184(2):265–275. https://doi.org/10.1007/s10549-020-05849-2

Ho AS, Ochoa A, Jayakumaran G, Zehir A, Valero Mayor C, Tepe J et al (2019) Genetic hallmarks of recurrent/metastatic adenoid cystic carcinoma. J Clin Invest 129(10):4276–4289. https://doi.org/10.1172/jci128227

Hoppe S, Meder L, Gebauer F, Ullrich RT, Zander T, Hillmer AM et al (2022) Trophoblast cell surface antigen 2 (TROP2) as a predictive bio-marker for the therapeutic efficacy of Sacituzumab Govitecan in adenocarcinoma of the esophagus. Cancers (Basel) 14(19):4789

Humtsoe JO, Kim HS, Jones L, Cevallos J, Boileau P, Kuo F et al (2022) Development and characterization of MYB-NFIB fusion expression in adenoid cystic carcinoma. Cancers (Basel) 14(9). https://doi.org/10.3390/cancers14092263

Hutchinson L (2010) Targeted therapies: PARP inhibitor olaparib is safe and effective in patients with BRCA1 and BRCA2 mutations. Nat Rev Clin Oncol 7(10): 549

Iams WT, Mackay M, Ben-Shachar R, Drews J, Manghnani K, Hockenberry AJ et al (2024) Concurrent tissue and circulating tumor DNA molecular profiling to detect guideline-based targeted mutations in a multicancer cohort. JAMA Netw Open 7(1):e2351700. https://doi.org/10.1001/jamanetworkopen.2023.51700

Issa-Nummer Y, Darb-Esfahani S, Loibl S, Kunz G, Nekljudova V, Schrader I et al (2013) Prospective validation of immunological infiltrate for prediction of response to neoadjuvant chemotherapy in HER2-negative breast cancer–a substudy of the neoadjuvant GeparQuinto trial. PLoS One 8(12):e79775

Jaspers JE, Kersbergen A, Boon U, Sol W, van Deemter L, Zander SA et al (2013) Loss of 53BP1 causes PARP inhibitor resistance in Brca1-mutated mouse mammary tumors. Cancer Discov 3(1):68–81. https://doi.org/10.1158/2159-8290.Cd-12-0049

Jiang YZ, Ma D, Suo C, Shi J, Xue M, Hu X et al (2019) Genomic and transcriptomic landscape of triple-negative breast cancers: subtypes and treatment strategies. Cancer Cell 35(3):428–40.e5. https://doi.org/10.1016/j.ccell.2019.02.001

Ke L, Li S, Cui H (2022) The prognostic role of tumor mutation burden on survival of breast cancer: a systematic review and meta-analysis. BMC Cancer 22(1):1185. https://doi.org/10.1186/s12885-022-10284-1

Kim J, Geyer FC, Martelotto LG, Ng CK, Lim RS, Selenica P et al (2018) MYBL1 rearrangements and MYB amplification in breast adenoid cystic carcinomas lacking the MYB-NFIB fusion gene. J Pathol 244(2):143–150. https://doi.org/10.1002/path.5006

Klouch KZ, Stern M-H, Trabelsi-Grati O, Kiavue N, Cabel L, Silveira AB et al (2022) Microsatellite instability detection in breast cancer using drop-off droplet digital PCR. Oncogene 41(49):5289–5297. https://doi.org/10.1038/s41388-022-02504-6

Kobayashi Y, Chhoeu C, Li J, Price KS, Kiedrowski LA, Hutchins JL et al (2022) Silent mutations reveal therapeutic vulnerability in RAS Q61 cancers. Nature 603(7900):335–342. https://doi.org/10.1038/s41586-022-04451-4

Krings G, Joseph NM, Bean GR, Solomon D, Onodera C, Talevich E et al (2017) Genomic profiling of breast secretory carcinomas reveals distinct genetics from other breast cancers and similarity to mammary analog secretory carcinomas. Mod Pathol 30(8):1086–1099. https://doi.org/10.1038/modpathol.2017.32

Laetsch TW, DuBois SG, Mascarenhas L, Turpin B, Federman N, Albert CM et al (2018) Larotrectinib for paediatric solid tumours harbouring NTRK gene fusions: phase 1 results from a multicentre, open-label, phase 1/2 study. Lancet Oncol 19(5):705–714. https://doi.org/10.1016/s1470-2045(18)30119-0

Lazard T, Bataillon G, Naylor P, Popova T, Bidard FC, Stoppa-Lyonnet D et al (2022) Deep learning identifies morphological patterns of homologous recombination deficiency in luminal breast cancers from whole slide images. Cell Rep Med 3(12):100872. https://doi.org/10.1016/j.xcrm.2022.100872

Lee JY, Schizas M, Geyer FC, Selenica P, Piscuoglio S, Sakr RA et al (2019) Lobular carcinomas in situ display Intralesion genetic heterogeneity and clonal evolution in the progression to invasive lobular carcinoma. Clin Cancer Res 25(2):674–686. https://doi.org/10.1158/1078-0432.Ccr-18-1103

Lehal R, Zaric J, Vigolo M, Urech C, Frismantas V, Zangger N et al (2020) Pharmacological disruption of the Notch transcription factor complex. Proc Natl Acad Sci USA 117(28):16292–16301. https://doi.org/10.1073/pnas.1922606117

Lehmann BD, Bauer JA, Chen X, Sanders ME, Chakravarthy AB, Shyr Y et al (2011) Identification of human triple-negative breast cancer subtypes and preclinical models for selection of targeted therapies. J Clin Invest 121(7):2750–2767

Li CI, Anderson BO, Daling JR, Moe RE (2003) Trends in incidence rates of invasive lobular and ductal breast carcinoma. JAMA 289(11):1421–1424

Li A, Keck JM, Parmar S, Patterson J, Labrie M, Creason AL et al (2021) Characterizing advanced breast cancer heterogeneity and treatment resistance through serial biopsies and comprehensive analytics. NPJ Precis Oncol 5(1):28. https://doi.org/10.1038/s41698-021-00165-4

Lin Q-Q, Sun J-L, Wang F, Zhang H-Z, Zhou G, Xi Q (2023) Current understanding of adenoid cystic carcinoma in the gene expression and targeted therapy. Holist Integr Oncol 2(1):7

Lindström LS, Karlsson E, Wilking UM, Johansson U, Hartman J, Lidbrink EK et al (2012) Clinically used breast cancer markers such as estrogen receptor, progesterone receptor, and human epidermal growth factor receptor 2 are unstable throughout tumor progression. J Clin Oncol 30(21):2601–2608. https://doi.org/10.1200/jco.2011.37.2482

Litjens G, Bandi P, Ehteshami Bejnordi B, Geessink O, Balkenhol M, Bult P et al (2018) 1399 H&E-stained sentinel lymph node sections of breast cancer patients: the CAMELYON dataset. Gigascience 7(6). https://doi.org/10.1093/gigascience/giy065

Liu YL, Choi C, Lee SM, Zhong X, Hibshoosh H, Kalinsky K et al (2018) Invasive lobular breast carcinoma: pleomorphic versus classical subtype, associations and prognosis. Clin Breast Cancer 18(2):114–120

Liu L, Matsunaga Y, Tsurutani J, Akashi-Tanaka S, Masuda H, Ide Y et al (2020) BRCAness as a prognostic indicator in patients with early breast cancer. Sci Rep 10(1):21173

Liu Y, Han D, Parwani AV, Li Z (2023) Applications of artificial intelligence in breast pathology. Arch Pathol Lab Med 147(9):1003–1013. https://doi.org/10.5858/arpa.2022-0457-RA

Lluch A, González-Angulo AM, Casadevall D, Eterovic AK, Martínez de Dueñas E, Zheng X et al (2019) Dynamic clonal remodelling in breast cancer metastases is associated with subtype conversion. Eur J Cancer 120:54–64. https://doi.org/10.1016/j.ejca.2019.07.003

Lord CJ, Ashworth A (2016) BRCAness revisited. Nat Rev Cancer 16(2):110–120

Luo C, Zhong X, Fan Y, Wu Y, Zheng H, Luo T (2022) Clinical characteristics and survival outcome of patients with estrogen receptor low positive breast cancer. Breast 63:24–28. https://doi.org/10.1016/j.breast.2022.03.002

Malik SS, Zia A, Mubarik S, Masood N, Rashid S, Sherrard A et al (2020) Correlation of MLH1 polymorphisms, survival statistics, in silico assessment and gene downregulation with clinical outcomes among breast cancer cases. Mol Biol Rep 47:683–692

Mandelker D, Kumar R, Pei X, Selenica P, Setton J, Arunachalam S et al (2019) The landscape of somatic genetic alterations in breast cancers from CHEK2 germline mutation carriers. JNCI Cancer Spectr 3(2):pkz027. https://doi.org/10.1093/jncics/pkz027

Marchiò C, Weigelt B, Reis-Filho JS (2010) Adenoid cystic carcinomas of the breast and salivary glands (or 'The strange case of Dr Jekyll and Mr Hyde' of exocrine gland carcinomas). J Clin Pathol 63(3):220–228. https://doi.org/10.1136/jcp.2009.073908

Marra A, Safonov A, Drago J (2022) Genomic characterization of primary and metastatic HER2-low breast cancers. In: Proceedings of the 2022 San Antonio Breast Cancer Symposium 2022, pp 6–10

Masood S, Davis C, Kubik MJ (2012) Changing the term "breast tumor resembling the tall cell variant of papillary thyroid carcinoma" to "tall cell variant of papillary breast carcinoma". Adv Anat Pathol 19(2):108–110. https://doi.org/10.1097/PAP.0b013e318249d090

Masse J, Truntzer C, Boidot R, Khalifa E, Perot G, Velasco V et al (2020) Solid-type adenoid cystic carcinoma of the breast, a distinct molecular entity enriched in NOTCH and CREBBP mutations. Mod Pathol 33(6):1041–1055. https://doi.org/10.1038/s41379-019-0425-3

McCart Reed AE, Kalinowski L, Simpson PT, Lakhani SR (2021) Invasive lobular carcinoma of the breast: the increasing importance of this special subtype. Breast Cancer Res 23(1):6. https://doi.org/10.1186/s13058-020-01384-6

Metaxas GI, Tsiambas E, Marinopoulos S, Adamopoulou M, Spyropoulou D, Falidas E et al (2023) DNA mismatch repair system imbalances in breast adenocarcinoma. Cancer Diagn Progn 3(2):169–174. https://doi.org/10.21873/cdp.10197

Middha S, Zhang L, Nafa K, Jayakumaran G, Wong D, Kim HR et al (2017) Reliable pan-cancer microsatellite instability assessment by using targeted next-generation sequencing data. JCO Precis Oncol 2017. https://doi.org/10.1200/po.17.00084

Miglietta F, Griguolo G, Bottosso M, Giarratano T, Lo Mele M, Fassan M et al (2022) HER2-low-positive breast cancer: evolution from primary tumor to residual disease after neoadjuvant treatment. NPJ Breast Cancer 8(1):66. https://doi.org/10.1038/s41523-022-00434-w

Modi S, Jacot W, Yamashita T, Sohn J, Vidal M, Tokunaga E et al (2022) Trastuzumab deruxtecan in previously treated HER2-low advanced breast cancer. N Engl J Med 387(1):9–20. https://doi.org/10.1056/NEJMoa2203690

Möller S, Mucci LA, Harris JR, Scheike T, Holst K, Halekoh U et al (2016) The heritability of breast cancer among women in the Nordic twin study of cancer. Cancer Epidemiol Biomarkers Prev 25(1):145–150. https://doi.org/10.1158/1055-9965.Epi-15-0913

Moon J, Kitty I, Renata K, Qin S, Zhao F, Kim W (2023) DNA damage and its role in cancer therapeutics. Int J Mol Sci 24(5):4741

Mouabbi JA, Meric-Bernstam F, Khorkova S, Turova P, Kotlov N, Chernyshov K et al (2023) Differential genomic and transcriptomic analysis of invasive lobular and ductal carcinomas. American Society of Clinical Oncology

Nadelman CM, Leslie KO, Fishbein MC (2006) "Benign," metastasizing adenomyoepithelioma of the breast: a report of 2 cases. Arch Pathol Lab Med 130(9):1349–1353. https://doi.org/10.5858/2006-130-1349-bmaotb

Nagayama A, Vidula N, Ellisen L, Bardia A (2020) Novel antibody-drug conjugates for triple negative breast cancer. Ther Adv Med Oncol 12:1758835920915980. https://doi.org/10.1177/1758835920915980

Navas LE, Carnero A (2021) NAD(+) metabolism, stemness, the immune response, and cancer. Signal Transduct Target Ther 6(1):2. https://doi.org/10.1038/s41392-020-00354-w

Ng CKY, Piscuoglio S, Geyer FC, Burke KA, Pareja F, Eberle CA et al (2017) The landscape of somatic genetic alterations in metaplastic breast carcinomas. Clin Cancer Res 23(14):3859–3870. https://doi.org/10.1158/1078-0432.CCR-16-2857

Nguyen B, Veys I, Leduc S, Bareche Y, Majjaj S, Brown DN et al (2019) Genomic, transcriptomic, epigenetic, and immune profiling of mucinous breast cancer. J Natl Cancer Inst 111(7):742–746. https://doi.org/10.1093/jnci/djz023

Nishimura T, Kakiuchi N, Yoshida K, Sakurai T, Kataoka TR, Kondoh E et al (2023) Evolutionary histories of breast cancer and related clones. Nature 620(7974):607–614. https://doi.org/10.1038/s41586-023-06333-9

Nones K, Johnson J, Newell F, Patch AM, Thorne H, Kazakoff SH et al (2019) Whole-genome sequencing reveals clinically relevant insights into the aetiology of familial breast cancers. Ann Oncol 30(7):1071–1079. https://doi.org/10.1093/annonc/mdz132

Ortiz MMO, Andrechek ER (2023) Molecular characterization and landscape of breast cancer models from a multi-omics perspective. J Mammary Gland Biol Neoplasia 28(1):12. https://doi.org/10.1007/s10911-023-09540-2

Orvieto E, Maiorano E, Bottiglieri L, Maisonneuve P, Rotmensz N, Galimberti V et al (2008) Clinicopathologic characteristics of invasive lobular carcinoma of the breast: results of an analysis of 530 cases from a single institution. Cancer 113(7):1511–1520. https://doi.org/10.1002/cncr.23811

Paakkola NM, Karakatsanis A, Mauri D, Foukakis T, Valachis A (2021) The prognostic and predictive impact of low estrogen receptor expression in early breast cancer: a systematic review and meta-analysis. ESMO Open 6(6):100289. https://doi.org/10.1016/j.esmoop.2021.100289

Pareja F, D'Alfonso TM (2020) Neuroendocrine neoplasms of the breast: a review focused on the updated World Health Organization (WHO) 5th edition morphologic classification. Breast J 26(6):1160–1167. https://doi.org/10.1111/tbj.13863

Pareja F, Geyer FC, Marchiò C, Burke KA, Weigelt B, Reis-Filho JS (2016) Triple-negative breast cancer: the importance of molecular and histologic subtyping, and recognition of low-grade variants. NPJ Breast Cancer 2:16036. https://doi.org/10.1038/npjbcancer.2016.36

Pareja F, Lee JY, Brown DN, Piscuoglio S, Gularte-Merida R, Selenica P et al (2019) The genomic landscape of mucinous breast cancer. J Natl Cancer Inst 111(7):737–741. https://doi.org/10.1093/jnci/djy216

Pareja F, Brown DN, Lee JY, Da Cruz PA, Selenica P, Bi R et al (2020a) Whole-exome sequencing analysis of the progression from non-low-grade ductal carcinoma in situ to invasive ductal carcinoma. Clin Cancer Res 26(14):3682–3693. https://doi.org/10.1158/1078-0432.CCR-19-2563

Pareja F, Ferrando L, Lee SSK, Beca F, Selenica P, Brown DN et al (2020b) The genomic landscape of metastatic histologic special types of invasive breast cancer. NPJ Breast Cancer 6:53. https://doi.org/10.1038/s41523-020-00195-4

Pareja F, da Silva EM, Frosina D, Geyer FC, Lozada JR, Basili T et al (2020c) Immunohistochemical analysis of IDH2 R172 hotspot mutations in breast papillary neoplasms: applications in the diagnosis of tall cell carcinoma with reverse polarity. Mod Pathol 33(6):1056–1064. https://doi.org/10.1038/s41379-019-0442-2

Pareja F, Toss MS, Geyer FC, da Silva EM, Vahdatinia M, Sebastiao APM et al (2020d) Immunohistochemical assessment of HRAS Q61R mutations in breast adenomyoepitheliomas. Histopathology 76(6):865–874. https://doi.org/10.1111/his.14057

Pareja F, Weigelt B, Reis-Filho JS (2021) Problematic breast tumors reassessed in light of novel molecular data. Mod Pathol 34(Suppl 1):38–47. https://doi.org/10.1038/s41379-020-00693-7

Pareja F, Vahdatinia M, Marchio C, Lee SSK, Da Cruz PA, Derakhshan F et al (2022) Neuroendocrine tumours of the breast: a genomic comparison with mucinous breast cancers and neuroendocrine tumours of other anatomic sites. J Clin Pathol 75(1):10–17. https://doi.org/10.1136/jclinpath-2020-207052

Persson M, Andrén Y, Mark J, Horlings HM, Persson F, Stenman G (2009) Recurrent fusion of MYB and NFIB transcription factor genes in carcinomas of the breast and head and neck. Proc Natl Acad Sci USA 106(44):18740–18744. https://doi.org/10.1073/pnas.0909114106

Piscuoglio S, Ng CKY, Geyer FC, Burke KA, Cowell CF, Martelotto LG et al (2017) Genomic and transcriptomic heterogeneity in metaplastic carcinomas of the breast. NPJ Breast Cancer 3:48. https://doi.org/10.1038/s41523-017-0048-0

Poon IK, Tsang JY, Li J, Chan SK, Shea KH, Tse GM (2020) The significance of highlighting the oestrogen receptor low category in breast cancer. Br J Cancer 123(8):1223–1227. https://doi.org/10.1038/s41416-020-1009-1

Prat J, Ribé A, Gallardo A (2005) Hereditary ovarian cancer. Hum Pathol 36(8):861–870

Privitera AP, Barresi V, Condorelli DF (2021) Aberrations of chromosomes 1 and 16 in breast cancer: a framework for cooperation of transcriptionally dysregulated genes. Cancers 13(7):1585

Prokopcova J, Kleibl Z, Banwell CM, Pohlreich P (2007) The role of ATM in breast cancer development. Breast Cancer Res Treat 104:121–128

Qu Y, Qin S, Yang Z, Li Z, Liang Q, Long T et al (2023) Targeting the DNA repair pathway for breast cancer therapy: beyond the molecular subtypes. Biomed Pharmacother 169:115877. https://doi.org/10.1016/j.biopha.2023.115877

Raheem F, Karikalan SA, Batalini F, El Masry A, Mina L (2023) Metastatic ER+ breast cancer: mechanisms of resistance and future therapeutic approaches. Int J Mol Sci 24(22):16198

Rakha EA, Pareja FG (2021) New advances in molecular breast cancer pathology. Semin Cancer Biol 72:102–113. https://doi.org/10.1016/j.semcancer.2020.03.014

Razavi P, Chang MT, Xu G, Bandlamudi C, Ross DS, Vasan N et al (2018) The genomic landscape of endocrine-resistant advanced breast cancers. Cancer Cell 34(3):427–38.e6. https://doi.org/10.1016/j.ccell.2018.08.008

Reina-Campos M, Moscat J, Diaz-Meco M (2017) Metabolism shapes the tumor microenvironment. Curr Opin Cell Biol 48:47–53. https://doi.org/10.1016/j.ceb.2017.05.006

Reis-Filho JS, Pusztai L (2011) Gene expression profiling in breast cancer: classification, prognostication, and prediction. Lancet 378(9805):1812–1823. https://doi.org/10.1016/s0140-6736(11)61539-0

Richard F, Majjaj S, Venet D, Rothé F, Pingitore J, Boeckx B et al (2020) Characterization of stromal tumor-infiltrating lymphocytes and genomic alterations in metastatic lobular breast cancer. Clin Cancer Res 26(23):6254–6265

Riedlinger GM, Joshi S, Hirshfield KM, Barnard N, Ganesan S (2021) Targetable alterations in invasive pleomorphic lobular carcinoma of the breast. Breast Cancer Res 23:1–8

Roberts SA, Gordenin DA (2014) Hypermutation in human cancer genomes: footprints and mechanisms. Nat Rev Cancer 14(12):786–800. https://doi.org/10.1038/nrc3816

Rooper LM, Agaimy A, Assaad A, Bal M, Eugene H, Gagan J et al (2023) Recurrent IDH2 mutations in salivary gland striated duct adenoma define an expanded histologic Spectrum distinct from Canalicular adenoma. Am J Surg Pathol 47(3):333–343. https://doi.org/10.1097/PAS.0000000000002004

Rosa-Rosa JM, Caniego-Casas T, Leskela S, Cristobal E, González-Martínez S, Moreno-Moreno E et al (2019) High frequency of ERBB2 activating mutations in invasive lobular breast carcinoma with pleomorphic features. Cancers (Basel) 11(1). https://doi.org/10.3390/cancers11010074

Ross DS, Pareja F (2021) Molecular pathology of breast tumors: diagnostic and actionable genetic alterations. Surg Pathol Clin 14(3):455–471. https://doi.org/10.1016/j.path.2021.05.009

Russo L, Maltese A, Betancourt L, Romero G, Cialoni D, De la Fuente L et al (2019) Locally advanced breast cancer: tumor-infiltrating lymphocytes as a predictive factor of response to neoadjuvant chemotherapy. Eur J Surg Oncol 45(6):963–968. https://doi.org/10.1016/j.ejso.2019.01.222

Ryan CJ, Devakumar LPS, Pettitt SJ, Lord CJ (2023) Complex synthetic lethality in cancer. Nat Genet 55(12):2039–2048. https://doi.org/10.1038/s41588-023-01557-x

Salgado R, Denkert C, Campbell C, Savas P, Nuciforo P, Aura C et al (2015) Tumor-infiltrating lymphocytes and associations with pathological complete response and event-free survival in HER2-positive early-stage breast cancer treated with Lapatinib and Trastuzumab: a secondary analysis of the NeoALTTO trial. JAMA Oncol 1(4):448–454. https://doi.org/10.1001/jamaoncol.2015.0830

Sammons S, Raskina K, Danziger N, Alder L, Schrock AB, Venstrom JM et al (2022) APOBEC mutational signatures in hormone receptor-positive human epidermal growth factor receptor 2-negative breast cancers are associated with poor outcomes on CDK4/6 inhibitors and endocrine therapy. JCO Precis Oncol 6:e2200149. https://doi.org/10.1200/po.22.00149

Savas P, Salgado R, Denkert C, Sotiriou C, Darcy PK, Smyth MJ et al (2016) Clinical relevance of host immunity in breast cancer: from TILs to the clinic. Nat Rev Clin Oncol 13(4):228–241. https://doi.org/10.1038/nrclinonc.2015.215

Schrijver WAME, Suijkerbuijk KPM, van Gils CH, van der Wall E, Moelans CB, van Diest PJ (2018) Receptor conversion in distant breast cancer metastases: a systematic review and meta-analysis. JNCI J Natl Cancer Inst 110(6):568–580. https://doi.org/10.1093/jnci/djx273

Schrodi S, Braun M, Andrulat A, Harbeck N, Mahner S, Kiechle M et al (2021) Outcome of breast cancer patients with low hormone receptor positivity: analysis of a 15-year population-based cohort. Ann Oncol 32(11):1410–1424. https://doi.org/10.1016/j.annonc.2021.08.1988

Schwartz CJ, da Silva EM, Marra A, Gazzo AM, Selenica P, Rai VK et al (2022a) Morphologic and genomic characteristics of breast cancers occurring in individuals with lynch syndrome. Clin Cancer Res 28(2):404–413. https://doi.org/10.1158/1078-0432.CCR-21-2027

Schwartz CJ, Brogi E, Marra A, Da Cruz Paula AF, Nanjangud GJ, da Silva EM et al (2022b) The clinical behavior and genomic features of the so-called adenoid cystic carcinomas of the solid variant with basaloid features. Mod Pathol 35(2):193–201. https://doi.org/10.1038/s41379-021-00931-6

Schwartz CJ, Ruiz J, Bean GR, Sirohi D, Joseph NM, Hosfield EM et al (2023) Triple-negative apocrine carcinomas: toward a unified group with shared molecular features and clinical behavior. Mod Pathol 36(5):100125. https://doi.org/10.1016/j.modpat.2023.100125

Schwartz CJ, Khorsandi N, Blanco A, Mukhtar RA, Chen YY, Krings G (2024) Clinicopathologic and genetic analysis of invasive breast carcinomas in women with germline CHEK2 variants. Breast Cancer Res Treat 204(1):171–179. https://doi.org/10.1007/s10549-023-07176-8

Setton J, Selenica P, Mukherjee S, Shah R, Pecorari I, McMillan B et al (2021) Germline RAD51B variants confer susceptibility to breast and ovarian cancers deficient in homologous recombination. NPJ Breast Cancer 7(1):135. https://doi.org/10.1038/s41523-021-00339-0

Shamir ER, Chen YY, Krings G (2020) Genetic analysis of pleomorphic and florid lobular carcinoma in situ variants: frequent ERBB2/ERBB3 alterations and clonal relationship to classic lobular carcinoma in situ and invasive lobular carcinoma. Mod Pathol 33(6):1078–1091. https://doi.org/10.1038/s41379-019-0449-8

Shamir ER, Bean GR, Schwartz CJ, Vohra P, Wang A, Allard GM et al (2023) Solid-basaloid adenoid cystic carcinoma of the breast: an aggressive subtype enriched for Notch pathway and chromatin modifier mutations with MYB overexpression. Mod Pathol 36(12):100324. https://doi.org/10.1016/j.modpat.2023.100324

Shukla N, Roberts SS, Baki MO, Mushtaq Q, Goss PE, Park BH et al (2017) Successful targeted therapy of refractory pediatric ETV6-NTRK3 fusion-positive secretory breast carcinoma. JCO Precis Oncol 2017. https://doi.org/10.1200/PO.17.00034

Simpson P, Reis-Filho J, Lambros M, Jones C, Steele D, Mackay A et al (2008) Molecular profiling pleomorphic lobular carcinomas of the breast: evidence for a common molecular genetic pathway with classic lobular carcinomas. J Pathol 215(3):231–244

Sivakumar S, Jin DX, Tukachinsky H, Murugesan K, McGregor K, Danziger N et al (2022) Tissue and liquid biopsy profiling reveal convergent tumor evolution and therapy evasion in breast cancer. Nat Commun 13(1):7495. https://doi.org/10.1038/s41467-022-35245-x

Skálová A, Vanecek T, Sima R, Laco J, Weinreb I, Perez-Ordonez B et al (2010) Mammary analogue secretory carcinoma of salivary glands, containing the ETV6-NTRK3 fusion gene: a hitherto undescribed salivary gland tumor entity. Am J Surg Pathol 34(5):599–608. https://doi.org/10.1097/PAS.0b013e3181d9efcc

Smid M, Schmidt MK, Prager-van der Smissen WJC, Ruigrok-Ritstier K, Schreurs MAC, Cornelissen S et al (2023) Breast cancer genomes from CHEK2 c.1100delC mutation carriers lack somatic TP53 mutations and display a unique structural variant size distribution profile. Breast Cancer Res 25(1):53. https://doi.org/10.1186/s13058-023-01653-0

Sokol ES, Feng YX, Jin DX, Basudan A, Lee AV, Atkinson JM et al (2019) Loss of function of NF1 is a mechanism of acquired resistance to endocrine therapy in lobular breast cancer. Ann Oncol 30(1):115–123. https://doi.org/10.1093/annonc/mdy497

Sołek JM, Braun M, Kalwas M, Jesionek-Kupnicka D, Romańska HM (2020) Adenoid cystic carcinoma of the breast - an uncommon malignancy with unpredictable clinical behaviour. A case series of three patients. Contemp Oncol (Pozn) 24(4):263–265. https://doi.org/10.5114/wo.2020.99025

Song F, Tarantino P, Garrido-Castro A, Lynce F, Tolaney SM, Schlam I (2024) Immunotherapy for early-stage triple negative breast cancer: is earlier better? Curr Oncol Rep. https://doi.org/10.1007/s11912-023-01487-1

Steiner DF, MacDonald R, Liu Y, Truszkowski P, Hipp JD, Gammage C et al (2018) Impact of deep learning assistance on the histopathologic review of lymph nodes for metastatic breast cancer. Am J Surg Pathol 42(12):1636

Sun J, Meng H, Yao L, Lv M, Bai J, Zhang J et al (2017) Germline mutations in cancer susceptibility genes in a large series of unselected breast cancer patients. Clin Cancer Res 23(20):6113–6119. https://doi.org/10.1158/1078-0432.Ccr-16-3227

Tarantino P, Gupta H, Hughes ME, Files J, Strauss S, Kirkner G et al (2023) Comprehensive genomic characterization of HER2-low and HER2-0 breast cancer. Nat Commun 14(1):7496. https://doi.org/10.1038/s41467-023-43324-w

Tarragó-Celada J, Cascante M (2021) Targeting the metabolic adaptation of metastatic cancer. Cancers (Basel) 13(7). https://doi.org/10.3390/cancers13071641

Tierno D, Grassi G, Scomersi S, Bortul M, Generali D, Zanconati F et al (2023) Next-generation sequencing and triple-negative breast cancer: insights and applications. Int J Mol Sci 24(11). https://doi.org/10.3390/ijms24119688

Tille JC, Vieira AF, Saint-Martin C, Djerroudi L, Furhmann L, Bidard FC et al (2020) Tumor-infiltrating lymphocytes are associated with poor prognosis in invasive lobular breast carcinoma. Mod Pathol 33(11):2198–2207. https://doi.org/10.1038/s41379-020-0561-9

Tognon C, Knezevich SR, Huntsman D, Roskelley CD, Melnyk N, Mathers JA et al (2002) Expression of the ETV6-NTRK3 gene fusion as a primary event in human secretory breast carcinoma. Cancer Cell 2(5):367–376. https://doi.org/10.1016/s1535-6108(02)00180-0

Topatana W, Juengpanich S, Li S, Cao J, Hu J, Lee J et al (2020) Advances in synthetic lethality for cancer therapy: cellular mechanism and clinical translation. J Hematol Oncol 13(1):118. https://doi.org/10.1186/s13045-020-00956-5

Trinh A, Gil Del Alcazar CR, Shukla SA, Chin K, Chang YH, Thibault G et al (2021) Genomic alterations during the in situ to invasive ductal breast carcinoma transition shaped by the immune system. Mol Cancer Res 19(4):623–635

Tung NM, Robson ME, Ventz S, Santa-Maria CA, Nanda R, Marcom PK et al (2020) TBCRC 048: phase II study of olaparib for metastatic breast cancer and mutations in homologous recombination-related genes. J Clin Oncol 38(36):4274–4282

Turashvili G, Brogi E (2017) Tumor heterogeneity in breast cancer. Front Med (Lausanne) 4:227. https://doi.org/10.3389/fmed.2017.00227

Turner NC, Reis-Filho JS (2006) Basal-like breast cancer and the BRCA1 phenotype. Oncogene 25(43):5846–5853. https://doi.org/10.1038/sj.onc.1209876

Tutt ANJ, Garber JE, Kaufman B, Viale G, Fumagalli D, Rastogi P et al (2021) Adjuvant olaparib for patients with BRCA1- or BRCA2-mutated breast cancer. N Engl J Med 384(25):2394–2405. https://doi.org/10.1056/NEJMoa2105215

Valenza C, Taurelli Salimbeni B, Santoro C, Trapani D, Antonarelli G, Curigliano G (2023) Tumor infiltrating lymphocytes across breast cancer subtypes: current issues for biomarker assessment. Cancers (Basel) 15(3). https://doi.org/10.3390/cancers15030767

Van Baelen K, Geukens T, Maetens M, Tjan-Heijnen V, Lord CJ, Linn S et al (2022) Current and future diagnostic and treatment strategies for patients with invasive lobular breast cancer. Ann Oncol 33(8):769–785. https://doi.org/10.1016/j.annonc.2022.05.006

van der Groep P, van der Wall E, van Diest PJ (2011) Pathology of hereditary breast cancer. Cell Oncol (Dordr) 34(2):71–88. https://doi.org/10.1007/s13402-011-0010-3

van Seijen M, Lips EH, Thompson AM, Nik-Zainal S, Futreal A, Hwang ES et al (2019) Ductal carcinoma in situ: to treat or not to treat, that is the question. Br J Cancer 121(4):285–292

Varley J (2003) Germline TP53 mutations and Li-Fraumeni syndrome. Hum Mutat 21(3):313–320

Villegas SL, Nekljudova V, Pfarr N, Engel J, Untch M, Schrodi S et al (2021) Therapy response and prognosis of patients with early breast cancer with low positivity for hormone receptors - an analysis of 2765 patients from neoadjuvant clinical trials. Eur J Cancer 148:159–170. https://doi.org/10.1016/j.ejca.2021.02.020

Vogel A, Haupts A, Kloth M, Roth W, Hartmann N (2024) A novel targeted NGS panel identifies numerous homologous recombination deficiency (HRD)-associated gene mutations in addition to known BRCA mutations. Diagn Pathol 19(1):9. https://doi.org/10.1186/s13000-023-01431-8

Voorwerk L, Sanders J, Keusters MS, Balduzzi S, Cornelissen S, Duijst M et al (2023) Immune landscape of breast tumors with low and intermediate estrogen receptor expression. NPJ Breast Cancer 9(1):39. https://doi.org/10.1038/s41523-023-00543-0

Wang L, Geng H, Liu Y, Liu L, Chen Y, Wu F et al (2023) Hot and cold tumors: immunological features and the therapeutic strategies. MedComm (2020) 4(5):e343. https://doi.org/10.1002/mco2.343

Weigelt B, Bi R, Kumar R, Blecua P, Mandelker DL, Geyer FC et al (2018) The landscape of somatic genetic alterations in breast cancers from ATM germline mutation carriers. J Natl Cancer Inst 110(9):1030–1034. https://doi.org/10.1093/jnci/djy028

Weisman PS, Ng CK, Brogi E, Eisenberg RE, Won HH, Piscuoglio S et al (2016) Genetic alterations of triple negative breast cancer by targeted next-generation sequencing and correlation with tumor morphology. Mod Pathol 29(5):476–488. https://doi.org/10.1038/modpathol.2016.39

WHO Classification of Tumours Editorial Board: WHO Classification of Tumours, 5th Edition, Volume 2. Breast Tumours (2019)

Willis J, Lefterova MI, Artyomenko A, Kasi PM, Nakamura Y, Mody K et al (2019) Validation of microsatellite instability detection using a comprehensive plasma-based genotyping panel. Clin Cancer Res 25(23):7035–7045

Willmann L, Schlimpert M, Hirschfeld M, Erbes T, Neubauer H, Stickeler E et al (2016) Alterations of the exo- and endometabolite profiles in breast cancer cell lines: a mass spectrometry-based metabolomics approach. Anal Chim Acta 925:34–42. https://doi.org/10.1016/j.aca.2016.04.047

Wilson JR, Bateman AC, Hanson H, An Q, Evans G, Rahman N et al (2010) A novel HER2-positive breast cancer phenotype arising from germline TP53 mutations. J Med Genet 47(11):771–774. https://doi.org/10.1136/jmg.2010.078113

Wolff AC, Hammond MEH, Allison KH, Harvey BE, Mangu PB, Bartlett JMS et al (2018) Human epidermal growth factor receptor 2 testing in breast cancer: American Society of Clinical Oncology/College of American Pathologists Clinical Practice Guideline Focused Update. J Clin Oncol 36(20):2105–2122. https://doi.org/10.1200/jco.2018.77.8738

Xian Z, Quinones AK, Tozbikian G, Zynger DL (2017) Breast cancer biomarkers before and after neoadjuvant chemotherapy: does repeat testing impact therapeutic management? Hum Pathol 62:215–221. https://doi.org/10.1016/j.humpath.2016.12.019

Xu J, Bao H, Wu X, Wang X, Shao YW, Sun T (2019) Elevated tumor mutation burden and immunogenic activity in patients with hormone receptor-negative or human epidermal growth factor receptor 2-positive breast cancer. Oncol Lett 18(1):449–455. https://doi.org/10.3892/ol.2019.10287

Yamaguchi R, Tanaka M, Yano A, Tse GM, Yamaguchi M, Koura K et al (2012) Tumor-infiltrating lymphocytes are important pathologic predictors for neoadjuvant chemotherapy in patients with breast cancer. Hum Pathol 43(10):1688–1694. https://doi.org/10.1016/j.humpath.2011.12.013

Yang X, Leslie G, Doroszuk A, Schneider S, Allen J, Decker B et al (2020) Cancer risks associated with germline PALB2 pathogenic variants: an international study of 524 families. J Clin Oncol 38(7):674

Yao L, Chen J, Ma W (2023) Decoding TROP2 in breast cancer: significance, clinical implications, and therapeutic advancements. Front Oncol 13. https://doi.org/10.3389/fonc.2023.1292211

Yates LR, Gerstung M, Knappskog S, Desmedt C, Gundem G, Van Loo P et al (2015) Subclonal diversification of primary breast cancer revealed by multiregion sequencing. Nat Med 21(7):751–759. https://doi.org/10.1038/nm.3886

Yoon KH, Park Y, Kang E, Kim EK, Kim JH, Kim SH et al (2022) Effect of estrogen receptor expression level and hormonal therapy on prognosis of early breast cancer. Cancer Res Treat 54(4):1081–1090. https://doi.org/10.4143/crt.2021.890

Yoshida A, Hayashi N, Suzuki K, Takimoto M, Nakamura S, Yamauchi H (2017) Change in HER2 status after neoadjuvant chemotherapy and the prognostic impact in patients with primary breast cancer. J Surg Oncol 116(8):1021–1028. https://doi.org/10.1002/jso.24762

Yu KD, Cai YW, Wu SY, Shui RH, Shao ZM (2021) Estrogen receptor-low breast cancer: biology chaos and treatment paradox. Cancer Commun (Lond) 41(10):968–980. https://doi.org/10.1002/cac2.12191

Yu J, Guo Z, Wang L (2023) Progress and challenges of immunotherapy predictive biomarkers for triple negative breast cancer in the era of single-cell multi-omics. Life (Basel) 13(5). https://doi.org/10.3390/life13051189

Zatreanu D, Robinson HMR, Alkhatib O, Boursier M, Finch H, Geo L et al (2021) Polθ inhibitors elicit BRCA-gene synthetic lethality and target PARP inhibitor resistance. Nat Commun 12(1):3636. https://doi.org/10.1038/s41467-021-23463-8

Zhang X, Li J, Yang Q, Wang Y, Li X, Liu Y et al (2020) Tumor mutation burden and JARID2 gene alteration are associated with short disease-free survival in locally advanced triple-negative breast cancer. Ann Transl Med 8(17):1052

Zheng F, Yue C, Li G, He B, Cheng W, Wang X et al (2016) Nuclear AURKA acquires kinase-independent transactivating function to enhance breast cancer stem cell phenotype. Nat Commun 7:10180. https://doi.org/10.1038/ncomms10180

Zhong E, Scognamiglio T, D'Alfonso T, Song W, Tran H, Baek I et al (2019) Breast tumor resembling the tall cell variant of papillary thyroid carcinoma: molecular characterization by next-generation sequencing and histopathological comparison with tall cell papillary carcinoma of thyroid. Int J Surg Pathol 27(2):134–141. https://doi.org/10.1177/1066896918800779

Zhu S, Lu Y, Fei X, Shen K, Chen X (2023) Pathological complete response, category change, and prognostic significance of HER2-low breast cancer receiving neoadjuvant treatment: a multicenter analysis of 2489 cases. Br J Cancer 129(8):1274–1283. https://doi.org/10.1038/s41416-023-02403-x

14 E-Cadherin-Mediated Cell–Cell Adhesion and Invasive Lobular Breast Cancer

Esme Bullock and Valerie G. Brunton

Abstract

E-cadherin is a transmembrane protein and central component of adherens junctions (AJs). The extracellular domain of E-cadherin forms homotypic interactions with E-cadherin on adjacent cells, facilitating the formation of cell–cell adhesions, known as AJs, between neighbouring cells. The intracellular domain of E-cadherin interacts with α-, β- and p120-catenins, linking the AJs to the actin cytoskeleton. Functional AJs maintain epithelial tissue identity and integrity. Transcriptional downregulation of E-cadherin is the first step in epithelial-to-mesenchymal transition (EMT), a process essential in development and tissue repair, which, in breast cancer, can contribute to tumour progression and metastasis. In addition, loss-of-function mutations in E-cadherin are a defining feature of invasive lobular breast cancer (also known as invasive lobular carcinoma (ILC)), the second most common histological subtype of breast cancer. ILC displays a discohesive, single-file invasive growth pattern due to the loss of functional AJs. Despite being so prevalent, until recently there has been limited ILC-focused research and historically ILC patients have often been excluded from clinical trials. Despite displaying a number of good prognostic indicators, such as low grade and high rates of estrogen receptor positivity, ILC patients tend to have similar or poorer outcomes relative to the most common subtype of breast cancer, invasive ductal carcinoma (IDC). In ILC, E-cadherin loss promotes hyperactivation of growth factor receptors, in particular insulin-like growth factor 1 receptor, anoikis resistance and synthetic lethality with ROS1 inhibition. These features introduce clinical vulnerabilities that could potentially be exploited to improve outcomes for ILC patients, for whom there are currently limited tailored treatments available.

Keywords

E-cadherin · Adherens junctions · Rho GTPases · Actomyosin · Invasive lobular cancer · Anoikis · Epithelial-to-mesenchymal transition

Key Points

- E-cadherin-mediated cell–cell adhesion signalling is critical in normal tissue development
- E-cadherin-mediated AJs serve as key signalling hubs controlling actomyosin

E. Bullock · V. G. Brunton (✉)
Cancer Research UK Scotland Centre (Edinburgh), Institute of Genetics & Cancer, University of Edinburgh, Edinburgh, UK
e-mail: v.brunton@ed.ac.uk

T. Sørlie, R. B. Clarke (eds.), *A Guide to Breast Cancer Research*, Advances in Experimental Medicine and Biology 1464, https://doi.org/10.1007/978-3-031-70875-6_14

contractility and epithelial tissue integrity
- E-cadherin is essential for mammary gland development
- ILC is a distinct histological subtype that is defined by a loss of E-cadherin
- Loss of E-cadherin in breast epithelial cells co-operates with oncogenes, tumour suppressors and actin regulators to promote development of ILC
- Loss of E-cadherin provides cellular vulnerabilities that can be exploited for therapeutic benefit with a number of ongoing clinical trials in ILC

14.1 Introduction

Intercellular adherens junctions (AJs) are fundamental structures within epithelial cells required to maintain tissue integrity. The cadherin–catenin complex is the major component of AJs allowing cells to adhere to adjacent cells and contributing to morphogenesis and tissue repair in epithelial tissues. Classical cadherins are a family of transmembrane proteins that enable calcium-dependent cell–cell adhesion: they include *CDH1* (E-cadherin), *CDH2* (N-cadherin), *CDH3* (P-cadherin), *CDH4* (R-cadherin) and *CDH15* (M-Cadherin). Here we will focus on E-cadherin, which plays a critical role in normal mammary gland development. E-cadherin expression is a defining feature of epithelial identity, and loss of E-cadherin expression is associated with epithelial-to-mesenchymal transition (EMT), a process that occurs during development but is also implicated in breast cancer progression and metastasis. E-cadherin loss is also a defining feature of a histological subtype of breast cancer called invasive lobular carcinoma (ILC). We will cover the latest findings in ILC research that are defining the impact of loss of E-cadherin on the unique behaviour of this breast cancer subtype.

14.2 Adherens Junctions

14.2.1 Structure

E-cadherin is a transmembrane glycoprotein that contains five calcium-dependent extracellular domains that mediate calcium-dependent homotypic cell–cell adhesions. The carboxy-terminal cytoplasmic domain of E-cadherin interacts with α-, β- and p120-catenin, and this complex is essential for the integrity of the AJs, linking them to the intracellular actin and microtubule networks (Fig. 14.1). α-catenin binds F-actin and forms a heterodimer with β-catenin, which binds to the cytoplasmic tail of E-cadherin. The resulting mechanical tension and actomyosin contractility co-operates with the homophilic interactions of the E-cadherin extracellular domains to support E-cadherin clustering and the formation of stable AJs. α-catenin also binds other actin-binding proteins such as vinculin in an actomyosin force-dependent manner, leading to further strengthening of AJ stability. p120-catenin binds E-cadherin at the juxtamembrane region of E-cadherin and stabilises E-cadherin at the cell surface by inhibiting its endocytosis and internalisation. Further details on the molecular interactions within AJs, and the formation of E-cadherin-mediated cell–cell adhesions are provided in these excellent review articles (Mege and Ishiyama 2017; Lecuit and Yap 2015; Katsuno-Kambe and Yap 2020; Zhang et al. 2023).

Glossary

Actomyosin network: Complex of actin and myosin that forms part of the cellular cytoskeleton and is responsible for contraction within cells.

Adherens junctions: Multiprotein adhesion complexes present in epithelial cells that support intercellular adhesion.

Anoikis: A Greek word meaning homelessness, used to describe cell death induced by loss of cellular adhesion to the extracellular matrix (ECM).

Epithelial-to-mesenchymal transition: A reversible process where epithelial cells lose their epithelial identity and undergo multiple biochemical changes to acquire a mesenchymal cell phenotype. The reverse process is termed mesenchymal-to-epithelial transition (MET).

Extracellular matrix: Non-cellular component of tissues composed of multiple macromolecules that provide structural support for tissues.

Dormancy: A process whereby disseminated tumour cells seed and remain quiescent (or dormant) at secondary sites for many years before progressing to form metastases.

Mechanosensing: Cellular response to mechanical stimuli.

RhoGTPases: A family of small signalling G-proteins involved in control of actin.

Sleeping Beauty transposon system: Insertional mutagenesis system utilising synthetic DNA transposon that moves from one genomic location to another by a cut-and-paste mechanism to introduce precise DNA sequences into the genome. Used for unbiased genetic cancer screens in mice.

Synthetic lethality: A genetic interaction where the simultaneous occurrence of two genetic events leads to cell or organism death (lethality), but where the single genetic perturbations are non-lethal.

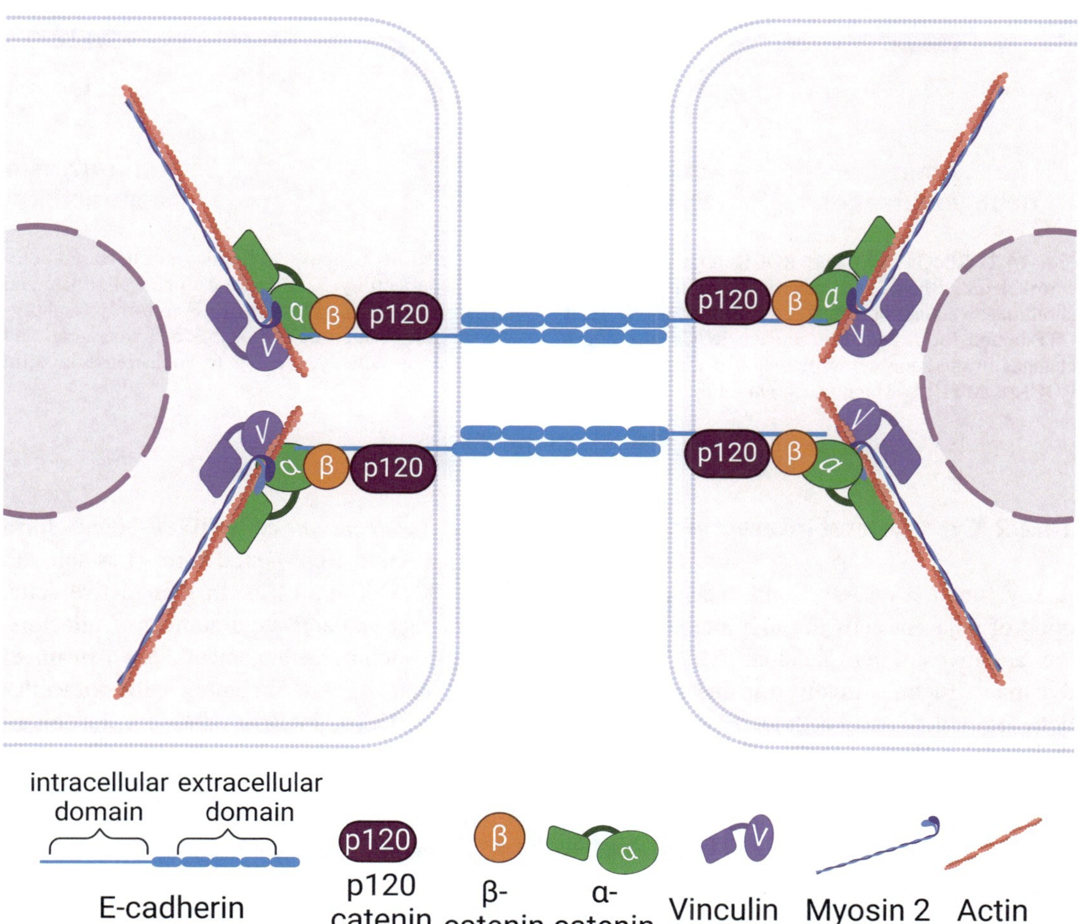

Fig. 14.1 Adherens junctions (AJs). Main structural components of E-cadherin-mediated cell–cell AJs

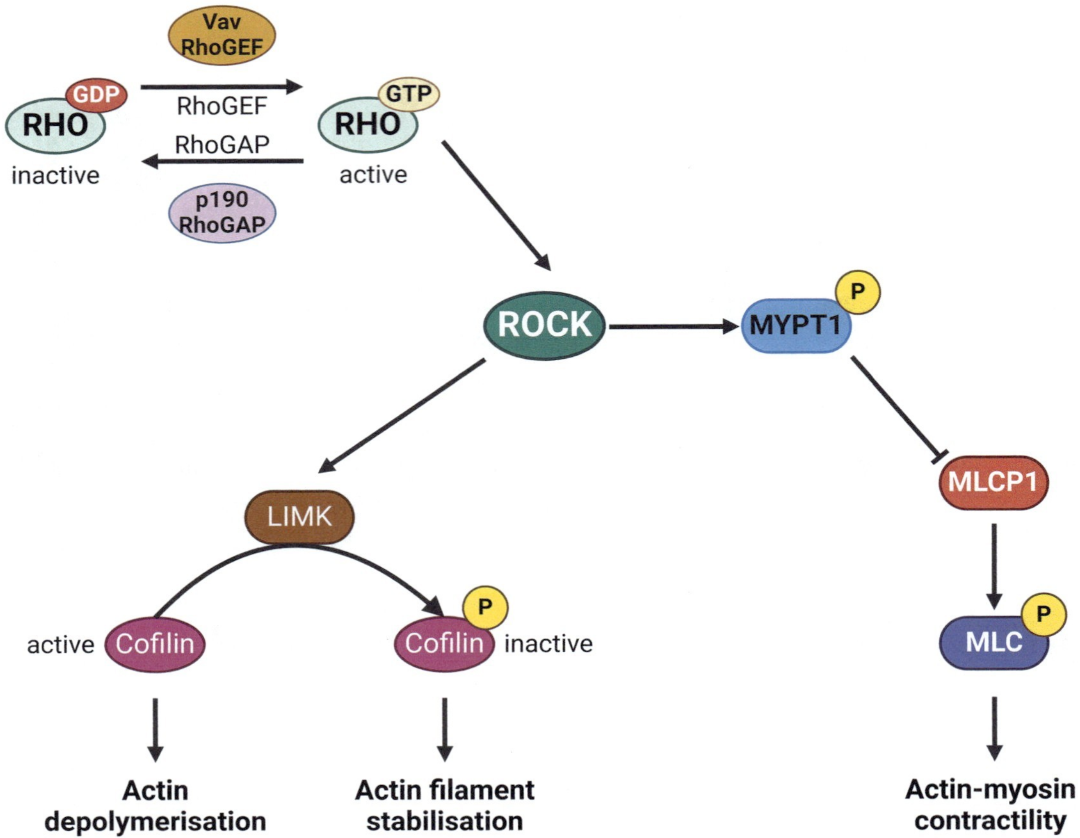

Fig. 14.2 RhoGTPases and ROCK regulate the actin cytoskeleton. RhoGTPase activity is controlled by the coordinated action of RhoGEFs and RhoGAPs. In its GTP-bound form, Rho can activate ROCK, leading to changes in the actin cytoskeleton. A major substrate of ROCK is MYPT1, which leads, via inhibition of MLCP, to increased MLC phosphorylation and increased acto-myosin contractility. ROCK can also phosphorylate and activate LIM-kinase (LIMK). LIMK in turn phosphorylates cofilin, inhibiting its actin-depolymerising and actin-severing activity, leading to an increase in actin filaments

14.2.2 Cytoskeletal Interactions

A key function of AJs is the mechanical coupling of adjacent cells through interactions with the actomyosin cytoskeleton. AJs are highly dynamic structures involved in mechanosensing both from their extracellular environment and from cell-intrinsic mechanical cues. In this way, epithelial cells can resist mechanical stresses and contribute to normal tissue homeostasis. AJs are also signalling hubs that regulate the actomyosin network. Rho GTPases are a family of G-proteins that act as molecular switches cycling between an active GTP-bound form and an inactive GDP-bound form (Lawson and Ridley 2018) (Fig. 14.2). In their active state, they interact and activate a number of effectors, leading to actin rearrangements downstream of extracellular signals, including cell–extracellular matrix (ECM) integrin adhesion, transmembrane tyrosine kinase receptors and G-protein coupled receptors. At AJs, the cadherin–catenin complex also acts to co-ordinate the activity of Rho activators (guanine nucleotide exchange factors (GEFs)) and inactivators (GTPase-activating proteins (GAPs)), and AJ stability depends on myosin II-mediated actomyosin contractility and the co-ordinated activity of the Rho GTPases RhoA, Rac1 and Cdc42. p120-catenin plays an important role in the co-ordinated control of Rho GTPase activity (Schackmann et al. 2013): it can bind directly to RhoA and suppress its activity, or it can recruit other Rho regulatory proteins, including p190RhoGAP and myosin phosphatase interacting protein (MRIP). p120-catenin also interacts with the RhoGEF Vav, resulting in activation of Rac1 and Cdc42 and inactivation of RhoA. One of the main downstream effectors of RhoA is Rho-associated kinase (ROCK), a serine/threonine kinase which plays a major role in mediating rearrangements of the actomyosin cytoskeleton via phosphorylation of the myosin light chain (MLC) (Fig. 14.2). AJs also promote actin assembly by recruiting actin regulators, including the Arp2/3 complex and formins, which nucleate and polymerise actin at sites of E-cadherin-mediated adhesion. This is regulated in part by the recruitment of Arp2/3 regulators such as WAVE2, N-WASP and cortactin, which together promote actin nucleation and AJ stability. The associations between RhoGTPases and actin regulators at AJs are required for actomyosin contractility, although different RhoGTPase effectors have been shown to have opposing effects on AJ integrity (Sahai and Marshall 2002), highlighting the complexity of the signalling pathways involved and the likely cell context dependence of their effects.

14.3 Invasive Lobular Carcinoma

ILC is a histological subtype of breast cancer that is defined by loss of AJs, most frequently due to inactivating mutations in *CDH1* (E-cadherin) (Mouabbi et al. 2022). They are characterised by small, discohesive tumour cells infiltrating into the surrounding stroma in a single-file pattern; thus, classical ILC lacks the cohesive structure that is usually observed in invasive ductal carcinoma (IDC) (Fig. 14.3). This growth pattern is attributed to the early loss of E-cadherin and contributes to difficulties in detection of ILC, as tumours do not classically form a lump, rather presenting as dimpled or 'orange-peel'-like skin. ILC accounts for 10%–15% of breast cancer diagnoses and is the second most common histological subtype of breast cancer, after IDC (also known as invasive breast cancer of no special type (NST)) (Mouabbi et al. 2022). Histologically, ILC is classified into subtypes that refer to different growth patterns and organisation of tumour cells within the breast tissue. These include classical, trabecular, pleomorphic, alveolar, tubulolobular, solid, signet ring cell carcinoma and solid mixed lobular carcinoma, with classical ILC being the most prevalent (Christgen et al. 2021).

The vast majority of ILC tumours are luminal A, with low proliferation, low grade and high expression of estrogen receptor (ER) (Ciriello et al. 2015; Desmedt et al. 2016; Iorfida et al. 2012). However, non-classical ILC

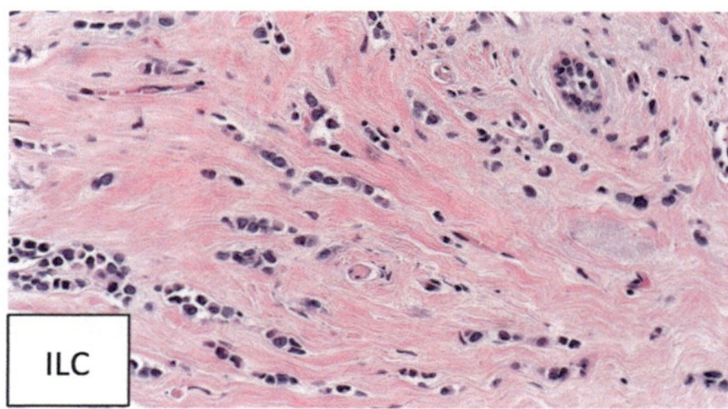

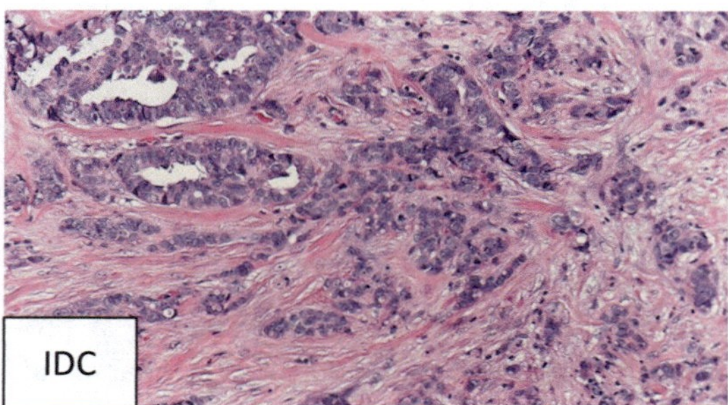

Fig. 14.3 ILC and IDC are morphologically distinct. Representative images of haematoxylin and eosin (H&E)-stained ILC and IDC. Images from https://pathology.jhu.edu/breast/types-of-breast-cancer/

morphological subtypes are more frequently classified as luminal B, particularly the more aggressive pleomorphic subtype (Iorfida et al. 2012). Very few ILC patients are classed as HER2+ (2%–5%) (Ciriello et al. 2015), and most HER2+ tumours are non-classical subtypes. HER2+ ILC has been shown to have the poorest outcomes relative to luminal and triple-negative ILC (TN-ILC), though these analyses included HER2-positive patients from the period before HER2-targeted therapies were routinely used (Iorfida et al. 2012; Okines et al. 2022). TN-ILC patients represent roughly 5% of all ILC patients and 1% of all triple-negative breast cancer (TNBC) patients (Okines et al. 2022; Dalenc et al. 2022; Joshi et al. 2023). However, TN-ILC tumours are often found to be luminal-like rather than basal and to have a poorer response to chemotherapy than TN-IDC tumours (Joshi et al. 2023; Tubiana-Hulin et al. 2006).

ILC tumours have been further categorised into three transcriptomic subtypes based on gene expression (Ciriello et al. 2015). The 'proliferative' subtype is defined by high expression of cell cycle genes and proteins and has the poorest rates of overall survival (OS) of the three. 'Immune-related' tumours have high expression of immune modulatory genes and macrophage-related signatures. The 'reactive-like' subtype is defined by high levels of stromal-related signalling and has significantly lower rates of proliferation and improved OS compared to the proliferative subtype of ILC. Profiling of immune cell populations showed that tumour-infiltrating lymphocytes were significantly lower in ILC compared to IDC and that macrophages are the predominant immune cells in ILC (Desmedt et al. 2018; Onkar et al. 2023). Macrophages within ILC and IDC have divergent phenotypes, with more of the infiltrating macrophages in ILC having a pro-tumourigenic M2-like phenotype (Onkar et al. 2023). Due to the discohesive growth pattern of ILC, they have a much higher stromal content than IDC, and differences in ECM proteins and cancer-associated fibroblast populations between ILC and IDC have been described (Batra et al. 2023; Gomez-Cuadrado et al. 2022; Nakagawa et al. 2016; Park et al. 2016; Westhoff et al. 2020). To date, it is not fully understood what the significance of the unique make-up of the tumour microenvironment in ILC is. However, enrichment of ECM proteins, including the collagen modifying enzyme lysyl oxidase-like 1 (LOXL1), has been reported in ILC, and treatment with a LOX inhibitor was able to decrease tumour growth and metastasis in mice (Sflomos et al. 2021a). The ability to target the ECM environment in ILC provides exciting new potential therapeutic opportunities. Understanding more about the complex interplay between tumour cells and the surrounding microenvironment in ILC, and how it impacts the biology of the disease, will be important going forward.

ILC and IDC tumours both metastasise to the brain, bone, lung and liver, common metastatic sites for breast cancer. However, ILC tumours have a higher rate of metastasis to peritoneum, ovaries and gastrointestinal tract and are less likely to metastasise to the lungs and liver than IDC tumours (Mathew et al. 2017). Metastases to these unusual sites appear to be due to ILC tumour cell intrinsic features, as this metastatic pattern is recapitulated in intraductal xenograft mouse models of human ILC cell lines and in genetically engineered mouse models of ILC (Sflomos et al. 2021b). The molecular mechanisms driving this tropism are not known. Figure 14.4 summarises the key differences between ILC and IDC.

14.3.1 E-cadherin Alterations in Human ILC

E-cadherin loss is responsible for the discohesive growth pattern seen in ILC, and the majority of ILCs lack membranous E-cadherin expression. E-cadherin immunohistochemistry is used to help in the diagnosis of ILC, but in a small number of cases where there is aberrant E-cadherin expression (weak cytoplasmic staining), the identification of cytoplasmic rather than membranous p120-catenin staining can help with a positive diagnosis (Christgen et al. 2021). The lack of E-cadherin expression is mainly due to loss-of-

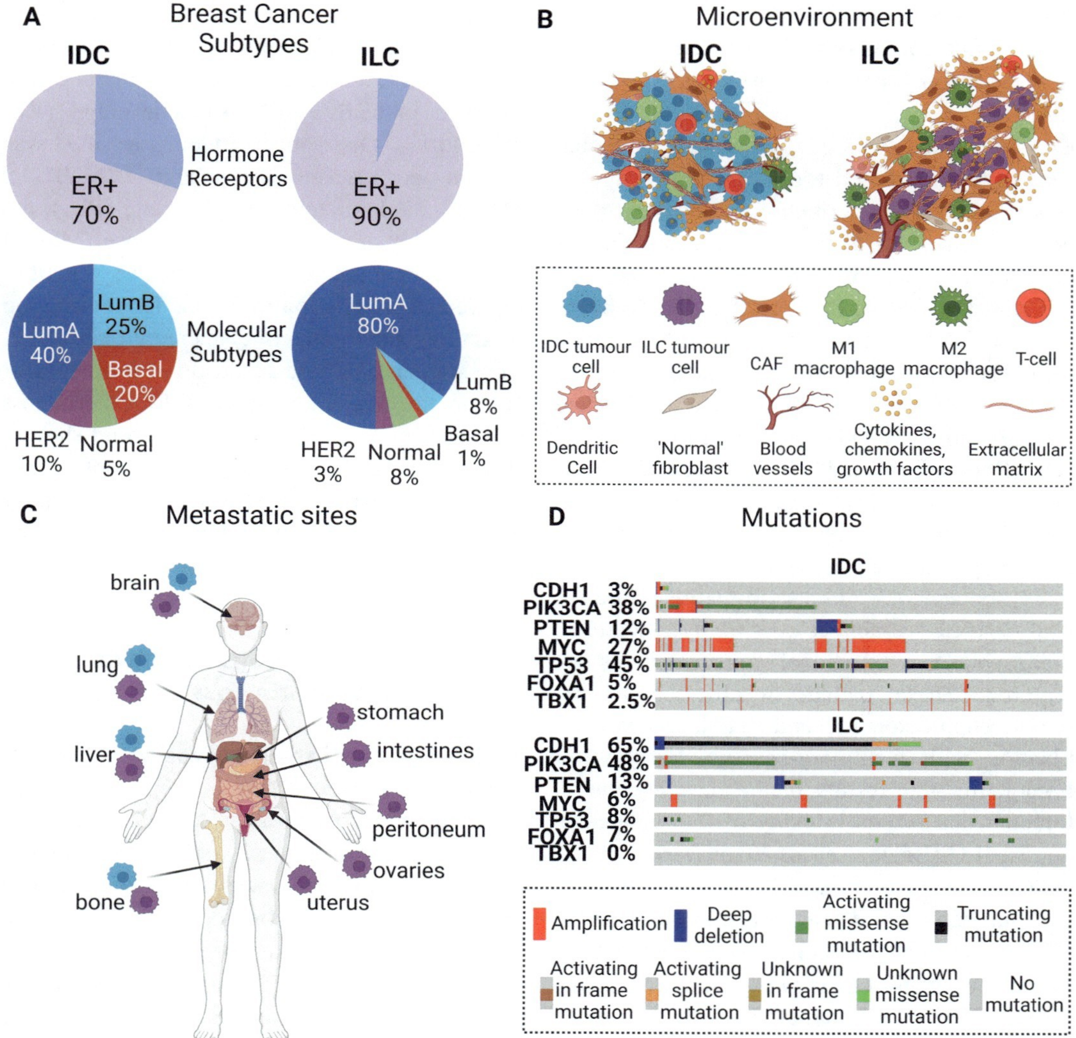

Fig. 14.4 Key differences between ILC and IDC. (**a**) The majority of ILC are ER-positive luminal A tumours. (**b**) The tumour microenvironment differs in ILC and IDC with ILC having higher numbers of CAFs and different immune cell populations. (**c**) ILCs have different preferred sites of metastatic spread compared to IDC. (**d**) ILCs are characterised by loss-of-function mutations in *CDH1* and have a higher incidence of *PIK3CA*, and lower incidence of *MYC* and *TP53* mutations than IDC tumours

function somatic mutations accompanied by loss of heterozygosity of the remaining wild-type *CDH1* allele on chromosome 16q22.1, with promoter methylation only occurring rarely (Ciriello et al. 2015; Desmedt et al. 2016). Epigenetic silencing by hypermethylation of the *CDH1* gene promoter has only been reported in rare cases and does not appear to play a significant role in downregulation of E-cadherin expression in ILC. This genetic and epigenetic control of E-cadherin expression in ILC contrasts what is seen in IDC which lack E-cadherin expression, where somatic mutations are rare and hypermethylation of the *CDH1* promoter is more prevalent. Interestingly, germline-inactivating *CDH1* mutations are responsible for hereditary diffuse gastric cancer (HDGC), and there is an increased risk of ILC in HDGC families. Subsequently, germline *CDH1* mutations have also been identified in ILC in the absence of HDGC (Masciari et al. 2007).

14.3.2 E-cadherin in ILC Development: Evidence from Mouse Studies

E-cadherin is expressed by luminal epithelial cells in the breast and forms AJs between adjacent cells, which are critical for mammary gland development. Loss of E-cadherin leads to a loss of epithelial architecture and morphogenesis (Shamir et al. 2014; Boelens et al. 2016) but is not associated with the dissemination of single cells. Rather in mice, loss of E-cadherin in the mammary gland limits epithelial cell survival and leads to apoptosis and clearance of the epithelial cells (Boussadia et al. 2002; Derksen et al. 2011). Studies in genetically engineered mouse models have shown that inactivation of E-cadherin in the mammary gland of mice is not sufficient to promote spontaneous tumour formation (Boelens et al. 2016; Boussadia et al. 2002; Derksen et al. 2006), but that additional genetic drivers are required. These include inactivation of the tumour suppressors p53 and PTEN, and, in combination with mammary-specific depletion of E-cadherin, this results in the development of tumours that resemble many of the features of human ILC (Boelens et al. 2016; Derksen et al. 2006; Annunziato et al. 2016). Phosphatase and TENsin homolog deleted on chromosome 10 (PTEN) is a dual-specificity phosphatase and key negative regulator of the phosphatidylinositol-3-kinase (PI3K)/AKT signalling pathway, which controls cell growth, proliferation and survival, and is a critical regulator of tumour development (Lee et al. 2018). Activating mutations in AKT also synergise with E-cadherin to induce ILC formation (Annunziato et al. 2016), further supporting the importance of the PI3K/AKT signalling pathway in the genesis of ILC. Activation of the PI3K pathway rescues the apoptosis induced by E-cadherin loss in mouse mammary epithelium.

In addition to co-operation with oncogenes and tumour suppressor genes, loss of E-cadherin also co-operates with actin regulators to enable ILC formation. In normal mammary epithelial cells, loss of E-cadherin induces ROCK-dependent phosphorylation of MLC and actomyosin contractility, which reduces their adhesion and survival, thereby preventing tumour formation (Schipper et al. 2019). In an insertional mutagenesis screen using the *Sleeping Beauty* transposon system in mice with mammary-specific inactivation of *Cdh1*, a number of actin regulators were identified in the ILC tumours that developed (Kas et al. 2017). One actin regulator identified was myosin phosphatase target subunit 1 (MYPT1). MYPT1 binds protein phosphatase 1 (PP1), the catalytic subunit of MLC phosphatase (MLCP) and reduces actomyosin contractility by facilitating dephosphorylation of MLC. This relaxation of actomyosin contractility increased cell adhesion and survival and could drive formation of ILC in mice in the context of E-cadherin loss (Schipper et al. 2019). The same group showed that apoptosis stimulating protein of p53-2 (ASPP2) also reduced actomyosin contractility and was required for the initiation of ILC formation in mice (Schipper et al. 2020).

14.3.3 Functional Consequences of E-cadherin Loss

14.3.3.1 Migration and Invasion

Early studies showed that E-cadherin could act as a suppressor of invasion and that inhibition of E-cadherin function was sufficient to induce the dissociation and invasion of epithelial cancer cells (Birchmeier and Behrens 1994). However, this is too simplistic and dependent on the cellular context; E-cadherin can also promote migration and invasion (Shamir and Ewald 2015). Unlike in ILC, loss of E-cadherin in many IDC breast cancers is linked with transcriptional downregulation of E-cadherin expression. This is often associated with a process called EMT, which, for many years, has been proposed to be an important driver of epithelial cancer progression (Thiery 2002; Sun and Ma 2024) (Fig. 14.5). EMT was first identified during embryonic development, where epithelial cells lose their cell–cell contacts and adopt a mesenchymal migratory and invasive phenotype in response to cues from the external environment. This is associated with the loss of E-cadherin and the concomitant acquisition of mesenchymal markers, including N-cadherin and vimentin. EMT is triggered by pleiotropic signals and is controlled by transcription factors including SNAIL, SLUG, TWIST and ZEB1/2 and miRNAs. The classical description of EMT as a

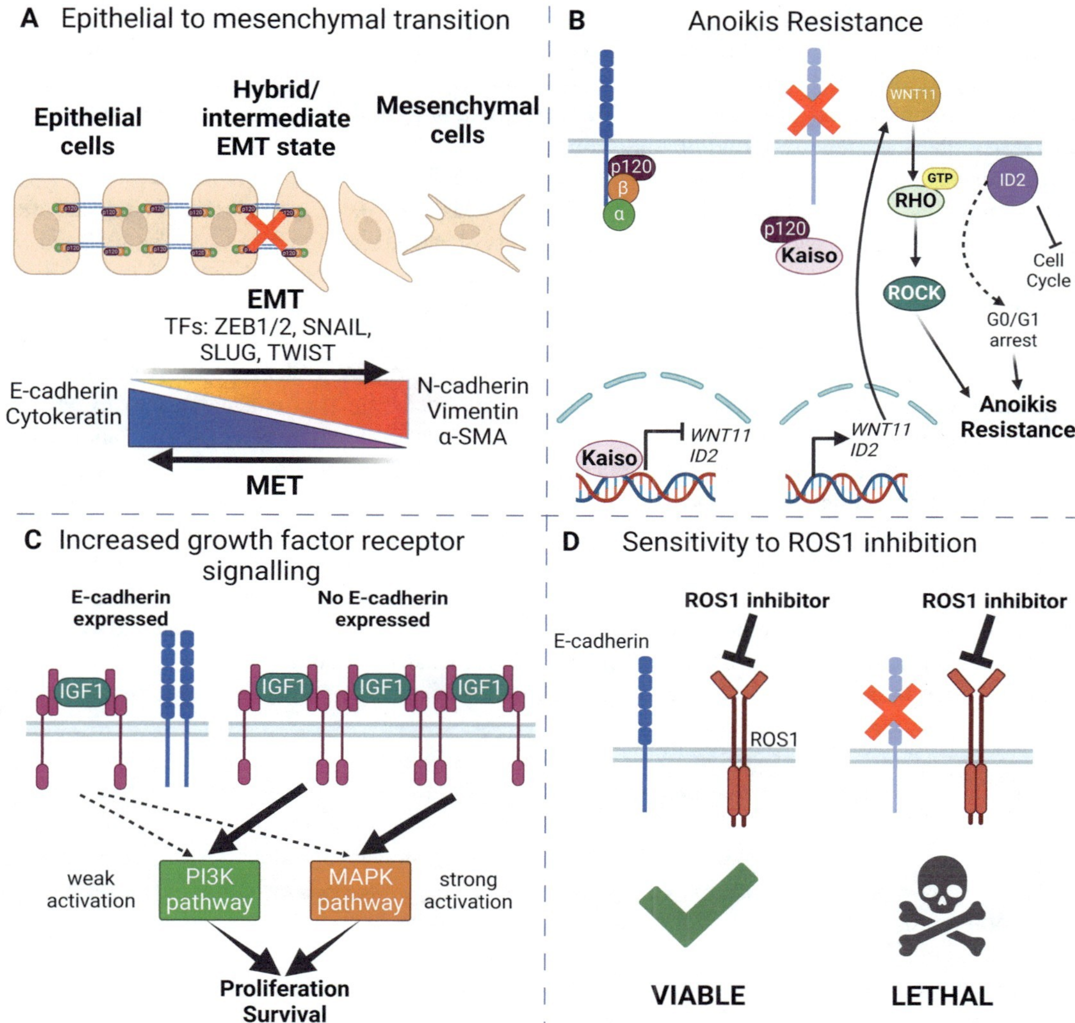

Fig. 14.5 Consequences of E-cadherin loss in tumours. (**a**) Transcriptional downregulation of E-cadherin leads to an EMT, with a loss of epithelial cell markers and acquisition of mesenchymal markers leading to more migratory and invasive cells. These are highly plastic states and tumours can exist in hybrid/intermediate EMT states and can also undergo a MET, reverting back to an epithelial-like phenotype. (**b**) E-cadherin-deficient cells are resistant to anchorage-independent-induced cell death known as anoikis. Loss of E-cadherin leads to a translocation of p120-catenin from the membrane to the cytoplasm, and it can shuttle to the nucleus, where it binds to the transcriptional repressor Kaiso, preventing its repression of genes including *WNT11* and *ID2*. Signalling downstream of WNT11 and ID2 promotes anoikis resistance via RhoGTPase activation and cell cycle arrest. (**c**) Loss of E-cadherin leads to increased growth factor signalling. The exact mechanisms are not known, but loss of E-cadherin can regulate the amount of growth factor receptors that are available at the cell surface for ligand binding, resulting in increased pathway activation. (**d**) Synthetic lethal interaction between E-cadherin loss and inhibition of the receptor tyrosine kinase ROS1 leads to increased cell death in E-cadherin-deficient cells

two-state process has now been revised with an understanding that cells are highly plastic and can transition through intermediate EMT states and frequently undergo a partial EMT programme, where they express both epithelial and mesenchymal markers (Nieto et al. 2016). Although EMT can promote invasion and metastasis, most metastases consist of epithelial cells which are presumed to have undergone a mesenchymal-to-epithelial transition (MET), whereby they regain their epithelial traits. However, there are a number of reports in mouse models demonstrating that metastatic spread is dependent on repression of EMT, supporting a cell- and tissue-dependent mechanism in driving the disparate effects of EMT on tumour progression (Aouad et al. 2023). EMT also plays an important role in controlling the dormancy of disseminated tumour cells at metastatic sites, and restoration of an epithelial phenotype via reexpression of E-cadherin and MET can promote escape from dormancy and the outgrowth of metastatic cells (Aouad et al. 2022).

In non-malignant breast epithelial cells, E-cadherin loss alters cytoskeletal organisation and adhesion, but is insufficient to induce an EMT (Chen et al. 2014), and early E-cadherin loss in the context of ILC development in mice is not sufficient to induce EMT (Derksen et al. 2006). This is consistent with data in human ILC, where despite the loss of E-cadherin, ILC retain the morphological features associated with epithelial cells and do not demonstrate the co-ordinated alteration of multiple EMT markers, as seen in other breast cancer subtypes (McCart Reed et al. 2016). The characteristic single-file invasive growth pattern in ILC is therefore unlikely to be aligned with an EMT, although a partial or hybrid EMT state cannot be ruled out.

14.3.3.2 Resistance to Anoikis

Anoikis is a type of apoptosis that is induced after loss of cell adhesion to the ECM. Cell–ECM interactions are generally mediated by integrin receptors, which form multimolecular scaffolding and signalling complexes called focal adhesions (see Box: Integrin-Dependent Focal Adhesions). In normal cells, integrin engagement to ECM proteins initiates pro-survival signals, and anoikis is a physiological defence mechanism that is required for development and tissue homeostasis. However, cancer cells are resistant to anoikis, and the resulting survival advantage is a recognised hallmark of cancer cells, playing an important role in their metastatic dissemination (Hanahan and Weinberg 2011; Khan et al. 2022).

Integrin-Dependent Focal Adhesions

Integrins are transmembrane receptors for extra-cellular ligands including ECM proteins. They consist of α- and β-subunit heterodimers: there are 18 α- and 8 β-subunits that can combine to form 24 different integrin heterodimers that have overlapping functions with respect to ligand binding and downstream signalling. Integrins undergo both inside-out and outside-in signalling, where they act as signalling hubs, transmitting signals between the interior of the cell and the extracellular environment to regulate adhesion, while extracellular ligand binding can activate intracellular signalling pathways (Kadry and Calderwood 1862). Integrin activation occurs through a multistep process: initially, the intracellular adaptor proteins kindlin and talin are recruited to the integrin cytoplasmic tails, which leads to a conformational change in the integrin heterodimer that drives external ligand engagement and connection with the intracellular actin cytoskeleton. This promotes full integrin activation and the formation of focal adhesions, which are multi-protein complexes that tether cells to the ECM. Focal adhesions are dynamic structures made up of a large number of cytoskeletal and signalling molecules including the non-receptor tyrosine kinases SRC and focal adhesion kinase (FAK), which initiate downstream signalling (Horton et al. 2015). These complex and dynamic structures play important roles in many cellular processes, and, in cancer, have been implicated in all aspects of tumour development and progression including cancer initiation and proliferation, increased migration and invasion, extravasation and anchorage-independent survival and formation of the metastatic niche (Hamidi and Ivaska 2018). Extensive crosstalk exists between E-cadherin-mediated AJs and integrin-mediated cell–ECM adhesion complexes and their association with the actin cytoskeleton, with many of the same molecules present in both adhesion types. This crosstalk helps to fine-tune the dynamic interplay between cells and the surrounding environment and controls diverse cellular processes such as polarity and migration (Mui et al. 2016).

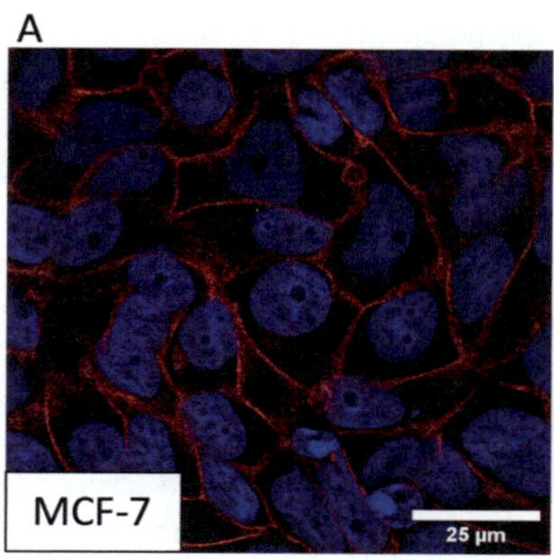

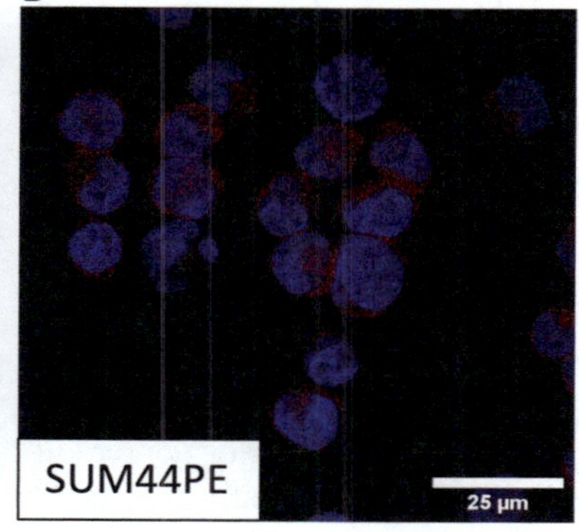

Fig. 14.6 Cellular p120-catenin localisation is dependent on E-cadherin at AJs. Immunofluorescence images of p120-catenin (red) in E-cadherin-expressing MCF-7 IDC cells (**a**) and E-cadherin-deficient SUM44PE ILC cells (**b**). Nuclei stained with DAPI (blue). Note the cytoplasmic localisation of p120-catenin in the E-cadherin-deficient SUM44PE cells

E-cadherin loss renders cells more resistant to anoikis (Derksen et al. 2006), with ILC cell lines being far more resistant to anoikis in anchorage-independent conditions compared to E-cadherin-positive IDC cell lines (Tasdemir et al. 2018, 2020). In cells lacking functional E-cadherin and AJs, p120-catenin is released from the AJ and relocalised from its juxtamembrane position to the cytoplasm (Fig. 14.6). Cytoplasmic p120-catenin promotes anoikis resistance via inhibition of actomyosin contractility and activation of Rho/ROCK signalling (Schackmann et al. 2011). p120-catenin shuttles from the cytoplasm to the nucleus, and within the nucleus it binds to the transcriptional repressor Kaiso. *Wnt11* is a direct and p120-catenin-dependent Kaiso target gene that regulates ILC anoikis resistance through the autocrine activation of RhoA (van de Ven et al. 2015). In addition, E-cadherin loss promotes the expression of inhibitor of DNA binding 2 (Id2) proteins due to a direct p120-catenin/Kaiso-dependent transcriptional de-repression (Ratze et al. 2022). Id2 is essential for anoikis resistance in models of ILC, where it promotes a CDK4/6-dependent G0/G1 cell cycle arrest (Fig. 14.5).

14.3.3.3 Increased Growth Factor Signalling

In breast cancer cell lines, loss of E-cadherin leads to increased insulin-like growth factor 1 (IGF-1) pathway activation through the IGF-1 receptor (IGF-1R) (Elangovan et al. 2022; Erdem et al. 2016; Nagle et al. 2018; Teo et al. 2018). IGF-1 signalling plays a crucial role in breast cancer growth, survival and metastasis (Christopoulos et al. 2015; Farabaugh et al. 2015). The IGF-1R is a transmembrane receptor that belongs to the receptor tyrosine kinase family, and it consists of two extracellular α-subunits and two transmembrane β-subunits. Upon IGF-1 binding, IGF-1R undergoes conformational changes, which trigger the autophosphorylation and activation of its tyrosine kinase domain, leading to downstream activation of signalling pathways via the insulin receptor substrate 1 adaptor protein (IRS-1). E-cadherin regulates the amount of IGF1-R available for ligand binding at the cell surface, resulting in increased pathway activation. The two predominant IGF-1 responsive pathways are the PI3K/AKT pathway, and the rapidly accelerated fibrosarcoma (RAF) kinase/mitogen-activated protein kinase (RAF/MAPK) pathway, which can both provide proliferative and survival signals (Christopoulos et al. 2015; Farabaugh et al. 2015) (Fig. 14.5). Forced expression of E-cadherin in a breast cancer cell line was able to attenuate signalling via IGF-1 and also epidermal growth factor (EGF), suggesting that increased growth factor signalling may be a more general consequence of E-cadherin loss (Qian et al. 2004).

14.4 Clinical Implications of E-cadherin Loss

14.4.1 Current Treatment Options and Outcomes for ILC

Although ILC tumours display a number of features considered to be good prognostic indicators, including low grade, slow proliferation and high ER expression, generally ILC patients have been shown to have either similar or poorer outcomes relative to IDC patients (Batra et al. 2023; Adachi et al. 2016; Arpino et al. 2004; Chen et al. 2017; Korhonen et al. 2013; Timbres et al. 2021; Dayan et al. 2023). Generally, in the short term, ILC patients have better OS than IDC patients, possibly due to the slow-growing nature of ILC tumours. However, in longer-term analyses (up to 20 years), ILC patients have been shown to have poorer outcomes than IDC patients (Chen et al. 2017; Pestalozzi et al. 2008; Rakha et al. 2008; Oesterreich et al. 2022), potentially reflecting the higher rate of late recurrences in ILC. A recent retrospective analysis of a French multicentre cohort demonstrated poorer OS for metastatic ILC patients with matched clinical characteristics to metastatic IDC patients (Dalenc et al. 2022), although OS for TN-ILC patients was better, OS for HER2+ ILC was similar to that of IDC and OS of ER+/PR+/HER2− was worse than that of IDC. However, another study found no differences in survival between metastatic ILC and IDC patients (Thill et al. 2023), though there was a shorter median OS for ILC patients approaching significance.

Numerous studies have shown that ILC patients have decreased response rates to chemotherapy and poorer OS compared to chemotherapy-treated IDC patients (reviewed in Van Baelen et al. (2022)). Despite the large size of ILC tumours at diagnosis, the vast majority of ILC tumours are low-grade with slow rates of proliferation, which could account for this discrepancy in chemotherapy response between ILC and IDC. However, when comparing stage-matched ILC and IDC patients treated with chemotherapy, ILC patients still have decreased OS, suggesting that other ILC phenotypes may influence chemotherapy response.

As the vast majority (90%–95%) of ILC tumours are ER+, the first-line treatment is with endocrine-targeted therapy. Several studies have shown that response rates differ between ILC and IDC patients and also between different treatments. For example, in the Breast International Group (BIG) 1–98 trial, while there was no difference in OS or disease-free survival (DFS) for IDC patients treated with either the selective estrogen modulator tamoxifen or the aromatase inhibitor letrozole, ILC patients treated with tamoxifen had a significantly worse OS and DFS than those treated with letrozole (Metzger Filho et al. 2015). Tamoxifen-treated ILC patients also had a far worse outcome than both tamoxifen- and letrozole-treated IDC patients. In vitro studies have shown that ILC cell lines respond differently from IDC cell lines to estrogen- and endocrine-targeted therapies. An ILC-specific estrogen responsive set of genes has been identified, and ILC cell lines have been shown to be more tamoxifen-resistant than IDC cell lines (Nardone et al. 2022; Sottnik et al. 2021). In vitro models of tamoxifen resistance in ILC cell lines have identified a number of resistance mechanisms, including upregulation of fatty acid metabolism (Du et al. 2018), increased expression of the ILC-specific estrogen response gene *WNT4*, leading to increased proliferation and mammalian target of rapamycin (mTOR) activation (Sikora et al. 2016), and the ILC-specific interaction between ERα and a co-regulator, mediator of DNA damage checkpoint 1 (MDC1) (Sottnik et al. 2021).

A chromatin state unique to ILC, driven by the pioneer factor FOXA1, has also been shown to promote tamoxifen resistance by allowing the retention of ERα at promoters that are lost in tamoxifen-treated IDC cells (Nardone et al. 2022). This chromatin state was found to be independent of E-cadherin expression and to specifically associate with worse outcomes in luminal A ILC but not IDC, highlighting another unique feature of ILC cell lines that requires further exploration.

14.4.2 New Potential Treatment Options for ILC

Several studies have shown strong associations between IGF-1R pathway activation and clinical outcomes in breast cancer patients (Creighton et al. 2008; Law et al. 2008; Litzenburger et al. 2011), and a number of approaches to target the IGF-1/IGF-1R signalling axis have been developed. These include IGF-1-neutralising antibodies, anti-IGF-1R antibodies and dual insulin receptor (IR)/IGF-1R tyrosine kinase inhibitors (Ianza et al. 2021; Lee et al. 2022). Although these have been trialled extensively in a range of tumour types, including breast cancer, the results have been disappointing, either due to a lack of efficacy resulting from activation of compensatory signalling pathways linked to systemic effects on insulin secretion, or metabolic toxicity. Attempts to identify molecular markers that would predict sensitivity to targeting IGF-1/IGF-1R signalling identified increased sensitivity to IGF-1 activation in cell lines that had lost E-cadherin (see Sect. 14.3.3.3). Furthermore, in clinical datasets, increased levels of phosphorylated IGF-1R and downstream pathway activation were found in ILC compared to IDC tumours. In addition, increased levels of IGF-1 and IGF-2 ligands in ILC compared to IDC tumours have been reported (Nakagawa et al. 2016; Nagle et al. 2018; Teo et al. 2018). Together, this suggests that ILC tumours may be more dependent on IGF-1 signalling for their proliferation and survival, providing a potential therapeutic opportunity for the treatment of patients with ILC. In support of this, loss of E-cadherin can sensitise cells to treatment with IGF-1R and PI3K inhibitors (Elangovan et al. 2022; Nagle et al. 2018; Teo et al. 2018).

After *CDH1* mutations, activating point mutations in *PIK3CA* are the most common mutations in ILC, being more prevalent in ILC than in IDC (Fig. 14.4). Over half of ILC tumours have mutually exclusive activating mutations in *PIK3CA* and *AKT1* or inactivating mutations in *PTEN*, leading to persistent activation of the PI3K/AKT pathway (Ciriello et al. 2015; Desmedt et al. 2016). PI3K-targeted therapies have been shown to modestly increase progression-free survival in metastatic breast cancer, particularly in *PIK3CA*-mutated tumours, though with high rates of side effects and resistance. Several trials are currently ongoing, investigating the combination of PI3K-targeted drugs with CDK4/6 inhibitors and endocrine therapies in metastatic ER+/HER2− breast cancer (Fuso et al. 2022). To date no studies have specifically investigated or reported on the response of ILC tumours to PI3K-targeted therapies. However, due to the high frequency of *PIK3CA* and *PTEN* mutations in ILC and hyperactivation of the pathway, PI3K-targeted therapy is an attractive potential therapeutic option for ILC.

Loss of E-cadherin can also lead to increased growth factor-mediated PI3K pathway activation in the absence of *PIK3CA* or *PTEN* mutations, leading to sensitivity to AKT inhibitors (Teo et al. 2018). Thus, such targeted therapies may provide benefit in a wider cohort of ILC patients. Other clinically actionable genomic alterations in ILC have been identified in a small number of cases and include *BRCA1* and *BRCA2* mutations, *HER2* amplification and *NTRK1-3* fusions, with evidence of further genomic alterations that may provide potential new treatment options (Van Baelen et al. 2022).

Synthetic lethality screening (see Box: Synthetic Lethality), to identify lethal genetic interactions with E-cadherin loss, identified the tyrosine kinase ROS1 (Bajrami et al. 2018) (Fig. 14.5). Using isogeneic E-cadherin-deficient breast cancer cells, synthetic lethality was identified in a siRNA sensitivity screen targeting >1000 cell-cycle control genes, kinase-coding genes or DNA repair-related genes. A small-molecule inhibitor screen also identified ROS1 inhibitors as candidate synthetic lethal drugs, with sensitivity to ROS1 inhibitors being validated in a range of breast cancer cell lines with defective E-cadherin expression. ROS1 inhibitors showed activity in multiple models of ILC, supporting clinical trials with this class of drug in ILC patients (see Sect. 14.4.3). ROS1 inhibitors induced mitotic abnormalities and multinucleation in E-cadherin-defective cells, which was associated with a defect in cytokinesis and aberrant p120-catenin phosphorylation, which controls actomyosin contractility during mitosis.

Synthetic Lethality

This refers to a genetic interaction where the simultaneous occurrence of two genetic events leads to cell or organism death (lethality), but where the single genetic perturbations are non-lethal. Initially, the term referred to an incompatibility between pairs of mutations in *Drosophila* and was first proposed as a potential drug discovery tool in 1997 (Hartwell et al. 1997). In the context of cancer, it refers to a situation where inactivation of one gene by deletion or mutation renders cells exceptionally sensitive to the perturbation of another gene or its protein product by pharmacological inhibition. In principle, this would lead to selective killing of tumour cells harbouring specific mutations, while normal cells are spared the effect of the drug (Huang et al. 2020).

The first example of a clinically actionable synthetic lethality was the treatment of BRCA1- or BRCA2-deficient tumours with poly(ADP-ribose) polymerase (PARP) inhibitors (Lord and Ashworth 2017). Normally, PARP activity is not essential, but in the absence of *BRCA* gene function, PARP activity is critical for cell survival. In clinical trials, PARP inhibitors can elicit significant and sustained antitumor responses in patients with *BRCA1* or *-2* mutant tumours and have now been licenced for use in *BRCA*-mutated ovarian and breast cancers. However, true synthetic lethal interactions are very rare, and often those that have been identified in the preclinical setting have been difficult to translate into the clinical setting due to the complexity of the genetic interactions and the influence of the surrounding tumour environment (Ryan et al. 2023).

14.4.3 ILC-Specific Clinical Trials

The ongoing ROSALINE (NCT04551495) and ROLo (NCT03620643) trials are both focused on targeting the tyrosine kinase ROS1, the inhibition of which has shown synthetic lethality with E-cadherin loss in vitro and to reduce growth of primary E-cadherin negative tumours in vivo (Bajrami et al. 2018). The ROSALINE trial is using a combination of the ROS1 inhibitor entrectinib and endocrine therapy in early-stage ER+ ILC (Agostinetto et al. 2022) whereas ROLo is using the ROS1 inhibitor crizotinib either alone or in combination with fulvestrant in metastatic ILC (NCT03620643). The PELOPS trial (NCT02764541) is also ongoing, and is looking at response to the CDK4/6 inhibitor palbociclib in combination with either tamoxifen or letrozole in ILC and IDC patients. The recently reported GELATo trial demonstrated partial response or stable disease in 6 out of 23 metastatic ILC patients treated with carboplatin and the immune checkpoint inhibitor atezolizumab (anti-PD-L1) (Voorwerk et al. 2023). However, four out of six responsive tumours were triple-negative ILC, representing a relatively small population of ILC patients.

14.5 Conclusions

E-cadherin-mediated AJs are critical for epithelial cell integrity linking the actin cytoskeleton to mechanical stimuli through a complex network of signalling and regulator proteins. However, in breast cancer, E-cadherin expression is often lost either through loss-of-function truncating mutations, which are characteristic of ILC, or via transcriptional downregulation of E-cadherin mediated via an EMT program, as is common in IDC. Loss of E-cadherin is a key marker of EMT and although it promotes a more invasive and migratory phenotype, not all breast cancers are required to undergo EMT to metastasise and the mechanism governing the disparate effects of EMT on cancer progression are still be uncovered.

In ILC. the positive prognostic factors associated with ILC do not translate into improved survival compared to IDC patients. This emphasises the need for ILC to be treated as a disease distinct from IDC, with more ILC-focused research and trials required. Historically, ILC patients have either been excluded from clinical trials or results for ILC patients have not been reported separately from those of IDC patients, with both subtypes combined in an ER+ or luminal group. In trials in the metastatic setting, proportionally fewer ILC patients are included, often due to the diffuse growth pattern of ILC metastases in more unusual metastatic sites, making 'measurable disease' more difficult to determine (Abel et al. 2021). However, there is now considerable evidence from in vitro studies and analyses of trials where ILC-specific data is available, showing that ILC and IDC tumours have differing responses to therapies. Progress in the development of ILC-specific therapies has been hampered by the scarcity of good preclinical models to predict the efficacy of novel treatments. This is partly due to the lower incidence of ILC and fewer ILC patients in clinical trials, along with the intrinsic characteristics of ILC that make it difficult to grow ILC tumours following transplantation into mice, or grow as organoids. For example, the loss of Ecadherin expression and lack of AJs impede proper 3D formation, development and expansion of noncohesive ILC organoids. However, considerable efforts are being made to develop, characterise and refine ILC models (Sflomos et al. 2021b), which will provide further understanding of the complex biology and help identify new therapeutic targets. The ability to harness vulnerabilities resulting from the disruption of E-cadherin-mediated AJs has the exciting potential to provide personalised therapies for ILC patients in the future.

References

Abel MK et al (2021) Decreased enrollment in breast cancer trials by histologic subtype: does invasive lobular carcinoma resist RECIST? NPJ Breast Cancer 7(1):139

Adachi Y et al (2016) Comparison of clinical outcomes between luminal invasive ductal carcinoma and luminal invasive lobular carcinoma. BMC Cancer 16:248

Agostinetto E et al (2022) ROSALINE: a phase II, neoadjuvant study targeting ROS1 in combination with endocrine therapy in invasive lobular carcinoma of the breast. Future Oncol 18(22):2383–2392

Annunziato S et al (2016) Modeling invasive lobular breast carcinoma by CRISPR/Cas9-mediated somatic genome editing of the mammary gland. Genes Dev 30(12):1470–1480

Aouad P et al (2022) Epithelial-mesenchymal plasticity determines estrogen receptor positive breast cancer dormancy and epithelial reconversion drives recurrence. Nat Commun 13(1):4975

Aouad P et al (2023) Tumor dormancy: EMT beyond invasion and metastasis. Genesis 62:e23552

Arpino G et al (2004) Infiltrating lobular carcinoma of the breast: tumor characteristics and clinical outcome. Breast Cancer Res 6(3):R149–R156

Bajrami I et al (2018) E-cadherin/ROS1 inhibitor synthetic lethality in breast cancer. Cancer Discov 8(4):498–515

Batra H et al (2023) Exploration of cancer associated fibroblasts phenotypes in the tumor microenvironment of classical and pleomorphic invasive lobular carcinoma. Front Oncol 13:1281650

Birchmeier W, Behrens J (1994) Cadherin expression in carcinomas: role in the formation of cell junctions and the prevention of invasiveness. Biochim Biophys Acta 1198(1):11–26

Boelens MC et al (2016) PTEN loss in E-cadherin-deficient mouse mammary epithelial cells rescues apoptosis and results in development of classical invasive lobular carcinoma. Cell Rep 16(8):2087–2101

Boussadia O et al (2002) E-cadherin is a survival factor for the lactating mouse mammary gland. Mech Dev 115(1–2):53–62

Chen A et al (2014) E-cadherin loss alters cytoskeletal organization and adhesion in non-malignant breast cells but is insufficient to induce an epithelial-mesenchymal transition. BMC Cancer 14:552

Chen Z et al (2017) Invasive lobular carcinoma of the breast: a special histological type compared with invasive ductal carcinoma. PLoS One 12(9):e0182397

Christgen M et al (2021) Lobular breast cancer: histomorphology and different concepts of a special spectrum of tumors. Cancers (Basel) 13(15)

Christopoulos PF, Msaouel P, Koutsilieris M (2015) The role of the insulin-like growth factor-1 system in breast cancer. Mol Cancer 14:43

Ciriello G et al (2015) Comprehensive molecular portraits of invasive lobular breast cancer. Cell 163(2): 506–519

Creighton CJ et al (2008) Insulin-like growth factor-I activates gene transcription programs strongly associated with poor breast cancer prognosis. J Clin Oncol 26(25):4078–4085

Dalenc F et al (2022) Impact of lobular versus ductal histology on overall survival in metastatic breast cancer: a French retrospective multicentre cohort study. Eur J Cancer 164:70–79

Dayan D et al (2023) Effect of histological breast cancer subtypes invasive lobular versus non-special type on survival in early intermediate-to-high-risk breast carcinoma: results from the SUCCESS trials. Breast Cancer Res 25(1):153

Derksen PW et al (2006) Somatic inactivation of E-cadherin and p53 in mice leads to metastatic lobular mammary carcinoma through induction of anoikis resistance and angiogenesis. Cancer Cell 10(5):437–449

Derksen PW et al (2011) Mammary-specific inactivation of E-cadherin and p53 impairs functional gland development and leads to pleomorphic invasive lobular carcinoma in mice. Dis Model Mech 4(3):347–358

Desmedt C et al (2016) Genomic characterization of primary invasive lobular breast cancer. J Clin Oncol 34(16):1872–1881

Desmedt C et al (2018) Immune infiltration in invasive lobular breast cancer. J Natl Cancer Inst 110(7): 768–776

Du T et al (2018) Key regulators of lipid metabolism drive endocrine resistance in invasive lobular breast cancer. Breast Cancer Res 20(1):106

Elangovan A et al (2022) Loss of E-cadherin induces IGF1R activation and reveals a targetable pathway in invasive lobular breast carcinoma. Mol Cancer Res 20(9):1405–1419

Erdem C et al (2016) Proteomic screening and lasso regression reveal differential signaling in insulin and insulin-like growth factor I (IGF1) pathways. Mol Cell Proteomics 15(9):3045–3057

Farabaugh SM, Boone DN, Lee AV (2015) Role of IGF1R in breast cancer subtypes, stemness, and lineage differentiation. Front Endocrinol (Lausanne) 6:59

Fuso P et al (2022) PI3K inhibitors in advanced breast cancer: the past, the present, new challenges and future perspectives. Cancers (Basel) 14(9)

Gomez-Cuadrado L et al (2022) Characterisation of the stromal microenvironment in lobular breast cancer. Cancers (Basel) 14(4)

Hamidi H, Ivaska J (2018) Every step of the way: integrins in cancer progression and metastasis. Nat Rev Cancer 18(9):533–548

Hanahan D, Weinberg RA (2011) Hallmarks of cancer: the next generation. Cell 144(5):646–674

Hartwell LH et al (1997) Integrating genetic approaches into the discovery of anticancer drugs. Science 278(5340):1064–1068

Horton ER et al (2015) Definition of a consensus integrin adhesome and its dynamics during adhesion complex assembly and disassembly. Nat Cell Biol 17(12):1577–1587

Huang A et al (2020) Synthetic lethality as an engine for cancer drug target discovery. Nat Rev Drug Discov 19(1):23–38

Ianza A et al (2021) Role of the IGF-1 axis in overcoming resistance in breast cancer. Front Cell Dev Biol 9:641449

Iorfida M et al (2012) Invasive lobular breast cancer: subtypes and outcome. Breast Cancer Res Treat 133(2):713–723

Joshi U et al (2023) Clinical outcomes and prognostic factors in triple-negative invasive lobular carcinoma of the breast. Breast Cancer Res Treat 200(2):217–224

Kadry YA, Calderwood DA (1862) Chapter 22: Structural and signaling functions of integrins. Biochim Biophys Acta Biomembr 2020(5):183206

Kas SM et al (2017) Insertional mutagenesis identifies drivers of a novel oncogenic pathway in invasive lobular breast carcinoma. Nat Genet 49(8):1219–1230

Katsuno-Kambe H, Yap AS (2020) Endocytosis, cadherins and tissue dynamics. Traffic 21(3):268–273

Khan SU, Fatima K, Malik F (2022) Understanding the cell survival mechanism of anoikis-resistant cancer cells during different steps of metastasis. Clin Exp Metastasis 39(5):715–726

Korhonen T et al (2013) The impact of lobular and ductal breast cancer histology on the metastatic behavior and long term survival of breast cancer patients. Breast 22(6):1119–1124

Law JH et al (2008) Phosphorylated insulin-like growth factor-i/insulin receptor is present in all breast cancer subtypes and is related to poor survival. Cancer Res 68(24):10238–10246

Lawson CD, Ridley AJ (2018) Rho GTPase signaling complexes in cell migration and invasion. J Cell Biol 217(2):447–457

Lecuit T, Yap AS (2015) E-cadherin junctions as active mechanical integrators in tissue dynamics. Nat Cell Biol 17(5):533–539

Lee YR, Chen M, Pandolfi PP (2018) The functions and regulation of the PTEN tumour suppressor: new modes and prospects. Nat Rev Mol Cell Biol 19(9):547–562

Lee JS, Tocheny CE, Shaw LM (2022) The insulin-like growth factor signaling pathway in breast cancer: an elusive therapeutic target. Life (Basel) 12(12)

Litzenburger BC et al (2011) High IGF-IR activity in triple-negative breast cancer cell lines and tumorgrafts correlates with sensitivity to anti-IGF-IR therapy. Clin Cancer Res 17(8):2314–2327

Lord CJ, Ashworth A (2017) PARP inhibitors: synthetic lethality in the clinic. Science 355(6330):1152–1158

Masciari S et al (2007) Germline E-cadherin mutations in familial lobular breast cancer. J Med Genet 44(11):726–731

Mathew A et al (2017) Distinct pattern of metastases in patients with invasive lobular carcinoma of the breast. Geburtshilfe Frauenheilkd 77(6):660–666

McCart Reed AE et al (2016) An epithelial to mesenchymal transition programme does not usually drive the phenotype of invasive lobular carcinomas. J Pathol 238(4):489–494

Mege RM, Ishiyama N (2017) Integration of cadherin adhesion and cytoskeleton at adherens junctions. Cold Spring Harb Perspect Biol 9(5):a028738

Metzger Filho O et al (2015) Relative effectiveness of letrozole compared with tamoxifen for patients with lobular carcinoma in the BIG 1-98 trial. J Clin Oncol 33(25):2772–2779

Mouabbi JA et al (2022) Invasive lobular carcinoma: an understudied emergent subtype of breast cancer. Breast Cancer Res Treat 193(2):253–264

Mui KL, Chen CS, Assoian RK (2016) The mechanical regulation of integrin-cadherin crosstalk organizes cells, signaling and forces. J Cell Sci 129(6): 1093–1100

Nagle AM et al (2018) Loss of E-cadherin enhances IGF1-IGF1R pathway activation and sensitizes breast cancers to anti-IGF1R/InsR inhibitors. Clin Cancer Res 24(20):5165–5177

Nakagawa S et al (2016) Tumor microenvironment in invasive lobular carcinoma: possible therapeutic targets. Breast Cancer Res Treat 155(1):65–75

Nardone A et al (2022) A distinct chromatin state drives therapeutic resistance in invasive lobular breast cancer. Cancer Res 82(20):3673–3686

Nieto MA et al (2016) EMT: 2016. Cell 166(1):21–45

Oesterreich S et al (2022) Clinicopathological features and outcomes comparing patients with invasive ductal and lobular breast cancer. J Natl Cancer Inst 114(11):1511–1522

Okines A et al (2022) Clinical outcomes in patients with triple negative or HER2 positive lobular breast cancer: a single institution experience. Breast Cancer Res Treat 192(3):563–571

Onkar S et al (2023) Immune landscape in invasive ductal and lobular breast cancer reveals a divergent macrophage-driven microenvironment. Nat Cancer 4(4):516–534

Park CK, Jung WH, Koo JS (2016) Expression of cancer-associated fibroblast-related proteins differs between invasive lobular carcinoma and invasive ductal carcinoma. Breast Cancer Res Treat 159(1):55–69

Pestalozzi BC et al (2008) Distinct clinical and prognostic features of infiltrating lobular carcinoma of the breast: combined results of 15 International Breast Cancer Study Group clinical trials. J Clin Oncol 26(18):3006–3014

Qian X et al (2004) E-cadherin-mediated adhesion inhibits ligand-dependent activation of diverse receptor tyrosine kinases. EMBO J 23(8):1739–1748

Rakha EA et al (2008) Invasive lobular carcinoma of the breast: response to hormonal therapy and outcomes. Eur J Cancer 44(1):73–83

Ratze MAK et al (2022) Loss of E-cadherin leads to Id2-dependent inhibition of cell cycle progression in metastatic lobular breast cancer. Oncogene 41(21):2932–2944

Ryan CJ et al (2023) Complex synthetic lethality in cancer. Nat Genet 55(12):2039–2048

Sahai E, Marshall CJ (2002) ROCK and Dia have opposing effects on adherens junctions downstream of Rho. Nat Cell Biol 4(6):408–415

Schackmann RC et al (2011) Cytosolic p120-catenin regulates growth of metastatic lobular carcinoma through Rock1-mediated anoikis resistance. J Clin Invest 121(8):3176–3188

Schackmann RC et al (2013) p120-catenin in cancer - mechanisms, models and opportunities for intervention. J Cell Sci 126(Pt 16):3515–3525

Schipper K et al (2019) Rebalancing of actomyosin contractility enables mammary tumor formation upon loss of E-cadherin. Nat Commun 10(1):3800

Schipper K et al (2020) Truncated ASPP2 drives initiation and progression of invasive lobular carcinoma via distinct mechanisms. Cancer Res 80(7):1486–1497

Sflomos G et al (2021a) Intraductal xenografts show lobular carcinoma cells rely on their own extracellular matrix and LOXL1. EMBO Mol Med 13(3):e13180

Sflomos G et al (2021b) Atlas of lobular breast cancer models: challenges and strategic directions. Cancers (Basel) 13(21)

Shamir ER, Ewald AJ (2015) Adhesion in mammary development: novel roles for E-cadherin in individual and collective cell migration. Curr Top Dev Biol 112:353–382

Shamir ER et al (2014) Twist1-induced dissemination preserves epithelial identity and requires E-cadherin. J Cell Biol 204(5):839–856

Sikora MJ et al (2016) WNT4 mediates estrogen receptor signaling and endocrine resistance in invasive lobular carcinoma cell lines. Breast Cancer Res 18(1):92

Sottnik JL et al (2021) Mediator of DNA damage checkpoint 1 (MDC1) is a novel estrogen receptor coregulator in invasive lobular carcinoma of the breast. Mol Cancer Res 19(8):1270–1282

Sun Y, Ma L (2024) A milestone in epithelial-mesenchymal transition. Nat Cell Biol 26(1):29–30

Tasdemir N et al (2018) Comprehensive phenotypic characterization of human invasive lobular carcinoma cell lines in 2D and 3D cultures. Cancer Res 78(21):6209–6222

Tasdemir N et al (2020) Proteomic and transcriptomic profiling identifies mediators of anchorage-independent growth and roles of inhibitor of differentiation proteins in invasive lobular carcinoma. Sci Rep 10(1):11487

Teo K et al (2018) E-cadherin loss induces targetable autocrine activation of growth factor signalling in lobular breast cancer. Sci Rep 8(1):15454

Thiery JP (2002) Epithelial-mesenchymal transitions in tumour progression. Nat Rev Cancer 2(6):442–454

Thill M et al (2023) Treatment and outcome in metastatic lobular breast cancer in the prospective German research platform OPAL. Breast Cancer Res Treat 198(3):545–553

Timbres J et al (2021) Survival outcomes in invasive lobular carcinoma compared to oestrogen receptor-positive invasive ductal carcinoma. Cancers (Basel) 13(12)

Tubiana-Hulin M et al (2006) Response to neoadjuvant chemotherapy in lobular and ductal breast carcinomas: a retrospective study on 860 patients from one institution. Ann Oncol 17(8):1228–1233

Van Baelen K et al (2022) Current and future diagnostic and treatment strategies for patients with invasive lobular breast cancer. Ann Oncol 33(8):769–785

van de Ven RA et al (2015) Nuclear p120-catenin regulates the anoikis resistance of mouse lobular breast cancer cells through Kaiso-dependent Wnt11 expression. Dis Model Mech 8(4):373–384

Voorwerk L et al (2023) PD-L1 blockade in combination with carboplatin as immune induction in metastatic lobular breast cancer: the GELATO trial. Nat Cancer 4(4):535–549

Westhoff CC et al (2020) Prognostic relevance of the loss of stromal CD34 positive fibroblasts in invasive lobular carcinoma of the breast. Virchows Arch 477(5):717–724

Zhang N et al (2023) Dynamics and functions of E-cadherin complexes in epithelial cell and tissue morphogenesis. Mar Life Sci Technol 5(4): 585–601

Part V

Signaling Pathways

Therese Sørlie and Robert Clarke

Signaling pathways play pivotal roles in breast development, cancer initiation, progression, and metastasis. In this part, we examine three key signaling mechanisms shaping the landscape of breast cancer: hormone signaling, the RANK/RANKL pathway, and metabolic reprogramming.

In Chap. 15, Cathrin Brisken and her colleague at Ecole Polytechnique Fédérale de Lausanne (EPFL), Switzerland, explain how hormones, including estrogens, progesterone, and testosterone, intricately regulate normal breast development and are implicated in breast cancer pathogenesis. Estrogens are established drivers of estrogen receptor-positive (ER+) breast cancers, while the roles of progesterone receptor (PR) and androgen receptor (AR) signaling remain under scrutiny. Insights from preclinical models shed light on the interplay between hormone receptors and their context-dependent roles in breast cancer, offering valuable lessons and highlighting current challenges in understanding hormone action.

In Chap. 16, Eva González-Suárez and her colleagues at Centro Nacional de Investigaciones Oncológicas (CNIO), Madrid, Spain, describe how the RANK pathway has emerged as a promising target in breast cancer therapeutics, with denosumab, an anti-RANKL drug, showing potential benefits. RANK signaling mediates mammary gland development and influences breast cancer initiation and progression by regulating cell proliferation, stem cell fate, and tumor microenvironment interactions. This chapter explores the multifaceted roles of the RANK pathway in immunity, inflammation, and tumor immune surveillance. Discussions encompass the therapeutic implications of targeting RANK signaling, including its effects on tumor cell intrinsic behavior, sensitivity to therapy, and modulation of the tumor microenvironment, offering insights into ongoing clinical trials and future directions.

T. Sørlie
Oslo, Norway

R. Clarke
Manchester, UK

In Chap. 17, Yibin Kang and his colleague at Princeton University, USA, propose that metabolic dysregulation is increasingly recognized as a hallmark of cancer, including breast cancer, impacting initiation, progression, and metastasis. This chapter illuminates the diverse metabolic phenotypes observed in different molecular subtypes of breast cancer, elucidating their implications for therapeutic strategies. The intricate interplay between cancer cells and the tumor microenvironment shapes metabolic adaptations, influencing nutrient uptake, utilization, and interactions with stromal and immune components. Understanding the metabolic reprogramming orchestrated by oncogenes, tumor suppressors, and signaling pathways provides insights into the dynamic processes driving breast cancer progression and metastasis, paving the way for innovative therapeutic interventions tailored to distinct metabolic vulnerabilities.

In conclusion, the exploration of signaling pathways in breast cancer reveals the intricate interplay between hormonal regulation, microenvironmental signaling, and metabolic reprogramming. Understanding these pathways at various levels, from molecular mechanisms to clinical implications, offers invaluable insights into breast cancer initiation and progression and guides therapeutic strategies.

Hormone Signaling in Breast Development and Cancer

15

Andrea Agnoletto and Cathrin Brisken

Abstract

Hormones control normal breast development and function. They also impinge on breast cancer (BC) development and disease progression in direct and indirect ways. The major ovarian hormones, estrogens and progesterone, have long been established as key regulators of mammary gland development in rodents and linked to human disease. However, their roles have been difficult to disentangle because they act on multiple tissues and can act directly and indirectly on different cell types in the breast, and their receptors interact at different levels within the target cell. Estrogens are well-recognized drivers of estrogen receptor-positive (ER+) breast cancers, and the ER is successfully targeted in ER+ disease. The role of progesterone receptor (PR) as a potential target to be activated or inhibited is debated, and androgen receptor (AR) signaling has emerged as a potentially interesting pathway to target on the stage.

In this chapter, we discuss hormone signaling in normal breast development and in cancer, with a specific focus on the key sex hormones: estrogen, progesterone, and testosterone. We will highlight the complexities of endocrine control mechanisms at the organismal, tissue, cellular, and molecular levels. As we delve into the mechanisms of action of hormone receptors, their interplay and their context-dependent roles in breast cancer will be discussed. Drawing insights from new preclinical models, we will describe the lessons learned and the current challenges in understanding hormone action in breast cancer.

Keywords

Steroid hormones · Hormone receptors · Estrogen receptor · Progesterone receptor · Androgen receptor

Key Points

- Reproductive hormones control the normal breast development and impinge on breast carcinogenesis at multiple levels.
- The major ovarian hormones estrogen and progesterone drive different stages of mammary epithelial cell expansion acting through sensor cells.
- Exposures to endogenous and exogenous hormones and hormonally active substances contribute to breast cancer risk.

A. Agnoletto (✉) · C. Brisken
Swiss Institute for Experimental Cancer Research, School of Life Sciences, Ecole Polytechnique Fédérale de Lausanne, Lausanne, Switzerland
e-mail: andrea.agnoletto@epfl.ch; cathrin.brisken@epfl.ch

T. Sørlie, R. B. Clarke (eds.), *A Guide to Breast Cancer Research*, Advances in Experimental Medicine and Biology 1464, https://doi.org/10.1007/978-3-031-70875-6_15

- Estrogen, progesterone, and androgen actions are mediated by nuclear hormone receptors that act as ligand-activated transcription factors.
- The activity of hormone receptor signaling is affected by multiple signaling pathways, and the outcome of hormone signaling is highly context-dependent.

15.1 Introduction

In 1896, George Beatson first reported that surgical removal of the ovaries resulted in breast tumor regression, linking ovarian function to breast tumor growth well before estrogens and progesterone were identified (Beatson 1896). Epidemiological studies have since revealed that a woman's reproductive history with changing endocrine milieus affects her risk of developing breast cancer. Similarly, exposures to exogenous hormones through hormonal contraception and hormone replacement therapy are associated with increased breast cancer risk. Clinically, it is well established that the course of the disease depends on whether a woman is premenopausal, pregnant, or menopaused. In these different physiological states, different therapeutic approaches are required.

Various experimental approaches have been taken to address how hormones impinge on breast cancer development and how this can be exploited therapeutically, and this will be reviewed here considering multiple levels of complexity. First and foremost, linked to the physiological role of hormones at the organismal level, they elicit changes in multiple organs that may directly and indirectly affect different cell types in the breast and in different cell types of a breast tumor. These systemic effects have largely been studied in rodent models.

Second, hormones elicit complex intra- and intercellular signaling both in normal breast epithelial cells and breast cancer cells. For the former, the field has largely relied on genetic studies in mouse models. In these, we always need to consider the developmental stage and physiologic state in which a hormone acts. For studying the latter, a small number of hormone-sensitive breast cancer cell lines have served as the workhorses for research. Yet these simplified models of human cancers, with their limitations, have allowed researchers to reveal a plethora of mechanisms, and multiple ramifications of hormone signaling have been revealed.

Another level of complexity comes from the fact that the expression of the ER itself is altered during tumorigenesis. In fact, one of the earliest signs of premalignancy is the increased ER expression in luminal cells and the loss of the variegated pattern of expression of ER in the luminal epithelial cells that is characteristic of the normal breast epithelium (Lee et al. 2006).

In recent decades, as different subtypes of breast cancer have been characterized, it has become apparent that endocrine factors are more important in the genesis of tumors that are ER+ or PR+ than of hormone-insensitive breast cancers (Huang et al. 2000), largely represented by triple-negative breast cancers. In clinical practice, a tumor is defined as ER+ by immunohistochemistry when at least 1% of the tumor cells express the ER; these represent more than 70% of all cases. Experimentally, these tumors were difficult to study because few genetically engineered mouse models (GEMMs) develop ER+ mammary carcinomas, and ER+ BC cells were difficult to xenograft. With the demonstration that ER+ BC cells can readily be established by grafting them into the milk ducts, the number of ER+ models has been increasing, leading to new insights that will be discussed here (Richard et al. 2016; Sflomos et al. 2016).

Exposure to endocrine disruptors that induce changes in breast development already in utero has mostly been studied in rodent models. As rodent models do not correctly reflect the different subtypes observed in humans as discussed below, we can only speculate whether they may globally contribute to increased prevalence or predispose to specific tumor subtypes. Exposure to endocrine disruptors which may already occur in utero can have lasting impact through epigenetic changes that alter the development and the gland's susceptibility for the disease (Soto and Sonnenschein 2010). The difficulty of defining exposures, the complexity of interactions between different compounds, and the fact that exposures are pervasive make it challenging to determine effects and will not be discussed here.

Box 15.1 Type of Hormones: Steroids, Modified Amino Acids, Proteins, and Peptides

Hormones (from the Greek "to arouse, to excite") are mediators for intercellular as well as interorgan communication. They travel across the whole body through the bloodstream, thereby reaching distant tissues, and exert their action over a spread of timescales. Hormones can be divided in several classes based on their chemical origin.

Lipid-based hormones, more commonly known as steroid hormones, include the sex hormones estradiol, progesterone, and testosterone, as well as vitamin D and the stress hormone cortisol. Given their uncharged and lipophilic nature, they passively cross lipid bilayers and typically do not require transporters. Their action is mediated by nuclear hormone receptors.

A second type are amino acid-based hormones. Well-known examples are thyroid hormones, derived from the amino acid tyrosine and involved in the regulation of body metabolism, as well as melatonin, which is derived from tryptophan and regulates the circadian rhythm.

A third major group of hormones are protein hormones, of different sizes and complexities. Prolactin, a large polypeptide (199 amino acids) produced by the pituitary, stimulates milk production in the breast, and the 96-amino-acid-long luteinizing hormone, also from the pituitary, triggers ovulation in females and testosterone production in males. Peptide hormones typically range from 3 to 100 amino acids in length and comprise insulin, which is produced in the pancreas and regulates glucose concentration homeostasis, and oxytocin ("the love hormone") that is released at the level of the brain and is involved in social behaviors as well as in facilitating childbirth and milk letdown reflex. Both protein and peptide hormones bind to specific receptors on the surface of target cells to initiate signaling cascades.

Finally, gases and various hydrophobic molecules can act as hormones. They are produced as specific sites and exert their action by crossing the cell membrane and binding to intracellular receptors. One such example is nitric oxide that is involved in a plethora of biological processes, ranging from the regulation of immune response, to control of vascular tone and blood flow, and to the modulation of cellular metabolic rates.

While the female sex hormones estrogens and progesterone primarily drive breast development and are best studied in breast cancer, many other hormones fine-tune breast development and may impinge on breast cancer onset and progression.

15.2 Role of Hormones in Breast Development

The importance of ovarian hormones (i.e., estrogen, progesterone) in breast cancer development relates to the biology of the breast and their key role in breast development and function. The breast is a unique organ in that it undergoes most of its development after birth as a function of reproductive needs. For this, the breast retains plasticity and is able to undergo extensive cell proliferation and differentiation followed by involution with every pregnancy in the adult organism.

While there are species-specific features in reproductive physiology, breast anatomy, and tissue composition, the basic endocrine control mechanisms in terms of which hormones are involved, their sequential and stage-specific roles, the way they affect intercellular communication, as well as the major downstream signaling pathways appear to be evolutionarily conserved. Most of our understanding of breast development and how hormones control it throughout a woman's reproductive life is gleaned from experimental studies in rodents, and we need to remember that not every finding translates to humans one-to-one.

Mammary gland development begins with the appearance of placodes in the ventral skin in female embryos along the milk line, which are controlled by epithelial-mesenchymal interactions. These placodes grow into buds that give rise to rudimentary ductal trees, which are embedded in a pad of adipose tissue that is morphologically distinct from the remaining subcutaneous fat and readily detectable at birth. The number of buds on the milk line that will persist and develop into mammary glands depends on the typical litter size of a species.

Until puberty, the mammary glands grow isometrically with the rest of the body. At this stage, the ovaries produce only trace amounts of the sex steroids, and the prepubertal part of development is largely considered hormone independent. However, a quantitative examination of the ductal trees in infant female mice with germline deletions of estrogen receptor (ER) or progesterone receptor (PR) genes revealed that they are smaller and less complex compared to those of their wild-type counterparts (Lydon et al. 1995; Cagnet et al. 2018). This observation may be attributed to the role of these two hormones in regulating stem cell function already prior to puberty (Rajaram et al. 2015).

With the onset of puberty and the increased secretion of follicle-stimulating hormone (FSH) and luteinizing hormone (LH) from the pituitary gland, the ovarian follicles begin to mature and produce significant levels of estrogens. These drive the outgrowth of the ducts into the surrounding fatty stroma. The concomitant growth of the mammary fat pad is termed thelarche in prepubescent girls. Subsequently, maturation of the hypothalamic-pituitary axis results in cyclic release of FSH and LH and ovulatory cycles. Progesterone (P4) is secreted by the corpora lutea in the ovary following the release of the egg. Two phases of the ovulatory menstrual cycle can clearly be distinguished in humans: the preovulatory phase, characterized by an estradiol (E2) peak, and the postovulatory/luteal phase, characterized by a smaller E2 and a large P4 peak (Fig. 15.1).

The analysis of GEMMs with germline deletion of either *Esr1* or *Pgr* (the genes encoding for ER and PR, respectively), combined with powerful tissue recombination techniques, allowed us to dissect gene function specifically in the mammary epithelium and in the mammary fat pad from indirect, systemic effects of receptor loss during mammary gland development (Brisken and O'Malley 2011). It emerged that estrogens play a pivotal role in driving ductal outgrowth. *Pgr*, which itself is a target of ER, is induced and PR signaling seconds the E2 driven growth by activating stem cells and their niches (Haslam and Shyamala 1979; Rajaram et al. 2015; Ataca et al. 2020). As mice reach sexual maturity, a rudimentary ductal system is established throughout the mammary fat pad through dichotomous branching. In adult mice, E2 is supplanted by P4 as the major mitogen. Repeated estrous cycles lead to recurrent activation of PR signaling during diestrus, the postovulatory phase of the estrous cycle in mice. This cyclic activation of PR results in the ductal system gaining complexity through side branches which bud from preexisting ducts at a 90-degree angle. This phenomenon is enhanced during pregnancy and critical for the increase in functional surface. During the last third of pregnancy, small sac-like structures called alveoli start forming along the ductal system. Luminal cells in the alveoli will differentiate into milk-secreting cells, a process that requires epithelial prolactin receptor signaling (Brisken et al. 1999).

Thus, through partly sequential and largely cooperative actions of the three major female reproductive hormones, the mammary functional surface is expanded, and the mammary gland enabled to secrete copious amounts of milk that

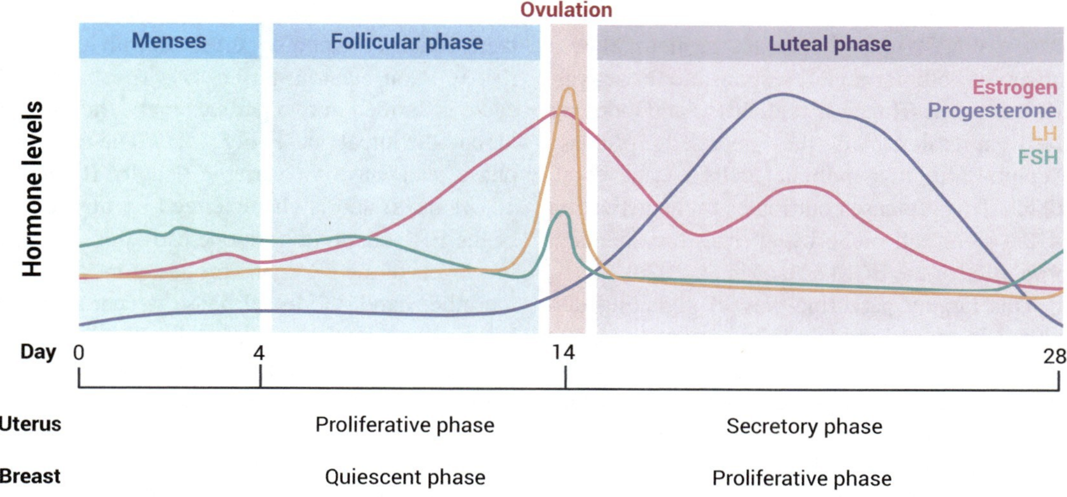

Fig. 15.1 Hormone levels throughout the menstrual cycle and effect on reproductive tissues. The cycle begins with the menstrual phase, characterized by the shedding of the uterine linings. During the follicular phase, the FSH produced by the pituitary gland stimulates the growth of the ovarian follicles, which in turn produce estrogen, the dominant ovarian hormone of this phase. During this period, cell proliferation occurs within the uterus, while the breast remains quiescent. As the cycle progresses, estrogen levels drop, and a surge of LH triggers ovulation. In the luteal phase, the ruptured follicle transforms into the corpus luteum and starts producing progesterone, which is the dominant hormone in this phase. During the luteal phase, the uterus produces glycogen-rich secretions, and the breast experiences an increased rate of cell proliferation. If fertilization does not occur, both estrogen and progesterone levels decrease, leading to menstruation

ensure the survival of the pups. In addition, pituitary growth hormone (GH) is required for the entire process as shown by classical hormone ablation and replacement experiments in mice and rats (Lyons 1958; Nandi 1958). Both prolactin and GH are also synthesized in the mammary epithelium, the latter downstream of PR signaling and implicated in local control. Many more hormones impinge on the breast epithelium and other cells directly and indirectly, fine-tuning various biological processes. These include thyroid hormones, testosterone, and leptin.

During pregnancy, notable transformations occur not only within the epithelial cells themselves but also in the composition of the adjacent adipose tissue. These alterations are accompanied by systemic metabolic changes. However, the precise understanding of the endocrine mechanisms governing these processes still awaits disentangling.

In orchestrating the development and functional differentiation of the mammary gland, the ovarian hormones act on a subset of luminal epithelial cells that typically co-express ER, PR, and AR, dubbed “hormone sensor cells” (Duss et al. 2007). In response to fluctuations in hormone levels, these sensor cells directly modulate gene expression, leading to the production of various secreted factors. These factors, in turn, impact neighboring luminal and myoepithelial cells, resulting in complex changes in cellular interactions, extracellular matrix (ECM) composition, and interactions with stromal cells. These intricate modifications are essential for the profound developmental changes that occur within the mammary gland (for further review, see Brisken and Scabia 2020).

Key downstream mediators have been identified using genetic tools in mice. For instance, during pubertal outgrowth, E2-induced cell proliferation is mediated by factors such as amphiregulin (Ciarloni et al. 2007) and fibroblast growth factors (FGFs) (Lu et al. 2008). Cyclin D1 is involved in cell-intrinsic proliferation of the sensor cells, while RANKL plays a role in paracrine proliferation downstream of progesterone (Fernandez-Valdivia et al. 2009; Beleut et al. 2010). WNT4 is an important mediator downstream of both hormones, responsible for activating stem cells (Rajaram et al. 2015) and inducing the expression of the secreted protease Adamts18 in myoepithelial cells (Ataca et al. 2020). This protease contributes to the activation of the stem cell niche by altering the chemical properties of the ECM (Ataca et al. 2020).

This largely paracrine way of signaling discerned in mouse models is important to ensure that the behavior of multiple cell types is coordinated. This tissue organizational principle is conserved across species, and evidence has accumulated that RANKL is similarly important in the human breast (Lim et al. 2010; Tanos et al. 2013). Both *RANKL* and *WNT4* were also shown to follow a menstrual cycle-related expression in the human breast epithelium (Pardo et al. 2014). Importantly, one of the earliest hallmarks of premalignant lesions is the loss of patterned HR expression (Lee et al. 2006). The gradient in ER expression is important for correct signaling in the normal mammary epithelium. The differential importance of AF-1 versus AF-2 mediated signaling (see below) depending on ER expression levels is lost early during breast carcinogenesis (Cagnet et al. 2018). Instead of the characteristic variegated pattern of HR expression, the ER is uniformly expressed at high levels in the luminal epithelial cells of hyperplastic enlarged lobular unit (Lee et al. 2006). While cell proliferation in human adult breast epithelium mainly occurs in the HR negative cells, in ER+ breast cancers, ER+ cells proliferate (Clarke et al. 1997; Shoker et al. 1999).

15.3 Hormone Exposures and Breast Cancer Risk

15.3.1 Reproductive Factors

Epidemiological studies have shown that the risk of developing breast cancer rises with early menarche and late menopause, which together lengthen the woman's exposure to ovarian hormones (Pike et al. 1983; Colditz et al. 2004; Hanamura et al. 2021). Shorter duration of the menstruation cycles also correlates with increased risk (Olsson et al. 1983, 1987). The menstrual cycle is divided in two parts, namely, the follicular and the luteal phase (Fig. 15.1). The follicular phase can have a variable length (typically 10–21 days) and is characterized by high levels of the ER-activating hormone estradiol (E2) and low levels of the PR ligand progesterone (P4). On the other hand, the luteal phase is characterized by the opposite hormonal profile (high P4 and low E2) and is associated with increased breast epithelial cell proliferation (Brisken and Scabia 2020).

Having children raises the risk of getting breast cancer for up to 15 years after the baby is born, but it becomes protective over the long run (Yuasa and MacMahon 1970; Schedin 2006; Nelson et al. 2012). For instance, each individual pregnancy with childbirth is associated with an 11% decrease in the risk of developing breast cancer. This is specific for hormone receptor-positive breast cancers (Ma et al. 2006). However, this effect is reduced if the first pregnancy occurs after the age of 30. Breastfeeding has protective effects on breast cancer risk, as reported by a collective analysis of epidemiological studies from different countries (Yuasa and MacMahon 1970; Hanamura et al. 2021). In addition, a longer duration of lactation correlates with lower breast cancer risk (Laamiri et al. 2015). The mechanisms underlying the reduced risk of breast cancer in parous women have been proposed to derive from both the enhanced differentiation of the mammary cells associated with lactation and the decreased hormone exposure associated with gestation (Russo et al. 2005).

15.3.2 Exposures to Exogenous Hormones and Hormonally Active Compounds

The consumption of oral contraceptives, composed of combinations of estrogen and progestins (i.e., synthetic progesterone analogs), is associated with a 1.5-fold increase in breast cancer risk (Nelson et al. 2012). Similarly, hormone replacement therapy (HRT) has been postulated to increase the risk of hormone receptor-positive breast cancer in postmenopausal women (Colditz et al. 2004). Weak or no association with breast cancer risk was found when HRT was administered as estradiol alone (Opatrny et al. 2008; Mastorakos et al. 2021). However, combined HRT in which estrogen and a synthetic progestin are coadministered is linked to a greater incidence of breast cancer compared to estrogen alone. In contrast, natural progesterone showed no statistically significant increase in the likelihood of developing breast cancer (Fournier et al. 2008).

15.4 Steroid Hormone Receptors: Structure and General Principles of Signaling

The members of the steroid hormone receptor family comprise ER, PR, AR, glucocorticoid receptor (GR), and mineralocorticoid receptor (MR). They share a common structure composed of six modular domains, named from A to F (Fig. 15.2). Functionally, starting from the N-terminus are found the amino terminal domain (NTD, A/B region) and the central DNA binding domain (DBD, C region), linked by a hinge region (D) to the C-terminal ligand-binding domain (LBD, E/F region) (Helsen et al. 2012). The NTD and LBD are also known as activation function 1 and 2 (AF-1 and AF-2), and these domains are responsible for the transcriptional activation of the receptor. The DBD contains two zinc finger motifs, each identified by an α-helix containing a group of four cysteines, coordinating the binding with a zinc atom (Kumar and Thompson 1999; Aranda and Pascual 2001). Zinc-coordinating DNA motifs are commonly found in DNA-interacting proteins and mediate binding of the receptor with the major groove of the double helix. These two modules, although similar, are characterized by unique biochemical features that confer specialized functions in the action of nuclear hormone receptors. The first subdomain contains the so-called P box, a series of three to four amino acids that mediates the site-specific recognition of the receptor at the DNA level (Kumar and Thompson 1999). The second zinc finger motif is less involved in DNA binding but participates in receptor homodimerization (Helsen et al. 2012).

The biological function of steroid hormone receptors is further determined by the carboxy-terminal LBD. This part is less conserved than the DBD and is composed of 12 α-helices connected by loop regions. In the inactive receptor conformation, the DBD is masked by heat-shock proteins (Aranda and Pascual 2001). The docking of the ligand to the hormone receptor initiates extensive conformational remodeling that induces dissociation of the receptor from the heat-shock proteins, dimerization, nuclear translocation, and the repositioning of helix 12 over the hydrophobic pocket in the ligand-binding domain, thereby creating a new surface for the binding of transcriptional coregulators (Needham et al. 2000). The other domains are less conserved and participate in conformational changes induced upon ligand binding.

Steroid hormone receptors bind to DNA directly via their DNA binding domain (DBD) recognizing receptor-specific DNA sequences, the response elements (REs). REs are typically located in proximity to the target genes and consist of three parts, namely, a five- to six-nucleotide sequence, followed by a spacer of variable length,

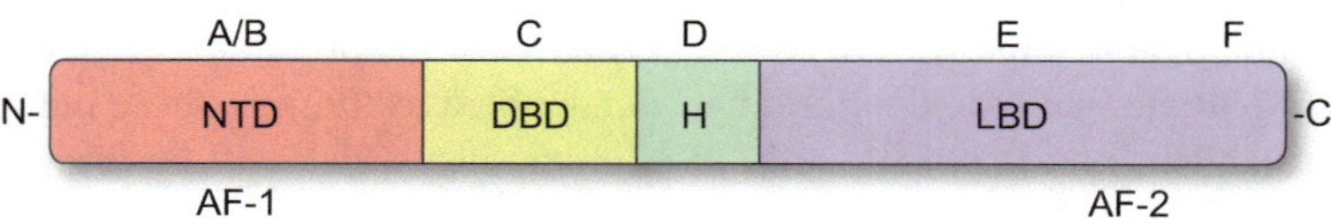

Fig. 15.2 The basic structure of steroid hormone receptors. Six modular domains are named from A to F from the N-terminus to the C-terminus. The functional domains are known as *NTD* N-terminal domain, *DBD* DNA binding domain, *H* hinge region, *LBD* ligand-binding domain, *AF-1 and AF-2* activation function 1 and 2

and a direct or inverse repeat of the initial five to six nucleotides. The presence of two recognition sequences within the RE is essential, since most nuclear receptors act in the forms of homo- or heterodimers (Helsen et al. 2012).

The gene expression regulation exerted by the activation of a given hormone receptor can vary across different tissues and cell types. A compelling hypothesis is that this results from epigenetic differences as well as expression of distinct sets of transcriptional cofactors, which can determine the specificity of the transcriptional response elicited by a hormonal stimulation (Gertz et al. 2013). Additionally, the transcriptional response initiated by hormones usually takes place in multiple steps (Groshong et al. 1997; Hsu et al. 2019). The direct stimulation of a relatively small number of target genes occurs rapidly and constitutes the primary response. A delayed secondary response is then initiated by the protein products of the primary target genes. As a further level of complexity, some of the proteins produced in the primary response may inhibit the transcription of primary response genes, thereby limiting the hormone-induced response (Drabovich et al. 2016). The same process can continue over multiple rounds of gene induction and repression carried on by consecutive series of target genes. In this way, a simple hormonal trigger can cause a very complex change in the pattern of cellular gene expression.

Finally, posttranslational modifications (PTMs) play a crucial role in the modulation of steroid hormone receptors. These modifications, including phosphorylation, acetylation, ubiquitination, and SUMOylation, impact on the activity and stability of hormone receptors, thereby contributing to cell-specific gene regulation (Faus and Haendler 2006). Another significant modification is the palmitoylation of hormone receptors. This modification enables these receptors to bind to the cellular membrane (Marino and Ascenzi 2006). Membrane-bound hormone receptors can establish noncanonical cellular responses by activating intracellular signaling cascades, often resulting in the regulation of a distinguished set of genes compared to those transcribed based on the classical nuclear receptor mechanism (Gagniac et al. 2020).

15.5 Molecular Mechanisms of Individual Hormone Receptors

Extensive insights about the molecular mechanisms underlying hormone receptors signaling have been gained from in vitro studies using breast cancer cell lines. In the early 1970s, cells derived from the pleural effusion of a 69-year-old patient with metastatic disease were successfully established in cell culture, generating the first hormone receptor-positive breast cancer cell line, MCF-7 (Soule et al. 1973). Soon after, MCF-7 cells have been used to demonstrate that ER+ breast cancer cells rely on estrogens to sustain their growth and can be inhibited by tamoxifen (Lippman and Bolan 1975), becoming the workhorse of the research community. Ten years after their establishment, the isolation of the estrogen receptor (ERα) from MCF-7 cells marked a significant milestone for our further understanding of hormone receptors (Greene et al. 1986). For five decades, breast cancer cell lines have been extensively used to study hormone action and have yielded detailed insights into the biochemistry of hormone-dependent pathways at the cellular level.

Following the characterization of MCF-7, several hormone receptor-positive cell lines, such as T47D, HCC1428, and ZR-75-1, have been established and characterized, expanding the number of cell line models for investigating hormone-dependent mechanisms (Dai et al. 2017). Cell lines are simple to maintain and provide a robust platform for rapidly examining the effects of hormone signaling on cell proliferation, migration, and gene expression in vitro. Despite the undoubted usefulness, these models have several limitations, which will be discussed later in this chapter.

15.5.1 Estrogen Receptor

There are two types of estrogen receptors: the estrogen receptor alpha (ERα, encoded by *ESR1*) and estrogen receptor beta (ERβ, encoded by *ESR2*). ERα (hereinafter referred to as ER) is the primary mediator of estrogens' physiological effects in the breast and therapeutic target in hormone receptor-positive breast cancers. The full-length ER is a protein of a molecular weight of 67 kDa, composed of 595 amino acids.

According to the classical model of action of ER, the binding of estrogens with the LBD induces a conformational change that leads to the detachment from the heat-shock proteins associated with the hinge region and consequent exposure of the nuclear localization signal (NLS). Ligand-bound ER forms strong dimers through mutual interaction of monomers in the E regions in the LBD (Brzozowski et al. 1997). Once translocated to the nucleus, ER dimers directly bind the DNA with the zinc fingers located in the DBD, recognizing two palindromic consensus sequences "AGGTCA" spaced by three nucleotides, known as estrogen response elements (EREs) (Schwabe et al. 1993). Alternatively, ER can interact with the DNA indirectly by associating to other transcriptional coregulators such as AP-1, p300, and SP-1 through protein-protein interactions (Kushner et al. 2000; Safe 2001). The full transcriptional activation of the receptor is achieved when AF-1 and AF-2 work synergistically (Kumar et al. 2011). The investigation of mutant forms of the ER has demonstrated that AF-1 displays transcriptional activity also in unliganded ER, whereas AF-2 function is strictly dependent on the binding of ER with its ligand (Tora et al. 1989; Kato et al. 1995; Rogatsky et al. 1999). On the chromatin, ER localizes distal to transcription start sites and binds mostly to cis-regulatory enhancer regions (Carroll et al. 2006; Farcas et al. 2021). These regions function as hubs that attract transcription factors, chromatin remodelers, and coregulators, which together orchestrate the ER-driven transcriptome. Upon modulating gene transcription, ER is rapidly degraded (Reid et al. 2003). This involves its ubiquitination by enzymes that associate with ER transcriptional complex on the chromatin, followed by the ER nuclear export and degradation by the proteosome in the cytosolic compartment (Calligé and Richard-Foy 2006). Studies using breast cancer cell lines have shown that ER modulates the expression of proliferation-related genes such as *CCND1*, *PGR*, *MYC*, and *BCL-2*, either by direct binding to EREs on the chromatin or by indirect binding assisted by transcriptional coregulators such as AP-1 (Petz et al. 2002; Cicatiello et al. 2004; Wang et al. 2011; Cheng et al. 2018). Both the canonical and ligand-independent functions of ER are regulated by a plethora of posttranslational modifications, which influence its activity and stability (reviewed in Le Romancer et al. 2011). These include phosphorylation, ubiquitylation, SUMOylation, palmitoylation, acetylation, methylation, and glycosylation. Multiple cellular pathways converge in fine-tuning the activity of ER through PTMs, and their alterations play a significant role in breast cancer. One example is the regulation of ER by the cytoplasmic kinase glycogen synthase kinase-3 (GSK3), which acts downstream of numerous signaling pathways and modulates ER ligand-dependent activity by phosphorylation of multiple serine residues (Medunjanin et al. 2005).

15.5.1.1 Deregulation of ER Chromatin Interactors in Breast Cancer

To date, more than 400 coregulators that interact with the ER have been identified (Lonard and O'Malley 2012; Altwegg and Vadlamudi 2021). Their expression levels as well as the epigenetic context determine the tissue specificity of ER action on gene expression (Gertz et al. 2013). The ER chromatin binding profile is tightly linked to the activity of the pioneer factors FOXA1 and GATA3 (Hoch et al. 1999; Hurtado et al. 2011) (Fig. 15.3). This special class of transcription factors can bind the chromatin of condensed nucleosomes and facilitate the association of other transcription factors to the DNA. Whereas ER mutations are rare in primary breast cancer, GATA3 and FOXA1 are more commonly mutated or amplified (Usary et al. 2004; Ciriello et al. 2015). Deregulations of pioneer factors such as FOXA1 and GATA3 have been implicated in

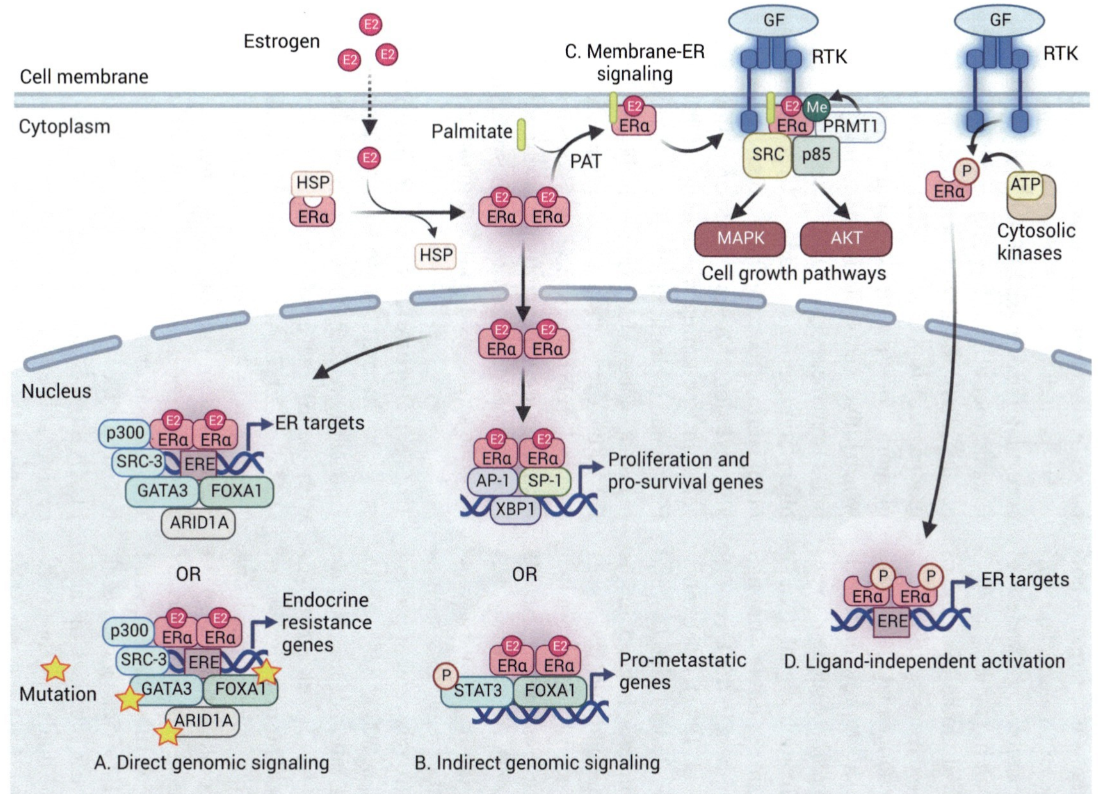

Fig. 15.3 ER mechanisms of action. (**a**) Direct genomic signaling. The pioneer factors FOXA1 and GATA3 and the SWI/SNF complex component ARID1A assist ER in binding to estrogen response elements (EREs) on the DNA. Recruitment of p300 and SRC-3 increases the chromatin accessibility to activate transcription of ER target genes. Mutations in FOXA1, GATA3, or ARID1A result in gene expression programs that are associated with endocrine resistance. (**b**) Indirect genomic signaling. ER binds to chromatin regions lacking EREs by indirect interaction via the transcription cofactors AP-1 and SP-1. The presence of XBP1 redirects ER binding to specific genomic loci by coordinating chromatin unfolding. Indirect ER transcriptional activity in breast cancer results in the expression of proliferation and pro-survival genes. (**c**) Membrane-ER signaling. Palmytoilation of ER performed by palmitoyl acyl transferases (PATs) allows the docking to the cell membrane. Membrane-bound ER associates with several receptor tyrosine kinases (RTKs) in response to growth factors. Upon methylation by the methyltransferase PRMT1, membrane-ER interacts with SRC and the PI3K subunit p85 to enhance the signaling cascades of the cell growth pathways MAPK and AKT. (**d**) Ligand-independent signaling. Unliganded ER can be activated by phosphorylation events regulated by RTKs and cytosolic kinases. Through these PTMs, ER can translocate to the nucleus and regulate gene transcription in unliganded form

breast cancer progression and endocrine resistance by altering the ERα dependent transcriptional output in cell lines and patient samples (Dydensborg et al. 2009; Yan et al. 2010; Hurtado et al. 2011; Ross-Innes et al. 2012; Fu et al. 2016, 2019; Razavi et al. 2018). Steroid receptor coactivator 3 (SRC-3) is one of the first coregulators found involved in breast carcinogenesis and is found amplified in about 10% of patients or overexpressed in 60% of breast cancers (Anzick et al. 1997). Studies in HeLa and MCF-7 cell lines showed that SRC-3 directly interacts with ER and cooperates with the histone acetyltransferase p300 and the arginine methyltransferase CARM-1 to form a core complex that relaxes the chromatin and increases the accessibility of target genes (Kraus and Kadonaga 1998; Carascossa et al. 2010). By modulating ectopic expression of SRC-3 in the keratinocyte cell line HaCaT, which has a very low baseline SRC-3 expression, it has been demonstrated that the SRC-3 abundance influences the capability of liganded ER to upregulate cell cycle-related genes such as cyclin D1 (Planas-Silva et al. 2001). Activator protein 1 (AP-1) is a dimeric transcription factor composed of proteins from the Jun and Fos families. AP-1 regulates the gene expression in response to stimuli such as growth factors and cytokines. In multidrug resistant strains of MCF-7 cells, activated AP-1 recruits ER to regulate genes lacking EREs, mediating a pro-survival effect (Daschner et al. 1999). Inactivating mutations of ARID1A, a component of the SWI/SNF chromatin remodeling complex that interacts with ER, are detected in 12% of metastatic ER+ breast cancer patients and are associated to worse prognosis and endocrine resistance (Pereira et al. 2016; Yates et al. 2017). Preclinical studies using MCF-7 pointed that the loss of ARID1A induces the downregulation of a luminal gene expression signature and confers resistance to tamoxifen and fulvestrant by enhancing a basal-like (ER-negative) transcriptome (Nagarajan et al. 2020; Xu et al. 2020). X-box binding protein 1 (XBP1) is a basic leucine zipper transcription factor involved in unfolded protein response and regulation of cell survival and apoptosis. XBP1 is a direct transcriptional target of ER and is upregulated in breast cancer cells (Davies et al. 2008; Sengupta et al. 2010). Experiments performed in 293 T, MDA-MB-435, and Chinese hamster ovary (CHO) cells indicate that ER and XBP1 physically interact and that XBP1 enhances ER transcriptional activity by orchestrating a large-scale chromatin unfolding (Ding et al. 2003; Fang et al. 2004). This ER-XBP1 cross talk has been linked to pro-survival mechanisms that confer resistance to ER-targeted breast cancer therapies (Barua et al. 2020). Furthermore, it has been demonstrated that upon interleukin 6 (IL6) signaling activation, the signal transducer and activator of transcription 3 (STAT3) associates with the ER/FOXA1 complex on the chromatin in T47D cells (Siersbæk et al. 2020). The STAT3/ER/FOXA1 transcriptional complex activates a subset of shared enhancer regions under the control of STAT3 and independently to ER/FOXA1, resulting in a gene expression program associated with breast cancer metastasis.

15.5.1.2 Non-genomic Functions of ER

While ER primarily functions as a transcription factor by regulating gene expression through genomic mechanisms, it can furthermore influence cellular processes through non-genomic or extranuclear signaling pathways (Fig. 15.3). Interestingly, even though it does not contain transmembrane domains, a fraction of ER is associated with the plasma membrane (Razandi et al. 1999). This is made possible by the palmitoylation of the cysteine residue 447 operated by palmitoyl acyl transferases (PATs) (Acconcia et al. 2005). Via the palmitoylated cysteine, ER docks to the plasma membrane on the cytoplasmic side. The membrane-bound ER is essential for the intercellular communication in the mouse mammary epithelium (Gagniac et al. 2020). It enables the rapid, non-genomic effects of estrogens by direct interactions with signal transducers downstream of growth factor receptors. Activation of non-genomic ER signaling in MCF-7 involves its methylation on the arginine residue 260 by a cytoplasmic complex constituted by the methyltransferase PRMT1 associated with the insulin-like growth factor receptor (IGFR) in response to exogenous IGF-1 (Le

Romancer et al. 2008). Upon E2 binding, methylated ER physically associates with the protein kinase SRC and the p85 subunit of PI3-kinase (Migliaccio et al. 1996; Castoria et al. 2001). This triggers the activation of both MAPK and AKT pathways, resulting in rapid induction of cell cycle entry. The epidermal growth factor receptor HER2 has also been shown to interact with ER in the cytoplasm of HER2-overexpressing MCF-7 cells, resulting in amplification of ERK1/2 activity (Yang et al. 2004). Furthermore, multiple studies on breast cancer cell lines reported that growth factor receptors and cytosolic kinases can trigger the ligand-independent activation of the ER through posttranslational modifications (reviewed in Shupnik 2004). These non-genomic mechanisms provide additional avenues for ER signaling and contribute to the complex regulation of breast cancer cell behavior. It is important to note that the distinction between genomic and non-genomic mechanisms of ER signaling is not clear-cut, as these pathways work in conjunction to mediate the cellular responses to hormones.

15.5.2 Progesterone Receptor

Together with ER, PR expression is an established biomarker to characterize the breast cancer subtype and determine the treatment decisions. PR is considered a favorable prognostic factor in breast cancer. This is partially because PR is a transcriptional target of ER, and its expression is indicative of active ER signaling and response to endocrine therapies.

PR is encoded by a single gene (*PGR*), but its transcription occurs from two separate promoters, resulting in the expression of two PR isoforms, known as PR-A and PR-B. The two isoforms are structurally identical, except that PR-A is lacking 164 amino acids at its N-terminus. Despite the similarity, at a functional level, PR-A and PR-B display distinct effects on gene modulation. PR-B is the main mediator of progesterone-dependent gene transcription, whereas PR-A lacks intrinsic transactivation properties but is able to inhibit the activity of PR-B as well as other steroid hormone receptors (Wen et al. 1994). Interestingly, the ratio of PR-A/PR-B increases from normal to malignant breast epithelial cells, implying that the relative expression of the two isoforms may play a role in breast carcinogenesis (Mote et al. 2002). A multitude of posttranslational modifications that regulate PR have been identified, including phosphorylation, acetylation, ubiquitination, and SUMOylation (reviewed in Abdel-Hafiz and Horwitz 2014). These modifications serve as molecular switches that modulate ligand-dependent and ligand-independent functions of PR. The PR cistrome has considerable overlap with the chromatin binding profiles of ER and androgen receptor (AR), as elegantly demonstrated by chromatin-immunoprecipitation sequencing (ChIP-seq) of patient samples (Severson et al. 2018).

15.5.2.1 Insights of PR Action in Breast Cancer from Cell Lines

While the role of PR in the normal mouse mammary gland development is well documented, its action on breast cancer is multifaceted and less understood. Experiments in cultured T47D and MCF-7 cells indicate that PR activation with the synthetic progestin R5020 has no effect on cell growth when administered alone, but it inhibits cell proliferation in the presence of 1 nM estradiol, suggesting that PR interferes with ER signaling (Vignon et al. 1983; Gill et al. 1987) (Fig. 15.4). At the same time, exposure to the antiprogestins such as mifepristone and onapristone results in a cytostatic effect in the same cell lines, both in the presence and in the absence of estradiol, suggesting a separate, ER-independent mechanism of PR (Gill et al. 1987; Classen et al. 1993).

The inhibitory effect of PR on estrogen-induced proliferation is likely the consequence of direct PR interaction with ER, as observed in MCF-7 and T47D cells, which leads to repositioning of ER on the chromatin and results in a weakening of the expression of proliferation-related genes (Mohammed et al. 2015). On the other hand, potentiation of ER signaling has been observed by overexpressing PR-B in the PR-low breast cancer cell line MCF-7, resulting in the

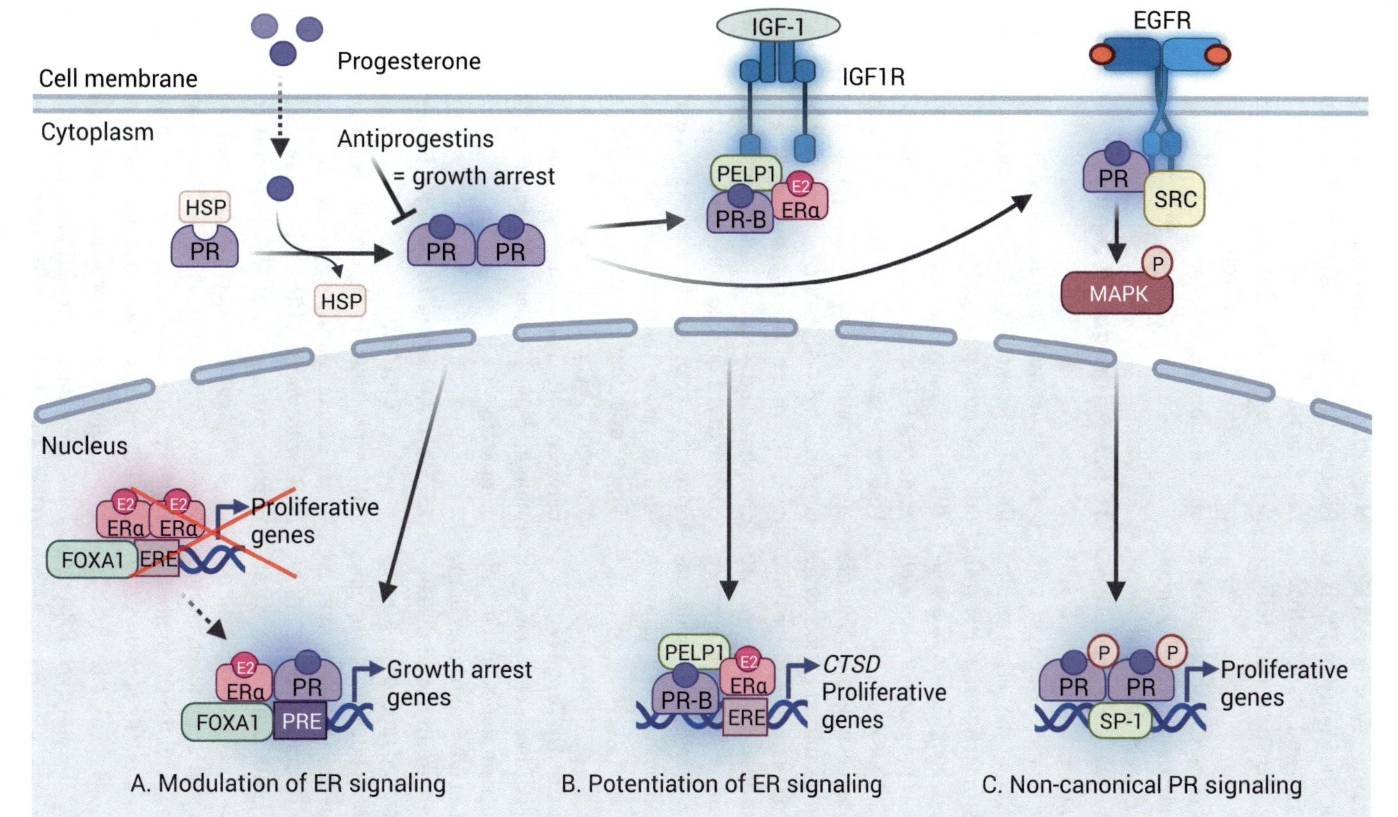

Fig. 15.4 PR mechanisms of action. (**a**) PR inhibits estrogen-induced proliferation by associating with ER on the chromatin and redirecting ER away from its canonical target, resulting in a different set of ER-regulated genes and growth arrest. (**b**) The PR isoform PR-B forms a protein complex with the growth factor receptor IGF1R, the ER cofactor and signal transducer PELP1, and ER. The PR/ER/PELP1 complex translocates to the nucleus and upregulates ER targets such as *CTSD* and proliferation-related genes. (**c**) PR acts as a scaffold for intracellular components and associates with the tyrosine kinase receptor EGFR and the cytosolic kinase SRC, activating the MAPK signaling cascade. In turn, PR is phosphorylated by intracellular kinases, translocates to the nucleus, and associates to SP-1 to upregulate noncanonical PR target genes associated with cell proliferation

upregulation of ER targets such as *CTSD* (encoding cathepsin D) and stimulation of cell growth in response to estradiol and insulin-like growth factor 1 (IGF1) (Daniel et al. 2015). Mechanistically, this has been attributed to the ability of PR-B to form a complex with ER and its coactivator PELP1 downstream of the activated IGF1R (Daniel et al. 2015).

Moreover, PR also acts as a scaffold protein that interacts with several intracellular components to activate rapid signaling pathways (reviewed in Daniel et al. 2009). For instance, in T47D, progestin-stimulated PR activates EGFR and MAPK signaling cascade, which in turn induces the phosphorylation of the serine residue 345 of PR, triggering the interaction of PR with SP-1 on the chromatin and the initiation of a non-canonical gene expression program driving cell proliferation (Faivre et al. 2008).

Collectively, this evidence indicates that the two *PGR* isoforms can either inhibit or cooperate with ER, resulting in the negative or positive modulation of the estrogen-induced growth depending on the cellular context. Moreover, alternative PR signaling mechanisms independent of ER can sustain cell proliferation of breast cancer cells.

15.5.2.2 PR as a Therapeutic Target

PR has been proposed as a therapeutic target in breast cancer, and both its stimulation and inhibition have been evaluated in clinical trials. On the one hand, studies reported an improved disease-free survival in women with advanced ER+ breast cancer treated with the synthetic PR agonist medroxyprogesterone acetate (MPA) or megestrol acetate (Megace) (Pannuti et al. 1979; Alexieva-figusch et al. 1980; Izuo et al. 1981; Ingle et al. 1982; Muss et al. 2016). On the other hand, several trials reported significant clinical benefits in patients treated with the PR inhibitors mifepristone and onapristone (Robertson et al. 1999; Cottu et al. 2018; Lewis et al. 2020; Bartlett et al. 2022; Elía et al. 2023). Moreover, PR inhibition with ulipristal acetate is currently being evaluated for the prevention of breast cancer in high-risk patients (Howell et al. 2022). The relative abundance of PR-A and PR-B has been identified as an important predictive factor for the response to antiprogestins in breast cancer treatment (Rojas et al. 2017; Abascal et al. 2022; Elía et al. 2023). Given this bidirectional potential for PR targeting, the exploration of context-specific behaviors in breast cancer and patient heterogeneity becomes the next step to elucidate which tumors benefit more from either PR stimulation or its inhibition.

15.5.3 Androgen Receptor

AR is structurally and functionally a close relative of ER and PR and is considered a major driver of prostate cancer (Taplin 2007; Tan et al. 2015). As many as 90% of ER+ breast cancers express AR (Lea et al. 1989; Moinfar et al. 2003; Park et al. 2009). Moreover, AR is expressed in approximately 60% of HER2-positive breast cancers and in 30–45% of triple-negative breast cancers. The role of AR signaling in breast cancer is complex, and several factors contribute to this complexity. For example, the impact of AR on breast cancer progression can vary depending on breast cancer subtype and the context of the tumor microenvironment (Chen et al. 2020; Yamaguchi et al. 2021) (Fig. 15.5). The cross talk between AR and other signaling pathways, including the ER pathway, further adds to this complexity.

15.5.3.1 AR Signaling in ER+ Breast Cancer

AR expression in hormone receptor-positive breast cancers, similarly to ER and PR, is associated with more differentiated, less aggressive tumors (Moinfar et al. 2003), and it is an independent predictor of both overall and disease-free survival (Peters et al. 2009; Kensler et al. 2019b). However, it has been also reported that a higher AR:ER ratio is associated with more aggressive breast cancer, worse prognosis, and higher risk to fail in response to traditional endocrine therapy (Cochrane et al. 2014; Rangel et al. 2018). This suggests that not only AR expression but also its stoichiometry with ER can differentially impact breast cancer progression. Functionally, the pro-

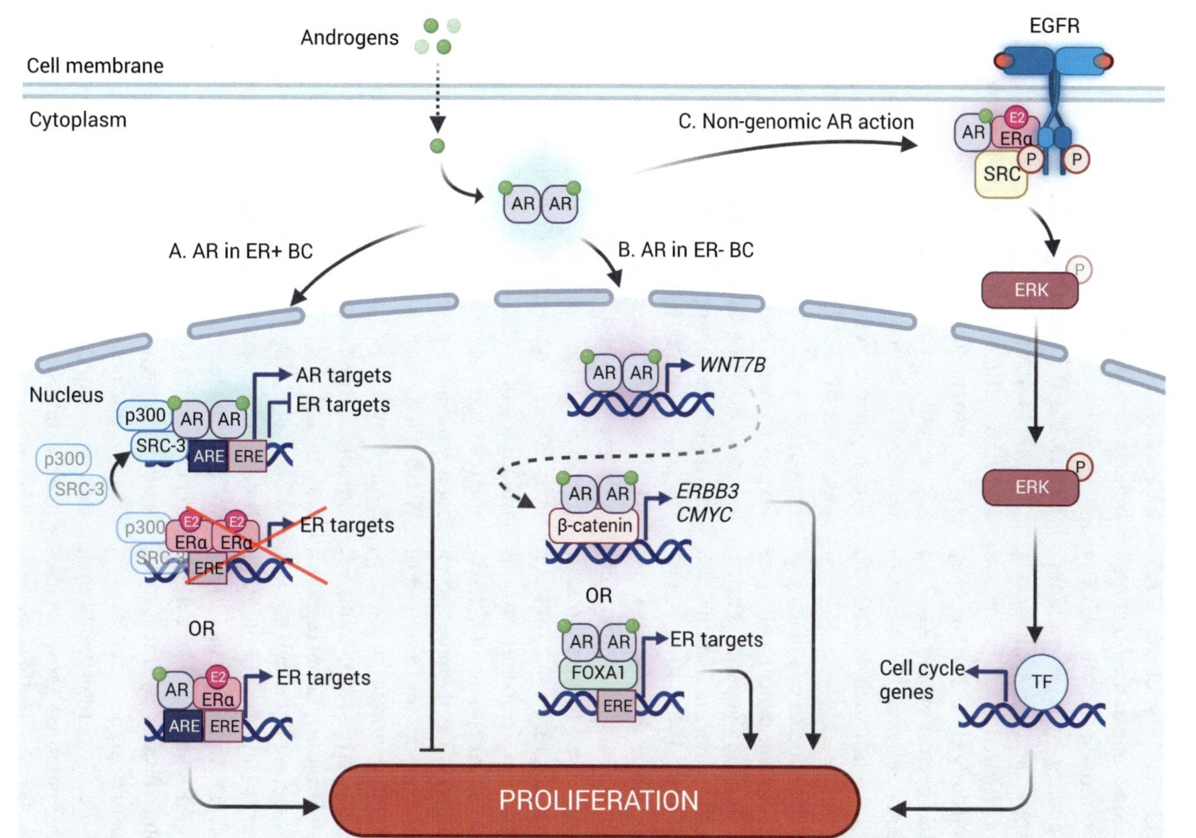

Fig. 15.5 AR mechanisms of action. (**a**) In ER+ BC, AR can either increase or decrease the hormone-dependent transcriptional program, depending on the cellular context. Upon ligand with androgens, AR translocates to the nucleus and binds to both AR and ER target DNA regions. ER signaling can be suppressed through the sequestration by AR of the shared transcriptional cofactors p300 and SRC-3. Alternatively, AR can cooperate with ER on the chromatin to upregulate ER target genes and cell proliferation. (**b**) In ER- BC, AR upregulates the expression of the WNT receptor ligand *WNT7B*. Downstream of activated WNT signaling, AR physically associates with β-catenin on the chromatin to upregulate the expression of the proliferative genes *ERBB3* and *MYC*. In molecular apocrine BC, AR relies on FOXA1 on the chromatin to sustain the expression of ER target genes. (**c**) AR/ER complex associates with the epidermal growth factor receptor (EGFR) and the kinase SRC to activate the induced cell proliferation through the MAPK/ERK pathway

posed protective role of AR on hormone receptor-positive breast cancer can be explained by several mechanisms. First, experiments on multiple breast cancer cell lines have shown that AR can bind a large proportion of ER target genes on the chromatin, and this competition results in a decreased ER signaling (Peters et al. 2009; Hickey et al. 2021). Second, due to the functional similarity of the two hormone receptors, AR can further suppress ER signaling by reprogramming ER and FOXA1 cistrome and by sequestering transcriptional cofactors shared by ER, such as p300 and SRC-3 (Ponnusamy et al. 2019; Hickey et al. 2021). Lastly, it has been shown in ZR-75-1 cells that AR can directly activate the transcription of tumor suppressor genes such as *ZBTB16* (Hickey et al. 2021).

On the other side of the spectrum, studies performed on several ER+ breast cancer cell lines have reported that AR signaling supports growth of ER+ breast cancer cells, whereas its inhibition reduces it (Di Monaco et al. 1993; Birrell et al. 1995; Di Monaco et al. 1995). Recent work has demonstrated that AR inhibition with enzalutamide, an AR antagonist used to treat prostate cancer, results in growth suppression of ER+ cell lines, including tamoxifen resistant strains (Cochrane et al. 2014; D'Amato et al. 2016). Mechanistic studies in MCF-7 cells have shown that AR can directly activate the transcription of ER target genes through genomic binding in response to estradiol, as well as enhancing ER nuclear translocation and transcriptional response by AR-ER physical interaction in the cell nucleus (Birrell et al. 1995; Panet-Raymond et al. 2000; Cochrane et al. 2014; D'Amato et al. 2016). Similar to ER and PR, AR can modulate cellular signaling in non-genomic fashion by direct interaction with cytoplasmic signal transducers. Experiments on MCF-7 cells demonstrated that, upon stimulation with epidermal growth factor (EGF), an AR:ER complex physically associates with the cytoplasmic kinase SRC to trigger ERK pathway, resulting in the induction of cell cycle progression (Migliaccio et al. 2005; Ciupek et al. 2015). AR antagonists, as well as decoy peptides that prevent AR-SRC association in MCF-7cells, were proven to reduce the signal transduction of EGF and the downstream effect on proliferation (Migliaccio et al. 2005, 2007). Thus, depending on the preclinical models used and the experimental conditions, AR stimulates or inhibits cellular proliferation. Multiple factors, including the diverse proteins that interact with AR and the fine balance of cell signaling, may determine the final biological outcome.

15.5.3.2 AR Signaling in ER- Breast Cancer

Just like in ER+ breast cancers, the role of AR as a prognostic factor is inconsistent in ER-negative breast tumors. Several studies have reported a better prognosis in triple-negative breast cancers expressing high levels of AR (Asano et al. 2017; Kucukzeybek et al. 2018). However, a large study of 4147 women with invasive breast cancer concluded that AR was associated with a 62% increase in breast cancer mortality compared to ER−/AR- patients (Kensler et al. 2019a). Others have reported that AR positivity is associated with worse clinical outcome in both HER2+/ER- and TNBC patients (Qu et al. 2013; Bozovic-Spasojevic et al. 2017; Feng et al. 2017). Functionally, multiple lines of preclinical research have explored the role and potential druggability of AR in hormone receptor-negative breast cancer. In the ER-/HER2+ cell line, MDA-MB-453, AR has been shown to promote cell growth by transcriptionally upregulating the WNT/β-catenin pathway ligand *WNT7B* (Ni et al. 2011). Following WNT signaling activation, the stabilized β-catenin associates with AR on the chromatin to upregulate *ERBB3* (encoding HER3) and *MYC*, leading to further induction of growth signaling pathways (Ni et al. 2011; Huang et al. 2017). Furthermore, a subset of ER−/AR+ tumors, termed "molecular apocrine," exhibit a gene expression profile that shares similarities with hormone-sensitive breast cancer, despite lacking ER expression (Farmer et al. 2005; Doane et al. 2006; Robinson et al. 2011). It is postulated that molecular apocrine breast tumors rely on AR and FOXA1 to mimic ER in sustaining hormone-dependent signaling and cell proliferation (Robinson et al. 2011).

Preclinical studies performed in multiple AR+ TNBC cell lines showed that they grow in response to androgens and that androgen blockage with first- and second-generation AR inhibitors can reduce cell proliferation and invasion (Barton et al. 2015, 2017).

15.5.3.3 AR in Endocrine Resistance

Several lines of research have shown that AR signaling can, at least in some contexts, compensate for the loss of ER signaling induced by ER-targeting compounds, leading to resistance to endocrine therapy. Transcriptomic profiling of patient tumors revealed that AR expression is increased in samples from metastatic endocrine resistant tumors compared to tamoxifen (an ER antagonist) sensitive primary tumors (Cui et al. 2006; De Amicis et al. 2010). In MCF-7 cells, overexpression of AR was shown to confer resistance to tamoxifen, and AR inhibition with bicalutamide restored the growth inhibitory effect of tamoxifen (De Amicis et al. 2010). Moreover, whereas tamoxifen leads to a downregulation of ER target genes in *wild-type* MCF-7 cells, it results in the induction of ER target genes such as *CCND1* in AR overexpressing cells, suggesting that AR can assist a tamoxifen-dependent ER stimulation (Ciupek et al. 2015). A similar outcome has been described in AR-overexpressing cells resistant to aromatase inhibitors, where it was found that AR interaction with ER results in the constitutive activation of the growth factor receptor IGF1R and downstream AKT signaling, representing an escape survival mechanism to endocrine therapy (Rechoum et al. 2014). Experiments inducing AR knockdown in endocrine resistant ER+ cell lines suggested that AR supports growth via noncanonical AR signaling, as pharmacological AR inhibition did not phenocopy the same antiproliferative effect (Ming Chia et al. 2019). In support of this hypothesis, SUMOylation of AR by Hsp27 has been reported in acquired and intrinsic endocrine resistant MCF-7 cells, leading to a constitutively active form of AR that is resistant to canonical pharmacological inhibition (Bahnassy et al. 2020). In contrast to these findings, in vitro studies on MCF-7 and ZR-75-1 cells have demonstrated that AR activation with androgens, as well its overexpression, can inhibit the estrogen-induced proliferation of these ER+ breast cancer cells (Peters et al. 2009; Hickey et al. 2021). A plausible explanation is that the impact of AR is reliant on specific cellular contexts, such as the level of AR expression (i.e., endogenous versus ectopic expression) or the presence of adequate estradiol milieu.

15.5.3.4 AR in Breast Cancer Metastasis

Whereas the molecular drivers of breast cancer metastasis are not well understood, recent evidence points to a possible role of AR in regulating cell viability and organ-specific tropism of disseminated cells. The expression of AR and its constitutively active splicing variant AR-v7 were found to be more expressed in circulating tumor cells isolated from ER+ breast cancer patients with bone metastasis compared to those derived from patients with metastases in other soft tissues (Lu and Luo 2013; Aceto et al. 2018). Studies on TNBC cell lines have indicated that blocking AR may effectively hinder the proliferation and dissemination of tumor cells of this subtype (Barton et al. 2017). Using TNBC cell lines as experimental model, it has been shown that AR favors the metastatic process via a positive feedback loop with TGFβ pathway, resulting in cancer stem cell-like traits, as well as protection against cell death mediated by cell detachment, supporting the viability of disseminated cells (Rosas et al. 2021). The efficacy of inhibiting both TGFβ and AR pathways was found to be more effective in cells under anchorage-independent conditions, suggesting their potential utility as combinatory targets for the treatment of triple-negative breast cancers. Additionally, preclinical evidence points to a direct regulation of AR in regulating epithelial-to-mesenchymal transition (EMT). It has been shown that both hormone receptor-positive and hormone receptor-negative breast cancer cell lines exposed to the pure AR agonist dihydrotestosterone (DHT) display increased invasion and migration (Feng et al. 2017). This is associated with a downregulation of the epithelial marker E-cadherin and upregulation of mesenchymal markers, such as vimentin and fibronectin. At the molecular level, it has been proposed that AR and the histone demethylase LSD1 bind regulatory regions of EMT genes on the chromatin to modulate gene transcription (Amente et al. 2010, 2013).

15.6 Preclinical Models to Study Hormone Action: Challenges and New Perspectives

15.6.1 Rodent Models of Estrogen Receptor-Positive Breast Cancer

The study of hormone signaling in breast cancer has been hindered by the scarcity of preclinical models. GEMMs are generally powerful tools to study mammary carcinogenesis in vivo. Yet, for reasons that are not fully understood, they mostly develop ER-negative tumors, when most human breast cancers are ER+.

Chemically induced mammary carcinogenesis in rats has been a useful model for studying breast cancer. Chemical agents such as 7,12-dimethylbenz(a)anthracene (DMBA) and N-methyl-N-nitrosourea (MNU) have been shown to induce tumor formation in rats with a single administration (Russo and Russo 1996). The time required for tumor development typically falls within the range of 8–21 weeks, with incidences close to 100% (Russo and Russo 1996). Compared to mice, rats are considered more similar to humans in terms of mammary gland anatomy and histological characteristic of the mammary epithelium (Singh et al. 2000; Russo et al. 2015). Chemically induced tumors in rats are hormone receptor positive and are sensitive to estrogen levels (Thompson et al. 1998). Additionally, pregnancy significantly reduces the incidence of mammary tumors in rats, similarly to humans (Thordarson et al. 1995). One drawback associated with rat models is their limited suitability for genetic manipulation compared to mice. Moreover, the use of chemical carcinogens can result in multiple genetic alterations that may not reflect the spontaneous disease.

15.6.2 Limitations of Cell Line Models

Most of our mechanistic knowledge of hormone signaling in breast cancer is derived from studies on the few cell lines that express hormone receptors. Cell lines simplify experimental models by providing a homogeneous population of cells that can be easily cultured and maintained in the laboratory. This simplification facilitates the examination of specific molecular and cellular events related to hormone signaling. While breast cancer cell lines have provided a wealth of valuable insights into hormone action, they have some limitations. Most breast cancer cell lines are derived from pleural or peritoneal effusions, i.e., from advanced, metastatic tumors, and hence may not fully represent the features and heterogeneity of primary tumors. Importantly, during the isolation process, they were selected for their ability to grow as monolayers on plastic, which poorly recapitulates the in vivo physiology (Holliday and Speirs 2011). Although breast cancer cell lines retain the major genomic hallmarks of their tumor subtype, they are subject to genetic drift and can progressively differ from the original tumor from which they were derived (Dai et al. 2017). Experimentally, individual hormones are typically added to hormone-deprived cell culture media to investigate the downstream effects. However, in physiological contexts, breast cancer cells are concomitantly exposed to multiple hormones and growth factors, which result in a complex interplay between the different hormone receptors to modulate the cell states (Mohammed et al. 2015; D'Amato et al. 2016; Hickey et al. 2021; Shamseddin et al. 2021; Scabia et al. 2022).

15.6.3 Xenograft Models and Tissue Context

Some of the limitations of in vitro-grown breast cancer cell lines can be overcome by xenografting the cells in mice. This is typically performed by injecting millions of cells in the mammary fat pad of immunocompromised mice. However, only few ER+ breast cancer cell lines can be engrafted successfully, and they require exogenous estradiol supplementation for their growth. This constraint results in estradiol levels, higher than those found in postmenopausal women. It has been shown the cells engrafted into the mammary gland adipose stroma have induced TGFβ/SLUG signaling and tend to differentiate toward basal cells, resulting in reduced hormone receptor expression and partial loss of their luminal identity (Sflomos et al. 2016).

15.6.4 Insights from Patient-Derived Xenografts

Patient-derived xenografts (PDXs) involve the transplantation of tumor tissue from a patient into immunodeficient mice. PDXs are attractive models for breast cancer research as they better capture the full spectrum of the disease compared to cell lines (Dobrolecki et al. 2016; Scabia et al. 2022). Similar to cell line xenografts, the use of PDXs has long been a challenge due to the low engraftment rate of ER+ PDXs in the mammary fat pad. Direct injection of BC cells into the mammary ducts, the site of origin of breast cancer (Behbod et al. 2009; Sflomos et al. 2016), a method known as mouse intraductal model (MIND), has significantly improved the engraftment success rate of both PDXs and cell lines, with engraftment rates exceeding 90% and the ability of grafts to grow without the need for estradiol supplementation (Haricharan et al. 2016; Sflomos et al. 2016). Intraductally injected tumors retain hormone receptor expression and faithfully replicate various aspects of the human disease in vivo, including the histological pattern of the original tumor, the transition from in situ to invasive disease, and the capacity to metastasize to relevant organs (Fiche et al. 2019; Aouad et al. 2021; Sflomos et al. 2021; Hong et al. 2022; Scabia et al. 2022).

The MIND method has also enabled the in vivo investigation of human primary normal breast epithelial cells (Shamseddin et al. 2021) and thus offers a novel avenue for studying all stages of human breast tumorigenesis in vivo and evaluating the impact of exogenous hormones on the proliferation of breast epithelial tissue, with the caveat that the host is immunocompromised. Notably, recent research has tested the effect of commonly prescribed synthetic progestins on the proliferation of human breast epithelial cells grafted in the murine mammary ducts (Shamseddin et al. 2021). Growth-stimulatory effects were observed with progestins that display binding affinity to AR besides PR, referred to as "androgenic" progestins (Louw-du Toit et al. 2017; Shamseddin et al. 2021). These findings point to a cooperation between PR and AR in mediating the tumor promoting effects of androgenic progestins.

The utilization of patient-derived intraductal xenografts of ER+ BC has also unveiled an intricate level of complexity in the tumor response to ovarian hormones. Individual PDXs exposed to physiological levels of E2 and P4 exhibited different sensitivity to either E2 or P4 alone or their combination, ultimately influencing tumor growth in distinct ways (Scabia et al. 2022). While most tumors responded with increased growth to E2, when exposed to progesterone, some PDXs increased proliferation while others did not. Transcriptomic profiling of the responders and nonresponders indicated that PDXs that respond to progesterone with increased tumor growth display low baseline MYC and AR activity, as well as enhanced interferon alpha (IFNα) signaling. These findings suggest that the nonresponders are characterized by high baseline activity of PR related pathways. Progesterone combined with estradiol increased the metastatic spread of PDXs in vivo compared to estrogen alone, even when the growth of the primary tumor mass was inhibited. This evidence highlights the significance of considering the metastatic disease in preclinical studies, as it is ultimately the factor that renders cancer fatal, shifting the focus beyond tumor growth alone. Moreover, these observations suggest that a personalized approach to endocrine therapy may be necessary.

15.7 Sex Hormones as Regulators of the Tumor Microenvironment

Breast cancer hormonal regulation is mediated by both cell autonomous and non-cell autonomous mechanisms. Specifically, the latter include all those interactions that participate in the modulation of the stromal and immune cells located in the vicinity of the tumor, collectively forming the so-called tumor microenvironment (TME).

The major TME cell types are cancer-associated fibroblasts, which are directly recruited by tumor cells. Among other functions, they are responsible for the production and secretion of the extracellular matrix (ECM), which in turn mediates both mechanical and molecular signaling onto the tumor cells. A second constituent of the TME includes innate and adaptive immune cells, such as T cells, B cells, neutrophils, natural killer cells, dendritic cells, and macrophages, that can be instructed by malignant cells to support tumor progression. Finally, the vasculature surrounding and infiltrating the tumor mass determines the local availability of nutrients and oxygen and is therefore a crucial factor in the evolution of the tumorigenic process.

As discussed above, hormone-dependent cellular cross talks play key roles in the proper development and physiology of the normal breast. This signaling remains a fundamental component also in its malignant counterpart, where it contributes to modeling the TME, ultimately favoring tumor growth.

For instance, analysis of breast adipose stromal cells has shown that the expression of aromatase—the enzyme involved in estrogen biosynthesis through the conversion of androgens—is overall higher in breast cancer compared to the normal breast. This difference likely arises from the activation of alternative promoters that regulate the aromatase expression, specifically in fibroblasts (Agarwal et al. 1996; Santen et al. 2009). It has been postulated that breast cancer cells can modulate the aromatase promoter usage in fibroblasts by secreting immunomodulatory molecules such as prostaglandin E2 (Zhao et al. 1996). Downstream of the augmented aromatase activity, an increased production of estrogen at these sites fuels estrogen-mediated signaling within cancer cells, leading to enhanced tumor proliferation.

The hormone receptor status of the breast tumor is key in determining the profile and the extent of immune cell infiltration (reviewed in Hargrove-Wiley and Fingleton 2023). For instance, the balance of estrogen and progesterone signaling influences the number as well as the transcriptional state of tumor-associated macrophages, ultimately favoring the development of an immuno-permissive environment (reviewed in Miller and Hunt 1996). Hormone-dependent immune modulation can be exerted both indirectly, through hormone-dependent production of immunomodulatory mediators by cancer cells, and directly in a cell autonomous manner. For instance, tumor-associated macrophages (TAMs) express AR, and in vivo experiment on tumor-bearing mice suggested that increased androgen production by breast cancer cell can modulate the surrounding TAMs toward an immunotolerant phenotype (Yamaguchi et al. 2021).

Finally, hormone signaling also modulates the composition and production of the breast ECM that in turn contributes to determine mammographic density and tissue stiffness. Experiments on GEMMs demonstrated that higher stiffness promotes tumor growth and invasion via integrin signaling (Levental et al. 2009). Interestingly, combined HRT has been associated with an increased breast density, which is itself an important risk factor for breast cancer (Azam et al. 2020). Murine breast cancer models showed that estrogen signaling can facilitate breast cancer progression and metastasis also via inducing increased stromal production ECM components as well as via altering collagen fiber alignment, finally leading to increased stiffness (Jallow et al.

2019). On the other hand, increased collagen deposition can in turn enhance estrogen signaling within tumor cells and favor tumor growth (Jallow et al. 2019), suggesting the existence of a positive feedback loop.

15.8 Conclusions

The understanding of hormone signaling and the advancement of endocrine therapies have improved prevention and treatment of breast cancer. Nevertheless, numerous questions remain unanswered regarding the role of hormone signaling in the normal and malignant breast tissue. The precise molecular mechanisms that determine the change in hormone receptor expression patterns in early breast tumorigenesis as well as the switch from a paracrine to a cell-intrinsic hormonal action have not been clearly defined yet. Moreover, hormone-induced cellular signaling can elicit divergent biological outcomes, to the point where the same hormonal stimulation has been shown to either facilitate or hinder breast cancer growth. In order to better choose when to stimulate or inhibit hormone receptors to treat breast cancer patients, it is crucial to fully understand the complex interaction between hormone signaling pathways in the different breast cancer subtypes and their implication in the contexts of endocrine therapy and resistance.

It is still puzzling how the combined action of hormone receptors with partially overlapping functions can either stimulate or inhibit tumor proliferation through genomic and non-genomic signaling. Possibly, context-specific interactions between hormone receptors and their transcriptional networks might contribute to these effects. Therefore, the elucidation of hormone receptor cross talk on the chromatin, as well as their interactions with cytosolic signaling transducers, warrants further investigation. Better modeling of inter-patient variability is required for the identification of predictive biomarkers and the development of novel personalized therapies. This goal strictly requires the implementation of new approaches, as well as the refinement of the existing preclinical models to faithfully recapitulate human disease.

Intraductal patient-derived xenografts (PDXs) have provided valuable insights into the individualized response of patients to hormones within a physiologically relevant environment. However, their full potential is limited by the use of immunocompromised mice as hosts. Consequently, the intricate interplay between cancer cells and the immune system, which plays a prominent role in tumor growth, metastasis, and therapeutic response in humans, remains poorly understood (Standish et al. 2008). The ongoing advancements in developing immunocompetent xenograft models will open up the potential to study how hormones modulate the interactions between tumor cells and the immune system (Kalscheuer et al. 2012; Basel et al. 2018; Stripecke et al. 2020).

References

Abascal MF et al (2022) Progesterone receptor isoform ratio dictates antiprogestin/progestin effects on breast cancer growth and metastases: A role for NDRG1. Int J Cancer 150(9):1481–1496. https://doi.org/10.1002/IJC.33913

Abdel-Hafiz HA, Horwitz KB (2014) Post-translational modifications of the progesterone receptors. J Steroid Biochem Mol Biol 140:80–89. https://doi.org/10.1016/J.JSBMB.2013.12.008

Acconcia F et al (2005) Palmitoylation-dependent estrogen receptor alpha membrane localization: regulation by 17beta-estradiol. Mol Biol Cell 16(1):231–237. https://doi.org/10.1091/MBC.E04-07-0547

Aceto N et al (2018) AR expression in breast cancer CTCs associates with bone metastases. Mol Cancer Res 16(4):720–727. https://doi.org/10.1158/1541-7786.MCR-17-0480

Agarwal VR et al (1996) Use of alternative promoters to express the aromatase cytochrome P450 (CYP19) gene in breast adipose tissues of cancer-free and breast cancer patients. J Clin Endocrinol Metab 81(11):3843–3849. https://doi.org/10.1210/JCEM.81.11.8923826

Alexieva-figusch J et al (1980) Progestin therapy in advanced breast cancer: megestrol acetate-an evaluation of 160 treated cases. Cancer 46:2369–2372. https://doi.org/10.1002/1097-0142

Altwegg KA, Vadlamudi RK (2021) Role of estrogen receptor coregulators in endocrine resistant breast cancer. Explor Target Anti-tumor Ther 2(4):385. https://doi.org/10.37349/ETAT.2021.00052

Amente S et al (2010) LSD1-mediated demethylation of histone H3 lysine 4 triggers Myc-induced transcription. Oncogene 29(25):3691–3702. https://doi.org/10.1038/onc.2010.120

Amente S, Lania L, Majello B (2013) The histone LSD1 demethylase in stemness and cancer transcription programs. Biochim Biophys Acta (BBA) - Gene Regul Mech 1829(10):981–986. https://doi.org/10.1016/J.BBAGRM.2013.05.002

Anzick SL et al (1997) AIB1, a steroid receptor coactivator amplified in breast and ovarian cancer. Science 277(5328):965–968. https://doi.org/10.1126/SCIENCE.277.5328.965/ASSET/5BA0D9A2-728B-4E77-84F2-E000C019AEEC/ASSETS/GRAPHIC/SE3375589004.JPEG

Aouad P et al. (2021) Epithelial-mesenchymal plasticity determines estrogen receptor positive (ER+) breast cancer dormancy and reacquisition of an epithelial state drives awakening. doi: https://doi.org/10.1101/2021.07.22.453458

Aranda A, Pascual A (2001) Nuclear hormone receptors and gene expression. Physiol Rev 81(3):1269–1304. https://doi.org/10.1152/PHYSREV.2001.81.3.1269

Asano Y et al (2017) Expression and clinical significance of androgen receptor in triple-negative breast cancer. Cancers 9(1). https://doi.org/10.3390/CANCERS9010004

Ataca D et al (2020) The secreted protease Adamts18 links hormone action to activation of the mammary stem cell niche. Nat Commun 11(1):1571. https://doi.org/10.1038/s41467-020-15357-y

Azam S et al (2020) Mammographic density change and risk of breast cancer. J Natl Cancer Inst 112(4): 391–399. https://doi.org/10.1093/JNCI/DJZ149

Bahnassy S et al (2020) Constitutively active androgen receptor supports the metastatic phenotype of endocrine-resistant hormone receptor-positive breast cancer. Cell Commun Signal 18(1):1–11. https://doi.org/10.1186/S12964-020-00649-Z/FIGURES/6

Bartlett TE et al (2022) Antiprogestins reduce epigenetic field cancerization in breast tissue of young healthy women. Genome Med 14(1):1–18. https://doi.org/10.1186/S13073-022-01063-5/FIGURES/6

Barton VN et al (2015) Multiple molecular subtypes of triple-negative breast cancer critically rely on androgen receptor and respond to enzalutamide in vivo. Mol Cancer Therap 14(3):769–778. https://doi.org/10.1158/1535-7163.MCT-14-0926/8810/P/MULTIPLE-MOLECULAR-SUBTYPES-OF-TRIPLE-NEGATIVE

Barton VN et al (2017) Androgen receptor supports an anchorage-independent, cancer stem cell-like population in triple-negative breast cancer. Cancer Res 77(13):3455. https://doi.org/10.1158/0008-5472.CAN-16-3240

Barua D, Gupta A, Gupta S (2020) Targeting the IRE1-XBP1 axis to overcome endocrine resistance in breast cancer: opportunities and challenges. Cancer Lett 486:29–37. https://doi.org/10.1016/J.CANLET.2020.05.020

Basel MT et al (2018) Developing a xenograft human tumor model in immunocompetent mice. Cancer Lett 412:256–263. https://doi.org/10.1016/J.CANLET.2017.10.009

Beatson GT (1896) On the treatment of inoperable cases of carcinoma of the mamma: suggestions for a new method of treatment, with illustrative cases. Transactions 15:153–179. Accessed: 19 May 2023

Behbod F et al (2009) An intraductal human-in-mouse transplantation model mimics the subtypes of ductal carcinoma in situ. Breast Cancer Res 11(5):R66. https://doi.org/10.1186/bcr2358

Beleut M et al (2010) Two distinct mechanisms underlie progesterone-induced proliferation in the mammary gland. Proc Natl Acad Sci USA 107:2989–2994. https://doi.org/10.1073/pnas.0915148107

Birrell SN et al (1995) Androgens induce divergent proliferative responses in human breast cancer cell lines. J Steroid Biochem Mol Biol 52(5):459–467. https://doi.org/10.1016/0960-0760(95)00005-K

Bozovic-Spasojevic I et al (2017) The prognostic role of androgen receptor in patients with early-stage breast cancer: a metaanalysis of clinical and gene expression data. Clin Cancer Res 23(11):2702–2712. https://doi.org/10.1158/1078-0432.CCR-16-0979/128539/AM/THE-PROGNOSTIC-ROLE-OF-ANDROGEN-RECEPTOR-IN

Brisken C, O'Malley B (2011) Hormone action in the mammary gland. Cold Spring Harb Perspect Biol 2:a003178. https://doi.org/10.1101/cshperspect.a003178

Brisken C, Scabia V (2020) 90 years of progesterone: progesterone receptor signaling in the normal breast and its implications for cancer. J Mol Endocrinol 65(1):T81–T94. https://doi.org/10.1530/JME-20-0091

Brisken C et al (1999) Prolactin controls mammary gland development via direct and indirect mechanisms. Dev Biol 210:96–106. https://doi.org/10.1006/dbio.1999.9271

Brzozowski AM et al (1997) Molecular basis of agonism and antagonism in the oestrogen receptor. Nature 389(6652):753–758. https://doi.org/10.1038/39645

Cagnet S et al (2018) Oestrogen receptor α AF-1 and AF-2 domains have cell population-specific functions in the mammary epithelium. Nat Commun 9(1):4723. https://doi.org/10.1038/s41467-018-07175-0

Calligé M, Richard-Foy H (2006) Ligand-Induced Estrogen Receptor α Degradation by the Proteasome: New Actors? Nuclear Receptor Signal 4(1):nrs.04004. https://doi.org/10.1621/nrs.04004

Carascossa S et al (2010) CARM1 mediates the ligand-independent and tamoxifen-resistant activation of the estrogen receptor alpha by cAMP. Genes Dev 24(7):708–719. https://doi.org/10.1101/GAD.568410

Carroll JS et al (2006) Genome-wide analysis of estrogen receptor binding sites. Nat Genet 38(11):1289–1297. https://doi.org/10.1038/NG1901

Castoria G et al (2001) PI3-kinase in concert with Src promotes the S-phase entry of oestradiol-stimulated

MCF-7 cells. EMBO J 20(21):6050–6059. https://doi.org/10.1093/EMBOJ/20.21.6050

Chen M et al (2020) Androgen receptor in breast cancer: from bench to bedside. Front Endocrinol 11:573. https://doi.org/10.3389/FENDO.2020.00573/BIBTEX

Cheng M, Michalski S, Kommagani R (2018) Role for growth regulation by estrogen in breast cancer 1 (GREB1) in hormone-dependent cancers. Int J Mol Sci 19(9). https://doi.org/10.3390/IJMS19092543

Ciarloni L, Mallepell S, Brisken C (2007) Amphiregulin is an essential mediator of estrogen receptor alpha function in mammary gland development. Proc Natl Acad Sci USA 104:5455–5460. https://doi.org/10.1073/pnas.0611647104

Cicatiello L et al (2004) Estrogens and progesterone promote persistent CCND1 gene activation during G1 by inducing transcriptional derepression via c-Jun/c-Fos/estrogen receptor (progesterone receptor) complex assembly to a distal regulatory element and recruitment of cyclin D1 to its own gene promoter. Mol Cell Biol 24(16):7260–7274. https://doi.org/10.1128/MCB.24.16.7260-7274.2004

Ciriello G et al (2015) Comprehensive molecular portraits of invasive lobular breast cancer. Cell 163(2):506–519. https://doi.org/10.1016/J.CELL.2015.09.033

Ciupek A et al (2015) Androgen receptor promotes tamoxifen agonist activity by activation of EGFR in ERα-positive breast cancer. Breast Cancer Res Treat 154(2):225–237. https://doi.org/10.1007/S10549-015-3609-7/FIGURES/5

Clarke RB et al (1997) Dissociation between steroid receptor expression and cell proliferation in the human breast. Cancer Res 57:4987–4991

Classen S et al (1993) Effect of onapristone and medroxyprogesterone acetate on the proliferation and hormone receptor concentration of human breast cancer cells. J Steroid Biochem Mol Biol 45(4):315–319. https://doi.org/10.1016/0960-0760(93)90348-Z

Cochrane DR et al (2014) Role of the androgen receptor in breast cancer and preclinical analysis of enzalutamide. Breast Cancer Res 16(1). https://doi.org/10.1186/bcr3599

Colditz GA et al (2004) Risk factors for breast cancer according to estrogen and progesterone receptor status. J Natl Cancer Inst 96(3):218–228. https://doi.org/10.1093/JNCI/DJH025

Cottu PH et al (2018) Phase I study of onapristone, a type I antiprogestin, in female patients with previously treated recurrent or metastatic progesterone receptor-expressing cancers. PLoS One 13(10). https://doi.org/10.1371/JOURNAL.PONE.0204973

Cui Y et al (2006) Elevated expression of mitogen-activated protein kinase phosphatase 3 in breast tumors: a mechanism of tamoxifen resistance. Cancer Res 66(11):5950–5959. https://doi.org/10.1158/0008-5472.CAN-05-3243

D'Amato NC et al (2016) Cooperative dynamics of AR and ER activity in breast cancer. Mol Cancer Res 14(11):1054–1067. https://doi.org/10.1158/1541-7786.mcr-16-0167

Dai X et al (2017) Breast cancer cell line classification and its relevance with breast tumor subtyping. J Cancer 8(16):3131. https://doi.org/10.7150/JCA.18457

Daniel AR, Knutson TP, Lange CA (2009) Signaling inputs to progesterone receptor gene regulation and promoter selectivity. Mol Cell Endocrinol 308:47–52. https://doi.org/10.1016/j.mce.2009.01.004

Daniel AR et al (2015) Progesterone receptor-B enhances estrogen responsiveness of breast cancer cells via scaffolding PELP1- and estrogen receptor-containing transcription complexes. Oncogene 34(4):506. https://doi.org/10.1038/ONC.2013.579

Daschner PJ et al (1999) Increased AP-1 activity in drug resistant human breast cancer MCF-7 cells. Breast Cancer Res Treat 53(3):229–240. https://doi.org/10.1023/A:1006138803392

Davies MPA et al (2008) Expression and splicing of the unfolded protein response gene XBP-1 are significantly associated with clinical outcome of endocrine-treated breast cancer. Int J Cancer 123(1):85–88. https://doi.org/10.1002/IJC.23479

De Amicis F et al (2010) Androgen receptor overexpression induces tamoxifen resistance in human breast cancer cells. Breast Cancer Res Treat 121(1):1. https://doi.org/10.1007/S10549-009-0436-8

Di Monaco M et al (1993) The antiandrogen flutamide inhibits growth of mcf-7 human breast-cancer cell-line. Int J Oncol 2(4):653–656. https://doi.org/10.3892/IJO.2.4.653

Di Monaco M et al (1995) Inhibitory effect of hydroxyflutamide plus tamoxifen on oestradiol-induced growth of MCF-7 breast cancer cells. J Cancer Res Clin Oncol 121:710–714

Ding L et al (2003) Ligand-independent activation of estrogen receptor α by XBP-1. Nucl Acids Res 31(18):5266–5274. https://doi.org/10.1093/NAR/GKG731

Doane AS et al (2006) An estrogen receptor-negative breast cancer subset characterized by a hormonally regulated transcriptional program and response to androgen. Oncogene 25(28):3994–4008. https://doi.org/10.1038/SJ.ONC.1209415

Dobrolecki LE et al (2016) Patient-derived xenograft (PDX) models in basic and translational breast cancer research. Cancer Metastasis Rev 35:547–573. https://doi.org/10.1007/s10555-016-9653-x

Drabovich AP et al (2016) Dynamics of protein expression reveals primary targets and secondary messengers of estrogen receptor alpha signaling in MCF-7 breast cancer cells. Mol Cell Proteomics 15(6):2093–2107. https://doi.org/10.1074/MCP.M115.057257

Duss S et al (2007) An oestrogen-dependent model of breast cancer created by transformation of normal human mammary epithelial cells. Breast Cancer Res 9:R38. https://doi.org/10.1186/bcr1734

Dydensborg AB et al (2009) 'GATA3 inhibits breast cancer growth and pulmonary breast cancer metastasis. Oncogene 28(29):2634–2642. https://doi.org/10.1038/onc.2009.126

Elía A et al (2023) Beneficial effects of mifepristone treatment in patients with breast cancer selected by the progesterone receptor isoform ratio: results from the MIPRA trial. Clin Cancer Res 29(5):866. https://doi.org/10.1158/1078-0432.CCR-22-2060

Faivre EJ et al (2008) Progesterone receptor rapid signaling mediates serine 345 phosphorylation and tethering to specificity protein 1 transcription factors. Mol Endocrinol 22(4):823–837. https://doi.org/10.1210/ME.2007-0437

Fang Y et al (2004) XBP-1 increases ERα transcriptional activity through regulation of large-scale chromatin unfolding. Biochem Biophys Res Commun 323(1):269–274. https://doi.org/10.1016/J.BBRC.2004.08.100

Farcas AM et al (2021) Genome-wide estrogen receptor activity in breast cancer. Endocrinology 162(2). https://doi.org/10.1210/ENDOCR/BQAA224

Farmer P et al (2005) Identification of molecular apocrine breast tumours by microarray analysis. Oncogene 24(29):4660–4671. https://doi.org/10.1038/sj.onc.1208561

Faus H, Haendler B (2006) Post-translational modifications of steroid receptors. Biomed Pharmacother 60(9):520–528. https://doi.org/10.1016/J.BIOPHA.2006.07.082

Feng J et al (2017) Androgen and AR contribute to breast cancer development and metastasis: an insight of mechanisms. Oncogene 36(20):2775–2790. https://doi.org/10.1038/ONC.2016.432

Fernandez-Valdivia R et al (2009) The RANKL signaling axis is sufficient to elicit ductal side-branching and alveologenesis in the mammary gland of the virgin mouse. Dev Biol 328(1):127–139. https://doi.org/10.1016/J.YDBIO.2009.01.019

Fiche M et al (2019) Intraductal patient-derived xenografts of estrogen receptor α-positive breast cancer recapitulate the histopathological spectrum and metastatic potential of human lesions. J Pathol 247(3):287–292. https://doi.org/10.1002/path.5200

Fournier A, Berrino F, Clavel-Chapelon F (2008) Unequal risks for breast cancer associated with different hormone replacement therapies: results from the E3N cohort study. Breast Cancer Res Treat 107(1):103–111. https://doi.org/10.1007/s10549-007-9523-x

Fu X et al (2016) FOXA1 overexpression mediates endocrine resistance by altering the ER transcriptome and IL-8 expression in ER-positive breast cancer. Proc Natl Acad Sci U S A 113(43):E6600–E6609. https://doi.org/10.1073/PNAS.1612835113/SUPPL_FILE/PNAS.1612835113.SD01.XLSX

Fu X et al (2019) FOXA1 upregulation promotes enhancer and transcriptional reprogramming in endocrine-resistant breast cancer. Proc Natl Acad Sci U S A 116(52):26823–26834. https://doi.org/10.1073/PNAS.1911584116/SUPPL_FILE/PNAS.1911584116.SD05.XLSX

Gagniac L et al (2020) Membrane expression of the estrogen receptor ERα is required for intercellular communications in the mammary epithelium. Development (Cambridge) 147(5). https://doi.org/10.1242/DEV.182303/VIDEO-1

Gertz J et al (2013) Distinct properties of cell type-specific and shared transcription factor binding sites. Mol Cell 52(1):25–36. https://doi.org/10.1016/J.MOLCEL.2013.08.037

Gill PG et al (1987) Difference between R5020 and the antiprogestin RU486 in antiproliferative effects on human breast cancer cells. Breast Cancer Res Treat 10(1):37–45. https://doi.org/10.1007/BF01806133/METRICS

Greene GL et al (1986) Sequence and expression of human estrogen receptor complementary DNA. Science 231(4742):1150–1154. https://doi.org/10.1126/SCIENCE.3753802

Groshong SD et al (1997) Biphasic regulation of breast cancer cell growth by progesterone: role of the cyclin-dependent kinase inhibitors, p21 and p27Kip1. Mol Endocrinol 11(11):1593–1607. https://doi.org/10.1210/MEND.11.11.0006

Hanamura T et al (2021) Reproductive factors and breast cancer risk according to joint estrogen and progesterone receptor status: a meta-analysis of epidemiological studies. Breast Cancer Res 13(3):1–11. https://doi.org/10.1073/pnas.0600089103

Hargrove-Wiley E, Fingleton B (2023) Sex hormones in breast cancer immunity. Cancer Res 83(1):12–19. https://doi.org/10.1158/0008-5472.CAN-22-1829

Haricharan S, Lei J, Ellis M (2016) Mammary ductal environment is necessary for faithful maintenance of estrogen signaling in ER+ breast cancer. Cancer Cell:249–250. https://doi.org/10.1016/j.ccell.2016.02.017

Haslam SZ, Shyamala G (1979) Effect of oestradiol on progesterone receptors in normal mammary glands and its relationship with lactation. Biochem J 182:127–131

Helsen C et al (2012) Structural basis for nuclear hormone receptor DNA binding. Mol Cell Endocrinol 348(2):411–417. https://doi.org/10.1016/J.MCE.2011.07.025

Hickey TE et al (2021) The androgen receptor is a tumor suppressor in estrogen receptor-positive breast cancer. Nat Med 27(2):310–320. https://doi.org/10.1038/S41591-020-01168-7

Hoch RV et al (1999) Gata-3 is expressed in association with estrogen receptor in breast cancer. Int J Cancer (Pred Oncol) 84:122–128. https://doi.org/10.1002/(SICI)1097-0215(19990420)84:2

Holliday DL, Speirs V (2011) Choosing the right cell line for breast cancer research. Breast Cancer Res 13(4):1–7. https://doi.org/10.1186/BCR2889/COMMENTS

Hong Y et al (2022) Mouse-INtraDuctal (MIND): an in vivo model for studying the underlying mechanisms of DCIS malignancy. J Pathol 256(2):186–201. https://doi.org/10.1002/PATH.5820

Howell S et al (2022) Abstract P1-10-01: Results from the breast cancer - anti progestin prevention study 1 (BC-APPS1) trial - a novel approach in breast cancer prevention. Cancer Res 82(4_Supplement):P1-10–01. https://doi.org/10.1158/1538-7445.SABCS21-P1-10-01

Hsu SP et al (2019) Progesterone up-regulates p27 through an increased binding of the progesterone receptor-A-p53 protein complex onto the non-canonical p53 binding motif in HUVEC. J Steroid Biochem Mol Biol 185:163–171. https://doi.org/10.1016/J.JSBMB.2018.08.011

Huang WY et al (2000) Hormone-related factors and risk of breast cancer in relation to estrogen receptor and progesterone receptor status. Am J Epidemiol 151(7):703–714. https://doi.org/10.1093/OXFORDJOURNALS.AJE.A010265

Huang R et al (2017) Androgen receptor expression and bicalutamide antagonize androgen receptor inhibit β-catenin transcription complex in estrogen receptor-negative breast cancer. Cell Physiol Biochem 43(6):2212–2225. https://doi.org/10.1159/000484300

Hurtado A et al (2011) FOXA1 is a key determinant of estrogen receptor function and endocrine response. Nat Genet 43(1):27–33. https://doi.org/10.1038/NG.730

Ingle JN et al (1982) Randomized clinical trial of megestrol acetate versus tamoxifen in paramenopausal or castrated women with advanced breast cancer. Am J Clin Oncol 5(2):155–160. https://doi.org/10.1097/00000421-198204000-00062

Izuo M, Iino Y, Endo K (1981) Oral high-dose medroxyprogesterone acetate (MAP) in treatment of advanced breast cancer - A preliminary report of clinical and experimental studies. Breast Cancer Res Treat 1(2):125–130. https://doi.org/10.1007/BF01805865/METRICS

Jallow F et al (2019) Dynamic interactions between the extracellular matrix and estrogen activity in progression of ER+ breast cancer. Oncogene 38(43):6913–6925. https://doi.org/10.1038/s41388-019-0941-0

Kalscheuer H et al (2012) A model for personalized in vivo analysis of human immune responsiveness. Sci Transl Med 4(125). https://doi.org/10.1126/SCITRANSLMED.3003481/SUPPL_FILE/4-125RA30_SM.PDF

Kato S et al (1995) Activation of the estrogen receptor through phosphorylation by mitogen-activated protein kinase. Science (New York, N.Y.) 270(5241):1491–1494. https://doi.org/10.1126/SCIENCE.270.5241.1491

Kensler KH, Poole EM et al (2019a) Androgen receptor expression and breast cancer survival: results from the nurses' health studies. J Natl Cancer Inst 111(7):700. https://doi.org/10.1093/JNCI/DJY173

Kensler KH, Regan MM et al (2019b) Prognostic and predictive value of androgen receptor expression in postmenopausal women with estrogen receptor-positive breast cancer: Results from the Breast International Group Trial 1-98. Breast Cancer Res 21(1):30. https://doi.org/10.1186/s13058-019-1118-z

Kraus WL, Kadonaga JT (1998) p300 and estrogen receptor cooperatively activate transcription via differential enhancement of initiation and reinitiation. Genes Dev 12(3):331. https://doi.org/10.1101/GAD.12.3.331

Kucukzeybek BB et al (2018) Prognostic significance of androgen receptor expression in HER2-positive and triple-negative breast cancer. Polish J Pathol 69(2):157–168. https://doi.org/10.5114/PJP.2018.76699

Kumar R, Thompson EB (1999) The structure of the nuclear hormone receptors. Steroids 64(5):310–319. https://doi.org/10.1016/S0039-128X(99)00014-8

Kumar R et al (2011) The dynamic structure of the estrogen receptor. J Amino Acids 2011:1–7. https://doi.org/10.4061/2011/812540

Kushner PJ et al (2000) Estrogen receptor pathways to AP-1. J Steroid Biochem Mol Biol 74(5):311–317. https://doi.org/10.1016/S0960-0760(00)00108-4

Laamiri FZ et al (2015) Risk factors for breast cancer of different age groups: Moroccan data? Open J Obstet Gynecol 5(2):79–87. https://doi.org/10.4236/OJOG.2015.52011

Le Romancer M et al (2008) Regulation of estrogen rapid signaling through arginine methylation by PRMT1. Mol Cell 31(2):212–221. https://doi.org/10.1016/J.MOLCEL.2008.05.025

Le Romancer M et al (2011) Cracking the estrogen receptor's posttranslational code in breast tumors. Endocr Rev 32(5):597–622. https://doi.org/10.1210/ER.2010-0016

Lea OA, Kvinnsland S, Thorsen T (1989) Improved measurement of androgen receptors in human breast cancer. Cancer Res 49(24 Part 1)

Lee S et al (2006) Hormones, receptors, and growth in hyperplastic enlarged lobular units: early potential precursors of breast cancer. Breast Cancer Res 8(1):R6. https://doi.org/10.1186/BCR1367

Levental KR et al (2009) Matrix crosslinking forces tumor progression by enhancing integrin signaling. Cell 139(5):891–906. https://doi.org/10.1016/j.cell.2009.10.027

Lewis JH et al (2020) Onapristone extended release: safety evaluation from phase I–II studies with an emphasis on hepatotoxicity. Drug Saf 43(10):1045–1055. https://doi.org/10.1007/S40264-020-00964-X/FIGURES/2

Lim E et al (2010) Transcriptome analyses of mouse and human mammary cell subpopulations reveal multiple conserved genes and pathways. Breast Cancer Res 12(2):R21. https://doi.org/10.1186/bcr2560

Lippman ME, Bolan G (1975) Oestrogen-responsive human breast cancer in long term tissue culture. Nature 256(5518):592–593. https://doi.org/10.1038/256592A0

Lonard DM, O'Malley BW (2012) Nuclear receptor coregulators: modulators of pathology and therapeutic targets. Nat Rev Endocrinol 8(10):598–604. https://doi.org/10.1038/NRENDO.2012.100

Louw-du Toit R et al (2017) Comparing the androgenic and estrogenic properties of progestins used in contraception and hormone therapy. Biochem Biophys Res Commun 491(1):140–146. https://doi.org/10.1016/J.BBRC.2017.07.063

Lu C, Luo J (2013) Decoding the androgen receptor splice variants. Transl Androl Urol 2(3):178–186. https://doi.org/10.3978/J.ISSN.2223-4683.2013.09.08

Lu P et al (2008) Genetic mosaic analysis reveals FGF receptor 2 function in terminal end buds during mammary gland branching morphogenesis. Dev Biol 321(1):77–87. https://doi.org/10.1016/J.YDBIO.2008.06.005

Lydon JP et al (1995) Mice lacking progesterone receptor exhibit pleiotropic reproductive abnormalities. Genes Dev 9(18):2266–2278. https://doi.org/10.1101/GAD.9.18.2266

Lyons WR (1958) Hormonal synergism in mammary growth. Proc R Soc Lond B Biol Sci 149(936):303–325. https://doi.org/10.1098/rspb.1958.0071

Ma H et al (2006) Reproductive factors and breast cancer risk according to joint estrogen and progesterone receptor status: a meta-analysis of epidemiological studies. Breast Cancer Res 8(4). https://doi.org/10.1186/BCR1525

Marino M, Ascenzi P (2006) Steroid hormone rapid signaling: the pivotal role of S-palmitoylation. IUBMB Life 58(12):716–719. https://doi.org/10.1080/15216540601019485

Mastorakos G et al (2021) Progestins and the risk of breast cancer. Acta Endocrinologica Foundation 17(1):90. https://doi.org/10.4183/AEB.2021.90

Medunjanin S et al (2005) Glycogen synthase kinase-3 interacts with and phosphorylates estrogen receptor α and is involved in the regulation of receptor activity. J Biol Chem 280(38):33006–33014. https://doi.org/10.1074/jbc.M506758200

Migliaccio A et al (1996) Tyrosine kinase/p21ras/MAP-kinase pathway activation by estradiol-receptor complex in MCF-7 cells. EMBO J 15(6):1292. https://doi.org/10.1002/j.1460-2075.1996.tb00471.x

Migliaccio A et al (2005) Steroid receptor regulation of epidermal growth factor signaling through Src in breast and prostate cancer cells: steroid antagonist action. Cancer Res 65(22):10585–10593. https://doi.org/10.1158/0008-5472.CAN-05-0912

Migliaccio A et al (2007) Inhibition of the SH3 domain-mediated binding of Src to the androgen receptor and its effect on tumor growth. Oncogene 26(46):6619–6629. https://doi.org/10.1038/sj.onc.1210487

Miller L, Hunt JS (1996) Sex steroid hormones and macrophage function. Life Sci 59(1):1–14. https://doi.org/10.1016/0024-3205(96)00122-1

Ming Chia K, Portman N, Laven-Law G (2019) Non-canonical AR activity facilitates endocrine resistance in breast cancer Mechanisms of sex hormone signalling and the emergence of resistance to hormonal therapies used in the treatment of breast and prostate cancer. Acquir Mutations Immune Dis. https://doi.org/10.1530/ERC-18-0333

Mohammed H et al (2015) Progesterone receptor modulates ERα action in breast cancer. Nature 523(7560):313–317. https://doi.org/10.1038/NATURE14583

Moinfar F et al (2003) Androgen receptors frequently are expressed in breast carcinomas: potential relevance to new therapeutic strategies. Cancer 98(4):703–711. https://doi.org/10.1002/cncr.11532

Mote PA et al (2002) Loss of co-ordinate expression of progesterone receptors A and B is an early event in breast carcinogenesis. Breast Cancer Res Treat 72(2):163–172. https://doi.org/10.1023/A:1014820500738

Muss HB et al (2016) Megestrol acetate versus tamoxifen in advanced breast cancer: 5-year analysis--a phase III trial of the Piedmont Oncology Association. J Clin Oncol 6(7):1098–1106. https://doi.org/10.1200/JCO.1988.6.7.1098

Nagarajan S et al (2020) ARID1A influences HDAC1/BRD4 activity, intrinsic proliferative capacity and breast cancer treatment response. Nat Genet 52(2):187. https://doi.org/10.1038/S41588-019-0541-5

Nandi S (1958) Endocrine control of mammary-gland development and function in the C3H/He Crgl mouse. J Natl Cancer Inst 21(6):1039–1063. https://doi.org/10.1093/JNCI/21.6.1039

Needham M et al (2000) Differential interaction of steroid hormone receptors with LXXLL motifs in SRC-1a depends on residues flanking the motif. J Steroid Biochem Mol Biol 72(1–2):35–46. https://doi.org/10.1016/S0960-0760(00)00027-3

Nelson HD et al (2012) Risk factors for breast cancer for women aged 40 to 49 years: a systematic review and meta-analysis. Ann Intern Med 156(9):635–648. https://doi.org/10.7326/0003-4819-156-9-201205010-00006

Ni M et al (2011) Targeting androgen receptor in estrogen receptor-negative breast cancer. Cancer cell 20(1):119–131. https://doi.org/10.1016/J.CCR.2011.05.026

Olsson HR, Landin-Olsson M, Gullberg B (1983) Retrospective assessment of menstrual cycle length in patients with breast cancer, in patients with benign breast disease, and in women without breast disease. J Natl Cancer Inst 70(1):17–20. https://doi.org/10.1093/JNCI/70.1.17

Olsson H, Ranstam M, Landin Olsson J (1987) The number of menstrual cycles prior to the first full term pregnancy an important risk factor of breast cancer? Acta Oncol 26(5):387–389. https://doi.org/10.3109/02841868709104365

Opatrny L et al (2008) Hormone replacement therapy use and variations in the risk of breast cancer. Int J Obstet Gynaecol 115(2):169–175. https://doi.org/10.1111/J.1471-0528.2007.01520.X

Panet-Raymond V et al (2000) Interactions between androgen and estrogen receptors and the effects on their transactivational properties. Mol Cell Endocrinol 167(1–2):139–150. https://doi.org/10.1016/S0303-7207(00)00279-3

Pannuti F et al (1979) Prospective, randomized clinical trial of two different high dosages of medroxyprogesterone acetate (MAP) in the treatment of metastatic breast cancer. Eur J Cancer (1965) 15(4):593–601. https://doi.org/10.1016/0014-2964(79)90097-5

Pardo I et al (2014) Next-generation transcriptome sequencing of the premenopausal breast epithelium using specimens from a normal human breast tissue bank. Breast Cancer Res 16:R26. https://doi.org/10.1186/bcr3627

Park S et al (2009) Expression of androgen receptors in primary breast cancer. Ann Oncol 21(3):488–492. https://doi.org/10.1093/annonc/mdp510

Pereira B et al (2016) The somatic mutation profiles of 2,433 breast cancers refine their genomic and transcriptomic landscapes. Nat Commun 7(1):1–16. https://doi.org/10.1038/ncomms11479

Peters AA et al (2009) Androgen receptor inhibits estrogen receptor-α activity and is prognostic in breast cancer. Cancer Res 69(15):6131–6140. https://doi.org/10.1158/0008-5472.CAN-09-0452

Petz LN et al (2002) Estrogen receptor α and activating protein-1 mediate estrogen responsiveness of the progesterone receptor gene in MCF-7 breast cancer cells. Endocrinology 143(12):4583–4591. https://doi.org/10.1210/EN.2002-220369

Pike MC et al (1983) "Hormonal" risk factors, "Breast tissue age" and the age-incidence of breast cancer. Nature 303(5920):767–770. https://doi.org/10.1038/303767a0

Planas-Silva MD et al (2001) AIB1 enhances estrogen-dependent induction of cyclin D1 expression. Cancer Res 61:3858–3862

Ponnusamy S et al (2019) Androgen receptor is a non-canonical inhibitor of wild-type and mutant estrogen receptors in hormone receptor-positive breast cancers. iScience 21:341–358. https://doi.org/10.1016/j.isci.2019.10.038

Qu Q et al (2013) The impact of androgen receptor expression on breast cancer survival: a retrospective study and meta-analysis. PLoS One 8(12):e82650. https://doi.org/10.1371/JOURNAL.PONE.0082650

Rajaram RD et al (2015) Progesterone and Wnt4 control mammary stem cells via myoepithelial crosstalk. EMBO J 34(5):641–652. https://doi.org/10.15252/embj.201490434

Rangel N et al (2018) The role of the AR/ER ratio in ER-positive breast cancer patients. Endocr Relat Cancer 25(3):163–172. https://doi.org/10.1530/ERC-17-0417

Razandi M et al (1999) Cell membrane and nuclear estrogen receptors (ERs) originate from a single transcript: studies of ERα and ERβ expressed in Chinese hamster ovary cells. Mol Endocrinol 13(2):307–319. https://doi.org/10.1210/MEND.13.2.0239

Razavi P et al (2018) The genomic landscape of endocrine-resistant advanced breast cancers. Cancer Cell 34(3):427–438.e6. https://doi.org/10.1016/J.CCELL.2018.08.008

Rechoum Y et al (2014) AR collaborates with ERα in aromatase inhibitor-resistant breast cancer. Breast Cancer Res Treat 147(3):473–485. https://doi.org/10.1007/S10549-014-3082-8/FIGURES/6

Reid G et al (2003) Cyclic, proteasome-mediated turnover of unliganded and liganded ERα on responsive promoters is an integral feature of estrogen signaling. Mol Cell 11(3):695–707. https://doi.org/10.1016/S1097-2765(03)00090-X

Richard E et al (2016) The mammary ducts create a favourable microenvironment for xenografting of luminal and molecular apocrine breast tumours. J Pathol. https://doi.org/10.1002/path.4772

Robertson JFR et al (1999) Onapristone, a progesterone receptor antagonist, as first-line therapy in primary breast cancer. Eur J Cancer 35(2):214–218. https://doi.org/10.1016/S0959-8049(98)00388-8

Robinson JLL et al (2011) Androgen receptor driven transcription in molecular apocrine breast cancer is mediated by FoxA1. EMBO J 30(15):3019–3027. https://doi.org/10.1038/emboj.2011.216

Rogatsky I, Trowbridge JM, Garabedian MJ (1999) Potentiation of human estrogen receptor alpha transcriptional activation through phosphorylation of serines 104 and 106 by the cyclin A-CDK2 complex. J Biol Chem 274(32):22296–22302. https://doi.org/10.1074/JBC.274.32.22296

Rojas PA et al (2017) Progesterone receptor isoform ratio: a breast cancer prognostic and predictive factor for antiprogestin responsiveness. J Natl Cancer Inst 109(7). https://doi.org/10.1093/JNCI/DJW317

Rosas E et al (2021) A positive feedback loop between TGFβ and androgen receptor supports triple-negative breast cancer anoikis resistance. Endocrinology 162(2). https://doi.org/10.1210/ENDOCR/BQAA226

Ross-Innes CS et al (2012) Differential oestrogen receptor binding is associated with clinical outcome in breast cancer. Nature 481:389–393. https://doi.org/10.1038/nature10730

Russo J, Russo IH (1996) Experimentally induced mammary tumors in rats. Breast Cancer Res Treat 39(1):7–20. https://doi.org/10.1007/BF01806074

Russo J et al (2005) The protective role of pregnancy in breast cancer. Breast Cancer Res 7(3):131. https://doi.org/10.1186/BCR1029

Russo MV et al (2015) A new mouse avatar model of non-small cell lung cancer. Front Oncol 5:52. https://doi.org/10.3389/fonc.2015.00052

Safe S (2001) Transcriptional activation of genes by 17 beta-estradiol through estrogen receptor-Sp1 interactions. Vitam Horm 62:231–252. https://doi.org/10.1016/S0083-6729(01)62006-5

Santen RJ et al (2009) History of aromatase: saga of an important biological mediator and therapeutic target. Endocr Rev 30(4):343–375. https://doi.org/10.1210/ER.2008-0016

Scabia V et al (2022) Estrogen receptor positive breast cancers have patient specific hormone sensitivities and rely on progesterone receptor. Nat Commun 13(1):1–15. https://doi.org/10.1038/s41467-022-30898-0

Schedin P (2006) Pregnancy-associated breast cancer and metastasis. Nat Commun 6(4):281–291. https://doi.org/10.1038/nrc1839

Schwabe JWR et al (1993) The crystal structure of the estrogen receptor DNA-binding domain bound to DNA: how receptors discriminate between their response elements. Cell 75(3):567–578. https://doi.org/10.1016/0092-8674(93)90390-C

Sengupta S et al (2010) Estrogen regulation of X-box binding protein-1 and its role in estrogen induced growth of breast and endometrial cancer cells. Horm Mol Biol Clin Investig 2(2):235. https://doi.org/10.1515/HMBCI.2010.025

Severson TM et al (2018) Characterizing steroid hormone receptor chromatin binding landscapes in male and female breast cancer. Nat Commun 9(1):482. https://doi.org/10.1038/s41467-018-02856-2

Sflomos G et al (2016) A preclinical model for ERα-positive breast cancer points to the epithelial microenvironment as determinant of luminal phenotype and hormone response. Cancer Cell 29(3):407–422. https://doi.org/10.1016/J.CCELL.2016.02.002

Sflomos G et al (2021) Intraductal xenografts show lobular carcinoma cells rely on their own extracellular matrix and LOXL1. EMBO Mol Med 13(3):e13180. https://doi.org/10.15252/emmm.202013180

Shamseddin M et al (2021) Contraceptive progestins with androgenic properties stimulate breast epithelial cell proliferation. EMBO Mol Med 13(7). https://doi.org/10.15252/EMMM.202114314

Shoker BS et al (1999) Estrogen receptor-positive proliferating cells in the normal and precancerous breast. Am J Pathol 155(6):1811. https://doi.org/10.1016/S0002-9440(10)65498-3

Shupnik MA (2004) Crosstalk between steroid receptors and the c-Src-receptor tyrosine kinase pathways: implications for cell proliferation. Oncogene 23(48):7979–7989. https://doi.org/10.1038/sj.onc.1208076

Siersbæk R et al (2020) IL6/STAT3 signaling hijacks ER enhancers to drive breast cancer metastasis. Cancer Cell 38(3):412. https://doi.org/10.1016/J.CCELL.2020.06.007

Singh M, McGinley JN, Thompson HJ (2000) A comparison of the histopathology of premalignant and malignant mammary gland lesions induced in sexually immature rats with those occurring in the human. Lab Investig 80(2):221–231. https://doi.org/10.1038/labinvest.3780025

Soto AM, Sonnenschein C (2010) Environmental causes of cancer: endocrine disruptors as carcinogens. Nat Rev Endocrinol 6(7):363–370. https://doi.org/10.1038/nrendo.2010.87

Soule HD et al (1973) A human cell line from a pleural effusion derived from a breast carcinoma. J Natl Cancer Inst 51(5):1409–1416. https://doi.org/10.1093/JNCI/51.5.1409

Standish LJ et al (2008) Breast Cancer and the Immune System. J Soc Integr Oncol 6(4):158. https://doi.org/10.2310/7200.2008.0027

Stripecke R et al (2020) Innovations, challenges, and minimal information for standardization of humanized mice. EMBO Mol Med 12(7):e8662. https://doi.org/10.15252/EMMM.201708662

Tan ME et al (2015) Androgen receptor: structure, role in prostate cancer and drug discovery. Acta Pharmacol Sin:3–23. https://doi.org/10.1038/aps.2014.18

Tanos T et al (2013) Progesterone/RANKL is a major regulatory axis in the human breast. Sci Transl Med 5(182):182ra55. https://doi.org/10.1126/scitranslmed.3005654

Taplin ME (2007) Drug insight: role of the androgen receptor in the development and progression of prostate cancer. Nat Clin Pract Oncol, pp 236–244. https://doi.org/10.1038/ncponc0765

Thompson HJ et al (1998) Ovarian hormone dependence of pre-malignant and malignant mammary gland lesions induced in pre-pubertal rats by 1-methyl-1-nitrosourea. Carcinogenesis 19(3):383–386. https://doi.org/10.1093/CARCIN/19.3.383

Thordarson G et al (1995) Refractoriness to mammary tumorigenesis in parous rats: is it caused by persistent changes in the hormonal environment or permanent biochemical alterations in the mammary epithelia? Carcinogenesis 16(11):2847–2853. https://doi.org/10.1093/CARCIN/16.11.2847

Tora L et al (1989) The human estrogen receptor has two independent nonacidic transcriptional activation functions. Cell 59(3):477–487. https://doi.org/10.1016/0092-8674(89)90031-7

Usary J et al (2004) Mutation of GATA3 in human breast tumors. Oncogene 23(46):7669–7678. https://doi.org/10.1038/sj.onc.1207966

Vignon F et al (1983) Antiestrogenic effect of R5020, a synthetic progestin in human breast cancer cells in culture. J Clin Endocrinol Metab 56(6):1124–1130. https://doi.org/10.1210/JCEM-56-6-1124

Wang C et al (2011) Estrogen induces c-myc gene expression via an upstream enhancer activated by the estrogen receptor and the AP-1 transcription factor. Mol Endocrinol (Baltimore, Md.) 25(9):1527–1538. https://doi.org/10.1210/ME.2011-1037

Wen DX et al (1994) The A and B isoforms of the human progesterone receptor operate through distinct signaling pathways within target cells. Mol Cell Biol 14(12):8356. https://doi.org/10.1128/MCB.14.12.8356

Xu G et al (2020) ARID1A determines luminal identity and therapeutic response in estrogen-receptor-positive breast cancer. Nat Genet 52(2):198–207. https://doi.org/10.1038/s41588-019-0554-0

Yamaguchi M et al (2021) Androgens enhance the ability of intratumoral macrophages to promote breast cancer progression. Oncol Rep 46(3):1–11. https://doi.org/10.3892/OR.2021.8139/HTML

Yan W et al (2010) GATA3 inhibits breast cancer metastasis through the reversal of epithelial-mesenchymal transition. J Biol Chem 285(18):14042. https://doi.org/10.1074/JBC.M110.105262

Yang Z, Barnes CJ, Kumar R (2004) Human epidermal growth factor receptor 2 status modulates subcellular localization of and interaction with estrogen receptor α in breast cancer cells. Clin Cancer Res 10(11):3621–3628. https://doi.org/10.1158/1078-0432.CCR-0740-3

Yates LR et al (2017) Genomic evolution of breast cancer metastasis and relapse. Cancer Cell 32(2):169–184.e7. https://doi.org/10.1016/J.CCELL.2017.07.005

Yuasa S, MacMahon B (1970) Lactation and reproductive histories of breast cancer patients in Tokyo, Japan. Bull World Health Organ 42:195–204

Zhao Y et al (1996) Estrogen biosynthesis proximal to a breast tumor is stimulated by PGE2 via cyclic AMP, leading to activation of promoter II of the CYP19 (aromatase) gene. Endocrinology 137(12):5739–5742. https://doi.org/10.1210/ENDO.137.12.8940410

RANK/RANKL Signaling Pathway in Breast Development and Cancer

16

Gema Pérez-Chacón, Patricia G. Santamaría, Jaime Redondo-Pedraza, and Eva González-Suárez

Abstract

RANK pathway has attracted increasing interest as a promising target in breast cancer, given the availability of denosumab, an anti-RANKL drug. RANK signaling mediates progesterone-driven regulation of mammary gland development and favors breast cancer initiation by controlling mammary cell proliferation and stem cell fate. RANK activation promotes luminal mammary epithelial cell senescence, acting as an initial barrier to tumorigenesis but ultimately facilitating tumor progression and metastasis. Comprehensive analyses have demonstrated that RANK protein expression is an independent biomarker of poor prognosis in postmenopausal and estrogen receptor-negative breast cancer patients. RANK pathway also has multiple roles in immunity and inflammation, regulating innate and adaptive responses. In the tumor microenvironment, RANK and RANKL are expressed by different immune cell populations and contribute to the regulation of tumor immune surveillance, mainly driving immunosuppressive effects.

Herein, we discuss the preventive and therapeutic potential of targeting RANK signaling in breast cancer given its tumor cell intrinsic and extrinsic effects. RANKL inhibition has been shown to induce mammary tumor cell differentiation and an antitumor immune response. Moreover, loss of RANK signaling increases sensitivity of breast cancer cells to chemotherapy, targeted therapies such as HER2 and CDK4/6 inhibitors, and immunotherapy. Finally, we describe clinical trials of denosumab for breast cancer prevention, such as those ongoing in women with high risk of developing breast cancer, large phase III clinical trials where the impact of adjuvant denosumab on disease-free survival has been assessed, and window trials to evaluate the immunomodulatory effects of denosumab in breast cancer and other solid tumors.

Keywords

RANKL · RANK · Denosumab · Mammary gland · Breast cancer · Immunotherapy

Gema Pérez-Chacón and Patricia G. Santamaría contributed equally with all other contributors.

G. Pérez-Chacón · P. G. Santamaría · J. Redondo-Pedraza
Molecular Oncology, Spanish National Cancer Research Centre (CNIO), Madrid, Spain

E. González-Suárez (✉)
Molecular Oncology, Spanish National Cancer Research Centre (CNIO), Madrid, Spain

Oncobell, Bellvitge Biomedical Research Institute (IDIBELL), L'Hospitalet de Llobregat, Barcelona, Spain
e-mail: egsuarez@idibell.cat; egonzalez@cnio.es

T. Sørlie, R. B. Clarke (eds.), *A Guide to Breast Cancer Research*, Advances in Experimental Medicine and Biology 1464, https://doi.org/10.1007/978-3-031-70875-6_16

Key Points

- RANK/RANKL signaling is the main paracrine mediator of the proliferative and pro-tumorigenic action of progesterone in the mammary gland, regulating mammary gland development and promoting breast cancer initiation.
- Ectopic RANK expression induces senescence in mammary luminal cells, resulting in enhanced stemness and delayed tumor onset but increased tumor aggressiveness.
- RANK and RANKL are expressed in the tumor microenvironment and can regulate tumor immunity at multiple levels.
- RANK pathway inhibition in breast tumors can induce tumor cell differentiation, enhance the antitumor immune response, and improve the therapeutic benefit of immune checkpoint inhibitors.
- RANK protein expression is more frequent in hormone receptor-negative breast tumors and associates with poor prognosis, particularly in postmenopausal women.
- Denosumab is a promising drug for breast cancer prevention and, in combination with immunotherapy, for the treatment of breast cancer and other solid tumors.

16.1 Introduction

Breast cancer is the most commonly diagnosed cancer among women and the leading cause of cancer-related death worldwide in this population (Sung et al. 2021). Breast cancer incidence has been rising globally, and it is estimated that in 2040, the number of newly diagnosed breast cancer cases will increase by over 40% (Arnold et al. 2022). Survival rates have notably improved during the last decades, mostly due to the implementation of mammography screening programs and adjuvant therapies. More recently, the development of highly effective targeted therapies, promptly introduced in the clinical practice for early and advanced disease settings, has profoundly improved outcomes. An unparalleled integration of data from multi-omics approaches have revealed distinct breast cancer subtypes [reviewed in Harbeck et al. (2019)] and highlighted the relevance of the tumor microenvironment, including the immune and stromal compartments [reviewed in Nolan et al. (2023)]. However, breast cancer remains a fatal disease and a global burden due to metastatic dissemination and the emergence of therapy resistance, ongoing challenges in the field [reviewed in Nolan et al. (2023)]. A better understanding of the genetic alterations and disentanglement of the molecular mechanisms governing the different breast cancer subtypes is crucial for the development of superior and effective therapeutic strategies and their translation into precision medicine.

Signal transduction dysregulation, usually resulting from genetic alterations, is a crucial process in the development and progression of cancer. In breast cancer, a number of signaling networks, including ovarian steroid hormones, ERBB2/HER2, PI3K-AKT, MAPK, FGFR, NOTCH, and JAK-STAT [reviewed in Nolan et al. (2023)], have been associated with different aspects of the development of the disease, including tumor cell proliferation, progression, and metastasis. In this chapter, we have focused on the RANK/RANKL/OPG signaling axis, a pathway classically related to bone remodeling that has been demonstrated to play a significant role in breast cancer.

16.2 RANK, RANKL, and OPG: Members of the TNF Family of Ligands and Receptors

The tumor necrosis factor (TNF) ligand and receptor (TNFR) superfamilies (TNFSF and TNFRSF) contain 19 ligands and 29 receptors, respectively, which regulate numerous cell functions including cell proliferation, death, or differentiation. Members of these families regulate immune responses, hematopoiesis, and morphogenesis, being also involved in bone resorption and osteoporosis, inflammation, autoimmune diseases, and tumorigenesis [reviewed in Aggarwal (2003)].

All but two TNF ligands are type II transmembrane proteins with a C-terminal extracellular domain, single transmembrane domain, and N-terminal intracellular domain. The C-terminal domain, known as the TNF homology domain, has 20–30% amino acid identity among the family members and is responsible for binding to the receptor. Most members of the TNFSF are released from the cell surface by proteases to produce soluble ligands that signal via their receptors, although less efficiently than the membrane-bound forms.

The TNF receptors are type I transmembrane proteins, containing an extracellular amino-terminal ectodomain with several cysteine-rich domains (CRDs), a single transmembrane domain, and an intracellular carboxy-terminal domain, responsible for recruiting the cytoplasmic signal transduction proteins. The receptors can be classified into three groups based on their domains and functions: (I) death receptors (DRs) that contain an intracellular death domain (DD) and activate apoptosis; (II) TNFR-associated factor (TRAF)-interacting receptors that interact with members of the TRAF family; and (III) decoy receptors (DcRs) that act as TNFSF ligand inhibitors with no intracellular binding partners [reviewed in Aggarwal (2003), Vanamee and Faustman (2018)].

Signaling is activated only when a trimeric ligand (noncovalent homotrimer) binds three monomers of the receptor, which preassemble on the cell surface. The conformational changes brought upon ligand binding and activation in the transmembrane and intracellular regions of the receptor promote the recruitment of downstream signaling partners, believed to be facilitated through complex hexagonal oligomeric structures. Current models propose that TNFRSF members are prearranged as trimers on the surface, while two monomers from adjacent trimers form antiparallel dimers that bury the ligand-binding site and represent the "non-signaling" resting state of the receptor (Vanamee and Faustman 2018). Receptor activation in the absence of ligand, although less likely to occur, has also been reported for some TNFRSF members (Boldin et al. 1995), as discussed below.

The focus of this chapter is the receptor activator of NFKB (RANK) and its ligand RANKL, TNF(R)SF members best known for their essential role in bone remodeling (Wada et al. 2006). This signaling node also involves osteoprotegerin (OPG), a decoy receptor lacking a transmembrane domain and secreted as a soluble domain that binds and sequesters RANKL, therefore hindering RANK activation (Fig. 16.1a).

RANK pathway regulates multiple biological aspects ranging from bone physiology, immunity, and mammary gland development. Besides, RANK signaling is implicated in the onset and progression of breast cancer (Kong et al. 1999; Fata et al. 2000; Gonzalez-Suarez et al. 2010; Schramek et al. 2010; Nolan et al. 2016; Yoldi et al. 2016; Ciscar et al. 2023), and accumulating evidence suggests that RANK/RANKL interactions between tumor cells and the tumor microenvironment could be determinant for immune surveillance (Tan et al. 2011; Smyth et al. 2016; Ahern et al. 2017, 2018a, b; Liede et al. 2018; Gomez-Aleza et al. 2020).

We summarize here the involvement of RANK pathway in the regulation of bone metabolism, detailing the characteristics and functions of RANK/RANKL/OPG axis members (Fig. 16.1b, c) and focusing on their relevant role in the immune system and mammary gland biology, breast cancer, and tumor immunity.

16.2.1 RANK

RANK, with ~620 amino acids and 85% homology between mouse and human homologs, has four tandem CRDs in the N-terminal domain and five cytoplasmic TRAF binding domains that bind different adaptor proteins including TRAFs (Aggarwal 2003). The cytoplasmic domain (comprising amino acids 232–616) shares no significant homology with other TNFRSF mem-

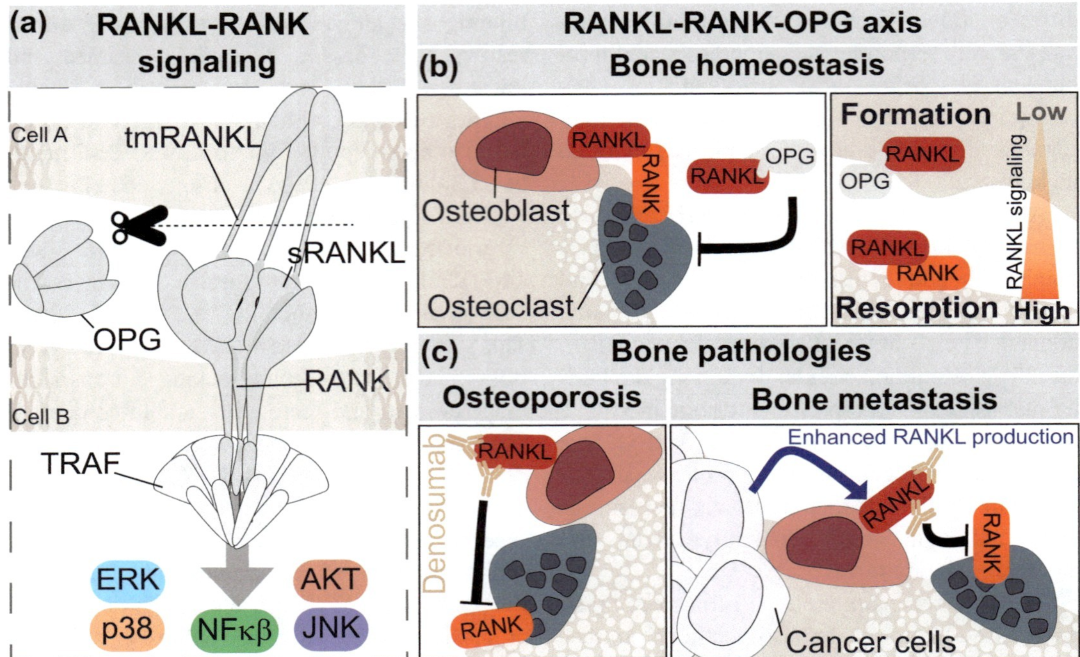

Fig. 16.1 Signaling and physiological role of the RANK/RANKL/OPG axis. (**a**) Transmembrane (tm)RANKL and cleaved soluble (s)RANKL bind to RANK receptor, triggering receptor activation, and TRAF-mediated signaling through NFKB, AKT, JNK, ERK, and p38 proteins. Osteoprotegerin (OPG) is the RANKL decoy receptor. OPG regulates RANK/RANKL signaling by sequestering RANKL and preventing its binding to RANK receptor and, therefore, downstream signaling. (**b**) RANK/RANKL/OPG axis is essential in bone physiology. In the bone, osteoblasts express RANKL and OPG while RANK is expressed by osteoclasts. A tight regulation of the RANK/RANKL/OPG axis is required to maintain the physiological balance between bone formation and resorption. Activation of RANK/RANKL signaling drives osteoclast-mediated bone resorption, whereas RANKL sequestration by OPG decreases RANK/RANKL signaling favoring bone formation. (**c**) Denosumab, a human monoclonal antibody against RANKL, is used in the clinic to inhibit RANK/RANKL signaling for the treatment of osteoporosis and bone-related events such as the exacerbated bone resorption promoted by metastatic cancer cells

bers but contains a pre-ligand assembly domain (PLAD) present in TNFRSF members and required for receptor preassembly on the surface of the cell (Aggarwal 2003; Vanamee and Faustman 2018). RANK downstream signaling is mediated through the activation of JNK, ERK, p38, AKT, and NFKB signaling pathways that in turn regulate multiple biological processes [reviewed in Rao et al. (2018)] (Fig. 16.1a). Early experiments on bone metabolism demonstrated that extracellular binding of RANKL, the only known biological ligand for RANK, results in osteoclastogenesis from progenitor cells and the activation of mature osteoclasts (Wada et al. 2006; Leibbrandt and Penninger 2008; Liu et al. 2010).

RANK is expressed in myeloid cells including monocytes, macrophages, and dendritic cells (DCs) and in osteoclasts and osteoclast progenitors (Rao et al. 2018). Besides regulating bone metabolism by controlling osteoclast development, RANK pathway is involved in physiological processes within the immune system (Dougall et al. 1999; Kong et al. 1999); therefore, RANK/RANKL/OPG mediate the interaction between the skeletal and immune systems and are considered key players in osteoimmunology (Nakashima and Takayanagi 2009). As discussed in detail in this chapter, RANK is also expressed in the mammary epithelium, where it regulates mammary gland development and is involved in the onset and progression of breast cancer [reviewed in Gonzalez-Suarez and Sanz-Moreno (2016), Rao et al. (2018)].

In humans, mutations in the gene encoding RANK (*TNFSF11A*) have been associated with different skeletal disorders such as Paget's disease of the bone (Albagha et al. 2010; Chung et al. 2010a, b) or autosomal-recessive osteopetrosis (Guerrini et al. 2008; Pangrazio et al. 2012). Besides, human patients with *TNFSF11A* mutations show partial defects in B cell maturation (Guerrini et al. 2008), likely due to a perturbed bone marrow environment (Rao et al. 2018).

Alternative splice variants of human RANK have been described, affecting the extracellular (Sirinian et al. 2013) or cytoplasmic domains (Papanastasiou et al. 2012), with altered RANKL binding and signaling abilities. One of them, named RANK-c, lacking the transmembrane domain and most of the intracellular domain, was found to be upregulated in human breast cancer cell lines and tissues and shown to behave as a dominant negative regulator by inhibiting NFKB activation by RANK (Papanastasiou et al. 2012).

Rank and *Rankl* null mice are osteopetrotic, lack lymph nodes, have impaired B cell development (Dougall et al. 1999; Kong et al. 1999), and do not lactate due to defective alveolar development (Fata et al. 2000; Gonzalez-Suarez et al. 2010).

In vitro results have demonstrated that RANK cytoplasmic domain interacts with most TRAF proteins with different affinities through two independent TRAF binding regions: amino acids 544–616 that enable binding to TRAF1, TRAF2, TRAF3, TRAF5, and TRAF6; and amino acids 340–421, specific for TRAF6 (Galibert et al. 1998; Hsu et al. 1999). Although it is not yet clear whether RANK may signal through TRAF-independent mechanisms, in vitro evidence suggests that TRAF6 is the main downstream RANK binding protein triggering NFKB activity and osteoclastogenesis. *Traf6* knockout mice also exhibit osteopetrosis (Lomaga et al. 1999), but they do not lack osteoclasts as *Rank* and *Rankl* null mice (Dougall et al. 1999, Kong et al. 1999). Moreover, none of the *Traf* knockouts with osteopetrotic phenotypes show deficient lymph node formation. This fact, together with subtle phenotypic differences between *Rank* and *Rankl* knockout mice such as the development and function of the thymus, normal in *Rank* but impaired in *Rankl* null mice (Dougall et al. 1999), indicates that RANK acts through a complex signal transduction pathway, determined by expression levels, temporal and spatial context, and presence and availability of upstream and downstream effectors.

An important issue with relevant implications in cancer is that, at least in vitro, ectopic overexpression of RANK leads to ligand-independent NFKB signaling (Dougall et al. 1999; Palafox et al. 2012), similar to other TNFRSF members (Boldin et al. 1995).

16.2.2 RANKL

RANKL is the type II transmembrane protein TNFSF11. It was first identified in the late 1990s by Wong et al. (Wong et al. 1997a, b) in activated T lymphocytes and termed tumor necrosis factor (TNF)-related activation-induced cytokine (TRANCE). At the same time, Anderson et al. identified the expression of the gene in mature DCs and was designated as RANKL (Anderson et al. 1997). Later on, two additional groups isolated RANKL from myelomonocytic and bone marrow stromal cell lines as a factor of osteoclastogenesis, referring to it as osteoprotegerin ligand (OPGL) (Lacey et al. 1998) and osteoclast differentiation factor (ODF) (Yasuda et al. 1998).

In bone tissue, RANKL is expressed mainly by osteoblasts and osteocytes (Nakashima et al. 2011; Xiong et al. 2011), although other cell types have been described to express it, including preosteoblastic marrow stromal cells and megakaryocytes (Eghbali-Fatourechi et al. 2003, Bord et al. 2004). RANKL expression can be regulated by various osteoactive factors, such as glucocorticoids, vitamin D3, and TNFα, among others (Yasuda et al. 1998; Hofbauer et al. 1999a, b; Masuyama et al. 2006). Regarding the immune system, in addition to the increased expression in activated T cells and DCs (Anderson et al. 1997; Wong et al. 1997a, b), RANKL has been detected in B cells upon stimulation (Titanji 2017).

Three alternative splicing isoforms of RANKL have been described in both mice and humans (Ikeda et al. 2001). In mice, besides the canonical isoform Rankl1 (316 amino acids), two new isoforms have been detected: Rankl2 (287 amino acids) and Rankl3 (199 amino acids). Rankl1 is a membrane-anchored protein (tmRankl1) with an extracellular domain at the carboxy-terminus (Nakashima et al. 2012), sharing a close homology to other TNFSF members such as Trail, Fasl, and Tnfa (Wong et al. 1997a, b). Additionally, the extracellular ectodomain of the canonical isoform can be shed by specific enzymes or by alternative splicing to produce a soluble form (sRankl1), which has been suggested to have more potent activity than the transmembrane isoform (Nakashima et al. 2000). Depending on the context, the proteolytic cleavage of Rankl1 is carried out by proteins belonging to two different families, a disintegrin and metalloprotease domain (ADAM) family and matrix metalloproteinase (MMP) family. Rankl1 is detected in the endoplasmic reticulum, Golgi network, and cytoplasmic and membrane regions (Ikeda et al. 2001). In relation to the noncanonical isoforms, Rankl2 is characterized by having a shorter intracellular domain and is predominantly detected in the endoplasmic reticulum and Golgi network, whereas Rankl3 lacks both the intracellular and transmembrane domains and has been proposed to be a soluble isoform that accumulates in the cytoplasm (Ikeda et al. 2003). Regarding human RANKL isoforms, RANKL1, RANKL2, and RANKL3 are composed of 317, 270, and 244 amino acids, respectively. Like mouse Rankl, the full-length transmembrane RANKL1 presents intracellular, transmembrane, and extracellular domains, while RANKL3 contains only the extracellular domain. In contrast to murine Rankl2, the sequence that encodes the human RANKL2 intracellular domain is completely deleted (Suzuki et al. 2004). RANKL1 is detected in the membrane of human cells, unlike RANKL2 and RANKL3.

In addition to RANK, leucine-rich repeat-containing G protein-coupled receptor 4 (LGR4), a 951-amino-acid transmembrane receptor belonging to the group B of the LGR family, has been reported as a receptor for RANKL (Luo et al. 2016). LGR4 is also expressed on osteoclasts and competes with RANK for binding to RANKL, although through different domains. This LGR4-RANKL interaction activates the Gq protein alpha subunit, which triggers intracellular calcium release, resulting in NFATc1 inhibition and the suppression of the canonical RANK pathway during osteoclast differentiation. More recently, additional experiments have demonstrated that the interaction of LGR4 with R-spondin-2 and Rankl promotes osteoclastic premetastatic niche formation, favoring bone metastasis (Yue et al. 2022).

16.2.3 OPG

The decoy receptor osteoprotegerin (OPG) is the TNFRSF member 11B (TNFRSF11B) (Simonet et al. 1997), also known as osteoclastogenesis inhibitory factor (OCIF) (Tsuda et al. 1997), TNF receptor-like molecule 1 (TR1) (Tan et al. 1997; Kwon et al. 1998), or follicular DC-derived receptor-1 (FDCR-1) (Yun et al. 1998). OPG is a secreted glycoprotein produced by osteoblasts and bone marrow stromal cells that binds RANKL (Boyce and Xing 2007; Okamoto et al. 2017). *OPG* gene encodes a full-length glycoprotein of 401 amino acids, which is cleaved by signal peptidase to a 380-amino-acid form containing 7 functional domains: 4 cysteine-rich domains (CRD) at the amino-terminus, crucial for the interaction with RANKL, and 2 death domain-homologous (DDH) tandem regions, and 1 heparin-binding domain plus a cysteine residue at the carboxyl-terminus, all essential for the dimerization of OPG (Schneeweis et al. 2005). Human and mouse OPG proteins share 85% identity in their amino acid sequences (Simonet et al. 1997).

Although OPG binds to RANKL with high affinity, it also binds with a lower affinity to lymphotoxin alpha (LTα) and tumor necrosis factor-related apoptosis-inducing ligand (TRAIL), among others [reviewed in Baud'huin et al. (2013)]. The regulation of the levels of OPG is essential for the bone health. OPG protects from excessive bone resorption by binding RANKL and preventing the activation of RANK signaling pathway. For that, the balance between OPG and RANKL is determinant for osteoclast functions, and the alteration of this ratio can result in pathological bone states. Indeed, OPG-deficient mice show a severe decrease in bone density and vascular calcification (Bucay et al. 1998; Mizuno et al. 1998), and OPG-overexpressing transgenic mice the protein present a marked osteopetrosis (Simonet et al. 1997).

16.3 Role of RANK/RANKL Signaling Pathway in Biological Processes

16.3.1 Bone Metabolism

16.3.1.1 Osteoclasts, Osteoblasts, Osteocytes, and NFKB Activation

RANK/RANKL pathway has been broadly characterized in the bone (Fig. 16.1b), where it plays a key role in maintaining the balance between bone formation, driven by osteoblasts, and bone resorption, driven by osteoclasts (Dougall et al. 1999; Kong et al. 1999; Fata et al. 2000; Gonzalez-Suarez and Sanz-Moreno 2016). Osteoblasts, which can further differentiate into osteocytes, are mesenchymal cells that secrete the main components of the bone such as collagen, hydroxylapatite, and osteocalcin, among others (Kong et al. 1999). Osteocytes are the principal source of RANKL in the bone (Nakashima et al. 2011), while osteoclasts are RANK+ cells that derive from hematopoietic precursors within the bone marrow. Upon RANK activation, they reabsorb bone tissue, liberating calcium and participating in homeostatic bone remodeling processes (Dougall et al. 1999, Kong et al. 1999, Fata et al. 2000, Gonzalez-Suarez and Sanz-Moreno 2016).

The relevance of RANK signaling in bone remodeling is strongly supported by the phenotype of murine *Rank* or *Rankl* full-body knockouts, which present severe osteopetrosis and absence of osteoclasts (Dougall et al. 1999; Kong et al. 1999). In the same line, overexpression of OPG also results in severe osteopetrosis (Simonet et al. 1997). Classical in vitro functional studies demonstrate that RANKL and myeloid colony-stimulating factor are sufficient to generate osteoclasts from myeloid progenitors. Osteoclasts are characterized by the expression of tartrate-resistant acid phosphatase (TRAP) 5b, enzyme involved in bone matrix degradation and considered a good marker for monitoring bone resorption (Dougall et al. 1999; Kong et al. 1999; Fata et al. 2000; Takayanagi et al. 2000; Nakamura et al. 2006; Ju et al. 2008).

Studies with osteoclasts have revealed that RANK signaling can activate both canonical and noncanonical NFKB pathways, main downstream effectors of RANK-mediated bone resorption (Locksley et al. 2001; Wada et al. 2006; Boyce and Xing 2007). Data from genetically engineered mouse models of key members of the canonical and noncanonical NFKB pathways, as well as results from in vitro studies, suggest that the main mediator of osteoclast differentiation and function is canonical NFKB signaling, while the noncanonical pathway has redundant effects to those of other inflammatory pathways and may have alternative regulatory functions in bone homeostasis [reviewed in Novack (2011)].

RANK secreted in extracellular vesicles from osteoclasts has been described to activate reverse signaling through membrane-bound RANKL in osteoblasts (Ikebuchi et al. 2018; Ma et al. 2019), which could also play a role in bone homeostasis and other physiological settings. Regarding OPG, it is secreted by osteoblasts in response to several cytokines and growth factors such as WNT, TGFβ, and INFγ (Theoleyre et al. 2004; Glass II et al. 2005), in order to sequester RANKL and block RANK pathway activation. Therefore, the levels of RANKL and OPG, differently regulated in physiological and pathological conditions, control bone metabolism, impacting on the balance between bone resorption and formation.

16.3.1.2 Osteoporosis

One of the major contributors to postmenopausal osteoporosis, characterized by low bone mass and bone tissue deterioration, is the loss of ovarian function to supply estrogen and progesterone, steroid hormones that influence bone metabolism through the RANK/RANKL/OPG axis. In vitro and in vivo evidences indicate that sex hormones directly regulate OPG (Hofbauer et al. 1999a, b; Nakashima et al. 2000; Saika et al. 2001; Bord et al. 2003) and RANKL levels (Streicher et al. 2017). Therefore, the drop in sex hormone levels after menopause leads to a reduction in OPG and an increase in RANKL, exacerbating RANK signaling in the bone and promoting bone resorption and osteoporosis. The relevance of RANK signaling in age-related osteoporosis is confirmed by the fact that antibodies directed against RANKL abrogate bone mass loss in ovariectomized mice and in women with postmenopausal osteoporosis [reviewed in Miyazaki et al. (2014)] (Fig. 16.1c).

16.3.1.3 Bone Metastasis

The bone is the most frequent site for metastasis for many cancers, notably for breast cancer (70%), but also prostate, lung, kidney, and multiple myeloma (Body et al. 2017; Hernandez et al. 2018). Bone metastases often lead to skeletal morbidity, reducing overall survival (OS) and promoting reduced mobility and poor quality of life, with associated substantial medical costs (Macedo et al. 2017). Breast cancer patients diagnosed with bone metastases show a median survival from 3 to 5 years (Coleman et al. 2020).

Skeletal metastases result from the interaction between tumor cells and cells in the bone microenvironment. Within the bone, tumor cells may remain quiescent for years before resuming proliferation and causing overt bone metastasis, promoting bone destruction via RANK-driven activation of osteoclast-mediated osteolysis. When tumor cells reach the bone, they release multiple cytokines and factors including IL1β, IL6, IL8, IL11, IL17, macrophage inflammatory protein-1α (MIP1α), TNFα, parathyroid hormone-related protein (PTHrP), prostaglandin E2 (PGE2), CXCL13, DKK-1, or EGF, which lead to upregulation of RANKL and/or decrease in local OPG expression in the bone stroma [reviewed in Dougall et al. (2014)]. Indeed, RANKL+ stromal cells are found at the tumor/bone interface adjacent to osteoclasts and associated with tumor-induced osteolysis (Nannuru et al. 2009).

RANK is the common signaling pathway, employed by diverse tumor cell types, for tumor-induced osteolysis, contributing to early tumor colonization and progression of bone metastasis. The local increase of the RANKL/OPG ratio leads to overactivation of RANK signaling in osteoclasts, causing locally aggressive osteolytic bone destruction, contributing to skeletal morbidity and early tumor colonization and progression. Bone resorption releases cytokines and growth factors that further stimulate tumor cell proliferation and survival, resulting in a positive feedback loop, the so-called vicious cycle (Ell and Kang 2012). Tumor cells themselves can express OPG or RANKL, directly exacerbating bone resorption. However, experimental evidence indicates that tumor-expressed RANKL has relatively minimal or variable contributions to bone metastasis in vivo (Dougall et al. 2014). In fact, tumor-associated bone destruction in bone metastasis models from multiple tumor types is prevented by pharmacological inhibition of RANKL [reviewed in Roodman and Dougall (2008)], irrespective of the expression of RANK/RANKL/OPG by tumor or stromal cells (Fig. 16.1c).

16.3.2 RANK/RANKL Signaling in Mammary Gland Biology

The mammary gland is a highly specialized organ modeled during embryogenesis that, unlike most vertebrate organs, undergoes major morphogenesis postnatally. Extensive mammary gland development occurs at the onset of puberty in response to the release of ovarian hormones, driven by specified mammary epithelium. Since the essential function of the mammary gland is the production of milk to nourish the offspring, the final developmental fate of the mammary gland is completed only when pregnancy and lactation occur. The estrous cycles and pregnancy dictate changes in the physiological levels of steroid hormones, estrogen and progesterone, promoting epithelial proliferation and apoptosis, underlying the extensive mammary gland tissue remodeling occurring during each reproductive round (Fata et al. 2001; Fu et al. 2020).

The adult mammary gland is composed of two mammary epithelial cell (MEC) lineages organized into an inner layer of luminal epithelial cells and an outer layer of myoepithelial cells with contractile properties (Howard and Gusterson 2000). The current view is that after birth, basal and unipotent luminal progenitors are responsible for mammary gland development; basal progenitors will maintain the myoepithelial lineage, whereas luminal progenitors will give rise to two luminal cell subsets: the hormone-sensing lineage, expressing estrogen and progesterone receptors (ER+/PR+), and the hormone receptor-negative lineage (ER-/PR-), which will differentiate into the secretory alveolar lineage upon pregnancy. Within luminal cell progenitors, ER+ and ER− cells are maintained by distinct pools of lineage-restricted stem cells during puberty and adulthood (Van Keymeulen et al. 2017). Multipotent mammary stem cells (MaSCs) will be active mostly during embryogenesis, becoming quiescent after birth (Watson and Khaled 2020) but being able to reactivate bipotency upon certain circumstances (Centonze et al. 2020).

RANK/RANKL pathway plays a crucial role in mammary gland development (Fata et al. 2000; Gonzalez-Suarez et al. 2007; Schramek et al. 2010; Rocha et al. 2023), with progesterone being the main upstream regulator of the pathway (Beleut et al. 2010; Joshi et al. 2010) (Fig. 16.2a, b). After the rise of estrogen at the beginning of the menstrual cycle in humans, paralleled by the murine estrous cycle, progesterone levels peak, inducing RANKL expression in ER+/PR+ luminal cells. RANKL acts in a paracrine fashion on the adjacent PR-, RANK-expressing mammary progenitor cells, driving the mitogenic expansion of basal and luminal progenitor cells, a mechanism essential to expand the mammary epithelium and form milk-secreting acini during pregnancy (Asselin-Labat et al. 2010; Beleut et al. 2010; Joshi et al. 2010) (Fig. 16.2c). In fact, progesterone induces two proliferation bursts: a cell-autonomous small wave that results in the self-expansion of PR+ cells leading to increased levels of PR targets such as cyclin D1 and RANKL, and a second large wave that relies on RANKL to elicit proliferation of PR- cells by paracrine mechanisms (Beleut et al. 2010).

The regulation of mammary progenitor cell proliferation by the RANK/RANKL pathway appears to be universal across mammals (Sigl et al. 2016). Mouse models with constitutive and epithelium-specific Rank deletion display defective alveologenesis and lactation failure due to impaired MEC proliferation and differentiation (Fata et al. 2000; Gonzalez-Suarez et al. 2010; Joshi et al. 2015; Rocha et al. 2023) (Fig. 16.2). Whereas PR or prolactin receptor null mice show multiple reproductive abnormalities (Lydon et al. 1995; Ormandy et al. 1997), full-body Rankl depletion phenocopies Rank deficiency in mammary glands, confirming that Rankl signaling through Rank is essential for pregnancy-induced mammary gland morphogenesis (Fata et al. 2000; Rocha et al. 2023). In fact, local administration of recombinant Rankl restores lactation and lobuloalveolar development in pregnant *Rankl* knockout mice (Fata et al. 2000). Interrogating mammary cell lineage-specific Rank loss-of-function mouse models, we recently unveiled that basal Rank deletion does not have a major impact on mammary gland development, whereas the loss of luminal Rank results in lactation failure. Phenotypic and lineage tracing experiments demonstrated that Rank signaling is required for the maintenance of luminal progenitors, preventing early mammary alveolar differentiation and renewal during lactation/involution cycles. Moreover, in the presence of Rank-depleted dysfunctional luminal cells, basal Rank signaling ensures mammary gland homeostasis by reactivating basal cell bipotency, usually restricted to embryogenesis (Rocha et al. 2023).

Rank pathway activation in transgenic mice by the overexpression of Rank under the control of the mouse mammary tumor virus (MMTV) promoter also impairs functional development of

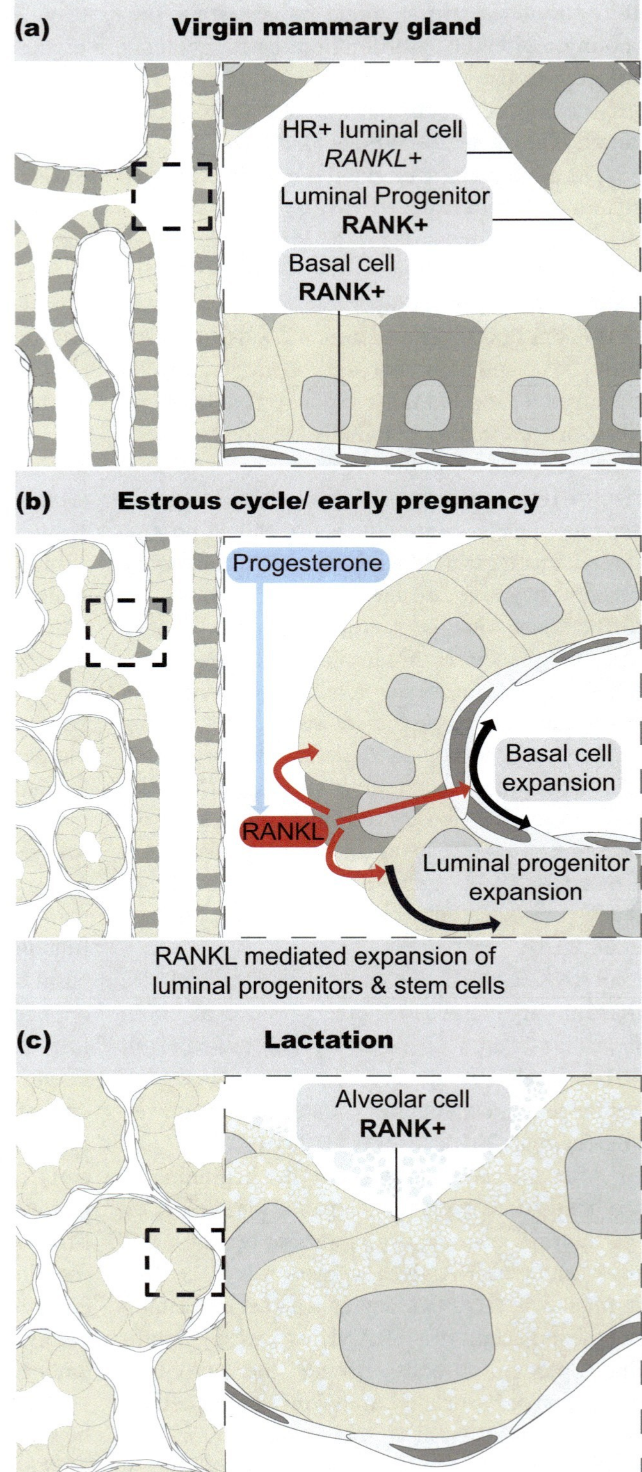

Fig. 16.2 RANK signaling is essential for mammary gland development. (**a**) Mammary epithelial cells differentially express RANK and RANKL. In the virgin mammary gland, hormone-sensing (HR+) luminal cells express RANKL, while luminal progenitors and basal cells express RANK. (**b**) RANK/RANKL pathway is the main paracrine mediator of the proliferative action of progesterone in the mammary gland. During the estrous cycle and in early pregnancy, progesterone levels peak, inducing RANKL expression in HR+ luminal cells. RANKL acts in a paracrine fashion on the adjacent luminal progenitor and basal cells, driving their expansion. (**c**) RANK/RANKL-mediated cross talk is essential for the expansion and differentiation of the mammary epithelium to generate milk-proficient glands during pregnancy and lactation

mammary alveoli, leading to lactation failure accompanied by sustained mammary epithelial proliferation during pregnancy (Gonzalez-Suarez et al. 2007). Further studies showed that pharmacological inhibition of Rank signaling at mid-pregnancy results in premature lactogenesis through the interference with prolactin/Stat5 signaling (Cordero et al. 2016). Mechanistically, progesterone-mediated induction of Rankl during early pregnancy supports epithelial expansion and alveolar morphogenesis, whereas Rankl-mediated inhibition of Stat5 hinders the expression of milk proteins during pregnancy. Therefore, restricting Rank signaling activity at midgestation allows Stat5 phosphorylation and activation and lactogenic differentiation (Cordero et al. 2016).

Also, the cross talk between the mammary epithelium and stroma is key for mammary gland architecture and function, contributing to mammary development from midgestation to the final stages of development during pregnancy and lactation. The stroma is composed of multiple cell types such as fibroblasts, adipocytes, endothelial and myeloid cells, and extracellular matrix components like collagens and metalloproteinases. Stromal cells and proteins are tightly regulated throughout the mammary gland developmental stages and control key stages such as epithelial side branching and involution after lactation (Wiseman and Werb 2002). Besides, it is well established that the stiffness of the extracellular matrix influences tissue development and cancer. Intriguingly, in mouse models with high mechano-transduction promoted by integrins, high extracellular matrix stiffness leads to an expansion of mammary epithelial progenitors by regulating progesterone-induced RANK signaling (Northey et al. 2022).

In the next sections, we will dissect the involvement of RANK/RANKL signaling in the early steps and progression of breast tumorigenesis as well as its role on the immune and tumor environment, discussing possible therapy approaches to tackle RANK pathway in order to improve clinical outcome.

16.3.3 RANK/RANKL Signaling and the Complex Regulation of the Immune System

In the last decades, RANK/RANKL signaling axis has gained relevance for its role in the regulation of the immune system. This pathway contributes not only to lymphoid organogenesis and to establishing central and peripheral tolerance but also plays a multifactorial role in the development, maintenance, and function of different immune populations, regulating immunity and inflammation (Dougall et al. 1999; Theill et al. 2002). Moreover, accumulating evidence indicates that RANK-RANKL interactions between tumor cells and the tumor microenvironment are determinant for tumor immunosurveillance (Ahern et al. 2018b; Gomez-Aleza and Gonzalez-Suarez 2021).

16.3.3.1 The Role of RANK/RANKL in Immune Cell Development and Function

RANK/RANKL/OPG axis plays a pivotal role in the development and function of the thymus, in particular in establishing central and peripheral immune tolerance. During negative and positive selection, thymic epithelial cells (TECs) provide the suitable conditions to guarantee the production of self-tolerant and functionally competent T cells (Takaba and Takayanagi 2017). Thymocytes that undergo positive selection in the inner cortex of the thymus upregulate RANKL (Josien et al. 1999; Rossi et al. 2007; Hikosaka et al. 2008; Roberts et al. 2012), which is indispensable for the proliferation and maturation of medullary TECs (mTECs) and for the formation of the thymic medulla. On the other hand, RANK expression has been identified in different subsets of mTECs (McCarthy et al. 2015), where it induces the activation of both canonical and noncanonical NFKB signaling pathways. The activation of NFKB results in the expression of the autoimmune regulator (AIRE) transcription factor (Haljasorg et al. 2015). AIRE triggers promiscuous transcription of thousands of tissue-specific antigens (TSAs) that are processed into peptides to be presented on MHC molecules to eliminate self-reactive T cells and avoid autoimmune responses. Indeed, RANK deficiency in TECs promotes the onset of autoimmunity, inducing the production of autoantibodies directed against different tissues (Rossi et al. 2007).

RANK/RANKL signaling has also a relevant role in the development of secondary lymphoid organs. In the spleen of *Rank* and *Rankl* knockout mice, a decrease of mature B cells is detected (Dougall et al. 1999; Kong et al. 1999). Also, a slight increase of mature neutrophils and no variation in the number of T cells and macrophages are found in *Rank* null mice, in contrast to *Rankl* knockout mice, where there is an upregulation of the number of nonactivated T cells (Kong et al. 1999). In the same line, lymph node development is tightly controlled [reviewed in Eckert et al. (2019)], in part by RANK/RANKL signaling pathway. Indeed, *Rank* and *Rankl*-deficient mice lack lymph nodes and have defective Peyer's patches and cryptopatches (Dougall et al. 1999; Kong et al. 1999). *Rankl* null mice present a strong reduction in lymphoid tissue inducer cell number in mesenteric lymph nodes at birth, impairing the development of lymph nodes but not of Peyer's patches (Kim et al. 2000).

Further experiments using a Tg(*Itgax-Cre*);*Tnfrsf11af/f* mouse model, where Rank is deleted in DCs as well as in CD11c$^+$ macrophage subpopulations, have emphasized the importance of RANK/RANKL signaling axis in orchestrating splenic immune responses (Habbeddine et al. 2017). In the spleen, Rank expression in DCs is crucial for the priming and activation of CD8$^+$ T cells and for the development of CD11c$^+$ CD169$^+$ macrophages in the splenic marginal zone. Interestingly, Rankl expression is essential for the differentiation, maintenance, and function of subcapsular and medullary CD169$^+$ sinusoidal macrophages in murine lymph nodes. During early age or after activation of innate immunity, the activation of Rankl in lymphatic endothelial cells is key to create an appropriate microenvironment for sinusoidal macrophage recruitment and development (Camara et al. 2019, 2022).

All these data support the importance of RANK/RANKL signaling in the development and function of primary and secondary lymphoid organs, as well as in the maintenance of certain immune subpopulations like splenic and lymph node CD169$^+$ macrophages.

16.3.3.2 RANK/RANKL Signaling in the Tumor Immune Microenvironment

RANK/RANKL pathway has a key role in the regulation of innate and adaptive tumor immune responses. Various cell types in the tumor microenvironment express RANK/RANKL influencing tumor immune surveillance. RANK can be expressed in DCs, natural killer (NK) cells, and macrophages, whereas RANKL can be expressed on CD4$^+$ and CD8$^+$ T cells upon activation (Josien et al. 1999). Also, RANK/RANKL pathway controls the development and function of DCs. Culturing RANK-expressing DCs with RANKL leads to a higher survival of DCs and a prolonged interaction of DC-T cells in vitro, supporting the role of RANK pathway in the efficient priming and activation of T cells (Anderson et al. 1997; Wong et al. 1997a, b; Josien et al. 1999). RANK-RANKL interaction can potentially promote or suppress immunity depending on the context. In a cancer context, DCs can interact with RANKL-expressing tumor cells, resulting in a tolerogenic effect (Demoulin et al. 2015).

Studies in *Rankl*$^{-/-}$ chimeric mouse models demonstrate a role of Rankl in the development of B cell precursors (Kong et al. 1999). However, although B cells can potentially express Rank (Yun et al. 1998), mouse Rank deletion specifically in B cells determined that Rank is not important for their development and function (Perlot and Penninger 2012).

NK cells derived from the bone marrow also express RANK (Atkins et al. 2006), which is upregulated under an immunosuppressive microenvironment. NK cells play an important role in tumor immunosurveillance. In acute myeloid leukemia (AML), in which 75% of patients express RANKL, the interaction between RANKL expressed in malignant cells and RANK expressed in NK cells induces a reverse signaling and the release of soluble factors that impair NK cell function, generating a "vicious cycle" (Schmiedel et al. 2013). Moreover, NK cells cocultured with RANKL-expressing AML cells show reduced INFγ release and cytotoxicity, recovered in the presence of denosumab (Schmiedel et al. 2013b). A similar interaction is observed in other two RANKL-expressing hematological diseases, multiple myeloma and chronic lymphocytic leukemia, where the use of a RANK construct to inhibit RANK/RANKL signaling has shown a reactivation of NK cell function (Schmiedel et al. 2013c). In solid tumors, platelet-derived RANKL has been described to inhibit the activity of normal NK cells against cancer cells through the interaction with RANK, facilitating the tumor immune evasion (Clar et al. 2019). All these observations suggest that RANK could be an additional inhibitory receptor of NK activity.

RANK expressed in macrophages also plays a role in tumor contexts, inducing a vicious cycle similar to that described for NK cells. RANKL has the capacity of recruiting monocytes that express RANK (Breuil et al. 2003) and then differentiate into macrophages in the tumor tissue. Tumor-associated macrophages (TAMs) accumulate in the tumor microenvironment and acquire mainly an immunosuppressive phenotype, known as M2-like TAMs that favor tumor development. In breast carcinoma, RANKL can be produced by Treg lymphocytes (Tan et al. 2011), responsible for recruiting monocytes to the tumor. Here, M2-like TAMs induce Treg cell proliferation, probably mediated by several soluble factors (Fujimura et al. 2015). In fact, the expression of RANK has been shown to co-localize with M2-like markers (CD163, ARG1, and CD206) in extramammary Paget's disease, and RANK-expressing macrophages are suggested to recruit Tregs to the lesions (Fujimura et al. 2012; Kambayashi et al. 2015).

These data indicate that direct or indirect RANK-RANKL interactions mediated by immune cells have a crucial role in the development of tumors, and targeting RANK/RANKL signaling pathway represents a promising strategy to be addressed in the treatment of breast cancer but also of other hematological and solid tumors.

16.4 RANK/RANKL Signaling in Breast Cancer

The developing mammary gland displays many of the properties associated with tumor progression, such as invasion, ability to initiate cell proliferation throughout its lifetime, resistance to apoptosis during lactation to prevent premature involution, and angiogenic remodeling. Multiple results support that tumors originate from progenitor cells or from cells that reacquire characteristics of stem/progenitor cells [reviewed in Celia-Terrassa (2018)], although the level of complexity within the mammary epithelium suggests that one or more cell types contribute to the development of breast cancer. Hence, breast cancer progression relies on co-opting the stroma and perverting the cross talk between the mammary epithelia and its microenvironment to foster instructive and permissive signals for tumorigenesis (Wiseman and Werb 2002).

RANK signaling deregulation contributes to the initiation and progression of mammary tumorigenesis, as anticipated due to its crucial role in mammary gland biology, controlling stem cell expansion and proliferation, as well as different aspects of the immune system. Therefore, RANK has emerged as an attractive target for breast cancer treatment as will be discussed below.

16.4.1 RANK/RANKL Signaling in Breast Cancer Initiation

16.4.1.1 Rank Signaling in Mouse Mammary Tumorigenesis

Molecular profiling and histopathological analysis have been crucial to disentangle breast cancer heterogeneity, allowing to identify the intrinsic breast cancer subtypes, which have had a profound and positive impact on patient stratification and treatment selection [reviewed in Nolan et al. (2023)]. Putative epithelial cells of origin for each breast tumor subtype are similar to adult progenitor stem cells, as unveiled from comprehensive transcriptomic analyses and studies of mouse mammary stem cells (Lim et al. 2009; Molyneux et al. 2010; Santagata and Ince 2014;

Visvader and Stingl 2014; Nguyen et al. 2018; Fu et al. 2020; Bach et al. 2021; Gray et al. 2022).

In mice, Rank pathway promotes mammary tumorigenesis. The overexpression of Rank in the mammary gland, under the MMTV promoter, MMTV-Rank or Rank$^{+/tg}$ mice, which drives Rank expression mainly to the luminal compartment, favors spontaneous adenocarcinomas characterized by the presence of bipotent epithelial cell progenitors (Gonzalez-Suarez et al. 2010; Pellegrini et al. 2013). Mechanistically, the constitutive activation of Rank signaling in the mammary gland expands the basal and luminal compartments, increasing MaSCs and luminal progenitors and altering the distribution of the luminal cell subsets. In fact, Rank expression interferes with the commitment of the alveolar lineage subpopulation, underlying the impaired alveologenesis and lactation failure seen in Rank$^{+/tg}$ mice (Gonzalez-Suarez et al. 2007).

Loss-of-function approaches also demonstrated the pro-tumorigenic role of Rank pathway in mouse models. Pharmacological inhibition of Rankl using Rank-Fc in "wild-type" mice prevents chemically induced mammary carcinogenesis by the synthetic progestin, medroxyprogesterone acetate (MPA), and the chemical mutagen 7,12-dimethylbenz[a]anthracene (DMBA) (Gonzalez-Suarez et al. 2010). The loss of Rank within the mammary epithelium (MMTV-driven) markedly delays mammary tumor onset, reduces tumor incidence, and increases survival upon MPA/DMBA treatments, hindering progestin-driven epithelial cell proliferation and impairing the expansion of stem-like MECs (Schramek et al. 2010). However, the protective effect is less severe than the one achieved with systemic Rankl inhibition, suggesting a pro-tumorigenic role for Rank beyond the mammary epithelium.

Mammary tumor onset upon chemical carcinogenesis is also impaired by the loss of epithelial Rank, once more confirming the relevance of Rank pathway in regulating mammary cell stemness (Schramek et al. 2010). Conversely, Rank$^{+/tg}$ mice treated with MPA/DMBA show faster tumor onset and increased incidence of premalignant and malignant lesions, which is reversed by the pharmacological treatment with Rank-Fc to inhibit Rankl (Gonzalez-Suarez et al. 2010). In contrast with the complete tumor protection observed in a wild-type background, Rankl inhibition is not able to fully prevent breast carcinogenesis in Rank$^{+/tg}$ mice, which may be indicative of a pro-tumorigenic role for Rank independent of Rankl. While in preneoplastic lesions (hyperplasias and mammary intraepithelial neoplasias) Rankl inhibition markedly reduces cell proliferation, in established breast adenocarcinomas, proliferation is independent of Rankl. In breast tumor cells, Rank pathway inhibition leads to an increase in tumor cell apoptosis, in line with a pro-survival role of Rank signaling in cancer cells (Jones et al. 2006). These studies provided compelling evidence for the involvement of Rank pathway in hormone-induced mammary tumorigenesis, consistent with a crucial role of Rank signaling in mammary gland development in response to sex hormones.

In oncogene-driven mouse models such as the Neu transgenic mice (MMTV-Neu, Neu), a spontaneous mouse model of mammary tumorigenesis driven by Neu oncogene, the rat homolog for HER2, Rank-Fc treatment reduces significantly the total number of tumors as well as lung metastatic burden (Gonzalez-Suarez et al. 2010). In contrast, in the more aggressive MMTV-NeuT model, where the Neu oncogene is constitutively active in the breast tissue, the mammary-specific deletion of Rank does not decrease tumor incidence (Schramek et al. 2010). These apparent conflicting results could reflect different experimental settings, such as mouse lines and background, or epithelial versus systemic effects of Rank signaling, but already pointed to an involvement of Rank pathway in spontaneous breast tumorigenesis besides hormone and carcinogenic-driven cancer. Complementary studies in PyMT transgenic mice (MMTV-PyMT, PyMT), an aggressive oncogene-driven mouse model that spontaneously develops mammary tumors, showed that Rank genetic deletion increases tumor latency and decreases tumor incidence and lung colonization as well as the pool of cancer stem cells (Yoldi et al. 2016).

Recent evidence indicates that extracellular matrix stiffness and mechano-signaling modulate progesterone-induced RANKL signaling in MECs, at least in part by enhancing ERK-mediated phosphorylation of progesterone receptor, potentiating mammary tumorigenesis in an oncogenic context (Northey et al. 2022).

Analyses of Rank and Rankl expression during tumor progression in Neu and PyMT oncogenic models showed that Rank protein is detected in non-transformed mammary glands, and its expression increases in mammary hyperplasias and adenocarcinomas. Regarding Rankl, it is undetected in PyMT and Neu malignant lesions but present in early preneoplastic lesions (Gonzalez-Suarez et al. 2010; Schramek et al. 2010; Yoldi et al. 2016), in line with the loss of hormone receptor expression during breast tumorigenesis (Lin et al. 2003). These differences in Rank and Rankl protein expression in breast tumors have important implications for the approaches considered for the prevention and treatment of breast cancer, as will be discussed in detail in the following sections.

The genetic inactivation of *Rank* in mice with double deletion of *Brca1* and *p53* in the mammary epithelium (K5Cre) decreases proliferation of MECs as well as the development of low and high-grade intraepithelial neoplasias and invasive carcinomas (Sigl et al. 2016). A similar protective effect is observed in a mouse model where *Rank*, *Brca1*, and *p53* deletions are driven by Wap-Cre. In these mice, Rank depletion delays tumor onset and reduces tumor incidence, impairing progression to high-grade tumors. In addition, the pharmacological inhibition of Rankl using RANK-Fc treatment in a mouse model that only lacks *Brca1* prevents the development of preneoplastic mammary lesions. In *Brca1/p53*-mutated mammary glands, Rank signaling controls the expansion and function of progenitor cells (Sigl et al. 2016), establishing a link between Rank pathway and *Brca1*-driven breast cancer. In a similar mouse model with mammary gland-specific *Brca1* deletion and heterozygous for *p53*, the mammary tumors developed show high expression of Rank, but not Rankl, whereas Rank signaling inhibition using denosumab attenuates tumor growth (Nolan et al. 2016). Both studies include relevant analyses in clinical samples from *BRCA1/2* mutation carriers, detailed below, leading to propose the targeting of RANK pathway to prevent or delay breast cancer.

16.4.1.2 RANK and Risk of Developing Breast Cancer: *BRCA1/2* Mutation Carriers and Women with High Mammographic Density

Two independent studies highlighted in 2016 the relevance of RANK pathway in the molecular mechanism contributing to breast tumorigenesis in *BRCA1/2* mutation carriers (Nolan et al. 2016; Sigl et al. 2016), supporting the use of denosumab as a prevention strategy in these high-risk women.

Sigl and coauthors observed high levels of RANK protein expression in breast tumors from *BRCA1/2* mutation carriers that show a similar pattern of RANKL expression. In these tumors, only RANK expression significantly correlates with higher grade. Besides, women with *BRCA1* mutation display single-nucleotide variants at the RANK locus that may modify their risk of developing breast cancer (Sigl et al. 2016).

Nolan and collaborators assessed RANK expression in epithelial cell subsets in mammoplasties from healthy women and in prophylactic mastectomies from *BRCA1/2* mutation carriers, finding that RANK expression was restricted to the luminal progenitor subpopulation in preneoplastic tissue. In *BRCA1* mutation carriers, RANK expression confers proliferation and clonogenic capacity in premalignant stages, whereas *BRCA1*-mutated triple-negative breast tumors show higher RANK expression but not RANKL. *BRCA1*-mutated ex vivo organoids display an exacerbated proliferative response to progesterone, confirming the crucial role for the RANK pathway in *BRCA1*-associated breast tumorigenesis (Nolan et al. 2016).

Breast density is considered one of the risk factors for the development of breast cancer. In line with mouse evidence indicating that increased stiffness leads to progesterone-driven increase in Rankl, the stiff breast tissue from women with high mammographic density shows high RANKL expression and elevated RANK signaling (Toriola et al. 2017; Northey et al. 2022), suggesting these women may benefit from the preventive action of denosumab to reduce breast cancer risk.

16.4.2 RANK in Breast Cancer Progression: Tumor Cell Intrinsic and Extrinsic Effects

16.4.2.1 Rank Signaling and Mammary Epithelium Senescence and Stemness

When Rank (Rank$^{+/tg}$) is constitutively expressed in the presence of PyMT or Neu oncogenes, these mice develop luminal-like mammary gland multifocal adenocarcinomas and lung metastasis, similar to single PyMT and Neu mice (Muller et al. 1988; Guy et al. 1992; Maglione et al. 2001; Herschkowitz et al. 2007). Surprisingly, the expression of Rank in the context of PyMT and Neu oncogenes remarkably delays tumor initiation and decreases tumor incidence in double transgenic mice while paradoxically promoting tumor aggressiveness once tumors are established, endorsing tumor stemness and lung colonization (Benitez et al. 2021). Analyses of PyMT Rank$^{+/tg}$ and Neu Rank$^{+/tg}$ mouse models reveal that Rank expression interferes with mammary cell fate already in preneoplastic mammary glands, altering the distribution of basal and luminal epithelial subpopulations (Cordero et al. 2023). In fact, Rank expression promotes a similar disturbance of the epithelial cell hierarchy as described in single Rank$^{+/tg}$ mice (Pellegrini et al. 2013; Benitez et al. 2021), demonstrating that PyMT and Neu oncogenes do not favor further alterations in the distribution of epithelial subsets, at least not during the initial tumorigenic stages. In particular, Rank expression in these oncogene-driven mouse models decreases the frequency of luminal progenitor subpopulations and, importantly, restrains luminal as well as basal mammary epithelial tumor initiation potential. Therefore, the expression of Rank hinders tumor formation independently of the tumor cell of origin in preneoplastic mammary glands. On the other hand, upon tumor establishment, Rank expression in PyMT and Neu oncogenic backgrounds enhances tumor aggressiveness and lung metastatic colonization, in part through the accumulation of luminal progenitors and embryonic-like bipotent epithelial cells (Benitez et al. 2021; Cordero et al. 2023).

Studies of Rank overexpression in non-transformed mammary epithelia provided the key to understand the mechanisms underlying the dual role of Rank in delaying tumorigenesis but promoting tumor aggressiveness in oncogenic contexts (Fig. 16.3). Whereas *Rank* null MECs show reduced proliferation and stemness (Fata et al. 2000; Gonzalez-Suarez et al. 2010; Yoldi et al. 2016), the activation of Rank signaling promotes senescence (Benitez et al. 2021), which in turn restrains tumorigenesis similarly to what is seen upon genetically or pharmacologically depleting Rank pathway (Yoldi et al. 2016). Indeed, Rank overexpression in mouse and human MECs, as well as in breast cancer cells, interferes with their differentiation and promotes an accumulation of stem and progenitor cell subpopulations (Gonzalez-Suarez et al. 2007; Palafox et al. 2012; Pellegrini et al. 2013; Cordero et al. 2016; Yoldi et al. 2016). In PyMT Rank$^{+/tg}$ and Neu Rank$^{+/tg}$ mice, high levels of senescence were already detected in hyperplastic lesions and early mammary intraepithelial neoplasias (Fig. 16.3a). This Rank-dependent induction of senescence in vivo was reproduced in vitro, upon Rank ectopic expression in MECs derived from single PyMT or Neu mice. The administration of Rankl also induced senescence in these oncogenic contexts, demonstrating that Rank signaling is a potent driver of senescence in the mouse mammary gland, which is dependent on the presence of p16 (Ink4a)/p19 (Arf) tumor suppressors. Although Rank-induced senescence is restricted to the luminal cell compartment, it drives stemness features not only in luminal but also in basal epithelial cells, indicative of a paracrine mechanism through the senescence-associated secretory phenotype (SASP) from luminal senescent cells (Fig. 16.3a). The use of senolytic agents targeting senescent cells demonstrated the requirement of senescence for Rank-induced stemness, ultimately contributing to the enhanced aggressiveness of established tumors from PyMT Rank$^{+/tg}$ mice, characterized by faster tumor growth, higher lung metastatic burden, and increased tumor- and metastasis-initiating cells (Benitez et al. 2021, Cordero et al. 2023). Consequently, Rank expression in the mammary

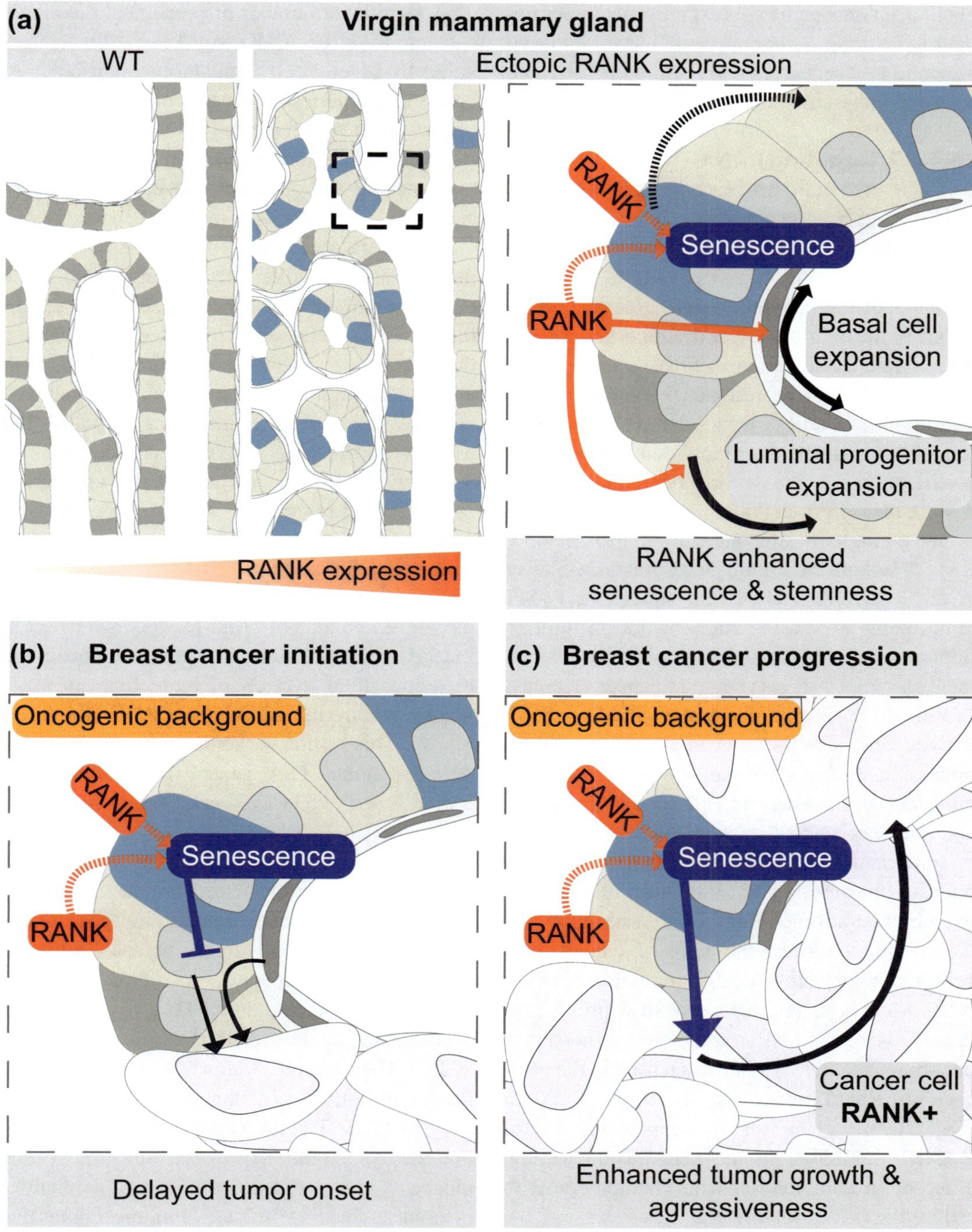

Fig. 16.3 Ectopic RANK signaling activation in the mammary gland drives senescence, a double-edged sword in breast cancer initiation and progression. (**a**) Constitutive RANK signaling activation in the luminal mammary epithelia induces senescence and promotes an accumulation of luminal progenitor and basal stem cell populations. (**b**) In oncogenic backgrounds (such as PyMT/Neu mouse models), high levels of RANK-driven senescence are detected in preneoplastic stages, which delay tumor onset and decrease tumor incidence. (**c**) Once tumors are established, RANK-induced senescence enhances tumor aggressiveness, endorsing tumor growth, stemness, and lung metastasis

gland in an oncogenic context prevents tumor initiation favoring senescence, and Rank-induced premalignant senescent cells prime cancer stemness and metastatic potential (Fig. 16.3b, c).

16.4.2.2 Targeting RANK-Driven Intrinsic and Extrinsic Effects in Breast Cancer

As detailed above, compelling preclinical evidence demonstrates that RANKL is the main mediator of the pro-tumorigenic role of progesterone in the mammary gland, supporting the key role of RANK signaling in breast cancer initiation (Fig. 16.4a). Regarding its therapeutic potential, initial studies have demonstrated that Rank-Fc treatment does not reduce tumor cell proliferation in breast adenocarcinomas and, despite that tumor cell apoptosis is induced, this is not enough to attenuate tumor growth once Rank$^{+/tg}$ tumors are established (Gonzalez-Suarez et al. 2010). Transplantation studies of PyMT tumor cells, expressing Rank or not, in limiting dilution assays, confirmed Rank pathway involvement in tumor cell survival and cancer stemness (Yoldi et al. 2016). *Rank* null PyMT tumor-derived cells show a reduced ability to grow as tumorspheres and give rise to novel tumors and lung metastasis when transplanted in syngeneic and immunodeficient mice (Yoldi et al. 2016).

Importantly, not only *Rank* genetic deletion but also pharmacological inhibition of Rankl by the administration of Rank-Fc in a neoadjuvant-like setting decrease the pool of cancer stem cells, inducing lactogenic differentiation of tumor cells. Moreover, an increased susceptibility to taxanes is found in Rank-depleted tumor cells, denoting a putative benefit when used in the presence of Rankl inhibitors (Yoldi et al. 2016) (Fig. 16.4b). These results support the use of RANKL inhibitors in the neoadjuvant setting, alone or in combination with chemotherapy, to reduce the risk of relapse and metastasis.

Besides the intrinsic effect of RANK pathway in the development of breast cancer, RANK has also a fundamental extrinsic role through the modulation of the tumor microenvironment, mainly the immune system, as discussed above.

A significant number of preclinical data indicate that RANK/RANKL signaling pathway triggered by several cell populations contributes to create an immunosuppressive microenvironment [reviewed in Ahern et al. (2018a)], opening the possibility that modulation of Rank signaling may prevent and/or revert this immunosuppression (Fig. 16.4c, d).

One of the strategies addressed is by blocking the central T cell tolerance as many of the TSAs expressed in the thymus are also expressed in tumor cells. Hence, the removal of autoreactive thymocytes by negative selection might also eliminate a high-affinity T cell clone capable of tackling tumor cells. It has been proposed that transiently blocking the central tolerance by depleting mTECs or modulating the expression of *Aire* could represent a strategy to generate a repertoire of T lymphocytes recognizing malignant cells. Blocking RANK/RANKL signaling could be a promising approach given its role in the development of Aire-expressing mTECs. Indeed, anti-RANKL treatment has demonstrated to reduce total mTECs in more than an 80%, mainly mature mTEC subsets (MHC IIhi Aire$^+$, >90%). This results in the downregulation of the Aire-dependent TSA gene expression and the decrease of Foxp3+ Treg cells (Waterfield et al. 2014).

An alternative strategy is the coadministration of RANKL inhibitors with immune checkpoint inhibitors. *Rank* genetic deletion in PyMT mammary tumor cells leads to an increase in tumor-infiltrating leukocytes, tumor-infiltrating lymphocytes (TILs), and CD8$^+$ T cells and a decrease in myeloid cells (Gomez-Aleza et al. 2020). The delayed tumor onset observed in Rank null tumors is mediated by T cells, specifically by CD8$^+$ T cells, as demonstrated in depletion assays. Rank expression in tumor cells induces the release of pro-inflammatory cytokines, leading to an immunosuppressive microenvironment favorable for myeloid cells, which induces neutrophil survival and impairs T cell proliferation (Fig. 16.4c). In fact, Rankl pharmacological inhibition, although unable to attenuate tumor growth when used as single therapy, improves the response to CTLA4 and PD1

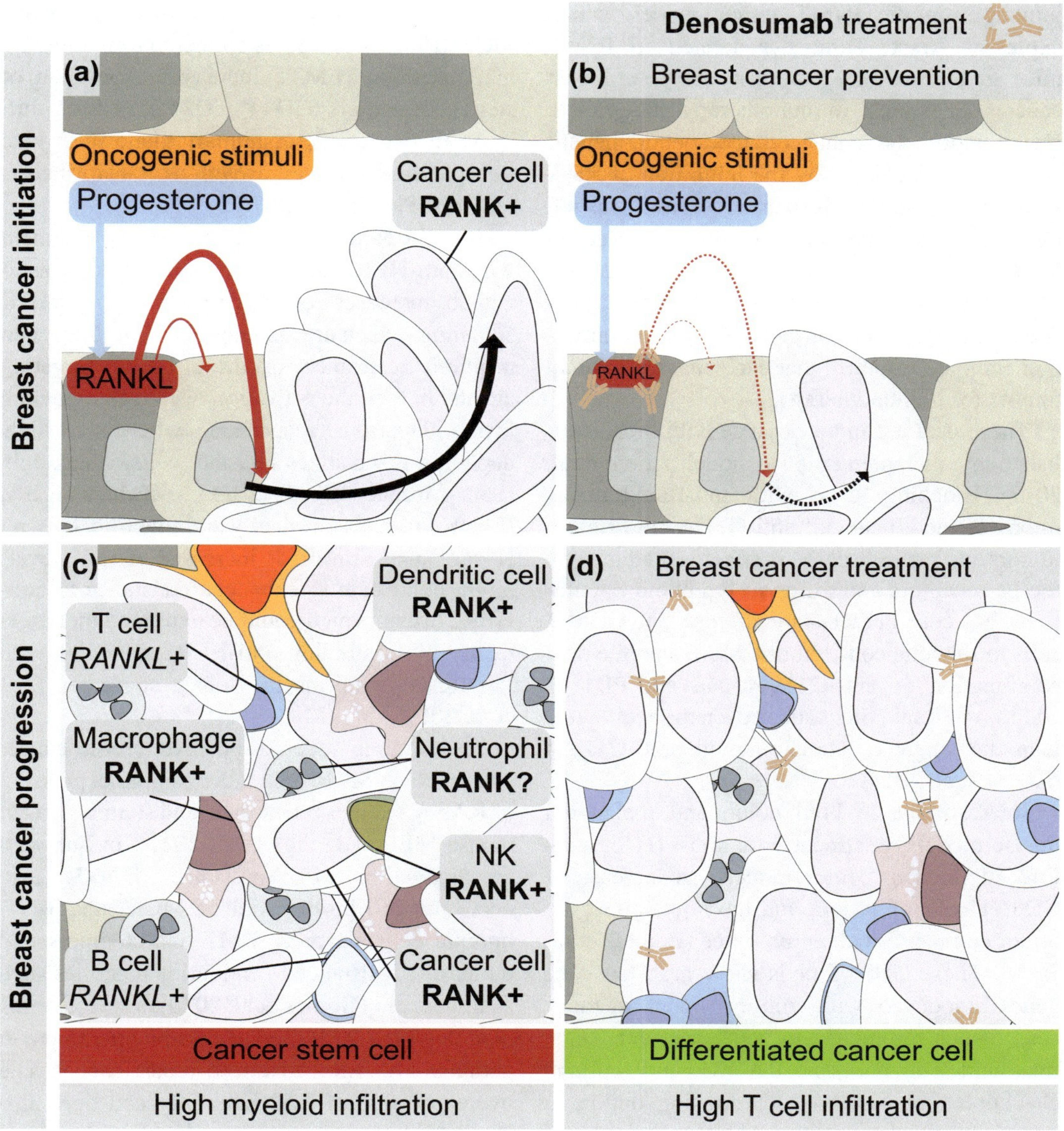

Fig. 16.4 RANK/RANKL pathway promotes breast cancer initiation and progression modulating cancer stemness and tumor immunity. Denosumab, a fully human anti-RANKL antibody, is a promising drug for breast cancer prevention and treatment. (**a**) Exacerbated RANK pathway activation due to increased progesterone signaling coupled with chemical oncogenic stimuli leads to mammary tumor development. (**b**) Pharmacological inhibition of RANKL prevents or attenuates mammary tumorigenesis highlighting the value of denosumab for breast cancer prevention. (**c**) RANK/RANKL interaction between tumor and immune cells regulates tumor immune surveillance. The cross talk between breast cancer cells and the indicated immune cell subsets, expressing RANK or RANKL, leads to an expansion of the cancer stem cell pool as well as an immunosuppressive microenvironment favorable for myeloid cells. (**d**) RANKL pharmacological inhibition impacts both breast tumor cells and their immune microenvironment favoring tumor cell differentiation and increasing tumor-infiltrating lymphocytes. Therefore, the use of denosumab in combination with immunotherapy is regarded as an encouraging approach for breast cancer treatment

inhibitors in the PyMT tumor model, which expresses Rank. Tumors generated in PyMT mice are luminal-like tumors, a subtype of breast cancer for which immunotherapy has failed. Interestingly, the enhanced therapeutic benefit seems to be mediated by the inhibition of Rank signaling in tumor cells themselves, as it was not observed when the combination was used in *Rank* null tumors (Gomez-Aleza et al. 2020). These findings indicate that loss of Rank signaling in mammary tumor cells leads to an antitumor immune response that can sensitize luminal tumors for immunotherapy.

These data are in accordance with those published in a melanoma mouse model (Ahern et al. 2017). Blocking Rankl with anti-Rankl mAbs improves the efficacy of anti-CTLA4 in primary tumors and metastases. This effect is mediated by the Fc receptors and different lymphoid populations, NK cells in metastatic disease, and $CD8^+$ T cells in subcutaneous tumors. Moreover, the dual combination of anti-CTLA4 and anti-PD1 in addition to Rankl blockade is even more effective than the single combination with anti-CTLA4 (Ahern et al. 2018).

Interestingly, in both colon and melanoma mouse models, treatment with anti-PD1 or anti-CTLA4 in *Aire*$^{-/-}$ mice induces an increase of $CD8^+$ T cell infiltration and the rejection of the tumor compared with *Aire*$^{+/+}$ mice (Benitez et al. 2020). These $CD8^+$ T cells show high levels of genes associated with tumor-resident memory cells, which are related to better survival. Thus, treatment with both anti-RANKL and immune checkpoint inhibitors is a promising option to induce the blocking of the central tolerance and the modulation of the tumor microenvironment.

16.4.3 RANK Pathway in Human Breast Cancer Progression

16.4.3.1 RANK in Human Breast Cancer Cell Lines and Treatment Resistance

RANK overexpression in a panel of human breast cancer cell lines, with mutated or methylated *BRCA1*, induces stemness and endorses tumorigenesis and metastasis (Palafox et al. 2012). Forced expression of RANK in non-transformed MCF10A cells promotes epithelial to mesenchymal transition (EMT), increased expression of stem cell markers ($CD44^+$ $CD24^-$), and the ability to regenerate the mammary gland in in vivo transplantation assays, as well as transformation features (Palafox et al. 2012).

In HER2+ breast cancer cell lines, treatment with anti-HER2 drugs, lapatinib and/or trastuzumab, increases RANK expression and RANK signaling, which are also higher in cell lines with acquired resistance to these HER2 targeting agents. In fact, the activation of RANK signaling favors lapatinib resistance, whereas RANK depletion resensitizes resistant cells to lapatinib (Sanz-Moreno et al. 2021). Mechanistically, RANK interacts physically and functionally with HER2, suggesting that increased RANK levels might contribute to enhanced resistance to anti-HER2 drugs, which could be exploited therapeutically by combining anti-HER2 therapies with RANK targeting, as previously suggested (Zoi et al. 2019).

In hormone receptor-positive breast cancer cells such as MCF7 cells, the ectopic expression of RANK induces senescence and stemness, as in mouse MECs (Benitez et al. 2021). In line with the induction of senescence, RANK also decreases cell proliferation in MCF7 and T47D luminal cells, favoring EMT and stemness and increasing resistance to endocrine therapies such as fulvestrant (Gomes et al. 2020), a selective ER modulator (SERM) used as first-line treatment in patients with ER+ advanced breast cancer. The overexpression of RANK in ER+ cell lines also slowed down tumor cell proliferation in orthotopic assays, in contrast with the observations from mouse and human tumors, in which RANK is associated with higher proliferation index. The observation that RANK overexpression decreases proliferation in luminal breast cells and tumors inspired further studies of interactions between RANK signaling and cell-cycle targeting drugs in the context of luminal breast cancer.

Indeed, it has been recently proposed that RANK signaling mediates resistance to cyclin-dependent kinase 4/6 inhibitors (CDK4/6i) (Gomes et al. 2023) that, combined with endocrine therapy, are current first-line treatment for advanced ER+ HER2- breast tumors. The overexpression of RANK in luminal MCF7 and T47D cells drives intrinsic resistance to several CDK4/6i, whereas pharmacological RANK pathway inhibition using OPG-Fc (RANKL neutralizing antibody) or RANK-Fc restores sensitivity in xenograft models. Moreover, the inhibition of RANK pathway prevents and delays acquired resistance to CDK4/6i, associated with aberrant interferon (IFN)-response in tumor cells, highlighting the clinical value of combining CDK4/6i with RANK pathway inhibitors (Gomes et al. 2023).

16.4.3.2 RANK/RANKL Expression in Breast Tumors and Its Association with Prognosis

The analysis of RANK protein expression in human breast cancer has been hindered by the scarce availability of specific and well-characterized antihuman RANK antibodies. Up to now, just one antibody has been widely accepted in the research community, N1H8 from Amgen, which is not sufficiently sensitive nor commercialized. Worryingly, this antibody on occasion fails to detect RANK in breast tumor samples, even when further functional analyses confirm active RANK expression (Gomez-Aleza et al. 2020). Hence, progress for clinically targeting RANK pathway in breast cancer patients has been dragged by the absence of superior research and diagnostic tools to identify RANK+ patients.

Initial analyses of RANK and RANKL in a subgroup of human adenocarcinomas established high levels of RANK in tumors lacking ER and PR expression and in tumors with high proliferation index and pathological grade, associating high RANK/RANKL gene expression with metastatic tumors (Gonzalez-Suarez et al. 2010; Palafox et al. 2012). Further analyses of breast cancer data from The Cancer Genome Atlas (TCGA) project (Cancer Genome Atlas 2012) determined that *RANK* gene expression in luminal tumors correlates with signatures that characterize mammary stem cells and luminal progenitors as well as senescence (Pellegrini et al. 2013; Benitez et al. 2021). In luminal A and basal-like breast intrinsic subtypes, RANK is associated with altered mammary differentiation (Palafox et al. 2012). Altogether, these results confirmed the observations in Rank gain- and loss-of-function mouse models.

The first analysis of RANK and RANKL expression by immunohistochemistry in a large cohort of patients with primary invasive breast cancer was published by Pfitzner and collaborators in 2014 (Pfitzner et al. 2014). RANK/RANKL expression was assessed in 601 FFPE biopsies of primary breast carcinoma from pretreated patients enrolled in the GeparTrio neoadjuvant study (2357 study participants) (von Minckwitz et al. 2008). These analyses confirmed previous indications associating increased RANK expression with high tumor grade and lack of hormone receptor expression (Palafox et al. 2012). Therefore, shorter disease-free survival (DFS) and OS were found in patients with higher levels of RANK expression, although RANK expression was not an independent prognostic and predictive factor. This study also confirmed previous data regarding RANKL expression in breast tumors (Gonzalez-Suarez et al. 2010), which was rarely detected in patients' tumor samples and not associated with any clinical parameter (Pfitzner et al. 2014). Unlike in the normal mammary gland, where RANKL is expressed in ER+ cells, RANKL is rarely found in ER+ tumor cells and mostly restricted to a subset of luminal A-like tumors (Azim et al. 2015), but has been found in the stroma surrounding the tumor (including TILs and fibroblast-like cells) (Gonzalez-Suarez et al. 2010). RANK expression was also found in the stroma including in immune cells: macrophages, DCs, and NK cells (Ahern et al. 2018b).

Previous studies in smaller cohorts showed related results, associating high RANK expression in 93 breast cancer patients with higher risk of developing bone metastasis and shorter skeletal DFS (Santini et al. 2011). Furthermore, in 102 metastatic breast cancer patients, RANK expression was significantly correlated with young age at diagnosis (Azim et al. 2015), and in patients with bone metastasis, with short progression-free survival (PFS) (Zhang et al. 2012). Pregnant patients showed increased RANKL expression on tumor and adjacent normal tissue, as seen in normal breast, and patients with slow proliferative tumors expressed higher levels of RANKL (Azim et al. 2015). Although there are some discrepancies regarding the frequency of RANK expression in the mentioned studies, most likely attributed to different experimental approaches, altogether they established that breast cancer patients expressing RANK show poorer prognosis and survival, probably due to the higher frequency of RANK expression in hormone receptor-negative breast cancer.

More recently, the expression of RANK and RANKL proteins was evaluated in >2000 breast cancer samples from four independent tissue-microarray (TMA) collections, two of them containing all breast cancer subtypes and two with only ER- tumors. Again, in the two general cohorts, RANK expression was significantly associated with ER/PR negativity, triple-negative breast cancer (TNBC) subtype, and poor prognosis (Ciscar et al. 2023). Importantly, when the ER- breast cancer cohort was specifically analyzed (around 400 samples), RANK expression was associated with poor distal metastasis-free survival (DMFS) and breast cancer-specific survival (BCSS). Moreover, patients with ER-RANK-expressing tumors after adjuvant chemotherapy showed poorer survival than those lacking RANK (Ciscar et al. 2023). These results are clinically relevant given the heterogeneity and poor prognosis of ER- tumors and the lack of targeted therapies. Considering that RANK is more frequently expressed in ER- tumors, RANK can become a biomarker of prognosis and a therapeutic target in ER- breast cancer.

One of the limitations of this study was that the samples from the general cohorts analyzed were collected more than 20 years ago, which would result in an underestimation of RANK detection by immunohistochemistry. The lower frequency of RANK+ samples detected within the ER+ cohort prevented associations with clinicopathological parameters in this subtype. Future studies are required to determine the clinical relevance of RANK as biomarker or therapeutic target in ER+ breast cancer.

Indeed, in tumors from luminal breast cancer patients treated with CDK4/6i and enrolled in the NeoPalAna neoadjuvant clinical trial, RANK signaling activation, measured by the upregulation of RANK metagene, which contains the top 100 *RANK*-correlated genes, predicts resistance to CDK4/6i treatment (Gomes et al. 2023).

In 151 patients from the PAMELA phase II clinical trial (Llombart-Cussac et al. 2017), RANK expression was higher in hormone receptor-negative tumor samples, confirming previous data. RANK expression, but not RANKL, was significantly associated with the basal-like breast cancer subtype, followed by the HER2-enriched subtype. Moreover, patients treated with lapatinib and trastuzumab, HER2-targeted agents, showed increased RANK levels ($n = 151$), whereas RANK protein expression was higher in residual samples from trastuzumab-resistant patients ($n = 22$) compared to treatment of naïve patients ($n = 67$) (Sanz-Moreno et al. 2021). These data suggest that RANK upregulation, but not RANKL, might underlie the emergence of resistance against anti-HER2 drugs, assessed by in vitro studies detailed above.

16.4.3.3 RANK and Menopausal Status

Pre- and postmenopausal breast cancers have distinct causes and molecular features, and menopausal status has a strong influence on breast cancer prevention, detection, prognosis, and therapeutic management of breast cancer patients (Heer et al. 2020). The loss of ovarian function, which curtails the supply of estrogen and progesterone after menopause, causes important systemic metabolic alterations as well as inflammatory responses, influencing postmenopausal breast cancer (Boonyaratanakornkit and Pateetin 2015). These alterations might underlie the association of obesity with postmenopausal breast cancer prognosis, worse in hormone receptor-positive breast tumors [reviewed in Garcia-Estevez et al. (2021)].

Interestingly, in the general cohorts of postmenopausal breast cancer, but not in premenopausal, RANK expression in tumor cells is associated with worse survival in univariate as well as in multivariate analysis (Ciscar et al. 2023). When menopausal status is considered in the ER- breast tumor cohort, RANK expression also associates with poorer survival in postmenopausal, but not premenopausal, patients.

These observations are counterintuitive, given the role of RANKL acting as a mediator of progesterone in the mammary gland, implying a more prominent role of RANK signaling in breast cancer in premenopausal women. However, gene expression data suggest that, although the frequency of RANK protein expression in breast tumor cells is not associated with the menopausal status, RANK signaling seems to be more active in tumors from postmenopausal women than in those from younger women. A similar scenario is observed in the bone, where overactivation of RANK signaling pathway after menopause disrupts the balance between bone resorption and bone formation, resulting in osteoporosis.

These results demonstrate that RANK expression is an independent biomarker of poor prognosis in postmenopausal breast cancer patients, particularly in those with ER- breast cancer. Moreover, they open the possibility for new combinatory treatments with RANK pathway inhibitors such as denosumab in postmenopausal breast cancer patients. The meta-analysis by the Early Breast Cancer Clinical Trialists' Collaborative Group supports the idea that adjuvant treatment of early breast cancer might be more efficacious with the addition of a bone-modifying agent, particularly in postmenopausal women, or in combination with ovarian function suppression (Chukir et al. 2019; Perrone and Gravina 2020). It cannot be ruled out that RANK also acts a predictive biomarker in ER+ breast cancer, specifically in postmenopausal ER+ breast cancer. Indeed, results from the *ABCSG-18* trial reveal that adjuvant denosumab reduces the risk of clinical fractures and improves DFS of hormone receptor-positive postmenopausal breast cancer patients receiving aromatase inhibitors (Gnant et al. 2019, 2022).

16.4.3.4 RANK and RANKL in Patient-Derived Xenografts

Patient-derived xenograft (PDX) models recapitulate the complexity and heterogeneity of breast cancer and have emerged as superior preclinical tools to address clinically relevant questions, from the identification of novel biomarkers and therapeutic targets to the understanding of clonal dynamics and evolution during tumor progression and the emergence of resistance mechanisms upon therapy. The implementation of co-clinical trials involving PDXs and patients has now become a reality (Byrne et al. 2017). In breast cancer, hundreds of stably transplantable PDX models representing the three main subtypes are widely available through consortiums and collaborations—their number increases daily (Whittle et al. 2015; Dobrolecki et al. 2016; Byrne et al. 2017). RANK and RANKL gene and protein expression patterns in breast cancer PDX models recapitulate those found in clinical collections, with RANK being more frequently found in breast cancer cells than RANKL (Ciscar et al. 2023). Moreover, studies ex vivo and in vivo using RANKL and RANK-Fc demonstrate the functionality of physiological levels of RANK signaling in breast cancer PDXs and their ability to modulate tumor cell proliferation, survival, stemness, metabolism, and immunity. While RANKL inhibition shows a modest ability to attenuate tumor growth when used as single agent, an improved response to taxanes is observed in several RANK+ TNBC and in one *BRCA1*-mutant breast cancer PDX, being able to eradicate tumor relapses in some PDX models (Nolan et al. 2016; Ciscar et al. 2023). Of note, studies in PDXs are most probably underestimating the response to RANKL inhibition given its important role regulating immunosurveillance. Future studies in these well-characterized RANK+ PDXs using state-of-the-art therapies will help select the combination partner for denosumab in breast cancer and the subset of breast cancer patients who may benefit from these treatments.

16.5 Targeting RANK/RANKL Signaling Pathway for the Prevention and/or Treatment of Breast Cancer

The effect of RANKL inhibition in mouse models has been first evaluated in preclinical studies using Fc fusion proteins, Fc-OPG, OPG-Fc, and RANK-Fc. But these Fc fusion proteins show a series of disadvantages that led to the development of a more proficient RANKL inhibitor, denosumab (AMG-162, Amgen) (Lacey et al. 2012). Denosumab is a fully synthetic human monoclonal antibody (IgG_2) that binds to and inhibits human soluble and membrane RANKL with high affinity and specificity (Fig. 16.1c), not recognizing rodent Rankl (McClung et al. 2006). Denosumab shares the pharmacological attributes of OPG but has a substantial longer half-life, allowing treatments with lower frequency of administration (Bekker et al. 2001; Kostenuik 2005).

In 2010, denosumab was approved by the US Food and Drug Administration (FDA) (https://www.fda.gov/) for the treatment of osteoporosis due to its potent antiresorptive activity. Months later, it was approved for the prevention of skeletal-related events (SREs) in patients with bone metastasis from solid tumors and for the treatment of bone loss in patients with prostate or breast cancer undergoing hormone ablation therapy. Subsequent approvals by the FDA are related with the management of bone loss conditions, such as metastatic bone disease or prevention of fractures associated with cancer therapies. Indeed, denosumab is the second most used drug for SREs after alendronate, and more than a half of the clinical trials approved for denosumab have been conducted to study its therapeutic potential in osteoporosis and bone-related diseases. In May 2010, the use of denosumab in Europe was approved by the European Medicines Agency (EMA) (https://www.ema.europa.eu/en). Nowadays, denosumab is commercialized in over 80 countries worldwide.

Although anti-RANKL treatment has been recently proposed as a novel approach for preventing and treating breast cancer and metastases, up to now, denosumab has not been approved for the prevention or treatment of any type of cancer.

16.5.1 Use of Denosumab in Breast Cancer Prevention

Women at high risk of developing breast cancer are a heterogeneous group including women with high-risk germline mutation/s, such as in *BRCA1/2*, but also those with other nongenetic risk factors, like women with high mammographic density. The most effective preventive strategy particularly used for *BRCA1* mutation carriers includes preventive mastectomy. Preventive therapy with SERMs like tamoxifen and aromatase inhibitors (AIs) has also demonstrated to reduce the incidence of breast cancer in healthy postmenopausal women and the risk for breast cancer in high-risk premenopausal women (Cuzick et al. 2013). SERMs work as ER antagonists in breast tissue, blocking the effect of estrogen and hindering the proliferation of malignant cells. In addition, they act as agonists in other tissues such as the bone, preventing osteoporosis. More recently, AIs have been shown to reduce the risk of developing breast cancer in postmenopausal women, although they are not approved by the FDA for this indication (Goss and Wu 2007; Richardson et al. 2007; Cigler et al. 2011; Goss et al. 2011; Cuzick et al. 2020). Conversely, hormone replacement therapies, particularly those combining estrogen and progesterone, indicated to relieve the symptoms of menopause, have been linked epidemiologically to the onset and incidence of breast cancer (Rossouw et al. 2002; Beral and Million Women Study 2003).

Thus, pilot clinical trials have been conducted with the objective of preventing breast cancer by antagonizing progesterone with selective PR modulators (SPRMs) in women at increased familial breast cancer risk.

In the phase II pilot prevention study of *BC-APPS1* (NCT02408770) with antiprogestin ulipristal acetate (UA), a reduction of the percentage of median Ki67, luminal progenitor population, and breast density are observed after UA treatment (Howell et al. 2022). In the same line, mifepristone (*NCT01898312*), another SPRM, reduces the mitotic age as well as the proportion of luminal progenitor cells and, interestingly, the number of mutations of the *TP53* gene (Bartlett et al. 2022). These data support the use of SPRMs for primary prevention of breast cancer, including those tumors with poor prognosis.

Similarly, based on RANKL being the main mediator of the pro-tumorigenic role of progesterone in the mammary gland and its distinct biology in *BRCA1*-mutated mammary cells (Gonzalez-Suarez et al. 2010; Schramek et al. 2010; Nolan et al. 2016; Sigl et al. 2016; Yoldi et al. 2016), the proof-of-concept pilot *BRCA-D* clinical trial (ACTRN12614000694617) was started in Australia a decade ago to study the preventive effect of denosumab in both *BRCA1*- and *BRCA2*-mutated patients. A total of 32 patients were recruited and the study was completed. Preliminary results reported a lower proliferation of tumor cells in three patients treated with denosumab, as measured by Ki67 expression in breast histologically normal tissue (Nolan et al. 2016). This trial was the foundation for a larger clinical trial conducted in Australia and led by the Austrian Breast Cancer Study Group (ABCSG), the *BRCA-P* trial (BCT 1801/ABCSG 50), which studies the effect of denosumab on preventing breast cancer in women with *BRCA1* germline mutations. The clinical trial involves five additional countries, Germany, Israel, Spain, the United Kingdom, and the United States. It is a randomized, double-blind phase III study in which denosumab-treated patients received denosumab subcutaneously every 6 months for up to 5 years in the absence of disease progression or unacceptable toxicity. The primary endpoint is to analyze the effect of denosumab in the risk of developing any type of breast cancer, ductal carcinoma in situ or invasive. Among the secondary endpoints, whether denosumab leads to a reduction of the risk of other gynecological tumors, clinical fractures, or benign breast lesions, will be analyzed. First results are expected in 2026–2033.

Breast density is considered one of the risk factors for the development of breast cancer, and RANKL expression has been associated with a higher mammographic density (Toriola et al. 2017). In this regard, the *TRIDENT* clinical trial (NCT04067726) is a randomized phase II trial aimed to analyze the effect of denosumab on mammographic density in premenopausal women with dense breasts. A total of 210 women are enrolled in this study, who are randomized in placebo and denosumab arms. Women in the denosumab arm are administrated with 60-mg subcutaneous denosumab at two time points: baseline and 6 months. As an additional endpoint, the study proposes to analyze the changes in the expression of RANKL pathway genes in response to denosumab treatment. A previous early phase I study of the same group completed in 2018 (*NCT03629717*) has been used to establish the bases of *TRIDENT* trial.

16.5.2 Denosumab as a Candidate for the Treatment of Breast Cancer

According to ClinicalTrials.gov, denosumab has been included in almost 300 clinical trials up to July 2023, a third of them involving patients with cancer and over 30 trials directed at breast cancer patients. Although most of these clinical trials are focused on reducing bone-related events, some of them include endpoints beyond SREs and have enrolled a remarkable number of patients.

In the *ABCSG-18* clinical trial (NCT00556374), the effect of denosumab in postmenopausal patients with early-stage hormone receptor-positive breast cancer treated with nonsteroidal AI adjuvant therapy is investigated. Here, 3425 postmenopausal hormone-positive breast cancer patients are randomized in placebo and denosumab groups. Denosumab-treated patients are subcutaneously administered with 60-mg doses every 6 months until the end of the study. Results indicate that denosumab delays the appearance of clinical fractures by increasing bone mass density (Gnant et al. 2019, 2022). In addition, denosumab administration does not induce an added toxicity. Importantly, it is the first clinical trial in breast cancer patients describing that adjuvant denosumab increases both DFS and OS in postmenopausal women with breast cancer receiving AIs, supporting the anticipated benefit of denosumab in postmenopausal breast cancer expressing RANK and suggested in (Ciscar et al. 2023). However, in this trial, RANK expression has not been measured, and patients are not stratified according to this parameter, a crucial limitation of the study.

Another study addressing the effect of adjuvant denosumab in DFS as a secondary endpoint is the *D-CARE* clinical trial (NCT01077154), where 4509 patients are enrolled. This trial has been designed to test whether denosumab in combination with standard-of-care adjuvant or neoadjuvant chemotherapy would increase

BMFS in women with high-risk early breast cancer. Women are randomized in control and denosumab groups, and denosumab group is subcutaneously treated with 120-mg denosumab every 4 weeks for 6 months and then once every 3 months for 4.5 years. Unfortunately, in *D-CARE*, denosumab does not improve neither BMFS nor DFS in women with early-stage high-risk breast cancer versus placebo independently of the subgroup studied (Coleman et al. 2020), in contrast to the *ABCSG-18* trial, where differences in DFS are observed (Gnant et al. 2019, 2022). However, the effects of denosumab on the incidence and timing of appearance of first clinical fractures were similar to those observed in the ABCSG-18 study. Discrepancies observed in the clinical outcome between both trials might be explained by differences in patients enrolled in the corresponding study and in treatment regimens. In the *D-CARE* study, patients are unselected and heterogeneous in terms of tumor biology, RANK/RANKL expression levels, tumor type, and menopausal status. They show tumors in stage II or III with lymph node metastasis and are treated with chemotherapy and hormonal therapy, whereas patients in the *ABCSG-18* trial are all postmenopausal—most of them present grade II tumors and are treated with AIs. In addition, the unusual number of patients withdrawing the informed consent in *D-CARE* (>10%) and the unexpected lower number of events for efficacy endpoints could have affected the results in this study.

Another study with a high number of recruited breast cancer patients is the *GeparX* clinical trial (NCT02682693), which includes 780 patients. This is a multicenter, prospective, 2 × 2 randomized, open-label phase IIb study in which denosumab is used in the neoadjuvant setting. Here, 120-mg denosumab are subcutaneously administrated every 4 weeks for six cycles to patients with two different nab-paclitaxel regimens in combination with trastuzumab and pertuzumab (for HER2+ patients) or carboplatin (for TNBC patients) or an epirubicin plus cyclophosphamide regimen (combined with HER2 inhibitors for HER2+ patients). One of the co-primary endpoints in GeparX trial is to measure the pathological complete response (pCR) rates to study the benefit of adding denosumab in combination with the mentioned chemotherapy. Treatment with denosumab does not improve the pCR rate, irrespective of the breast cancer subtype analyzed (Blohmer et al. 2022). Notably, as a secondary endpoint, it is proposed to study the interaction of denosumab treatment with RANK expression. Interestingly, although patients showing tumors with a higher RANK expression have a significantly higher pCR rate than those with low RANK expression, the clinical benefit of denosumab concerning RANK expression is not clear. These significant differences might be related to the higher frequency of RANK expression in ER- tumors, which show higher pCR rates after chemotherapy (Liedtke et al. 2008).

Recently, our group have published the results obtained from the *D-BEYOND* clinical trial (NCT01864798) (Gomez-Aleza et al. 2020), a prospective, single-arm phase IIa trial in newly diagnosed, early-stage breast cancer, where 24 premenopausal women received 2 doses of single agent denosumab (120 mg) after diagnosis. Here, the primary endpoint has not been reached, as no effect in proliferation is observed when the biopsy and surgery samples were compared. However, upon analyzing the composition of the tumor immune infiltrate as a secondary objective, an increase in the percentage of TILs, specifically $CD8^+$ T cells, is observed after RANKL inhibition with denosumab, in line with the results in the mouse models (Gomez-Aleza et al. 2020). Remarkably, all tumors except one are ER+, a subtype of breast tumors known for being immunologically cold. Moreover, patients responding to denosumab show a higher RANK signaling activation in the tumors and RANKL levels in serum. These results are pending to be confirmed in the ongoing window-of-opportunity study, the *D-BIOMARK* clinical trial (NCT03691311). Sixty breast cancer patients pre- and postmenopausal, with early HER2- breast cancer scheduled for primary surgery, were randomized in a 2:1 ratio to receive two doses of 120-mg denosumab on days 1 and 8 after diagnosis versus no treatment before surgery. Primary endpoints will address the putative antiproliferative, proapoptotic role of denosumab in paired biopsy/surgical specimens. Exploratory endpoints include the analyses of denosumab as immunomodulator and the identification of biomarkers of response to denosumab in breast cancer. Results obtained from these clinical trials will open new perspectives for breast cancer treatment, supporting the use of denosumab in combination with immunotherapy in breast cancer. The immunomodulatory effect of denosumab in combination with immunotherapy is being tested in other tumors as discussed in the next section.

16.5.3 Potential Use of Denosumab as an Immunomodulator in Other Solid Tumors

Immune checkpoint blockade using monoclonal antibodies such as anti-CTLA4 or anti-PD1/PDL1 has revolutionized the treatment of highly immunogenic tumors including melanoma and non-small cell lung cancer (NSCLC) [reviewed in Huang and Zappasodi (2022), Lahiri et al. (2023)]. This new line of treatment has resulted in better outcomes and in the reduction of side effects compared with chemotherapy. However, results in breast cancer have shown modest results to date. In contrast to other tumors, breast cancer, and luminal tumors in particular, exhibit a low immune infiltration and a poor response to immunotherapy. Only limited success has been achieved in TNBC patients using the anti-PD1 inhibitor pembrolizumab in combination with chemotherapy (*KEYNOTE-355*, NCT02819518) (Cortes et al. 2022). In fact, results derived from this trial have led to the approval of pembrolizumab for the treatment of TNBC, opening a promising area in breast cancer treatment. However, new strategies involving immunotherapy need to be developed for the treatment of low-infiltrated cancers, such as compounds able to modulate the immune infiltration and improve the immunotherapy effects. Given its immune-related effects, denosumab is not only being considered as a candidate to be used as an immunomodulator in the treatment of breast cancer but also in other solid tumors (Table 16.1). Some of these clinical trials are focused on analyzing the capacity of denosumab to modulate the immune system and increase the efficacy of immunotherapy, in particular in melanoma and lung cancer (Box 16.1). Results from these trials will pave the way for similar combinations in breast cancer and other tumors.

Table 16.1 Examples of clinical trials evaluating denosumab as an immunomodulator in solid tumors

Cancer type	ID	*N*	Phase	Use of denosumab
Melanoma	NCT03620019	25	II	Denosumab alone or in combination with anti-PD1 agent (nivolumab)
	NCT03161756 (CHARLI)	72	Ib/II	Denosumab in combination with anti-PD1 (nivolumab) and/or anti-CTLA4 (ipilimumab) agents
Lung cancer	NCT03669523 (DENIVOS)	82	II	Denosumab in combination with anti-PD1 agent (nivolumab)
	ACTRN12618001121257 (POPCORN)	30	Ib/II	Denosumab in combination with anti-PD1 agent (nivolumab)
	NCT02129699 (SPLENDOUR)	514	III	Denosumab in combination with platinum-based doublet chemotherapy
	NCT01951586	226	II	Denosumab in combination with platinum-based doublet chemotherapy
Pancreas cancer	NCT04907851 (PORCUPINE2)	80	II	Denosumab in combination with WNT signaling inhibitors
Thyroid cancer	NCT03732495 (LENVOS)	35	II	Denosumab combined with lenvatinib (tyrosine kinase inhibitor)
Renal cancer	NCT03280667 (KEYPAD)	59	II	Denosumab in combination with PD1 agent (pembrolizumab)

Box 16.1 Clinical trials combining denosumab and immunotherapy in melanoma and lung cancer

In melanoma, two studies have been conducted using denosumab with immune checkpoint inhibitors. The clinical trial *NCT03620019* is a single-arm, phase II study analyzing the immune-mediated mechanism of action of denosumab (120 mg) alone or in combination with nivolumab (anti-PD1) in 25 patients with unresectable (or resectable) stage III or distant metastatic PD-1/PD-L1 inhibitor-naïve cutaneous melanoma (AJCC stage III/IV). This study has been completed and results are now available in ClinicalTrials.gov. In the phase Ib/II *CHARLI* clinical trial (NCT03161756) of 72 patients with unresectable or metastatic melanoma, denosumab is combined with anti-PD1 agent (nivolumab) or with nivolumab plus anti-CTLA4 agent (ipilimumab). Endpoints in this trial are focused on describing the effect of both combinations in survival parameters, as well as on characterizing tumor immune populations and mechanisms of activity and resistance. This trial was estimated to conclude by the end of 2023, but no results are yet available.

Regarding lung cancer, an Australian phase Ib/II translational trial in resectable non-small cell lung cancer (NSCLC) (*POPCORN*, ACTRN12618001121257) has been completed, recruiting 28 patients with the aim of analyzing the neoadjuvant effect of denosumab in combination with nivolumab (Ahern et al. 2019). Patients are randomized in nivolumab or nivolumab plus denosumab arms (120 mg every 2 weeks) before surgery. The primary endpoint is to define the pharmacodynamic effect, activity, and safety of the combination compared with single treatment studying TCR clonality, transcriptomic profile changes, and immune biomarkers. Secondary endpoints include survival parameters such as DFS or OS. In other line, the phase II *DENIVOS* trial (NCT03669523) is evaluating the combination of denosumab plus nivolumab as a second-line therapy in stage IV NSCLC patients with bone metastases. Doses of 120-mg denosumab are subcutaneously administrated every 4 weeks in combination with 240-mg nivolumab every 2 weeks for a maximum of 2 years. This study only considers the analysis of survival parameters and SREs, but not changes concerning the immune system.

16.6 Conclusions

It may take decades until the extent of success of the breast cancer prevention trials with denosumab will be known, but the strong biology underlining the design of these trials holds out hope for many women with hereditary breast cancer and other high-risk populations. Based on the results gathered from clinical trials, denosumab seems to have a low benefit as a single agent in the treatment of breast cancer, but strong preclinical and clinical evidence support its use in combination with other approved drugs. It is important to consider that most of the clinical trials using denosumab do not categorize patients according to RANK/RANKL protein expression levels. For that, further explorative analyses in new clinical trials are necessary to decipher the best setting in which denosumab has a potential benefit and to identify biomarkers of response to denosumab to select the breast cancer patients who can benefit from the treatment. Interestingly, denosumab capacity to modulate the immune system places it as a promising compound to be used in combination with immunotherapy regimens such as checkpoint inhibitor agents. Overall, RANK pathway is intimately involved in breast cancer, from tumor initiation to tumor immune control, supporting the use of RANK/RANKL signaling inhibitors for breast cancer prevention but also for breast cancer treatment, most likely in combination with other drugs as chemotherapeutics, targeted therapies, and immunotherapies. Therefore, RANK pathway inhibitors as denosumab represent a valuable option for more effective and personalized combination treatments in breast cancer.

References

Aggarwal BB (2003) Signalling pathways of the TNF superfamily: a double-edged sword. Nat Rev Immunol 3(9):745–756

Ahern E, Harjunpaa H, Barkauskas D, Allen S, Takeda K, Yagita H, Wyld D, Dougall WC, Teng MWL, Smyth MJ (2017) Co-administration of RANKL and CTLA4 antibodies enhances lymphocyte-mediated antitumor immunity in mice. Clin Cancer Res 23(19):5789–5801

Ahern E, Harjunpaa H, O'Donnell JS, Allen S, Dougall WC, Teng MWL, Smyth MJ (2018a) RANKL blockade improves efficacy of PD1-PD-L1 blockade or dual PD1-PD-L1 and CTLA4 blockade in mouse models of cancer. Onco Targets Ther 7(6):e1431088

Ahern E, Smyth MJ, Dougall WC, Teng MWL (2018b) Roles of the RANKL-RANK axis in antitumour immunity - implications for therapy. Nat Rev Clin Oncol 15(11):676–693

Ahern E, Cubitt A, Ballard E, Teng MWL, Dougall WC, Smyth MJ, Godbolt D, Naidoo R, Goldrick A, Hughes BGM (2019) Pharmacodynamics of Pre-Operative PD1 checkpoint blockade and receptor activator of NFkB ligand (RANKL) inhibition in non-small cell lung cancer (NSCLC): study protocol for a multicentre, open-label, phase 1B/2, translational trial (POPCORN). Trials 20(1):753

Albagha OM, Visconti MR, Alonso N, Langston AL, Cundy T, Dargie R, Dunlop MG, Fraser WD, Hooper MJ, Isaia G, Nicholson GC, del Pino Montes J, Gonzalez-Sarmiento R, di Stefano M, Tenesa A, Walsh JP, Ralston SH (2010) Genome-wide association study identifies variants at CSF1, OPTN and TNFRSF11A as genetic risk factors for Paget's disease of bone. Nat Genet 42(6):520–524

Anderson DM, Maraskovsky E, Billingsley WL, Dougall WC, Tometsko ME, Roux ER, Teepe MC, DuBose RF, Cosman D, Galibert L (1997) A homologue of the TNF receptor and its ligand enhance T-cell growth and dendritic-cell function. Nature 390(6656):175–179

Arnold M, Morgan E, Rumgay H, Mafra A, Singh D, Laversanne M, Vignat J, Gralow JR, Cardoso F, Siesling S, Soerjomataram I (2022) Current and future burden of breast cancer: global statistics for 2020 and 2040. Breast 66:15–23

Asselin-Labat ML, Vaillant F, Sheridan JM, Pal B, Wu D, Simpson ER, Yasuda H, Smyth GK, Martin TJ, Lindeman GJ, Visvader JE (2010) Control of mammary stem cell function by steroid hormone signalling. Nature 465(7299):798–802

Atkins GJ, Kostakis P, Vincent C, Farrugia AN, Houchins JP, Findlay DM, Evdokiou A, Zannettino AC (2006) RANK Expression as a cell surface marker of human osteoclast precursors in peripheral blood, bone marrow, and giant cell tumors of bone. J Bone Miner Res 21(9):1339–1349

Azim HA Jr, Peccatori FA, Brohee S, Branstetter D, Loi S, Viale G, Piccart M, Dougall WC, Pruneri G, Sotiriou C (2015) RANK-ligand (RANKL) expression in young breast cancer patients and during pregnancy. Breast Cancer Res 17:24

Bach K, Pensa S, Zarocsinceva M, Kania K, Stockis J, Pinaud S, Lazarus KA, Shehata M, Simoes BM, Greenhalgh AR, Howell SJ, Clarke RB, Caldas C, Halim TYF, Marioni JC, Khaled WT (2021) Time-resolved single-cell analysis of Brca1 associated mammary tumourigenesis reveals aberrant differentiation of luminal progenitors. Nat Commun 12(1):1502

Bartlett TE, Evans I, Jones A, Barrett JE, Haran S, Reisel D, Papaikonomou K, Jones L, Herzog C, Pashayan N, Simoes BM, Clarke RB, Evans DG, Ghezelayagh TS, Ponandai-Srinivasan S, Boggavarapu NR, Lalitkumar PG, Howell SJ, Risques RA, Radestad AF, Dubeau L, Gemzell-Danielsson K, Widschwendter M (2022) Antiprogestins reduce epigenetic field cancerization in breast tissue of young healthy women. Genome Med 14(1):64

Baud'huin M, Duplomb L, Teletchea S, Lamoureux F, Ruiz-Velasco C, Maillasson M, Redini F, Heymann MF, Heymann D (2013) Osteoprotegerin: multiple partners for multiple functions. Cytokine Growth Factor Rev 24(5):401–409

Bekker PJ, Holloway D, Nakanishi A, Arrighi M, Leese PT, Dunstan CR (2001) The effect of a single dose of osteoprotegerin in postmenopausal women. J Bone Miner Res 16(2):348–360

Beleut M, Rajaram RD, Caikovski M, Ayyanan A, Germano D, Choi Y, Schneider P, Brisken C (2010) Two distinct mechanisms underlie progesterone-induced proliferation in the mammary gland. Proc Natl Acad Sci USA 107(7):2989–2994

Benitez AA, Khalil-Aguero S, Nandakumar A, Gupta NT, Zhang W, Atwal GS, Murphy AJ, Sleeman MA, Haxhinasto S (2020) Absence of central tolerance in Aire-deficient mice synergizes with immune-checkpoint inhibition to enhance antitumor responses. Commun Biol 3(1):355

Benitez S, Cordero A, Santamaria PG, Redondo-Pedraza J, Rocha AS, Collado-Sole A, Jimenez M, Sanz-Moreno A, Yoldi G, Santos JC, De Benedictis I, Gomez-Aleza C, Da Silva-Alvarez S, Troule K, Gomez-Lopez G, Alcazar N, Palmero I, Collado M, Serrano M, Gonzalez-Suarez E (2021) RANK links senescence to stemness in the mammary epithelia, delaying tumor onset but increasing tumor aggressiveness. Dev Cell 56(12):1727–1741 e1727

Beral V, C. Million Women Study (2003) Breast cancer and hormone-replacement therapy in the Million Women Study. Lancet 362(9382):419–427

Blohmer JU, Link T, Reinisch M, Just M, Untch M, Stotzer O, Fasching PA, Schneeweiss A, Wimberger

P, Seiler S, Huober J, Thill M, Jackisch C, Rhiem K, Solbach C, Hanusch C, Seither F, Denkert C, Engels K, Nekljudova V, Loibl S, Gbg and B. Ago (2022) Effect of denosumab added to 2 different nab-paclitaxel regimens as neoadjuvant therapy in patients with primary breast cancer: the geparx 2 x 2 randomized clinical trial. JAMA Oncol 8(7):1010–1018

Body JJ, Quinn G, Talbot S, Booth E, Demonty G, Taylor A, Amelio J (2017) Systematic review and meta-analysis on the proportion of patients with breast cancer who develop bone metastases. Crit Rev Oncol Hematol 115:67–80

Boldin MP, Mett IL, Varfolomeev EE, Chumakov I, Shemer-Avni Y, Camonis JH, Wallach D (1995) Self-association of the "death domains" of the p55 tumor necrosis factor (TNF) receptor and Fas/APO1 prompts signaling for TNF and Fas/APO1 effects. J Biol Chem 270(1):387–391

Boonyaratanakornkit V, Pateetin P (2015) The role of ovarian sex steroids in metabolic homeostasis, obesity, and postmenopausal breast cancer: molecular mechanisms and therapeutic implications. Biomed Res Int 2015:140196

Bord S, Ireland DC, Beavan SR, Compston JE (2003) The effects of estrogen on osteoprotegerin, RANKL, and estrogen receptor expression in human osteoblasts. Bone 32(2):136–141

Bord S, Frith E, Ireland DC, Scott MA, Craig JI, Compston JE (2004) Synthesis of osteoprotegerin and RANKL by megakaryocytes is modulated by oestrogen. Br J Haematol 126(2):244–251

Boyce BF, Xing L (2007) Biology of RANK, RANKL, and osteoprotegerin. Arthritis Res Ther 9(Suppl 1):S1

Breuil V, Schmid-Antomarchi H, Schmid-Alliana A, Rezzonico R, Euller-Ziegler L, Rossi B (2003) The receptor activator of nuclear factor (NF)-kappaB ligand (RANKL) is a new chemotactic factor for human monocytes. FASEB J 17(12):1751–1753

Bucay N, Sarosi I, Dunstan CR, Morony S, Tarpley J, Capparelli C, Scully S, Tan HL, Xu W, Lacey DL, Boyle WJ, Simonet WS (1998) osteoprotegerin-deficient mice develop early onset osteoporosis and arterial calcification. Genes Dev 12(9):1260–1268

Byrne AT, Alferez DG, Amant F, Annibali D, Arribas J, Biankin AV, Bruna A, Budinska E, Caldas C, Chang DK, Clarke RB, Clevers H, Coukos G, Dangles-Marie V, Eckhardt SG, Gonzalez-Suarez E, Hermans E, Hidalgo M, Jarzabek MA, de Jong S, Jonkers J, Kemper K, Lanfrancone L, Maelandsmo GM, Marangoni E, Marine JC, Medico E, Norum JH, Palmer HG, Peeper DS, Pelicci PG, Piris-Gimenez A, Roman-Roman S, Rueda OM, Seoane J, Serra V, Soucek L, Vanhecke D, Villanueva A, Vinolo E, Bertotti A, Trusolino L (2017) Interrogating open issues in cancer precision medicine with patient-derived xenografts. Nat Rev Cancer 17(4):254–268

Camara A, Cordeiro OG, Alloush F, Sponsel J, Chypre M, Onder L, Asano K, Tanaka M, Yagita H, Ludewig B, Flacher V, Mueller CG (2019) Lymph Node Mesenchymal and Endothelial Stromal Cells Cooperate via the RANK-RANKL Cytokine Axis to Shape the Sinusoidal Macrophage Niche. Immunity 50(6):1467–1481 e1466

Camara A, Lavanant AC, Abe J, Desforges HL, Alexandre YO, Girardi E, Igamberdieva Z, Asano K, Tanaka M, Hehlgans T, Pfeffer K, Pfeffer S, Mueller SN, Stein JV, Mueller CG (2022) CD169(+) macrophages in lymph node and spleen critically depend on dual RANK and LTbetaR signaling. Proc Natl Acad Sci USA 119(3)

Cancer Genome Atlas, N (2012) Comprehensive molecular portraits of human breast tumours. Nature 490(7418):61–70

Celia-Terrassa T (2018) Mammary stem cells and breast cancer stem cells: molecular connections and clinical implications. Biomedicines 6(2)

Centonze A, Lin S, Tika E, Sifrim A, Fioramonti M, Malfait M, Song Y, Wuidart A, Van Herck J, Dannau A, Bouvencourt G, Dubois C, Dedoncker N, Sahay A, de Maertelaer V, Siebel CW, Van Keymeulen A, Voet T, Blanpain C (2020) Heterotypic cell-cell communication regulates glandular stem cell multipotency. Nature 584(7822):608–613

Chukir T, Liu Y, Farooki A (2019) Antiresorptive agents' bone-protective and adjuvant effects in postmenopausal women with early breast cancer. Br J Clin Pharmacol 85(6):1125–1135

Chung PY, Beyens G, Boonen S, Papapoulos S, Geusens P, Karperien M, Vanhoenacker F, Verbruggen L, Fransen E, Van Offel J, Goemaere S, Zmierczak HG, Westhovens R, Devogelaer JP, Van Hul W (2010a) The majority of the genetic risk for Paget's disease of bone is explained by genetic variants close to the CSF1, OPTN, TM7SF4, and TNFRSF11A genes. Hum Genet 128(6):615–626

Chung PY, Beyens G, Riches PL, Van Wesenbeeck L, de Freitas F, Jennes K, Daroszewska A, Fransen E, Boonen S, Geusens P, Vanhoenacker F, Verbruggen L, Van Offel J, Goemaere S, Zmierczak HG, Westhovens R, Karperien M, Papapoulos S, Ralston SH, Devogelaer JP, Van Hul W (2010b) Genetic variation in the TNFRSF11A gene encoding RANK is associated with susceptibility to Paget's disease of bone. J Bone Miner Res 25(12):2592–2605

Cigler T, Richardson H, Yaffe MJ, Fabian CJ, Johnston D, Ingle JN, Nassif E, Brunner RL, Wood ME, Pater JL, Hu H, Qi S, Tu D, Goss PE (2011) A randomized, placebo-controlled trial (NCIC CTG MAP.2) examining the effects of exemestane on mammographic breast density, bone density, markers of bone metabolism and serum lipid levels in postmenopausal women. Breast Cancer Res Treat 126(2):453–461

Ciscar M, Trinidad EM, Perez-Chacon G, Alsaleem M, Jimenez M, Jimenez-Santos MJ, Perez-Montoyo H, Sanz-Moreno A, Vethencourt A, Toss M, Petit A, Soler-Monso MT, Lopez V, Gomez-Miragaya J, Gomez-Aleza C, Dobrolecki LE, Lewis MT, Bruna A, Mouron S, Quintela-Fandino M, Al-Shahrour F, Martinez-Aranda A, Sierra A, Green AR, Rakha E, Gonzalez-Suarez E (2023) RANK is a poor prognosis marker and a therapeutic target in ER-negative postmenopausal breast cancer. EMBO Mol Med 15(4):e16715

Clar KL, Hinterleitner C, Schneider P, Salih HR, Maurer S (2019) Inhibition of NK reactivity against solid tumors by platelet-derived RANKL. Cancers (Basel) 11(3)

Coleman RE, Croucher PI, Padhani AR, Clezardin P, Chow E, Fallon M, Guise T, Colangeli S, Capanna R, Costa L (2020) Bone metastases. Nat Rev Dis Primers 6(1):83

Cordero A, Pellegrini P, Sanz-Moreno A, Trinidad EM, Serra-Musach J, Deshpande C, Dougall WC, Pujana MA, Gonzalez-Suarez E (2016) Rankl impairs lactogenic differentiation through inhibition of the prolactin/Stat5 pathway at midgestation. Stem Cells 34(4):1027–1039

Cordero A, Santamaria PG, Gonzalez-Suarez E (2023) Rank ectopic expression in the presence of Neu and PyMT oncogenes alters mammary epithelial cell populations and their tumorigenic potential. J Mammary Gland Biol Neoplasia 28(1):2

Cortes J, Rugo HS, Cescon DW, Im SA, Yusof MM, Gallardo C, Lipatov O, Barrios CH, Perez-Garcia J, Iwata H, Masuda N, Torregroza Otero M, Gokmen E, Loi S, Guo Z, Zhou X, Karantza V, Pan W, Schmid P, Investigators K (2022) Pembrolizumab plus chemotherapy in advanced triple-negative breast cancer. N Engl J Med 387(3):217–226

Cuzick J, Sestak I, Bonanni B, Costantino JP, Cummings S, DeCensi A, Dowsett M, Forbes JF, Ford L, LaCroix AZ, Mershon J, Mitlak BH, Powles T, Veronesi U, Vogel V, Wickerham DL, SERM Chemoprevention of Breast Cancer Overview Group (2013) Selective oestrogen receptor modulators in prevention of breast cancer: an updated meta-analysis of individual participant data. Lancet 381(9880):1827–1834

Cuzick J, Sestak I, Forbes JF, Dowsett M, Cawthorn S, Mansel RE, Loibl S, Bonanni B, Evans DG, Howell A, I.-I. investigators (2020) Use of anastrozole for breast cancer prevention (IBIS-II): long-term results of a randomised controlled trial. Lancet 395(10218):117–122

Demoulin SA, Somja J, Duray A, Guenin S, Roncarati P, Delvenne PO, Herfs MF, Hubert PM (2015) Cervical (pre)neoplastic microenvironment promotes the emergence of tolerogenic dendritic cells via RANKL secretion. Onco Targets Ther 4(6):e1008334

Dobrolecki LE, Airhart SD, Alferez DG, Aparicio S, Behbod F, Bentires-Alj M, Brisken C, Bult CJ, Cai S, Clarke RB, Dowst H, Ellis MJ, Gonzalez-Suarez E, Iggo RD, Kabos P, Li S, Lindeman GJ, Marangoni E, McCoy A, Meric-Bernstam F, Piwnica-Worms H, Poupon MF, Reis-Filho J, Sartorius CA, Scabia V, Sflomos G, Tu Y, Vaillant F, Visvader JE, Welm A, Wicha MS, Lewis MT (2016) Patient-derived xenograft (PDX) models in basic and translational breast cancer research. Cancer Metastasis Rev 35(4):547–573

Dougall WC, Glaccum M, Charrier K, Rohrbach K, Brasel K, De Smedt T, Daro E, Smith J, Tometsko ME, Maliszewski CR, Armstrong A, Shen V, Bain S, Cosman D, Anderson D, Morrissey PJ, Peschon JJ, Schuh J (1999) RANK is essential for osteoclast and lymph node development. Genes Dev 13(18):2412–2424

Dougall WC, Holen I, Gonzalez Suarez E (2014) Targeting RANKL in metastasis. Bonekey Rep 3:519

Eckert N, Permanyer M, Yu K, Werth K, Forster R (2019) Chemokines and other mediators in the development and functional organization of lymph nodes. Immunol Rev 289(1):62–83

Eghbali-Fatourechi G, Khosla S, Sanyal A, Boyle WJ, Lacey DL, Riggs BL (2003) Role of RANK ligand in mediating increased bone resorption in early postmenopausal women. J Clin Invest 111(8):1221–1230

Ell B, Kang Y (2012) SnapShot: bone metastasis. Cell 151(3):690–690 e691

Fata JE, Kong YY, Li J, Sasaki T, Irie-Sasaki J, Moorehead RA, Elliott R, Scully S, Voura EB, Lacey DL, Boyle WJ, Khokha R, Penninger JM (2000) The osteoclast differentiation factor osteoprotegerin-ligand is essential for mammary gland development. Cell 103(1):41–50

Fata JE, Chaudhary V, Khokha R (2001) Cellular turnover in the mammary gland is correlated with systemic levels of progesterone and not 17beta-estradiol during the estrous cycle. Biol Reprod 65(3):680–688

Fu NY, Nolan E, Lindeman GJ, Visvader JE (2020) Stem cells and the differentiation hierarchy in mammary gland development. Physiol Rev 100(2):489–523

Fujimura T, Kambayashi Y, Hidaka T, Hashimoto A, Haga T, Aiba S (2012) Comparison of Foxp3+ regulatory T cells and CD163+ macrophages in invasive and non-invasive extramammary Paget's disease. Acta Derm Venereol 92(6):625–628

Fujimura T, Kambayashi Y, Furudate S, Asano M, Kakizaki A, Aiba S (2015) Receptor activator of NF-kappaB ligand promotes the production of CCL17 from RANK+ M2 macrophages. J Invest Dermatol 135(11):2884–2887

Galibert L, Tometsko ME, Anderson DM, Cosman D, Dougall WC (1998) The involvement of multiple tumor necrosis factor receptor (TNFR)-associated factors in the signaling mechanisms of receptor activator of NF-kappaB, a member of the TNFR superfamily. J Biol Chem 273(51):34120–34127

Garcia-Estevez L, Cortes J, Perez S, Calvo I, Gallegos I, Moreno-Bueno G (2021) Obesity and breast cancer: a paradoxical and controversial relationship influenced by menopausal status. Front Oncol 11:705911

Glass DA II, Bialek P, Ahn JD, Starbuck M, Patel MS, Clevers H, Taketo MM, Long F, McMahon AP, Lang RA, Karsenty G (2005) Canonical Wnt signaling in differentiated osteoblasts controls osteoclast differentiation. Dev Cell 8(5):751–764

Gnant M, Pfeiler G, Steger GG, Egle D, Greil R, Fitzal F, Wette V, Balic M, Haslbauer F, Melbinger-Zeinitzer E, Bjelic-Radisic V, Jakesz R, Marth C, Sevelda P, Mlineritsch B, Exner R, Fesl C, Frantal S, Singer CF, Austrian Breast and Colorectal Cancer Study Group (2019) Adjuvant denosumab in postmenopausal patients with hormone receptor-positive breast cancer (ABCSG-18): disease-free survival results from a randomised, double-blind, placebo-controlled, phase 3 trial. Lancet Oncol 20(3):339–351

Gnant M, Frantal S, Pfeiler G, Steger GG, Egle D, Greil R, Fitzal F, Wette V, Balic M, Haslbauer F, Melbinger E, Bjelic-Radisic V, Artner-Matuscheck S, Kainberger F, Ritter M, Rinnerthaler G, Sevelda P, Bergh J, Kacerovsky-Strobl S, Suppa C, Brunner C, Deutschmann C, Gampenrieder SP, Fohler H, Jakesz R, Fesl C, Singer C, for the Austrian Brest and Colorectal Canser Study Group (2022) Long-term outcomes of adjuvant denosumab in breast cancer. New Engl J Med Evidence 1(12)

Gomes I, de Almeida BP, Damaso S, Mansinho A, Correia I, Henriques S, Cruz-Duarte R, Vilhais G, Felix P, Alves P, Corredeira P, Barbosa-Morais NL, Costa L, Casimiro S (2020) Expression of receptor activator of NFkB (RANK) drives stemness and resistance to therapy in ER+HER2- breast cancer. Oncotarget 11(19):1714–1728

Gomes I, Gallego-Paez LM, Jimenez M, Santamaria PG, Mansinho A, Sousa R, Abreu C, Suarez EG, Costa L, Casimiro S (2023) Co-targeting RANK pathway treats and prevents acquired resistance to CDK4/6 inhibitors in luminal breast cancer. Cell Rep Med 101120

Gomez-Aleza C, Gonzalez-Suarez E (2021) Inhibition of RANK signaling as a potential immunotherapy in breast cancer. Onco Targets Ther 10(1):1923156

Gomez-Aleza C, Nguyen B, Yoldi G, Ciscar M, Barranco A, Hernandez-Jimenez E, Maetens M, Salgado R, Zafeiroglou M, Pellegrini P, Venet D, Garaud S, Trinidad EM, Benitez S, Vuylsteke P, Polastro L, Wildiers H, Simon P, Lindeman G, Larsimont D, Van den Eynden G, Velghe C, Rothe F, Willard-Gallo K, Michiels S, Munoz P, Walzer T, Planelles L, Penninger J, Azim HA Jr, Loi S, Piccart M, Sotiriou C, Gonzalez-Suarez E (2020) Inhibition of RANK signaling in breast cancer induces an anti-tumor immune response orchestrated by CD8+ T cells. Nat Commun 11(1):6335

Gonzalez-Suarez E, Sanz-Moreno A (2016) RANK as a therapeutic target in cancer. FEBS J 283(11):2018–2033

Gonzalez-Suarez E, Branstetter D, Armstrong A, Dinh H, Blumberg H, Dougall WC (2007) RANK overexpression in transgenic mice with mouse mammary tumor virus promoter-controlled RANK increases proliferation and impairs alveolar differentiation in the mammary epithelia and disrupts lumen formation in cultured epithelial acini. Mol Cell Biol 27(4):1442–1454

Gonzalez-Suarez E, Jacob AP, Jones J, Miller R, Roudier-Meyer MP, Erwert R, Pinkas J, Branstetter D, Dougall WC (2010) RANK ligand mediates progestin-induced mammary epithelial proliferation and carcinogenesis. Nature 468(7320):103–107

Goss P, Wu M (2007) Application of aromatase inhibitors in endocrine responsive breast cancers. Breast 16(Suppl 2):S114–S119

Goss PE, Ingle JN, Ales-Martinez JE, Cheung AM, Chlebowski RT, Wactawski-Wende J, McTiernan A, Robbins J, Johnson KC, Martin LW, Winquist E, Sarto GE, Garber JE, Fabian CJ, Pujol P, Maunsell E, Farmer P, Gelmon KA, Tu D, Richardson H, Investigators NCMS (2011) Exemestane for breast-cancer prevention in postmenopausal women. N Engl J Med 364(25):2381–2391

Gray GK, Li CM, Rosenbluth JM, Selfors LM, Girnius N, Lin JR, Schackmann RCJ, Goh WL, Moore K, Shapiro HK, Mei S, D'Andrea K, Nathanson KL, Sorger PK, Santagata S, Regev A, Garber JE, Dillon DA, Brugge JS (2022) A human breast atlas integrating single-cell proteomics and transcriptomics. Dev Cell 57(11):1400–1420 e1407

Guerrini MM, Sobacchi C, Cassani B, Abinun M, Kilic SS, Pangrazio A, Moratto D, Mazzolari E, Clayton-Smith J, Orchard P, Coxon FP, Helfrich MH, Crockett JC, Mellis D, Vellodi A, Tezcan I, Notarangelo LD, Rogers MJ, Vezzoni P, Villa A, Frattini A (2008) Human osteoclast-poor osteopetrosis with hypogammaglobulinemia due to TNFRSF11A (RANK) mutations. Am J Hum Genet 83(1):64–76

Guy CT, Cardiff RD, Muller WJ (1992) Induction of mammary tumors by expression of polyomavirus middle T oncogene: a transgenic mouse model for metastatic disease. Mol Cell Biol 12(3):954–961

Habbeddine M, Verthuy C, Rastoin O, Chasson L, Bebien M, Bajenoff M, Adriouch S, den Haan JMM, Penninger JM, Lawrence T (2017) Receptor activator of NF-kappaB orchestrates activation of antiviral memory CD8 T cells in the spleen marginal zone. Cell Rep 21(9):2515–2527

Haljasorg U, Bichele R, Saare M, Guha M, Maslovskaja J, Kond K, Remm A, Pihlap M, Tomson L, Kisand K, Laan M, Peterson P (2015) A highly conserved NF-kappaB-responsive enhancer is critical for thymic expression of Aire in mice. Eur J Immunol 45(12):3246–3256

Harbeck N, Penault-Llorca F, Cortes J, Gnant M, Houssami N, Poortmans P, Ruddy K, Tsang J, Cardoso F (2019) Breast cancer. Nat Rev Dis Primers 5(1):66

Heer E, Harper A, Escandor N, Sung H, McCormack V, Fidler-Benaoudia MM (2020) Global burden and trends in premenopausal and postmenopausal breast cancer: a population-based study. Lancet Glob Health 8(8):e1027–e1037

Hernandez RK, Wade SW, Reich A, Pirolli M, Liede A, Lyman GH (2018) Incidence of bone metastases in patients with solid tumors: analysis of oncology electronic medical records in the United States. BMC Cancer 18(1):44

Herschkowitz JI, Simin K, Weigman VJ, Mikaelian I, Usary J, Hu Z, Rasmussen KE, Jones LP, Assefnia S, Chandrasekharan S, Backlund MG, Yin Y, Khramtsov AI, Bastein R, Quackenbush J, Glazer RI, Brown PH, Green JE, Kopelovich L, Furth PA, Palazzo JP, Olopade OI, Bernard PS, Churchill GA, Van Dyke T, Perou CM (2007) Identification of conserved gene expression features between murine mammary carcinoma models and human breast tumors. Genome Biol 8(5):R76

Hikosaka Y, Nitta T, Ohigashi I, Yano K, Ishimaru N, Hayashi Y, Matsumoto M, Matsuo K, Penninger JM, Takayanagi H, Yokota Y, Yamada H, Yoshikai Y, Inoue J, Akiyama T, Takahama Y (2008) The cytokine RANKL produced by positively selected thymocytes fosters medullary thymic epithelial cells that express autoimmune regulator. Immunity 29(3):438–450

Hofbauer LC, Khosla S, Dunstan CR, Lacey DL, Spelsberg TC, Riggs BL (1999a) Estrogen stimulates gene expression and protein production of osteoprotegerin in human osteoblastic cells. Endocrinology 140(9):4367–4370

Hofbauer LC, Lacey DL, Dunstan CR, Spelsberg TC, Riggs BL, Khosla S (1999b) Interleukin-1beta and tumor necrosis factor-alpha, but not interleukin-6, stimulate osteoprotegerin ligand gene expression in human osteoblastic cells. Bone 25(3):255–259

Howard BA, Gusterson BA (2000) Human breast development. J Mammary Gland Biol Neoplasia 5(2):119–137

Howell S, Greenhalgh A, Pedley R, Alghamdi S, Caruso A, Ansari M, Moreira T, Astlet S, Maxwell A, Lim Y, Brookes H, Idries F, Howell A, Evans DG, Sherratt M, Gilmore A, Harkness E, Khaled W, Twigger A-J, Clarke R, Simoes B (2022) Abstract P1-10-01: results from the breast cancer - anti progestin prevention study 1 (BC-APPS1) trial - a novel approach in breast cancer prevention. Cancer Res 82:P1-10-01

Hsu H, Lacey DL, Dunstan CR, Solovyev I, Colombero A, Timms E, Tan HL, Elliott G, Kelley MJ, Sarosi I, Wang L, Xia XZ, Elliott R, Chiu L, Black T, Scully S, Capparelli C, Morony S, Shimamoto G, Bass MB, Boyle WJ (1999) Tumor necrosis factor receptor family member RANK mediates osteoclast differentiation and activation induced by osteoprotegerin ligand. Proc Natl Acad Sci USA 96(7):3540–3545

Huang AC, Zappasodi R (2022) A decade of checkpoint blockade immunotherapy in melanoma: understanding the molecular basis for immune sensitivity and resistance. Nat Immunol 23(5):660–670

Ikebuchi Y, Aoki S, Honma M, Hayashi M, Sugamori Y, Khan M, Kariya Y, Kato G, Tabata Y, Penninger JM, Udagawa N, Aoki K, Suzuki H (2018) Coupling of bone resorption and formation by RANKL reverse signalling. Nature 561(7722):195–200

Ikeda T, Kasai M, Utsuyama M, Hirokawa K (2001) Determination of three isoforms of the receptor activator of nuclear factor-kappaB ligand and their differential expression in bone and thymus. Endocrinology 142(4):1419–1426

Ikeda T, Kasai M, Suzuki J, Kuroyama H, Seki S, Utsuyama M, Hirokawa K (2003) Multimerization of the receptor activator of nuclear factor-kappaB ligand (RANKL) isoforms and regulation of osteoclastogenesis. J Biol Chem 278(47):47217–47222

Jones DH, Nakashima T, Sanchez OH, Kozieradzki I, Komarova SV, Sarosi I, Morony S, Rubin E, Sarao R, Hojilla CV, Komnenovic V, Kong YY, Schreiber M, Dixon SJ, Sims SM, Khokha R, Wada T, Penninger JM (2006) Regulation of cancer cell migration and bone metastasis by RANKL. Nature 440(7084):692–696

Joshi PA, Jackson HW, Beristain AG, Di Grappa MA, Mote PA, Clarke CL, Stingl J, Waterhouse PD, Khokha R (2010) Progesterone induces adult mammary stem cell expansion. Nature 465(7299):803–807

Joshi PA, Waterhouse PD, Kannan N, Narala S, Fang H, Di Grappa MA, Jackson HW, Penninger JM, Eaves C, Khokha R (2015) RANK signaling amplifies WNT-responsive mammary progenitors through R-SPONDIN1. Stem Cell Reports 5(1):31–44

Josien R, Wong BR, Li HL, Steinman RM, Choi Y (1999) TRANCE, a TNF family member, is differentially expressed on T cell subsets and induces cytokine production in dendritic cells. J Immunol 162(5):2562–2568

Ju JH, Cho ML, Moon YM, Oh HJ, Park JS, Jhun JY, Min SY, Cho YG, Park KS, Yoon CH, Min JK, Park SH, Sung YC, Kim HY (2008) IL-23 induces receptor activator of NF-kappaB ligand expression on CD4+ T cells and promotes osteoclastogenesis in an autoimmune arthritis model. J Immunol 181(2):1507–1518

Kambayashi Y, Fujimura T, Furudate S, Asano M, Kakizaki A, Aiba S (2015) The possible interaction between receptor activator of nuclear factor kappa-B ligand expressed by extramammary paget cells and its ligand on dermal macrophages. J Invest Dermatol 135(10):2547–2550

Kim D, Mebius RE, MacMicking JD, Jung S, Cupedo T, Castellanos Y, Rho J, Wong BR, Josien R, Kim N, Rennert PD, Choi Y (2000) Regulation of peripheral lymph node genesis by the tumor necrosis factor family member TRANCE. J Exp Med 192(10):1467–1478

Kong YY, Yoshida H, Sarosi I, Tan HL, Timms E, Capparelli C, Morony S, Oliveira-dos-Santos AJ, Van G, Itie A, Khoo W, Wakeham A, Dunstan CR, Lacey DL, Mak TW, Boyle WJ, Penninger JM (1999) OPGL is a key regulator of osteoclastogenesis, lymphocyte development and lymph-node organogenesis. Nature 397(6717):315–323

Kostenuik PJ (2005) Osteoprotegerin and RANKL regulate bone resorption, density, geometry and strength. Curr Opin Pharmacol 5(6):618–625

Kwon BS, Wang S, Udagawa N, Haridas V, Lee ZH, Kim KK, Oh KO, Greene J, Li Y, Su J, Gentz R, Aggarwal BB, Ni J (1998) TR1, a new member of the tumor necrosis factor receptor superfamily, induces fibroblast proliferation and inhibits osteoclastogenesis and bone resorption. FASEB J 12(10):845–854

Lacey DL, Timms E, Tan HL, Kelley MJ, Dunstan CR, Burgess T, Elliott R, Colombero A, Elliott G, Scully S, Hsu H, Sullivan J, Hawkins N, Davy E, Capparelli C, Eli A, Qian YX, Kaufman S, Sarosi I, Shalhoub V, Senaldi G, Guo J, Delaney J, Boyle WJ (1998) Osteoprotegerin ligand is a cytokine that regulates osteoclast differentiation and activation. Cell 93(2):165–176

Lacey DL, Boyle WJ, Simonet WS, Kostenuik PJ, Dougall WC, Sullivan JK, San Martin J, Dansey R (2012) Bench to bedside: elucidation of the OPG-RANK-RANKL pathway and the development of denosumab. Nat Rev Drug Discov 11(5):401–419

Lahiri A, Maji A, Potdar PD, Singh N, Parikh P, Bisht B, Mukherjee A, Paul MK (2023) Lung cancer immunotherapy: progress, pitfalls, and promises. Mol Cancer 22(1):40

Leibbrandt A, Penninger JM (2008) RANK/RANKL: regulators of immune responses and bone physiology. Ann N Y Acad Sci 1143:123–150

Liede A, Hernandez RK, Wade SW, Bo R, Nussbaum NC, Ahern E, Dougall WC, Smyth MJ (2018) An observational study of concomitant immunotherapies and denosumab in patients with advanced melanoma or lung cancer. Onco Targets Ther 7(12):e1480301

Liedtke C, Mazouni C, Hess KR, Andre F, Tordai A, Mejia JA, Symmans WF, Gonzalez-Angulo AM, Hennessy B, Green M, Cristofanilli M, Hortobagyi GN, Pusztai L (2008) Response to neoadjuvant therapy and long-term survival in patients with triple-negative breast cancer. J Clin Oncol 26(8):1275–1281

Lim E, Vaillant F, Wu D, Forrest NC, Pal B, Hart AH, Asselin-Labat ML, Gyorki DE, Ward T, Partanen A, Feleppa F, Huschtscha LI, Thorne HJ, kConFab, Fox SB, Yan M, French JD, Brown MA, Smyth GK, Visvader JE, Lindeman GJ (2009) Aberrant luminal progenitors as the candidate target population for basal tumor development in BRCA1 mutation carriers. Nat Med 15(8):907–913

Lin EY, Jones JG, Li P, Zhu L, Whitney KD, Muller WJ, Pollard JW (2003) Progression to malignancy in the polyoma middle T oncoprotein mouse breast cancer model provides a reliable model for human diseases. Am J Pathol 163(5):2113–2126

Liu C, Walter TS, Huang P, Zhang S, Zhu X, Wu Y, Wedderburn LR, Tang P, Owens RJ, Stuart DI, Ren J, Gao B (2010) Structural and functional insights of RANKL-RANK interaction and signaling. J Immunol 184(12):6910–6919

Llombart-Cussac A, Cortes J, Pare L, Galvan P, Bermejo B, Martinez N, Vidal M, Pernas S, Lopez R, Munoz M, Nuciforo P, Morales S, Oliveira M, de la Pena L, Pelaez A, Prat A (2017) HER2-enriched subtype as a predictor of pathological complete response following trastuzumab and lapatinib without chemotherapy in early-stage HER2-positive breast cancer (PAMELA): an open-label, single-group, multicentre, phase 2 trial. Lancet Oncol 18(4):545–554

Locksley RM, Killeen N, Lenardo MJ (2001) The TNF and TNF receptor superfamilies: integrating mammalian biology. Cell 104(4):487–501

Lomaga MA, Yeh WC, Sarosi I, Duncan GS, Furlonger C, Ho A, Morony S, Capparelli C, Van G, Kaufman S, van der Heiden A, Itie A, Wakeham A, Khoo W, Sasaki T, Cao Z, Penninger JM, Paige CJ, Lacey DL, Dunstan CR, Boyle WJ, Goeddel DV, Mak TW (1999) TRAF6 deficiency results in osteopetrosis and defective interleukin-1, CD40, and LPS signaling. Genes Dev 13(8):1015–1024

Luo J, Yang Z, Ma Y, Yue Z, Lin H, Qu G, Huang J, Dai W, Li C, Zheng C, Xu L, Chen H, Wang J, Li D, Siwko S, Penninger JM, Ning G, Xiao J, Liu M (2016) LGR4 is a receptor for RANKL and negatively regulates osteoclast differentiation and bone resorption. Nat Med 22(5):539–546

Lydon JP, DeMayo FJ, Funk CR, Mani SK, Hughes AR, Montgomery CA Jr, Shyamala G, Conneely OM, O'Malley BW (1995) Mice lacking progesterone receptor exhibit pleiotropic reproductive abnormalities. Genes Dev 9(18):2266–2278

Ma Q, Liang M, Wu Y, Ding N, Duan L, Yu T, Bai Y, Kang F, Dong S, Xu J, Dou C (2019) Mature osteoclast-derived apoptotic bodies promote osteogenic differentiation via RANKL-mediated reverse signaling. J Biol Chem 294(29):11240–11247

Macedo F, Ladeira K, Pinho F, Saraiva N, Bonito N, Pinto L, Goncalves F (2017) Bone Metastases: An Overview. Oncol Rev 11(1):321

Maglione JE, Moghanaki D, Young LJ, Manner CK, Ellies LG, Joseph SO, Nicholson B, Cardiff RD, MacLeod CL (2001) Transgenic Polyoma middle-T mice model premalignant mammary disease. Cancer Res 61(22):8298–8305

Masuyama R, Stockmans I, Torrekens S, Van Looveren R, Maes C, Carmeliet P, Bouillon R, Carmeliet G (2006) Vitamin D receptor in chondrocytes promotes osteoclastogenesis and regulates FGF23 production in osteoblasts. J Clin Invest 116(12):3150–3159

McCarthy NI, Cowan JE, Nakamura K, Bacon A, Baik S, White AJ, Parnell SM, Jenkinson EJ, Jenkinson WE, Anderson G (2015) Osteoprotegerin-mediated homeostasis of Rank+ thymic epithelial cells does not limit Foxp3+ regulatory T cell development. J Immunol 195(6):2675–2682

McClung MR, Lewiecki EM, Cohen SB, Bolognese MA, Woodson GC, Moffett AH, Peacock M, Miller PD, Lederman SN, Chesnut CH, Lain D, Kivitz AJ, Holloway DL, Zhang C, Peterson MC, Bekker PJ, AMG 162 Bone Loss Study Group (2006) Denosumab in postmenopausal women with low bone mineral density. N Engl J Med 354(8):821–831

Miyazaki T, Tokimura F, Tanaka S (2014) A review of denosumab for the treatment of osteoporosis. Patient Prefer Adherence 8:463–471

Mizuno A, Amizuka N, Irie K, Murakami A, Fujise N, Kanno T, Sato Y, Nakagawa N, Yasuda H, Mochizuki S, Gomibuchi T, Yano K, Shima N, Washida N, Tsuda E, Morinaga T, Higashio K, Ozawa H (1998) Severe osteoporosis in mice lacking osteoclastogenesis inhibitory factor/osteoprotegerin. Biochem Biophys Res Commun 247(3):610–615

Molyneux G, Geyer FC, Magnay FA, McCarthy A, Kendrick H, Natrajan R, Mackay A, Grigoriadis A, Tutt A, Ashworth A, Reis-Filho JS, Smalley MJ (2010) BRCA1 basal-like breast cancers originate from luminal epithelial progenitors and not from basal stem cells. Cell Stem Cell 7(3):403–417

Muller WJ, Sinn E, Pattengale PK, Wallace R, Leder P (1988) Single-step induction of mammary adenocarcinoma in transgenic mice bearing the activated c-neu oncogene. Cell 54(1):105–115

Nakamura ES, Koizumi K, Kobayashi M, Saitoh Y, Arita Y, Nakayama T, Sakurai H, Yoshie O, Saiki I (2006) RANKL-induced CCL22/macrophage-derived chemokine produced from osteoclasts potentially promotes the bone metastasis of lung cancer expressing its receptor CCR4. Clin Exp Metastasis 23(1):9–18

Nakashima T, Takayanagi H (2009) Osteoimmunology: crosstalk between the immune and bone systems. J Clin Immunol 29(5):555–567

Nakashima T, Kobayashi Y, Yamasaki S, Kawakami A, Eguchi K, Sasaki H, Sakai H (2000) Protein expression and functional difference of membrane-bound and soluble receptor activator of NF-kappaB ligand: modulation of the expression by osteotropic factors and cytokines. Biochem Biophys Res Commun 275(3):768–775

Nakashima T, Hayashi M, Fukunaga T, Kurata K, Oh-Hora M, Feng JQ, Bonewald LF, Kodama T, Wutz A, Wagner EF, Penninger JM, Takayanagi H (2011) Evidence for osteocyte regulation of bone homeostasis through RANKL expression. Nat Med 17(10):1231–1234

Nakashima T, Hayashi M, Takayanagi H (2012) New insights into osteoclastogenic signaling mechanisms. Trends Endocrinol Metab 23(11):582–590

Nannuru KC, Futakuchi M, Sadanandam A, Wilson TJ, Varney ML, Myers KJ, Li X, Marcusson EG, Singh RK (2009) Enhanced expression and shedding of receptor activator of NF-kappaB ligand during tumor-bone interaction potentiates mammary tumor-induced osteolysis. Clin Exp Metastasis 26(7):797–808

Nguyen QH, Pervolarakis N, Blake K, Ma D, Davis RT, James N, Phung AT, Willey E, Kumar R, Jabart E, Driver I, Rock J, Goga A, Khan SA, Lawson DA, Werb Z, Kessenbrock K (2018) Profiling human breast epithelial cells using single cell RNA sequencing identifies cell diversity. Nat Commun 9(1):2028

Nolan E, Vaillant F, Branstetter D, Pal B, Giner G, Whitehead L, Lok SW, Mann GB, C. Kathleen Cuningham Foundation Consortium for Research into Familial Breast, Rohrbach K, Huang LY, Soriano R, Smyth GK, Dougall WC, Visvader JE, Lindeman GJ (2016) RANK ligand as a potential target for breast cancer prevention in BRCA1-mutation carriers. Nat Med 22(8):933–939

Nolan E, Lindeman GJ, Visvader JE (2023) Deciphering breast cancer: from biology to the clinic. Cell 186(8):1708–1728

Northey JJ, Yui Y, Hayward M-K, Stashko C, Kai F, Mouw JK, Thakar D, Lakins JN, Ironside AJ, Samson S, Mukhtar RA, Hwang ES, Weaver VM (2022) Mechanosensitive hormone signaling promotes mammary progenitor expansion and breast cancer progression. bioRxiv: 2022.2004.2019.487741

Novack DV (2011) Role of NF-kappaB in the skeleton. Cell Res 21(1):169–182

Okamoto K, Nakashima T, Shinohara M, Negishi-Koga T, Komatsu N, Terashima A, Sawa S, Nitta T, Takayanagi H (2017) Osteoimmunology: the conceptual framework unifying the immune and skeletal systems. Physiol Rev 97(4):1295–1349

Ormandy CJ, Camus A, Barra J, Damotte D, Lucas B, Buteau H, Edery M, Brousse N, Babinet C, Binart N, Kelly PA (1997) Null mutation of the prolactin receptor gene produces multiple reproductive defects in the mouse. Genes Dev 11(2):167–178

Palafox M, Ferrer I, Pellegrini P, Vila S, Hernandez-Ortega S, Urruticoechea A, Climent F, Soler MT, Munoz P, Vinals F, Tometsko M, Branstetter D, Dougall WC, Gonzalez-Suarez E (2012) RANK induces epithelial-mesenchymal transition and stemness in human mammary epithelial cells and promotes tumorigenesis and metastasis. Cancer Res 72(11):2879–2888

Pangrazio A, Cassani B, Guerrini MM, Crockett JC, Marrella V, Zammataro L, Strina D, Schulz A, Schlack C, Kornak U, Mellis DJ, Duthie A, Helfrich MH, Durandy A, Moshous D, Vellodi A, Chiesa R, Veys P, Lo Iacono N, Vezzoni P, Fischer A, Villa A, Sobacchi C (2012) RANK-dependent autosomal recessive osteopetrosis: characterization of five new cases with novel mutations. J Bone Miner Res 27(2):342–351

Papanastasiou AD, Sirinian C, Kalofonos HP (2012) Identification of novel human receptor activator of nuclear factor-kB isoforms generated through alternative splicing: implications in breast cancer cell survival and migration. Breast Cancer Res 14(4):R112

Pellegrini P, Cordero A, Gallego MI, Dougall WC, Munoz P, Pujana MA, Gonzalez-Suarez E (2013) Constitutive activation of RANK disrupts mammary cell fate leading to tumorigenesis. Stem Cells 31(9):1954–1965

Perlot T, Penninger JM (2012) Development and function of murine B cells lacking RANK. J Immunol 188(3):1201–1205

Perrone F, Gravina A (2020) Denosumab in early breast cancer: negative data and a call to action. Lancet Oncol 21(1):5–6

Pfitzner BM, Branstetter D, Loibl S, Denkert C, Lederer B, Schmitt WD, Dombrowski F, Werner M, Rudiger T, Dougall WC, von Minckwitz G (2014) RANK expression as a prognostic and predictive marker in breast cancer. Breast Cancer Res Treat 145(2):307–315

Rao S, Cronin SJF, Sigl V, Penninger JM (2018) RANKL and RANK: from mammalian physiology to cancer treatment. Trends Cell Biol 28(3):213–223

Richardson H, Johnston D, Pater J, Goss P (2007) The National Cancer Institute of Canada Clinical Trials Group MAP.3 trial: an international breast cancer prevention trial. Curr Oncol 14(3):89–96

Roberts NA, White AJ, Jenkinson WE, Turchinovich G, Nakamura K, Withers DR, McConnell FM, Desanti GE, Benezech C, Parnell SM, Cunningham AF, Paolino M, Penninger JM, Simon AK, Nitta T, Ohigashi I, Takahama Y, Caamano JH, Hayday AC, Lane PJ, Jenkinson EJ, Anderson G (2012) Rank signaling links the development of invariant gammadelta T cell progenitors and Aire(+) medullary epithelium. Immunity 36(3):427–437

Rocha AS, Collado-Sole A, Grana-Castro O, Redondo-Pedraza J, Soria-Alcaide G, Cordero A, Santamaria PG, Gonzalez-Suarez E (2023) Luminal rank loss decreases cell fitness leading to basal cell bipotency in parous mammary glands. Nat Commun 14(1):6213

Roodman GD, Dougall WC (2008) RANK ligand as a therapeutic target for bone metastases and multiple myeloma. Cancer Treat Rev 34(1):92–101

Rossi SW, Kim MY, Leibbrandt A, Parnell SM, Jenkinson WE, Glanville SH, McConnell FM, Scott HS, Penninger JM, Jenkinson EJ, Lane PJ, Anderson G (2007) RANK signals from CD4(+)3(−) inducer cells regulate development of Aire-expressing epithelial cells in the thymic medulla. J Exp Med 204(6):1267–1272

Rossouw JE, Anderson GL, Prentice RL, LaCroix AZ, Kooperberg C, Stefanick ML, Jackson RD, Beresford SA, Howard BV, Johnson KC, Kotchen JM, Ockene J, I. Writing Group for the Women's Health Initiative (2002) Risks and benefits of estrogen plus progestin in healthy postmenopausal women: principal results From the Women's Health Initiative randomized controlled trial. JAMA 288(3):321–333

Saika M, Inoue D, Kido S, Matsumoto T (2001) 17beta-estradiol stimulates expression of osteoprotegerin by a mouse stromal cell line, ST-2, via estrogen receptor-alpha. Endocrinology 142(6):2205–2212

Santagata S, Ince TA (2014) Normal cell phenotypes of breast epithelial cells provide the foundation of a breast cancer taxonomy. Expert Rev Anticancer Ther 14(12):1385–1389

Santini D, Schiavon G, Vincenzi B, Gaeta L, Pantano F, Russo A, Ortega C, Porta C, Galluzzo S, Armento G, La Verde N, Caroti C, Treilleux I, Ruggiero A, Perrone G, Addeo R, Clezardin P, Muda AO, Tonini G (2011) Receptor activator of NF-kB (RANK) expression in primary tumors associates with bone metastasis occurrence in breast cancer patients. PLoS One 6(4):e19234

Sanz-Moreno A, Palomeras S, Pedersen K, Morancho B, Pascual T, Galvan P, Benitez S, Gomez-Miragaya J, Ciscar M, Jimenez M, Pernas S, Petit A, Soler-Monso MT, Vinas G, Alsaleem M, Rakha EA, Green AR, Santamaria PG, Mulder C, Lemeer S, Arribas J, Prat A, Puig T, Gonzalez-Suarez E (2021) RANK signaling increases after anti-HER2 therapy contributing to the emergence of resistance in HER2-positive breast cancer. Breast Cancer Res 23(1):42

Schmiedel BJ, Grosse-Hovest L, Salih HR (2013) A "vicious cycle" of NK-cell immune evasion in acute myeloid leukemia mediated by RANKL? Onco Targets Ther 2(5):e23850

Schmiedel BJ, Nuebling T, Steinbacher J, Malinovska A, Wende CM, Azuma M, Schneider P, Grosse-Hovest L, Salih HR (2013b) Receptor activator for NF-kappaB ligand in acute myeloid leukemia: expression, function, and modulation of NK cell immunosurveillance. J Immunol 190(2):821–831

Schmiedel BJ, Scheible CA, Nuebling T, Kopp HG, Wirths S, Azuma M, Schneider P, Jung G, Grosse-Hovest L, Salih HR (2013c) RANKL expression, function, and therapeutic targeting in multiple myeloma and chronic lymphocytic leukemia. Cancer Res 73(2):683–694

Schneeweis LA, Willard D, Milla ME (2005) Functional dissection of osteoprotegerin and its interaction with receptor activator of NF-kappaB ligand. J Biol Chem 280(50):41155–41164

Schramek D, Leibbrandt A, Sigl V, Kenner L, Pospisilik JA, Lee HJ, Hanada R, Joshi PA, Aliprantis A, Glimcher L, Pasparakis M, Khokha R, Ormandy CJ, Widschwendter M, Schett G, Penninger JM (2010) Osteoclast differentiation factor RANKL controls development of progestin-driven mammary cancer. Nature 468(7320):98–102

Sigl V, Owusu-Boaitey K, Joshi PA, Kavirayani A, Wirnsberger G, Novatchkova M, Kozieradzki I, Schramek D, Edokobi N, Hersl J, Sampson A, Odai-Afotey A, Lazaro C, Gonzalez-Suarez E, Pujana MA, Cimba F, Heyn H, Vidal E, Cruickshank J, Berman H, Sarao R, Ticevic M, Uribesalgo I, Tortola L, Rao S, Tan Y, Pfeiler G, Lee EY, Bago-Horvath Z, Kenner L, Popper H, Singer C, Khokha R, Jones LP, Penninger JM (2016) RANKL/RANK control Brca1 mutation. Cell Res 26(7):761–774

Simonet WS, Lacey DL, Dunstan CR, Kelley M, Chang MS, Luthy R, Nguyen HQ, Wooden S, Bennett L, Boone T, Shimamoto G, DeRose M, Elliott R, Colombero A, Tan HL, Trail G, Sullivan J, Davy E, Bucay N, Renshaw-Gegg L, Hughes TM, Hill D, Pattison W, Campbell P, Sander S, Van G, Tarpley J, Derby P, Lee R, Boyle WJ (1997) Osteoprotegerin: a novel secreted protein involved in the regulation of bone density. Cell 89(2):309–319

Sirinian C, Papanastasiou AD, Zarkadis IK, Kalofonos HP (2013) Alternative splicing generates a truncated isoform of human TNFRSF11A (RANK) with an altered capacity to activate NF-kappaB. Gene 525(1):124–129

Smyth MJ, Yagita H, McArthur GA (2016) Combination anti-CTLA-4 and anti-RANKL in metastatic melanoma. J Clin Oncol 34(12):e104–e106

Streicher C, Heyny A, Andrukhova O, Haigl B, Slavic S, Schuler C, Kollmann K, Kantner I, Sexl V, Kleiter M, Hofbauer LC, Kostenuik PJ, Erben RG (2017) Estrogen regulates bone turnover by targeting RANKL expression in bone lining cells. Sci Rep 7(1):6460

Sung H, Ferlay J, Siegel RL, Laversanne M, Soerjomataram I, Jemal A, Bray F (2021) Global cancer statistics 2020: GLOBOCAN estimates of incidence and mortality worldwide for 36 cancers in 185 countries. CA Cancer J Clin 71(3):209–249

Suzuki J, Ikeda T, Kuroyama H, Seki S, Kasai M, Utsuyama M, Tatsumi M, Uematsu H, Hirokawa K (2004) Regulation of osteoclastogenesis by three human RANKL isoforms expressed in NIH3T3 cells. Biochem Biophys Res Commun 314(4):1021–1027

Takaba H, Takayanagi H (2017) The mechanisms of T cell selection in the thymus. Trends Immunol 38(11):805–816

Takayanagi H, Ogasawara K, Hida S, Chiba T, Murata S, Sato K, Takaoka A, Yokochi T, Oda H, Tanaka K, Nakamura K, Taniguchi T (2000) T-cell-mediated regulation of osteoclastogenesis by signalling cross-talk between RANKL and IFN-gamma. Nature 408(6812):600–605

Tan KB, Harrop J, Reddy M, Young P, Terrett J, Emery J, Moore G, Truneh A (1997) Characterization of a novel TNF-like ligand and recently described TNF ligand and TNF receptor superfamily genes and their constitutive and inducible expression in hematopoietic and non-hematopoietic cells. Gene 204(1-2):35–46

Tan W, Zhang W, Strasner A, Grivennikov S, Cheng JQ, Hoffman RM, Karin M (2011) Tumour-infiltrating regulatory T cells stimulate mammary cancer metastasis through RANKL-RANK signalling. Nature 470(7335):548–553

Theill LE, Boyle WJ, Penninger JM (2002) RANK-L and RANK: T cells, bone loss, and mammalian evolution. Annu Rev Immunol 20:795–823

Theoleyre S, Wittrant Y, Tat SK, Fortun Y, Redini F, Heymann D (2004) The molecular triad OPG/RANK/RANKL: involvement in the orchestration of pathophysiological bone remodeling. Cytokine Growth Factor Rev 15(6):457–475

Titanji K (2017) Beyond antibodies: B cells and the OPG/RANK-RANKL pathway in health, non-HIV disease and HIV-induced bone loss. Front Immunol 8:1851

Toriola AT, Dang HX, Hagemann IS, Appleton CM, Colditz GA, Luo J, Maher CA (2017) Increased breast tissue receptor activator of nuclear factor-kappaB ligand (RANKL) gene expression is associated with higher mammographic density in premenopausal women. Oncotarget 8(43):73787–73792

Tsuda E, Goto M, Mochizuki S, Yano K, Kobayashi F, Morinaga T, Higashio K (1997) Isolation of a novel cytokine from human fibroblasts that specifically inhibits osteoclastogenesis. Biochem Biophys Res Commun 234(1):137–142

Van Keymeulen A, Fioramonti M, Centonze A, Bouvencourt G, Achouri Y, Blanpain C (2017) Lineage-restricted mammary stem cells sustain the development, homeostasis, and regeneration of the estrogen receptor positive lineage. Cell Rep 20(7):1525–1532

Vanamee ES, Faustman DL (2018) Structural principles of tumor necrosis factor superfamily signaling. Sci Signal 11(511)

Visvader JE, Stingl J (2014) Mammary stem cells and the differentiation hierarchy: current status and perspectives. Genes Dev 28(11):1143–1158

von Minckwitz G, Kummel S, Vogel P, Hanusch C, Eidtmann H, Hilfrich J, Gerber B, Huober J, Costa SD, Jackisch C, Loibl S, Mehta K, Kaufmann M, German Breast G (2008) Intensified neoadjuvant chemotherapy in early-responding breast cancer: phase III randomized GeparTrio study. J Natl Cancer Inst 100(8):552–562

Wada T, Nakashima T, Hiroshi N, Penninger JM (2006) RANKL-RANK signaling in osteoclastogenesis and bone disease. Trends Mol Med 12(1):17–25

Waterfield M, Khan IS, Cortez JT, Fan U, Metzger T, Greer A, Fasano K, Martinez-Llordella M, Pollack JL, Erle DJ, Su M, Anderson MS (2014) The transcriptional regulator Aire coopts the repressive ATF7ip-MBD1 complex for the induction of immunotolerance. Nat Immunol 15(3):258–265

Watson CJ, Khaled WT (2020) Mammary development in the embryo and adult: new insights into the journey of morphogenesis and commitment. Development 147(22)

Whittle JR, Lewis MT, Lindeman GJ, Visvader JE (2015) Patient-derived xenograft models of breast cancer and their predictive power. Breast Cancer Res 17(1):17

Wiseman BS, Werb Z (2002) Stromal effects on mammary gland development and breast cancer. Science 296(5570):1046–1049

Wong BR, Josien R, Lee SY, Sauter B, Li HL, Steinman RM, Choi Y (1997a) TRANCE (tumor necrosis factor [TNF]-related activation-induced cytokine), a new TNF family member predominantly expressed in T cells, is a dendritic cell-specific survival factor. J Exp Med 186(12):2075–2080

Wong BR, Rho J, Arron J, Robinson E, Orlinick J, Chao M, Kalachikov S, Cayani E, Bartlett FS 3rd, Frankel WN, Lee SY, Choi Y (1997b) TRANCE is a novel ligand of the tumor necrosis factor receptor family that activates c-Jun N-terminal kinase in T cells. J Biol Chem 272(40):25190–25194

Xiong J, Onal M, Jilka RL, Weinstein RS, Manolagas SC, O'Brien CA (2011) Matrix-embedded cells control osteoclast formation. Nat Med 17(10):1235–1241

Yasuda H, Shima N, Nakagawa N, Yamaguchi K, Kinosaki M, Mochizuki S, Tomoyasu A, Yano K, Goto M, Murakami A, Tsuda E, Morinaga T, Higashio K, Udagawa N, Takahashi N, Suda T (1998) Osteoclast differentiation factor is a ligand for osteoprotegerin/osteoclastogenesis-inhibitory factor and is identical to TRANCE/RANKL. Proc Natl Acad Sci USA 95(7):3597–3602

Yoldi G, Pellegrini P, Trinidad EM, Cordero A, Gomez-Miragaya J, Serra-Musach J, Dougall WC, Munoz P, Pujana MA, Planelles L, Gonzalez-Suarez E (2016) RANK signaling blockade reduces breast cancer recurrence by inducing tumor cell differentiation. Cancer Res 76(19):5857–5869

Yue Z, Niu X, Yuan Z, Qin Q, Jiang W, He L, Gao J, Ding Y, Liu Y, Xu Z, Li Z, Yang Z, Li R, Xue X, Gao Y, Yue F, Zhang XH, Hu G, Wang Y, Li Y, Chen G, Siwko S, Gartland A, Wang N, Xiao J, Liu M, Luo J (2022) RSPO2 and RANKL signal through LGR4 to regulate osteoclastic premetastatic niche formation and bone metastasis. J Clin Invest 132(2)

Yun TJ, Chaudhary PM, Shu GL, Frazer JK, Ewings MK, Schwartz SM, Pascual V, Hood LE, Clark EA (1998) OPG/FDCR-1, a TNF receptor family member, is expressed in lymphoid cells and is up-regulated by ligating CD40. J Immunol 161(11):6113–6121

Zhang L, Teng Y, Zhang Y, Liu J, Xu L, Qu J, Hou K, Yang X, Liu Y, Qu X (2012) Receptor activator for nuclear factor kappa B expression predicts poor prognosis in breast cancer patients with bone metastasis but not in patients with visceral metastasis. J Clin Pathol 65(1):36–40

Zoi I, Karamouzis MV, Xingi E, Sarantis P, Thomaidou D, Lembessis P, Theocharis S, Papavassiliou AG (2019) Combining RANK/RANKL and ERBB-2 targeting as a novel strategy in ERBB-2-positive breast carcinomas. Breast Cancer Res 21(1):132

17 Metabolic Reprogramming and Adaption in Breast Cancer Progression and Metastasis

Qianying Zuo and Yibin Kang

Abstract

Recent evidence has revealed that cancer is not solely driven by genetic abnormalities but also by significant metabolic dysregulation. Cancer cells exhibit altered metabolic demands and rewiring of cellular metabolism to sustain their malignant characteristics. Metabolic reprogramming has emerged as a hallmark of cancer, playing a complex role in breast cancer initiation, progression, and metastasis. The different molecular subtypes of breast cancer exhibit distinct metabolic genotypes and phenotypes, offering opportunities for subtype-specific therapeutic approaches. Cancer-associated metabolic phenotypes encompass dysregulated nutrient uptake, opportunistic nutrient acquisition strategies, altered utilization of glycolysis and TCA cycle intermediates, increased nitrogen demand, metabolite-driven gene regulation, and metabolic interactions with the microenvironment. The tumor microenvironment, consisting of stromal cells, immune cells, blood vessels, and extracellular matrix components, influences metabolic adaptations through modulating nutrient availability, oxygen levels, and signaling pathways. Metastasis, the process of cancer spread, involves intricate steps that present unique metabolic challenges at each stage. Successful metastasis requires cancer cells to navigate varying nutrient and oxygen availability, endure oxidative stress, and adapt their metabolic processes accordingly. The metabolic reprogramming observed in breast cancer is regulated by oncogenes, tumor suppressor genes, and signaling pathways that integrate cellular signaling with metabolic processes. Understanding the metabolic adaptations associated with metastasis holds promise for identifying therapeutic targets to disrupt the metastatic process and improve patient outcomes. This chapter explores the metabolic alterations linked to breast cancer metastasis and highlights the potential for targeted interventions in this context.

Keywords

Breast cancer · Metabolism · Metastasis · Epithelial-mesenchymal transition (EMT) · Circulating tumor cells (CTCs) · Metastatic colonization

Q. Zuo · Y. Kang (✉)
Department of Molecular Biology, Princeton University, Princeton, NJ, USA

Ludwig Institute for Cancer Research Princeton Branch, Princeton, NJ, USA
e-mail: ykang@princeton.edu

T. Sørlie, R. B. Clarke (eds.), *A Guide to Breast Cancer Research*, Advances in Experimental Medicine and Biology 1464, https://doi.org/10.1007/978-3-031-70875-6_17

Key Points

- EMT is a critical step in tumor invasion, involving the gradual transformation of cells with varying degrees of epithelial and mesenchymal characteristics. Glucose metabolism, acetyl-CoA, 2-HG, and creatine play critical roles in regulating EMT and cancer metastasis.
- CTCs are key intermediates in breast cancer metastasis and are linked to lower patient survival rates. CTCs have stemlike properties, promoting tumor growth, and adapt to oxidative stress to evade cell death while circulating in the bloodstream.
- Metastatic colonization relies on metastasis-initiating cells (MICs) or cancer stem cells (CSCs), with organ-specific traits influencing successful establishment in distant organs. The tumor microenvironment and immune cell interactions play critical roles in facilitating metastasis.
- Metabolic adaptations in breast cancer cells, such as the preferential reliance on aerobic glycolysis and altered glucose metabolism, support their rapid proliferation and survival.
- Dysregulated lipid metabolism is a prominent feature in breast cancer, with increased emphasis on lipogenesis, enhanced lipolysis, and augmented lipid uptake by cancer cells. These alterations support vital cellular functions, promote tumor growth, and contribute to aggressiveness.

17.1 Introduction

In recent years, a growing body of evidence has shed light on the fact that cancer is not solely driven by genetic abnormalities but also by significant metabolic dysregulation. Cancer cells exhibit elevated metabolic demands and undergo rewiring of cellular metabolism to sustain their malignant characteristics. Oncogenic signaling pathways have been found to actively participate in energy regulation and anabolism to support the rapid proliferation and spread of tumors (Wishart 2015). This recognition has led to the concept of cancer as a metabolic disease, with metabolic reprogramming emerging as a hallmark of cancer (Hanahan 2022). Within the context of breast cancer, metabolic reprogramming plays a complex and influential role in tumor initiation, progression, and metastasis (Monaco 2017; Yousuf et al. 2022; Geck and Toker 2016; Chen et al. 2007; McDonnell et al. 2014; Jin et al. 2022).

Breast cancer, known for its heterogeneity, encompasses four main intrinsic molecular subtypes: luminal A, luminal B, HER2-positive, and triple-negative breast cancer (TNBC). Each of these subtypes possesses distinct characteristics in terms of proliferation rates, metastatic potential, as well as unique metabolic genotypes and phenotypes. For instance, TNBC cells exhibit specific metabolic traits characterized by heightened hypoxic conditions and dynamic mitochondrial processes (Han et al. 2015). On the other hand, luminal B breast cancer demonstrates elevated glutamine metabolic activity compared to other subtypes (Craze et al. 2018). These metabolic differences not only underscore the diverse nature of breast cancer but also highlight the potential for subtype-specific therapeutic approaches targeting metabolic vulnerabilities.

Thompson et al. categorized cancer-associated metabolic phenotypes into six hallmarks, including dysregulated nutrient uptake, utilization of opportunistic nutrient acquisition strategies, utilization of glycolysis and TCA cycle intermediates for biosynthesis and NADPH production, increased nitrogen demand, alterations in metabolite-driven gene regulation, and metabolic interactions with the microenvironment (Pavlova and Thompson 2016; Pavlova et al. 2022). Thus, it is important to recognize that metabolic changes in breast cancer are not solely dictated by intrinsic factors within cancer cells. The complex interplay between cancer cells and the tumor microenvironment further shapes and influences metabolic adaptations. The tumor microenvironment, consisting of stromal cells, immune cells, blood vessels, and extracellular matrix components, plays a critical role in modulating nutrient availability, oxygen levels, and metabolic signaling pathways. This dynamic interaction between cancer cells and the microenvironment can fuel or inhibit metabolic reprogramming, impacting tumor growth, invasion, and metastasis.

Metastasis, the process by which cancer spreads from the primary tumor to distant sites, encompasses a series of intricate steps. These sequential events begin with local invasion into the tumor-associated stroma, followed by intravasation into the hematopoietic and lymphatic systems or peritoneum. Cancer cells then navigate the challenging environment of circulation, evading immune surveillance and enduring shear stress. Upon successful survival in the bloodstream, cancer cells face the daunting task of extravasation, breaching the endothelial barrier and infiltrating premetastatic niches in distant organs. Finally, the colonization of these niches allows cancer cells to establish metastatic lesions (Lambert et al. 2017). Notably, each step of the metastatic cascade presents distinct metabolic challenges for cancer cells. Metastatic sites often exhibit varying nutrient and oxygen availability, necessitating adaptations in cellular metabolism to meet the energy demands of tumor cells. Moreover, the dynamic microenvironment of distant organs can subject cancer cells to heightened oxidative stress, further impacting their metabolic processes. The ability of cancer cells to successfully navigate these metabolic hurdles is crucial for their survival and proliferation at metastatic sites (Schild et al. 2018). The metabolic reprogramming observed in breast cancer is driven by a complex network of regulatory mechanisms. Oncogenes and tumor suppressor genes, such as TP53 and PTEN, actively participate in metabolic regulation, influencing key metabolic pathways and enzymes (Kurose et al. 2002; Kim et al. 2015; Walsh et al. 2006). Signaling pathways, such as PI3K/AKT/mTOR and AMPK, play a critical role in integrating cellular signaling with metabolic processes, sensing nutrient availability, and regulating metabolic flux (LaPensee et al. 2008; Makino et al. 1998; McCall et al. 1992). Importantly, there is cross talk between metabolic pathways and cell signaling, creating a tightly regulated network that governs the metabolic fate of cancer cells.

This chapter aims to explore the metabolic adaptations associated with metastasis, as unraveling these processes can provide valuable insights into potential therapeutic targets. By targeting the metabolic alterations involved in metastasis, we can potentially disrupt the metastatic process and improve patient outcomes.

17.2 Metabolic Rewiring on Metastatic Signaling Cascades

Metastasis is the complex process of spreading of cancer cells from the primary tumor to distant sites, involving local invasion, entry into circulation, survival in the bloodstream, breaching the endothelial barrier, and colonizing distant organs to form metastatic lesions (Lambert et al. 2017). The impact of metabolic reprogramming on breast cancer metastasis is of particular significance. Metabolic alterations have been implicated in various steps of the metastatic cascade, including EMT, cancer cell migration, invasion, and colonization of distant organs. Metabolic adaptations during metastatic colonization enable cancer cells to survive and thrive in foreign microenvironments with limited nutrient availability and harsh conditions. Understanding the metabolic drivers of metastasis and the unique metabolic dependencies of disseminated cancer cells holds promise for developing targeted therapies to combat metastatic breast cancer. Metabolic reprogramming in the breast cancer metastatic cascade is summarized in Fig. 17.1 and described below.

17.2.1 The Initial Trigger: EMT to Facilitate Tumor Invasion

EMT is an initiating step in the metastatic cascades where cells undergo a transformation, losing their epithelial characteristics and adopting mesenchymal features (Nieto et al. 2016; De

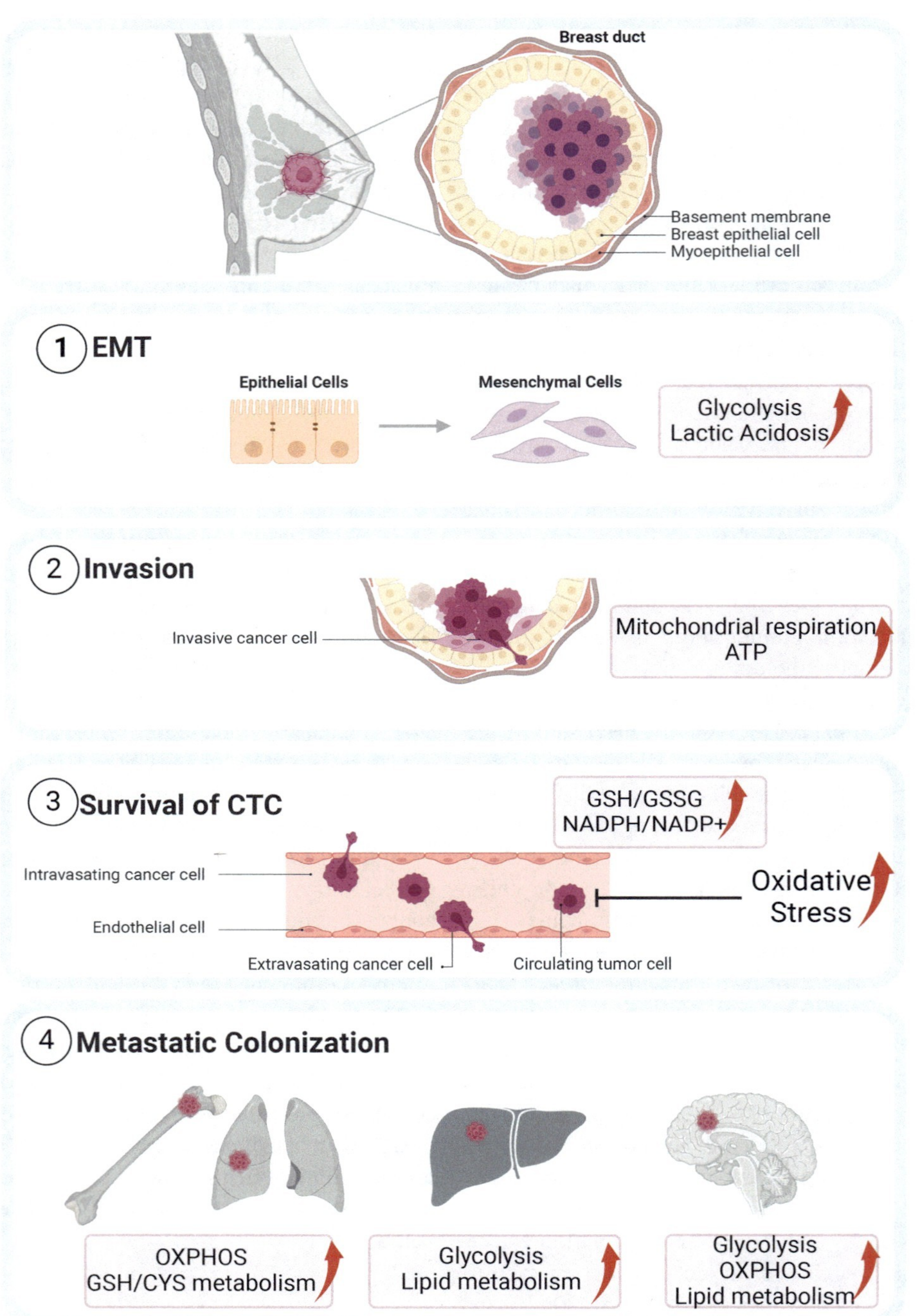

Fig. 17.1 Metabolic reprogramming in the breast cancer metastatic cascade. During EMT, highly migratory, mesenchymal cells primarily utilize glycolysis and generate lactic acidosis. Mitochondrial respiration, leading to increased ATP production, correlates with enhanced migratory and invasive capacities. Circulating cancer cells utilize heightened antioxidant defense mechanisms to counteract reactive oxygen species (ROS) by increasing the levels of glutathione (GSH) and nicotinamide adenine dinucleotide phosphate (NADPH). Metastatic breast cancer growth in different tissues requires metabolic adaptations due to variations in nutrient availability. These adaptations are necessary for tumor progression in bone, lung, liver, and brain microenvironments

Craene and Berx 2013). Traditionally, EMT has been considered a binary process, dividing cells into distinct epithelial and mesenchymal populations. This classification is often based on the loss of the epithelial markers such as E-cadherin and the acquisition of the mesenchymal marker such as vimentin (Puisieux et al. 2014). EMT is predominantly regulated by specific transcription factors, including the Snail family of zinc-finger transcription factors (SNAIL1/2), zinc-finger E-box-binding (ZEB1/2), and basic helix-loop-helix transcription factors (TWIST1/2). These transcription factors play a crucial role in repressing epithelial marker genes while promoting the expression of mesenchymal markers (Lamouille et al. 2014). Additionally, factors within the tumor microenvironment, such as inflammation and hypoxia, can serve as triggers for initiating EMT (Bertolini et al. 2022; Azimi et al. 2019). Adipose tissue within the breast cancer microenvironment also influences tumor progression through the secretion of adipokines, particularly IL-6. Adipocyte-derived IL-6 activates EMT in breast cancer cells via the STAT3 pathway, promoting increased migration, invasion, and aggressive behavior of the cancer cells (Gyamfi et al. 2018; Siersbæk et al. 2020). This intricate regulatory network involving transcription factors and microenvironmental cues orchestrates the process of EMT in a coordinated manner.

Recent studies have revealed a more nuanced understanding of EMT. Rather than a binary process, EMT occurs gradually, encompassing multiple cellular states. These states exhibit varying levels of epithelial and mesenchymal markers, along with intermediate morphological, transcriptional, and epigenetic characteristics that bridge the gap between epithelial and mesenchymal cells (Pastushenko et al. 2018). In the context of breast cancer research, extensive investigations have been conducted on the expression of epithelial and mesenchymal markers. Notably, certain breast cancer cell lines demonstrate a unique phenomenon where both markers are co-expressed within the same cells. This discovery suggests the existence of hybrid EMT states, which are associated with enhanced invasion and migration abilities (Bronsert et al. 2014; Zhang et al. 2014; Hendrix et al. 1997). In breast cancer cells, such as MDA-MB-231, the relationship between glucose metabolism and EMT impacts cell migration. Highly migratory mesenchymal cells preferentially use glycolysis, while weakly migratory epithelial cells rely on mitochondrial respiration. Modulating glucose metabolism or EMT can alter these phenotypes, highlighting the connection between EMT, glucose metabolism, and migration in cancer cells (Schwager et al. 2022). LeBleu et al. showed that migratory and invasive capacities in murine mammary cancer cells are specifically biased toward mitochondrial respiration, resulting in heightened ATP production (LeBleu et al. 2014).

During prolonged treatment with tyrosine kinase inhibitors (TKIs), cancer cells dependent on EGFR or MET showed a metabolic shift toward increased glycolysis and lactate production. Lactate, when secreted, plays a crucial role in instructing cancer-associated fibroblasts to produce hepatocyte growth factor (HGF) through a nuclear factor κB-dependent pathway. The elevated HGF levels then activate MET-dependent signaling in cancer cells, leading to sustained resistance against TKIs (Apicella et al. 2018). This new perspective sheds light on the complexity and clinical implications of EMT in cancer progression. For example, researchers have found that exploiting cancer cell plasticity can be a therapeutic strategy by inducing the transformation of EMT-derived breast cancer cells into mature and nondividing fat cells (adipocytes) using MEK inhibitors and the antidiabetic drug rosiglitazone (Ishay-Ronen et al. 2019). This approach leads to the suppression of primary tumor invasion and the formation of metastases.

Acetyl-CoA, a central and versatile metabolic intermediate and critical signaling molecule, holds significance at the convergence of fatty acid synthesis, ATP production, and protein acetylation. Cytosolic and nuclear acetyl-CoA levels are regulated by four metabolic pathways: direct synthesis from acetate and CoA via acetyl-CoA synthetase (ACSS), conversion from citrate to acetyl-CoA by ATP citrate lyase (ACLY), catabolism to acetate and CoA by acyl-CoA thioesterase (ACOT), and irreversible carboxylation from acetyl-CoA to malonyl-CoA by acetyl-CoA carboxylase (ACC) (Guertin and Wellen 2023; He et al. 2023). Regarding clinical associations with expression, increased ACSS2 expression is linked to reduced survival specifically in triple-negative breast cancer (Miller et al. 2021). Similarly, elevated ACLY expression, serving as a recurrence biomarker, is associated with lower survival in breast cancers (Chen et al. 2020). ACC1 phosphorylation, mediated by TGFβ-activated kinase 1 (TAK1) and influenced by leptin and TGFβ signaling, plays a key role. Inhibiting ACC1 increases acetyl-CoA levels, leading to Smad2 activation and promoting EMT and metastasis. ACC1 deficiency worsens tumor recurrence after primary tumor removal, and ACC1 phosphorylation levels correlate with metastatic potential in breast cancer patients (Rios Garcia et al. 2017).

2-Hydroxyglutarate (2-HG) is an oncometabolite found in tumors with IDH1/2 mutations. These mutations disrupt the normal function of IDH1/2 enzymes, which convert isocitrate to α-ketoglutarate (α-KG) in the TCA cycle. Instead, the mutated enzymes promote the conversion of α-KG to 2-HG, resulting in abnormally high 2-HG levels (5–35 mM) (Sasaki et al. 2012). Notarangelo et al. demonstrated that elevated levels of 2HG directly inhibited lactate dehydrogenase in mouse CD8+ T cells. This inhibition altered glucose metabolism in the T cells, resulting in impaired proliferation, reduced cytotoxicity and interferon-γ signaling, as well as diminished ability to eliminate target cells (Notarangelo et al. 2022). The discovery that 2HG levels are increased in breast cancer, even in the absence of IDH mutations and driven by glutamine anaplerosis, has raised the possibility that 2HG levels may be elevated in various malignancies that do not necessarily possess mutated IDH (Wise et al. 2008; Colvin et al. 2016). 2-HG also induces ZEB1-mediated EMT (Colvin et al. 2016; Larsen et al. 2016), which contributes to breast cancer cell spread. ZEB1 modulates ERα (estrogen receptor alpha)-mediated transcription shortly after EMT induction in breast cancer cells, even when they remain epithelial. This interaction between ZEB1 and ERα may influence metastatic breast cancer cells' preference for bone tissue, supported by ex vivo and xenograft studies (Mohammadi Ghahhari et al. 2022). Besides, breast cell EMT leads to heightened glutamine demand for fatty acid synthesis, impacting its role in glutathione biosynthesis and increasing cellular sensitivity to mTOR (mammalian target of rapamycin) inhibitors (Karvelsson et al. 2021).

Furthermore, the absence of 2-HG dehydrogenases leads to an increase in 2-HG levels by inhibiting its conversion back to α-KG (Dang et al. 2009). α-KG acts as a metastasis suppressor by counteracting the effects of 2-HG. The α-KG dehydrogenase complex plays a crucial role in regulating cellular α-KG levels by converting it to succinyl-CoA. Increased expression of α-KG dehydrogenase in breast cancer leads to diminished α-KG levels and oncogenic properties. Conversely, inhibiting this enzyme promotes α-KG accumulation, resulting in limiting cell migration and epithelial-mesenchymal transition, particularly in lung metastasis formation of 4T1 breast cancer cells (Atlante et al. 2018). Recent research revealed that supplementing αKG externally inhibits tumor growth and metastasis in triple-negative breast cancer. This metabolic switch from glycolytic to oxidative metabolism reduces glycolytic enzymes, increases succinate dehydrogenase and fumarate hydratase, and decreases fumarate and succinate levels, ultimately destabilizing HIF-1α, a key protein involved in tumor progression (Tseng et al. 2018).

Creatine, a popular muscle-building supplement, has been found to promote colorectal and breast cancer metastasis and reduce mouse survival. The enzyme glycine amidinotransferase (GATM), the rate-limiting enzyme for creatine synthesis, is upregulated in liver metastases. Increased dietary intake or de novo synthesis of creatine through GATM enhances cancer metastasis by activating Snail and Slug expression via MPS1-mediated Smad2 and Smad3 phosphorylation. Inhibiting GATM or MPS1 suppresses cancer metastasis and improves survival by reducing Snail and Slug expression (Zhang et al. 2021).

17.2.2 Survival of Circulating Tumor Cells (CTCs)

CTCs are cancer cells that slough off the primary site and extravasate into and circulate in the bloodstream. A higher count of CTCs is linked to an increased risk of breast cancer metastasis and is associated with lower survival rates in patients (Cristofanilli et al. 2019; Bidard et al. 2014). While it is estimated that as many as 10^6 cancer cells per gram of tumor tissue are released into the bloodstream, the metastatic efficiency of CTCs is relatively low, with estimates ranging around 0.01% (Butler and Gullino 1975; Merino et al. 2019). Although most CTCs perish while circulating, a small number can survive and initiate tumor growth at secondary sites. Emerging research indicates that CTCs undergo changes in response to the dynamic biophysical conditions in the bloodstream, including fluid shear stress (FSS), oxidative stress, and escape immunosurveillance to survive (Liu et al. 2017; Krol et al. 2021; Lin et al. 2021; Alix-Panabières and Pantel 2014). In a clinical setting, the combination of total CTC count and the proportion of mesenchymal CTCs can be utilized to monitor therapeutic resistance and predict prognosis in breast cancer patients. This criterion holds significant value in determining survival differences and guiding treatment decisions (Guan et al. 2019; Horimoto et al. 2018). In a breast cancer model involving brain metastasis, it has been proposed that hemodynamic shear flow can stimulate the upregulation of stemness-related genes in CTCs, enabling their survival in the presence of shear flow conditions (Jin et al. 2018). Nicola Aceto's research found that most CTCs enter the bloodstream during sleep in breast cancer patients and mouse models. CTCs formed during rest are prone to metastasize, whereas those from the active phase lack metastatic potential, challenging conventional views (Diamantopoulou et al. 2022). Overall, CTCs have been proposed as a prognostic tool for monitoring metastasis and evaluating the effectiveness of chemotherapy and immunotherapy (Smerage et al. 2014; Papadaki et al. 2020; Krebs et al. 2014).

17.2.2.1 Stemness of CTCs

Numerous prior studies have identified a subset of highly aggressive CTCs in various types of cancer. These CTCs possess "stemness" characteristics, which encompass their ability for self-renewal and promotion of tumor growth. A minority of CTCs establish close interactions with platelets, neutrophils, macrophages, myeloid-derived suppressor cells (MDSCs), or cancer-associated fibroblasts (CAFs) as a strategy to evade the immune system and enhance their survival (Rejniak 2016; Garrido-Navas et al. 2019). The downregulation of ERK and GSK3β signaling pathways, leading to an EMT-like transition in CTCs, may facilitate the transformation of CTCs into stemlike CTCs with enhanced abilities for sphere formation and initiation of tumor growth (Choi et al. 2019). In breast cancer, the presence of CD44+/CD24−/low and aldehyde dehydrogenase 1 (ALDH1) + cell phenotypes is associated with stemness. Theodoropoulos et al. examined the expression of CD44, CD24, and ALDH1 in CTCs from 30 metastatic breast cancer patients. They found that 35.2% of 1439 CTCs were CD44+/CD24−/low and 17.7% of 238 CTCs were ALDH1high/CD24−/low, indicating the presence of stemlike properties in CTCs (Theodoropoulos et al. 2010). Lactate dehydrogenase-A (LDHA) is commonly upregulated in various cancers and plays a significant role in CSCs (Mishra and Banerjee 2019). Inhibiting the process of fermentative glycolysis, in which LDHA is involved, reduces the tumor-initiating capacity of CSCs. Moreover, suppressing LDHA through knockdown or pharmacological inhibition has been shown to decrease cancer stemness, as evidenced by decreased tumorsphere formation and reduced expression of CD24/CD44 markers (Xie et al. 2014). Furthermore, a cell line called CTC-3, derived from the peripheral blood cells of a breast cancer patient, exhibited more aggressive growth compared to the commonly used MCF-7 breast cancer cell line. Gene profiling of CTC-3 cells revealed higher expression of stemness markers compared to MCF-7 cells (Zhao et al. 2019).

17.2.2.2 Oxidative Stress

CTCs that underwent a partial mesenchymal transition while maintaining their epithelial characteristics demonstrated the highest capacity for forming lung metastases. On the other hand, CTCs that fully embraced a mesenchymal state showed limited ability to form metastases (Liu et al. 2019). Another study revealed that the loss of extracellular matrix in non-tumorigenic human mammary epithelial cells (MCF10A) resulted in increased production of reactive oxygen species (ROS) (Schafer et al. 2009). A prospective study involving 39 patients diagnosed with invasive breast cancer discovered that most CTCs displayed a diverse range of characteristics (heterogeneous phenotypes). Among the detectable samples (24 out of 39), 22 exhibited a phenomenon called EMT plasticity (Tashireva et al. 2021). Furthermore, breast cancer cells exposed to fluid shear stress (FSS), isolated from stage III breast cancer patients, displayed an upregulation of genes encoding antioxidant enzymes like superoxide dismutase, catalase, and glutathione peroxidase. This upregulation potentially supports the survival of cancer cells within the circulatory system (Choi et al. 2019). In a study by Ma et al., it was demonstrated that exposing MDA-MB-231 cells to FSS at magnitudes of 5, 15, and 30 dyn/cm^2 resulted in elevated production of hydrogen peroxide and increased migration of cancer cells (Ma et al. 2017). Additionally, oxidative stress was found to enhance the transition of circulating tumor cells to a phenotype negative for the HER2 protein, a characteristic associated with aggressive breast cancers (Jordan et al. 2016).

To evade cell death induced by detachment from the extracellular matrix, cancer cells employ increased antioxidant defense mechanisms while circulating in the bloodstream (Piskounova et al. 2015; Grossmann 2002). Metabolism of lactate and pyruvate potentially contributes to the resistance of matrix-detached cells against ROS. In patients with aggressive metastatic breast cancer, higher levels of pyruvate were detected in the serum compared to patients with early-stage breast cancer (Jobard et al. 2014). Disrupting the intracellular conversion of pyruvate to oxaloacetate in cultured breast cancer cells led to a decrease in the NADPH/NADP+ and glutathione (GSH)/glutathione disulfide (GSSG) ratios, indicating a reduced capacity for ROS scavenging, and consequently resulted in elevated oxidative stress (Wilmanski et al. 2017).

17.2.3 Metastatic Colonization

The final stage of metastasis entails the proliferation and establishment of cancer cells in distant organs. Metastasis-initiating cells (MICs) or cancer stem cells (CSCs) play a crucial role in this process. They possess metabolic adaptability to thrive in diverse microenvironments, as well as the capacity for self-renewal and sustained tumorigenesis, distinguishing them from non-CSCs that cannot initiate tumorigenesis. CSCs exhibit distinct metabolic programs that contribute to the maintenance of their stemness characteristics. Additionally, the outgrowth of a metastatic colony involves a phenotypic reversion of cells from a mesenchymal to an epithelial state, referred to as the mesenchymal-epithelial transition. This process, akin to the EMT, involves significant metabolic rewiring (Massague and Obenauf 2016). Clinical observations indicate that the process of metastatic colonization is highly inefficient, where most cells perish and only a minority manage to establish macrometastases. This inefficiency cannot be solely attributed to a scarcity of cancer stem cells capable of initiating metastasis, as most breast cancer stem cells reaching the lungs undergo apoptosis (Malanchi et al. 2012). Similarly, breast cancer cells infiltrating the brain are prone to cell death (Heyn et al. 2006). In the case of disseminated tumor cells (DTCs) that survive after infiltrating distant organs, such as the bone marrow, they can persist for years in individuals with cancer. However, only approximately half of these DTCs progress to overt metastasis (Braun et al. 2005).

17.2.3.1 Overt Metastasis

Metastasis, the ultimate stage of cancer progression leading to organ infiltration, is the primary cause of cancer-related mortality. However, the process of establishing metastatic colonies in distant organs is highly selective, with only a small fraction of cancer cells overcoming the barriers and achieving successful colonization. Metastasis in breast cancer occurs in several sites, with bone, liver, lung, and brain being the most frequent locations. Among stage IV breast cancer patients, bone metastasis is the most prevalent (68.8%), followed by lung (16.0%), liver (13.3%), and brain (1.9%) (Gong et al. 2017). Each organ presents unique challenges for cancer cells, requiring distinct mechanisms for metastatic colonization. While breaking growth-inhibitory or immune barriers can initiate aggressive metastatic outgrowth in certain organs, the composition and structure of tissues differ significantly among organs, resulting in organ-specific metastatic traits that govern successful colonization (Obenauf and Massagué 2015). A recent study in breast cancer patients found that elevated levels of circulating miR-122 microRNA (miR-122) can predict metastatic progression in early-stage breast cancer. The study further revealed that cancer-secreted miR-122 can be transferred to normal cells in premetastatic niches, leading to the suppression of glucose utilization in those cells. This metabolic alteration allows cancer cells to meet their high energy demands during metastatic growth (Fong et al. 2015). Specialized niches serve as the residence for adult stem cells, offering crucial cues to maintain a delicate equilibrium between the proliferation and quiescence of stem cells, as well as the balance between self-renewal and differentiation.

Breast cancer metastasis commonly occurs in the bone, representing the most frequent site of metastatic spread (Chen et al. 2018). The receptor CXCR4, which binds to the chemokine CXCL12, serves as both a marker and mediator of breast cancer metastasis to bone marrow sites enriched with CXCL12 (Muller et al. 2001). Breast tumors that have a mesenchymal stroma that secretes CXCL12 tend to favor the selection of cancer cell populations that are responsive to CXCL12. These CXCL12-responsive cancer cells exhibit a predisposition to survive and establish themselves within the bone marrow (Zhang et al. 2013). Furthermore, both hypoxia through HIF-1α and TGF-β signaling can independently induce the expression of vascular endothelial growth factor (VEGF) and CXCR4, contributing to the promotion of breast cancer bone metastases (Dunn et al. 2009). Furthermore, bone metastasis-derived patient-derived xenografts (PDXs) exhibited heightened activation of the OXPHOS signature (AIFM1, NDUFV1, NDUFAB1, NDUFA7, NDUFS6, and MRPS12) as well as several TCA cycle intermediates compared to the corresponding breast primary tumors (PT). This heightened activation is associated with poorer survival outcomes in breast cancer patients (El-Botty et al. 2023). Studies have demonstrated that mTOR signaling plays a crucial role in stimulating mitochondrial biogenesis and activating OXPHOS (Morita et al. 2013). This is also evidenced by elevated levels of gamma-glutamyl amino acids and other metabolites from the glutathione and cysteine pathways, indicating increased resistance to oxidative stress. The higher levels of GSH may contribute to chemoresistance by enhancing the cells' ability to reduce oxidative stress (Bansal and Simon 2018).

Breast cancer cells that metastasize to the lungs have been found to produce the extracellular matrix protein tenascin C. This protein is deposited in the developing colony and serves to enhance signaling pathways such as Notch and Wnt (Oskarsson et al. 2011). Additionally, breast cancer stem cells can secrete TGF-β, which stimulates stromal fibroblasts to produce periostin. Periostin acts as a binding partner for tenascin C and facilitates the recruitment of Wnt factors (Malanchi et al. 2012). Moreover, cancer cells secrete enzymes called LOX and PLOD2, which promote the cross-linking of collagen and result in a stiffer extracellular matrix. This, in turn, amplifies integrin-focal adhesion signaling and promotes the process of metastasis (Gilkes et al. 2013). Importantly, breast cancer cells exhibiting elevated levels of PGC-1α, a transcriptional coactivator involved in upregulating oxidative phosphorylation and mitochondrial biogenesis, have a propensity for preferential metastasis to specific tissues, including the lung and bone (Andrzejewski et al. 2017). Research using TNBC PDX tumors revealed that lung metastases exhibited a higher expression of genes related to mitochondrial OXPHOS compared to the corresponding PT (Davis et al. 2020).

The processes of fatty acid uptake, synthesis, and modification play a pivotal role in facilitating the colonization of the metastatic niche, employing multiple mechanisms. Lipid accumulation in the liver due to obesity or nonalcoholic fatty liver disease (NAFLD) can contribute to the promotion of metastasis, and the presence of NAFLD activates triglyceride lipolysis in hepatocytes adjacent to tumors. This activation facilitates breast-to-liver metastasis (Li et al. 2020a). CD36, a receptor for fatty acids, plays a role in facilitating the uptake of long-chain fatty acids. Notably, $CD36^{high}$ CSCs exhibit heightened consumption of environmental palmitic acid which enhanced their tumor-initiating capacity in distant sites. Metastasis of $CD36^{high}$ CSCs can be induced by palmitate or a high-fat diet, whereas blocking CD36 with neutralizing antibodies hampers tumor metastasis. This suggests that the elevated utilization of fatty acids, which serve as energy-dense fuel, may enhance the survival of CSCs within the distant metastatic niche (Pascual et al. 2017). The enzyme fatty acid amide hydrolase (FAAH) serves as a predictor of long-term survival in patients with luminal breast cancer. It plays a significant role in impeding tumor progression and lung metastasis in both cell and mouse models of breast cancer (Tundidor et al. 2023). In addition, Dupuy et al. found that breast cancer liver metastases depend on a HIF-1α/(pyruvate dehydrogenase kinase-1) PDK1-dependent axis for their intrinsic metabolic reprogramming, leading to their successful colonization and growth in the liver. Efficient formation of liver metastases requires PDK1, and human liver metastases show elevated levels of PDK1 expression (Dupuy et al. 2015).

Breast cancers growing in the brain show higher fatty acid synthesis compared to tumors at other sites. The brain environment has low lipid levels, necessitating de novo fatty acid synthesis for tumor growth. Inhibiting FASN genetically or pharmacologically suppresses breast cancer growth in the brain (Ferraro et al. 2021). High levels of fatty acid-binding protein 7 (FABP7) support a glycolytic phenotype and storage of lipid droplets, enabling cancer cell adaptation and survival in the brain microenvironment, which is associated with lower survival rates and increased incidence of brain metastases in HER2+ breast cancer patients. Additionally, FABP7 is essential for the upregulation of key metastatic genes and pathways, such as integrin-Src and VEGFA (Cordero et al. 2019). In latent brain metastatic (Lat) cells, fragmented mitochondrial puncta support fatty acid oxidation (FAO) for cellular bioenergetics and redox homeostasis. Parida et al. reported that reducing dynamin-related protein 1 (DRP1), which enriches Lat cells and restricts mitochondrial plasticity led to elevated lipid droplet accumulation, impaired FAO, and reduced metastasis (Parida et al. 2023).

17.2.3.2 Metastasis and Tumor Microenvironments: Immune Cell Interactions

Metastasis is the spread of cancer cells to distant sites, facilitated by the tumor microenvironment (TME) comprising cells, blood vessels, and signaling molecules. The TME promotes tumor growth, and angiogenesis influences immune responses and facilitates cancer cell invasion and migration. It includes various nonmalignant stromal cells like endothelial cells, adipocytes, fibroblasts, immune cells, and extracellular matrix proteins (Baghban et al. 2020). In an antitumor immune response, various immune cells like natural killer (NK) cells, CD8+ and CD4+ T cells, and dendritic cells (DCs) play a role. However, elements within the TME can manipulate these cells to become pro-tumorigenic. As the tumor grows, it faces limitations due to increased hypoxia and reduced metabolic substrates, leading to the activation of HIF-1 and HIF-2 and triggering angiogenesis. This process involves the production of pro-angiogenic growth factors like VEGF (Liu et al. 2023; Carmeliet and Jain 2000; Radomska-Lesniewska et al. 2021). Understanding and targeting the TME is crucial for combating metastasis.

Breast cancer cells employ various mechanisms to promote metastasis. They produce colony-stimulating factor 1 (CSF1) to recruit tumor-associated macrophages, which serve as a source of epidermal growth factor (EGF) (Wyckoff et al. 2004). M2-like tumor-associated macrophages (TAMs) have the highest capacity for intratumoral glucose uptake. This increased glucose uptake drives hexosamine biosynthetic pathway-dependent O-GlcNAcylation, leading to enhanced cancer metastasis and chemoresistance (Shi et al. 2022). Breast cancer cells secrete CXCL1 to attract myeloid precursors, which act as a source of calprotectin (S100A8/9) for MAPK activation (Acharyya et al. 2012). Contact between vascular cell adhesion molecule 1 (VCAM1) on breast cancer cells in the lungs and α4 integrins on stromal monocytes and macrophages triggers PI3K-AKT signaling in the cancer cells (Chen et al. 2011). Neutrophil extracellular trap formation (NETosis), a neutrophil function, plays a crucial role in promoting breast cancer liver metastasis. Different populations of pro-metastatic neutrophils exhibit high metabolic adaptability, facilitating the formation of liver metastases (Hsu et al. 2019). Similarly, neutrophils in the premetastatic lung acquire a lipid-laden phenotype through interactions with lung mesenchymal cells, facilitated by the repression of adipose triglyceride lipase (ATGL) activity. These lipid-loaded neutrophils transfer lipids to metastatic tumor cells, promoting their survival and proliferation and fueling breast cancer lung metastasis (Li et al. 2020b). Besides, lung-resident mesenchymal cells (MCs) accumulate neutral lipids through interleukin-1β (IL-1β)-induced hypoxia-inducible lipid droplet-associated (HILPDA), suppressing ATGL activity. These lipid-laden MCs transfer lipids to tumor cells and NK cells via vesicles, promoting tumor cell survival and proliferation while impairing NK cell function. Targeting IL-1β improves the efficacy of NK cell immunotherapy in mitigating breast cancer lung metastasis (Gong et al. 2022).

17.3 Metabolic and Signaling Pathways Supporting Tumor Biomass Production

Metabolic alterations in breast cancer extend beyond basic energy production and nutrient utilization. They encompass a diverse array of processes that influence various aspects of cellular metabolism. These include not only glucose metabolism, which plays a crucial role in fueling cancer cell growth, but also lipid metabolism, involved in membrane synthesis and signaling pathways, as well as amino acid metabolism, which contributes to protein synthesis and cellular functions. The intricate interplay between these metabolic pathways in breast cancer highlights the complexity of the disease and provides potential avenues for targeted therapeutic interventions. The main metabolic pathways in breast cancer cells are summarized in Fig. 17.2 and described below.

17.3.1 Glucose Metabolism

17.3.1.1 Glycolysis

Under normal cellular function, glucose acts as a stimulant for pancreatic β cells, triggering the release of insulin. This insulin release facilitates the uptake of glucose into cells, where it can be utilized as an energy source (Haythorne et al. 2019). During rapid cell proliferation, normal cells activate specific signaling pathways to suppress oxidative phosphorylation (OXPHOS) and promote glycolysis and anabolic metabolism in response to growth signals. Cancer cells exploit this mechanism, known as the "Warburg effect," wherein they preferentially rely on aerobic glycolysis even in the presence of oxygen (Warburg 1956). This altered glucose metabolism allows cancer cells, including breast cancer cells, to efficiently generate adenosine triphosphate (ATP) and metabolic intermediates to support their rapid proliferation (Vander Heiden et al. 2009). Extensive research has demonstrated that cancer cells exhibit an increased dependency on blood glucose, driven by the need for rapid cell growth. Moreover, glucose has been found to influence tumor cell proliferation directly or indirectly, as evidenced by the higher incidence of breast cancer in diabetic and obese populations. This observation supports the notion that a low-carbohydrate diet could potentially restrict or impede tumor growth (Gluschnaider et al. 2014). Specifically, studies on MCF-7 and T47D breast cancer cells, as well as MCF-10A breast epithelial cells, have

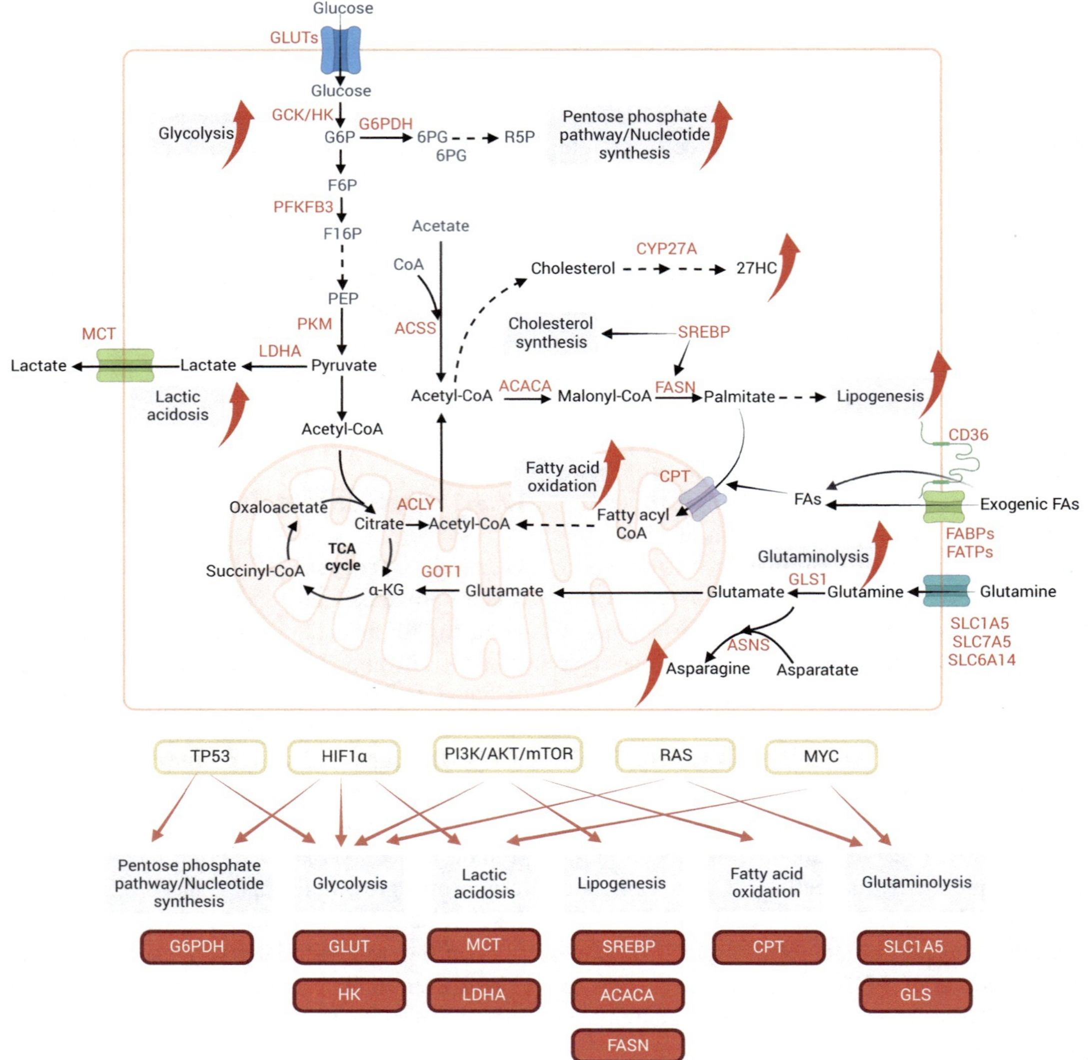

Fig. 17.2 Metabolic pathways in breast cancer cells. Highlighted is the enhanced metabolism of glucose, amino acids, and lipids for providing essential building blocks and energy for rapid cell division and sustaining tumor growth. These pathways are subject to regulation by oncogenes and other factors, promoting a highly proliferative state

shown that reducing glucose concentrations significantly inhibits cell proliferation (Maldonado et al. 2021). Additionally, in vivo experiments have indicated that mice fed sugar-rich diets display a higher burden of liver metastatic ER+ breast cancer, whereas mice fed high-fat/low-sugar diets exhibit lower tumor burden despite being obese (Zuo et al. 2022). Collectively, these findings suggest that glucose intake may serve as a growth stimulus for primary and metastatic tumors.

Interestingly, tumors exhibit dual metabolic characteristics, as tumor cells can switch from aerobic glycolysis to an OXPHOS phenotype in the presence of lactic acidosis with overexpressed MCT1 (Wu et al. 2016; Pinheiro et al. 2011). In normal conditions, lactate and pyruvate serve as circulating redox buffers that maintain NADH/NAD balance across cells and tissues (Rabinowitz and Enerbäck 2020). The hypoxic conditions within breast tumors lead to elevated production of reactive oxygen species (ROS) (Vaupel et al. 2007). In response, hypoxia-inducible factor 1 (HIF-1) activates glucose metabolism and the pentose phosphate pathway (PPP) to detoxify ROS and maintain redox homeostasis (Semenza 2017; Aykin-Burns et al. 2009; Lee and Yoon 2015). Glycolysis minimizes mitochondrial ROS production, while the PPP generates ROS-detoxifying molecule, NADPH through enzymes like glucose-6-phosphate dehydrogenase (G6PD) and 6-phosphogluconolactonase (6PGL), assisting cancer cells in coping with oxidative stress (Salazar 2018; Patra and Hay 2014). Notably, the HER2 subtype exhibits a higher expression of G6PD and 6PGL, suggesting increased PPP activity compared to other subtypes (Choi et al. 2018). Moreover, elevated levels of G6PD and transketolase (TKT) are associated with decreased overall survival and relapse-free survival in breast cancer (Benito et al. 2017). The reverse Warburg effect or metabolic coupling suggests that glycolytic metabolism in the tumor stroma sustains adjacent cancer cells, which explains the paradoxical observation of high mitochondrial respiration and low glycolysis rates in certain tumor cells (Pavlides et al. 2009; Wilde et al. 2017). The metabolic phenotypes also vary across breast cancer subtypes, with luminal subtypes exhibiting metabolically inactive reverse Warburg/null phenotypes, while TNBC is associated with metabolically active Warburg/mixed phenotypes (Choi et al. 2013a). Osteogenic differentiation of human breast cancer cells triggers the activation of both the TGF-β/Smad signaling pathway and the MAPK pathway, promoting the progression of EMT. Additionally, this differentiation process leads to a metabolic shift toward enhancing OXPHOS (Hu et al. 2020).

17.3.1.2 Glucose Transporters and Regulated Enzymes

Glucose transporters, including GLUT1–GLUT6 and GLUT12, play a crucial role in transporting glucose into breast cancer cells (Rogers et al. 2003; Garrido et al. 2013; Godoy et al. 2006; Shin and Koo 2021). Overexpression of GLUT1 and GLUT3 is often observed in aggressive tumors and is associated with increased glucose uptake (Tian et al. 2004; Zhang et al. 2017). In breast cancer, elevated levels of GLUT1 have been linked to high histologic grade, enhanced proliferation, poor differentiation, and unfavorable prognosis (Pinheiro et al. 2011; Krzeslak et al. 2012). Interestingly, the expression of GLUT1 is particularly high in TNBC, indicating a highly active metabolic state in this subtype (Choi et al. 2013b; Wu et al. 2020). Additionally, key glycolysis-related enzymes like hexokinase (HK) (Hennipman et al. 1988; Yang et al. 2018), 6-phosphofructo-2-kinase/fructose-2, 6-biphosphatase 3 (PFKFB3) (O'Neal et al. 2016), pyruvate kinase M2 (PKM2) (Lin et al. 2015), and lactate dehydrogenase-A (LDHA) (Zhao et al. 2009) are significantly activated in breast cancer and contribute to cancer growth and progression. Glucose also directly promotes tumor cell proliferation through the insulin/insulin-like growth factor 1 (IGF1)/ phosphoinositide 3-kinase (PI3K) signaling pathway, leading to increased levels of free IGF-1 that stimulate cell growth and proliferation (Cully et al. 2006; Klement and Kämmerer 2011). Activation of the PI3K signaling pathway exerts a cascade of events within breast cancer cells. This includes the phosphorylation and activation of Akt, which in turn activates the mTOR. The activation of mTOR plays a crucial role in inducing aerobic glycolysis by upregulating key factors such as KRAS, MYC, and hypoxia-inducible factor 1 (HIF-1). PIK3CA gene mutations are common in estrogen receptor (ER)-positive breast cancer. While isoform-specific PI3K inhibitors are used, resistance remains a challenge (Razavi et al. 2018). Persistent FOXM1 expression posttreatment is a biomarker of resistance to PI3Kα inhibition in ER+ breast cancer. FOXM1 promotes lactate dehydrogenase (LDH) expression but not hexokinase 2 (HK-II) (Ros et al. 2020). Moreover, the upregulation of GLUTs facilitates increased glucose uptake, enabling cancer cells to meet their heightened metabolic demands (Ghanavat et al. 2021; Abdel-Wahab et al. 2019). Furthermore, insulin stimulation triggers a response that involves the release of interleukin 6 (IL-6) and tumor necrosis factor α (TNF-α). These cytokines contribute to the intricate interplay between metabolic signaling and tumor microenvironment, potentially influencing cancer cell behavior and progression (LaPensee et al. 2008; Makino et al. 1998; McCall et al. 1992). These molecular interactions highlight the complex and interconnected nature of metabolic pathways and cytokine signaling in breast cancer.

The reliance on glucose by tumor cells can be targeted through interventions like the fasting-mimicking diet or ketogenic diet (low-carbohydrate diets), which provide alternative fuel sources such as fat and protein that cannot be utilized by "glycolytic, Warburg-like phenotype" tumors (Tan-Shalaby 2017). Numerous animal studies across different cancer types have demonstrated the effectiveness of the low-carbohydrate diet in inhibiting tumor growth, either alone or in combination with other therapies (Allen et al. 2013; Abdelwahab et al. 2012; Fokidis et al. 2015; Ho et al. 2011, 2014; Martuscello et al. 2016; Hopkins et al. 2018; Caffa et al. 2020). In a mouse model of metastatic 4T1 mammary tumors, the combined intervention of a low-carbohydrate/high-protein diet and a cyclooxygenase-2 inhibitor leads to a significant reduction in breast cancer lung metastasis (Morita et al. 2013). Similarly, in HER2-negative early breast cancer, the fasting-mimicking diet, in conjunction with chemotherapy, demonstrates the capacity to enhance tumor cell death and mitigate chemotherapy-induced DNA damage in T-lymphocytes (Vernieri et al. 2020; de Groot et al. 2020). These findings offer promise for improving treatment outcomes and minimizing chemotherapy-related adverse effects in individuals with HER2-negative breast cancer.

17.3.2 Lipid Metabolism

Dysregulated lipid metabolism is a prevalent characteristic observed in breast cancer, which encompasses various alterations in lipogenic processes, lipolysis, and lipid uptake. This dysregulation is driven by the increased demand for lipids to sustain vital cellular functions such as membrane synthesis, energy storage, and the production of signaling molecules (Simeone et al. 2021). In breast cancer cells, there is a heightened emphasis on lipogenesis, the de novo synthesis of fatty acids, to support the rapid proliferation and growth of tumor cells. Additionally, enhanced lipolysis, the breakdown of stored triglycerides, provides a crucial source of fatty acids that can be utilized as an energy substrate by cancer cells. Moreover, breast cancer cells exhibit an augmented capacity for lipid uptake, enabling them to scavenge external sources of lipids from the surrounding microenvironment, to be used in fatty acid uptake/transport (CD36, FATPs, and FABPs), lipolysis (LIPE), and lipid peroxidation (AKR1C1) (Koundouros and Poulogiannis 2020; Marino et al. 2020).

17.3.2.1 Lipogenesis

Studies have revealed that increased lipogenesis is observed in breast cancers (Gong et al. 2021; Luo et al. 2021; Rajput et al. 2023). Peroxisome proliferator-activated receptor alpha (PPARα), a transcriptional factor regulating lipid metabolism, plays a significant role in breast cancer. PPARα impacts the cell cycle, apoptosis, and the tumor microenvironment by controlling genes involved in lipogenesis, fatty acid oxidation, activation, and uptake. It also modulates signaling pathways like NF-κB and PI3K/AKT/mTOR to regulate inflammation and angiogenesis in the tumor microenvironment (Qian et al. 2023). Investigations have revealed positive correlations between tumor burden and hepatic fat accumulation, insulin levels, and liver IL-6, while an inverse correlation was observed with adiponectin (Healy et al. 2015; Bechmann et al. 2012).

The expression of fatty acid synthase (FASN), a key enzyme essential for de novo fatty acid synthesis using malonyl-CoA, is elevated in breast cancer and leads to metastasis (Okada et al. 2023; Santos and Schulze 2012; Wang et al. 2001; Menendez and Lupu 2007; Giro-Perafita et al. 2017). The lipogenic transcription factor Sterol Regulatory Element-Binding Protein (SREBP)-1 plays a role in the regulation of FASN expression by binding to the promoter site of the FASN gene (Donnelly et al. 2009). Hypoxic conditions in breast tumor cells lead to the upregulation of the FASN gene, which is mediated by the activation of AKT and SREBP-1 (Furuta et al. 2008). Visfatin, an adipokine, promotes breast cancer growth by impacting glucose, lipid, and protein metabolism. It activates key signaling pathways, including EGFR, AKT, and GSK3β, in MCF-7 cells. Additionally, visfatin activates SREBP-1 and its target genes, leading to excessive lipid deposition and cell growth. Inhibiting or silencing SREBP-1 effectively counters the visfatin-induced metabolic changes in MCF-7 cells (Rajput et al. 2023). Obesity-related factors and growth factors activate Src, leading to enhanced lipin-1 phosphorylation and increased tumor growth. Moreover, increased lipogenesis, driven by phosphorylation of lipin-1 by the Src kinase, promotes glycerolipid synthesis and contributes to the malignancy of breast cancer. Human breast tumors exhibit elevated levels of phosphorylated lipin-1, which correlate with tumor size, lymph node metastasis, recurrence, and patient survival (Song et al. 2020).

The dysregulation of lipid metabolism plays a crucial role in the growth, survival, and aggressiveness of breast cancer cells, underscoring its significance in tumor progression. Highly expressed lipogenic enzymes such as ATP citrate lyase (ACLY), acetyl-Coenzyme A carboxylase alpha (ACACA), and FASN in TNBC contribute to the synthesis of membrane phospholipids, signaling molecules, protein modifications, and energy required for rapid proliferation (Simeone et al. 2021; Jones and Infante 2015; Park et al. 2022). However, targeting these enzymes directly as therapeutic interventions raises concerns due to their essential roles in early embryonic development and embryonic lethality observed in knockout mouse models (Beigneux et al. 2004; Abu-Elheiga et al. 2005; Chirala et al. 2003). A recent study has identified NFYAv1 as a variant that promotes the transcription of key lipogenic enzymes ACACA and FASN, enhancing the malignant behavior of TNBC. Notably, Nfyav1-deficient mice did not exhibit developmental abnormalities, suggesting NFYAv1 is a potentially safe therapeutic target for TNBC (Okada et al. 2023).

17.3.2.2 Fatty Acid Oxidation

Fatty acid oxidation, also known as β-oxidation, is a metabolic process where fatty acids are broken down in the mitochondria to produce acetyl coenzymes for energy production in the TCA cycle (Chang 2023). Elevated levels of free fatty acids (FFAs) have been associated with breast cancer and shown to promote tumor growth and metastasis (Senzaki et al. 1998; Bani et al. 1986; Wicha et al. 1979; Zuo et al. 2021). In obesity, higher concentrations of free IGF-1 have been observed compared to lean individuals, potentially influenced by insulin-related effects (Nam et al. 1997). Impaired insulin sensitivity in obesity diminishes its ability to inhibit lipolysis, leading to increased levels of FFAs in the bloodstream (Pasarica et al. 2010). Moreover, obese individuals tend to exhibit higher plasma concentrations of free fatty acids relative to those who are lean (Opie and Walfish 1963). Madak-Erdogan et al. demonstrated that circulating FFAs, especially palmitic acid, derived from dietary intake or adipose tissue can activate both the ERα and mTOR pathways in estrogen-positive breast cancer cells. This activation leads to increased proliferation and aggressiveness of cancer cells, particularly in postmenopausal women who are obese (Madak-Erdogan et al. 2019). Fatty acid translocase/CD36 is a crucial membrane glycoprotein responsible for importing fatty acids from adipocytes into breast cancer cells. It directly interacts with FABP4 to regulate fatty acid import, transport, and metabolism. Inhibiting CD36 and FABP4 induces apoptosis in breast cancer cells (Gyamfi et al. 2021). The rate-limiting enzyme for fatty acid oxidation is carnitine palmitoyl transferase 1 (CPT1), responsible for facilitating the translocation of activated fatty acids to the inner mitochondrial membrane.

Recent studies have provided evidence supporting the role of FAO, regulated by the key enzyme CPT1, as the primary energy source driving metastatic breast cancer progression (Han et al. 2021; Ruidas et al. 2022). Fast-recurrence tumors undergo a metabolic shift from glycolysis to mitochondrial metabolism, relying on fatty acids as the primary energy source. In contrast, slow-recurrence tumors exhibit a combination of glycolysis and mitochondrial metabolism. This metabolic reprogramming was observed in a Her2+/Neu breast cancer model throughout the stages of tumor regression, dormancy, and recurrence. Targeting the metabolic changes with a CPT1 inhibitor, etomoxir, during regression prolongs overall survival, highlighting the potential of metabolism-targeted therapies at specific time points in breast cancer treatment (Madonna et al. 2022). Furthermore, in TNBC cells, cannabinoid receptor type 1 (CB1) is involved in regulating fatty acid metabolism through stearoyl-CoA desaturase 1 (SCD1) and fatty acyl desaturase 2 (FADS2). The inhibition of CB1 sensitizes TNBC cells to ferroptosis by regulating fatty acid metabolism via PI3K/AKT and MAPK signaling pathways (Li et al. 2022).

17.3.2.3 Cholesterol

Hypercholesterolemia increases the risk of ER-positive breast cancers and reduces the effectiveness of endocrine therapies. The primary metabolite of cholesterol, 27-hydroxycholesterol (27HC), acts as an ER and liver X receptor (LXR) ligand, promoting tumor growth and metastasis in mouse models. This effect requires conversion of cholesterol to 27HC by the enzyme CYP27A1. Human breast cancer specimens with high-grade tumors showed elevated CYP27A1 expression in both tumor cells and tumor-associated macrophages. Lowering cholesterol levels or inhibiting CYP27A1 conversion to 27HC may offer a potential strategy to prevent and treat breast cancer (Nelson et al. 2013). In addition, 27HC, an oxysterol, promotes breast cancer metastasis through its effects on myeloid immune cells. It increases the number of polymorphonuclear neutrophils and γδ-T cells at distal metastatic sites while reducing the number of cytotoxic CD8+ T-lymphocytes. Thus, 27-hydroxycholesterol acts as a biochemical mediator of metastatic effects in hypercholesterolemia (Baek et al. 2017).

17.3.3 Amino Acid Metabolism

The dysregulated metabolism of amino acids serves as a crucial source for protein synthesis and impacts redox homeostasis, cellular signaling, and immune modulation. Research has revealed the involvement of transport systems, stromal cells, gene silencing, and redox homeostasis in facilitating cancer cells' acquisition of amino acids to support their proliferative capacity.

17.3.3.1 Glutamine

Glutamine, the most abundant circulating amino acid, plays a multifaceted role in cellular energy production, proliferation, and various physiological processes such as nucleotide synthesis, pH balance, redox balance, signaling, and detoxification (Hosios et al. 2016; Fan et al. 2013). Interestingly, cancer cells, such as those in the NCI-60 cell lines, exhibit excessive glutamine consumption, far exceeding the amount needed for protein synthesis and surpassing the utilization of other amino acids (i.e., serine, leucine) (Brunk et al. 2018; Jain et al. 2012). Some cancer cells develop a dependency on glutamine, known as "glutamine addiction" (Wise and Thompson 2010), particularly observed in TNBC and ER+ metastatic breast cancer subtypes. These cancer cells are sensitive to drugs targeting glutamine-related pathways due to their upregulated expression of key genes involved in glutamine utilization (van Geldermalsen et al. 2016; Gross et al. 2014; Cotul et al. 2020). Oncogenic transcription factors like c-MYC and RAS play a crucial role in enhancing cancer cell glutamine metabolism by upregulating glutamine transporters (e.g., ASCT2/SLC1A5) and enzymes involved in glutamine-to-glutamate conversion (e.g., GLS-1) (Eberhardy and Farnham 2001; Perez-Escuredo et al. 2016). Additionally, the overexpression of SLC1A5, SLC7A5, and SLC6A14 in TNBC contributes to increased glutamine metabolism, fostering tumor growth (van Geldermalsen et al. 2016). TNBC cells exhibit enhanced TCA cycle fluxes and replenishment of intermediates through their preferential utilization of glutamine in single-pass glutaminolysis, enabling the oxidation of glucose while preserving glutamine nitrogen (Quek et al. 2022).

17.3.3.2 Asparagine

Asparagine, a nonessential amino acid, plays a significant role in cancer biology. Upregulation of asparagine synthetase (ASNS), the enzyme responsible for de novo synthesis of asparagine, has been observed in various cancers (Lomelino et al. 2017). In a study by Knott et al., ASNS was identified as a top essential gene for breast cancer cell migration and lung metastasis. Silencing ASNS reduced intracellular asparagine levels, suppressing cell invasion, which could be rescued by exogenous asparagine. Asparagine was found to promote epithelial-mesenchymal transition (EMT) through TWIST upregulation. Treatment with L-asparaginase or dietary restriction of asparagine suppressed breast cancer metastasis, while excessive dietary asparagine or ASNS ectopic expression exacerbated metastasis, specifically affecting metastatic progression without impacting primary tumor growth (Knott et al. 2018). ASNS deprivation also significantly inhibited the growth of breast cancer cells ZR-75-30 and MDA-MB-231 (Yang et al. 2014). Furthermore, asparagine promotes the expression of glutamine synthetase (GLUL), enabling de novo glutamine biosynthesis, which sustains cell proliferation and protein synthesis (Pavlova et al. 2018). Asparagine-mediated promotion of GLUL helps tumor cell survival in low-glutamine environments of distant organs, facilitating metastatic outgrowth (Luo et al. 2018).

17.4 Conclusions

The interplay between cellular metabolism and the complex process of metastasis is particularly relevant in the context of breast cancer. Breast cancer cells exhibit distinct metabolic adaptations to fulfill their specific nutritional requirements during invasion and metastasis. Moreover, they have developed mechanisms to overcome environmental stresses encountered in the circulation and metastatic microenvironments. To advance our understanding and develop effective strategies against breast cancer metastasis, future preclinical studies should consider the intricate tumor microenvironment. This holistic approach will allow for the validation of potential targets and contribute to the identification of novel molecular markers that can suppress breast cancer metastasis specifically. To fully exploit the potential of metabolic and antimetastatic modulators, future clinical trials in breast cancer should incorporate comprehensive biomarker analyses. These analyses can help unravel the metastatic proteomic, transcriptomic, and metabolomic markers that are specific to breast cancer, enabling the identification of patient subsets that are most likely to benefit from targeted treatments.

Given the strong association between the metastatic cascade and metabolic pathways in breast cancer, a combination approach that targets both metastatic signaling and metabolic regulators holds great promise. The development of rational drug combinations, which integrate metabolic inhibitors, antimetastatic agents, and traditional chemotherapeutics, can lead to synergistic inhibition of breast cancer metastasis. This multifaceted approach has the potential to significantly impact the management and treatment outcomes of breast cancer, paving the way for improved patient care in the future.

References

Abdelwahab MG et al (2012) The ketogenic diet is an effective adjuvant to radiation therapy for the treatment of malignant glioma. PLoS One 7(5)

Abdel-Wahab AF, Mahmoud W, Al-Harizy RM (2019) Targeting glucose metabolism to suppress cancer progression: prospective of anti-glycolytic cancer therapy. Pharmacol Res 150:104511

Abu-Elheiga L et al (2005) Mutant mice lacking acetyl-CoA carboxylase 1 are embryonically lethal. Proc Natl Acad Sci USA 102(34):12011–12016

Acharyya S et al (2012) A CXCL1 paracrine network links cancer chemoresistance and metastasis. Cell 150(1):165–178

Alix-Panabières C, Pantel K (2014) Challenges in circulating tumour cell research. Nat Rev Cancer 14(9):623–631

Allen BG et al (2013) Ketogenic diets enhance oxidative stress and radio-chemo-therapy responses in lung cancer xenografts. Clin Cancer Res 19(14):3905–3913

Andrzejewski S et al (2017) PGC-1alpha promotes breast cancer metastasis and confers bioenergetic flexibility against metabolic drugs. Cell Metab 26(5):778–787 e5

Apicella M et al (2018) Increased lactate secretion by cancer cells sustains non-cell-autonomous adaptive resistance to MET and EGFR targeted therapies. Cell Metab 28(6):848–865 e6

Atlante S et al (2018) alpha-ketoglutarate dehydrogenase inhibition counteracts breast cancer-associated lung metastasis. Cell Death Dis 9(7):756

Aykin-Burns N et al (2009) Increased levels of superoxide and H2O2 mediate the differential susceptibility of cancer cells versus normal cells to glucose deprivation. Biochem J 418(1):29–37

Azimi I et al (2019) ORAI1 and ORAI3 in breast cancer molecular subtypes and the identification of ORAI3 as a hypoxia sensitive gene and a regulator of hypoxia responses. Cancers 11(2):208

Baek AE et al (2017) The cholesterol metabolite 27 hydroxycholesterol facilitates breast cancer metastasis through its actions on immune cells. Nat Commun 8(1):864

Baghban R et al (2020) Tumor microenvironment complexity and therapeutic implications at a glance. Cell Commun Signal 18:1–19

Bani I et al (1986) Plasma lipids and prolactin in patients with breast cancer. Br J Cancer 54(3):439

Bansal A, Simon MC (2018) Glutathione metabolism in cancer progression and treatment resistance. J Cell Biol 217(7):2291–2298

Bechmann LP et al (2012) The interaction of hepatic lipid and glucose metabolism in liver diseases. J Hepatol 56(4):952–964

Beigneux AP et al (2004) ATP-citrate lyase deficiency in the mouse. J Biol Chem 279(10):9557–9564

Benito A et al (2017) Glucose-6-phosphate dehydrogenase and transketolase modulate breast cancer cell metabolic reprogramming and correlate with poor patient outcome. Oncotarget 8(63):106693

Bertolini I et al (2022) NFκB activation by hypoxic small extracellular vesicles drives oncogenic reprogramming in a breast cancer microenvironment. Oncogene 41(17):2520–2525

Bidard FC et al (2014) Clinical validity of circulating tumour cells in patients with metastatic breast cancer: a pooled analysis of individual patient data. Lancet Oncol 15(4):406–414

Braun S et al (2005) A pooled analysis of bone marrow micrometastasis in breast cancer. N Engl J Med 353(8):793–802

Bronsert P et al (2014) Cancer cell invasion and EMT marker expression: a three-dimensional study of the human cancer-host interface. J Pathol 234(3):410–422

Brunk E et al (2018) Recon3D enables a three-dimensional view of gene variation in human metabolism. Nat Biotechnol 36(3):272–281

Butler TP, Gullino PM (1975) Quantitation of cell shedding into efferent blood of mammary adenocarcinoma. Cancer Res 35(3):512–516

Caffa I et al (2020) Fasting-mimicking diet and hormone therapy induce breast cancer regression. Nature 583(7817):620–624

Carmeliet P, Jain RK (2000) Angiogenesis in cancer and other diseases. Nature 407(6801):249–257

Chang JS (2023) Recent insights into the molecular mechanisms of simultaneous fatty acid oxidation and synthesis in brown adipocytes. Front Endocrinol (Lausanne) 14:1106544

Chen EI et al (2007) Adaptation of energy metabolism in breast cancer brain metastases. Cancer Res 67(4):1472–1486

Chen Q, Zhang XH-F, Massagué J (2011) Macrophage binding to receptor VCAM-1 transmits survival signals in breast cancer cells that invade the lungs. Cancer Cell 20(4):538–549

Chen W et al (2018) Organotropism: new insights into molecular mechanisms of breast cancer metastasis. NPJ Precis Oncol 2(1):4

Chen Y et al (2020) ACLY: A biomarker of recurrence in breast cancer. Pathol Res Pract 216(9):153076

Chirala SS et al (2003) Fatty acid synthesis is essential in embryonic development: fatty acid synthase null mutants and most of the heterozygotes die in utero. Proc Natl Acad Sci 100(11):6358–6363

Choi J et al (2013a) Metabolic interaction between cancer cells and stromal cells according to breast cancer molecular subtype. Breast Cancer Res 15:1–20

Choi J, Jung WH, Koo JS (2013b) Metabolism-related proteins are differentially expressed according to the molecular subtype of invasive breast cancer defined by surrogate immunohistochemistry. Pathobiology 80(1):41–52

Choi J, Kim E-S, Koo JS (2018) Expression of pentose phosphate pathway-related proteins in breast cancer. Dis Markers 2018

Choi HY et al (2019) Hydrodynamic shear stress promotes epithelial-mesenchymal transition by downregulating ERK and GSK3β activities. Breast Cancer Res 21:1–20

Colvin H et al (2016) Oncometabolite D-2-hydroxyglurate directly induces epithelial-mesenchymal transition and is associated with distant metastasis in colorectal cancer. Sci Rep 6(1):36289

Cordero A et al (2019) FABP7 is a key metabolic regulator in HER2+ breast cancer brain metastasis. Oncogene 38(37):6445–6460

Cotul EK et al (2020) Combined targeting of estrogen receptor alpha and Exportin 1 in metastatic breast cancers. Cancers (Basel) 12(9)

Craze ML et al (2018) MYC regulation of glutamine–proline regulatory axis is key in luminal B breast cancer. Br J Cancer 118(2):258–265

Cristofanilli M et al (2019) The clinical use of circulating tumor cells (CTCs) enumeration for staging of metastatic breast cancer (MBC): international expert consensus paper. Crit Rev Oncol Hematol 134:39–45

Cully M et al (2006) Beyond PTEN mutations: the PI3K pathway as an integrator of multiple inputs during tumorigenesis. Nat Rev Cancer 6(3):184–192

Dang L et al (2009) Cancer-associated IDH1 mutations produce 2-hydroxyglutarate. Nature 462(7274):739–744

Davis RT et al (2020) Transcriptional diversity and bioenergetic shift in human breast cancer metastasis revealed by single-cell RNA sequencing. Nat Cell Biol 22(3):310–320

De Craene B, Berx G (2013) Regulatory networks defining EMT during cancer initiation and progression. Nat Rev Cancer 13(2):97–110

de Groot S et al (2020) Fasting mimicking diet as an adjunct to neoadjuvant chemotherapy for breast cancer in the multicentre randomized phase 2 DIRECT trial. Nat Commun 11(1):1–9

Diamantopoulou Z et al (2022) The metastatic spread of breast cancer accelerates during sleep. Nature 607(7917):156–162

Donnelly C et al (2009) Conjugated linoleic acid (CLA) inhibits expression of the Spot 14 (THRSP) and fatty acid synthase genes and impairs the growth of human breast cancer and liposarcoma cells. Nutr Cancer 61(1):114–122

Dunn LK et al (2009) Hypoxia and TGF-β drive breast cancer bone metastases through parallel signaling pathways in tumor cells and the bone microenvironment. PLoS One 4(9):e6896

Dupuy F et al (2015) PDK1-dependent metabolic reprogramming dictates metastatic potential in breast cancer. Cell Metab 22(4):577–589

Eberhardy SR, Farnham PJ (2001) c-Myc mediates activation of the cad promoter via a post-RNA polymerase II recruitment mechanism. J Biol Chem 276(51):48562–48571

El-Botty R et al (2023) Oxidative phosphorylation is a metabolic vulnerability of endocrine therapy and palbociclib resistant metastatic breast cancers. Nat Commun 14(1):4221

Fan J et al (2013) Glutamine-driven oxidative phosphorylation is a major ATP source in transformed mammalian cells in both normoxia and hypoxia. Mol Syst Biol 9(1):712

Ferraro GB et al (2021) Fatty acid synthesis is required for breast cancer brain metastasis. Nat Cancer 2(4):414–428

Fokidis HB et al (2015) A low carbohydrate, high protein diet suppresses intratumoral androgen synthesis and slows castration-resistant prostate tumor growth in mice. J Steroid Biochem Mol Biol 150:35–45

Fong MY et al (2015) Breast-cancer-secreted miR-122 reprograms glucose metabolism in premetastatic niche to promote metastasis. Nat Cell Biol 17(2):183–194

Furuta E et al (2008) Fatty acid synthase gene is up-regulated by hypoxia via activation of Akt and sterol regulatory element binding protein-1. Cancer Res 68(4):1003–1011

Garrido P et al (2013) 17beta-estradiol activates glucose uptake via GLUT4 translocation and PI3K/Akt signaling pathway in MCF-7 cells. Endocrinology 154(6):1979–1989

Garrido-Navas C et al (2019) Cooperative and escaping mechanisms between circulating tumor cells and blood constituents. Cells 8(11):1382

Geck RC, Toker A (2016) Nonessential amino acid metabolism in breast cancer. Adv Biol Regul 62:11–17

Ghanavat M et al (2021) Digging deeper through glucose metabolism and its regulators in cancer and metastasis. Life Sci 264:118603

Gilkes DM et al (2013) Procollagen lysyl hydroxylase 2 is essential for hypoxia-induced breast cancer metastasis. Mol Cancer Res 11(5):456–466

Giro-Perafita A et al (2017) Fatty acid synthase expression and its association with clinico-histopathological features in triple-negative breast cancer. Oncotarget 8(43):74391–74405

Gluschnaider U et al (2014) Long-chain fatty acid analogues suppress breast tumorigenesis and progression. Cancer Res 74(23):6991–7002

Godoy A et al (2006) Differential subcellular distribution of glucose transporters GLUT1-6 and GLUT9 in human cancer: ultrastructural localization of GLUT1 and GLUT5 in breast tumor tissues. J Cell Physiol 207(3):614–627

Gong Y et al (2017) Impact of molecular subtypes on metastatic breast cancer patients: a SEER population-based study. Sci Rep 7:45411

Gong M et al (2021) Identification of a lipid metabolism-associated gene signature predicting survival in breast cancer. Int J General Med:9503–9513

Gong Z et al (2022) Lipid-laden lung mesenchymal cells foster breast cancer metastasis via metabolic reprogramming of tumor cells and natural killer cells. Cell Metab 34(12):1960–1976 e9

Gross MI et al (2014) Antitumor activity of the glutaminase inhibitor CB-839 in triple-negative breast cancer. Mol Cancer Ther 13(4):890–901

Grossmann J (2002) Molecular mechanisms of "detachment-induced apoptosis—Anoikis". Apoptosis 7:247–260

Guan X et al (2019) The prognostic and therapeutic implications of circulating tumor cell phenotype detection based on epithelial-mesenchymal transition markers in the first-line chemotherapy of HER2-negative metastatic breast cancer. Cancer Commun (Lond) 39(1):1

Guertin DA, Wellen KE (2023) Acetyl-CoA metabolism in cancer. Nat Rev Cancer 23(3):156–172

Gyamfi J et al (2018) Interleukin-6/STAT3 signalling regulates adipocyte induced epithelial-mesenchymal transition in breast cancer cells. Sci Rep 8(1):8859

Gyamfi J et al (2021) Interaction between CD36 and FABP4 modulates adipocyte-induced fatty acid import and metabolism in breast cancer. NPJ Breast Cancer 7(1):129

Han XJ et al (2015) Mitochondrial dynamics regulates hypoxia-induced migration and antineoplastic activity of cisplatin in breast cancer cells. Int J Oncol 46(2):691–700

Han J et al (2021) MSC-induced lncRNA AGAP2-AS1 promotes stemness and trastuzumab resistance through regulating CPT1 expression and fatty acid oxidation in breast cancer. Oncogene 40(4):833–847

Hanahan D (2022) Hallmarks of cancer: new dimensions. Cancer Discov 12(1):31–46

Haythorne E et al (2019) Diabetes causes marked inhibition of mitochondrial metabolism in pancreatic beta-cells. Nat Commun 10(1):2474

He W, Li Q, Li X (2023) Acetyl-CoA regulates lipid metabolism and histone acetylation modification in cancer. Biochim Biophys Acta Rev Cancer 1878(1):188837

Healy ME et al (2015) Dietary effects on liver tumor burden in mice treated with the hepatocellular carcinogen diethylnitrosamine. J Hepatol 62(3):599–606

Hendrix MJ et al (1997) Experimental co-expression of vimentin and keratin intermediate filaments in human breast cancer cells results in phenotypic interconversion and increased invasive behavior. Am J Pathol 150(2):483–495

Hennipman A et al (1988) Glycolytic enzyme activities in breast cancer metastases. Tumour Biol 9(5):241–248

Heyn C et al (2006) In vivo MRI of cancer cell fate at the single-cell level in a mouse model of breast cancer metastasis to the brain. Magn Reson Med 56(5):1001–1010

Ho VW et al (2011) A low carbohydrate, high protein diet slows tumor growth and prevents cancer initiation. Cancer Res 71(13):4484–4493

Ho VW et al (2014) A low carbohydrate, high protein diet combined with celecoxib markedly reduces metastasis. Carcinogenesis 35(10):2291–2299

Hopkins BD et al (2018) Suppression of insulin feedback enhances the efficacy of PI3K inhibitors. Nature 560(7719):499–503

Horimoto Y et al (2018) Analysis of circulating tumour cell and the epithelial mesenchymal transition (EMT) status during eribulin-based treatment in 22 patients with metastatic breast cancer: a pilot study. J Transl Med 16(1):1–8

Hosios AM et al (2016) Amino acids rather than glucose account for the majority of cell mass in proliferating mammalian cells. Dev Cell 36(5):540–549

Hsu BE et al (2019) immature low-density neutrophils exhibit metabolic flexibility that facilitates breast cancer liver metastasis. Cell Rep 27(13):3902–3915 e6

Hu Y et al (2020) OXPHOS-dependent metabolic reprogramming prompts metastatic potential of breast cancer cells under osteogenic differentiation. Br J Cancer 123(11):1644–1655

Ishay-Ronen D et al (2019) Gain fat—lose metastasis: converting invasive breast cancer cells into adipocytes inhibits cancer metastasis. Cancer Cell 35(1): 17–32. e6

Jain M et al (2012) Metabolite profiling identifies a key role for glycine in rapid cancer cell proliferation. Science 336(6084):1040–1044

Jin J et al (2018) Hemodynamic shear flow regulates biophysical characteristics and functions of circulating breast tumor cells reminiscent of brain metastasis. Soft Matter 14(47):9528–9533

Jin L et al (2022) Lactate receptor HCAR1 regulates cell growth, metastasis and maintenance of cancer-specific energy metabolism in breast cancer cells. Mol Med Rep 26(2)

Jobard E et al (2014) A serum nuclear magnetic resonance-based metabolomic signature of advanced metastatic human breast cancer. Cancer Lett 343(1):33–41

Jones SF, Infante JR (2015) Molecular pathways: fatty acid synthase. Clin Cancer Res 21(24): 5434–5438

Jordan NV et al (2016) HER2 expression identifies dynamic functional states within circulating breast cancer cells. Nature 537(7618):102–106

Karvelsson ST et al (2021) EMT-derived alterations in glutamine metabolism sensitize mesenchymal breast cells to mTOR inhibition. Mol Cancer Res 19(9):1546–1558

Kim G et al (2015) SOCS3-mediated regulation of inflammatory cytokines in PTEN and p53 inactivated triple negative breast cancer model. Oncogene 34(6):671–680

Klement RJ, Kämmerer U (2011) Is there a role for carbohydrate restriction in the treatment and prevention of cancer? Nutr Metab 8(1):1–16

Knott SRV et al (2018) Asparagine bioavailability governs metastasis in a model of breast cancer. Nature 554(7692):378–381

Koundouros N, Poulogiannis G (2020) Reprogramming of fatty acid metabolism in cancer. Br J Cancer 122(1):4–22

Krebs MG et al (2014) Molecular analysis of circulating tumour cells—biology and biomarkers. Nat Rev Clin Oncol 11(3):129–144

Krol I et al (2021) Detection of clustered circulating tumour cells in early breast cancer. Br J Cancer 125(1):23–27

Krzeslak A et al (2012) Expression of GLUT1 and GLUT3 glucose transporters in endometrial and breast cancers. Pathol Oncol Res 18(3):721–728

Kurose K et al (2002) Frequent somatic mutations in PTEN and TP53 are mutually exclusive in the stroma of breast carcinomas. Nat Genet 32(3):355–357

Lambert AW, Pattabiraman DR, Weinberg RA (2017) Emerging biological principles of metastasis. Cell 168(4):670–691

Lamouille S, Xu J, Derynck R (2014) Molecular mechanisms of epithelial–mesenchymal transition. Nat Rev Mol Cell Biol 15(3):178–196

LaPensee CR, Hugo ER, Ben-Jonathan N (2008) Insulin stimulates interleukin-6 expression and release in LS14 human adipocytes through multiple signaling pathways. Endocrinology 149(11):5415–5422

Larsen JE et al (2016) ZEB1 drives epithelial-to-mesenchymal transition in lung cancer. J Clin Invest 126(9):3219–3235

LeBleu VS et al. (2014) PGC-1alpha mediates mitochondrial biogenesis and oxidative phosphorylation in cancer cells to promote metastasis. Nat Cell Biol 16(10): 992–1003, 1–15

Lee M, Yoon J-H (2015) Metabolic interplay between glycolysis and mitochondrial oxidation: The reverse Warburg effect and its therapeutic implication. World J Biol Chem 6(3):148

Li Y et al (2020a) Hepatic lipids promote liver metastasis. JCI Insight 5(17)

Li P et al (2020b) Lung mesenchymal cells elicit lipid storage in neutrophils that fuel breast cancer lung metastasis. Nat Immunol 21(11):1444–1455

Li P et al (2022) Inhibition of cannabinoid receptor type 1 sensitizes triple-negative breast cancer cells to ferroptosis via regulating fatty acid metabolism. Cell Death Dis 13(9):808

Lin Y et al (2015) High expression of pyruvate kinase M2 is associated with chemosensitivity to epirubicin and 5-fluorouracil in breast cancer. J Cancer 6(11):1130

Lin D et al (2021) Circulating tumor cells: biology and clinical significance. Signal Transduct Target Ther 6(1):404

Liu Q et al (2017) Factors involved in cancer metastasis: a better understanding to "seed and soil" hypothesis. Mol Cancer 16:1–19

Liu X et al (2019) Epithelial-type systemic breast carcinoma cells with a restricted mesenchymal transition are a major source of metastasis. Sci Adv 5(6):eaav4275

Liu ZL et al (2023) Angiogenic signaling pathways and anti-angiogenic therapy for cancer. Signal Transduct Target Ther 8(1):198

Lomelino CL et al (2017) Asparagine synthetase: function, structure, and role in disease. J Biol Chem 292(49):19952–19958

Luo M, Brooks M, Wicha MS (2018) Asparagine and glutamine: co-conspirators fueling metastasis. Cell Metab 27(5):947–949

Luo H et al (2021) Increased lipogenesis is critical for self-renewal and growth of breast cancer stem cells: impact of omega-3 fatty acids. Stem Cells 39(12):1660–1670

Ma S et al (2017) Hemodynamic shear stress stimulates migration and extravasation of tumor cells by elevating cellular oxidative level. Cancer Lett 388:239–248

Madak-Erdogan Z et al (2019) Free fatty acids rewire cancer metabolism in obesity-associated breast cancer via estrogen receptor and mTOR signaling. Cancer Res 79(10):2494–2510

Madonna MC et al (2022) In vivo metabolic imaging identifies lipid vulnerability in a preclinical model of Her2+/Neu breast cancer residual disease and recurrence. NPJ Breast Cancer 8(1):111

Makino T et al (1998) Circulating interleukin 6 concentrations and insulin resistance in patients with cancer. Br J Surg 85(12):1658–1662

Malanchi I et al (2012) Interactions between cancer stem cells and their niche govern metastatic colonization. Nature 481(7379):85–89

Maldonado R et al (2021) beta-hydroxybutyrate does not alter the effects of glucose deprivation on breast cancer cells. Oncol Lett 21(1):65

Marino N et al (2020) Upregulation of lipid metabolism genes in the breast prior to cancer diagnosis. NPJ Breast Cancer 6:50

Martuscello RT et al (2016) A supplemented high-fat low-carbohydrate diet for the treatment of glioblastoma. Clin Cancer Res 22(10):2482–2495

Massague J, Obenauf AC (2016) Metastatic colonization by circulating tumour cells. Nature 529(7586):298–306

McCall J, Tuckey J, Parry B (1992) Serum tumour necrosis factor alpha and insulin resistance in gastrointestinal cancer. Br J Surg 79(12):1361–1363

McDonnell DP et al (2014) Obesity, cholesterol metabolism, and breast cancer pathogenesis. Cancer Res 74(18):4976–4982

Menendez JA, Lupu R (2007) Fatty acid synthase and the lipogenic phenotype in cancer pathogenesis. Nat Rev Cancer 7(10):763–777

Merino D et al (2019) Barcoding reveals complex clonal behavior in patient-derived xenografts of metastatic triple negative breast cancer. Nat Commun 10(1):766

Miller KD et al (2021) Targeting ACSS2 with a transition-state mimetic inhibits triple-negative breast cancer growth. Cancer Res 81(5):1252–1264

Mishra D, Banerjee D (2019) Lactate dehydrogenases as metabolic links between tumor and stroma in the tumor microenvironment. Cancers 11(6):750

Mohammadi Ghahhari N et al (2022) Cooperative interaction between ERα and the EMT-inducer ZEB1 reprograms breast cancer cells for bone metastasis. Nat Commun 13(1):2104

Monaco ME (2017) Fatty acid metabolism in breast cancer subtypes. Oncotarget 8(17):29487–29500

Morita M et al (2013) mTORC1 controls mitochondrial activity and biogenesis through 4E-BP-dependent translational regulation. Cell Metab 18(5):698–711

Muller A et al (2001) Involvement of chemokine receptors in breast cancer metastasis. Nature 410(6824):50–56

Nam S et al (1997) Effect of obesity on total and free insulin-like growth factor (IGF)-1, and their relationship to IGF-binding protein (BP)-1, IGFBP-2, IGFBP-3, insulin, and growth hormone. Int J Obes Relat Metab Disord 21(5)

Nelson ER et al (2013) 27-Hydroxycholesterol links hypercholesterolemia and breast cancer pathophysiology. Science 342(6162):1094–1098

Nieto MA et al (2016) Emt: 2016. Cell 166(1):21–45

Notarangelo G et al (2022) Oncometabolite d-2HG alters T cell metabolism to impair CD8(+) T cell function. Science 377(6614):1519–1529

O'Neal J et al (2016) Inhibition of 6-phosphofructo-2-kinase (PFKFB3) suppresses glucose metabolism and the growth of HER2+ breast cancer. Breast Cancer Res Treat 160:29–40

Obenauf AC, Massagué J (2015) Surviving at a distance: organ-specific metastasis. Trends Cancer 1(1):76–91

Okada N et al (2023) NFYA promotes malignant behavior of triple-negative breast cancer in mice through the regulation of lipid metabolism. Commun Biol 6(1):596

Opie LH, Walfish PG (1963) Plasma free fatty acid concentrations in obesity. N Engl J Med 268(14):757–760

Oskarsson T et al (2011) Breast cancer cells produce tenascin C as a metastatic niche component to colonize the lungs. Nat Med 17(7):867–874

Papadaki MA et al (2020) Clinical relevance of immune checkpoints on circulating tumor cells in breast cancer. Cancers (Basel) 12(2)

Parida PK et al (2023) Limiting mitochondrial plasticity by targeting DRP1 induces metabolic reprogramming and reduces breast cancer brain metastases. Nat Cancer 4(6):893–907

Park JH et al (2022) Fatty acid synthetase expression in triple-negative breast cancer. J Pathol Transl Med 56(2):73–80

Pasarica M et al (2010) Reduced oxygenation in human obese adipose tissue is associated with impaired insulin suppression of lipolysis. J Clin Endocrinol Metabol 95(8):4052–4055

Pascual G et al (2017) Targeting metastasis-initiating cells through the fatty acid receptor CD36. Nature 541(7635):41–45

Pastushenko I et al (2018) Identification of the tumour transition states occurring during EMT. Nature 556(7702):463–468

Patra KC, Hay N (2014) The pentose phosphate pathway and cancer. Trends Biochem Sci 39(8):347–354

Pavlides S et al (2009) The reverse Warburg effect: aerobic glycolysis in cancer associated fibroblasts and the tumor stroma. Cell Cycle 8(23):3984–4001

Pavlova NN, Thompson CB (2016) The emerging hallmarks of cancer metabolism. Cell Metab 23(1): 27–47

Pavlova NN et al (2018) As extracellular glutamine levels decline, asparagine becomes an essential amino acid. Cell Metab 27(2):428–438 e5

Pavlova NN, Zhu J, Thompson CB (2022) The hallmarks of cancer metabolism: still emerging. Cell Metab 34(3):355–377

Perez-Escuredo J et al (2016) Lactate promotes glutamine uptake and metabolism in oxidative cancer cells. Cell Cycle 15(1):72–83

Pinheiro C et al (2011) GLUT1 and CAIX expression profiles in breast cancer correlate with adverse prognostic factors and MCT1 overexpression. Histol Histopathol 26(10):1279–1286

Piskounova E et al (2015) Oxidative stress inhibits distant metastasis by human melanoma cells. Nature 527(7577):186–191

Puisieux A, Brabletz T, Caramel J (2014) Oncogenic roles of EMT-inducing transcription factors. Nat Cell Biol 16(6):488–494

Qian Z et al (2023) The emerging role of PPAR-alpha in breast cancer. Biomed Pharmacother 161:114420

Quek LE et al (2022) Glutamine addiction promotes glucose oxidation in triple-negative breast cancer. Oncogene 41(34):4066–4078

Rabinowitz JD, Enerbäck S (2020) Lactate: the ugly duckling of energy metabolism. Nat Metab 2(7):566–571

Radomska-Lesniewska DM, Bialoszewska A, Kaminski P (2021) Angiogenic properties of NK cells in cancer and other angiogenesis-dependent diseases. Cells 10(7)

Rajput PK et al (2023) Visfatin-induced upregulation of lipogenesis via EGFR/AKT/GSK3beta pathway promotes breast cancer cell growth. Cell Signal 107:110686

Razavi P et al (2018) The genomic landscape of endocrine-resistant advanced breast cancers. Cancer Cell 34(3):427–438 e6

Rejniak KA (2016) Circulating tumor cells: when a solid tumor meets a fluid microenvironment. In: Systems biology of tumor microenvironment: quantitative modeling and simulations, pp 93–106

Rios Garcia M et al (2017) Acetyl-CoA carboxylase 1-dependent protein acetylation controls breast cancer metastasis and recurrence. Cell Metab 26(6): 842–855 e5

Rogers S et al (2003) Differential expression of GLUT12 in breast cancer and normal breast tissue. Cancer Lett 193(2):225–233

Ros S et al (2020) Metabolic imaging detects resistance to PI3Kalpha inhibition mediated by persistent FOXM1 expression in ER(+) breast cancer. Cancer Cell 38(4):516–533 e9

Ruidas B et al (2022) Quercetin: a silent retarder of fatty acid oxidation in breast cancer metastasis through steering of mitochondrial CPT1. Breast Cancer 29(4):748–760

Salazar G (2018) NADPH oxidases and mitochondria in vascular senescence. Int J Mol Sci 19(5)

Santos CR, Schulze A (2012) Lipid metabolism in cancer. FEBS J 279(15):2610–2623

Sasaki M et al (2012) IDH1(R132H) mutation increases murine haematopoietic progenitors and alters epigenetics. Nature 488(7413):656–659

Schafer ZT et al (2009) Antioxidant and oncogene rescue of metabolic defects caused by loss of matrix attachment. Nature 461(7260):109–113

Schild T et al (2018) Unique metabolic adaptations dictate distal organ-specific metastatic colonization. Cancer Cell 33(3):347–354

Schwager SC et al (2022) Link between glucose metabolism and epithelial-to-mesenchymal transition drives triple-negative breast cancer migratory heterogeneity. Iscience 25(10)

Semenza GL (2017) Hypoxia-inducible factors: coupling glucose metabolism and redox regulation with induction of the breast cancer stem cell phenotype. EMBO J 36(3):252–259

Senzaki H et al (1998) Dietary effects of fatty acids on growth and metastasis of KPL-1 human breast cancer cells in vivo and in vitro. Anticancer Res 18(3A):1621–1627

Shi Q et al (2022) Increased glucose metabolism in TAMs fuels O-GlcNAcylation of lysosomal Cathepsin B to promote cancer metastasis and chemoresistance. Cancer Cell 40(10):1207–1222 e10

Shin E, Koo JS (2021) Glucose metabolism and glucose transporters in breast cancer. Front Cell Dev Biol 9:728759

Siersbæk R et al (2020) IL6/STAT3 signaling hijacks estrogen receptor α enhancers to drive breast cancer metastasis. Cancer Cell 38(3):412–423.e9

Simeone P et al (2021) Expanding roles of De Novo lipogenesis in breast cancer. Int J Environ Res Public Health 18(7)

Smerage JB et al (2014) Circulating tumor cells and response to chemotherapy in metastatic breast cancer: SWOG S0500. J Clin Oncol 32(31):3483–3489

Song L et al (2020) Proto-oncogene Src links lipogenesis via lipin-1 to breast cancer malignancy. Nat Commun 11(1):5842

Tan-Shalaby J (2017) Ketogenic diets and cancer: emerging evidence. Fed Pract 34(Suppl 1):37S

Tashireva LA et al (2021) Heterogeneous manifestations of epithelial-mesenchymal plasticity of circulating tumor cells in breast cancer patients. Int J Mol Sci 22(5)

Theodoropoulos PA et al (2010) Circulating tumor cells with a putative stem cell phenotype in peripheral blood of patients with breast cancer. Cancer Lett 288(1):99–106

Tian M et al (2004) Expression of Glut-1 and Glut-3 in untreated oral squamous cell carcinoma compared with FDG accumulation in a PET study. Eur J Nucl Med Mol Imaging 31(1):5–12

Tseng CW et al (2018) Transketolase regulates the metabolic switch to control breast cancer cell metastasis via the alpha-ketoglutarate signaling pathway. Cancer Res 78(11):2799–2812

Tundidor I et al (2023) Identification of fatty acid amide hydrolase as a metastasis suppressor in breast cancer. Nat Commun 14(1):3130

van Geldermalsen M et al (2016) ASCT2/SLC1A5 controls glutamine uptake and tumour growth in triple-negative basal-like breast cancer. Oncogene 35(24):3201–3208

Vander Heiden MG, Cantley LC, Thompson CB (2009) Understanding the Warburg effect: the metabolic requirements of cell proliferation. Science 324(5930):1029–1033

Vaupel P, Hockel M, Mayer A (2007) Detection and characterization of tumor hypoxia using pO2 histography. Antioxid Redox Signal 9(8):1221–1235

Vernieri C et al (2020) Fasting-mimicking diet plus chemotherapy in breast cancer treatment. Nat Commun 11(1)

Walsh T et al (2006) Spectrum of mutations in BRCA1, BRCA2, CHEK2, and TP53 in families at high risk of breast cancer. JAMA 295(12):1379–1388

Wang Y et al (2001) Two-site ELISA for the quantitative determination of fatty acid synthase. Clin Chim Acta 304(1–2):107–115

Warburg O (1956) On the origin of cancer cells. Science 123(3191):309–314

Wicha MS, Liotta LA, Kidwell WR (1979) Effects of free fatty acids on the growth of normal and neoplastic rat mammary epithelial cells. Cancer Res 39(2 Part 1):426–435

Wilde L et al (2017) Metabolic coupling and the Reverse Warburg Effect in cancer: implications for novel biomarker and anticancer agent development. Semin Oncol 44(3):198–203

Wilmanski T et al (2017) Inhibition of pyruvate carboxylase by 1α, 25-dihydroxyvitamin D promotes oxidative stress in early breast cancer progression. Cancer Lett 411:171–181

Wise DR, Thompson CB (2010) Glutamine addiction: a new therapeutic target in cancer. Trends Biochem Sci 35(8):427–433

Wise DR et al (2008) Myc regulates a transcriptional program that stimulates mitochondrial glutaminolysis and leads to glutamine addiction. Proc Natl Acad Sci 105(48):18782–18787

Wishart DS (2015) Is cancer a genetic disease or a metabolic disease? EBioMedicine 2(6):478–479

Wu H, Ying M, Hu X (2016) Lactic acidosis switches cancer cells from aerobic glycolysis back to dominant oxidative phosphorylation. Oncotarget 7(26): 40621

Wu Q et al (2020) GLUT1 inhibition blocks growth of RB1-positive triple negative breast cancer. Nat Commun 11(1):4205

Wyckoff J et al (2004) A paracrine loop between tumor cells and macrophages is required for tumor cell migration in mammary tumors. Cancer Res 64(19):7022–7029

Xie H et al (2014) Targeting lactate dehydrogenase-a inhibits tumorigenesis and tumor progression in mouse models of lung cancer and impacts tumor-initiating cells. Cell Metab 19(5):795–809

Yang H et al (2014) Down-regulation of asparagine synthetase induces cell cycle arrest and inhibits cell proliferation of breast cancer. Chem Biol Drug Des 84(5):578–584

Yang T et al (2018) PIM2-mediated phosphorylation of hexokinase 2 is critical for tumor growth and paclitaxel resistance in breast cancer. Oncogene 37(45):5997–6009

Yousuf U et al (2022) Identification and analysis of dysregulated fatty acid metabolism genes in breast cancer subtypes. Med Oncol 39(12):256

Zhang XH et al (2013) Selection of bone metastasis seeds by mesenchymal signals in the primary tumor stroma. Cell 154(5):1060–1073

Zhang J et al (2014) TGF-β–induced epithelial-to-mesenchymal transition proceeds through stepwise activation of multiple feedback loops. Sci Signal 7(345):ra91

Zhang HL et al (2017) Blocking preferential glucose uptake sensitizes liver tumor-initiating cells to glucose restriction and sorafenib treatment. Cancer Lett 388:1–11

Zhang L, et al. (2021) Creatine promotes cancer metastasis through activation of Smad2/3. Cell Metab 33(6): 1111–1123. e4

Zhao Y et al (2009) Upregulation of lactate dehydrogenase A by ErbB2 through heat shock factor 1 promotes breast cancer cell glycolysis and growth. Oncogene 28(42):3689–3701

Zhao P et al (2019) Establishment and characterization of a CTC cell line from peripheral blood of breast cancer patient. J Cancer 10(24):6095–6104

Zuo Q et al (2021) Obesity and postmenopausal hormone receptor-positive breast cancer: epidemiology and mechanisms. Endocrinology 162(12)

Zuo Q et al (2022) Targeting metabolic adaptations in the breast cancer-liver metastatic niche using dietary approaches to improve endocrine therapy efficacy. Mol Cancer Res 20(6):923–937

Part VI

Metastasis and Immunity

This part sheds light on the intricate relationship between metastasis and the immune microenvironment in breast cancer. It examines cellular dormancy in metastatic breast cancer, emphasizing the influence of the tumor microenvironment on dormancy induction and reawakening, describes the multifaceted roles of myeloid cells in breast cancer progression, highlighting their contributions to tumor growth, dissemination, and immune modulation, and discusses the critical roles of immune cells in breast cancer metastasis, underscoring the potential for immune-based therapeutic strategies.

In Chap. 18, Momo Bentires-Alj and his colleagues from the University of Basel, Switzerland, explore the phenomenon of cellular dormancy in breast cancer metastasis, emphasizing the crucial role of the tumor microenvironment in influencing dormancy and subsequent reawakening. The chapter discusses the challenges in identifying dormant disseminated tumor cells (DTCs) and highlights the importance of understanding the cell-extrinsic mechanisms that regulate dormancy.

In Chap. 19, Shawn Zhang and his colleagues from Baylor College of Medicine, Houston, USA, shift the focus to the roles of myeloid cells in breast cancer progression. The chapter comprehensively reviews the diverse functions of tumor-associated myeloid cells, including their contributions to primary tumor growth, intravasation, dissemination, and colonization at metastatic sites. It also discusses therapeutic strategies targeting pro-tumoral myeloid cell subpopulations.

Finally, in Chap. 20, Bin-Zhi Qian and his colleague from Fudan University, Shanghai, China, delve further into the immune microenvironment in breast cancer metastasis, emphasizing its pivotal role in determining disease progression. By summarizing recent discoveries on immune cell heterogeneity and their implications for metastasis, this chapter highlights the potential for more precise treatment strategies.

Overall, these chapters underscore the complexity of metastasis and the critical influence of the immune microenvironment. By elucidating the mechanisms underlying metastasis and immune interactions, they pave the way for novel therapeutic approaches aimed at improving patient outcomes.

18 Microenvironmental Regulation of Dormancy in Breast Cancer Metastasis: "An Ally that Changes Allegiances"

Evrim Ceren Kabak, Sok Lin Foo, Maria Rafaeva, Ivan Martin, and Mohamed Bentires-Alj

Abstract

Breast cancer remission after treatment is sometimes long-lasting, but in about 30% of cases, there is a relapse after a so-called dormant state. Cellular cancer dormancy, the propensity of disseminated tumor cells (DTCs) to remain in a nonproliferative state for an extended period, presents an opportunity for therapeutic intervention that may prevent reawakening and the lethal consequences of metastatic outgrowth. Therefore, identification of dormant DTCs and detailed characterization of cancer cell-intrinsic and niche-specific [i.e., tumor microenvironment (TME) mediated] mechanisms influencing dormancy in different metastatic organs are of great importance in breast cancer. Several microenvironmental drivers of DTC dormancy in metastatic organs, such as the lung, bone, liver, and brain, have been identified using in vivo models and/or in vitro three-dimensional culture systems. TME induction and persistence of dormancy in these organs are mainly mediated by signals from immune cells, stromal cells, and extracellular matrix components of the TME. Alterations of the TME have been shown to reawaken dormant DTCs. Efforts to capitalize on these findings often face translational challenges due to limited availability of representative patient samples and difficulty in designing dormancy-targeting clinical trials. In this chapter, we discuss current approaches to identify dormant DTCs and provide insights into cell-extrinsic (i.e., TME) mechanisms driving breast cancer cell dormancy in distant organs.

Keywords

Dormancy · Quiescence · Breast cancer · Metastasis · Microenvironment · Niche · Disseminated tumor cells · Relapse

Evrim Ceren Kabak, Sok Lin Foo and Maria Rafaeva contributed equally with all other contributors.

E. C. Kabak
Laboratory of Tumor Heterogeneity, Metastasis and Resistance, Department of Biomedicine, University of Basel, University Hospital Basel, Basel, Switzerland

Department of Biomedicine, University Hospital Basel, University of Basel, Basel, Switzerland
e-mail: evrimceren.kabak@unibas.ch

S. L. Foo · M. Rafaeva · M. Bentires-Alj (✉)
Laboratory of Tumor Heterogeneity, Metastasis and Resistance, Department of Biomedicine, University of Basel, University Hospital Basel, Basel, Switzerland
e-mail: soklin.foo@unibas.ch; maria.rafaeva@unibas.ch; m.bentires-alj@unibas.ch

I. Martin
Department of Biomedicine, University Hospital Basel, University of Basel, Basel, Switzerland
e-mail: Ivan.Martin@usb.ch

T. Sørlie, R. B. Clarke (eds.), *A Guide to Breast Cancer Research*, Advances in Experimental Medicine and Biology 1464, https://doi.org/10.1007/978-3-031-70875-6_18

Key Points

- Clinical tumor latency is a dormant state of metastatic cancer cells (disseminated tumor cells) that is tightly influenced by cell-intrinsic and cell-extrinsic mechanisms.
- Dormant or quiescent cancer cells can be identified by a range of markers (e.g., NR2F1^{pos}, p27^{high}, Ki67^{neg}), failure to incorporate nucleotide analogs (e.g., BrdU, EdU), label retention (e.g., CFSE, PKH, DiL/DiD dyes, H2B-GFP TetON/OFF), or expression of fluorescent reporters (e.g., FUCCI, mVenus-p27K^{-}) in experimental models.
- Mechanisms of dormancy and reawakening in the lung, liver, bone, and brain depend on niche composition, with several of them being shared.
- Cell-extrinsic conditions associated with dormancy include environmental parameters (e.g., hypoxia, metabolites, stiffness), paracrine factors, long noncoding RNAs, and extracellular matrix proteins.

18.1 Introduction

Metastasis after apparently successful treatment of primary tumors is a critical threat in clinical oncology and the leading cause of cancer-related death among breast cancer (BC) patients. Clinical manifestation of metastasis differs between BC subtypes and can appear months to decades after the initial diagnosis. Hormone receptor (HR)-positive BCs, defined by expression of estrogen receptor (ER) and progesterone receptor (PR), tend to have a better prognosis than HR-negative BCs, which comprise triple-negative (TNBC) and HER2-positive BCs. HR-negative BCs generally recur within 2 years of surgery. In contrast, over half of HR-positive BCs recur at least 5 years after the initial diagnosis and primary tumor removal, with some cases extending beyond a two-decade timespan (Copson et al. 2013; Demicheli et al. 1996; Gomis and Gawrzak 2017; Pan et al. 2017; Pedersen et al. 2022). The long intervals before recurrence in BC are not congruent with the constant growth kinetics of cancer cells, which suggests a possible period of cancer dormancy in distant organs. Indeed, it was reported that circulating tumor cells (CTCs) can occur in BC patients without symptoms of disease up to 22 years after mastectomy (Meng et al. 2004). This prolonged latency again suggests a dormant stage of metastatic progression. Disseminated tumor cells (DTCs) arriving in distant organs either die, remain dormant, or readily form metastases. Strikingly, metastasis is diagnosed in certain organs more often than in others, depending on the BC subtype. Whereas TNBC and HER2-positive BC metastases are found more often in the brain and visceral organs such as the liver and lungs, ER-positive BC frequently develops metastases in bones, although in later stages they can be found in other organs (van Maaren et al. 2019). These observations raised the question of the selective factors and conditions within target organs that induce DTC dormancy versus overt metastases.

It has been proposed that a combination of cancer cell-intrinsic, cancer cell-extrinsic, and stochastic events contributes to the fate of DTCs. Cell-intrinsic mechanisms involve various cellular components, such as oncogenes, tumor suppressors, membrane proteins, signaling pathways, long noncoding RNAs, epithelial-mesenchymal transition (EMT) transcription factors, chromatin regulators, and mechanotransducers. Cell-extrinsic mechanisms, on the other hand, are a consequence of microenvironmental triggers such as stromal cells, extracellular matrix (ECM), immunosurveillance, or an angiogenic switch, as well as local biophysical and local or distant biochemical cues (Aguirre-Ghiso 2018; Montagner et al. 2020). Tumor dormancy at distant organs is the net effect of cell-intrinsic and cell-extrinsic mechanisms. Antineoplastic therapies (surgery, radiotherapy, chemotherapy, immunotherapy, hormonal therapy, and other more targeted therapies) may also drastically perturb not only the cancer cells but also the tumor microenvironment (TME). Antineoplastic therapies that target proliferating cells are a "double-edged sword": the proliferating cells are eliminated, but dormant cells resist therapy and may result in disease relapse and progression of an inexorable downhill course (Selli et al. 2019; Zhang et al. 2023; Zhao et al. 2023). Lifestyle (e.g., stress, smoking, diet, physical exercise) and biological (e.g., weight gain, aging, infections) factors may also contribute to the maintenance or reawakening of dormant cells, and their delineation is warranted. In this chapter, we review mechanisms regulating BC cell dormancy, focusing on crosstalk between dormant cancer cells and their de novo microenvironment.

18.2 Identification of Dormant DTCs

The clinical definition of dormancy is the prolonged period between primary tumor diagnosis and metastatic relapse at distant sites. This can occur at two levels: (i) cellular dormancy refers to a solitary cell or a small cluster of cells that survive in a quiescent, reversible, growth-arrested state for an extended period of time, and (ii) tumor mass dormancy refers to cancer cell proliferation that is offset by cell death due to immune surveillance and/or insufficient vascularization, such that there is no net change in cell number (Chambers et al. 2002; Fluegen et al. 2017; Ghajar 2015; Kang and Pantel 2013; Linde et al. 2016; Montagner and Sahai 2020; Phan and Croucher 2020; Polzer and Klein 2013).

Box 1

Here we offer guidance with a glossary of commonly used terms describing metastatic cancer cells:

DTCs (disseminated tumor cells)—cancer cells that infiltrate and survive at distant sites.

Quiescent DTCs—cancer cells in G0, cell cycle arrested. They may remain as such or resume proliferation due to a variety of cues. They share some features with senescent cells, and it is plausible that these cellular states transition in a quiescent-senescence continuum.

Dormant DTCs—cancer cells that can reversibly enter cell cycle progression from their prolonged quiescent state. They are often found as solitary cells.

Tumor mass dormancy—small cluster of cancer cells or micrometastases in equilibrium between cell proliferation and death.

Dormancy/latency (clinical)—the long lead time between treatment of the primary tumor and metastatic relapse at secondary sites.

Senescent DTCs—cancer cells that are nonreversibly (i.e., permanently) arrested in the G0 phase of the cell cycle. The permanence of arrest has been questioned by several recent studies. Senescence can be either oncogene-induced or therapy-induced and is driven mostly by a continuing DNA damage response.

Cancer stem cells (CSC)—this term was coined to describe tumorigenic cell subpopulations that (a) self-renew (i.e., form tumors when serially passaged at clonal cell doses) and (b) give rise to a new tumor that recapitulates the phenotypic heterogeneity of the parent tumor (Clarke and Fuller 2006; Kreso and Dick 2014).

To differentiate between dormant or other states of DTCs, a temporal characterization of the same cancer cell population is ideal but not necessary—a snapshot of marker expression (e.g., p27, Ki67) can provide information on a quiescent cell state that can be shown further to switch to proliferation following changes in microenvironmental cues.

While direct evidence for the existence of cellular or tumor mass dormancy in patients is lacking, several studies have detected DTCs in a solitary state in the bone marrow (BM) of BC patients with no evidence of metastatic disease (Borgen et al. 2018; Braun et al. 2000, 2005; Sanger et al. 2011), and the detection of DTCs in distant organs has been correlated with poor prognosis for many solid cancers (Braun et al. 2005; Pantel and Alix-Panabieres 2014). It is estimated that 30% of BC patients harbor DTCs at the time of cancer diagnosis (Braun et al. 2000; Sanger et al. 2011).

The dormancy status of patient-derived DTCs has been verified predominantly by the absence of markers of proliferation (i.e., Ki67, PCNA) and apoptosis (i.e., active caspases) (Akkoc et al. 2021; Clements and Johnson 2019; Fluegen et al. 2017). As Ki67 staining is positive in the nucleus at all phases of the cell cycle except in G0 arrest, Ki67^{neg} cells are considered nonproliferative. This suggests that, while Ki67 positivity identifies actively proliferating DTCs, Ki67 negativity may not accurately pinpoint dormant cells that are at the G0 and G0/G1 boundary (Borgen et al. 2018). In vitro and in vivo studies have also shown that a high activity ratio of the extracellular signal-regulated kinases ERK1/2 and p38 results in tumor growth and a low ratio corresponds to tumor dormancy (Gao et al. 2017). Moreover, an orphan nuclear receptor of the retinoic acid receptor family, Nuclear Receptor sub-

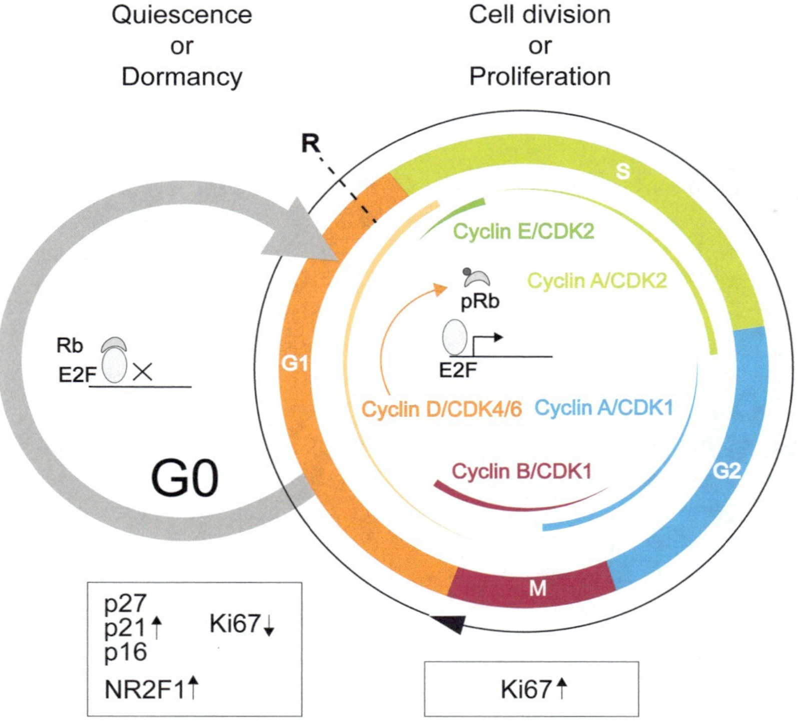

Fig. 18.1 Regulation of cell cycle progression and quiescent cell state. Cancer cell proliferation is regulated by CDKs, which form specific complexes with cyclins during different phases: Interphase—G1 (growth), S (replication), G2 (preparation); mitosis—M (cell division). This results in the transcription of certain genes and control of checkpoints/restriction: (R) point. In the G1 phase, the cyclin D/CDK4/6 complex hyperphosphorylates retinoblastoma susceptibility protein Rb, which then releases E2F transcriptional factor from the complex. In turn, E2F binds promoter regions of its targets, which results in mitosis (transcription of cyclin E and A, DNA polymerase, etc.). Proteins from INK4 (p16) and Cip/Kip (p21, p27) families are cyclin-CDK complex inhibitors in G0-early G1. Expression levels of certain proteins can be used to identify proliferative and quiescent cells—Ki67 increases during cell division, while p27, p21, p16, and NR2F1 increase in the quiescent state

family 2, group F, member 1 (NR2F1), was found upregulated in dormant DTCs in preclinical models and was used to stratify dormant DTCs in the BM of BC patients (Borgen et al. 2018). Patients with NR2F1^{high} DTCs experienced longer metastasis-free periods than patients with NR2F1^{low} DTCs. Further studies are required of NR2F1 as a potential marker for long-term quiescence (i.e., dormancy) in clinical settings, as this clinical study included only a limited number of patient samples, mainly within 3 years after diagnosis (Borgen et al. 2018).

Induction and maintenance of dormancy is a complex process mediated by intrinsic and extrinsic signaling mechanisms (Gomatou et al. 2021). Cell cycle arrest (G0) results from the activity of two families of cyclin-dependent kinase (CDK) inhibitors (CDKIs): (i) the inhibitor of the CDK 4 (INK4) family (i.e., p15, p16, p18, and p14ARF) at the beginning of entry into G1 and (ii) the Cip/Kip family (i.e., p21, p27, and p57), which impedes progression throughout the cell cycle. Increased p27 activity reduces the ability of CDKs to phosphorylate the retinoblastoma protein (Rb) (Fig. 18.1). In turn, hypophosphorylated Rb inhibits transcription factor E2F1, precluding expression of the target genes necessary for cell cycle progression. Hence, increased p27 expression is widely used as a marker of quiescence induction, and fluorescent p27 reporters are commonly used to track live cell entry and exit from quiescence (Oki et al. 2014). Fluorescent p21 reporters can also serve as a potential marker to identify and isolate quiescent cells. As p21 is also implicated in driving senescence, it is itself considered as a marker of senescent cells (Basu et al. 2022; Truskowski et al. 2023).

Numerous tools have been used to identify and isolate dormant DTCs. The nucleotide analog-based pulse-chase strategy is based on the incorporation of nucleotide analogs such as BrdU (5-bromo-2′-deoxyuridine) and EdU (5-ethynyl-2′-deoxyuridine) to pulse cancer cells in vitro or in vivo, followed by a chase phase, cell/tissue fixation, and staining with antibodies against BrdU or EdU. Proliferating cells exhibit high levels of incorporation of nucleotide analogs (i.e., BrdU or EdU), indicating ongoing DNA synthesis, whereas quiescent cells show low or no incorporation of the analogs (Basu et al. 2022). However, this technique precludes isolation of live quiescent DTCs for downstream analysis and functional studies due to the fixation step.

Label retention is one of the pulse-chase approaches that allows identification and purification of quiescent cells via fluorescent dyes that preferentially bind membrane or intracellular proteins (e.g., CellTrace or CFSE) or membrane lipids (e.g., PKH, DiD). While proliferating cells lose the fluorescent dyes, quiescent cells retain the label longer (Lawson et al. 2015; Regan et al. 2021; Yumoto et al. 2014). Inducible genetic systems (e.g., H2B-GFP Tet ON/OFF) for label retention assays have also been used to identify quiescent cells. H2B-GFP refers to a genetic construct in which the human histone H2B, a highly stable protein, is fused with a green fluorescent protein (GFP) and expressed (Tet ON) or suppressed (Tet OFF) under a doxycycline-inducible rtTA promoter. The H2B-GFP system enables identification of quiescent cells based on retention or loss of GFP fluorescence upon doxycycline treatment (Puig et al. 2018; Upadhaya et al. 2018).

An alternative approach is a fluorescent protein-based indicator system known as the fluorescent ubiquitination-based cell cycle indicator (FUCCI), which was developed to visualize and identify cell cycle phases of cells in real time (Sakaue-Sawano et al. 2008; Yano et al. 2020). In this system, G1 phase-specific proteolysis of Geminin and S/G2/M phase-specific proteolysis of Cdt1 are monitored using two different probes that consist of fusion proteins between the degrons of Geminin and Cdt1 and the fluorescent proteins. The FUCCI system differentially labels cells in G1 and those in S/G2/M, effectively allowing visualization of G1-S and M-G1 transitions (Oki et al. 2014). This system has led to increased understanding of the control of cancer dormancy, mainly by combining the probe with live-imaging techniques such as intravital imaging (Ohta et al. 2022; Yano et al. 2020). Although it has great potential for analyzing DTCs in a spatiotemporal manner, the system does not distinguish cells in G0 from those in G1, due to mutual expression of Cdt1 in both phases of the cycle (Basu et al. 2022).

18.3 Preconditions for Dormancy at Metastatic Sites

18.3.1 Regulation of Dormancy at the Primary Tumor Site

The initial step of metastatic seeding starts in the primary tumor, when cancer cells enter the blood and/or lymphatic vessels as a result of stromal invasion and intravasation. As this process can occur at early stages of tumor growth, it is plausible that the dormant or proliferative fates of DTCs may be primed by the TME at the primary site (Husemann et al. 2008). This is exemplified by increased expression of the dormancy marker NR2F1 and the stem cell/self-renewal marker SOX9 in cancer cells upon interaction with Tie2^{high} macrophages and blood vessel endothelial cells in the tumor. Subsequently, 40% of lung solitary DTCs originating from these tumors were double-positive, and expression of NR2F1 and SOX9 ceased in overt metastases. Consistently, downregulation of NR2F1 in cancer cells increased the number of metastatic foci in both spontaneous and experimental metastasis models (Borriello et al. 2022).

Other factors in the TME, such as hypoxia (i.e., decreased oxygen supply) due to undeveloped vasculature, also result in upregulation of dormancy markers in cancer cells. For instance, high levels of HIF1α/GLUT1 correlate significantly with upregulation of the dormancy markers NR2F1 and p27 (Fluegen et al. 2017). Furthermore, when cancer cells were exposed to normoxia or to hypoxia in vitro or in the chick chorioallantoic membrane (CAM) assay before being injected intravenously into mice, significantly more cells were retained in a dormant state in the lungs post-hypoxia compared to normoxia exposure. These results indicate the possible influence of the primary tumor TME in priming DTCs either by cell-cell interactions or by biochemical cues.

18.3.2 Regulation of Dormancy at Distant Sites by Systemic Factors

Tumor development inevitably has a systemic influence on distant organs of the body in which DTCs encounter compatible niches. Tumor-secreted factors such as cytokines and exosomes in the bloodstream can modify the microenvironment of distant organs (Baumann et al. 2022). Standard-of-care surgical removal of primary breast tumors was long considered to have a systemic effect on the body that may result in metastatic outbreaks. Earlier studies suggested the concept of "concomitant resistance," a biological situation wherein a growing primary tumor suppresses the growth of metastases. Several mechanisms have been proposed to explain this phenomenon (Galmarini et al. 2014): (i) the presence of the primary tumor triggers a specific immune response that, although not sufficient to effectively inhibit the primary tumor growth, can impede progression of smaller metastases (Franco et al. 1996); (ii) secretion by the primary tumor of antiangiogenic factors, such as thrombospondin (TSP), angiostatin or endostatin, inhibits vascularization and thus the growth of metastases (O'Reilly et al. 1994); (iii) the majority of essential nutrients for growth are used up by primary tumor metabolism, which starves metastases. The secretion from primary tumors of metabolic by-products such as *meta*-tyrosine and *ortho*-tyrosine, as a result of high metabolic activity, inhibits the mitogen-activated protein kinase (MAPK) pathway and inactivates signal transducer and activator of transcription 3 (STAT3), thereby inducing dormancy in DTCs at secondary sites (Ruggiero et al. 2012; Ruggiero et al. 2011). Moreover, removal of primary tumors in mice induced a wound-healing reaction, led to a systemic inflammatory response with the recruitment of myeloid cells (increased neutrophils and Ly6C^{high} monocytes in the blood), and increased metastases. Treatment with a perioperative nonsteroidal anti-inflammatory drug such as meloxicam mitigated this risk experimentally (Krall et al. 2018). Thus, suppression of inflammatory responses at the time of primary tumor removal may prevent reawakening of covert dormant DTCs. Clinical assessment of such a possibility is eagerly awaited.

18.4 Organ-Specific Regulation of Dormancy and Metastases

18.4.1 Lung-Specific Regulation

In the early 1900s, James Ewing proposed an alternative theory to Stephen Paget's "seed (DTCs) and soil (niches)" (1889) theory on organ-specific metastasis. Ewing suggested that physiological blood flow patterns solely regulate organ-specific metastasis. Anatomical and histological characteristics of certain organs, such as the lung, support Ewing's theory, especially in the case of BC (Akhtar et al. 2019; Ribatti et al. 2006). The lung is the first significant capillary bed that BC cells encounter after entering the bloodstream. Furthermore, 60–70% of metastatic BC patients who did not survive were diagnosed with lung metastasis (Liu et al. 2017). Growing evidence has shown that the two theories are complementary (Chambers et al. 2002; Chambers et al. 2000; Fidler 2001; Hart 1982; Massague and Obenauf 2016; Weiss et al. 1988; Wirtz et al. 2011). Although extravasation into lung tissue may occur easily, the transition of DTCs to micrometastases and progression to macrometastases (i.e., colonization) are a rate-limiting step that relies on the interaction between Paget's "seed" and "soil."

4T1 and 4T07 cells originated from a cell line (410) that was generated from a spontaneous metastatic nodule in the lung of immunocompetent BALB/c mice bearing a mammary tumor, and D2A1 and D2.OR cells were derived from murine mammary tumor D2 hyperplastic alveolar nodules of BALB/c mice. These cell lines are commonly used models in studies of mammary tumor dormancy in mice (Aslakson and Miller 1992; Morris et al. 1993). Once injected into the mammary fat pad of syngeneic BALB/c mice, these cells may further disseminate to the lungs. 4T1 and D2A1 cells form lung macrometastases, while 4T07 and D2.OR do not, despite being detectable in secondary organs such as the lung, at least within the time frame of the reported experiment (Aslakson and Miller 1992; Morris et al. 1993; Tallon de Lara et al. 2021). Thus, these cell lines are attractive for the study of dormancy.

Barkan et al. (2008) showed that mammary or BC cell lines that were either dormant (D2.OR and MCF-7) or proliferative (D2A1 and MDA-MB-231) in vivo proliferated similarly in a two-dimensional (2D) culture. In contrast, cells that were dormant in vivo remained in cell cycle arrest when cultured in 3D, as portrayed by elevated expression of p27 and p16. This highlights the relevance of 3D culture systems. They also showed that in activation from a dormant to a proliferative state, cancer cells rely on expression of fibronectin signaling through β1 integrin and the phosphorylation of myosin light chain (MLC) by MLC kinase (MLCK). This results in cytoskeletal reorganization with actin stress-fiber formation. When β1 integrin or MLCK was inhibited, the cells did not undergo transition from a quiescent to a proliferative state in vitro. Importantly, inhibition of MLCK also significantly reduced lung metastases. These findings indicate that the switch from dormancy to metastatic outgrowth may be epigenetically influenced downstream of signals emanating from the microenvironment (Barkan et al. 2008). Subsequent studies by Barkan et al. (2010) showed that induction of fibrosis, associated with deposition of type I collagen (COL-1), in the metastatic microenvironment could reawaken dormant DTCs and result in lung metastases. Using a 3D culture dormancy model, they demonstrated that the proliferative response to COL-1 is mediated through β1 integrin and requires Src and focal adhesion kinase (FAK) activation, ERK-dependent MLC phosphorylation by MLCK, and actin stress-fiber formation (Barkan et al. 2010).

Having previously discovered that changing the TME by induction of fibrosis with collagen and fibronectin deposition can reawaken dormant DTCs, Green's group used both in vivo and 3D in vitro models to examine the effect of Src family kinases (SFK) on this process. They found that inhibition of SFK signaling or reducing Src expression led to nuclear localization of p27, which prevented reawakening of dormant cells and formation of metastatic lesions. As SFK inhibition did not kill the dormant cells, since cell proliferation required activation of ERK1/2, The authors showed that a combination of SFK (AZD0530) and MEK1/2 (AZD6244) inhibitors induced apoptosis in tumor cells undergoing the dormant-to-proliferative switch and so delayed metastasis. This suggests that targeting SFK can prevent the COL-1-induced proliferative switch in dormant tumor cells and combining SFK inhibition with MEK1/2 inhibition may prevent BC recurrence (El Touny et al. 2014).

The microenvironment in the lung has also been shown to impact the dormant phenotype of DTCs. Using a gain-of-function cDNA screen, Gao et al. (2012) identified COCO (also known as DAND5), the antagonist for bone morphogenetic protein (BMP), as a potent mediator of dormancy reawakening through inhibition of lung-derived BMP. They also showed that COCO mediates organ-specific metastasis to the lung but not to the bone or to the brain, as the stroma in the lung contains high levels of bioactive BMP proteins. Their findings further suggest that BMP4 induces dormancy by repressing the two key cancer stem cell traits: self-renewal (as shown in vitro) and tumor initiation. While the study did not investigate the angiocrine source of BMP4, it is noteworthy that the dormant cells in this study were found exclusively on the lung microvasculature (Gao et al. 2012). Substantiating Gao's findings, autocrine BMP4 signaling by lung endothelium was subsequently shown in another study to induce lung-specific, calcineurin/NFATc1-dependent TSP1 expression, which is essential for alveolar lineage-specific bronchioalveolar stem cell differentiation (Lee et al. 2014).

Similarly, using murine and zebrafish models, as well as organotypic microvascular niches comprised of human cells, Ghajar et al. (2013) discovered that dormant DTCs originating from BC can exist close to the lung microvasculature. They also found that the microvasculature is a stable niche that sustains DTC quiescence through the endothelial-derived TSP1. However, this suppressive cue of TSP1 is lost in sprouting neovasculature, characterized by increased expression of pro-tumorigenic factors such as periostin (POSTN) and transforming growth factor-beta 1 (TGF-β1), which activate dormant DTCs and metastases (Ghajar et al. 2013).

Dormant DTCs in the lungs were shown to be influenced by interactions with epithelial cells, in particular alveolar type 1 (AT1) cells. AT1 cells can support the survival of D2.OR cells while inhibiting AT2 cells-induced proliferation. This interaction promotes the formation of fibronectin fibrils by dormant cells that trigger integrin-dependent pro-survival signals. RNA sequencing and dropout screening by Montagner et al. (2020) identified secreted frizzled-related protein 2 (SFRP2) as a pro-survival gene for dormant DTCs in the lungs. Interestingly, AT1 cells induce Sfrp2 expression in dormant DTCs, which in turn promotes deposition of fibronectin fibrils and mediates the formation of cellular protrusions, hence stimulating different signaling pathways important for DTC survival (Montagner et al. 2020).

One study used syngeneic ER-positive mouse models to assess DTCs in young and aged lungs or fibrotic microenvironments. Through transcriptional profiling, the study identified the platelet-derived growth factor C (PDGFC) as a crucial factor that is upregulated in aged and fibrotic lungs. This PDGFC^{high} environment promotes DTC proliferation and upregulates tumor cell *Pdgfc* expression, which leads to the accumulation of activated fibroblasts (i.e., high for PDGFRα) and increased metastatic outgrowth. Intriguingly, the expression of PDGF by disseminated ER-positive tumor cells in young mice in a PDGFC^{low} microenvironment was essential for the survival of DTCs. This highlights the potential of targeting PDGFC signaling to reduce the recurrence of ER-positive BC (Turrell et al. 2023). Pharmacological inhibition of PDGFRα or the PDGFC blocking antibody prevented reawakening of dormant cells, but whether it can also reduce established metastases remains to be tested. Nevertheless, interfering with this pathway may be relevant for halting metastases in high-risk patients.

Several studies have suggested that a pre-inflamed microenvironment in the lungs can enhance subsequent colonization by DTCs. Exploring an alternative scenario in which DTCs arrive in an initially normal lung microenvironment and thereafter experience pro-inflammatory signals, De Cock et al. (2016) showed that the inflamed tissue microenvironment released signals that spawn an EMT program in dormant DTCs and leads to active proliferation and metastases. They showed that tumor cells retrieved from lipopolysaccharide (LPS)-induced lung metastases expressed elevated levels of TWIST and ZEB1 EMT transcription factors. This finding is consistent with the causal association between the EMT program and metastatic outgrowth. As neutrophils are recruited in large numbers to the lungs following LPS treatment, and LPS activates neutrophils via toll-like receptor 4 signaling, the study further suggested that neutrophils facilitate LPS-induced metastatic outgrowth (De Cock et al. 2016).

It was also proposed that inflammation-evoked recruitment and activation of neutrophils resulted in neutrophil extracellular traps (NETs) that contributed to the reawakening of dormant DTCs in the lungs. Mechanistically, the data suggested that NET-associated proteases (matrix metalloproteinase 9 (MMP-9) and neutrophil elastase) remodeled the ECM by cleaving laminin and revealing an epitope that triggered proliferation of dormant DTCs through integrin activation and FAK/ERK/MLCK/YAP signaling (Albrengues et al. 2018).

Cancer progression is significantly influenced by interactions between cancer cells and the immune system. Using high-parametric single-cell profiling, Tallon de Lara et al. (2021) found a higher number of $CD39^{pos}$ $PD\text{-}1^{pos}$ $CD8^{pos}$ T cells in 4T07 tumors than in 4T1 tumors. They also showed that immunotherapy with anti-PD-1 reduced the number of 4T07 DTCs in the lungs in an orthotopic model, while adoptive transfer of purified $CD39^{pos}$ $PD\text{-}1^{pos}$ $CD8^{pos}$ T cells prevented metastatic outgrowth of intravenously injected 4T07 cells. In human BC, the frequency of $CD39^{pos}$ $PD\text{-}1^{pos}$ $CD8^{pos}$ T cells, but not the total $CD8^{pos}$ T cells, correlated with delayed metastatic relapse after tumor removal, emphasizing the significance of this population in BC progression. Furthermore, blocking antibodies revealed that dormancy conferred by $CD39^{pos}$ $PD\text{-}1^{pos}$ $CD8^{pos}$ T cells relied on tumor necrosis factor (TNF)-α and interferon (IFN)-γ (Tallon de Lara et al. 2021). For a summary of lung-specific cancer cell dormancy mechanisms, see Fig. 18.2 and Table 18.1.

18.4.2 Bone-Specific Regulation

DTCs are frequently found in the bone marrow (BM) of BC patients, including patients with no evidence of metastasis. The presence of DTCs in BM aspirates correlated with poor clinical outcomes, highlighting the importance of DTC detection for clinical decision-making (Braun et al. 2005).

The BM is home to hematopoietic stem cells (HSCs), which undergo tightly controlled differentiation and proliferation during hematopoiesis. HSCs reside in specialized niches within the BM without a defined spatial arrangement. These specialized niches, including the perivascular niche and endosteal niche, harbor and maintain the fate of HSCs (Muscarella et al. 2021). Growing evidence indicates that DTCs localized in these niches integrate microenvironmental signals that mediate dormancy and survival (Fig. 18.2) (Ghajar et al. 2013; Price et al. 2016).

The BM is a particularly permissive environment for cancer cell extravasation due to the presence of sinusoidal capillary beds with fenestrated endothelium (Azevedo et al. 2015). To address how DTCs traffic into the BM, Price et al. (2016) used intravital imaging of BM in a BC xenograft model and showed that dormant DTCs are predominantly localized in perisinusoidal vascular regions rich in E-selectin and stromal cell-derived factor 1 (SDF-1), also known as CXCL12. Using inhibitors of E-selectin and C-X-C chemokine receptor type 4 (CXCR4) (i.e., SDF-1 receptor), they demonstrated that E-selectin interactions are critical for DTC entry into the BM, while the SDF-1/CXCR4 interaction anchors DTCs to the microenvironment. The clinical relevance of these findings was examined by analysis of

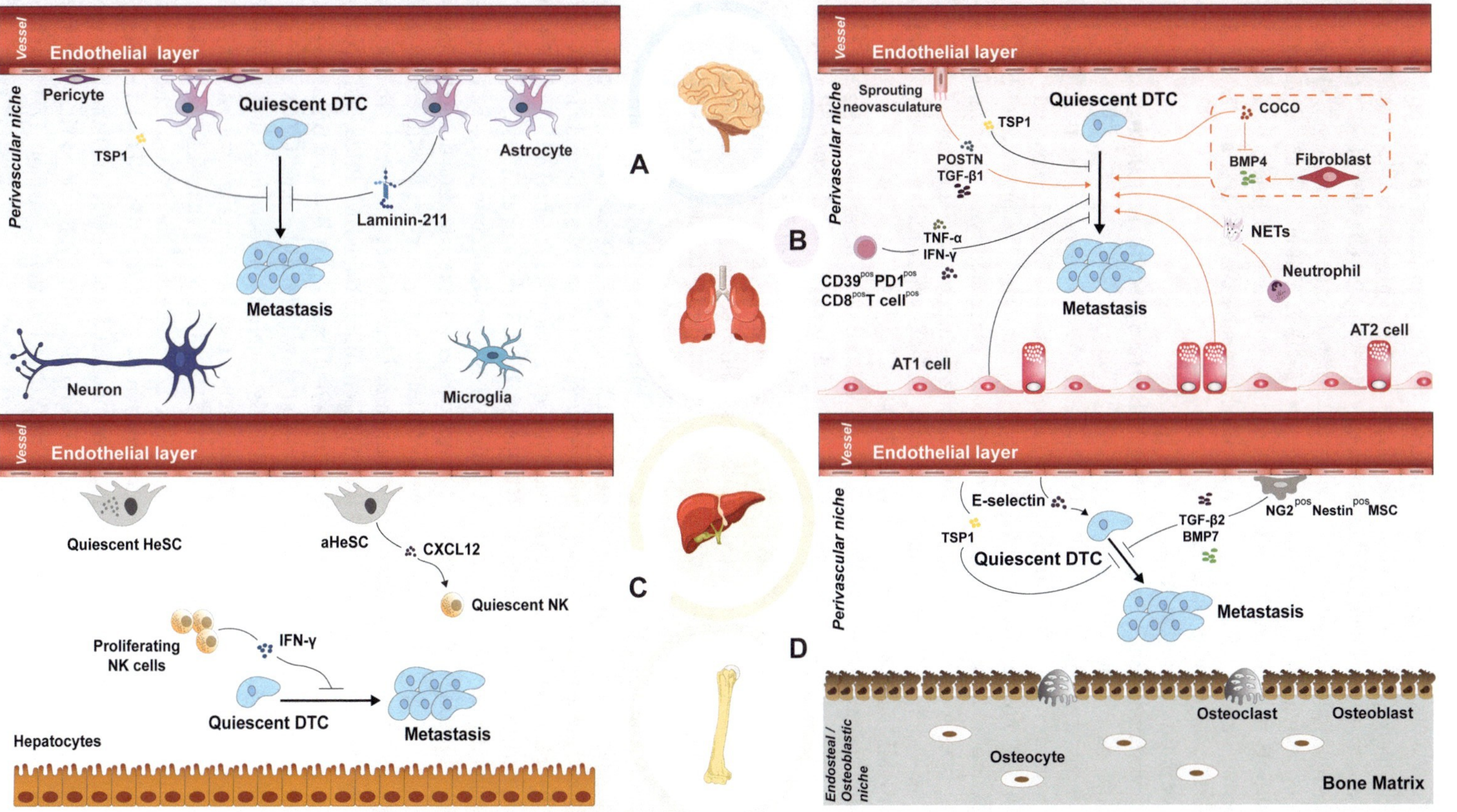

Fig. 18.2 Cell-extrinsic mechanisms controlling DTC dormancy and reawakening (i.e., metastases) in distant organs. (**a**) In the brain, astrocyte-deposited laminin-211 and endothelial-derived TSP1 induce BC DTC dormancy. (**b**) In the lung, BC DTC-secreted COCO, inflammation-induced NETs, and sprouting vasculature-secreted POSTN and TGF-ß1 stimulate metastatic outgrowth, while TNF-α and IFN-γ secreted by CD39^{pos} PD-1^{pos} CD8^{pos} T cells and endothelial-derived TSP1 sustain BC DTC dormancy. (**c**) In the liver, NK cells control BC DTC dormancy through IFN-γ secretion, while activated HeSCs enhance metastases by decreasing the proliferation of NK cells through CXCL12. (**d**) In the bone, E-selectin secreted by endothelial cells contributes to BC DTC proliferation, while endothelial-derived TSP1 and NG2^{pos} Nestin^{pos} MSC-derived TGF-β2 and BMP7 maintain dormancy of DTCs

Table 18.1 Summary of the studies which identified factors inducing breast cancer cell dormancy in metastatic organs

Category	Factor	Source	Metastatic site	Model (in vivo/in vitro)	References
Paracrine factors	BMP4	Epithelial and mesenchymal cells in lung niche	Lung	In vivo	Gao et al. (2012)
	BMP7	NG2^{pos} Nestin^{pos} MSC	Bone	In vivo	Nobre et al. (2021)
	DKK1	Sox2/9 high DTC	Lung	In vivo, in vitro	Malladi et al. (2016)
	E-selectin	Endothelial cells	Bone	In vivo	Price et al. (2016)
	IFN-γ	NK cells	Liver	In vivo	Correia et al. (2021)
	SFRP2	Dormant DTC	Lung	In vivo	Montagner et al. (2020)
	TGF-β2	NG2^{pos} Nestin^{pos} MSC	Bone	In vivo	Nobre et al. (2021)
lncRNA	NR2F1-AS-1 (NAS-1)	Dormant mesenchymal-like BC stem cell-like cells	Lung	In vivo	Liu et al. (2021)
ECM factors	Laminin-111, laminin-211, laminin-411, laminin-511	Perivascular niche	Lung	In vivo, in vitro	Albrengues et al. (2018)
	Laminin-211	Astrocytes	Brain	In vivo	Dai et al. (2022)
	TSP1	Endothelial cells	Lung, bone, brain	In vivo	Ghajar et al. (2013)

patient BM samples. This revealed that nonproliferative Ki67^{neg} DTCs are more likely to be found adjacent to sinusoids within the perivascular niche than to the endosteal surface (Price et al. 2016). An integrin-mediated interaction between DTCs, the von Willebrand factor (vWF), and vascular cell adhesion molecule 1 (VCAM1) was found to reduce the effect of chemotherapy on DTCs in the perivascular niche of the BM. Disrupting these interactions with integrin-blocking antibodies reduced DTC burden and prevented bone metastasis. Moreover, inhibiting β1 integrin and/or αVβ3 integrin sensitized DTCs to chemotherapy (Carlson et al. 2019).

BM mesenchymal stromal cells (MSCs) have been shown to enhance DTC dormancy in different ways. For example, secretion of MSC-derived exosomes consisting of distinct miRNA, such as miR222/miR223, induces tumor dormancy and therapy resistance in vitro (Bliss et al. 2016). Bartosh et al. (2016) generated 3D coculture spheroids using the hanging drop approach to recapitulate the cellular interactions of MSCs with MDA-MB-231 cancer cells (Bartosh 2017). They observed that MSCs sequentially surrounded the cancer cells, promoted the formation of cancer spheroids, and were internalized through a process known as cancer cell cannibalism. The cannibalism of MSCs enhanced survival of cancer cells deprived of nutrients and suppressed tumorigenicity, suggesting that the cancer cells entered dormancy.

A recent study from Aguirre-Ghiso's group revealed that periarteriolar BM-resident NG2^{pos} Nestin^{pos} MSCs enhance DTC dormancy by producing TGF-β2 and BMP7 and activating a quiescence pathway mediated by p38 and p27 via TGF-β receptor 3 (TGFBR3) and bone morphogenetic protein receptor type 2 (BMPR2). Genetic depletion of MSCs or a conditional knockout of TGF-β2 in MSCs using an NG2-CreER driver enhanced metastasis of otherwise dormant p27^{pos} Ki67^{neg} DTCs. Interestingly, NG2^{pos} Nestin^{pos} MSCs have also been shown to promote HSC quiescence in BM, suggesting that HSC dormancy niches may also control DTC dormancy (Nobre et al. 2021).

The endosteal niche is adjacent to the endosteum, which consists of primitive osteoblast-lineage cells such as MSCs and bone-lining cells (i.e., osteoblasts, osteocytes, and macrophages). The effect of osteoblasts in BC dormancy is more complex and depends on the dynamic remodeling capacity of the endosteal niche, which could induce proliferation of DTCs (Risson et al. 2020). Indeed, Zhang's group showed that osteoblast-lineage cells residing in the endosteal niche promote proliferation and early-stage localization of DTCs in BM. In the ex vivo osteogenic niche, luminal DTCs form heterotypic adherens-type junctions with osteoblast progenitors and osteoblasts, with E-cadherin on the cancer cell side and N-cadherin on the mesenchymal cell side. As the niche develops and the metastatic lesion progresses, the DTCs become enclosed by osteoblast-lineage cells, which leads to the development of functional gap junctions between the two cell types. DTCs are inefficient at absorbing calcium from the matrix, but those that receive calcium flux from osteogenic cells via the newly formed gap junctions have a growth advantage through mTOR signaling. Disruption of cadherins, gap junctions, or mTOR signaling decreases DTC colonization in the BM (Wang et al. 2018). Moreover, interaction of BC cells with osteoblasts or BM cells enhanced interleukin-1 beta (IL-1β) secretion by all cell types, resulting in expansion of the endosteal niche and cancer cell proliferation (Eyre et al. 2019; Tulotta et al. 2019). The results suggest that an endosteal niche partially influences the dormancy status of DTCs. However, it remains elusive how the signals from the endosteal surface impact individual DTCs and whether this depends on the precise cellular composition of the occupied endosteal niche (Clements and Johnson 2019). As DTCs are often preferentially home to HSC niches, their dormant or proliferative status is highly dependent on the microenvironmental cues in these environments. Nevertheless, no direct competition between BC cells and HSC niches has been reported to date.

BC metastasis to the BM is a frequent occurrence in ER-positive BC during late relapse. Using in vivo genome-wide short hairpin RNA screening, Gawrzak et al. (2018) identified the mitogen- and stress-activated kinase 1 (MSK1) as a potential inducer of metastatic dormancy in BC. Depletion of MSK1 in cancer cells down-regulated genes such as FOXA1 and GATA3 and increased metastasis-initiating potential (Gawrzak et al. 2018).

Another important aspect in DTC dormancy regulation is the effect of aging on the bone TME and DTCs (Risson et al. 2020; Singh et al. 2019). Age-associated changes in the bone secretome enhance proliferation of DTCs, HSCs, and MSCs (Singh et al. 2019). These studies revealed that PDGF signaling triggered bone-specific expansion of pericytes via remodeling of specialized type H blood vessels after therapy. On the contrary, reduction of blood flow inhibited pericyte expansion and endothelial PDGFB expression, which led to metastatic outgrowth and sensitization of proliferative cancer cells to radiation and chemotherapy (Fane and Weeraratna 2020; Singh et al. 2019). For a summary of the bone-specific cancer cell dormancy mechanisms, see Fig. 18.2 and Table 18.1.

Preclinical studies suggest that the bone microenvironment not only harbors a high number of DTCs but also facilitates metastasis of BC cells into multiple secondary organs. Using intra-iliac artery cell injection and an evolving barcoding system, it was proposed that epigenetic reprogramming promotes the metastatic bone microenvironment, which imparts stem cell-like properties to cancer cells that had disseminated from bone lesions to other organs (Kalhor et al. 2017; Yu et al. 2016). Additionally, they discovered that enhanced EZH2 activity is responsible for increased stemness and metastatic capacity. While this study revealed the impact of the bone microenvironment on the evolution of metastasis, the timing of the secondary metastasis that spread out of the initial bone lesions remained unanswered. Addressing this question experimentally and assessing its relevance in patients will determine the optimal therapeutic interventions in the adjuvant or metastatic setting (Zhang et al. 2021).

18.4.3 Liver-Specific Regulation

Ex vivo 3D microphysiological systems (MPSs) have been used to mimic the microenvironment, matrix, and cellular composition, as well as nutrient and gas flow of the metastatic niche. One such system, developed by Wheeler et al. (2014), is a human ex vivo hepatic MPS called LiverChip (Wheeler et al. 2014). The LiverChip was established with fresh human hepatocytes and non-parenchymal cells (NPCs), comprising endothelial, stromal, and immune cells, to create a TME with MCF-7 and MDA-MB-231 BC cell lines. This coculture system recapitulated some features of hepatic tissue, such as expression of liver-specific proteins and drug metabolism. They also showed that BC cells intercalate into the hepatic niche without interfering with hepatocyte activity, and a significant proportion of the cancer cells enter a quiescent state. However, the presence of NPCs altered the growth of MCF-7 and MDA-MB-231 cells in the hepatic niche, wherein the number of MDA-MB-231 cells was reduced but the number of MCF-7 cells increased. Analysis of cytokines, chemokines, and growth factors from LiverChip with NPC inclusion revealed that altered soluble signaling factors were involved in both the attenuation and outgrowth of the cancer cells. The lower number of MDA-MB-231 cells was associated with increased levels of follistatin and soluble HER2 (i.e., found in culture medium) as well as decreased levels of pro-inflammatory cytokines (e.g., IGFBP-1, MCP-1, MIP-1α, and IL-6) and cancer-promoting factors (e.g., uPA, osteopontin, EGF). Conversely, the increased number of MCF-7 cells was associated with elevated levels of cancer-promoting factors (e.g., osteopontin, soluble HER2, VEGF-A, uPA, and EGF) and pro-inflammatory cytokines (IL-6 and MCP-1). Nevertheless, the significance of these secreted factors for cancer cells remains to be investigated (Wheeler et al. 2014).

In a follow-up study, Clark et al. (2017) compared a LiverChip with softer PEGDa-SynKRGD hydrogel scaffolds that had a different interface with the tissue to the previously used LiverChip with polystyrene scaffolds. They incorporated donor-matched primary human hepatocytes and NPCs with MDA-MB-231 cancer cells to study the effect of matrix stiffness-induced inflammation on the occurrence of spontaneous dormancy in the ex vivo models. They showed that polystyrene-supported LiverChip treated with chemotherapies such as doxorubicin or cisplatin resulted in a dose-dependent elimination of the cancer cells. However, a differential response to chemotherapeutic treatment was observed in LiverChip using a softer hydrogel-based tissue interface with fibronectin-binding motifs. High doses of chemotherapy were minimally effective against the predominantly dormant MDA-MB-231 cancer cells. Interestingly, lower doses of chemotherapies seemed to induce proliferation (reawakening) of MDA-MB-231 cells. These findings highlight the importance of both mechanical and biochemical signals from the ECM in cancer cell dormancy (Clark et al. 2017).

CXCR3 ligands, CXCL9/10(IP-10)/11, have been implicated in several infectious and chronic diseases. In BC, the levels of IP-10 were highest in patients with TNBC and were correlated with shortened survival of patients with metastatic disease. Based on the significant increase in CXCR3 ligands, especially IP-10, during inflammation in the gut-liver MPS, Clark et al. (2021) further explored the effect of CXCR3 ligands in BC liver metastasis (Clark et al. 2021). Using a complex ex vivo all-human liver MPS model of dormant-emergent metastatic progression, they showed that CXCR3 ligands were significantly elevated in actively proliferating populations of MDA-MB-231 cancer cells but remained at levels like those of the tumor-free hepatic niche in populations with dormant MDA-MB-231 cancer cells. Stimulation of dormant MDA-MB-231 cancer cells with IP-10 in the ex vivo metastatic liver MPS model triggered their reawakening in a dose-dependent manner. However, when MDA-MB-231 cells were cultured alone (i.e., in the absence of the hepatic niche) and exposed to exogenous IP-10, no significant effect on the migratory, invasive, or proliferative behavior was observed. This implies that reawakening of cancer cells occurred indirectly, possibly via activation of the resident liver cells in the microenvironment (Clark et al. 2021).

Although much progress has been made in identifying genes and phenomena associated with BC metastasis to the liver, studies on BC dormancy in the liver remain scarce. Chemokines, such as IL-8 secreted by the hepatic stellate cells (HeSCs), and exosomes in the hepatic niche have been reported to either promote or halt the proliferation of BC cells in 2D coculture and MPS (Dioufa et al. 2017; Khazali et al. 2018). Using a spontaneous metastasis model of TNBC, our laboratory reported that cancer cells occupied different areas of the liver and existed as macrometastases or single quiescent cells. Transcriptomic analyses of the dormancy-associated milieus indicated an enrichment of genes related to a natural killer (NK) cell-mediated response. Indeed, the number and percentage of NK cells showed a descending gradient from the dormancy-associated stroma followed by stroma from tumor-free mice to the lowest in macrometastases-associated stroma. Depleting NK cells in mice bearing dormant DTCs increased the metastatic burden, while expanding them with IL-15 treatments in tumor-bearing mice reduced metastases. Moreover, the chemokine CXCL12 secreted by activated HeSCs decreased the proliferation of NK cells and contributed to metastatic outgrowth. Mechanistically, the study showed that NK cells influence BC dormancy in the liver by secretion of IFN-γ (Correia et al. 2021). These studies suggest that therapies aimed at normalizing the NK cell pool may prevent metastatic outgrowth in patients that present a high risk of relapse. Testing this interesting possibility is warranted. Moreover, our findings revive clinical interest in the use of CXCR4 inhibitors in the treatment of patients with cancer but suggest their application at earlier stages to prevent progression of dormant disease.

While most studies investigating BC dormancy in the liver have focused on TNBC models, it might be clinically relevant to determine whether ER-positive BC cells homing to the liver undergo the same dynamics, given that approximately 50% of ER-positive BC patients develop metastases in the liver (Chien et al. 2022). Moreover, a higher prevalence of liver metastases was found in patients with estrogen receptor 1 (ESR1) mutations. Nevertheless, the significance of these mutations in BC dormancy in the liver remains to be elucidated. For a summary of the liver-specific cancer cell dormancy mechanisms, see Fig. 18.2 and Table 18.1.

18.4.4 Brain-Specific Regulation

Among patients with metastatic BC, brain metastasis occurs in 32% of TNBC and 31% of HER2-positive subtypes but only in 15% of the ER-positive subtype (Kuksis et al. 2021). Outgrowth of metastases to a detectable size often occurs late in disease progression, when patients had other metastases diagnosed and were systemically treated. The brain is a highly compartmentalized organ, and metastasis can progress either in the parenchyma or in the leptomeninges layers covering the brain exposed to the cerebrospinal fluid circulation (Srinivasan et al. 2021). Mechanisms of dormancy in the brain are poorly understood and may include regulation both by the primary tumor and the local microenvironment. Using cellular iron oxide labeling visualized by magnetic resonance imaging (MRI), it was reported that the presence of MDA-MB-231 parental primary tumors in mice reduced brain metastases formed by intracardiac injection of MDA-MB-231-BR brain-tropic cells compared to tumor-lacking mice (Hamilton et al. 2016). Yet, the underlying mechanism remains undefined.

Cancer cells that colonize the brain are those that cross the blood-brain barrier-enforced capillaries, e.g., by MMP-9, neuropeptide substance P, and cathepsin S secretion that remodel the endothelial layer (Karreman et al. 2023; Rodriguez et al. 2014; Sevenich et al. 2014). They are then exposed to glial cells, primarily astrocytes, which results in a reactive state called gliosis that isolates metastasis from the normal tissue. Astrocytes secrete plasmin, which can cause either cancer cell death by a paracrine FasL signal or inactivate the L1CAM molecule that is important for the initial spreading of cancer cells along the vasculature. Anti-plasminogen activator serpins are secreted by surviving cancer cells (Valiente et al. 2014). Interaction of extravasated DTCs via the dystroglycan receptor with astrocyte-deposited laminin-211 suppresses their proliferation by downstream recruitment of YAP in the cytoplasm. In outgrowing metastasis, astrocytes endfeet were stripped from DTC-associated vessels (Dai et al. 2022). How this step emerges and whether other contacts with the ECM are important in this phenomenon remain unclear.

An astrocyte-evoked inflammatory response can also be pro-tumorigenic. Astrocytes cocultured with cancer cells increase IFN type I signaling (IFN-α,-β) and secrete C-C Motif Chemokine Ligand 2 (CCL2), which in turn recruits monocytic myeloid cells and fosters metastatic outgrowth (Ma et al. 2023). The presence of cancer cells can potentially reprogram populations of astrocytes, like the $STAT3^{pos}$ astrocytes discovered by Priego et al. (2018) that suppress $CD8^{pos}$ T cells and result in expansion of $CD74^{pos}$ macrophages/microglia and support of metastasis formation (Priego et al. 2018). Importantly, the brain niche has a metabolically different environment from other organs, where cancer cells compete with neurons for glucose. HER2-positive DTCs were found to remain dormant if they take up glutamine instead of glucose and maintain cellular redox homeostasis through the anionic amino acid transporter xCT. In contrast, aggressive cancer cells that form metastases were found to take up glucose and secrete lactate, which suppressed clustering and cytotoxicity of NK cells (Parida et al. 2022). Therefore, cell-intrinsic regulation of cancer cells can also mediate changes in the brain microenvironment favoring the switch from dormancy to metastasis. Other potential mechanisms involved in brain metastasis include vascular co-option and angiogenesis; acquisition of a neuron-like, GABAergic phenotype (Neman et al. 2014); and formation of pseudo-tripartite synapses between cancer cells and glutamatergic neurons (Zeng et al. 2019).

A microenvironmental factor, often overlooked in the brain, is its significantly softer mechanical properties compared to other organs. To study tumor cell cluster-brain interactions, Narkhede et al. (2020) used a biomaterial-based model with hyaluronic acid of varying stiffness to mimic the brain microenvironment and cell spheroids to mimic the cancer cell clusters. In this ex vivo study, they showed that MDA-MB-231-BR BC cell spheroids of varying diameter acquired a dormant phenotype in the soft hyaluronic acid-based cross-linked gels (0.4 kPa), whereas a size dependent switch between dormant and proliferative phenotypes was observed in stiffer hyaluronic hydrogels (4.5 kPa). They also reported that the matrix stiffness-driven dormancy was reversible by modulating the culture environment (Narkhede et al. 2020).

One of the limiting factors in studying dormancy in the brain is a lack of models—most of the experimental setups implement brain-tropic cell lines, preselected by cycles of in vivo passaging for brain metastases injected into aortic circulation (Miarka and Valiente 2021). This approach systematically induced brain metastases, whereas most of the spontaneous metastatic mouse models succumb due to disease progression in other organs. The alternative strategy was taken by Malladi et al. (2016) when, instead of isolating the brain-tropic clones, they generated latent clones from the brain by antibiotic resistance selection from macrometastases-free dissociated tissue (Malladi et al. 2016; Parida et al. 2022). This is one of the approaches for creating dormancy models, though with a focus on cell-intrinsic adaptations. For a summary of the brain-specific cancer cell dormancy mechanisms, see Fig. 18.2 and Table 18.1.

18.5 Shared Mechanisms of Dormancy Control

Metastasis is a systemic disease, with cancer cells arriving in multiple organs but being able to survive and grow in only a few. Cancer cell extravasation can be more challenging in the brain, where DTCs must cross the blood-brain barrier, while in the liver the presence of fenestrated capillaries readily allows extravasation of DTCs. The perivascular niche, composed of the endothelium, pericytes, and some organ-specific cell types, presents the first line of local niche to which DTCs get exposed. Spontaneously metastasizing BC cells often remain in a nonproliferative state when close to the vessels in the lung, bone, and brain (Ghajar et al. 2013). Work with ex vivo organotypic cultures modeling vasculature and stroma of the lung and the bone uncovered TSP1, a component of the ECM, as a shared upregulated protein deposited by endothelium that suppresses DTC proliferation. TSP1 is expressed by stabilized vasculature, to which cancer cells in the primary tumor are less likely to be exposed. Contrary to the initial suppression, sprouting neovascularization in metastatic sites leads to the accumulation of POSTN and TGF-β1 that reawaken dormant DTCs (Ghajar et al. 2013). This reawakening mechanism can be found across organs with sprouting neovascularization as a primary step in remodeling metastatic vasculature. However, since in the brain TNBC DTCs can grow along preexisting vasculature (vascular co-option) without inducing neovascularization, the mechanisms of reawakening may be different from those previously described in the lung and bone (Walchli et al. 2023).

Interplay between DTCs and immune cells (i.e., organ resident or infiltrating) upon extravasation presents another area with potentially shared mechanisms between metastatic organs. In a study by Malladi et al. (2016), a latency competent cancer (LCC) subclone of the HER2-positive cell line HCC1954 was shown to express the WNT inhibitor DKK1, which mediates cancer cell stemness by upregulation of SOX9 and SOX2 transcription factors. This clone downregulated the cell surface UL16-binding proteins (ULBP) as activators of NK cell-mediated cytotoxicity and receptors for cell death signals and hence escaped clearance by NK cells. Consistently, NK cell depletion resulted in permissive growth of metastasis in multiple organs (Malladi et al. 2016). This example shows that both cell-intrinsic and immune surveillance mechanisms are involved in the regulation of DTC dormancy.

18.6 Clinical Perspectives

The potential presence of dormant DTCs after primary tumor removal and initial treatments is an enduring worry, with the fear that these cells may reawaken and form life-threatening metastases. Three therapeutic strategies have been proposed to overcome this situation: (i) dormancy maintenance to prevent reawakening of dormant DTCs during the lifespan of the patient, (ii) reactivating dormant DTCs to sensitize them to cytotoxic chemotherapy, and (iii) eradicating dormant DTCs by specific targeting (Folkman and Kalluri 2004; Phan and Croucher 2020; Risson et al. 2020). For instance, adjuvant endocrine therapy has been offered for at least 5 years to early-stage ER-positive BC patients who are prone to late recurrence (Ramamoorthi et al. 2022). However, maintaining the disease in a dormant state indefinitely is difficult, because of drug toxicity and resistance arising in the cancer cells (Phan and Croucher 2020; Risson et al. 2020). The rationale behind the second strategy (i.e., reactivation of dormant DTCs) is that reentry of the cancer cells into G2/M will sensitize them to cytotoxic therapy. With this approach, dormant DTCs could be eradicated not only by targeting the dormant cells but also by suppressing microenvironmental signals that favor dormancy. For example, inhibiting integrin-mediated interactions between dormant DTCs and the perivascular niche has been shown to sensitize them to chemotherapy. Thus, combining integrin inhibitors with adjuvant therapy might effectively eradicate dormant DTCs and prevent metastasis (Carlson et al. 2019). The third approach (i.e., target dormant DTCs) is challenging as dormant DTCs do not respond to conventional cytotoxic therapies, which primarily target actively dividing cells. Furthermore, there is no currently approved method to identify patients who still harbor dormant DTCs after completion of adjuvant therapy. This also hampers monitoring of the effectiveness of such treatments. To overcome this limitation, the use of noninvasive assays, such as the detection of CTCs or cell-free DNA, could be useful for identifying patients with dormant DTCs. Increase in the sensitivity of currently available clinical imaging techniques (e.g., PET-CT, SPECT-CT, and MRI) is crucial for the detection of tumor mass but also of smaller clusters of cancer cells.

Despite offering a window of opportunity for intervention, targeting the dormant phase of cancer cells remains a major clinical challenge. Most studies on dormancy have been performed in preclinical animal models and limited analysis in human samples. Therefore, the translational potential of these discoveries remains to be proven. Furthermore, a dormancy-targeting clinical trial is perceived to be long, arduous, and costly, partly complicated by the lack of biomarkers for dormant DTCs or niches. Nevertheless, some clinical trials have been designed based on findings from cancer dormancy studies (Risson et al. 2020). These clinical trials focus primarily on the cell-autonomous mechanisms of cancer dormancy. As highlighted in this chapter, the cancer cell-TME interaction is integral for controlling cancer cell dormancy. Eradicating dormancy may require targeting not only the cancer cells but also the immune, stromal, vascular, and other cellular and extracellular matrix niches. Research addressing and validating these mechanisms of dormancy in human samples and testing them in patients with a high risk of recurrence will be key to designing therapeutic strategies toward long-lasting cure.

18.7 Conclusion

Metastasis is the fatal hallmark of cancer and cure of metastatic disease is rare. Therefore, preventing relapse by targeting cancer dormancy offers an attractive avenue for curing metastasis. As posited by Paget's "seed and soil" hypothesis and highlighted in this chapter, whether a cancer metastasizes to distant organs depends as much on the TME as on the cell-intrinsic properties of the cancer cells. In addition to animal models, various 3D culture approaches have been developed to study the mechanisms of dormancy and reawakening. Many studies have identified microenvironmental factors, such as the perivascular niche, components of the ECM, immune cells, and soluble factors that confer dormant properties on the cancer cells. However, these mechanisms are more likely to be tissue-specific than universal. This implies that niche-targeting therapy should be tailored to the specific niche within the organ of interest, as both the "dormant niche" and the "metastatic niche" could be present within the same organ. Understanding the heterogeneity between and within each organ is crucial to determining whether shared mechanisms of dormancy across organs can be exploited, either to sustain cancer dormancy or to eradicate dormant DTCs. Nevertheless, the major hurdle remaining is detecting dormant DTCs (e.g., by biomarker) before the findings in preclinical studies can be confirmed in humans. Continued research efforts focusing on unique characteristics of dormant cells and their microenvironment are necessary for developing personalized treatment strategies that can effectively target dormant cancer cells and their TME and ultimately lead to long-lasting cure.

References

Aguirre-Ghiso JA (2018) How dormant cancer persists and reawakens. Science 361(6409):1314–1315. https://doi.org/10.1126/science.aav0191

Akhtar M, Haider A, Rashid S, Al-Nabet ADMH (2019) Paget's "Seed and soil" theory of cancer metastasis: an idea whose time has come. Adv Anat Pathol 26(1):69–74. https://doi.org/10.1097/Pap.0000000000000219

Akkoc Y, Peker N, Akcay A, Gozuacik D (2021) Autophagy and cancer dormancy. Front Oncol 11:627023. https://doi.org/10.3389/fonc.2021.627023

Albrengues J, Shields MA, Ng D, Park CG, Ambrico A, Poindexter ME, Upadhyay P, Uyeminami DL, Pommier A, Kuttner V, Bruzas E, Maiorino L, Bautista C, Carmona EM, Gimotty PA, Fearon DT, Chang K, Lyons SK, Pinkerton KE et al (2018) Neutrophil extracellular traps produced during inflammation awaken dormant cancer cells in mice. Science 361(6409):1353. https://doi.org/10.1126/science.aao4227

Aslakson CJ, Miller FR (1992) Selective events in the metastatic process defined by analysis of the sequential dissemination of subpopulations of a mouse mammary-tumor. Cancer Res 52(6):1399–1405

Azevedo AS, Follain G, Patthabhiraman S, Harlepp S, Goetz JG (2015) Metastasis of circulating tumor cells: favorable soil or suitable biomechanics, or both? Cell Adhes Migr 9(5):345–356. https://doi.org/10.1080/19336918.2015.1059563

Barkan D, Kleinman H, Simmons JL, Asmussen H, Kamaraju AK, Hoenorhoff MJ, Liu ZY, Costes SV,

Cho EH, Lockett S, Khanna C, Chambers AF, Green JE (2008) Inhibition of metastatic outgrowth from single dormant tumor cells by targeting the cytoskeleton. Cancer Res 68(15):6241–6250. https://doi.org/10.1158/0008-5472.Can-07-6849

Barkan D, El Touny LH, Michalowski AM, Smith JA, Chu I, Davis AS, Webster JD, Hoover S, Simpson RM, Gauldie J, Green JE (2010) Metastatic growth from dormant cells induced by a Col-I-enriched fibrotic environment. Cancer Res 70(14):5706–5716. https://doi.org/10.1158/0008-5472.Can-09-2356

Bartosh TJ, Ullah M, Zeitouni S, Beaver J, Prockop DJ (2016) Cancer cells enter dormancy after cannibalizing mesenchymal stem/stromal cells (MSCs). Proc Natl Acad Sci USA 113(42):E6447-6456. https://doi.org/10.1073/pnas.1612290113

Bartosh TJ (2017) Cancer cell cannibalism and the SASP: ripples in the murky waters of tumor dormancy. Mol Cell Oncol 4(1):e1263715. https://doi.org/10.1080/23723556.2016.1263715

Basu S, Dong Y, Kumar R, Jeter C, Tang DG (2022) Slow-cycling (dormant) cancer cells in therapy resistance, cancer relapse and metastasis. Semin Cancer Biol 78:90–103. https://doi.org/10.1016/j.semcancer.2021.04.021

Baumann Z, Auf der Maur P, Bentires-Alj M (2022) Feed-forward loops between metastatic cancer cells and their microenvironment-the stage of escalation. EMBO Mol Med 14(6):e14283. https://doi.org/10.15252/emmm.202114283

Bliss SA, Sinha G, Sandiford OA, Williams LM, Engelberth DJ, Guiro K, Isenalumhe LL, Greco SJ, Ayer S, Bryan M, Kumar R, Ponzio NM, Rameshwar P (2016) Mesenchymal stem cell-derived exosomes stimulate cycling quiescence and early breast cancer dormancy in bone marrow. Cancer Res 76(19):5832–5844. https://doi.org/10.1158/0008-5472.CAN-16-1092

Borgen E, Rypdal MC, Sosa MS, Renolen A, Schlichting E, Lonning PE, Synnestvedt M, Aguirre-Ghiso JA, Naume B (2018) NR2F1 stratifies dormant disseminated tumor cells in breast cancer patients. Breast Cancer Res 20(1):120. https://doi.org/10.1186/s13058-018-1049-0

Borriello L, Coste A, Traub B, Sharma VP, Karagiannis GS, Lin Y, Wang Y, Ye X, Duran CL, Chen X, Friedman M, Sosa MS, Sun D, Dalla E, Singh DK, Oktay MH, Aguirre-Ghiso JA, Condeelis JS, Entenberg D (2022) Primary tumor associated macrophages activate programs of invasion and dormancy in disseminating tumor cells. Nat Commun 13(1):626. https://doi.org/10.1038/s41467-022-28076-3

Braun S, Pantel K, Muller P, Janni W, Hepp F, Kentenich CR, Gastroph S, Wischnik A, Dimpfl T, Kindermann G, Riethmuller G, Schlimok G (2000) Cytokeratin-positive cells in the bone marrow and survival of patients with stage I, II, or III breast cancer. N Engl J Med 342(8):525–533. https://doi.org/10.1056/NEJM200002243420801

Braun S, Vogl FD, Naume B, Janni W, Osborne MP, Coombes RC, Schlimok G, Diel IJ, Gerber B, Gebauer G, Pierga JY, Marth C, Oruzio D, Wiedswang G, Solomayer EF, Kundt G, Strobl B, Fehm T, Wong GY et al (2005) A pooled analysis of bone marrow micrometastasis in breast cancer. N Engl J Med 353(8):793–802. https://doi.org/10.1056/NEJMoa050434

Carlson P, Dasgupta A, Grzelak CA, Kim J, Barrett A, Coleman IM, Shor RE, Goddard ET, Dai J, Schweitzer EM, Lim AR, Crist SB, Cheresh DA, Nelson PS, Hansen KC, Ghajar CM (2019) Targeting the perivascular niche sensitizes disseminated tumour cells to chemotherapy. Nat Cell Biol 21(2):238–250. https://doi.org/10.1038/s41556-018-0267-0

Chambers AF, Naumov GN, Vantyghem SA, Tuck AB (2000) Molecular biology of breast cancer metastasis. Clinical implications of experimental studies on metastatic inefficiency. Breast Cancer Res 2(6):400–407. https://doi.org/10.1186/bcr86

Chambers AF, Groom AC, MacDonald IC (2002) Dissemination and growth of cancer cells in metastatic sites. Nat Rev Cancer 2(8):563–572. https://doi.org/10.1038/nrc865

Chien C, Raghavendra AS, Tripathy A, D., & A Madak-Erdogan, Z. (2022) ODP563 breast cancer with liver metastasis responds poorly to fulvestrant-based combination therapy and chemotherapy. J Endocr Soc 6(Supplement_1):A877–A878. https://doi.org/10.1210/jendso/bvac150.1816

Clark AM, Wheeler SE, Young CL, Stockdale L, Neiman JS, Zhao W, Stolz DB, Venkataramanan R, Lauffenburger D, Griffith L, Wells A (2017) A liver microphysiological system of tumor cell dormancy and inflammatory responsiveness is affected by scaffold properties. Lab Chip 17(1):156–168. https://doi.org/10.1039/c6lc01171c

Clark AM, Heusey HL, Griffith LG, Lauffenburger DA, Wells A (2021) IP-10 (CXCL10) Can Trigger Emergence of Dormant Breast Cancer Cells in a Metastatic Liver Microenvironment. *Frontiers*. Oncology 11. https://doi.org/10.3389/fonc.2021.676135

Clarke MF, Fuller M (2006) Stem cells and cancer: two faces of eve. Cell 124(6):1111–1115. https://doi.org/10.1016/j.cell.2006.03.011

Clements ME, Johnson RW (2019) Breast Cancer Dormancy in Bone. Curr Osteoporos Rep 17(5):353–361. https://doi.org/10.1007/s11914-019-00532-y

Copson E, Eccles B, Maishman T, Gerty S, Stanton L, Cutress RI, Altman DG, Durcan L, Simmonds P, Lawrence G, Jones L, Bliss J, Eccles D, Group PSS (2013) Prospective observational study of breast cancer treatment outcomes for UK women aged 18-40 years at diagnosis: the POSH study. J Natl Cancer Inst 105(13):978–988. https://doi.org/10.1093/jnci/djt134

Correia AL, Guimaraes JC, Auf der Maur P, De Silva D, Trefny MP, Okamoto R, Bruno S, Schmidt A, Mertz K, Volkmann K, Terracciano L, Zippelius A, Vetter

M, Kurzeder C, Weber WP, Bentires-Alj M (2021) Hepatic stellate cells suppress NK cell-sustained breast cancer dormancy. Nature 594(7864):566-+. https://doi.org/10.1038/s41586-021-03614-z

Dai J, Cimino PJ, Gouin KH 3rd, Grzelak CA, Barrett A, Lim AR, Long A, Weaver S, Saldin LT, Uzamere A, Schulte V, Clegg N, Pisarsky L, Lyden D, Bissell MJ, Knott S, Welm AL, Bielas JH, Hansen KC et al (2022) Astrocytic laminin-211 drives disseminated breast tumor cell dormancy in brain. Nat Cancer 3(1):25–42. https://doi.org/10.1038/s43018-021-00297-3

De Cock JM, Shibue T, Dongre A, Keckesova Z, Reinhardt F, Weinberg RA (2016) Inflammation triggers zeb1-dependent escape from tumor latency. Cancer Res 76(23):6778–6784. https://doi.org/10.1158/0008-5472.Can-16-0608

Demicheli R, Abbattista A, Miceli R, Valagussa P, Bonadonna G (1996) Time distribution of the recurrence risk for breast cancer patients undergoing mastectomy: further support about the concept of tumor dormancy. Breast Cancer Res Treat 41(2):177–185. https://doi.org/10.1007/BF01807163

Dioufa N, Clark AM, Ma B, Beckwitt CH, Wells A (2017) Bi-directional exosome-driven intercommunication between the hepatic niche and cancer cells. Mol Cancer 16. https://doi.org/10.1186/s12943-017-0740-6

El Touny LH, Vieira A, Mendoza A, Khanna C, Hoenerhoff MJ, Green JE (2014) Combined SFK/MEK inhibition prevents metastatic outgrowth of dormant tumor cells. J Clin Invest 124(1):156–168. https://doi.org/10.1172/Jci70259

Eyre R, Alferez DG, Santiago-Gomez A, Spence K, McConnell JC, Hart C, Simoes BM, Lefley D, Tulotta C, Storer J, Gurney A, Clarke N, Brown M, Howell SJ, Sims AH, Farnie G, Ottewell PD, Clarke RB (2019) Microenvironmental IL1beta promotes breast cancer metastatic colonisation in the bone via activation of Wnt signalling. Nat Commun 10(1):5016. https://doi.org/10.1038/s41467-019-12807-0

Fane M, Weeraratna AT (2020) How the ageing microenvironment influences tumour progression. Nat Rev Cancer 20(2):89–106. https://doi.org/10.1038/s41568-019-0222-9

Fidler IJ (2001) Seed and soil revisited: contribution of the organ microenvironment to cancer metastasis. Surg Oncol Clin N Am 10(2):257–269. vii–viiii

Fluegen G, Avivar-Valderas A, Wang Y, Padgen MR, Williams JK, Nobre AR, Calvo V, Cheung JF, Bravo-Cordero JJ, Entenberg D, Castracane J, Verkhusha V, Keely PJ, Condeelis J, Aguirre-Ghiso JA (2017) Phenotypic heterogeneity of disseminated tumour cells is preset by primary tumour hypoxic microenvironments. Nat Cell Biol 19(2):120–132. https://doi.org/10.1038/ncb3465

Folkman J, Kalluri R (2004) Cancer without disease. Nature 427(6977):787–787. https://doi.org/10.1038/427787a

Franco M, Bustuoabad OD, di Gianni PD, Goldman A, Pasqualini CD, Ruggiero RA (1996) A serum-mediated mechanism for concomitant resistance shared by immunogenic and non-immunogenic murine tumours. Br J Cancer 74(2):178–186. https://doi.org/10.1038/bjc.1996.335

Galmarini CM, Tredan O, Galmarini FC (2014) Concomitant resistance and early-breast cancer: should we change treatment strategies? Cancer Metastasis Rev 33(1):271–283. https://doi.org/10.1007/s10555-013-9449-1

Gao H, Chakraborty G, Lee-Lim AP, Mo QX, Decker M, Vonica A, Shen RL, Brogi E, Brivanlou AH, Giancotti FG (2012) The BMP inhibitor coco reactivates breast cancer cells at lung metastatic sites. Cell 150(4):764–779. https://doi.org/10.1016/j.cell.2012.06.035

Gao XL, Zhang M, Tang YL, Liang XH (2017) Cancer cell dormancy: mechanisms and implications of cancer recurrence and metastasis. Onco Targets Ther 10:5219–5228. https://doi.org/10.2147/OTT.S140854

Gawrzak S, Rinaldi L, Gregorio S, Arenas EJ, Salvador F, Urosevic J, Figueras-Puig C, Rojo F, Del Barco Barrantes I, Cejalvo JM, Palafox M, Guiu M, Berenguer-Llergo A, Symeonidi A, Bellmunt A, Kalafatovic D, Arnal-Estape A, Fernandez E, Mullauer B et al (2018) MSK1 regulates luminal cell differentiation and metastatic dormancy in ER(+) breast cancer. Nat Cell Biol 20(2):211–221. https://doi.org/10.1038/s41556-017-0021-z

Ghajar CM (2015) Metastasis prevention by targeting the dormant niche. Nat Rev Cancer 15(4):238–247. https://doi.org/10.1038/nrc3910

Ghajar CM, Peinado H, Mori H, Matei IR, Evason KJ, Brazier H, Almeida D, Koller A, Hajjar KA, Stainier DY, Chen EI, Lyden D, Bissell MJ (2013) The perivascular niche regulates breast tumour dormancy. Nat Cell Biol 15(7):807–817. https://doi.org/10.1038/ncb2767

Gomatou G, Syrigos N, Vathiotis IA, Kotteas EA (2021) Tumor dormancy: implications for invasion and metastasis. Int J Mol Sci 22(9). https://doi.org/10.3390/ijms22094862

Gomis RR, Gawrzak S (2017) Tumor cell dormancy. Mol Oncol 11(1):62–78. https://doi.org/10.1016/j.molonc.2016.09.009

Hamilton AM, Parkins KM, Murrell DH, Ronald JA, Foster PJ (2016) Investigating the impact of a primary tumor on metastasis and dormancy using MRI: new insights into the mechanism of concomitant tumor resistance. Tomography 2(2):79–84. https://doi.org/10.18383/j.tom.2016.00151

Hart IR (1982) 'Seed and soil' revisited: mechanisms of site-specific metastasis. Cancer Metastasis Rev 1(1):5–16. https://doi.org/10.1007/BF00049477

Husemann Y, Geigl JB, Schubert F, Musiani P, Meyer M, Burghart E, Forni G, Eils R, Fehm T, Riethmuller G, Klein CA (2008) Systemic spread is an early step in breast cancer. Cancer Cell 13(1):58–68. https://doi.org/10.1016/j.ccr.2007.12.003

Kalhor R, Mali P, Church GM (2017) Rapidly evolving homing CRISPR barcodes. Nat Methods 14(2):195–200. https://doi.org/10.1038/nmeth.4108

Kang Y, Pantel K (2013) Tumor cell dissemination: emerging biological insights from animal models and cancer patients. Cancer Cell 23(5):573–581. https://doi.org/10.1016/j.ccr.2013.04.017

Karreman MA, Bauer AT, Solecki G, Berghoff AS, Mayer CD, Frey K, Hebach N, Feinauer MJ, Schieber NL, Tehranian C, Mercier L, Singhal M, Venkataramani V, Schubert MC, Hinze D, Holzel M, Helfrich I, Schadendorf D, Schneider SW et al (2023) Active remodeling of capillary endothelium via cancer cell-derived MMP9 promotes metastatic brain colonization. Cancer Res 83(8):1299–1314. https://doi.org/10.1158/0008-5472.CAN-22-3964

Khazali AS, Clark AM, Wells A (2018) Inflammatory cytokine IL-8/CXCL8 promotes tumour escape from hepatocyte-induced dormancy. Br J Cancer 118(4):566–576. https://doi.org/10.1038/bjc.2017.414

Krall JA, Reinhardt F, Mercury OA, Pattabiraman DR, Brooks MW, Dougan M, Lambert AW, Bierie B, Ploegh HL, Dougan SK, Weinberg RA (2018) The systemic response to surgery triggers the outgrowth of distant immune-controlled tumors in mouse models of dormancy. Sci Transl Med 10(436). https://doi.org/10.1126/scitranslmed.aan3464

Kreso A, Dick JE (2014) Evolution of the cancer stem cell model. Cell Stem Cell 14(3):275–291. https://doi.org/10.1016/j.stem.2014.02.006

Kuksis M, Gao Y, Tran W, Hoey C, Kiss A, Komorowski AS, Dhaliwal AJ, Sahgal A, Das S, Chan KK, Jerzak KJ (2021) The incidence of brain metastases among patients with metastatic breast cancer: a systematic review and meta-analysis. Neuro-Oncology 23(6):894–904. https://doi.org/10.1093/neuonc/noaa285

Lawson MA, McDonald MM, Kovacic N, Hua Khoo W, Terry RL, Down J, Kaplan W, Paton-Hough J, Fellows C, Pettitt JA, Neil Dear T, Van Valckenborgh E, Baldock PA, Rogers MJ, Eaton CL, Vanderkerken K, Pettit AR, Quinn JM, Zannettino AC et al (2015) Osteoclasts control reactivation of dormant myeloma cells by remodelling the endosteal niche. Nat Commun 6:8983. https://doi.org/10.1038/ncomms9983

Lee JH, Bhang DH, Beede A, Huang TL, Stripp BR, Bloch KD, Wagers AJ, Tseng YH, Ryeom S, Kim CF (2014) Lung stem cell differentiation in mice directed by endothelial cells via a BMP4-NFATc1-thrombospondin-1 axis. Cell 156(3):440–455. https://doi.org/10.1016/j.cell.2013.12.039

Linde N, Fluegen G, Aguirre-Ghiso JA (2016) The relationship between dormant cancer cells and their microenvironment. Adv Cancer Res 132:45–71. https://doi.org/10.1016/bs.acr.2016.07.002

Liu Q, Zhang HF, Jiang XL, Qian CY, Liu ZQ, Luo DY (2017) Factors involved in cancer metastasis: a better understanding to "seed and soil" hypothesis. Mol Cancer 16. https://doi.org/10.1186/s12943-017-0742-4

Liu Y, Zhang P, Wu Q, Fang H, Wang Y, Xiao Y, Cong M, Wang T, He Y, Ma C, Tian P, Liang Y, Qin LX, Yang Q, Yang Q, Liao L, Hu G (2021) Long non-coding RNA NR2F1-AS1 induces breast cancer lung metastatic dormancy by regulating NR2F1 and DeltaNp63. Nat Commun 12(1):5232. https://doi.org/10.1038/s41467-021-25552-0

Ma W, Oliveira-Nunes MC, Xu K, Kossenkov A, Reiner BC, Crist RC, Hayden J, Chen Q (2023) Type I interferon response in astrocytes promotes brain metastasis by enhancing monocytic myeloid cell recruitment. Nat Commun 14(1):2632. https://doi.org/10.1038/s41467-023-38252-8

Malladi S, Macalinao DG, Jin X, He L, Basnet H, Zou Y, de Stanchina E, Massague J (2016) Metastatic latency and immune evasion through autocrine inhibition of WNT. Cell 165(1):45–60. https://doi.org/10.1016/j.cell.2016.02.025

Massague J, Obenauf AC (2016) Metastatic colonization by circulating tumour cells. Nature 529(7586):298–306. https://doi.org/10.1038/nature17038

Meng SD, Tripathy D, Frenkel EP, Shete S, Naftalis EZ, Huth JF, Beitsch PD, Leitch M, Hoover S, Euhus D, Haley B, Morrison L, Fleming TP, Herlyn D, Terstappen LWMM, Fehm T, Tucker TF, Lane N, Wang JQ, Uhr JW (2004) Circulating tumor cells in patients with breast cancer dormancy. Clin Cancer Res 10(24):8152–8162. https://doi.org/10.1158/1078-0432.Ccr-04-1110

Miarka L, Valiente M (2021) Animal models of brain metastasis. Neurooncol Adv 3(Suppl 5):v144–v156. https://doi.org/10.1093/noajnl/vdab115

Montagner M, Sahai E (2020) In vitro models of breast cancer metastatic dormancy. Front Cell Dev Biol 8:37. https://doi.org/10.3389/fcell.2020.00037

Montagner M, Bhome R, Hooper S, Chakravarty P, Qin X, Sufi J, Bhargava A, Ratcliffe CDH, Naito Y, Pocaterra A, Tape CJ, Sahai E (2020) Crosstalk with lung epithelial cells regulates Sfrp2-mediated latency in breast cancer dissemination. Nat Cell Biol 22(3):289-+. https://doi.org/10.1038/s41556-020-0474-3

Morris VL, Tuck AB, Wilson SM, Percy D, Chambers AF (1993) Tumor progression and metastasis in murine D2 hyperplastic alveolar nodule mammary-tumor cell-lines. Clin Exp Metastasis 11(1):103–112. https://doi.org/10.1007/Bf00880071

Muscarella AM, Aguirre S, Hao X, Waldvogel SM, Zhang XH (2021) Exploiting bone niches: progression of disseminated tumor cells to metastasis. J Clin Invest 131(6). https://doi.org/10.1172/JCI143764

Narkhede AA, Crenshaw JH, Crossman DK, Shevde LA, Rao SS (2020) An in vitro hyaluronic acid hydrogel based platform to model dormancy in brain metastatic breast cancer cells. Acta Biomater 107:65–77. https://doi.org/10.1016/j.actbio.2020.02.039

Neman J, Termini J, Wilczynski S, Vaidehi N, Choy C, Kowolik CM, Li H, Hambrecht AC, Roberts E, Jandial R (2014) Human breast cancer metastases to the brain display GABAergic properties in the neural niche. Proc Natl Acad Sci USA 111(3):984–989. https://doi.org/10.1073/pnas.1322098111

Nobre AR, Risson E, Singh DK, Di Martino JS, Cheung JF, Wang J, Johnson J, Russnes HG, Bravo-Cordero JJ,

Birbrair A, Naume B, Azhar M, Frenette PS, Aguirre-Ghiso JA (2021) Bone marrow NG2(+)/Nestin(+) mesenchymal stem cells drive DTC dormancy via TGFbeta2. Nat Cancer 2(3):327–339. https://doi.org/10.1038/s43018-021-00179-8

O'Reilly MS, Holmgren L, Shing Y, Chen C, Rosenthal RA, Moses M, Lane WS, Cao Y, Sage EH, Folkman J (1994) Angiostatin: a novel angiogenesis inhibitor that mediates the suppression of metastases by a Lewis lung carcinoma. Cell 79(2):315–328. https://doi.org/10.1016/0092-8674(94)90200-3

Ohta Y, Fujii M, Takahashi S, Takano A, Nanki K, Matano M, Hanyu H, Saito M, Shimokawa M, Nishikori S, Hatano Y, Ishii R, Sawada K, Machinaga A, Ikeda W, Imamura T, Sato T (2022) Cell-matrix interface regulates dormancy in human colon cancer stem cells. Nature 608(7924):784-+. https://doi.org/10.1038/s41586-022-05043-y

Oki T, Nishimura K, Kitaura J, Togami K, Maehara A, Izawa K, Sakaue-Sawano A, Niida A, Miyano S, Aburatani H, Kiyonari H, Miyawaki A, Kitamura T (2014) A novel cell-cycle-indicator, mVenus-p27K(−), identifies quiescent cells and visualizes G0-G1 transition. Sci Rep 4. https://doi.org/10.1038/srep04012

Pan H, Gray R, Braybrooke J, Davies C, Taylor C, McGale P, Peto R, Pritchard KI, Bergh J, Dowsett M, Hayes DF, Ebctcg. (2017) 20-Year risks of breast-cancer recurrence after stopping endocrine therapy at 5 years. N Engl J Med 377(19):1836–1846. https://doi.org/10.1056/NEJMoa1701830

Pantel K, Alix-Panabieres C (2014) Bone marrow as a reservoir for disseminated tumor cells: a special source for liquid biopsy in cancer patients. Bonekey Rep 3:584. https://doi.org/10.1038/bonekey.2014.79

Parida PK, Marquez-Palencia M, Nair V, Kaushik AK, Kim K, Sudderth J, Quesada-Diaz E, Cajigas A, Vemireddy V, Gonzalez-Ericsson PI, Sanders ME, Mobley BC, Huffman K, Sahoo S, Alluri P, Lewis C, Peng Y, Bachoo RM, Arteaga CL et al (2022) Metabolic diversity within breast cancer brain-tropic cells determines metastatic fitness. Cell Metab 34(1):90–105 e107. https://doi.org/10.1016/j.cmet.2021.12.001

Pedersen RN, Esen BO, Mellemkjaer L, Christiansen P, Ejlertsen B, Lash TL, Norgaard M, Cronin-Fenton D (2022) The incidence of breast cancer recurrence 10-32 years after primary diagnosis. J Natl Cancer Inst 114(3):391–399. https://doi.org/10.1093/jnci/djab/202

Phan TG, Croucher PI (2020) The dormant cancer cell life cycle. Nat Rev Cancer 20(7):398–411. https://doi.org/10.1038/s41568-020-0263-0

Polzer B, Klein CA (2013) Metastasis awakening: the challenges of targeting minimal residual cancer. Nat Med 19(3):274–275. https://doi.org/10.1038/nm.3121

Price TT, Burness ML, Sivan A, Warner MJ, Cheng R, Lee CH, Olivere L, Comatas K, Magnani J, Kim Lyerly H, Cheng Q, McCall CM, Sipkins DA (2016) Dormant breast cancer micrometastases reside in specific bone marrow niches that regulate their transit to and from bone. Sci Transl Med 8(340):340ra373. https://doi.org/10.1126/scitranslmed.aad4059

Priego N, Zhu L, Monteiro C, Mulders M, Wasilewski D, Bindeman W, Doglio L, Martinez L, Martinez-Saez E, Ramon YCS, Megias D, Hernandez-Encinas E, Blanco-Aparicio C, Martinez L, Zarzuela E, Munoz J, Fustero-Torre C, Pineiro-Yanez E, Hernandez-Lain A et al (2018) STAT3 labels a subpopulation of reactive astrocytes required for brain metastasis. Nat Med 24(7):1024–1035. https://doi.org/10.1038/s41591-018-0044-4

Puig I, Tenbaum SP, Chicote I, Arques O, Martinez-Quintanilla J, Cuesta-Borras E, Ramirez L, Gonzalo P, Soto A, Aguilar S, Eguizabal C, Caratu G, Prat A, Argiles G, Landolfi S, Casanovas O, Serra V, Villanueva A, Arroyo AG et al (2018) TET2 controls chemoresistant slow-cycling cancer cell survival and tumor recurrence. J Clin Invest 128(9):3887–3905. https://doi.org/10.1172/JCI96393

Ramamoorthi G, Kodumudi K, Gallen C, Zachariah NN, Basu A, Albert G, Beyer A, Snyder C, Wiener D, Costa RLB, Czerniecki BJ (2022) Disseminated cancer cells in breast cancer: Mechanism of dissemination and dormancy and emerging insights on therapeutic opportunities. Semin Cancer Biol 78:78–89. https://doi.org/10.1016/j.semcancer.2021.02.004

Regan JL, Schumacher D, Staudte S, Steffen A, Lesche R, Toedling J, Jourdan T, Haybaeck J, Mumberg D, Henderson D, Gyorffy B, Regenbrecht CRA, Keilholz U, Schafer R, Lange M (2021) RNA sequencing of long-term label-retaining colon cancer stem cells identifies novel regulators of quiescence. iScience 24(6):102618. https://doi.org/10.1016/j.isci.2021.102618

Ribatti D, Mangialardi G, Vacca A (2006) Stephen Paget and the 'seed and soil' theory of metastatic dissemination. Clin Exp Med 6(4):145–149. https://doi.org/10.1007/s10238-006-0117-4

Risson E, Nobre AR, Maguer-Satta V, Aguirre-Ghiso JA (2020) The current paradigm and challenges ahead for the dormancy of disseminated tumor cells. Nat Cancer 1(7):672–680. https://doi.org/10.1038/s43018-020-0088-5

Rodriguez PL, Jiang S, Fu Y, Avraham S, Avraham HK (2014) The proinflammatory peptide substance P promotes blood-brain barrier breaching by breast cancer cells through changes in microvascular endothelial cell tight junctions. Int J Cancer 134(5):1034–1044. https://doi.org/10.1002/ijc.28433

Ruggiero RA, Bruzzo J, Chiarella P, di Gianni P, Isturiz MA, Linskens S, Speziale N, Meiss RP, Bustuoabad OD, Pasqualini CD (2011) Tyrosine isomers mediate the classical phenomenon of concomitant tumor resistance. Cancer Res 71(22):7113–7124. https://doi.org/10.1158/0008-5472.CAN-11-0581

Ruggiero RA, Bruzzo J, Chiarella P, Bustuoabad OD, Meiss RP, Pasqualini CD (2012) Concomitant tumor resistance: the role of tyrosine isomers in the mechanisms of metastases control. Cancer Res 72(5):1043–1050. https://doi.org/10.1158/0008-5472.CAN-11-2964

Sakaue-Sawano A, Kurokawa H, Morimura T, Hanyu A, Hama H, Osawa H, Kashiwagi S, Fukami K, Miyata T, Miyoshi H, Imamura T, Ogawa M, Masai H, Miyawaki A (2008) Visualizing spatiotemporal dynamics of multicellular cell-cycle progression. Cell 132(3):487–498. https://doi.org/10.1016/j.cell.2007.12.033

Sanger N, Effenberger KE, Riethdorf S, Van Haasteren V, Gauwerky J, Wiegratz I, Strebhardt K, Kaufmann M, Pantel K (2011) Disseminated tumor cells in the bone marrow of patients with ductal carcinoma in situ. Int J Cancer 129(10):2522–2526. https://doi.org/10.1002/ijc.25895

Selli C, Turnbull AK, Pearce DA, Li A, Fernando A, Wills J, Renshaw L, Thomas JS, Dixon JM, Sims AH (2019) Molecular changes during extended neoadjuvant letrozole treatment of breast cancer: distinguishing acquired resistance from dormant tumours. Breast Cancer Res 21(1):2. https://doi.org/10.1186/s13058-018-1089-5

Sevenich L, Bowman RL, Mason SD, Quail DF, Rapaport F, Elie BT, Brogi E, Brastianos PK, Hahn WC, Holsinger LJ, Massague J, Leslie CS, Joyce JA (2014) Analysis of tumour- and stroma-supplied proteolytic networks reveals a brain-metastasis-promoting role for cathepsin S. Nat Cell Biol 16(9):876–888. https://doi.org/10.1038/ncb3011

Singh A, Veeriah V, Xi P, Labella R, Chen J, Romeo SG, Ramasamy SK, Kusumbe AP (2019) Angiocrine signals regulate quiescence and therapy resistance in bone metastasis. JCI Insight 4(13). https://doi.org/10.1172/jci.insight.125679

Srinivasan ES, Deshpande K, Neman J, Winkler F, Khasraw M (2021) The microenvironment of brain metastases from solid tumors. Neurooncol Adv 3(Suppl 5):v121–v132. https://doi.org/10.1093/noajnl/vdab121

Tallon de Lara P, Castanon H, Vermeer M, Nunez N, Silina K, Sobottka B, Urdinez J, Cecconi V, Yagita H, Attar FM, Hiltbrunner S, Glarner I, Moch H, Tugues S, Becher B, van den Broek M (2021) CD39(+)PD-1(+) CD8(+) T cells mediate metastatic dormancy in breast cancer. Nat Commun 12(1). https://doi.org/10.1038/s41467-021-21045-2

Truskowski K, Amend SR, Pienta KJ (2023) Dormant cancer cells: programmed quiescence, senescence, or both? Cancer Metastasis Rev 42(1):37–47. https://doi.org/10.1007/s10555-022-10073-z

Tulotta C, Lefley DV, Freeman K, Gregory WM, Hanby AM, Heath PR, Nutter F, Wilkinson JM, Spicer-Hadlington AR, Liu X, Bradbury SMJ, Hambley L, Cookson V, Allocca G, Kruithof de Julio M, Coleman RE, Brown JE, Holen I, Ottewell PD (2019) Endogenous production of IL1B by breast cancer cells drives metastasis and colonization of the bone microenvironment. Clin Cancer Res 25(9):2769–2782. https://doi.org/10.1158/1078-0432.CCR-18-2202

Turrell FK, Orha R, Guppy NJ, Gillespie A, Guelbert M, Starling C, Haider S, Isacke CM (2023) Age-associated microenvironmental changes highlight the role of PDGF-C in ER+ breast cancer metastatic relapse. Nat Cancer 4(4):468. https://doi.org/10.1038/s43018-023-00525-y

Upadhaya S, Reizis B, Sawai CM (2018) New genetic tools for the in vivo study of hematopoietic stem cell function. Exp Hematol 61:26–35. https://doi.org/10.1016/j.exphem.2018.02.004

Valiente M, Obenauf AC, Jin X, Chen Q, Zhang XH, Lee DJ, Chaft JE, Kris MG, Huse JT, Brogi E, Massague J (2014) Serpins promote cancer cell survival and vascular co-option in brain metastasis. Cell 156(5):1002–1016. https://doi.org/10.1016/j.cell.2014.01.040

van Maaren MC, de Munck L, Strobbe LJA, Sonke GS, Westenend PJ, Smidt ML, Poortmans PMP, Siesling S (2019) Ten-year recurrence rates for breast cancer subtypes in the Netherlands: a large population-based study. Int J Cancer 144(2):263–272. https://doi.org/10.1002/ijc.31914

Walchli T, Bisschop J, Carmeliet P, Zadeh G, Monnier PP, De Bock K, Radovanovic I (2023) Shaping the brain vasculature in development and disease in the single-cell era. Nat Rev Neurosci 24(5):271–298. https://doi.org/10.1038/s41583-023-00684-y

Wang H, Tian L, Liu J, Goldstein A, Bado I, Zhang W, Arenkiel BR, Li Z, Yang M, Du S, Zhao H, Rowley DR, Wong STC, Gugala Z, Zhang XH (2018) The osteogenic niche is a calcium reservoir of bone micrometastases and confers unexpected therapeutic vulnerability. Cancer Cell 34(5):823–839 e827. https://doi.org/10.1016/j.ccell.2018.10.002

Weiss L, Harlos JP, Torhorst J, Gunthard B, Hartveit F, Svendsen E, Huang WL, Grundmann E, Eder M, Zwicknagl M et al (1988) Metastatic patterns of renal carcinoma: an analysis of 687 necropsies. J Cancer Res Clin Oncol 114(6):605–612. https://doi.org/10.1007/BF00398185

Wheeler SE, Clark AM, Taylor DP, Young CL, Pillai VC, Stolz DB, Venkataramanan R, Lauffenburger D, Griffith L, Wells A (2014) Spontaneous dormancy of metastatic breast cancer cells in an all human liver microphysiologic system. Br J Cancer 111(12):2342–2350. https://doi.org/10.1038/bjc.2014.533

Wirtz D, Konstantopoulos K, Searson PC (2011) The physics of cancer: the role of physical interactions and mechanical forces in metastasis. Nat Rev Cancer 11(7):512–522. https://doi.org/10.1038/nrc3080

Yano S, Tazawa H, Kagawa S, Fujiwara T, Hoffman RM (2020) FUCCI real-time cell-cycle imaging as a guide for designing improved cancer therapy: a review of innovative strategies to target quiescent chemo-resistant cancer cells. Cancers 12(9). https://doi.org/10.3390/cancers12092655

Yu C, Wang H, Muscarella A, Goldstein A, Zeng HC, Bae Y, Lee BH, Zhang XH (2016) Intra-iliac artery injection for efficient and selective modeling of microscopic bone metastasis. J Vis Exp 115. https://doi.org/10.3791/53982

Yumoto K, Berry JE, Taichman RS, Shiozawa Y (2014) A novel method for monitoring tumor proliferation in vivo using fluorescent dye DiD. Cytometry A 85(6):548–555. https://doi.org/10.1002/cyto.a.22434

Zeng Q, Michael IP, Zhang P, Saghafinia S, Knott G, Jiao W, McCabe BD, Galvan JA, Robinson HPC, Zlobec I, Ciriello G, Hanahan D (2019) Synaptic proximity enables NMDAR signalling to promote brain metastasis. Nature 573(7775):526–531. https://doi.org/10.1038/s41586-019-1576-6

Zhang W, Bado IL, Hu J, Wan YW, Wu L, Wang H, Gao Y, Jeong HH, Xu Z, Hao X, Lege BM, Al-Ouran R, Li L, Li J, Yu L, Singh S, Lo HC, Niu M, Liu J et al (2021) The bone microenvironment invigorates metastatic seeds for further dissemination. Cell 184(9):2471–2486 e2420. https://doi.org/10.1016/j.cell.2021.03.011

Zhang Z, Tan Y, Huang C, Wei X (2023) Redox signaling in drug-tolerant persister cells as an emerging therapeutic target. EBioMedicine 89:104483. https://doi.org/10.1016/j.ebiom.2023.104483

Zhao Y, Lu T, Song Y, Wen Y, Deng Z, Fan J, Zhao M, Zhao R, Luo Y, Xie J, Hu B, Sun H, Wang Y, He S, Gong Y, Cheng J, Liu X, Yu L, Li J et al (2023) Cancer cells enter an adaptive persistence to survive radiotherapy and repopulate tumor. Adv Sci (Weinh) 10(8):e2204177. https://doi.org/10.1002/advs.202204177

19 The Roles of Myeloid Cells in Breast Cancer Progression

Charlotte Helena Rivas, Fengshuo Liu, and Xiang H.-F. Zhang

Abstract

This chapter reviews tumor-associated myeloid cells, including macrophages, neutrophils, and other innate immune cells, and their multifaceted roles in supporting breast cancer progression and metastasis. In primary tumors, myeloid cells play key roles in promoting tumor epithelial-mesenchymal transition (EMT) and invasion. They can facilitate intravasation (entry into the bloodstream) and colonization, disrupting the endothelial cell layer and reshaping the extracellular matrix. They can also stimulate angiogenesis, suppress immune cell responses, and enhance cancer cell adaptability. In the bloodstream, circulating myeloid cells enable the survival of disseminated tumor cells via immunosuppressive effects and physical shielding. At the metastatic sites, they prime the premetastatic niche, facilitate tumor cell extravasation, and support successful colonization and outgrowth. Mechanistically, myeloid cells enhance cancer cell survival, dormancy escape, proliferation, and mesenchymal-epithelial transition (MET). Nonetheless, substantial gaps in our understanding persist regarding the functional and spatiotemporal diversity, as well as the evolutionary patterns, of myeloid cells during metastatic progression. Myeloid cell plasticity and differential responses to therapies present key barriers to successful treatments. Identifying specific pro-tumoral myeloid cell subpopulations and disrupting their interactions with cancer cells represent promising therapeutic opportunities. Emerging evidence suggests combining immunomodulators or stromal normalizers with conventional therapies could help overcome therapy-induced immunosuppression and improve patient outcomes. Overall, further elucidating myeloid cell heterogeneity and function throughout the process of breast cancer progression and metastasis will enable more effective therapeutic targeting of these critical stromal cells.

Keywords

Myeloid cells · Tumor microenvironment · Metastasis · Breast cancer · Heterogeneity

Charlotte Helena Rivas and Fengshuo Liu contributed equally with all other contributors.

C. H. Rivas · F. Liu
Cancer and Cell Biology Program, Graduate School of Biomedical Sciences, San Antonio, TX, USA

X. H.-F. Zhang (✉)
Lester and Sue Smith Breast Center, Houston, TX, USA

Department of Molecular and Cellular Biology, Berkeley, CA, USA

Dan L. Duncan Comprehensive Cancer Center, Baylor College of Medicine, Houston, TX, USA
e-mail: xiangz@bcm.edu

T. Sørlie, R. B. Clarke (eds.), *A Guide to Breast Cancer Research*, Advances in Experimental Medicine and Biology 1464, https://doi.org/10.1007/978-3-031-70875-6_19

Key Points

1. Myeloid cell lineages originate from embryonic precursors or adult bone marrow progenitors, and their origin influences their heterogeneity and function in the tumor microenvironment.
2. Tumor-derived factors such as G-CSF and GM-CSF lead to systemic overproduction of myeloid cells and accumulation of pro-tumoral macrophages.
3. Tissue-resident macrophages are functionally diverse and can self-maintain independently of bone marrow progenitors but are partially replenished by circulating monocytes over time.
4. Tumor-associated myeloid cells promote primary tumor invasion and dissemination through mechanisms like extracellular matrix (ECM) remodeling, angiogenesis, immunosuppression, and modulating cancer cell plasticity while also facilitating extravasation and colonization of distant sites via endothelial disruption, matrix metalloproteinases (MMPs) production, creation of pre-metastatic niches, and supporting metastatic survival and outgrowth.
5. Combining immunomodulators or stromal normalizers with conventional cancer therapies may help overcome therapy-induced immunosuppression. Disrupting specific myeloid-cancer cell interactions remains a promising therapeutic strategy against metastasis.

19.1 Main Text

19.1.1 Myeloid Lineages in the Primary Tumor Ecosystem

The myeloid compartment is composed of a complex network of immune cells, and most have been reported to play fundamental roles in the solid tumor milieu. Most of the myeloid cells stem from bone marrow progenitors, with the exception of some populations of macrophages, which have a more intricate developmental origin. Due to their pivotal role within the tumor microenvironment, macrophages have garnered significant attention as potential therapeutic targets, albeit yielding only moderate success, in part due to their highly heterogeneous nature. We will explore these topics in more detail in the following sections.

19.1.1.1 Normal Myeloid Cell Functions in Homeostasis Maintenance

The myeloid compartment comprises macrophages, dendritic cells, monocytes, neutrophils, basophils, eosinophils, and mast cells. Macrophages, which are potent antigen-presenting immune cells that play a crucial role in organ homeostasis and inflammation, are a key component of the myeloid compartment and will be the primary focus of this section. Macrophages originate either from embryonic hematopoiesis (tissue-resident macrophages) or bone marrow progenitors postnatally (bone marrow-derived macrophages) (Davies et al. 2013). Myelopoiesis occurs in mammals through a stepwise process that begins during embryonic development by week 3–4 of gestation in humans (Traver et al. 2001). At this time, prior to the generation of definitive hematopoietic stem cells (HSCs) in the bone marrow, myeloid progenitors develop from the primitive ectoderm of the yolk sac (YS) and give rise to tissue-resident macrophages, which seed organs in three successive waves as depicted in Fig. 19.1 (De Kleer et al. 2014; Wu and Hirschi 2020). (1) The first wave, called *primitive hematopoiesis*, takes place in the extra-embryonic YS and produces primitive erythroblasts, megakaryocytes, and CSF-1R+ c-Myb- progenitors, which give rise to brain-resident macrophages, microglia (Wu and Hirschi 2020). (2) The second, called *the EMP wave*, takes place in the hemogenic endothelium in the YS and produces c-Myb+ hematopoietic progenitors named erythro-myeloid precursors (EMPs). EMPs give rise to YS macrophages, which differentiate into tissue-resident macrophages in the fetal liver, expand and then migrate to seed different tissues, such as

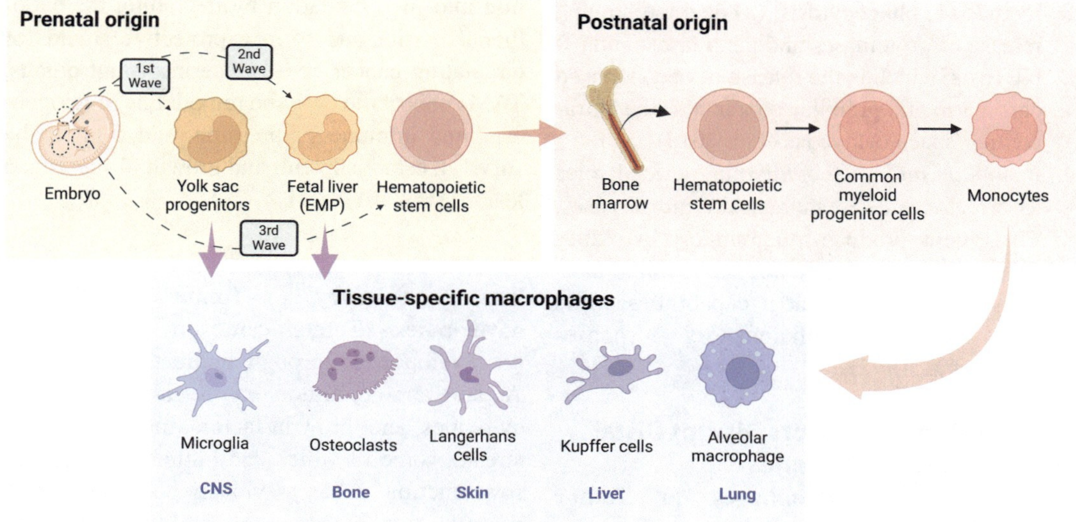

Fig. 19.1 Prenatally, tissue-resident macrophages are seeded across different tissues during embryonic development. Microglia, the brain-resident macrophages, arise during wave 1, while tissue-resident macrophages that colonize other tissues, such as the bone, skin, liver, or lung, arise during wave 2. Wave 3 gives rise to the hematopoietic stem cells that will colonize the bone marrow and establish the hematopoietic hierarchy. Postnatally, bone marrow-derived monocytes can replenish tissue-resident macrophages from different tissues

the lung (alveolar macrophages) and liver (Kupffer cells) (Wu and Hirschi 2020). (3) The third and last wave takes place in the hemogenic endothelium in the aorta-gonad-mesonephros (AGM) region and produces fetal hematopoietic stem and progenitor cells. These colonize the liver and establish definitive hematopoiesis in the bone marrow, mediated by self-renewing hematopoietic stem and progenitor cells as the ultimate precursors of the adult hematopoietic hierarchy (Wu and Hirschi 2020).

1. *Tissue-resident macrophages* can proliferate and self-renew during the lifetime of the organism, thus self-maintaining independently of bone marrow contribution during adulthood. However, tissue-resident macrophage turnover, at a rate specific to each organ, allows for their replenishment by bone marrow-derived monocytes, a postnatal macrophage precursor. Monocytes that are recruited into the tissue differentiate into macrophages and compete with tissue-resident macrophages for tissue colonization. These are primed by tissue cues to perform tissue-specific functions and acquire nearly identical transcriptomic profiles relative to embryonically derived macrophages (Guilliams et al. 2020). Macrophages are responsible for maintaining tissue integrity, and they accomplish this through a host of functions: removal of apoptotic cells, debris, and pathogens, tissue repair, and professional antigen presentation that can effectively and potently modulate pro- and anti-inflammatory signals (Gordon and Pluddemann 2017). The role of macrophages is complemented by other cells of the myeloid compartment, such as dendritic cells, neutrophils, basophils, and eosinophils.
2. *Dendritic cells* are antigen-presenting cells that play a vital role in establishing protective immunity. They phagocytize pathogens and induce adaptive immune responses by priming cells of the lymphoid compartment (CD4+ and CD8+ T cells and B cell) to eliciting memory formation (Liu 2016).
3. *Neutrophils* are the primary mediators of the rapid innate host defense and dominate the early stages of inflammation. The mechanisms these cells employ to fight infections

include (1) phagocytosis; (2) degranulation, a release of proteinases and peptidases; and (3) NETosis, which is the release of decondensed chromatin and granular contents to the extra-cellular space (Mayadas et al. 2014).

4. *Basophils and eosinophils* play crucial roles as effector cells in human allergic diseases. These cells produce inflammatory cytokines during allergic responses and exhibit anti-parasitic and bactericidal capabilities while also influencing inflammatory responses (Hirai et al. 1997).

19.1.1.2 Primary Tumors Disrupt Distal Myeloid Lineages

The Role of Macrophages in Tumor Progression Breast cancer is infiltrated by macrophages and monocytes. Monocytes are recruited to breast tumors through a complex interplay of molecular signals. One of the best-characterized cytokines responsible for monocyte-derived macrophage recruitment is the chemokine (C-C motif) ligand 2 (CCL2), also known as monocyte chemoattractant protein 1 (MCP-1). CCL2 is expressed by both stromal cells and tumor cells and is associated with poor prognosis in breast cancer (Hao et al. 2020). Monocytes in the tumor microenvironment can differentiate into tumor-associated macrophages (TAMs) and exert intricate pro-tumorigenic roles in breast cancer progression. TAMs can facilitate immune evasion by dampening effector-cell activity via the secretion of immunosuppressive cytokines, such as interleukin-10 (IL-10) and transforming growth factor-beta (TGF-β). They can also increase nutrient supply and tumor expansion by orchestrating neovascularization via the production of the vascular endothelial growth factor (VEGF) and fibroblast growth factor (FGF), key proteins involved in angiogenesis. TAMs play a multifaceted role in the metastatic cascade. Mechanistically, they contribute to ECM remodeling via MMPs, hence facilitating local tissue invasion and distant metastasis. They aid in the creation of a receptive pre-metastatic microenvironment by secreting factors that prepare distant tissues for cancer cell colonization. In addition, TAMs facilitate cancer cell intravasation into the circulation by degrading the endothelial barrier and form a protective shield for circulating cancer cells. Once in distant organs, TAMs contribute to tissue remodeling, angiogenesis, and immune suppression, and support the survival, establishment, and growth of metastatic lesions (Pollard 2004).

The Primary Tumor Disrupts Myelopoiesis Tumors can exert various effects on myelopoiesis through indirect mechanisms. As an example, tumors can release a variety of cytokines and growth factors into the bloodstream, some of which can influence bone marrow function. It has previously been shown that primary tumors have the ability to produce tumor-derived factors, like granulocyte colony-stimulating factor (G-CSF), through the activation of the mTOR signaling pathway, which is involved in gene transcription and protein synthesis regulation, thereby leading to the overproduction and accumulation of myeloid cells in the bone marrow, including monocytes that eventually infiltrate and support tumor progression (Welte et al. 2016; Hao et al. 2023).

19.1.1.3 Myeloid Cells Co-evolve with the Primary Tumor

Macrophages Facilitate EMT The role of the epithelial-to-mesenchymal transition (EMT) in tumor dissemination, survival, resistance, and stemness. EMT is a complex cellular program where epithelial cells lose their junctions and apical-basal polarity and undergo transformation into mesenchymal cells (Fleischmajer and Billingham 1968). This endows epithelial cells with mobility, allowing them to migrate to distant sites. EMT plays a fundamental role in normal biological processes during embryonic development and tissue wound repair (Fleischmajer and Billingham 1968). However, in recent years it has been identified as a hallmark of the metastatic cascade in various carcinomas, including breast cancer (Heerboth et al. 2015). Epithelial markers that allow cell-to-cell adhesion and junction formation, such as E-cadherin, are lost during EMT in breast cancer pathogenesis, while markers associated with mesenchymal features, such as N-cadherin and vimentin, are upregulated. Because of the increased migratory potential conferred by this program, EMT has been associated with higher metastatic potential and poor prognosis. TAMs have been shown to be the predominant myeloid compartment that infiltrates breast cancers, and they are known to play a pivotal role in driving EMT by secreting various factors (e.g., TGF-β, TNF-α, and IL-8) that activate key intracellular signaling pathways, including SMAD, MAPK, WNT/β-Catenin, NF-KB, and PI3K-AKT, that facilitate this transition (Li et al. 2022). The role of TGF-β in driving EMT has been widely investigated in the tumor milieu, revealing that TGF-β-induced SMADs bind to the promoters of the transcription factors SNAI1, TWIST1/TWIST2, and ZEB1, in this way increasing their expression and inducing EMT (Peinado et al. 2003). Specifically, these transcription factors are involved in repressing epithelial genes, hence facilitating the loss of cell adhesion molecules and increasing cell motility. Ultimately, in addition to enhancing migration, EMT can reduce the responsiveness of tumor cells to chemotherapy (Smith and Bhowmick 2016) and their vulnerability to cytotoxic cells (Akalay et al. 2013), while it also enhances tumor stemness (Roy et al. 2021), which increases the likelihood of recurrence.

19.1.2 The Role of Myeloid Cells in Breast Cancer Metastasis

Cancer metastasis entails the intricate process by which cancer cells detach from the primary tumor and journey to distant tissue, resulting in the initiation of new lesions. Metastatic lesions are the major cause of cancer-related deaths. While a small proportion of metastases are identified concurrently with primary tumors, a larger number arises metachronously, subsequent to the removal of the primary tumor. Albeit the existing standard of care is effective in addressing the primary tumor site, metastatic lesions in distant sites still present a considerable challenge for curability. Breast cancer metastasis exhibits tropism for specific organs, which is significantly influenced by the intricate interactions between tumor cells and host tissues. However, the underlying mechanisms are yet still obscure. This section aims to summarize our current knowledge of breast cancer metastasis with a specific focus on the role of myeloid cells in facilitating this process.

19.1.2.1 Primary Tumors Orchestrate Premetastatic Niches via Myeloid Cells

The concept of the premetastatic niche involves a sequence of molecular and cellular alterations in distant organs. These alterations prime the congenial soil for successful metastatic seeding prior to the arrival of disseminated tumor cells (Psaila and Lyden 2009). As shown in Fig. 19.2, the premetastatic niche is thought to consist largely of myeloid cells and their progenitors, which are known to be recruited at different stages of tumor progression and play a tumor protective role. Premetastatic niche formation primarily depends on tumor-derived soluble factors secreted by the primary tumor. Some of these factors include vascular endothelial growth factor (VEGFA), placental growth factor (PIGF) (Peinado et al. 2011; Kaplan et al. 2005), and extracellular vesicles (Hao et al. 2023). Furthermore, primary tumor can induce chronic inflammation in secondary organs, mimicking an immune response to an infection (Balkwill and Mantovani 2001). High infiltration of immune cells into the premetastatic niche disrupts the immune system's natural ability to mount an effective immune response, thus facilitating successful establishment of metastatic lesions. As an example, a recent study published on the ability of the primary breast tumor to stimulate the mobilization of CD11b+ myeloid cells to the lungs, thus establishing an immunosuppressive microenvironment that inhibits NK and T cell cytotoxic activity and enhances metastatic colonization success in lung tissue. Another study uncovered that lipid metabolites in lung-resident neutrophils make these cells a potent energy source that influences breast cancer lung metastasis (Li et al. 2020).

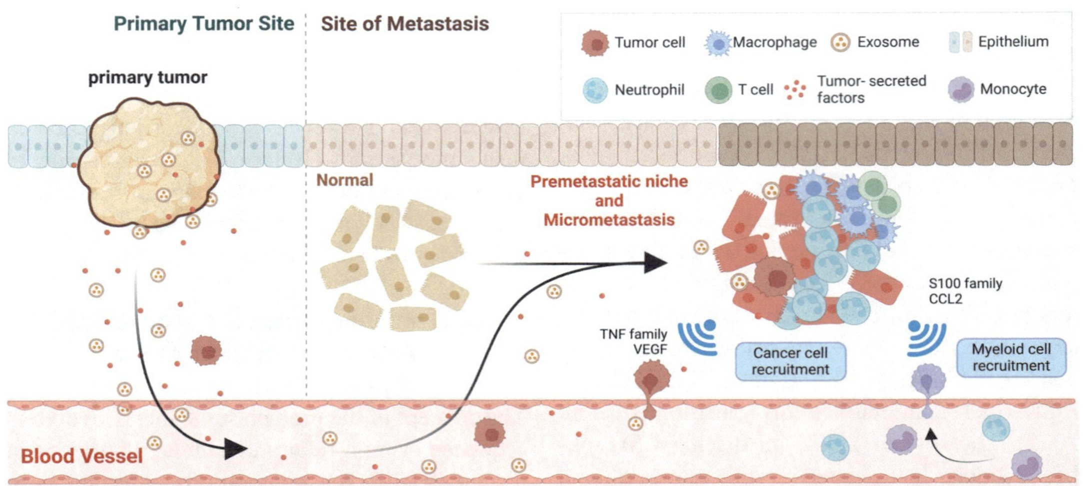

Fig. 19.2 The premetastatic niche refers to alterations in distant organs before tumor cell arrival that create a supportive environment for metastasis. Key mechanisms include recruitment of myeloid progenitor cells by factors secreted from the primary tumor like VEGFA and PIGF, which protect disseminated tumor cells; chronic inflammation mimicking infection to disrupt anti-tumor immunity; and substantial immune cells facilitating metastasis by inhibiting natural killer and T cell cytotoxicity. Recent evidence also uncovered lipid metabolites in lung neutrophils that act as an energy source driving breast cancer lung metastasis. Altogether the premetastatic niche disrupted immune surveillance and enabled metastatic colonization

19.1.2.2 Myeloid Cells Promote Tumor Dissemination and Intravasation

The metastatic process initiates during invasion of primary tumor cells into the surrounding tissue, followed by their entry into the bloodstream or lymphatic systems (Fig. 19.3). Successful progression in the metastatic cascade necessitates high intratumoral heterogeneity and disruption of the extracellular matrix (ECM) – two steps readily facilitated by the local immune tumor microenvironment (Lamouille et al. 2014; Lu et al. 2014). TANs and TAMs are one of the primary sources of matrix metalloproteinases (MMPs), which are key players in the degradation of the ECM (Clavel et al. 1992). Recent studies have also shown that TAMs and TANs have the ability to promote tumor cell invasion by additional mechanisms beyond MMP secretion. These include facilitating tumor cell-ECM interactions via secretion of osteonectin (SPARC) (Sangaletti et al. 2008), and further ECM remodeling via elastase (NE), cathepsins, and proteinase-3 (Sato et al. 2006; Tan et al. 2013) derives from TAMs and TANs, respectively.

Human breast cancer metastasis is predicted by the tumor microenvironment for metastasis (TMEM), which includes macrophages, endothelial cells, and tumor cells. In the TMEM, tumor cell intravasation is made possible by the development of invadopodia, which are formed in response to macrophage-tumor cell interaction (Condeelis and Pollard 2006; Rohan et al. 2014; Roh-Johnson et al. 2014). These interactions are driven by the formation of a paracrine loop that involves the growth factor (EGF) produced by macrophages and the colony-stimulating factor 1 (CSF1) produced by tumor cells. At TMEM locations, transient vascular permeability aids tumor cell circulation escape. A recent study reported that CSCs were observed to accumulate at the TMEM sites and in close contact with TAMs. These findings suggest that, although CSCs have a lower migration ability, they can efficiently intravasate through macrophage-endothelium connections (Harney et al. 2015; Sharma et al. 2021).

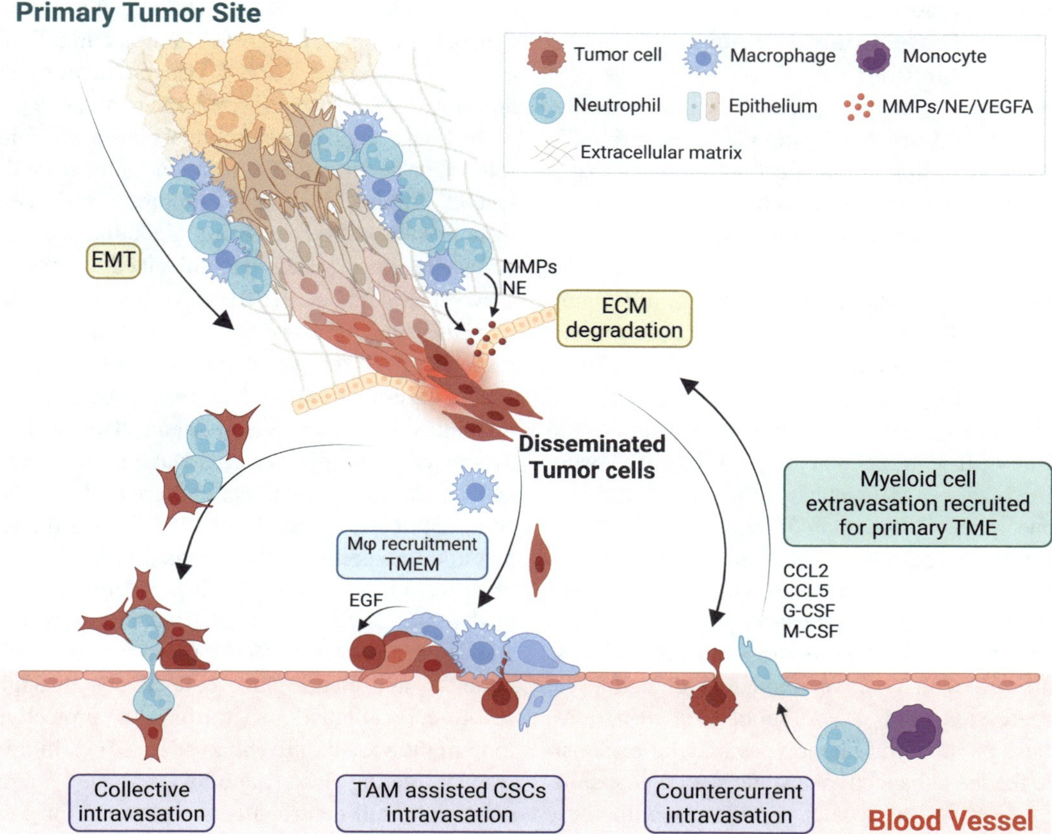

Fig. 19.3 Metastasis initiates when primary tumor cells gain invasive abilities and enter the bloodstream or lymphatic system, facilitated by epithelial-mesenchymal transition, cancer stem cells, and crosstalk with the tumor microenvironment including immune cells. To breach the extracellular matrix, primary tumors utilize matrix metalloproteinases secreted by tumor-associated macrophages and neutrophils. Metastatic site macrophages aid cancer cell intravasation through connections with endothelial cells and increased vascular permeability. Additional mechanisms include macrophages enhancing cell-matrix interactions via osteonectin, neutrophils remodeling the matrix, and Tie2+ macrophages promoting vascular leakiness to enable cancer cell escape into circulation. Overall, immune cells in the tumor microenvironment enable key steps of the metastatic cascade through matrix remodeling, vascular regulation, and direct physical interactions with tumor cells

In the polyomavirus middle T antigen overexpression (PyMT) model of breast cancer, TAMs can also increase blood vessel density through angiogenesis, which is in part driven by vascular endothelial growth factor A (VEGFA) production (Lin et al. 2007). A subset of Tie2+ TAMs can migrate to blood arteries where they can differentiate into perivascular macrophages that aid in vascular leakiness and the intravasation of cancer cells (Wyckoff et al. 2007; Mazzieri et al. 2011; Arwert et al. 2018). TANs also contribute to tumor cell intravasation but through distinct mechanisms. One hypothesis suggests that neutrophil migration creates tunnels in the ECM that allow tumor cells to escape and enter the vasculature. As neutrophils leave the main tumor site, tumor cells may also adhere to them and travel through the endothelium with them (Opdenakker and Van Damme 2004; Piccard et al. 2012). The mechanisms discussed above are summarized in Fig. 19.3.

19.1.2.3 Neutrophils Escort Disseminated Tumor Cell Circulation

The majority of the cancer cells that enter the blood vessel are Ki67+ circulating tumor cells (CSCs). Evading immune surveillance is a major challenge for circulating tumor cells (CTCs) to successfully arrive at a distal metastasis organ (Aramini et al. 2022). Figure 19.4 explains the reasons why myeloid cells are frequently found to form cell aggregates with disseminated tumor cells. In vitro studies first suggested that TANs facilitate the aggregation of breast cancer and colorectal cancer cells. Later, it was found that neutrophil extracellular traps (NETosis) were found to be associated with venous thrombi appearance in the lung (Demers et al. 2012). Further reports showed that the neutrophil-associated CTCs in the 4T1 mammary tumor model and breast cancer patients exhibited a pro-tumor gene expression profile, which is enriched with positive regulators of cell cycle progression and DNA replication programs. These pro-tumoral phenotypes may be responsible for the enhanced metastatic seeding capabilities seen in these cells. Consistent with these findings, antibody-mediated neutrophil blocking reduced metastatic incidence, while overexpression of the granulocyte colony-stimulating factor (G-CSF) increased TANs-CTCs clustering and enhanced metastasis. These findings highlight the significance of TANs-CTCs interactions in breast cancer metastasis (Szczerba et al. 2019).

In breast cancer, neutrophils play a twofold role in protecting CTCs from immune surveillance. Firstly, they can suppress NK cell responsiveness by dampening signaling via cell surface receptors, leading to enhanced tumor cell survival (Spiegel et al. 2016). Additionally, neutrophils shield tumor cells from anti-tumor T cell responses. Systemic expansion of T cell suppressive-neutrophils has been observed in mammary tumor models (Casbon et al. 2015). Moreover, neutrophils from melanoma and renal cell carcinoma patients show increased expression of ARG1, an inhibitor of T cell-mediated cytotoxic responses, while depletion of neutrophils restores cytotoxic T cell proliferation (Zea et al. 2005; De Santo et al. 2010). Notably, recent studies suggest that CTCs may activate both platelets and neutrophils collectively through cell-to-cell interactions, forming a protective loop in the vasculature (Shao et al. 2011), in this way facilitating clustering of disseminated tumor cells with both neutrophils and platelets for collective metastasis. This reciprocal activation may safeguard CTCs against mechanical and immune-regulated destruction during metastasis.

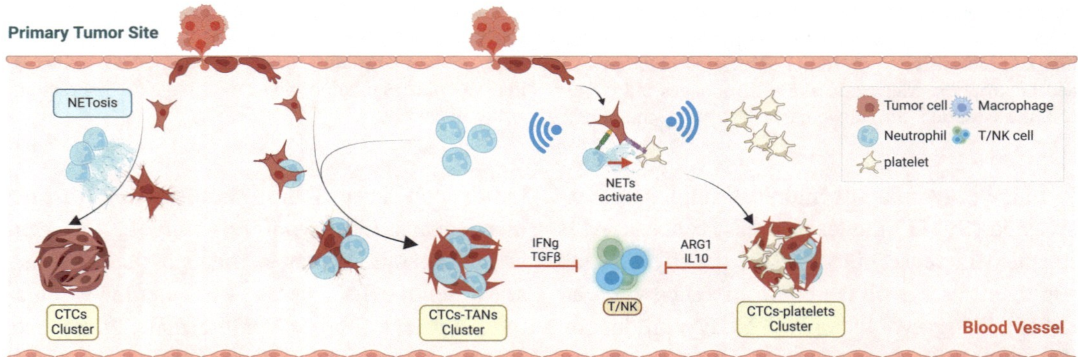

Fig. 19.4 Circulating tumor cells face immune surveillance as a major obstacle to successful metastasis but can evade immunity by clustering with myeloid cells. Neutrophils facilitate circulating tumor cell aggregation, enhance metastatic seeding through pro-tumor gene expression changes, and suppress NK and T cell cytotoxicity against tumor cells. Tumor cells can reciprocally activate platelets and neutrophils to form protective clusters in circulation. Therefore, interactions between disseminated tumor cells and myeloid cells like neutrophils enable collective metastasis and shield against immune destruction during transit

19.1.2.4 Myeloid Cells Assist Tumor Cell Extravasation and Distal Colonization

Surviving in circulation does not guarantee successful seeding. To enter distant organs, CTCs need to undergo a series of processes including adhesion, transendothelial migration, ECM degradation, and parenchymal invasion. Myeloid cells play important roles in these processes. Studies have shown that neutrophils co-localize with tumor cells at sites of metastasis, facilitating tumor cell adhesion and arrest. In the lung and liver, direct interactions between adherent neutrophils and circulating tumor cells (CTCs) enhance tumor cell adhesion and retention (Liang and Dong 2008; Huh et al. 2010). In experiments with aggressive mammary tumor models and human triple-negative breast cancer (TNBC) tumors, higher numbers of neutrophil-derived neutrophil extracellular traps (NETs) were observed in the lungs (Park et al. 2016). Induction of NETosis increased tumor cell adhesion to neutrophil monolayers, and inhibition of NET formation reduced this effect. Visualizations in murine models showed NETs wrapping around adherent tumor cells, trapping them at distant sites (Cools-Lartigue et al. 2013). NETosis was also associated with increased metastatic burden, while inhibition of NET formation reduced metastasis in various in vivo models (Park et al. 2016; Cools-Lartigue et al. 2013; Najmeh et al. 2017). In addition, the CTCs' transendothelial migration has been shown to be mediated through MMP-8/MMP-9 in neutrophils. Either inhibiting or knocking out MMP-8/MMP-9 on neutrophils reduced metastatic mammary tumor burden in mice (Spiegel et al. 2016).

In tumor immunology, monocytes are usually classified as pro-tumor classical monocytes ($CD14^{high}$ $CD16^{-}$ in humans or $Ly6C^{+}$ in mice) or anti-tumoral non-classical monocytes ($CD14^{+}$ $CD16^{high}$ in humans or $Ly6C^{low}$, in mice). Classical monocytes promote an invasive cancer cell phenotype when co-cultured with human breast cancer cells by boosting MMP-9, TNF, and growth factor production (Hiratsuka et al. 2002). Upon arrival at distal organs, most tumor cells may not proliferate immediately but rather enter a dormant status, referred to as quiescent tumor cells (Aguirre-Ghiso 2007). Quiescent tumor cells are often active, and via their active recruitment of circulating monocytes, they can facilitate tumor cell extravasation. Quiescent tumor cells attract monocytes through secretion of CCL2, a key ligand involved in $Ly6C^{+}$ monocyte recruitment. Monocytes enhance breast cancer cell extravasation into lung tissue via VEGFA production and MMP-9 synthesis (Kitamura et al. 2017). $Gr\text{-}1^{+}CD11b^{+}$ myeloid lineages also release MMP-9, which disrupts endothelial cell monolayers and increases permeability (Yan et al. 2010). Collectively, these findings suggest that both neutrophils and classical monocytes can influence endothelial permeability, potentially increasing cancer cell extravasation and metastasis (Fig. 19.5).

19.1.2.5 Tumors Thrive at the Metastatic Sites

Surviving and thriving in distal metastatic organs is the final step to successful metastatic colonization. Evidence suggests that many tumor cells are quiescent or dormant upon arrival; however, the underlying mechanisms involved in their awakening and outgrowth remain poorly understood. In melanoma models, inflammation has been one mechanism implicated in this process, where neutrophil-derived MMP-9 triggers angiogenesis in dormant micrometastasis, hence redirecting more nutrients and oxygen to the site of the lesion. Moreover, a recent study on breast and prostate cancer preclinical models found sustained systemic inflammation, leading to neutrophil infiltration and NET formation at the metastatic sites. NETs are known to remodel laminin, thereby activating integrin signaling and FAK/ERK/MLCK/YAP pathways and triggering proliferation of dormant cancer cells (Albrengues et al. 2018).

As mentioned previously, prior to the arrival of metastatic cancer cells at the distal site, myeloid cells participate in the formation of the premetastatic niche, which is a crucial step for successful metastatic growth. Neutrophils have been reported to accumulate in the lung prior to advanced tumor cell infiltration. Systemic disrup-

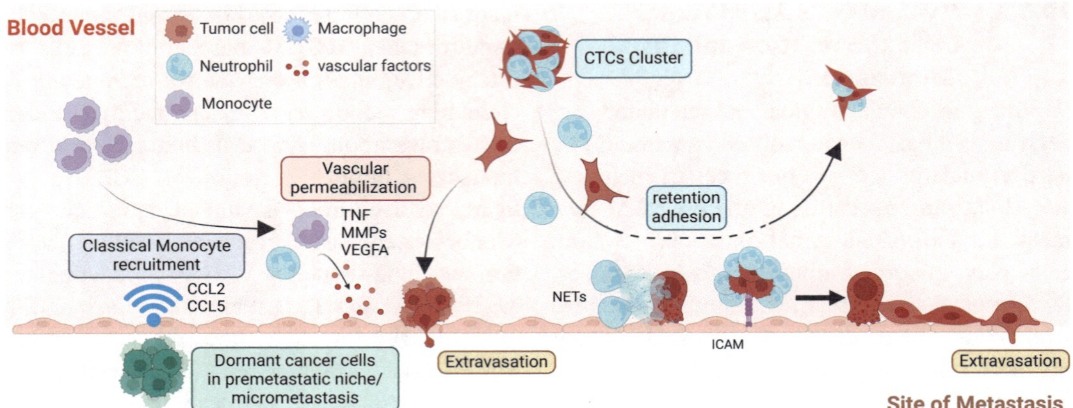

Fig. 19.5 After surviving circulation, circulating tumor cells rely on myeloid cells to successfully seed metastases through processes like adhesion, transendothelial migration, and tissue invasion. Neutrophils facilitate adhesion and arrest by trapping tumor cells in neutrophil extracellular traps, while their MMP-8/MMP-9 enables transendothelial migration. Classical monocytes also promote an invasive phenotype and extravasation through MMP-9 and factors like VEGFA. Therefore, interactions with myeloid cell populations are crucial for circulating tumor cells to complete later steps of the metastatic cascade after initial immune evasion

tion of the entire myelopoiesis has also been observed throughout both mouse and human breast malignancies (Hao et al. 2023). In human melanoma models, macrophage migration-inhibitory factors induce Kupffer cells expressing TGF-β to further recruit bone marrow-derived macrophages and upregulate fibronectin in the liver (Costa-Silva et al. 2015). It is reasonable to infer that tissue-resident myeloid lineages also play critical roles in breast cancer metastasis. Efforts have been made to study the mechanisms of how the myeloid lineage in the primary tumor affects the premetastatic niches remotely. For example, in KEP mammary tumors (breast cancer that overexpresses activated KRAS and ErbB2 while deactivating p53), tumor cell-derived CCL2 induced TAM accumulation and increased IL1-β secretion, in this way promoting immunosuppression at distant sites (Coffelt et al. 2015; Kersten et al. 2017).

Metastasis-associated macrophages (MAMs) have been identified as key players in eliciting and facilitating metastatic proliferation. Macrophage depletion has been shown to decrease metastatic burden, thus showcasing their significance in this process (Qian et al. 2009). Moreover, MAMs boost metastatic cell survival by promoting Akt activation in cancer cells, which endows them with protection against proapoptotic cytokines. Similarly, MAMs can form aggregates with circulating tumor cells via integrins, such as VCAM-1, in this way forming protective clusters that increase cancer cell survival success in the face of attrition during migration (Chen et al. 2011). Gr-1+ CD11b+ monocytes have also been linked to metastatic tumor cell establishment in the lung of breast tumor-bearing mice via PDGF-BB-induced angiogenesis (Hsu et al. 2019) and the generation of CCL9, which promotes tumor cell survival in mammary and melanoma tumor models (Yan et al. 2015). Another rate-limiting step in the metastatic cascade includes the mesenchymal-epithelial transition (MET), which is essential for cancer cells to regain proliferation capabilities. In vitro studies have shown that myeloid cell-conditioned media induces upregulation of E-cadherin and inhibits vimentin, thus favoring MET. In vivo depletion of myeloid cells leads to a failure of MET, accompanied by reduced metastatic tumor burden. Furthermore, it is known that macrophages in metastatic lungs may activate JAK-STAT6 signaling via IL-35 to induce MET in tumor cells. Albeit various mechanisms by which the myeloid compartment aids successful establishment of metastatic lesions have been elucidated, more in-

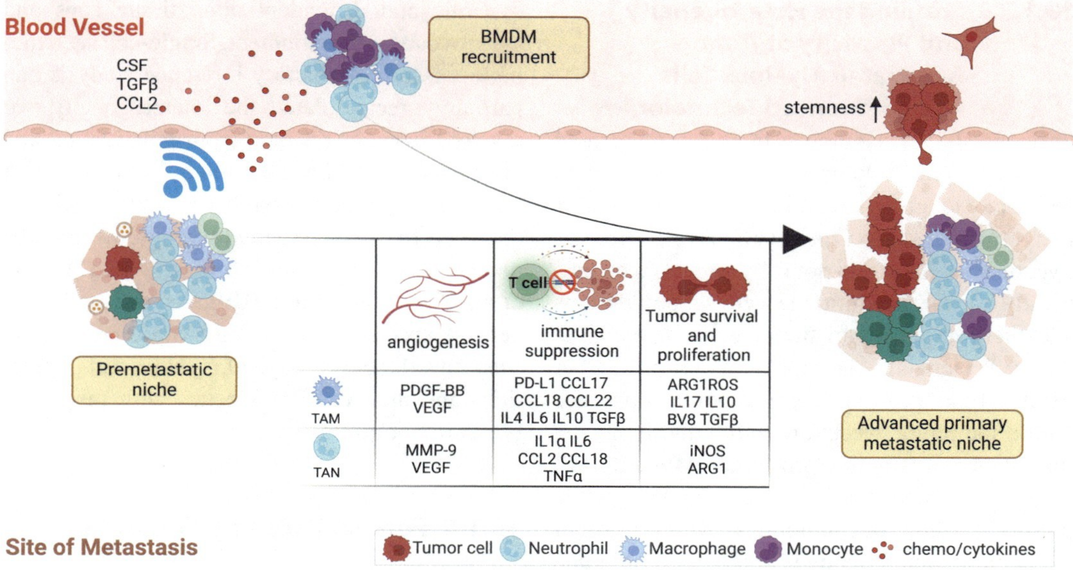

Fig. 19.6 After initial seeding, myeloid cells promote the awakening and outgrowth of previously dormant disseminated tumor cells at metastatic sites. Neutrophils can trigger dormant cell proliferation through MMP-9-induced angiogenesis and extracellular matrix remodeling. Additionally, metastasis-associated macrophages boost metastatic cell survival via AKT activation and VEGFR1/CSF1 signaling. Myeloid cells also facilitate mesenchymal-epithelial transition to regain proliferation capacity in tumor cells. Therefore, metastatic growth relies heavily on support from myeloid populations in the premetastatic niche

depth in vivo validation is needed (Gao et al. 2012; Lee et al. 2018) (Fig. 19.6).

19.1.3 Knowledge Gaps and Research Limitations

19.1.3.1 Myeloid Heterogeneity

Macrophage origin governs, in part, their functionality in the context of cancer. Several studies have highlighted the functional differences between tissue-resident macrophages and monocyte-derived macrophages, where tissue-resident macrophages have been associated with tumor-antagonizing properties (Nalio Ramos et al. 2022), while monocyte-derived macrophages have been unequivocally associated with tumor-supporting properties, particularly with facilitating metastatic colonization (Ma et al. 2020). Functional differences of macrophages in cancer arise in part from their cellular origin. Despite both tissue-resident macrophages and monocyte-derived macrophages display some degree of education by the tumor, tissue-resident macrophages, which inhabit and self-renew in tissues from embryonic development, feature restricted plasticity due to their prolonged tissue residence and imprinting by normal mammary tissue (Guilliams and Svedberg 2021). In stark contrast, bone marrow-derived monocytes, which progressively replenish embryonically derived macrophages in adulthood, exhibit remarkable plasticity, hence facilitating imprinting (Guilliams and Svedberg 2021) by the tumor and endowing them with potent pro-tumor functions. Previous studies have shown that the proportions of macrophage lineages in breast cancer are not static and that skewing the landscape towards monocyte-derived macrophage dominance accelerates tumor growth and metastasis. Understanding the functional heterogeneity of macrophages in breast cancer will establish the foundation for the rational finetuning of macrophage-centered therapies.

19.1.3.2 Profiling the Heterogeneity and Plasticity of Tumor-Associated Myeloid Cells Using Advanced Technologies

Previous studies have been limited by technical constraints and have only focused on individual cell types or groups identified by single or few markers, such as Gr-1 and Ly6C. While informative, these methods do not fully capture the complexity of various immune cell subpopulations and their responses to tumor cells or damage-induced signals. Macrophages, in particular, exhibit both pro- and anti-tumoral properties within the tumor. Recent research highlights the importance of targeting pro-tumoral functions of tumor-associated macrophages (TAMs) while preserving their anti-tumoral activities in order to achieve an effective anti-tumor immune response through checkpoint inhibition. The development of single-cell sequencing, a new generation of multichannel fluorescence-activated cell sorting (FACS), mass cytometry techniques such as CyTOF, and high-resolution multiplex immunohistochemical/fluorescent imaging hold promise in defining the heterogeneity of cancer-associated immune cells. These technologies have shed light on the evolution of tumors as they progress to a metastatic state and helped elucidate key differences between metastases and primary tumors. Collectively, these methods have expanded our technical repertoire to more thoroughly investigate immune population responses to immunotherapies or conventional treatments within their own specific "niches." Through the application of such techniques, unique immune cell subpopulations may be identified for the fine-tuning and optimization of myeloid-targeted modalities. This comprehensive approach has the potential to significantly advance our understanding of the immune response to cancer and pave the way for more effective and tailored therapeutic strategies.

Although these new technologies have become the top choices to determine the cellular identity/state in cancer progressions, they predominantly rely on capturing a snapshot of transcriptome profiling or cell surface markers. It is crucial to note that the polarization of myeloid cells is dynamic and dependent upon tissue cues and stage of cancer development. Single-cell sequencing accessorial trajectory inference analysis can partially recapitulate the heterogeneity of myeloid lineages resulted from polarization and differentiation. However, this is insufficient because trajectory inferences were originally designed for developmental biology, which may not be accurate in tumor contexts (La Manno et al. 2018; Cao et al. 2019). As such, comprehensive special-temporal studies are required to fully unveil the full scope of myeloid cell populations and their cellular kinetics with respect to breast tumor progression.

19.1.4 Perspectives and Conclusions

19.1.4.1 Targeting the Tumor Milieu at the Primary Tumor Site

Immune Checkpoint Inhibitors The presence of PD-L1 (programmed death ligand-1) on tumor cells, macrophages, or other cells of the tumor stroma can contribute to the establishment of an immunosuppressive tumor microenvironment, a mechanism by which the tumor can evade the immune response. PD-L1 interacts with the PD-1 receptor on effector immune cells, such as T or NK cells, leading to immune suppression and dampening the ability of lymphocytes to mount an effective anti-tumor response. The PD-1/PD-L1 axis is the most targeted immune checkpoint in breast cancer (Bastaki et al. 2020). Checkpoint inhibitors that block the interaction between PD-1 and PD-L1, such as pembrolizumab and atezolizumab, have been tested in clinical trials for advanced triple-negative breast cancer.

Myeloid-Targeted Therapies Anti-CSF1 (colony-stimulating factor 1) therapy is a type of macrophage-targeted treatment that focuses on blocking the CSF1/CSF1-receptor (CSF1R) axis by using monoclonal antibodies (Lin 2021). CSF1 is a cytokine that plays a fundamental role in the survival, proliferation, and differentiation of macrophages. Anti-CSF1/CSF1R targeted therapies work by blocking the interaction between CSF1 and CSF1-R, thereby decreasing macrophage numbers in the tumor. Other modalities have aimed to inhibit the CCL2/CCR2 chemokine axis to disrupt the chemokine-mediated recruitment of monocytes to the tumor microenvironment to ultimately reduce the number of TAMs (Fei et al. 2021). Despite dedicated attempts to enhance these treatments, the progress achieved has been relatively modest.

Therapy-Induced Tumor Microenvironment Alterations Cyclin-dependent kinases 4 and 6 (CDK4/CDK6) are fundamental players of cell cycle progression. Pharmacological CDK4/CDK6 inhibitors have shown promising clinical results against several types of solid tumors, including hormone receptor-positive, HER2-negative advanced breast cancer. These inhibitors cause cancer cell arrest by suppressing the phosphorylation of the retinoblastoma tumor suppressor protein and can significantly enhance anti-tumor immunity by increasing MHC-mediated tumor-antigen presentation; however, they have also been shown to suppress the proliferation of regulatory T cells (Goel et al. 2017). In contrast, PARP inhibitors (PARPi) have shown promising clinical results in BRCA-associated triple-negative breast cancer (TNBC). PARPi have been reported to reprogram macrophage metabolism in the tumor milieu, unveiling the potential benefits of combining PARPi with macrophage-directed therapies in TNBC (Mehta et al. 2021). Additionally, significant sex-specific differences in response to immune checkpoint blockade (ICB) therapies have been reported, revealing the role of estrogen via the Erα in promoting an immunosuppressive milieu in melanoma by inducing CD8+ T cell dysfunction, underscoring the ER signaling axis as a potential therapeutic target to enhance therapy efficacy of ICB (Chakraborty et al. 2021). While cancer therapies like chemotherapy, radiotherapy, and surgery aim to eliminate tumors, they may also inadvertently promote more aggressive disease by altering the tumor microenvironment. Radiotherapy, despite causing immunogenic cell death, recruits immunosuppressive myeloid cells that suppress cytotoxic T cell function (Demaria et al. 2005). Surgery can increase circulating tumor cells and systemic inflammation, supporting metastasis (Krall et al. 2018). Chemotherapy damages DNA but impairs antigen presentation and causes metabolic changes that deprive T cells of nutrients needed for activation. Abnormal tumor blood vessels are further damaged by therapy, worsening hypoxia, and metastasis. Cancer-associated fibroblasts and M2 macrophages repolarized by treatment secrete anti-inflammatory cytokines and remodel the extracellular matrix to suppress anti-tumor immune response (Kouidhi et al. 2018). Repeated therapies drive checkpoint molecule expression on cancer cells, dampening immune responses (Benavente et al. 2020). Combinational therapies include cytotoxic therapies and radiotherapies, and these can lead to secondary hematologic malignancies with more than 25% of patients developing therapy-related myeloid neoplasms (t-MN) (Bolton et al. 2020; Comen et al. 2020). As a result, the therapy-disturbed microenvironment allows tumors to evade immune surveillance, adapt metabolically, and progress. Understanding these mechanisms has led to combining standard therapies with immunomodulators and vascular/stromal normalizers to relieve immunosuppression and improve outcomes.

19.2 Conclusion

The myeloid compartment constitutes a highly heterogeneous group of immune cells that exhibit a wide array of functions crucial for tumor progression and distant colonization. The communication between tumor cells and myeloid cells involves a complex network of cytokines, chemokines, and other signaling pathways that influence myeloid cell polarization and function, and these may evolve throughout different stages of tumor progression. Therapeutic strategies targeting various aspects of the myeloid compartment have gained attention, aiming to shift the balance towards anti-tumor immunity, however, there is still significant potential for advancements.

Hence, a deeper understanding of the myeloid compartment's multifaceted roles in tumor progression is crucial for devising effective immunotherapies and personalized treatment strategies that harness the immune system's potential to combat cancer.

References

Aguirre-Ghiso JA (2007) Models, mechanisms and clinical evidence for cancer dormancy. Nat Rev Cancer 7:834–846

Akalay I et al (2013) Epithelial-to-mesenchymal transition and autophagy induction in breast carcinoma promote escape from T-cell-mediated lysis. Cancer Res 73:2418–2427

Albrengues J et al (2018) Neutrophil extracellular traps produced during inflammation awaken dormant cancer cells in mice. Science 361

Aramini B et al (2022) Cancer stem cells (CSCs), circulating tumor cells (CTCs) and their interplay with cancer associated fibroblasts (CAFs): a new world of targets and treatments. Cancers (Basel) 14

Arwert EN et al (2018) A unidirectional transition from migratory to perivascular macrophage is required for tumor cell intravasation. Cell Rep 23:1239–1248

Balkwill F, Mantovani A (2001) Inflammation and cancer: back to Virchow? Lancet 357:539–545

Bastaki S et al (2020) PD-L1/PD-1 axis as a potent therapeutic target in breast cancer. Life Sci 247:117437

Benavente S, Sanchez-Garcia A, Naches S, Esther LLM, Lorente J (2020) Therapy-induced modulation of the tumor microenvironment: new opportunities for cancer therapies. Front Oncologia 10:582884

Bolton KL et al (2020) Cancer therapy shapes the fitness landscape of clonal hematopoiesis. Nat Genet 52:1219–1226

Cao J et al (2019) The single-cell transcriptional landscape of mammalian organogenesis. Nature 566:496–502

Casbon AJ et al (2015) Invasive breast cancer reprograms early myeloid differentiation in the bone marrow to generate immunosuppressive neutrophils. Proc Natl Acad Sci USA 112:E566–E575

Chakraborty B, Byemerwa J, Shepherd J et al (2021) Inhibition of estrogen signaling in myeloid cells increases tumor immunity in melanoma. J Clin Invest 131(23):e151347. https://doi.org/10.1172/JCI151347

Chen Q, Zhang XH, Massague J (2011) Macrophage binding to receptor VCAM-1 transmits survival signals in breast cancer cells that invade the lungs. Cancer Cell 20:538–549

Clavel C, Polette M, Doco M, Binninger I, Birembaut P (1992) Immunolocalization of matrix metalloproteinases and their tissue inhibitor in human mammary pathology. Bull Cancer 79:261–270

Coffelt SB et al (2015) IL-17-producing gammadelta T cells and neutrophils conspire to promote breast cancer metastasis. Nature 522:345–348

Comen EA et al (2020) Evaluating clonal hematopoiesis in tumor-infiltrating leukocytes in breast cancer and secondary hematologic malignancies. J Natl Cancer Inst 112:107–110

Condeelis J, Pollard JW (2006) Macrophages: obligate partners for tumor cell migration, invasion, and metastasis. Cell 124:263–266

Cools-Lartigue J et al (2013) Neutrophil extracellular traps sequester circulating tumor cells and promote metastasis. J Clin Invest 123:3446–3458

Costa-Silva B et al (2015) Pancreatic cancer exosomes initiate pre-metastatic niche formation in the liver. Nat Cell Biol 17:816–826

Davies LC, Jenkins SJ, Allen JE, Taylor PR (2013) Tissue-resident macrophages. Nat Immunol 14:986–995

De Kleer I, Willems F, Lambrecht B, Goriely S (2014) Ontogeny of myeloid cells. Front Immunol 5: 423

De Santo C et al (2010) Invariant NKT cells modulate the suppressive activity of IL-10-secreting neutrophils differentiated with serum amyloid A. Nat Immunol 11:1039–1046

Demaria S et al (2005) Immune-mediated inhibition of metastases after treatment with local radiation and CTLA-4 blockade in a mouse model of breast cancer. Clin Cancer Res 11:728–734

Demers M et al (2012) Cancers predispose neutrophils to release extracellular DNA traps that contribute to cancer-associated thrombosis. Proc Natl Acad Sci USA 109:13076–13081

Fei L, Ren X, Yu H, Zhan Y (2021) Targeting the CCL2/CCR2 axis in cancer immunotherapy: one stone, three birds? Front Immunol 12:771210

Fleischmajer R; Billingham R E (ed.) (1968) Epithelial-mesenchymal interactions; 18th Hahnemann symposium. Williams & Wilkins, Baltimore

Gao D et al (2012) Myeloid progenitor cells in the pre-metastatic lung promote metastases by inducing mesenchymal to epithelial transition. Cancer Res 72:1384–1394

Goel S, DeCristo MJ, Watt AC et al (2017) CDK4/6 inhibition triggers anti-tumour immunity. Nature 548(7668):471–475. https://doi.org/10.1038/nature23465

Gordon S, Pluddemann A (2017) Tissue macrophages: heterogeneity and functions. BMC Biol 15:53

Guilliams M, Svedberg FR (2021) Does tissue imprinting restrict macrophage plasticity? Nat Immunol 22:118–127

Guilliams M, Thierry GR, Bonnardel J, Bajenoff M (2020) Establishment and maintenance of the macrophage niche. Immunity 52:434–451

Hao Q, Vadgama JV, Wang P (2020) CCL2/CCR2 signaling in cancer pathogenesis. Cell Commun Signal 18:82

Hao X et al (2023) Osteoprogenitor-GMP crosstalk underpins solid tumor-induced systemic immunosuppression and persists after tumor removal. Cell Stem Cell 30:648–664 e648

Harney AS et al (2015) Real-time imaging reveals local, transient vascular permeability, and tumor cell intravasation stimulated by TIE2hi macrophage-derived VEGFA. Cancer Discov 5:932–943

Heerboth S et al (2015) EMT and tumor metastasis. Clin Transl Med 4:6

Hirai K, Miyamasu M, Takaishi T, Morita Y (1997) Regulation of the function of eosinophils and basophils. Crit Rev Immunol 17:325–352

Hiratsuka S et al (2002) MMP9 induction by vascular endothelial growth factor receptor-1 is involved in lung-specific metastasis. Cancer Cell 2: 289–300

Hsu YL et al (2019) CXCL17-derived CD11b(+)Gr-1(+) myeloid-derived suppressor cells contribute to lung metastasis of breast cancer through platelet-derived growth factor-BB. Breast Cancer Res 21:23

Huh SJ, Liang S, Sharma A, Dong C, Robertson GP (2010) Transiently entrapped circulating tumor cells interact with neutrophils to facilitate lung metastasis development. Cancer Res 70:6071–6082

Kaplan RN et al (2005) VEGFR1-positive haematopoietic bone marrow progenitors initiate the pre-metastatic niche. Nature 438:820–827

Kersten K et al (2017) Mammary tumor-derived CCL2 enhances pro-metastatic systemic inflammation through upregulation of IL1beta in tumor-associated macrophages. Onco Targets Ther 6:e1334744

Kitamura T et al (2017) Monocytes differentiate to immune suppressive precursors of metastasis-associated macrophages in mouse models of metastatic breast cancer. Front Immunol 8:2004

Kouidhi S, Ben Ayed F, Benammar Elgaaied A (2018) Targeting tumor metabolism: a new challenge to improve immunotherapy. Front Immunol 9:353

Krall JA et al (2018) The systemic response to surgery triggers the outgrowth of distant immune-controlled tumors in mouse models of dormancy. Sci Transl Med 10

La Manno G et al (2018) RNA velocity of single cells. Nature 560:494–498

Lamouille S, Xu J, Derynck R (2014) Molecular mechanisms of epithelial-mesenchymal transition. Nat Rev Mol Cell Biol 15:178–196

Lee CC et al (2018) Macrophage-secreted interleukin-35 regulates cancer cell plasticity to facilitate metastatic colonization. Nat Commun 9:3763

Li P et al (2020) Lung mesenchymal cells elicit lipid storage in neutrophils that fuel breast cancer lung metastasis. Nat Immunol 21:1444–1455

Li X, Chen L, Peng X, Zhan X (2022) Progress of tumor-associated macrophages in the epithelial-mesenchymal transition of tumor. Front Oncol 12:911410

Liang S, Dong C (2008) Integrin VLA-4 enhances sialyl-Lewisx/a-negative melanoma adhesion to and extravasation through the endothelium under low flow conditions. Am J Physiol Cell Physiol 295:C701–C707

Lin CC (2021) Clinical development of colony-stimulating factor 1 receptor (CSF1R) inhibitors. J Immunother Precis Oncol 4:105–114

Lin EY et al (2007) Vascular endothelial growth factor restores delayed tumor progression in tumors depleted of macrophages. Mol Oncol 1:288–302

Liu K (2016) In Encyclopedia of cell biology, pp 741–749

Lu H et al (2014) A breast cancer stem cell niche supported by juxtacrine signalling from monocytes and macrophages. Nat Cell Biol 16:1105–1117

Ma RY et al (2020) Monocyte-derived macrophages promote breast cancer bone metastasis outgrowth. J Exp Med 217

Mayadas TN, Cullere X, Lowell CA (2014) The multifaceted functions of neutrophils. Annu Rev Pathol 9:181–218

Mazzieri R et al (2011) Targeting the ANG2/TIE2 axis inhibits tumor growth and metastasis by impairing angiogenesis and disabling rebounds of proangiogenic myeloid cells. Cancer Cell 19:512–526

Mehta AK, Cheney EM, Hartl CA et al (2021) Targeting immunosuppressive macrophages overcomes PARP inhibitor resistance in BRCA1-associated triple-negative breast cancer. Nat Cancer 2(1):66–82. https://doi.org/10.1038/s43018-020-00148-7

Najmeh S et al (2017) Neutrophil extracellular traps sequester circulating tumor cells via beta1-integrin mediated interactions. Int J Cancer 140:2321–2330

Nalio Ramos R et al (2022) Tissue-resident FOLR2(+) macrophages associate with CD8(+) T cell infiltration in human breast cancer. Cell 185:1189–1207 e1125

Opdenakker G, Van Damme J (2004) The countercurrent principle in invasion and metastasis of cancer cells. Recent insights on the roles of chemokines. Int J Dev Biol 48:519–527

Park J et al (2016) Cancer cells induce metastasis-supporting neutrophil extracellular DNA traps. Sci Transl Med 8:361ra138

Peinado H, Quintanilla M, Cano A (2003) Transforming growth factor beta-1 induces snail transcription factor in epithelial cell lines: mechanisms for epithelial mesenchymal transitions. J Biol Chem 278:21113–21123

Peinado H, Lavotshkin S, Lyden D (2011) The secreted factors responsible for pre-metastatic niche formation: old sayings and new thoughts. Semin Cancer Biol 21:139–146

Piccard H, Muschel RJ, Opdenakker G (2012) On the dual roles and polarized phenotypes of neutrophils in tumor development and progression. Crit Rev Oncol Hematol 82:296–309

Pollard JW (2004) Tumour-educated macrophages promote tumour progression and metastasis. Nat Rev Cancer 4:71–78

Psaila B, Lyden D (2009) The metastatic niche: adapting the foreign soil. Nat Rev Cancer 9:285–293

Qian B et al (2009) A distinct macrophage population mediates metastatic breast cancer cell extravasation, establishment and growth. PLoS One 4:e6562

Rohan TE et al (2014) Tumor microenvironment of metastasis and risk of distant metastasis of breast cancer. J Natl Cancer Inst 106

Roh-Johnson M et al (2014) Macrophage contact induces RhoA GTPase signaling to trigger tumor cell intravasation. Oncogene 33:4203–4212

Roy S, Sunkara RR, Parmar MY, Shaikh S, Waghmare SK (2021) EMT imparts cancer stemness and plasticity: new perspectives and therapeutic potential. Front Biosci (Landmark Ed) 26:238–265

Sangaletti S et al (2008) Macrophage-derived SPARC bridges tumor cell-extracellular matrix interactions toward metastasis. Cancer Res 68:9050–9059

Sato T et al (2006) Neutrophil elastase and cancer. Surg Oncol 15:217–222

Shao B et al (2011) Carcinoma mucins trigger reciprocal activation of platelets and neutrophils in a murine model of Trousseau syndrome. Blood 118: 4015–4023

Sharma VP et al (2021) Live tumor imaging shows macrophage induction and TMEM-mediated enrichment of cancer stem cells during metastatic dissemination. Nat Commun 12:7300

Smith BN, Bhowmick NA (2016) Role of EMT in metastasis and therapy resistance. J Clin Med 5

Spiegel A et al (2016) Neutrophils suppress intraluminal NK cell-mediated tumor cell clearance and enhance extravasation of disseminated carcinoma cells. Cancer Discov 6:630–649

Szczerba BM et al (2019) Neutrophils escort circulating tumour cells to enable cell cycle progression. Nature 566:553–557

Tan GJ, Peng ZK, Lu JP, Tang FQ (2013) Cathepsins mediate tumor metastasis. World J Biol Chem 4:91–101

Traver D et al (2001) Fetal liver myelopoiesis occurs through distinct, prospectively isolatable progenitor subsets. Blood 98:627–635

Welte T et al (2016) Oncogenic mTOR signalling recruits myeloid-derived suppressor cells to promote tumour initiation. Nat Cell Biol 18:632–644

Wu Y, Hirschi KK (2020) Tissue-resident macrophage development and function. Front Cell Dev Biol 8:617879

Wyckoff JB et al (2007) Direct visualization of macrophage-assisted tumor cell intravasation in mammary tumors. Cancer Res 67:2649–2656

Yan HH et al (2010) Gr-1+CD11b+ myeloid cells tip the balance of immune protection to tumor promotion in the premetastatic lung. Cancer Res 70:6139–6149

Yan HH et al (2015) CCL9 induced by TGFbeta signaling in myeloid cells enhances tumor cell survival in the premetastatic organ. Cancer Res 75:5283–5298

Zea AH et al (2005) Arginase-producing myeloid suppressor cells in renal cell carcinoma patients: a mechanism of tumor evasion. Cancer Res 65:3044–3048

20 Immune Microenvironment in Breast Cancer Metastasis

Bin-Zhi Qian and Ruo-Yu Ma

Abstract

Metastatic disease is the final stage of breast cancer that accounts for vast majority of patient death. Mounting data over recent years strongly support the critical roles of the immune microenvironment in determining breast cancer metastasis. The latest single-cell studies provide further molecular evidence illustrating the heterogeneity of this immune microenvironment. This chapter summarizes major discoveries on the role of various immune cells in metastasis progression and discusses future research opportunities. Studies investigating immune heterogeneity within primary breast cancer and across different metastasis target organs can potentially lead to more precise treatment strategies with improved efficacy.

Keywords

Metastasis · Immune microenvironment

B.-Z. Qian (✉) · R.-Y. Ma
Department of Oncology, Fudan University Shanghai Cancer Center, Zhangjiang-Fudan International Innovation Center, Shanghai Medical College, The Human Phenome Institute, Fudan University, Shanghai, China
e-mail: qianbinzhi@fudan.edu.cn

Key Points

- Immune microenvironment is essential in determining the metastasis cascade.
- Various immune cell types and subtypes have distinctive roles in breast cancer metastasis.
- Metastasis target organs have organ-specific immune responses towards metastasis.
- Immune microenvironment can be utilized to control metastatic disease.

20.1 Introduction

Metastasis, the dissemination of cancer cells from primary tumour to secondary organs, accounts for over 90% of breast cancer-associated patient death. The metastasis cascade contains a sequence of rate-limiting events including tumour cell invasion of the nearby tissue, entering microvasculature of the lymphatic and circulatory systems (intravasation), survival in the bloodstream, exiting from the blood vessel (extravasation) of target organs, survival in the foreign microenvironment, and, finally, adaptation to the metastasis microenvironment and the development into a visible secondary tumour (persistent growth) (Fidler 2003). Following Steven Paget's initial "seed and soil" hypothesis in 1889 (Paget 1889),

T. Sørlie, R. B. Clarke (eds.), *A Guide to Breast Cancer Research*, Advances in Experimental Medicine and Biology 1464, https://doi.org/10.1007/978-3-031-70875-6_20

numerous data strongly support that the host tissue microenvironment is critical for breast cancer metastasis.

Over the past 20 years, more and more studies indicated that the host immune compartment is a key component of the "soil" governing each step of the metastasis cascade (Kitamura et al. 2015a) (Fig. 20.1). This immune microenvironment contains almost all types of innate and adaptive immune cells, such as macrophages, neutrophils, dendritic cells, T cells, B cells, and natural killer (NK) cells (De Visser and Joyce 2023) (Fig. 20.1). Immunotherapies that target a variety of immune cells have been developed for the treatment of advanced cancer. Recent clinical trials, however, have demonstrated that these therapies have lim-

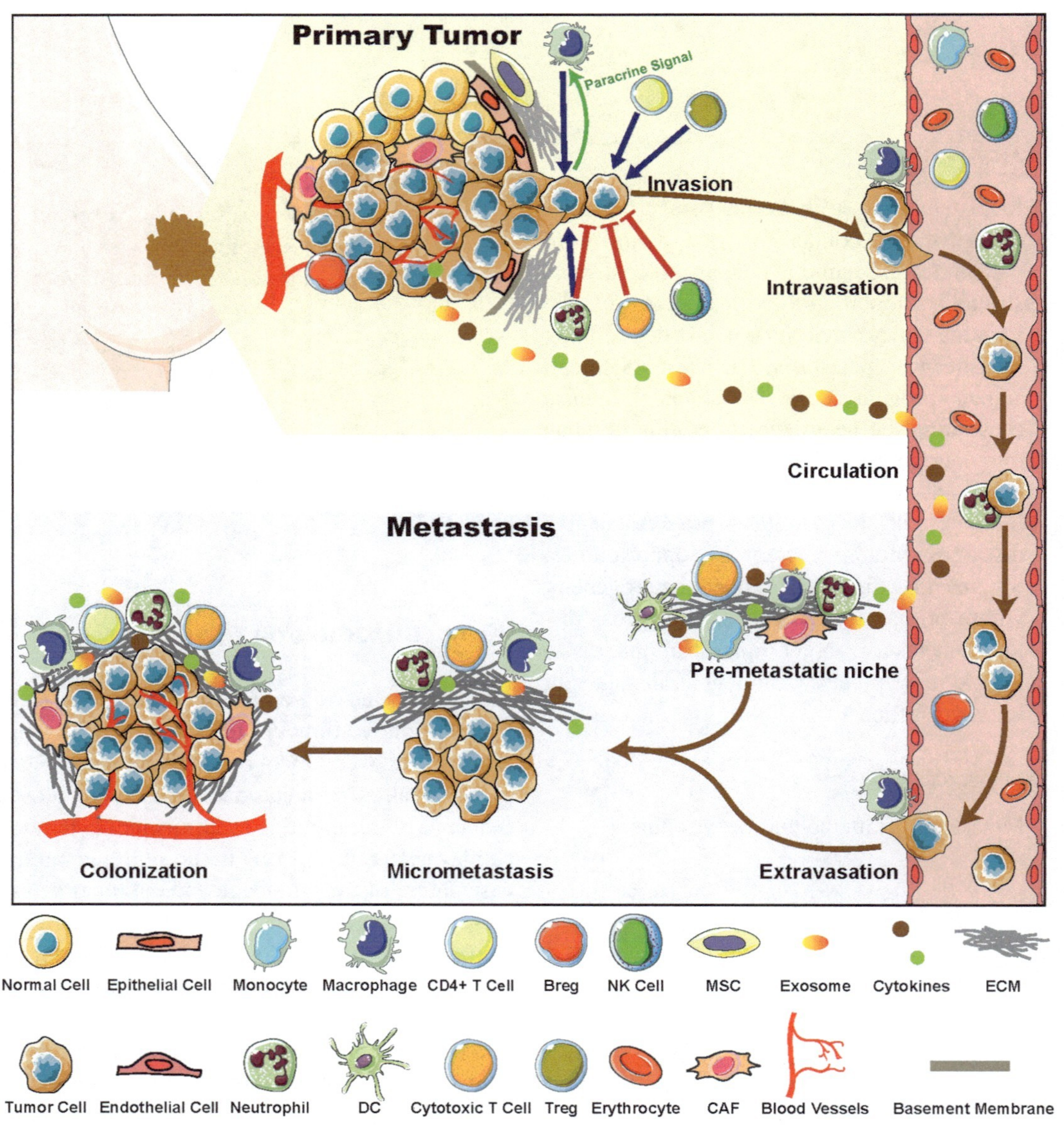

Fig. 20.1 Complex immune interaction in breast cancer metastasis. All types of immune cell types can involve in the various rate-limiting steps of the metastasis cascade. *Breg* regulatory B cells, *ECM* extracellular matrix, *DC* dendritic cells, *Treg* regulatory T cells, *MSC* mesenchymal stroma cells, *CAF* cancer-associated fibroblast

ited response rates and do not enhance survival of patients with metastatic breast cancer (Adams et al. 2019; Esteva et al. 2019). This indicates a significant lack of understanding of the intricate crosstalk among tumour cells and immune cells in the metastasis microenvironment. In this chapter, we will summarize major findings on the function of different immune cell types in breast cancer metastasis and discuss future challenges and research opportunities (Fig. 20.2).

20.1.1 Macrophages and Monocytes

Macrophage is the most abundant immune cells in breast cancer (Cassetta and Pollard 2018) and accounts for over 50% of tumour-infiltrating immune cells (Marelli et al. 2015). Enrichment of tumour-associated macrophages (TAMs) strongly correlates with poor prognostic features including tumour progression, metastasis, and therapy resistance (Denardo et al. 2011; Mahmoud et al. 2012).

Work pioneered by Pollard and colleagues, together with many others, has demonstrated potent tumour-promoting roles of macrophages in all rate-limiting steps of breast cancer metastasis (Kitamura et al. 2015a). In primary tumour site, TAMs were found to support the invasion of breast cancer cells through different mechanisms (Clark and Vignjevic 2015). TAMs can directly support tumour cell migration and invasion through a paracrine loop, in which colony-stimulating factor 1 (CSF1) secreted by tumour cells promotes macrophage reprogramming and infiltration, and in turn, epidermal growth factor (EGF) secreted by TAMs enhances tumour cell motility in spontaneous mouse mammary tumour model (Wyckoff et al. 2004; Goswami et al. 2005). Further investigations using patient samples indicated that tumour-secreted factors including CSF1 and TNFα can also promote the production of CCL8 from SIGLEC1^{hi} tissue-resident TAMs, which increased tumour cell invasion (Cassetta et al. 2019). TAMs were also reported being an important source of proteases including matrix metalloproteinases (MMPs), cathepsins, and serine proteases, which allowed the disruption of cell-cell junction and tumour cell invasion into surrounding tissues (Joyce and Pollard 2009). Moreover, researchers found that TAMs produce Wnt7b to induce the growth of new blood vessel, which significantly increases tumour cell invasion and metastasis (Yeo et al. 2014). In accordance with these preclinical findings, a higher fraction of macrophage and the expression of TAM markers were correlated with worse prognosis and vascular invasion in patients (Mahmoud et al. 2012; Miyasato et al. 2017). Using spatial transcriptomics technology, the latest studies revealed that *APOE*^{hi} lipid-associated macrophages (LAMs), located predominantly in the invasive tumour area, were positively correlated with T cell suppression, potentially through the high expression of PD-L1 and PD-L2. These data suggested the functional importance of the location of TAM subsets in breast cancer invasion (Wu et al. 2021b), which calls for further validation.

TAMs also play essential roles in the intravasation and extravasation processes of breast cancer metastasis. Using intravital imaging, a series of studies observed that monocyte-derived Tie2+ perivascular macrophages (Arwert et al. 2018) closely interacted with breast cancer cells (Wyckoff et al. 2007) and formed a micro-anatomical structure, which enhanced the permeability of blood vessels and allowed tumour cell intravasation. Similar micro-anatomic structure was identified in patient samples (Harney et al. 2015), and its abundance was correlated with distal metastasis (Rohan et al. 2014). Further studies indicated that blockade of perivascular macrophage activation through the Tie2 inhibitor rebastinib significantly reduced intravasation of tumour cells and inhibited metastasis growth in the PyMT breast cancer model, showing the importance of macrophages in tumour cell spreading (Harney et al. 2017).

Macrophages are a major immune compartment recruited in pre-metastatic niche of lung and bone in breast cancer models (Linde et al. 2018), which determines organ-specific metastasis preference (Peinado et al. 2017). Several studies suggested that primary tumour cells secreting chemoattractants such as C-C motif chemokine

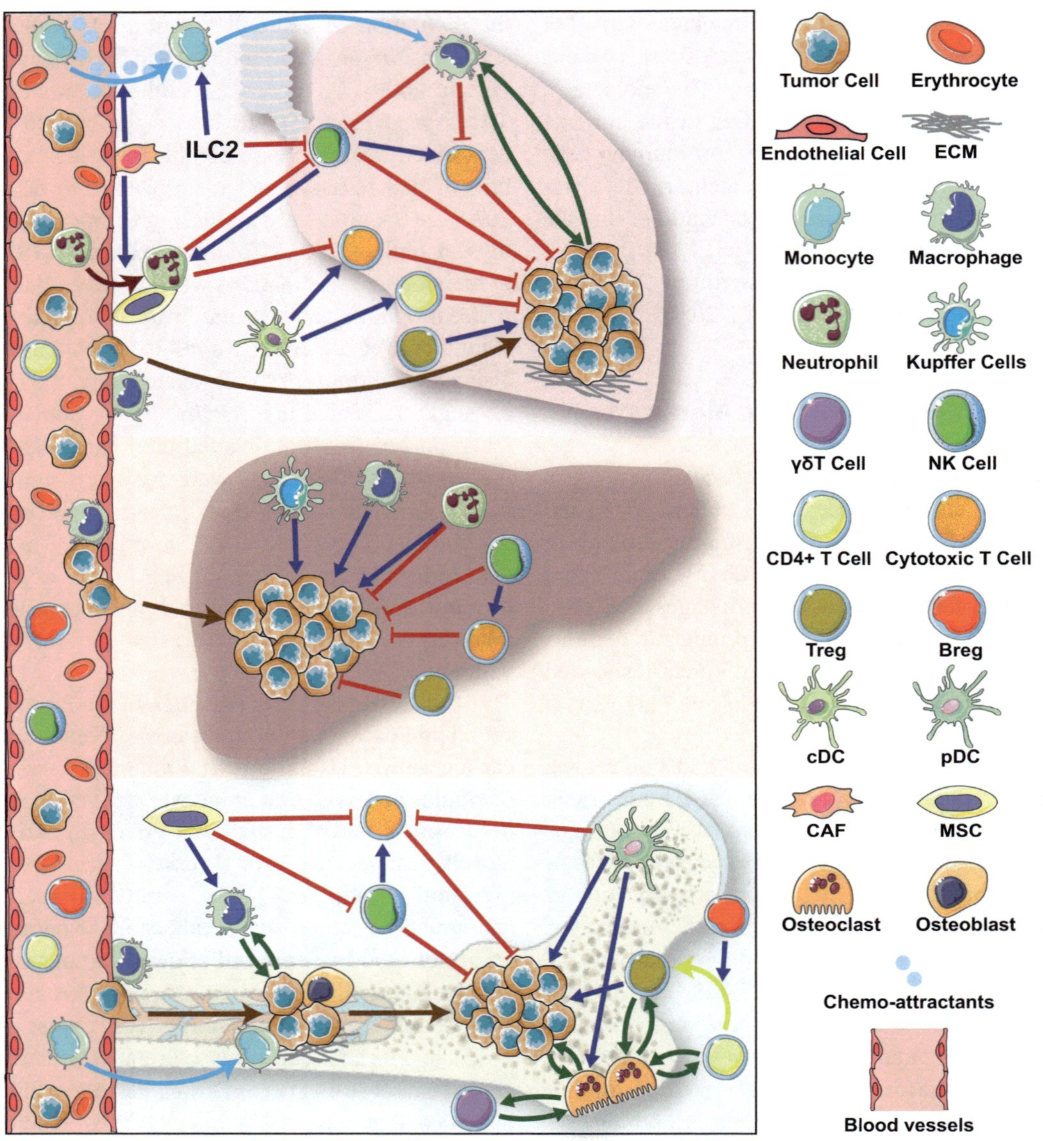

Fig. 20.2 Immune microenvironment regulates breast cancer distal metastasis. The three most frequent secondary sites for breast cancer distal metastasis are the bone, lung, and liver. Various immune cell interactions have been illustrated that regulate metastatic seeding and the persistent growth in these organs. Organ-specific immune responses may play a major role in determining the efficiency of distal metastasis. *ILC2* type 2 innate lymphoid cell

ligand 2 (CCL2) and S100 family proteins recruit circulating monocytes that differentiate into macrophages and support seeding and outgrowth of lung metastasis (Hiratsuka et al. 2006; Qian et al. 2011). Further studies revealed that breast cancer cells can produce various extracellular vesicles to modulate macrophages (Chen et al. 2022), which shapes tumour-promoting microenvironment by multiple mechanisms including generating immunosuppressive microenvironment through PD-L1 (Morrissey et al. 2021) and promoting angiogenesis through VEGF (Wang et al. 2023a) in lung tissues. Moreover, a recent paper indicated that the tumour-educated monocytes produced MMPs to disrupt the extracellular matrix (ECM), which helped cancer cells to exit blood vessels and invade lung tissues (Kim et al. 2019). Additionally, lysyl oxidase (LOX) was reported to recruit macrophages that produced MMP2 to cleave collagen and support pre-metastasis niche formation in liver and brain metastasis of breast cancer models and patient samples (Erler et al. 2009). Further studies demonstrated that LOX promoted bone metastasis through the activation of osteoclastogenesis in pre-metastatic lesions in 4T1 model (Cox et al. 2015).

At metastasis sites, macrophages have been identified as a multifunctional player supporting colonization or persistent growth. In lung metastasis, Qian et al. demonstrated that monocyte-derived macrophage was a major contributor promoting the extravasation, seeding, and persistent growth in PyMT-derived lung metastasis model. These macrophages were therefore termed as metastasis-associated macrophages (MAMs) (Qian et al. 2009). Further studies revealed that tumour cells recruit circulating inflammatory monocytes via CCL2-CCR2 signalling, which were the main source of MAMs (Qian et al. 2011). MAMs were reported to promote breast cancer cell survival through CCL3-CCR1 signalling (Kitamura et al. 2015b), and metastatic outgrowth through FMS-like tyrosine kinase 1 (FLT-1 or VEGFR1) mediated inflammatory response (Qian et al. 2015). Furthermore, MAMs supported tumour angiogenesis through the angiopoietin-1(Ang2)-Tie2 pathway in the lung metastasis of MMTV-PyMT model (Mazzieri et al. 2011). MAMs are also important for maintaining the stemness of metastatic cells. MAMs-derived CCL18 induce epithelial-mesenchymal transition (EMT) of tumour cells and enhance metastasis to the lung in multiple human breast cancer cell-derived models (Su et al. 2014). Interestingly, multiple factors control the recruitment and immune-suppressive function of MAMs which seem to be activated in tumour cells by cat eye syndrome chromosome region candidate 2 (CECR2), an acetyl-lysine reader and key epigenetic regulator (Zhang et al. 2022).

In bone metastasis, MAMs and bone-resident macrophages, especially osteoclasts, promote metastasis outgrowth through multiple mechanisms (Guo et al. 2024). Using a novel breast cancer bone metastasis model, MetBo2, in immune-proficient FVB background, a recent study illustrated that $CD204^{high}IL\text{-}4R^{high}$ macrophages, originating from $Ly6C^{+}CCR2^{+}$ inflammatory monocytes, are critical for metastatic outgrowth in an IL-4R-dependent manner (Ma et al. 2020). Another study illustrated that monocyte-/macrophage-CD137 (4-1BB) signal upregulated the expression of Fos-related antigen 1 (Fra1) and promoted macrophage migration and differentiation into osteoclasts, which promoted osteolysis and metastatic growth of breast cancer cells 4T1FL in allograft model (Jiang et al. 2019). Additionally, bone marrow macrophages can promote dormancy of breast cancer cells in the bone marrow through exosomes. Specifically, M2-like macrophages inhibit the proliferation of MDA-MB-231 and T47D breast cancer cells and promote drug resistance through forming gap junction-mediated intercellular communication with cancer stem cells, while exosomes from M1-like macrophages are capable of reversing dormancy by activating p65-NFkB signalling of breast cancer cells (Walker et al. 2019).

In brain metastasis, macrophages in general were reported to support breast cancer metastasis (Bowman et al. 2016; Gonzalez et al. 2022). A recent study indicated that blockade of MAM reprogramming using CSF1R and STAT5 inhibitors significantly reduced brain metastasis in MDA-BrM model (Klemm et al. 2021). Similar results were obtained in 4T1 and MDA-MB-231 brain metastasis model treated with CSF1R inhibitor PLX3397 (Wu et al. 2021a). Further studies indicated that the metastasis-promoting role of MAMs was P13K signalling-dependent. Pan-PI3K inhibitor buparlisib largely decreased MAM infiltration and reduced brain metastasis outgrowth in 4T1 model (Blazquez et al. 2018).

In brain metastasis, MAMs are heterogeneous with distinctive origins including monocyte-derived macrophages (MDMs), microglia, and central nervous system (CNS) border-associated macrophages (BAMs). In contrast to breast cancer metastases in other organs, only 5%–10% of MAMs in brain metastasis were originated from monocytes in 99LN-BrM model (Niesel et al. 2021). The role of MDM in brain metastasis is controversial. A recent study indicated a signalling cascade mediated by type I IFN derived from tumour-educated astrocyte stimulating tumour cell CCL2 expression which recruits monocytes to promote metastatic growth. This paper confirmed the critical metastasis-promoting role of MDM, at least in intracardiac injection models using E0771-Br and Yumm1.7-BrM cells (Ma et al. 2023). However, another study showed that genetic ablation of *Ccr2* did not affect brain metastasis outgrowth nor overall survival in E0771 model (Guldner et al. 2020). Microglia, a type of tissue-resident macrophage in the brain, was reported to promote metastasis. Microglia promotes the invasion of MCF7 breast cancer in brain tissue in a Wnt-dependent manner in an organotypic slice co-culture model (Pukrop et al. 2010). Furthermore, sc-RNAseq data revealed the immunosuppressive potential of LGALS1+ microglial cells in breast cancer patient samples (Zou et al. 2022). However, a few studies suggested an anti-tumour role of microglia. For example, in BCM2 and MBA-MD-231 model, metastatic tumour cells secrete neutrophin-3 to inhibit microglia activation and their immune surveillance in order to promote tumour cell invasion (Louie et al. 2012). Another recent study, using a microglia deficiency Csf1r$^{\Delta FIRE/\Delta FIRE}$ mice model, indicated that microglia enhanced the cytotoxicity of T and NK cells to suppress brain metastasis in MDA-MB-231-BR and E0771 models (Evans et al. 2023). BAMs were reported to support metastatic tumour cell extravasation across the blood-brain barrier (Sun and Jiang 2024). A CITE-seq analysis identified the existence of BAMs in E0771 breast cancer brain metastasis model (Guldner et al. 2020). However, specific function analysis is lacking.

MAMs play a metastasis-promoting role in liver metastasis models of breast cancer (Liu et al. 2022). In multiple in vivo models, MAMs secrete CCL18 to induce tumour cell EMT and liver metastasis (Chen et al. 2011; Su et al. 2014). A recent study characterized six MAM clusters in liver metastasis of six breast cancer patients using sc-RNAseq, including two distinct immunosuppressive MAMs marked by TREM2 and FCN3 expression, respectively. Among them, FCN3+ MAMs were unique for liver metastasis with high expression of MHC complex which may activate T cell through antigen presentation (Wang et al. 2024). Furthermore, GATA6+ resident peritoneal macrophages promote liver metastasis of 4T1 breast cancer model through PD-L1-mediated CD8+ T cell suppression (Hossain et al. 2022). Many studies have indicated that liver-resident macrophages, Kupffer cells, played a major role in extravasation, premetastatic niche formation, seeding, and the persistent growth of liver metastasis of several cancer types, including colon and pancreatic cancers (Keirsse et al. 2018). However, data evaluating the role of Kupffer cells in breast cancer liver metastasis were lacking.

Future studies on the role of distinctive macrophage subsets in various metastasis target organs are needed to improve our understanding of how macrophage heterogeneity may contribute to breast cancer metastasis.

20.1.2 Neutrophils

Neutrophils are a type of innate immune cells that rapidly respond to inflammatory signals in large numbers. Neutrophils participate in breast cancer metastasis by acting at both the primary tumour and the (pre)metastatic niche. In primary tumour models, neutrophils can release MMP9, S100A8/9, and BV8 to activate VEGF to promote angiogenesis (Shojaei et al. 2007). Laminin degradation by neutrophil-derived proteases, e.g. elastase and MMP9, and growth factors can assist tumour cell proliferation (Lerman and Hammes 2018). Neutrophils can also directly interact with cancer cells and promote their migration and invasion into surrounding tissues (Wu et al. 2020; Duits and De Visser 2021). Furthermore, inflammatory stimuli (e.g. IL-1β and TNF-α) can induce neutrophil c-MET expression and binding of HGF, leading to NO (nitric oxide) or elastase production and tumour cell killing (Finisguerra et al. 2015; Cui et al. 2021). Intriguingly, splenic neutrophils have been shown to contribute to the outgrowth of primary tumour and lung metastasis in 4T1 model through the creation of a glucose-deprived microenvironment in the white pulp, which induces T cell anergy by impairing pyruvate kinase M2 and its action on STAT5 (Wang et al. 2023b). Further investigation is needed to test if this can be a general mechanism.

More studies have focused on the role of neutrophils in distal metastasis. Tumour-secreted protease cathepsin C (CTSC)-PR3-IL-1β axis induced neutrophil production of reactive oxygen species and neutrophil extracellular traps (NETs), which were important for lung metastasis in multiple breast cancer models including 4T1, MDA-MB-231, LM2, and SCP28 (Xiao et al. 2021). Direct interactions between cancer cells and neutrophils or NETs can lead to tumour arrest in the vasculature and increase the efficiency of extravasation (McFarlane et al. 2021) and epithelial-mesenchymal transition, a pro-metastatic phenotype, of MCF7 human breast cancer cells (Martins-Cardoso et al. 2020). Another study indicated that NETs were abundant in the liver metastases of patients with breast and colon cancers and that serum NETs can predict the occurrence of liver metastases in patients with early-stage breast cancer. Mechanistically, NET-DNA acted as a chemotactic factor to attract cancer cells to form distant metastases in the livers or lungs. Transmembrane protein CCDC25 was suggested to act as a NET-DNA receptor that senses extracellular DNA and subsequently activated the ILK–β-parvin pathway to enhance cell motility. Furthermore, the expression of CCDC25 on cancer cells was closely associated with a poor prognosis in patients (Yang et al. 2020).

In pre-metastatic niche in 4T1 and MMTV-PyMT models, neutrophils were induced to accumulate neutral lipids upon interacting with mesenchymal cells. Lipids in these neutrophils were transported to metastatic tumour cells through a macropinocytosis-lysosome pathway, which promotes tumour cell survival and proliferation (Li et al. 2020a). Neutrophil-derived inflammatory molecules, such as S100A8, increased vascular permeability and extravasation (Kowanetz et al. 2010). Furthermore, recent studies suggested that lung-infiltrating neutrophils were reprogrammed by mesenchymal cells through PTGS2-PGE2 and robustly suppressed both T cells and NK cells to promote metastasis (Gong et al. 2023).

However, neutrophils can also aid tumour cell killing and inhibit metastasis. Neutrophils can use antibody-dependent cellular cytotoxicity (ADCC) to kill cancer cells (Matlung et al. 2018; Treffers et al. 2020). CCL2 produced by the primary tumour can activate neutrophils in the pre-metastatic niche (potential through monocytes) to produce hydrogen peroxide, providing an efficient tumour cell killing mechanism (Lavender et al. 2017; Hagerling et al. 2019). IFN-β was also shown to increase neutrophil anti-tumour potential by increasing NET capacity and cytotoxicity toward tumour cells (Andzinski et al. 2015). Interestingly, the function diversity of neutrophils can be partly dependent on the presence of NK cells. In NK cell-deficient mice, granulocyte colony-stimulating factor (G-CSF)-expanded neutrophils inhibited metastatic colonization of breast tumour cells in the lung. In contrast, in NK cell-competent mice, neutrophils facilitated metastatic colonization in the same models. Intriguingly, both modulatory effects are mediated by reactive oxygen species (ROS) (Li et al. 2020b). Therefore, the precise role of neutrophils in breast cancer metastasis remains controversial and is likely to be context-dependent.

CXCR1 and CXCR2 are important chemoattractant receptors for neutrophils. A phase I clinical trial (Study NCT02001974) on triple-negative metastatic breast cancer patients successfully evaluated the safety and pharmacokinetics of orally administered reparixin, an inhibitor of CXCR1 and CXCR2, in combination with paclitaxel. A current phase II study (Study NCT02370238) is evaluating the progression-free survival of newly diagnosed triple-negative breast cancer (TNBC) patients (newly diagnosed metastatic or relapsed following (neo)adjuvant chemotherapy) treated with reparixin in combination with paclitaxel vs. paclitaxel alone, whose results have not been published yet (Schott et al. 2017). Interestingly, neutrophils can naturally traffic to bone marrow and cross the bone marrow-blood barrier. Recent studies reported the use of neutrophils for targeted delivery of free cabazitaxel and drug-loaded poly(lactic-co-glycolic) acid nanoparticles to the bone marrow, which significantly inhibited metastatic growth (Luo et al. 2023). These studies suggested the therapeutic potential of utilizing neutrophils in treating breast cancer.

20.1.3 Dendritic Cell

Dendritic cells (DCs) are believed to be one of the major antigen-presenting cells. Recent studies indicated that Bruton's tyrosine kinase (BTK) inhibitor ibrutinib can induce the differentiation of monocytes to dendritic cells, enhancing antitumour Th1 and cytotoxic T lymphocyte (CTL) immune responses and suppressing metastasis in the E0771 model (Varikuti et al. 2020).

On the contrary, plasmacytoid dendritic cells (pDCs) have been shown to promote tumour growth and metastasis. In three immunocompetent mouse models of breast cancer bone metastasis, pDC and CD4+ T cell number increased with tumour burden, and pDC-derived osteolytic cytokines caused severe bone damage. Depletion of pDC though anti-PDAC-1 antibody resulted in decreased tumour burden and bone loss by activating tumour-specific CD8+ T cell (Sawant et al. 2012). More recent studies showed that pDC infiltration in breast cancer was associated with poor prognosis and promoted lymph node metastasis via the CXCR4/SDF-1 axis (Gadalla et al. 2019). Consistently, the density of LAMP3+ DCs was enriched in TNBCs and correlated with worse survival (Szpor et al. 2021). Further investigation is needed to better understand the pleotropic role of DCs in breast cancer metastasis.

20.1.4 B Cells

B cells are a type of adaptive immune cells that develop in bone marrow, where B cells and their precursors account for around 30% of all immune cells. Most B cells originate from haematopoiesis and are named B2 cells. Following activation by antigens, mature B cells function as cytotoxic cells by releasing various cytokines or differentiate into plasma cells to produce antibody. In contrast, regulatory B cells (Breg), a more recently identified B cell subset, were detected in bone marrow and displayed immunosuppressive function like Tregs (Rosser and Mauri 2015). Apart from these HSC-derived B cell subsets, bone marrow maintains a small population of B lineage cells originating from foetal liver, which are termed B1 cells. These B1 cells are a major resource of natural IgM antibody for inducing quick T cell-independent immune responses (Choi et al. 2012).

In localized breast cancer, B cells are the most abundant lymphocytes and account for 25%–40% of tumour-infiltrating lymphocytes (Nelson 2010). Several clinical studies indicated that accumulation of CD20+ tumour-infiltrating B cells was significantly correlated with better prognosis in all breast cancer subtypes (Coronella-Wood and Hersh 2003; Arias-Pulido et al. 2018). Furthermore, CD38+ tumour-infiltrating plasma cells and higher immunoglobulin (Ig) levels are favourable prognostic factors in TNBC (Yeong et al. 2018). However, B cells may play a supportive role in promoting breast cancer metastasis, especially in lymph node metastasis. A recent publication indicated that primary breast tumours induced the accumulation of B cells in lymph nodes, which promoted lymph node metastasis by secreting pathogenic IgG in PyMT and 4T1 breast cancer models (Gu et al. 2019). Consistently, 2 retrospective studies, with 134 and 124 breast cancer cases, respectively, found that the density of CD19+ B cells in tumours was positively correlated with lymph node metastasis and poor prognosis (Guan et al. 2016; Steenbruggen et al. 2023). Plasma cell abundance was correlated with worse overall survival in 97 cases of metastatic breast cancer (Wei et al. 2016).

Current preclinical data illustrated distinctive roles of B cell subsets in the tumour microenvironment (Laumont et al. 2022; Ramos et al. 2023). Among them, plasma cells are the only population capable of efficient antibody production, which mediates accurate tumour cell killing via ADCC. Indeed, plasma cells have been reported to infiltrate into tumour tissue and produce tumour antigen-specific Ig in several studies (Sharonov et al. 2020). Research demonstrated that IgG-producing plasma cells mediated humoral immune response against secreted/shed tumour glycoproteins (STGP) and promoted liver metastasis through monocyte activation in T47D breast cancer model (Nyhus et al. 2001). Bregs were reported to promote bone metastasis outgrowth by producing immunosuppressive cytokines such as IL-10 to convert anti-tumour CD4+ T cells to Tregs in various human breast cancer models (Olkhanud et al. 2011). Another study indicated that Bregs may also exert their immunosuppressive function by blocking the switch of memory B cells to plasma cells, which dampened antibody response and promoted breast cancer progression in patients (Pati et al. 2023). Additionally, research showed that $CD24^{hi}CD27^{+}$ Bregs promoted tumour cell EMT, stemness, and drug resistance in lymph node metastasis of multiple breast cancer models (Huang et al. 2023).

Genetic ablation of mature B cells enhanced anti-tumour response of T cells and reduced subcutaneous tumour growth in TS/A and EMT6 breast cancer models (Qin et al. 1998; Zhang et al. 2013). B cells were also found to interact with innate immune cells in the tumour microenvironment. Tumour-educated B cells selectively promoted breast cancer lymph node metastasis by HSPA4-targeting IgG (Gu et al. 2019). However, these potent tumour-promoting functions of mature B cells are yet to be confirmed in other metastatic target organs of breast cancer. In contrast, B1 cell-derived IgM induced tumour killing and protected mice from peritoneal metastasis in the TA3-Ha mammary carcinoma model (Haro et al. 2019). B cells were reported to produce tumour-specific isotype-switched antibodies and significantly reduced lung metastasis growth in preclinical models, suggesting B cells may have a role in tumour clearance (Guy et al. 2016).

Taken together, the current research suggests that B cells are a critical compartment of the immune microenvironment in metastatic breast cancer. Rituximab, an FDA-approved CD20 monoclonal antibody, showed no benefits in treating solid tumours, including breast cancer (Aklilu et al. 2004). Furthermore, patients receiving treatment showed high numbers of circulating tumour cells, suggesting a potential risk of increased metastasis (Neves and Kwok 2015; Pierpont et al. 2018). Future studies investigating the specific roles of B cell subsets in breast cancer metastasis may potentially improve B cell-targeting therapies in the clinic.

20.1.5 T Cells

T cells, or T lymphocytes, are a group of immune cells identified by their expression of surface T cell receptor (TCR). T cells originate from HSCs in bone marrow, which differentiate into T cell lineages under the regulation of transcription factor GATA3. These precursors migrate from bone marrow into the thymus for TCR rearrangement and selection and become naïve T cells that further differentiate into mature T cells in peripheral tissues. Based on the expression of TCR co-receptor, mature T cells are classified as CD8+ or CD4+ T cells. The CD8+ T cells are mainly responsible for inducing apoptosis of targeted cells such as cancer cells, thus are also termed as cytotoxic T cells (CTLs). The CD4+ T cells mainly modulate other immune cells and are further characterized as helper T cells (Th cells) or regulatory T cells (Tregs). Apart from the conventional adaptive T cell populations, recent studies identified rare populations of innate-like T cells, including both NKT and γδT cells, which express TCR but share molecular features and functions with innate immune cells. Similar to natural killer cells, natural killer T (NKT) cells can destroy target cells without prior antigen sensitization (Kriegsmann et al. 2018). Furthermore, recent studies identified a small group of T cells expressing γδ isoforms of TCR, instead of αβ TCR found on most T cells. Existing data indicate that these cells recognize antigens distinct from αβT cells. In addition, they are an important source of chemokines and cytokines to attract myeloid cells, suggesting their unique functions in immunomodulation, especially in autoimmune diseases (Vantourout and Hayday 2013).

In breast cancer, several studies confirmed the anti-tumour role of CD8+ T cells and their association with better clinical outcomes in all subtypes of breast cancer (Liu et al. 2012; Hou et al. 2018; Vihervuori et al. 2019). Conversely, CD4 and FOXP3 (Treg markers) expression were correlated with metastasis and poor prognosis (Xue et al. 2018; Matkowski et al. 2009). In addition, $CD25^{hi}$ Th17 cells were found to suppress CTL function and correlated with poor prognosis in local invasive breast cancer (Thibaudin et al. 2016). Therefore, T cells can be important regulators of breast cancer metastasis. Type 2 Th cells expressing IL-4 and IL-10 were found to support tumour growth by stimulating tumour-promoting cells like TAMs (Ellyard et al. 2007). Recent studies indicated that CD8 T cells predominately suppressed lung metastasis outgrowth in the 4T1 breast cancer model (Haider et al. 2020). Consistently, activation of tumour-specific CTLs largely prevented spontaneous lung metastasis in the same model (Hosoya et al. 2018). In contrast, accumulation of Tregs was linked with metastasis in breast cancer patients (Lal et al. 2013). Consistently, Tregs have been shown to promote lung and lymph node metastasis in various breast cancer models (Halvorsen et al. 2014).

Several studies suggested the critical roles of T cells in the seeding and colonization of breast cancer bone metastasis. Monteiro et al. found that knockdown of RANKL or IL-17 on T cells significantly promoted osteoclast-induced bone destruction before metastasis colonization in the 4T1 model, revealing T cells as a critical component in the pre-metastatic niche of the bone marrow (Monteiro et al. 2013). Indeed, Th17 (Sato et al. 2006) and FOXP3+ Tregs (Tan et al. 2011) can crosstalk with osteoclasts through the RANK-RANKL pathway, which is a key signalling pathway driving the differentiation of osteoclasts and bone homeostasis. Furthermore, γδT cells were reported to regulate osteoclastogenesis and bone resorption by producing pro-osteoclastogenic IL-6 or anti-osteoclastogenic IFN-γ dynamically (Phalke and Chiplunkar 2015). Osteoclasts in turn worked as antigen-presenting cells to activate T cells (Madel et al. 2019). Additionally, CD8+ T cells were found to reduce bone metastasis growth independent of osteolytic bone loss (Zhang et al. 2011). These data suggested that T cells could be a potential therapeutic target for bone metastatic breast cancer.

Several strategies have been developed to target T cells in breast cancer. Recent large-scale clinical trials have evaluated the effect of immune checkpoint in breast cancer patients as monotherapy or in combination with traditional treatments (Page et al. 2019). Although monotherapies had few benefits in patients with metastatic breast cancer, the combination of immunotherapy and chemotherapy or molecular-targeted therapies significantly enhanced patient survival and/or reduced adverse effects (Esteva et al. 2019). Trials also studied the therapeutic effect of chimeric antigen receptor-engineered T cells (CAR-T) in breast cancer patients (NCT04430595), which showed promising results in treating primary and progressive tumours in preclinical models (Martinez and Moon 2019). A recent study showed that the combination of CXCR4 inhibitor AMD3465 and an indoleamine 2,3-dioxygenase (IDO) inhibitor (D1MT) significantly inhibited bone metastasis growth in the 4T1 breast cancer model, by reducing the number of Tregs and enhancing the anti-tumour response of CTLs (Zhang et al. 2019). Of note, a case report showed that anti-PD-1 or anti-CTLA-4 therapy inhibited bone metastasis growth and bone-related events in patients of various cancer types (Te 2019). However, the therapeutic effect of T cell-targeting immunotherapy in patients with breast cancer bone metastasis remains inconclusive at the moment.

In summary, T cells can be a promising target for immunotherapy in metastatic breast cancer. However, further research understanding the distinctive roles of T cells in different metastasis loci is essential to maximize the therapeutic benefit.

20.1.6 Innate Lymphoid Cells

Innate lymphoid cells (ILCs) are a group of innate immune cells that belong to the lymphoid lineage but do not react in an antigen-specific fashion (Walker et al. 2013). Based on their cytokine production and transcription factor dependency, ILCs can be divided into three groups, Group 1–3, mirroring the nomenclature of T cell subsets (Lanier 2013). Group 1 ILCs, including ILC1 and NK cells, are characterized by their expression of T helper 1 (Th1) cytokines, typically IFN-γ. Group 2 ILCs express Th2 cytokines such as interleukin-4 (IL-4), IL-5, and IL-13. Group 3 ILCs produce Th17-associated cytokines IL-17 and IL-22. These differences lead to distinct immune-modulatory functions of the different ILC groups (Spits et al. 2013).

ILC1s have been reported to suppress tumour development in PyMT mouse mammary tumour models (Dadi et al. 2016). As a type of ILC1, NK cells have potent cytotoxic activity that lyses target cells directly via the production of perforin, granzyme B, and pro-inflammatory cytokines like IFN-γ. Their anti-tumour function was known for several decades (Rosenberg et al. 1972). NK cells can also lyse tumour cells through activation of T cells and antibody-dependent cell-mediated cytotoxicity. Thus, NK cell actively inhibits almost every step of tumour metastasis. For example, recent studies indicated that NK cells kept breast and lung cancer cells in quiescence in multiple metastasis target organs (Malladi et al. 2016). However, the cytotoxic functions of NK cells are often suppressed by tumour cells and the tumour microenvironment, (Pasero et al. 2016) including myeloid cells (Gabrilovich et al. 2012) and Tregs (Ghiringhelli et al. 2006; Jie et al. 2015). Of note, several clinical trials have tried to reactivate NK cells in order to treat late-stage metastatic tumours. Lirilumab, antibody blocking NK cell inhibitory receptors, the killer-cell immunoglobulin-like receptors (KIRs), has been tested in a clinical trial (NCT01714739), without reaching expected results due to side effects. Inhibition of the TAM tyrosine kinase receptors (Tyro3, Axl, and Mer) in NK cells may also potentiate their anti-metastatic potential (Paolino et al. 2014). A previous trial also tested adoptive transfer of human NK cells following pre-treatment with cytokine cocktail of IL-12, IL-15, and IL-18 in patients with acute myeloid leukaemia, without achieving the expected outcome (NCT01520558). Chimeric antigen receptor (CAR) has been explored to direct NK cell cytotoxicity more specifically toward cancer cells following autologous transfer of genetically engineered NK cells (Chu et al. 2013; Carlsten and Childs 2015; Schonfeld et al. 2015). More research efforts in both preclinical and clinical studies are needed in the coming years to fully utilize the anti-metastasis activity of NK cells in order to achieve clinical benefit.

Data on the role of other ILC populations in tumour are emerging. ILC2s were shown to promote tumour growth through IL-13 production and recruitment of myeloid cells and Tregs (Jovanovic et al. 2014; Qian 2017). Lung-resident ILC2s orchestrated the suppression of NK cell-mediated innate anti-tumour immunity, leading to increased lung metastases and mortality in multiple preclinical models. Mechanistically, this study showed that ILC2-derived IL-5 promoted eosinophil-mediated suppression of NK cells by restraining glucose metabolism (Schuijs et al. 2020). ILC2 may also promote lung metastasis in 4T1 breast cancer model through the recruitment of MDSCs by IL-33 (Ito et al. 2022) or IL-13 (Zhao et al. 2021). Thus, ILC2 may play important roles in the immune microenvironment of breast cancer metastasis.

Physiological function of ILC3 cells is involved in the suppression of bacteria-induced inflammation through IL-17 and/or IL-22 secretion and tissue homeostasis of the gastrointestinal tract (Zeng et al. 2019). Previous studies indicated that increased numbers of RORγt(+) ILC3 in human breast tumour samples correlated with an increased likelihood of lymph node metastasis. In 4T1.2 model, CCL21-mediated recruitment of ILC3 was proposed to promote cancer cell motility and lymph node metastasis through interaction with stromal cells and production of RANKL (Irshad et al. 2017). Recent sc-RNAseq studies identified NK cells and ILC3 as the prominent subpopulations of ILCs in lymph node metastasis from breast cancer patients (Rethacker et al. 2022). Together, these data suggest a specific role of ILC3 in lymph node metastasis, while the potential role of these cells in distal metastasis remains unknown.

20.1.7 Nonimmune Cells

Of note, nonimmune cells are important for the balance of the immune microenvironment. For example, cells of mesenchymal origin, most notably mesenchymal stem cells (MSCs) and fibroblasts, are important regulators of inflammatory response (Cai et al. 2021; Davidson et al. 2021). MSCs have potent immune-suppressive functions through inducible nitric oxide synthase (iNOS), indoleamine 2,3-dioxygenase (IDO), PGE2, IL-10, hemeoxygenase-1 (HO-1), programmed cell death 1 ligand 1 (PD-L1), and IL-6 (De Castro et al. 2019). MSCs can also recruit immune-suppressive macrophages to promote tumour growth through CCL2 secretion (Ren et al. 2012). Pro-inflammatory factors derived from cancer-associated fibroblasts (CAFs) have been shown to promote breast cancer progression (Sharon et al. 2015). In MMTV-PyMT and 4T1 models, CAF-derived IL-33 induced type-2 inflammation; recruited eosinophils, neutrophils, and inflammatory monocytes; and promoted lung metastasis (Shani et al. 2020). For a comprehensive summary of CAF function in breast cancer metastasis, please refer to a recent review by Li and colleagues (Li et al. 2023).

20.2 Conclusion

In summary, the immune microenvironment is hijacked to serve as a driving force for breast cancer metastasis. However, many immune cells have anti-tumour potential that can be elicited by the modulation of signalling pathways within these cells and/or of the cytokine environment. This provides an attractive therapeutic strategy to effectively treat metastatic breast cancer, alone or in combination with other therapeutic modalities.

Of note, even in aggressive tumours, only a minority of cancer cells are migratory as revealed by intravital imaging studies across multiple tumour models (Condeelis et al. 2005; Scheele et al. 2016). This may be partly caused by tumour cell plasticity (Beerling et al. 2016) and intrinsic heterogeneity (Pinner et al. 2009). Mounting evidence indicates that the immune microenvironment is also heterogeneous, which may be associated with heterogeneous tumour cell behaviour (Scheele et al. 2016).

With the advancement of single-cell omics technologies, more and more studies have characterized the heterogeneity of breast cancer immune microenvironment (Ali et al. 2020; Pal et al. 2021; Wu et al. 2021b; Andersson et al. 2021; McNamara et al. 2021; Liu et al. 2023). New immune cell subtypes and their spatial interaction with other cells are being characterized with unprecedented amounts of new data. Lots of data mining and validation efforts are still needed to further explore these single-cell and spatial omics data to reveal the mechanistic link between immune cell heterogeneity and metastasis. Future studies utilizing these data are warranted to identify novel mechanisms of cancer metastasis and inspire effective new therapies to eradicate this deadly disease.

Acknowledgement The authors would like to acknowledge Chengcheng Sun for creating illustrations. R.Y.M. is supported by the National Natural Science Foundation of China 82303476, Fellowship of China Postdoctoral Science Foundation 2021M700814, and International Postdoctoral Exchange Fellowship Program YJ20210251.

References

Adams S, Gatti-Mays ME, Kalinsky K, Korde LA, Sharon E, Amiri-Kordestani L, Bear H, McArthur HL, Frank E, Perlmutter J, Page DB, Vincent B, Hayes JF, Gulley JL, Litton JK, Hortobagyi GN, Chia S, Krop I, White J, Sparano J, Disis ML, Mittendorf EA (2019) Current landscape of immunotherapy in breast cancer: a review. JAMA Oncol

Aklilu M, Stadler WM, Markiewicz M, Vogelzang NJ, Mahowald M, Johnson M, Gajewski TF (2004) Depletion of normal B cells with rituximab as an adjunct to IL-2 therapy for renal cell carcinoma and melanoma. Ann Oncol 15:1109–1114

Ali HR, Jackson HW, Zanotelli VRT, Danenberg E, Fischer JR, Bardwell H, Provenzano E, Rueda OM, Chin S-F, Aparicio S, Caldas C, Bodenmiller B (2020) Imaging mass cytometry and multiplatform genomics define the phenogenomic landscape of breast cancer. Nat Cancer 1:163–175

Andersson A, Larsson L, Stenbeck L, Salmen F, Ehinger A, Wu SZ, Al-Eryani G, Roden D, Swarbrick A, Borg A, Frisen J, Engblom C, Lundeberg J (2021) Spatial deconvolution of HER2-positive breast cancer delineates tumor-associated cell type interactions. Nat Commun 12:6012

Andzinski L, Kasnitz N, Stahnke S, Wu CF, Gereke M, Ckritz-Blickwede VK, M., Schilling, B., Brandau, S., Weiss, S. & Jablonska, J. (2015) Type IIFNs induce anti-tumor polarization of tumor associated neutrophils in mice and human. Int J Cancer 138:1982–1993

Arias-Pulido H, Cimino-Mathews A, Chaher N, Qualls C, Joste N, Colpaert C, Marotti JD, Foisey M, Prossnitz ER, Emens LA, Fiering S (2018) The combined presence of CD20 + B cells and PD-L1 + tumor-infiltrating lymphocytes in inflammatory breast cancer is prognostic of improved patient outcome. Breast Cancer Res Treat 171:273–282

Arwert EN, Harney AS, Entenberg D, Wang Y, Sahai E, Pollard JW, Condeelis JS (2018) A unidirectional transition from migratory to perivascular macrophage is required for tumor cell intravasation. Cell Rep 23:1239–1248

Beerling E, Seinstra D, De Wit E, Kester L, Van Der Velden D, Maynard C, Schafer R, Van Diest P, Voest E, Van Oudenaarden A, Vrisekoop N, Van Rheenen J (2016) Plasticity between epithelial and mesenchymal states unlinks EMT from metastasis-enhancing stem cell capacity. Cell Rep 14:2281–2288

Blazquez R, Wlochowitz D, Wolff A, Seitz S, Wachter A, Perera-Bel J, Bleckmann A, Bei Barth T, Salinas G, Riemenschneider MJ, Proescholdt M, Evert M, Utpatel K, Siam L, Schatlo B, Balkenhol M, Stadelmann C, Schildhaus HU, Korf U, Reinz E, Wiemann S, Vollmer E, Schulz M, Ritter U, Hanisch UK, Pukrop T (2018) PI3K: a master regulator of brain metastasis-promoting macrophages/microglia. Glia 66:2438–2455

Bowman RL, Klemm F, Akkari L, Pyonteck SM, Sevenich L, Quail DF, Dhara S, Simpson K, Gardner EE, Iacobuzio-Donahue CA, Brennan CW, Tabar V, Gutin PH, Joyce JA (2016) Macrophage ontogeny underlies differences in tumor-specific education in brain malignancies. Cell Rep 17:2445–2459

Cai C, Zeng D, Gao Q, Ma L, Zeng B, Zhou Y, Wang H (2021) Decreased ferroportin in hepatocytes promotes macrophages polarize towards an M2-like phenotype and liver fibrosis. Sci Rep 11:13386

Carlsten M, Childs RW (2015) Genetic manipulation of NK cells for cancer immunotherapy: techniques and clinical implications. Front Immunol 6:266

Cassetta L, Pollard JW (2018) Targeting macrophages: therapeutic approaches in cancer. Nat Rev Drug Discov

Cassetta L, Fragkogianni S, Sims AH, Swierczak A, Forrester LM, Zhang H, Soong DYH, Cotechini T, Anur P, Lin EY, Fidanza A, Lopez-Yrigoyen M, Millar MR, Urman A, Ai Z, Spellman PT, Hwang ES, Dixon JM, Wiechmann L, Coussens LM, Smith HO, Pollard JW (2019) Human tumor-associated macrophage and monocyte transcriptional landscapes reveal cancer-specific reprogramming, biomarkers, and therapeutic targets. Cancer Cell 35:588–602 e10

Chen J, Yao Y, Gong C, Yu F, Su S, Chen J, Liu B, Deng H, Wang F, Lin L (2011) CCL18 from tumor-associated macrophages promotes breast cancer metastasis via PITPNM3. Cancer Cell 19:541–555

Chen X, Feng J, Chen W, Shao S, Chen L, Wan H (2022) Small extracellular vesicles: from promoting pre-metastatic niche formation to therapeutic strategies in breast cancer. Cell Commun Signal 20

Choi YS, Dieter JA, Rothaeusler K, Luo Z, Baumgarth N (2012) B-1 cells in the bone marrow are a significant source of natural IgM. Eur J Immunol 42:120–129

Chu J, Deng Y, Benson DM, He S, Hughes T, Zhang J, Peng Y, Mao H, Yi L, Ghoshal K, He X, Devine SM, Zhang X, Caligiuri MA, Hofmeister CC, Yu J (2013) CS1-specific chimeric antigen receptor (CAR)-engineered natural killer cells enhance in vitro and in vivo antitumor activity against human multiple myeloma. Leukemia 28:917–927

Clark AG, Vignjevic DM (2015) Modes of cancer cell invasion and the role of the microenvironment. Curr Opin Cell Biol 36:13–22

Condeelis J, Singer RH, Segall JE (2005) The great escape: when cancer cells hijack the genes for chemotaxis and motility. Annu Rev Cell Dev Biol 21:695–718

Coronella-Wood JA, Hersh EM (2003) Naturally occurring B-cell responses to breast cancer. Cancer Immunol Immunother 52:715–738

Cox TR, Rumney RM, Schoof EM, Perryman L, Hoye AM, Agrawal A, Bird D, Latif NA, Forrest H, Evans HR, Huggins ID, Lang G, Linding R, Gartland A, Erler JT (2015) The hypoxic cancer secretome induces pre-metastatic bone lesions through lysyl oxidase. Nature 522:106–110

Cui C, Chakraborty K, Tang XA, Zhou G, Schoenfelt KQ, Becker KM, Hoffman A, Chang Y-F, Blank A, Reardon CA, Kenny HA, Vaisar T, Lengyel E, Greene G, Becker L (2021) Neutrophil elastase selectively kills cancer cells and attenuates tumorigenesis. Cell 184:3163–3177.e21

Dadi S, Chhangawala S, Whitlock BM, Franklin RA, Luo CT, Oh SA, Toure A, Pritykin Y, Huse M, Leslie CS, Li MO (2016) Cancer immunosurveillance by tissue-resident innate lymphoid cells and innate-like T cells. Cell 164:365–377

Davidson S, Coles M, Thomas T, Kollias G, Ludewig B, Turley S, Brenner M, Buckley CD (2021) Fibroblasts as immune regulators in infection, inflammation and cancer. Nat Rev Immunol 21:704–717

De Castro LL, Lopes-Pacheco M, Weiss DJ, Cruz FF, Rocco PRM (2019) Current understanding of the immunosuppressive properties of mesenchymal stromal cells. J Mol Med 97:605–618

De Visser KE, Joyce JA (2023) The evolving tumor microenvironment: from cancer initiation to metastatic outgrowth. Cancer Cell 41:374–403

Denardo DG, Brennan DJ, Rexhepaj E, Ruffell B, Shiao SL, Madden SF, Gallagher WM, Wadhwani N, Keil SD, Junaid SA, Rugo HS, Hwang ES, Jirstrom K, West BL, Coussens LM (2011) Leukocyte complexity predicts breast cancer survival and functionally regulates response to chemotherapy. Cancer Discov 1:54–67

Duits DEM, De Visser KE (2021) Impact of cancer cell-intrinsic features on neutrophil behavior. Semin Immunol 57:101546

Ellyard JI, Simson L, Parish CR (2007) Th2-mediated anti-tumour immunity: friend or foe? Tissue Antigens 70:1–11

Erler JT, Bennewith KL, Cox TR, Lang G, Bird D, Koong A, Le QT, Giaccia AJ (2009) Hypoxia-induced lysyl oxidase is a critical mediator of bone marrow cell recruitment to form the premetastatic niche. Cancer Cell 15:35–44

Esteva FJ, Hubbard-Lucey VM, Tang J, Pusztai L (2019) Immunotherapy and targeted therapy combinations in metastatic breast cancer. Lancet Oncol 20:e175–e186

Evans KT, Blake K, Longworth A, Coburn MA, Insua-Rodr Guez J, McMullen TP, Nguyen QH, Ma D, Lev T, Hernandez GA, Oganyan AK, Orujyan D, Edwards RA, Pridans C, Green KN, Villalta SA, Blurton-Jones M, Lawson DA (2023) Microglia promote anti-tumour immunity and suppress breast cancer brain metastasis. Nat Cell Biol 25:1848–1859

Fidler IJ (2003) The pathogenesis of cancer metastasis: the 'seed and soil' hypothesis revisited. Nat Rev Cancer 3:453–458

Finisguerra V, Di Conza G, Di Matteo M, Serneels J, Costa S, Thompson AAR, Wauters E, Walmsley S, Prenen H, Granot Z, Casazza A, Mazzone M (2015) MET is required for the recruitment of anti-tumoural neutrophils. Nature 522:349–353

Gabrilovich DI, Ostrand-Rosenberg S, Bronte V (2012) Coordinated regulation of myeloid cells by tumours. Nat Rev Immunol 12:253–268

Gadalla R, Hassan H, Ibrahim SA, Abdullah MS, Gaballah A, Greve B, El-Deeb S, El-Shinawi M, Mohamed MM (2019) Tumor microenvironmental plasmacytoid dendritic cells contribute to breast cancer lymph node metastasis via CXCR4/SDF-1 axis. Breast Cancer Res Treat 174:679–691

Ghiringhelli F, Menard C, Martin F, Zitvogel L (2006) The role of regulatory T cells in the control of natural killer cells: relevance during tumor progression. Immunol Rev 214:229–238

Gong Z, Li Q, Shi J, Li P, Hua L, Shultz LD, Ren G (2023) Immunosuppressive reprogramming of neutrophils by lung mesenchymal cells promotes breast cancer metastasis. Sci Immunol 8

Gonzalez H, Mei W, Robles I, Hagerling C, Allen BM, Hauge Okholm TL, Nanjaraj A, Verbeek T, Kalavacherla S, Van Gogh M, Georgiou S, Daras M, Phillips JJ, Spitzer MH, Roose JP, Werb Z (2022) Cellular architecture of human brain metastases. Cell 185:729–745.e20

Goswami S, Sahai E, Wyckoff JB, Cammer M, Cox D, Pixley FJ, Stanley ER, Segall JE, Condeelis JS (2005) Macrophages promote the invasion of breast carcinoma cells via a colony-stimulating factor-1/epidermal growth factor paracrine loop. Cancer Res 65:5278–5283

Gu Y, Liu Y, Fu L, Zhai L, Zhu J, Han Y, Jiang Y, Zhang Y, Zhang P, Jiang Z, Zhang X, Cao X (2019) Tumor-educated B cells selectively promote breast cancer lymph node metastasis by HSPA4-targeting IgG. Nat Med 25:312–322

Guan H, Lan Y, Wan Y, Wang Q, Wang C, Xu L, Chen Y, Liu W, Zhang X, Li Y, Gu Y, Wang Z, Xie F (2016) PD-L1 mediated the differentiation of tumor-infiltrating CD19(+) B lymphocytes and T cells in Invasive breast cancer. Onco Targets Ther 5:e1075112

Guldner IH, Wang Q, Yang L, Golomb SM, Zhao Z, Lopez JA, Brunory A, Howe EN, Zhang Y, Palakurthi B, Barron M, Gao H, Xuei X, Liu Y, Li J, Chen DZ, Landreth GE, Zhang S (2020) CNS-native myeloid cells drive immune suppression in the brain metastatic niche through Cxcl10. Cell 183:1234–1248.e25

Guo J, Ma R-Y, Qian B-Z (2024) Macrophage heterogeneity in bone metastasis. J Bone Oncol 45:100598

Guy TV, Terry AM, Bolton HA, Hancock DG, Shklovskaya E, Fazekas DEST, Groth B (2016) Pro- and anti-tumour effects of B cells and antibodies in cancer: a comparison of clinical studies and preclinical models. Cancer Immunol Immunother 65:885–896

Hagerling C, Gonzalez H, Salari K, Wang C-Y, Lin C, Robles I, Van Gogh M, Dejmek A, Jirstr M, K. & Werb, Z. (2019) Immune effector monocyte–neutrophil cooperation induced by the primary tumor prevents metastatic progression of breast cancer. Proc Natl Acad Sci U S A 116:21704–21714

Haider MT, Smit DJ, Taipaleenmaki H (2020) The endosteal niche in breast cancer bone metastasis. Front Oncol 10:335

Halvorsen EC, Mahmoud SM, Bennewith KL (2014) Emerging roles of regulatory T cells in tumour progression and metastasis. Cancer Metastasis Rev 33:1025–1041

Harney AS, Arwert EN, Entenberg D, Wang Y, Guo P, Qian BZ, Oktay MH, Pollard JW, Jones JG, Condeelis JS (2015) Real-time imaging reveals local, transient vascular permeability, and tumor cell intravasation stimulated by TIE2hi macrophage-derived VEGFA. Cancer Discov 5:932–943

Harney AS, Karagiannis GS, Pignatelli J, Smith BD, Kadioglu E, Wise SC, Hood MM, Kaufman MD, Leary CB, Lu WP, Al-Ani G, Chen X, Entenberg D, Oktay MH, Wang Y, Chun L, De Palma M, Jones JG, Flynn DL, Condeelis JS (2017) The selective Tie2 inhibitor Rebastinib blocks recruitment and function of Tie2(Hi) macrophages in breast cancer and pancreatic neuroendocrine tumors. Mol Cancer Ther 16:2486–2501

Haro MA, Dyevoich AM, Phipps JP, Haas KM (2019) Activation of B-1 cells promotes tumor cell killing in the peritoneal cavity. Cancer Res 79:159–170

Hiratsuka S, Watanabe A, Aburatani H, Maru Y (2006) Tumour-mediated upregulation of chemoattractants and recruitment of myeloid cells predetermines lung metastasis. Nat Cell Biol 8:1369–1375

Hosoya T, Sato-Kaneko F, Ahmadi A, Yao S, Lao F, Kitaura K, Matsutani T, Carson DA, Hayashi T (2018) Induction of oligoclonal CD8 T cell responses against pulmonary metastatic cancer by a phospholipid-conjugated TLR7 agonist. Proc Natl Acad Sci U S A 115:E6836–E6844

Hossain M, Shim R, Lee W-Y, Sharpe AH, Kubes P (2022) Gata6+ resident peritoneal macrophages promote the growth of liver metastasis. Nat Commun 13

Hou Y, Nitta H, Wei L, Banks PM, Lustberg M, Wesolowski R, Ramaswamy B, Parwani AV, Li Z (2018) Pd-L1 expression and CD8-positive T cells are associated with favorable survival in HER2-positive invasive breast cancer. Breast J 24:911–919

Huang H, Yao Y, Shen L, Jiang J, Zhang T, Xiong J, Li J, Sun S, Zheng S, Jia F, Zhou J, Yu X, Chen W, Shen J, Xia W, Shao X, Wang Q, Huang J, Ni C (2023) CD24hiCD27+ bregs within metastatic lymph nodes promote multidrug resistance in breast cancer. Clin Cancer Res 29:5227–5243

Irshad S, Flores-Borja F, Lawler K, Monypenny J, Evans R, Male V, Gordon P, Cheung A, Gazinska P, Noor F, Wong F, Grigoriadis A, Fruhwirth GO, Barber PR, Woodman N, Patel D, Rodriguez-Justo M, Owen J, Martin SG, Pinder SE, Gillett CE, Poland SP, Ameer-Beg S, Mccaughan F, Carlin LM, Hasan U, Withers DR, Lane P, Vojnovic B, Quezada SA, Ellis P, Tutt ANJ, Ng T (2017) RORγt+ innate lymphoid cells promote lymph node metastasis of breast cancers. Cancer Res 77:1083–1096

Ito A, Akama Y, Satoh-Takayama N, Saito K, Kato T, Kawamoto E, Gaowa A, Park EJ, Takao M, Shimaoka M (2022) Possible metastatic stage-dependent ILC2 activation induces differential functions of MDSCs through IL-13/IL-13Rα1 Signaling during the Progression of Breast Cancer Lung Metastasis. Cancers 14:3267

Jiang P, Gao W, Ma T, Wang R, Piao Y, Dong X, Wang P, Zhang X, Liu Y, Su W, Xiang R, Zhang J, Li N (2019) CD137 promotes bone metastasis of breast cancer by enhancing the migration and osteoclast differentiation of monocytes/macrophages. Theranostics 9:2950–2966

Jie HB, Schuler PJ, Lee SC, Srivastava RM, Argiris A, Ferrone S, Whiteside TL, Ferris RL (2015) CTLA-4(+) regulatory T cells increased in cetuximab-treated head and neck cancer patients suppress NK cell cytotoxicity and correlate with poor prognosis. Cancer Res 75:2200–2210

Jovanovic IP, Pejnovic NN, Radosavljevic GD, Pantic JM, Milovanovic MZ, Arsenijevic NN, Lukic ML (2014) Interleukin-33/ST2 axis promotes breast cancer growth and metastases by facilitating intratumoral accumulation of immunosuppressive and innate lymphoid cells. Int J Cancer 134:1669–1682

Joyce JA, Pollard JW (2009) Microenvironmental regulation of metastasis. Nat Rev Cancer 9:239–252

Keirsse J, Van Damme H, Geeraerts X, Beschin A, Raes G, Van Ginderachter JA (2018) The role of hepatic macrophages in liver metastasis. Cell Immunol 330:202–215

Kim H, Chung H, Kim J, Choi DH, Shin Y, Kang YG, Kim BM, Seo SU, Chung S, Seok SH (2019) Macrophages-triggered sequential remodeling of endothelium-interstitial matrix to form pre-metastatic niche in microfluidic tumor microenvironment. Adv Sci (Weinh) 6:1900195

Kitamura T, Qian BZ, Pollard JW (2015a) Immune cell promotion of metastasis. Nat Rev Immunol 15:73–86

Kitamura T, Qian BZ, Soong D, Cassetta L, Noy R, Sugano G, Kato Y, Li J, Pollard JW (2015b) CCL2-induced chemokine cascade promotes breast cancer metastasis by enhancing retention of metastasis-associated macrophages. J Exp Med 212:1043–1059

Klemm F, Mockl A, Salamero-Boix A, Alekseeva T, Schaffer A, Schulz M, Niesel K, Maas RR, Groth M, Elie BT, Bowman RL, Hegi ME, Daniel RT, Zeiner PS, Zinke J, Harter PN, Plate KH, Joyce JA, Sevenich L (2021) Compensatory CSF2-driven macrophage activation promotes adaptive resistance to CSF1R inhibition in breast-to-brain metastasis. Nat Cancer 2:1086–1101

Kowanetz M, Wu X, Lee J, Tan M, Hagenbeek T, Qu X, Yu L, Ross J, Korsisaari N, Cao T, Bou-Reslan H, Kallop D, Weimer R, Ludlam MJC, Kaminker JS, Modrusan Z, Van Bruggen N, Peale FV, Carano R, Meng YG, Ferrara N (2010) Granulocyte-colony stimulating factor promotes lung metastasis through mobilization of Ly6G+Ly6C+ granulocytes. Proc Natl Acad Sci 107:21248–21255

Kriegsmann K, Kriegsmann M, Von Bergwelt-Baildon M, Cremer M, Witzens-Harig M (2018) NKT cells - new players in CAR cell immunotherapy? Eur J Haematol 101:750–757

Lal A, Chan L, Devries S, Chin K, Scott GK, Benz CC, Chen YY, Waldman FM, Hwang ES (2013) FOXP3-positive regulatory T lymphocytes and epithelial FOXP3 expression in synchronous normal, ductal carcinoma in situ, and invasive cancer of the breast. Breast Cancer Res Treat 139:381–390

Lanier LL (2013) Shades of grey--the blurring view of innate and adaptive immunity. Nat Rev Immunol 13:73–74

Laumont CM, Banville AC, Gilardi M, Hollern DP, Nelson BH (2022) Tumour-infiltrating B cells: immunological mechanisms, clinical impact and therapeutic opportunities. Nat Rev Cancer

Lavender N, Yang J, Chen S-C, Sai J, Johnson CA, Owens P, Ayers GD, Richmond A (2017) The Yin/Yan of

CCL2: a minor role in neutrophil anti-tumor activity in vitro but a major role on the outgrowth of metastatic breast cancer lesions in the lung in vivo. BMC Cancer 17

Lerman I, Hammes SR (2018) Neutrophil elastase in the tumor microenvironment. Steroids 133:96–101

Li P, Lu M, Shi J, Gong Z, Hua L, Li Q, Lim B, Zhang XHF, Chen X, Li S, Shultz LD, Ren G (2020a) Lung mesenchymal cells elicit lipid storage in neutrophils that fuel breast cancer lung metastasis. Nat Immunol 21:1444–1455

Li P, Lu M, Shi J, Hua L, Gong Z, Li Q, Shultz LD, Ren G (2020b) Dual roles of neutrophils in metastatic colonization are governed by the host NK cell status. Nat Communications 11

Li Y, Wang C, Huang T, Yu X, Tian B (2023) The role of cancer-associated fibroblasts in breast cancer metastasis. Front Oncology 13

Linde N, Casanova-Acebes M, Sosa MS, Mortha A, Rahman A, Farias E, Harper K, Tardio E, Reyes Torres I, Jones J, Condeelis J, Merad M, Aguirre-Ghiso JA (2018) Macrophages orchestrate breast cancer early dissemination and metastasis. Nat Commun 9:21

Liu S, Lachapelle J, Leung S, Gao D, Foulkes WD, Nielsen TO (2012) CD8+ lymphocyte infiltration is an independent favorable prognostic indicator in basal-like breast cancer. Breast Cancer Res 14:R48

Liu C, Mohan SC, Wei J, Seki E, Liu M, Basho R, Giuliano AE, Zhao Y, Cui X (2022) Breast cancer liver metastasis: Pathogenesis and clinical implications. Front Oncology 12

Liu YM, Ge JY, Chen YF, Liu T, Chen L, Liu CC, Ma D, Chen YY, Cai YW, Xu YY, Shao ZM, Yu KD (2023) Combined single-cell and spatial transcriptomics reveal the metabolic evolvement of breast cancer during early dissemination. Adv Science 10

Louie E, Chen XF, Coomes A, Ji K, Tsirka S, Chen EI (2012) Neurotrophin-3 modulates breast cancer cells and the microenvironment to promote the growth of breast cancer brain metastasis. Oncogene 32:4064–4077

Luo Z, Lu Y, Shi Y, Jiang M, Shan X, Li X, Zhang J, Qin B, Liu X, Guo X, Huang J, Liu Y, Wang S, Li Q, Luo L, You J (2023) Neutrophil hitchhiking for drug delivery to the bone marrow. Nat Nanotechnol 18:647–656

Ma RY, Zhang H, Li XF, Zhang CB, Selli C, Tagliavini G, Lam AD, Prost S, Sims AH, Hu HY, Ying T, Wang Z, Ye Z, Pollard JW, Qian BZ (2020) Monocyte-derived macrophages promote breast cancer bone metastasis outgrowth. J Exp Med 217

Ma W, Oliveira-Nunes MC, Xu K, Kossenkov A, Reiner BC, Crist RC, Hayden J, Chen Q (2023) Type I interferon response in astrocytes promotes brain metastasis by enhancing monocytic myeloid cell recruitment. Nat Communications 14

Madel MB, Ibanez L, Wakkach A, De Vries TJ, Teti A, Apparailly F, Blin-Wakkach C (2019) Immune function and diversity of osteoclasts in normal and pathological conditions. Front Immunol 10:1408

Mahmoud SM, Lee AH, Paish EC, Macmillan RD, Ellis IO, Green AR (2012) Tumour-infiltrating macrophages and clinical outcome in breast cancer. J Clin Pathol 65:159–163

Malladi S, Macalinao DG, Jin X, He L, Basnet H, Zou Y, De Stanchina E, Massague J (2016) Metastatic latency and immune evasion through autocrine inhibition of WNT. Cell 165:45–60

Marelli G, Allavena P, Erreni M (2015) Tumor-associated macrophages, multi-tasking cells in the cancer landscape. Cancer Res Front 1:149–161

Martinez M, Moon EK (2019) CAR T cells for solid tumors: new strategies for finding, infiltrating, and surviving in the tumor microenvironment. Front Immunol 10

Martins-Cardoso K, Almeida VH, Bagri KM, Rossi MID, Mermelstein CS, K Nig S, Monteiro RQ (2020) Neutrophil extracellular traps (NETs) promote pro-metastatic phenotype in human breast cancer cells through epithelial–mesenchymal transition. Cancers 12:1542

Matkowski R, Gisterek I, Halon A, Lacko A, Szewczyk K, Staszek U, Pudelko M, Szynglarewicz B, Szelachowska J, Zolnierek A (2009) The prognostic role of tumor-infiltrating CD4 and CD8 T lymphocytes in breast cancer. Anticancer Res 29:2445–2451

Matlung HL, Babes L, Zhao XW, Van Houdt M, Treffers LW, Van Rees DJ, Franke K, Schornagel K, Verkuijlen P, Janssen H, Halonen P, Lieftink C, Beijersbergen RL, Leusen JHW, Boelens JJ, Kuhnle I, Der Werff V, Ten Bosch J, Seeger K, Rutella S, Pagliara D, Matozaki T, Suzuki E, Der Houven M-V, Van Oordt CW, Van Bruggen R, Roos D, Van Lier RAW, Kuijpers TW, Kubes P, Van Den Berg TK (2018) Neutrophils kill antibody-opsonized cancer cells by trogoptosis. Cell Rep 23:3946–3959.e6

Mazzieri R, Pucci F, Moi D, Zonari E, Ranghetti A, Berti A, Politi LS, Gentner B, Brown JL, Naldini L, De Palma M (2011) Targeting the ANG2/TIE2 axis inhibits tumor growth and metastasis by impairing angiogenesis and disabling rebounds of proangiogenic myeloid cells. Cancer Cell 19:512–526

McFarlane AJ, Fercoq F, Coffelt SB, Carlin LM (2021) Neutrophil dynamics in the tumor microenvironment. J Clin Invest 131

McNamara KL, Caswell-Jin JL, Joshi R, Ma Z, Kotler E, Bean GR, Kriner M, Zhou Z, Hoang M, Beechem J, Zoeller J, Press MF, Slamon DJ, Hurvitz SA, Curtis C (2021) Spatial proteomic characterization of HER2-positive breast tumors through neoadjuvant therapy predicts response. Nat Cancer 2:400–413

Miyasato Y, Shiota T, Ohnishi K, Pan C, Yano H, Horlad H, Yamamoto Y, Yamamoto-Ibusuki M, Iwase H, Takeya M, Komohara Y (2017) High density of CD204-positive macrophages predicts worse clinical prognosis in patients with breast cancer. Cancer Sci 108:1693–1700

Monteiro AC, Leal AC, Goncalves-Silva T, Mercadante AC, Kestelman F, Chaves SB, Azevedo RB, Monteiro

JP, Bonomo A (2013) T cells induce pre-metastatic osteolytic disease and help bone metastases establishment in a mouse model of metastatic breast cancer. PLoS One 8:e68171

Morrissey SM, Zhang F, Ding C, Montoya-Durango DE, Hu X, Yang C, Wang Z, Yuan F, Fox M, Zhang H-G, Guo H, Tieri D, Kong M, Watson CT, Mitchell RA, Zhang X, McMasters KM, Huang J, Yan J (2021) Tumor-derived exosomes drive immunosuppressive macrophages in a pre-metastatic niche through glycolytic dominant metabolic reprogramming. Cell Metab 33:2040–2058.e10

Nelson BH (2010) Cd20+ B cells: the other tumor-infiltrating lymphocytes. J Immunol 185:4977–4982

Neves H, Kwok HF (2015) Recent advances in the field of anti-cancer immunotherapy. BBA Clin 3:280–288

Niesel K, Schulz M, Anthes J, Alekseeva T, Macas J, Salamero-Boix A, M Ckl A, Oberwahrenbrock T, Lolies M, Stein S, Plate KH, Reiss Y, R Del F, Sevenich L (2021) The immune suppressive microenvironment affects efficacy of radio-immunotherapy in brain metastasis. EMBO Mol Med 13

Nyhus JK, Wolford CC, Friece CR, Nelson BM, Sampsel JW, Barbera-Guillem E (2001) IgG-recognizing shed tumor-associated antigens can promote tumor invasion and metastasis. Cancer Immunol Immunother 50:361–372

Olkhanud PB, Damdinsuren B, Bodogai M, Gress RE, Sen R, Wejksza K, Malchinkhuu E, Wersto RP, Biragyn A (2011) Tumor-evoked regulatory B cells promote breast cancer metastasis by converting resting CD4(+) T cells to T-regulatory cells. Cancer Res 71:3505–3515

Page DB, Bear H, Prabhakaran S, Gatti-Mays ME, Thomas A, Cobain E, McArthur H, Balko JM, Gameiro SR, Nanda R, Gulley JL, Kalinsky K, White J, Litton J, Chmura SJ, Polley MY, Vincent B, Cescon DW, Disis ML, Sparano JA, Mittendorf EA, Adams S (2019) Two may be better than one: PD-1/PD-L1 blockade combination approaches in metastatic breast cancer. NPJ Breast Cancer 5:34

Paget S (1889) The distribution of secondary growths in cancer of the breast. Cancer Metastasis Rev 1:98

Pal B, Chen Y, Vaillant F, Capaldo BD, Joyce R, Song X, Bryant VL, Penington JS, Di Stefano L, Tubau Ribera N, Wilcox S, Mann GB, Kconfab, Papenfuss AT, Lindeman GJ, Smyth GK, Visvader JE (2021) A single-cell RNA expression atlas of normal, preneoplastic and tumorigenic states in the human breast. EMBO J 40:e107333

Paolino M, Choidas A, Wallner S, Pranjic B, Uribesalgo I, Loeser S, Jamieson AM, Langdon WY, Ikeda F, Fededa JP, Cronin SJ, Nitsch R, Schultz-Fademrecht C, Eickhoff J, Menninger S, Unger A, Torka R, Gruber T, Hinterleitner R, Baier G, Wolf D, Ullrich A, Klebl BM, Penninger JM (2014) The E3 ligase Cbl-b and TAM receptors regulate cancer metastasis via natural killer cells. Nature 507:508–512

Pasero C, Gravis G, Guerin M, Granjeaud S, Thomassin-Piana J, Rocchi P, Paciencia-Gros M, Poizat F, Bentobji M, Azario-Cheillan F, Walz J, Salem N, Brunelle S, Moretta A, Olive D (2016) Inherent and tumor-driven immune tolerance in the prostate microenvironment impairs natural killer cell antitumor activity. Cancer Res 76:2153–2165

Pati S, Mukherjee S, Dutta S, Guin A, Roy D, Bose S, Paul S, Saha S, Bhattacharyya S, Datta P, Chakraborty J, Sarkar DK, Sa G (2023) Tumor-associated CD19+CD39− B regulatory cells deregulate class-switch recombination to suppress antibody responses. Cancer Immunol Res 11:364–380

Peinado H, Zhang H, Matei IR, Costa-Silva B, Hoshino A, Rodrigues G, Psaila B, Kaplan RN, Bromberg JF, Kang Y, Bissell MJ, Cox TR, Giaccia AJ, Erler JT, Hiratsuka S, Ghajar CM, Lyden D (2017) Pre-metastatic niches: organ-specific homes for metastases. Nat Rev Cancer

Phalke SP, Chiplunkar SV (2015) Activation status of gammadelta T cells dictates their effect on osteoclast generation and bone resorption. Bone Rep 3:95–103

Pierpont TM, Limper CB, Richards KL (2018) Past, present, and future of Rituximab-the world's first oncology monoclonal antibody therapy. Front Oncol 8:163

Pinner S, Jordan P, Sharrock K, Bazley L, Collinson L, Marais R, Bonvin E, Goding C, Sahai E (2009) Intravital imaging reveals transient changes in pigment production and Brn2 expression during metastatic melanoma dissemination. Cancer Res 69:7969–7977

Pukrop T, Dehghani F, Chuang HN, Lohaus R, Bayanga K, Heermann S, Regen T, Van Rossum D, Klemm F, Schulz M, Siam L, Hoffmann A, Trumper L, Stadelmann C, Bechmann I, Hanisch UK, Binder C (2010) Microglia promote colonization of brain tissue by breast cancer cells in a Wnt-dependent way. Glia 58:1477–1489

Qian BZ (2017) Inflammation fires up cancer metastasis. Semin Cancer Biol 47:170–176

Qian B, Deng Y, Im JH, Muschel RJ, Zou Y, Li J, Lang RA, Pollard JW (2009) A distinct macrophage population mediates metastatic breast cancer cell extravasation, establishment and growth. PLoS One 4:e6562

Qian BZ, Li J, Zhang H, Kitamura T, Zhang J, Campion LR, Kaiser EA, Snyder LA, Pollard JW (2011) CCL2 recruits inflammatory monocytes to facilitate breast-tumour metastasis. Nature 475:222–225

Qian BZ, Zhang H, Li J, He T, Yeo EJ, Soong DY, Carragher NO, Munro A, Chang A, Bresnick AR, Lang RA, Pollard JW (2015) FLT1 signaling in metastasis-associated macrophages activates an inflammatory signature that promotes breast cancer metastasis. J Exp Med 212:1433–1448

Qin Z, Richter G, Schuler T, Ibe S, Cao X, Blankenstein T (1998) B cells inhibit induction of T cell-dependent tumor immunity. Nat Med 4:627–630

Ramos MJ, Lui AJ, Hollern DP (2023) The evolving landscape of B cells in cancer metastasis. Cancer Res 83:3835–3845

Ren G, Zhao X, Wang Y, Zhang X, Chen X, Xu C, Yuan ZR, Roberts AI, Zhang L, Zheng B, Wen T, Han Y, Rabson AB, Tischfield JA, Shao C, Shi Y (2012) CCR2-dependent recruitment of macrophages by tumor-educated mesenchymal stromal cells promotes tumor development and is mimicked by TNFalpha. Cell Stem Cell 11:812–824

Rethacker L, Boy M, Bisio V, Roussin F, Denizeau J, Vincent-Salomon A, Borcoman E, Sedlik C, Piaggio E, Toubert A, Dulphy N, Caignard A (2022) Innate lymphoid cells: NK and cytotoxic ILC3 subsets infiltrate metastatic breast cancer lymph nodes. Onco Targets Ther 11

Rohan TE, Xue X, Lin H-M, D'alfonso TM, Ginter PS, Oktay MH, Robinson BD, Ginsberg M, Gertler FB, Glass AG, Sparano JA, Condeelis JS, Jones JG (2014) Tumor microenvironment of metastasis and risk of distant metastasis of breast cancer. JNCI J Natl Cancer Inst 106

Rosenberg EB, Herberman RB, Levine PH, Halterman RH, Mccov JL, Wunderlich JR (1972) Lymphocyte cytotoxicity reactions to leukemia-associated antigens in identical twins. Int J Cancer 9:648–658

Rosser EC, Mauri C (2015) Regulatory B cells: origin, phenotype, and function. Immunity 42:607–612

Sato K, Suematsu A, Okamoto K, Yamaguchi A, Morishita Y, Kadono Y, Tanaka S, Kodama T, Akira S, Iwakura Y, Cua DJ, Takayanagi H (2006) Th17 functions as an osteoclastogenic helper T cell subset that links T cell activation and bone destruction. J Exp Med 203:2673–2682

Sawant A, Hensel JA, Chanda D, Harris BA, Siegal GP, Maheshwari A, Ponnazhagan S (2012) Depletion of plasmacytoid dendritic cells inhibits tumor growth and prevents bone metastasis of breast cancer cells. J Immunol 189:4258–4265

Scheele CLGJ, Maynard C, Van Rheenen J (2016) Intravital insights into heterogeneity, metastasis, and therapy responses. Trends Cancer 2:205–216

Schonfeld K, Sahm C, Zhang C, Naundorf S, Brendel C, Odendahl M, Nowakowska P, Bonig H, Kohl U, Kloess S, Kohler S, Holtgreve-Grez H, Jauch A, Schmidt M, Schubert R, Kuhlcke K, Seifried E, Klingemann HG, Rieger MA, Tonn T, Grez M, Wels WS (2015) Selective inhibition of tumor growth by clonal NK cells expressing an ErbB2/HER2-specific chimeric antigen receptor. Mol Ther 23:330–338

Schott AF, Goldstein LJ, Cristofanilli M, Ruffini PA, Mccanna S, Reuben JM, Perez RP, Kato G, Wicha M (2017) Phase Ib pilot study to evaluate reparixin in combination with weekly paclitaxel in patients with HER-2–negative metastatic breast cancer. Clin Cancer Res 23:5358–5365

Schuijs MJ, Png S, Richard AC, Tsyben A, Hamm G, Stockis J, Garcia C, Pinaud S, Nicholls A, Ros XR, Su J, Eldridge MD, Riedel A, Serrao EM, Rodewald H-R, Mack M, Shields JD, Cohen ES, McKenzie ANJ, Goodwin RJA, Brindle KM, Marioni JC, Halim TYF (2020) ILC2-driven innate immune checkpoint mechanism antagonizes NK cell antimetastatic function in the lung. Nat Immunol 21:998–1009

Shani O, Vorobyov T, Monteran L, Lavie D, Cohen N, Raz Y, Tsarfaty G, Avivi C, Barshack I, Erez N (2020) Fibroblast-derived IL33 facilitates breast cancer metastasis by modifying the immune microenvironment and driving type 2 immunity. Cancer Res 80:5317–5329

Sharon Y, Raz Y, Cohen N, Ben-Shmuel A, Schwartz H, Geiger T, Erez N (2015) Tumor-derived osteopontin reprograms normal mammary fibroblasts to promote inflammation and tumor growth in breast cancer. Cancer Res 75:963–973

Sharonov GV, Serebrovskaya EO, Yuzhakova DV, Britanova OV, Chudakov DM (2020) B cells, plasma cells and antibody repertoires in the tumour microenvironment. Nat Rev Immunol 20:294–307

Shojaei F, Wu X, Zhong C, Yu L, Liang X-H, Yao J, Blanchard D, Bais C, Peale FV, Van Bruggen N, Ho C, Ross J, Tan M, Carano RAD, Meng YG, Ferrara N (2007) Bv8 regulates myeloid-cell-dependent tumour angiogenesis. Nature 450:825–831

Spits H, Artis D, Colonna M, Diefenbach A, Di Santo JP, Eberl G, Koyasu S, Locksley RM, McKenzie AN, Mebius RE, Powrie F, Vivier E (2013) Innate lymphoid cells--a proposal for uniform nomenclature. Nat Rev Immunol 13:145–149

Steenbruggen TG, Wolf DM, Campbell MJ, Sanders J, Cornelissen S, Thijssen B, Salgado RA, Yau C, O-Grady N, Basu A, Bhaskaran R, Mittempergher L, Hirst GL, Coppe J-P, Kok M, Sonke GS, Van 'T Veer LJ, Horlings HM (2023) B-cells and regulatory T-cells in the microenvironment of HER2+ breast cancer are associated with decreased survival: a real-world analysis of women with HER2+ metastatic breast cancer. Breast Cancer Res 25

Su S, Liu Q, Chen J, Chen J, Chen F, He C, Huang D, Wu W, Lin L, Huang W, Zhang J, Cui X, Zheng F, Li H, Yao H, Su F, Song E (2014) A positive feedback loop between mesenchymal-like cancer cells and macrophages is essential to breast cancer metastasis. Cancer Cell 25:605–620

Sun R, Jiang H (2024) Border-associated macrophages in the central nervous system. J Neuroinflammation 21

Szpor J, Streb J, Glajcar A, Frączek P, Winiarska A, Tyrak KE, Basta P, Okoń K, Jach R, Hodorowicz-Zaniewska D (2021) Dendritic cells are associated with prognosis and survival in breast cancer. Diagnostics 11:702

Tan W, Zhang W, Strasner A, Grivennikov S, Cheng JQ, Hoffman RM, Karin M (2011) Tumour-infiltrating regulatory T cells stimulate mammary cancer metastasis through RANKL-RANK signalling. Nature 470:548–553

Te K (2019) Potential of targeting bone metastases with immunotherapies. Novel approaches in cancer study, 3

Thibaudin M, Chaix M, Boidot R, Vegran F, Derangere V, Limagne E, Berger H, Ladoire S, Apetoh L, Ghiringhelli F (2016) Human ectonucleotidase-expressing CD25(high) Th17 cells accumulate in breast cancer tumors and exert immunosuppressive functions. Onco Targets Ther 5:e1055444

Treffers LW, Ten Broeke T, Rösner T, Jansen JHM, Van Houdt M, Kahle S, Schornagel K, Verkuijlen PJJH, Prins JM, Franke K, Kuijpers TW, Van Den Berg TK, Valerius T, Leusen JHW, Matlung HL (2020) IgA-mediated killing of tumor cells by neutrophils is enhanced by CD47–SIRPα checkpoint inhibition. Cancer Immunol Res 8:120–130

Vantourout P, Hayday A (2013) Six-of-the-best: unique contributions of gammadelta T cells to immunology. Nat Rev Immunol 13:88–100

Varikuti S, Singh B, Volpedo G, Ahirwar DK, Jha BK, Saljoughian N, Viana AG, Verma C, Hamza O, Halsey G, Holcomb EA, Maryala RJ, Oghumu S, Ganju RK, Satoskar AR (2020) Ibrutinib treatment inhibits breast cancer progression and metastasis by inducing conversion of myeloid-derived suppressor cells to dendritic cells. Br J Cancer 122:1005–1013

Vihervuori H, Autere TA, Repo H, Kurki S, Kallio L, Lintunen MM, Talvinen K, Kronqvist P (2019) Tumor-infiltrating lymphocytes and CD8(+) T cells predict survival of triple-negative breast cancer. J Cancer Res Clin Oncol 145:3105–3114

Walker JA, Barlow JL, McKenzie AN (2013) Innate lymphoid cells--how did we miss them? Nat Rev Immunol 13:75–87

Walker ND, Elias M, Guiro K, Bhatia R, Greco SJ, Bryan M, Gergues M, Sandiford OA, Ponzio NM, Leibovich SJ, Rameshwar P (2019) Exosomes from differentially activated macrophages influence dormancy or resurgence of breast cancer cells within bone marrow stroma. Cell Death Dis 10:59

Wang Y, Li Y, Zhong J, Li M, Zhou Y, Lin Q, Zong S, Luo W, Wang J, Wang K, Wang J, Xiong L (2023a) Tumor-derived Cav-1 promotes pre-metastatic niche formation and lung metastasis in breast cancer. Theranostics 13:1684–1697

Wang Y, Xu M, Sun J, Li X, Shi H, Wang X, Liu B, Zhang T, Jiang X, Lin L, Li Q, Huang Y, Liang Y, Hu M, Zheng F, Zhang F, Sun J, Shi Y, Wang Y (2023b) Glycolytic neutrophils accrued in the spleen compromise anti-tumour T cell immunity in breast cancer. Nat Metab 5:1408–1422

Wang X, Zhou Y, Wu Z, Xie C, Xu W, Zhou Q, Yang D, Zhu D, Wang M-W, Wang L (2024) Single-cell transcriptomics reveals the role of antigen presentation in liver metastatic breast cancer. iScience 27:108896

Wei H, Fu P, Yao M, Chen Y, Du L (2016) Breast cancer stem cells phenotype and plasma cell-predominant breast cancer independently indicate poor survival. Pathol Res Pract 212:294–301

Wu L, Saxena S, Goel P, Prajapati DR, Wang C, Singh RK (2020) Breast cancer cell–neutrophil interactions enhance neutrophil survival and pro-tumorigenic activities. Cancers 12:2884

Wu AML, Gossa S, Samala R, Chung MA, Gril B, Yang HH, Thorsheim HR, Tran AD, Wei D, Taner E, Isanogle K, Yang Y, Dolan EL, Robinson C, Difilippantonio S, Lee MP, Khan I, Smith QR, Mcgavern DB, Wakefield LM, Steeg PS (2021a) Aging and CNS myeloid cell depletion attenuate breast cancer brain metastasis. Clin Cancer Res 27:4422–4434

Wu SZ, Al-Eryani G, Roden DL, Junankar S, Harvey K, Andersson A, Thennavan A, Wang C, Torpy JR, Bartonicek N, Wang T, Larsson L, Kaczorowski D, Weisenfeld NI, Uytingco CR, Chew JG, Bent ZW, Chan CL, Gnanasambandapillai V, Dutertre CA, Gluch L, Hui MN, Beith J, Parker A, Robbins E, Segara D, Cooper C, Mak C, Chan B, Warrier S, Ginhoux F, Millar E, Powell JE, Williams SR, Liu XS, O'toole S, Lim E, Lundeberg J, Perou CM, Swarbrick A (2021b) A single-cell and spatially resolved atlas of human breast cancers. Nat Genet 53:1334–1347

Wyckoff J, Wang W, Lin EY, Wang Y, Pixley F, Stanley ER, Graf T, Pollard JW, Segall J, Condeelis J (2004) A paracrine loop between tumor cells and macrophages is required for tumor cell migration in mammary tumors. Cancer Res 64:7022–7029

Wyckoff JB, Wang Y, Lin EY, Li JF, Goswami S, Stanley ER, Segall JE, Pollard JW, Condeelis J (2007) Direct visualization of macrophage-assisted tumor cell intravasation in mammary tumors. Cancer Res 67:2649–2656

Xiao Y, Cong M, Li J, He D, Wu Q, Tian P, Wang Y, Yang S, Liang C, Liang Y, Wen J, Liu Y, Luo W, Lv X, He Y, Cheng D-D, Zhou T, Zhao W, Zhang P, Zhang X, Xiao Y, Qian Y, Wang H, Gao Q, Yang Q-C, Yang Q, Hu G (2021) Cathepsin C promotes breast cancer lung metastasis by modulating neutrophil infiltration and neutrophil extracellular trap formation. Cancer Cell 39:423–437.e7

Xue D, Xia T, Wang J, Chong M, Wang S, Zhang C (2018) Role of regulatory T cells and CD8(+) T lymphocytes in the dissemination of circulating tumor cells in primary invasive breast cancer. Oncol Lett 16:3045–3053

Yang L, Liu Q, Zhang X, Liu X, Zhou B, Chen J, Huang D, Li J, Li H, Chen F, Liu J, Xing Y, Chen X, Su S, Song E (2020) DNA of neutrophil extracellular traps promotes cancer metastasis via CCDC25. Nature

Yeo EJ, Cassetta L, Qian BZ, Lewkowich I, Li JF, Stefater JA III, Smith AN, Wiechmann LS, Wang Y, Pollard JW, Lang RA (2014) Myeloid WNT7b mediates the angiogenic switch and metastasis in breast cancer. Cancer Res 74:2962–2973

Yeong J, Lim JCT, Lee B, Li H, Chia N, Ong CCH, Lye WK, Putti TC, Dent R, Lim E, Thike AA, Tan PH, Iqbal J (2018) High densities of tumor-associated plasma cells predict improved prognosis in triple negative breast cancer. Front Immunol 9:1209

Zeng B, Shi S, Ashworth G, Dong C, Liu J, Xing F (2019) ILC3 function as a double-edged sword in inflammatory bowel diseases. Cell Death Dis 10

Zhang K, Kim S, Cremasco V, Hirbe AC, Collins L, Piwnica-Worms D, Novack DV, Weilbaecher K, Faccio R (2011) CD8+ T cells regulate bone tumor burden independent of osteoclast resorption. Cancer Res 71:4799–4808

Zhang Y, Eliav Y, Shin SU, Schreiber TH, Podack ER, Tadmor T, Rosenblatt JD (2013) B lymphocyte inhibition of anti-tumor response depends on expansion of Treg but is independent of B-cell IL-10 secretion. Cancer Immunol Immunother 62:87–99

Zhang J, Pang Y, Xie T, Zhu L (2019) CXCR4 antagonism in combination with IDO1 inhibition weakens immune suppression and inhibits tumor growth in mouse breast cancer bone metastases. Onco Targets Ther 12:4985–4992

Zhang M, Liu ZZ, Aoshima K, Cai WL, Sun H, Xu T, Zhang Y, An Y, Chen JF, Chan LH, Aoshima A, Lang SM, Tang Z, Che X, Li Y, Rutter SJ, Bossuyt V, Chen X, Morrow JS, Pusztai L, Rimm DL, Yin M, Yan Q (2022) CECR2 drives breast cancer metastasis by promoting NF-kappaB signaling and macrophage-mediated immune suppression. Sci Transl Med 14:eabf5473

Zhao N, Zhu W, Wang J, Liu W, Kang L, Yu R, Liu B (2021) Group 2 innate lymphoid cells promote TNBC lung metastasis via the IL-13-MDSC axis in a murine tumor model. Int Immunopharmacol 99: 107924

Zou Y, Ye F, Kong Y, Hu X, Deng X, Xie J, Song C, Ou X, Wu S, Wu L, Xie Y, Tian W, Tang Y, Wong CW, Chen ZS, Xie X, Tang H (2022) The single-cell landscape of intratumoral heterogeneity and the immunosuppressive microenvironment in liver and brain metastases of breast cancer. Adv Science 10

Part VII

Subtypes, Treatment, and Resistance

Therese Sørlie and Robert Clarke

The final part provides a comprehensive exploration of breast cancer management, spanning intrinsic subtypes, targeted therapies, and resistance mechanisms.

In Chap. 21, Lajos Pusztai and his colleagues from the Yale School of Medicine, USA, and the University of Ulm, Germany, provide a detailed analysis of the clinical implications of breast cancer intrinsic subtypes. It underlines the genomic distinctions between estrogen receptor-positive (ER+) and estrogen receptor-negative (ER−) tumors, emphasizing their divergent clinical behaviors and therapeutic responses. Luminal cancers, characterized by ER expression, exhibit varying prognoses based on proliferation rates, with luminal B tumors showing higher recurrence risk and potential benefits from adjuvant chemotherapy. In contrast, basal-like cancers are uniformly highly proliferative, often requiring preoperative chemotherapy and immunotherapy for effective treatment. Additionally, HER2-enriched tumors, defined by HER2 gene amplification, present distinct therapeutic opportunities with HER2-targeted agents.

In Chap. 22, Sacha and Tony Howell from the Manchester Breast Centre, University of Manchester, UK, describe the evolution of estrogen receptor signaling-targeted therapies, elucidating the pivotal role of estrogen deprivation and selective estrogen receptor modulators in breast cancer treatment. It traces the development of these therapies over more than a century, highlighting advancements in endocrine therapy and the translation of novel compounds from advanced to early breast cancer settings. In addition, they provide a review of breast cancer prevention studies using endocrine agents and offer insights into their side effect profiles, providing a nuanced understanding of their clinical utility.

T. Sørlie
Oslo, Norway

R. Clarke
Manchester, UK

In Chap. 23, Luca Malorni and his colleagues from Hospital of Prato, Tuscany, Italy, focus on resistance to cyclin-dependent kinases 4 and 6 inhibitors in ER+ breast cancer. It examines the molecular mechanisms underlying resistance, including alterations in cell cycle-related genes and proteins, as well as dysregulation of nuclear and growth factor receptor signaling pathways. Despite substantial efforts to identify biomarkers and develop targeted therapeutic strategies, the management of resistance remains challenging. The chapter emphasizes the need for continued research to enhance patient stratification and to refine treatment approaches.

Finally, in Chap. 24, Rachel Schiff and her colleagues from Baylor College of Medicine, USA, address treatment of HER2-positive breast cancer, describing the transformative impact of HER2-targeted therapies on patient outcomes. However, pre-existing or emerging resistance of some HER2-positive tumors poses a significant clinical challenge, necessitating a deeper understanding of underlying mechanisms. From reactivation of HER receptors to deregulation of downstream signaling pathways, the chapter explores various resistance mechanisms and highlights ongoing efforts to develop new targeted agents and therapeutic approaches.

In conclusion, these chapters collectively convey the complexities of breast cancer management, emphasizing the importance of intrinsic subtype classification, targeted therapies, and resistance mechanisms in guiding treatment decisions. Elucidating the molecular underpinnings of breast cancer subtypes and their therapy-resistance pathways provides researchers and physicians invaluable insights that can inform the development of more effective therapeutic strategies, ultimately leading to improved patient outcomes.

21 Clinical Implications of Breast Cancer Intrinsic Subtypes

Alejandro Rios-Hoyo, Naing-Lin Shan, Philipp L. Karn, and Lajos Pusztai

Abstract

Estrogen receptor-positive (ER+) and estrogen receptor-negative (ER-) breast cancers have different genomic architecture and show large-scale gene expression differences consistent with different cellular origins, which is reflected in the luminal (i.e., ER+) versus basal-like (i.e., ER−) molecular class nomenclature. These two major molecular subtypes have distinct epidemiological risk factors and different clinical behaviors. Luminal cancers can be subdivided further based on proliferative activity and ER signaling. Those with a high expression of proliferation-related genes and a low expression of ER-associated genes, called luminal B, have a high risk of early recurrence (i.e., within 5 years), derive significant benefit from adjuvant chemotherapy, and may benefit from adding immunotherapy to chemotherapy. This subset of luminal cancers is identified as the genomic high-risk ER+ cancers by the MammaPrint, Oncotype DX Recurrence Score, EndoPredict, Prosigna, and several other molecular prognostic assays. Luminal A cancers are characterized by low proliferation and high ER-related gene expression. They tend to have excellent prognosis with adjuvant endocrine therapy. Adjuvant chemotherapy may not improve their outcome further. These cancers correspond to the genomic low-risk categories. However, these cancers remain at risk for distant recurrence for extended periods of time, and over 50% of distant recurrences occur after 5 years. Basal-like cancers are uniformly highly proliferative and tend to recur within 3–5 years of diagnosis. In the absence of therapy, basal-like breast cancers have the worst survival, but these also include many highly chemotherapy-sensitive cancers. Basal-like cancers are often treated with preoperative chemotherapy combined with an immune checkpoint inhibitor which results in 60–65% pathologic complete response rates that herald excellent long-term survival. Patients with residual cancer after neoadjuvant therapy can receive additional postoperative chemotherapy that improves their survival. Currently, there is no clinically actionable molecular subclassification for basal-like cancers, although cancers with high androgen receptor (AR)-related gene expression and those with high levels of immune infiltration have better prognosis, but currently their treatment is not different from

A. Rios-Hoyo · N.-L. Shan · L. Pusztai (✉)
Yale Cancer Center, Yale School of Medicine, New Haven, CT, USA
e-mail: alejandro.rioshoyo@yale.edu; nainglin.shan@yale.edu; lajos.pusztai@yale.edu

P. L. Karn
University of Ulm, Ulm, Germany
e-mail: philipp.karn@uni-ulm.de

T. Sørlie, R. B. Clarke (eds.), *A Guide to Breast Cancer Research*, Advances in Experimental Medicine and Biology 1464, https://doi.org/10.1007/978-3-031-70875-6_21

basal-like cancers in general. A clinically important, minor subset of breast cancers are characterized by frequent HER2 gene amplification and high expression of a few dozen genes, many residing on the HER2 amplicon. This is an important subset because of the highly effective HER2 targeted therapies which are synergistic with endocrine therapy and chemotherapy. The clinical behavior of HER2-enriched cancers is dominated by the underlying ER subtype. ER+/HER2-enriched cancers tend to have more indolent course and lesser chemotherapy sensitivity than their ER counterparts.

Keywords

Intrinsic subtypes · Breast cancer · Risk factors · Prognosis · Predictive · Breast cancer treatment

Key Points

- Luminal A tumors are strongly ER+ with low proliferation rate and have the best prognosis among breast cancers; however, their risk of recurrence extends over decades. These cancers derive little, or no, benefit from adjuvant chemotherapy and often retain an indolent clinical course and high endocrine treatment sensitivity even after metastatic recurrence.
- Luminal B tumors have higher proliferation rates and variable ER expression and may have lower endocrine therapy sensitivity but greater chemotherapy sensitivity. They comprise the molecularly high-risk ER+ cancers and often require adjuvant chemotherapy to maximize the chance of cure.
- Basal-like cancers are highly proliferative and tend to recur early, but many of these cancers are highly sensitive to chemotherapy. Molecular subsets exist within basal-like cancers, but these are not currently used in clinical decision-making. Adjuvant/neoadjuvant chemotherapy combined with immune checkpoint inhibitors has significantly improved the survival of basal-like breast cancers in the past decade.
- HER2-enriched breast cancers have unique sensitivity to HER2 targeted therapies and are predominantly comprised of HER2 gene-amplified cancers. Their prognosis and chemotherapy sensitivity are influenced by their ER status. The ER-/HER2-amplified cancers are the single most chemotherapy-sensitive type of breast cancer with pathologic complete response rates around 80% with preoperative chemotherapy plus HER2 targeted therapies.

21.1 Introduction

Molecular classification of breast cancer drew attention to the large-scale molecular differences between estrogen receptor-positive (ER+) and estrogen receptor-negative (ER-) cancers, resulting in a new way of conceptualizing and studying breast cancer. It also provided a new framework to interpret previously recognized prognostic markers and motivated the development of novel, more accurate prognostic gene signatures. Multiple different, partially overlapping molecular classification schemas were proposed by various academic groups, and these were superimposed on the already existing clinical classifications based on ER and human epidermal growth factor receptor 2 (HER2) protein expression, histologic grade, and proliferation metrics (e.g., Ki67 expression). Not surprisingly, the different classifications yielded partially discordant class assignments, even if each has demonstrated similar prognostic value. However, a broad consensus exists around four primary intrinsic molecular subtypes that can be distinguished on the basis of gene expression profiling, and these include luminal A, luminal B, HER2-enriched, and basal-like cancers (Perou et al. 2000; Sørlie et al. 2001; Herschkowitz et al. 2007; Sørlie et al. 2003; Hu et al. 2006). There is no standard clinical assay to assign molecular class to a newly diagnosed breast cancer. The closest is the Prosigna breast cancer prognostic gene signature assay by Veracyte Inc. that reports molecular subtype, but it is primarily a prognostic test for ER+ cancers. The St. Gallen International Expert Consensus on the Primary Therapy of Early Breast Cancer (Goldhirsch et al. 2011; Goldhirsch et al. 2013) also endorsed the use of various combinations of grade and ER, PR, HER2, and Ki67 immunohistochemistry results as surrogate to the mRNA-based molecular classification (Cardoso et al. 2019). Unfortunately, there is up to 30% discordance between immunohistochemistry-based and mRNA expression-based molecular class assignment (Yao et al. 2015; Prat et al. 2014).

In parallel with the molecular classification efforts, several independent prognostic gene signatures were also developed that took advantage of the large-scale gene expression differences between luminal A and B cancers. Almost all clinically validated multigene assays derive their prognostic value from quantifying proliferation and ER-related gene expressions (Tamimi et al. 2012). These tests were validated in either prospective clinical trials or archived tissues from large clinical trials and are now part of the routine assessment of newly diagnosed (ER+) breast cancers. In this chapter, we will use the four clinically relevant intrinsic subtypes as the conceptual framework to discuss the clinical behavior and treatment of breast cancers. While the day-to-day clinical management of breast cancer is guided by anatomical risk factors (i.e., tumor size, nodal status), ER and HER2 protein expression, and molecular prognostic assay, the intrinsic subtypes provide a coherent and biology-based interpretation of our treatment strategies.

21.2 Epidemiological and Genetic Risk Factors

Recognizing the distinct cellular origins of luminal and basal-like cancers allowed studying epidemiological risk factors separately for these two distinct disease types. Several well-recognized breast cancer risk factors confer risk for both subtypes, but notable differences also exist. Nulliparity is a risk factor for developing luminal cancers, whereas multiple early pregnancies, particularly if coupled with a lack or short duration of breastfeeding, are risk factors for basal-like cancers. There are also differences in genomic predisposition. Germline BRCA1 mutations are primarily associated with increased risk for basal-like cancers, whereas BRCA2 mutations confer equal risk for both luminal and basal-like cancers (Table 21.1) (Bazzi et al. 2023; Harbeck et al. 2019; Jung et al. 2022; Barnard et al. 2015; Łukasiewicz et al. 2021). Among women without high penetrance germline cancer predisposing mutations, distinct sets of germline single nucleotide polymorphisms (SNP) are associated with risk to develop basal-like and luminal breast cancer. Differences in risk factor prevalence partly explain the differences in breast cancer incidence in different parts of the world and across ancestry groups within countries.

21.3 Clinical Features of Intrinsic Subtypes

21.3.1 Luminal A

The term luminal cancer was derived from the unique cytokeratin expression in these tumors (CK7, CK8, CK18, CK19) that is similar to cytokeratin expression patterns in luminal epithelial cells of normal breast glands. Under morphological examination luminal A cancers tend to have strong homogenous ER and PR expression, low to intermediate histological grade, low nuclear pleomorphism, and low mitotic activity. Luminal A cancers are the most common type of breast cancer, accounting for approximately 50–60% of

Table 21.1 Risk factors associated with different intrinsic subtypes of breast cancer

	Luminal A	Luminal B	HER2-enriched	Basal-like
Clinical risk factors	Younger age at menarche Nulliparity Older age at first birth Older age at menopause Weight gain from 18 years of age Estrogen only and estrogen plus progestin hormone therapy as oral contraceptives and hormone replacement therapy Two first-degree relatives with breast cancer Prior benign breast disease Alcohol consumption	Younger age at menarche Weight gain from 18 years of age First-degree relatives with breast cancer Prior benign breast disease	Younger age at menarche Older age at menopause Two first-degree relatives with breast cancer Prior benign breast disease	Younger age at menarche Estrogen plus progestin hormone therapy as oral contraceptives Two first-degree relatives with breast cancer Prior benign breast disease *Inverse association with lactation and older age at first birth*
Genetic risk factors	*BRCA2*, *PALB2*, *CHEK2*, *ATM*, *NF1*, Cowden syndrome, hereditary diffuse gastric cancer syndrome, Peutz-Jegher syndrome	*BRCA2*, *PALB2*, *CHEK2*, *ATM*, *NF1*, Cowden syndrome, hereditary diffuse gastric cancer syndrome, Peutz-Jegher syndrome	*BRCA2*, *PALB2*, *ATM*, *NF1*, Cowden syndrome, hereditary diffuse gastric cancer syndrome, Peutz-Jegher syndrome, and Li-Fraumeni syndrome	*BRCA1*, *PALB2*, *ATM*, *NF1*, Cowden syndrome, hereditary diffuse gastric cancer syndrome, Peutz-Jegher syndrome

breast cancers, and the most prevalent in postmenopausal white women. On mammographic imaging, these tumors are spiculated masses associated with architectural distortion. Luminal A cancers have overall good prognosis, but the risk of distant recurrence extends over decades. Most luminal A cancers are assigned to low prognostic risk by Oncotype DX Recurrence Score, MammaPrint, and other multigene prognostic signatures. If metastatic recurrence develops, the most frequent initial site of recurrence is the bone, followed by the pleura and lymph nodes (Buonomo et al. 2017; Smid et al. 2008; Yersal 2014).

21.3.2 Luminal B

Luminal B tumors comprise approximately 25–30% of breast cancer and often have less than 100% ER positivity and negative progesterone receptor staining on immunohistochemistry. These tumors also have higher histologic grades and high mitotic counts. Many luminal B cancers are genomic high-risk when tested with multigene prognostic assays. On mammographic imaging, they present as masses with microlobulated or spiculated margins and are more likely to present with axillary lymph node involvement than luminal A tumors (Hu et al. 2006; Perou et al. 1999; Vuong et al. 2014). This subtype has a higher recurrence rate and a lower survival rate compared to luminal A tumors. Early relapses within a few years after diagnosis are more frequent, but the metastatic relapse patterns are similar to luminal A tumors with a predilection towards the bone, lung, pleura, and lymph nodes (Buonomo et al. 2017; Smid et al. 2008; Yersal 2014).

21.3.3 HER2-Enriched

HER2-enriched tumors represent 15–20% of breast cancers. They include both ER+ and ER- cancers, and the vast majority have HER2 gene amplification and correspond closely, but not perfectly, to cancers that are considered HER2 positive by conventional clinical assays. HER2-enriched cancers that are HER2 negative by clinical assays are treated as HER2-negative cancers guided by their estrogen receptor expression. The clinical behavior of HER2-enriched cancers is influenced by the underlying ER subtype; ER+/HER2-enriched cancers tend to have more indolent course and lesser chemotherapy sensitivity than their ER- counterparts. The ER-/HER2 gene-amplified HER2-enriched cancers are the most chemotherapy-sensitive breast cancer subtype. On imaging, HER2-enriched cancers may present as masses accompanied by pleomorphic calcifications or as calcifications alone that could be a sign of a rapidly growing tumor. Historically, HER2-enriched tumors had higher rates of recurrence than luminal cancers, but modern HER2 targeted therapies improved their survival dramatically, and these cancers are now considered among the most highly curable subtypes. Isolated recurrences in the brain are common compared to relapse in other organs sites and are consistent with the hypothesis that the central nervous system is a tumor sanctuary site, protected from systemic adjuvant therapies by the blood-brain barrier (Buonomo et al. 2017; Smid et al. 2008).

21.3.4 Basal-Like

Approximately 10–15% of breast cancers are basal-like tumors and correspond closely to triple-negative cancers (ER, PR, and HER2 negative) by immunohistochemistry (Koboldt et al. 2012; Weinstein et al. 2013). They express cytokeratins (CK5, CK6, CK14, CK17) that are typically seen in basal epithelial cells. They are high-grade, poorly differentiated tumors with high proliferation rate, often with signs of central necrosis attributed to rapid growth outstripping neovascularization leading to areas of necrosis within the tumor (Yersal 2014). On mammograms, the necrotic areas may appear as clusters of calcifications. Basal-like tumors tend to relapse within 2–3 years after the initial diagnosis and have a propensity to metastasize to multiple visceral organs as well as to the bone (Buonomo et al. 2017; Smid et al. 2008; Rakha et al. 2008). There is substantial further molecular heterogeneity within basal-like breast cancers, and several subclassification schemas exist, but these have limited clinical implications (Herschkowitz et al. 2007; Perou et al. 2010; Prat and Perou 2011). Basal-like cancers with high androgen receptor (AR)-related gene expression or with high levels of immune infiltration have better prognosis, whereas mesenchymal-enriched and claudin-low basal-like cancers tend to have lower chemotherapy sensitivity; however, their treatments are not different from basal-like cancers in general.

The original intrinsic molecular subtypes also included a normal-like breast cancer category. Subsequent analysis suggested that this group was mostly comprised of cancers with low tumor cellularity where transcriptomic signal was dominated by the presence of normal breast tissues (Elloumi et al. 2011). The normal-like category is no longer commonly used (Weigelt et al. 2010; Parker et al. 2009).

21.4 Within Tumor Cellular Heterogeneity and Plasticity of Molecular Subtypes

Single-cell transcriptomics allows cell level subtyping as opposed to bulk RNA-based molecular class assignment. Single-cell sequencing data suggest substantial, within tumor, cellular heterogeneity and plasticity of subtype assignment. In treatment-naïve patients, multiple different malignant phenotypes can be detected within the same tumor. A basal-like tumor on bulk profiling may contain cells that show features of HER2-enriched cancers, whereas luminal cancers often contain both luminal A and B type cancer cells. These observations are intriguing and may reflect genuine biological heterogeneity but could also be due to technical imprecisions and instability in class assignment. When breast cancer molecular subtypes were compared between paired primary and metastatic tissues, frequent molecular subtype conversions were also detected. Cancers that were luminal A at diagnosis converted to luminal B subtype in about 40% of metastatic lesions and to HER2-enriched subtype in about 13%. Cancers that were initially luminal B showed a 17% conversion rate to luminal A and 13% to HER2-enriched subtype in the metastatic sites (Wu et al. 2021; Chung et al. 2017; Cejalvo et al. 2017). Among HER2-enriched tumors, 23% underwent a conversion at the time of recurrence, with 15% converting to basal-like and 8% to luminal A. These findings could represent evolution of cancer under selective pressure, but some of these molecular subtype switches may also be due to technical limitations of class assignment that may be caused by the differing cellular composition (and therefore mRNA content) of biopsies from different organ sites (Cejalvo et al. 2017). Importantly, no study showed conversion of luminal cancers to basal-like cancers or vice versa, consistent with the assumption that these are fundamentally different types of cancers.

21.5 Prognostic Value of the Intrinsic Subtypes

The pure prognostic value of molecular class in the absence of any systemic therapy is difficult to determine since few patients receive no systemic adjuvant therapy in contemporary studies. Tumor size and nodal status also remain powerful independent prognostic factors that are often distributed differently across subtypes in convenience cohorts and confound prognostic associations. The largest study that attempted to define pure prognostic values of molecular class used the PAM50 assay and evaluated the prognosis of patients with node-negative breast cancer who received no systemic adjuvant therapy. It showed that luminal A tumors had the lowest relapse-free survival, whereas luminal B and HER2-enriched tumors had worse outcomes (Parker et al. 2009). Patients with basal-like tumors had intermediate prognosis, with high rates of early relapses within the first 3 years, after which annual risk of recurrence was lower than in luminal cancers (matched by clinical stage). The study also highlighted the independent prognostic value of tumor size and developed a combined clinical and genomic score to predict the risk of recurrence (ROR) in postmenopausal women. This PAM50-based ROR score is the basis of the commercially available Prosigna prognostic assay (Dowsett et al. 2013; Kjällquist et al. 2022). The Prosigna assay was also tested in tissues from clinical trials and demonstrated prognostic value in patients who received adjuvant endocrine therapy. Based on these results, it is endorsed by breast cancer practice guidelines as one of the several genomic prognostic assays that could be used in postmenopausal women with ER+/HER2-, node-negative breast cancer to assist in decision-making about the use of adjuvant chemotherapy (Cardoso et al. 2019; Andre et al. 2022; Gradishar et al. 2023). Patients with high ROR scores are candidates for adjuvant chemotherapy.

21.6 Association Between Chemotherapy Sensitivity and Intrinsic Subtypes

Several studies examined response to neoadjuvant (i.e., preoperative) chemotherapy in different intrinsic subtypes of breast cancer. A seminal study assessed pathologic complete response (pCR, defined as lack of any invasive cancer in the breast and lymph nodes after preoperative therapy) rates in stage I–III breast cancers treated with neoadjuvant chemotherapy and found that basal-like and HER2-enriched tumors had the highest pCR rates, whereas luminal A cancers had the lowest pCR rate (Rouzier et al. 2005). A subsequent larger study also reported low pCR rates in luminal cancers, 3% in luminal A tumors and 9% in luminal B tumors, and confirmed the high pCR rates in HER2-enriched and basal-like cancers, 46% and 42%, respectively (Prat et al. 2012). A pooled analysis of 6377 cancers treated with anthracycline-/taxane-based neoadjuvant chemotherapy and assigned to molecular subtypes based on immunohistochemistry results showed 6.4% pCR rate in luminal B/HER2- cancer, 11.2% in luminal B/HER2+ cancers treated without trastuzumab, and 31% in triple-negative cancers (von Minckwitz et al. 2012). HER2 positive and negative status was assigned using routine clinical criteria (i.e., HER2 gene-amplified or HER2 immunohistochemistry 3+ staining). These neoadjuvant studies also revealed that patients with HER2-enriched/HER2+ or with basal-like/triple-negative cancers that achieved a pCR have excellent long-term recurrence-free survival, while those with residual invasive cancer after neoadjuvant chemotherapy have poor prognosis (Carey et al. 2007). These observations provide the biological rationale for contemporary treatment strategies which aim to maximize pCR rates and improve outcome in those with residual disease through postoperative (i.e., adjuvant) therapy in triple-negative and HER2+ cancers.

All but the smallest of HER2+ and triple-negative cancers are treated with neoadjuvant chemotherapy (Pusztai et al. 2019). For larger HER2+ cancers, trastuzumab and pertuzumab are administered concurrent with chemotherapy, and about 50% of ER+/HER2+ cancers achieve a pCR with a third-generation chemotherapy regimen; pCR rates are even higher in ER-/HER2+ cancers, about 80% (Wuerstlein and Harbeck 2017). Equally important the KATHERINE clinical trial demonstrated that administration of 1 year of adjuvant ado-trastuzumab emtansine (Kadcyla™) improves recurrence-free survival in HER2+ patients who have residual disease after neoadjuvant therapy (von Minckwitz et al. 2018). The most effective neoadjuvant chemotherapy for triple-negative breast cancers includes a combination of pembrolizumab (anti-PD1 antibody) and paclitaxel/platinum followed by anthracycline/cyclophosphamide chemotherapy, which results in pCR rates of around 65% (Schmid et al. 2020). The CREATE-X trial demonstrated that in patients with triple-negative residual disease, six to eight cycles of adjuvant capecitabine improved survival (Masuda et al. 2017). Several clinical trials are testing novel, possibly more effective, adjuvant therapies for HER2+ and triple-negative breast cancers with residual disease after neoadjuvant therapy. The opportunity to receive additional therapy for patients who achieve less than the best response to standard chemotherapy is lost if patients undergo surgery first, which makes neoadjuvant chemotherapy the preferred strategy for HER2+ or triple-negative breast cancers. The substantial biological and clinical heterogeneity that exists within these subtypes motivates research to develop further subclassifications and composite biomarkers that could be used to refine personalized treatment selection. For example, among HER2-positive cancers, the subset of tumors that have HER2-enriched molecular class, high HER2 mRNA expression, and also HER2 gene copy number > 4, and are without PIK3CA mutation, can achieve pCR rates of 40–60% with dual HER2 targeted therapies (e.g., trastuzumab + pertuzumab or lapatinib) alone (without chemotherapy) (Prat et al. 2020).

Luminal cancers have substantially lower chemotherapy sensitivity than basal or HER2-enriched cancers that is apparent from the low pCR rates in neoadjuvant trials. However, a subset of these patients, largely but not completely corresponding to luminal B cancers, experience improved survival with adjuvant (or neoadjuvant) chemotherapy. Multiple mRNA expression-based prognostic assays were developed to identify ER+ cancers that derive benefit from adjuvant chemotherapy, including the Oncotype DX Recurrence Score, MammaPrint, EndoPredict, Prosigna ROR, Breast Cancer Index, and others (Andre et al. 2022). A subset of luminal B cancers has high immune cell infiltration and high programmed death ligand-1 (PD-L1) expression and corresponds to the ultra-high end of the MammaPrint risk score (i.e., MP High-2) (Pusztai et al. 2021; O'Meara et al. 2020). These luminal cancers show improved pCR rate when immune checkpoint inhibitors (durvalumab, pembrolizumab, nivolumab) are added to neoadjuvant chemotherapy. Ongoing randomized trials (KEYNOTE-756 [NCT03725059] and SWOG S2206 [NCT06058377]) are testing if the improved pCR rates will translate into improved recurrence free survival.

21.7 Endocrine Therapy for Luminal Cancer

Estrogen targeting endocrine therapy is a key component of treatment for all luminal cancers. However, neoadjuvant endocrine therapy trials showed differences in endocrine therapy sensitivity among ER+ breast cancers by molecular subtype. Since pCR is rare with neoadjuvant endocrine therapy, a proliferation arrest-based metric that combines residual tumor size, node status, and Ki67 and ER expression levels into a single preoperative endocrine prognostic index (PEPI) was developed as the measure of endocrine treatment response (Ellis et al. 2008). The ASCOSOG Z1031 clinical trial that tested neoadjuvant aromatase inhibitors (that inhibit estrogen production in non-ovarian tissues) in postmenopausal women with stage II–III, ER+/HER2-negative breast cancer found that luminal A tumors had better PEPI response (PEPI score 0 corresponds to the best response and predicts excellent prognosis) than luminal B tumors (27.1% vs. 10.7%) (Ellis et al. 2011). A minority of clinically ER+/HER2- cancers classify as HER2-enriched, and these cancers seem to be the least sensitive to preoperative endocrine therapy (Dunbier et al. 2011). Since the luminal A versus B classification relies heavily on capturing differences in proliferative activity, following neoadjuvant endocrine therapy, many luminal B tumors convert to luminal A tumors when molecular class is determined in both pre- and post-treatment samples, reflecting a decrease in proliferation. Consistent with the higher endocrine therapy sensitivity of luminal A cancers observed in the preoperative trials, these cancers also show the best long-term survival in adjuvant endocrine therapy trials (Gnant et al. 2013; Chia et al. 2012). More recently CDK 4/6 inhibitors (e.g., abemaciclib, ribociclib) were added to adjuvant endocrine therapy to reduce the risk of recurrence in clinically and genomically high-risk ER+/HER2- breast cancers. Formal analysis by molecular subtype has not been performed in the pivotal monarchE trial that established the role of abemaciclib as adjuvant therapy, but cancers with both low (<20%) and high (>20%) Ki67 expression benefited (Harbeck et al. 2021). While differences between prognoses and endocrine therapy sensitivity exist between luminal A and B cancers, both derive benefit from adjuvant endocrine therapy, and clinically high-risk luminal cancers also derive benefit from adjuvant CDK 4/6 inhibitors.

21.8 Intrinsic Subtypes in the Metastatic Setting

Most of the evidence regarding the prognostic and predictive value of the intrinsic subtypes of breast cancer comes from analysis of stage I–III breast cancers, but some studies also examined outcome in metastatic disease by molecular subtype. Combined analysis of the PALOMA-2 and PALOMA-3 studies that tested the CDK4/6 inhibitor palbociclib added to first-line or second-line endocrine therapy, respectively, in ER+/HER2- metastatic breast cancer showed that palbociclib improved progression-free survival in both luminal A and B cancers (Finn et al. 2020). However, progression-free survival was significantly longer in luminal A compared to luminal B cancers, and non-luminal cancers had the most rapid progression on therapy. Similar findings were reported from the MONALEESA clinical trials that tested ribociclib in combination with endocrine therapy in metastatic ER+/HER2- breast cancers. Most patients were classified into the luminal A or luminal B categories, comprising 46.8% and 24% of the study population, respectively. This study also found that the approximately 30% of patients who were classified as non-luminal cancers despite being clinically ER+ had the highest risk of disease progression and that the basal-like subtype had the shortest progression-free survival followed by HER2-enriched and luminal B subtypes (Prat et al. 2021). Importantly, both luminal A and B cancers had improved survival when ribociclib was added to endocrine therapy, but basal-like cancers did not. A meta-analysis of 2536 patients with ER+ metastatic breast cancer, treated with various endocrine therapies (tamoxifen, aromatase inhibitors, and fulvestrant) with and without other drugs (e.g., CDK 4/6 inhibitors, mTOR inhibitors, and tyrosine kinase inhibitors), confirmed that luminal A cancers had the best survival, followed by luminal B and non-luminal disease (Schettini et al. 2023). These results indicate that the fundamental biological and clinical characteristics of the molecular subtypes that were defined by studying newly diagnosed breast cancers carry over and continue to manifest themselves even after metastatic recurrence.

Inhibition of the PIK3CA (phosphatidylinositol-4,5-bisphosphate 3-kinase catalytic subunit alpha)-AKT (V-akt murine thymoma viral oncogene homolog/protein kinase-B)-mTOR (mammalian target of rapamycin) pathway emerged as a successful therapeutic strategy in metastatic breast cancers that harbor mutations in these genes. Activating mutations in PIK3CA can be detected in up to 45% of luminal A, 29% of luminal B, 39% of HER2-E, and 9% of basal-like tumors (Falato et al. 2023). The PIK3CA alpha subunit-specific inhibitor alpelisib was evaluated in combination with fulvestrant in the phase III SOLAR-1 trial that accrued patients with ER+/HER2-negative metastatic breast cancers with and without PIK3CA mutations and that had progressed on at least one previous line of endocrine therapy. The trial demonstrated significant improvement in progression-free survival in the PIK3CA mutant subset of cancers, with no improvement in the wild-type cancers (André et al. 2021). The AKT inhibitor capivasertib in combination with fulvestrant was tested in the CAPItello-291 trial that accrued ER+/HER2-negative metastatic breast cancer patients who had disease progression on previous aromatase inhibitor therapy (with or without a CDK4/6 inhibitor). This trial also demonstrated improved progression-free survival with AKT inhibition compared to fulvestrant alone, and benefit was largely, if not entirely, limited to cancer with mutations in either PIK3CA, AKT, or PTEN (phosphatase and tensin homolog) (Turner et al. 2023). The SOLAR-1 and CAPItello-291 trials have not yet reported efficacy by molecular subtype, but PIK3CA-AKT-PTEN alterations occur in all four subtypes with different frequencies. The BOLERO-2 trial evaluated the use of the mTOR inhibitor everolimus plus exemestane, compared to exemestane plus placebo in postmenopausal women with ER+/HER2-negative breast cancer, and prior exposure to nonsteroidal aromatase inhibitors. The trial demonstrated significant improvement in progression-free survival in the everolimus arm (Piccart et al. 2014). All molecular subtypes benefited, but luminal A and luminal B tumors had longer progression-free survival than non-luminal tumors, and interestingly, the HER2-enriched subtype, which had the worst prognosis with endocrine treatment alone, experienced the greatest relative benefit when exemestane was added to endocrine therapy (Prat et al. 2019).

In HER2-amplified/HER2-overexpressing metastatic breast cancers, the phase III HER2CLIMB trial evaluated the combination of tucatinib, trastuzumab, and capecitabine, compared to placebo, trastuzumab, and capecitabine. The three-drug combination improved both progression-free and overall survival (Curigliano et al. 2022). A unique aspect of this trial was that it allowed patients who had active or stable brain metastases. The central nervous system progression-free survival and overall survival were significantly better in the tucatinib group establishing a new standard of care for brain metastases (Lin et al. 2023). Whether treatment efficacy differed by molecular subtype has not been examined for this trial. A different strategy in the treatment of HER2-positive cancers includes the use of HER2-targeting antibody-drug conjugates, such as trastuzumab-emtansine (TDM1) and trastuzumab-deruxtecan (T-Dxd). The DESTINY-Breast03 trial compared T-Dxd versus TDM1 in patients with advanced HER2-positive breast cancer who progressed after taxane and trastuzumab therapy and demonstrated significantly longer progression-free and overall survival in the T-Dxd arm (Cortés et al. 2022). Remarkably, T-Dxd also showed efficacy in HER2-low breast cancers defined as HER2 1+ or 2+ by immunohistochemistry but without HER2 gene amplification (Modi et al. 2022). About 14% of these cancers are classified as HER2-enriched (Agostinetto et al. 2021). Molecular classification of cancers included in the trial found that T-Dxd improved outcome in luminal as well non-luminal HER2-low breast cancers (Modi et al. 2023).

Overall, results from multiple trials suggest that for molecularly targeted therapies, the genomic alteration itself is more important to determine treatment sensitivity than the molecular subtype.

21.9 Conclusions

Intrinsic subtyping of breast cancer provides a useful theoretical framework to study breast cancer and to understand the current treatment landscape. Recognizing that ER+ and ER- cancers are fundamentally different diseases allowed the discovery of distinct epidemiological risk factors for these two major subtypes. Understanding that metastatic patterns and annual hazards of recurrence differ between the subtypes led to designing separate clinical trials for ER+ and ER- cancers. Intrinsic subtyping as the name implies was derived from gene expression patterns that can define "naturally occurring" subsets of breast cancers. Several different intrinsic classification schemas can be generated from the same data by using different thresholds to define subgroups; however, smaller subsets in complex classifications tend to be unstable and may not correspond to any currently clinically meaningful subgroup. Current consensus considers four major subtypes as robust and clinically meaningful. Basal-like cancers differ from the rest of breast cancers by the expression of several thousand genes and are clinically characterized by the lack of ER, PR, and HER2 expression and the high risk of recurrence in the absence of adjuvant systemic therapy that reflects a propensity for early micrometastatic dissemination. Many of these cancers are also highly vulnerable to chemotherapy because of their rapid proliferation rate. Long-term survival of basal-like cancers improved significantly by implementing a preoperative chemotherapy followed by pathologic response-guided adjuvant therapy strategy. By virtue of frequent immune cell infiltration, these cancers also benefit from adding immune checkpoint inhibitors to neoadjuvant chemotherapy. Luminal cancers correspond to ER+ breast cancers and can be subdivided into two clinically important subsets. All other clinical prognostic variables kept equal, luminal A tumors have the best prognosis, but their outcome can be further improved by adjuvant endocrine therapy alone or in combination with CDK 4/6 inhibitors. Luminal B cancers more frequently have a high histologic grade, rapid proliferation, and more immune cell infiltration and, not unexpectedly, have a worse prognosis but somewhat greater chemotherapy sensitivity than luminal A cancers. The HER2-enriched subtype carries the transcriptional characteristics of HER2 gene-amplified cancers, but a substantial minority of these cancers are not HER2+ by conventional clinical assays.

In parallel with the unsupervised molecular classification efforts, other investigators pursued supervised prognostic marker development strategies. Supervised prognostic marker development involves a priori defining a classification challenge (e.g., which ER+ patients recur, or not, despite adjuvant endocrine therapy), selecting patients/samples that are best suited to find prognostic markers (e.g., patients who all received the same uniform adjuvant endocrine therapy and have detailed long-term follow-up), and identifying the molecular features that distinguish the two outcome groups (e.g., relapse vs. no-relapse). Many of these prospectively developed supervised multigene prognostic assays for ER+ cancers (Oncotype DX Recurrence Score, MammaPrint, EndoPredict, Prosigna ROR, Breast Cancer Index, etc.) provide robust, standardized, and reproducible prognostic risk estimates. The Oncotype DX Recurrence Score and MammaPrint were also shown to be able to identify ER+ patients whose survival improves with adjuvant chemotherapy in prospective clinical trials (O'Meara et al. 2020). Currently, these molecular assays rather than intrinsic subtyping guide adjuvant chemotherapy selection in ER+ breast cancers. Figure 21.1 summarizes treatment options for stage I–III breast cancers based on molecular assay results, intrinsic subtype, and clinical risk. There is only partial overlap between intrinsic subtypes, clinical ER/PR/HER2 pheno-

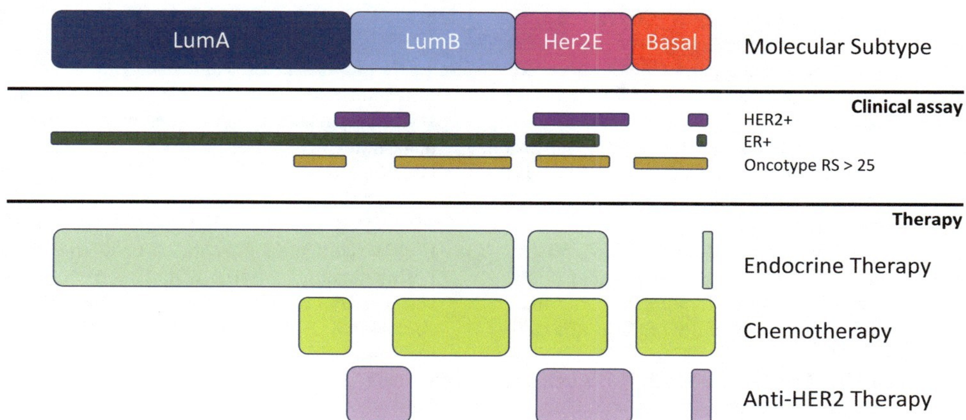

Fig. 21.1 Treatment options for stage I–III breast cancers based on molecular assay results, intrinsic subtype, and clinical risk. The figure illustrates the overlap between molecular subtype and clinical classification and shows how major treatment systemic modalities are applied across the different classification systems

type, and prognostic risk estimated by multigene assays. When different classifications provide concordant results, this is highly reassuring; however, physicians regularly encounter discordant results. For example, some luminal A cancers can have high recurrence score, and some HER2-enriched cancers have no HER2 gene amplification or HER2 protein overexpression; how to treat these discordant cases remains a challenge and would require new prospective studies to define the optimal treatment approach for these patients. Currently, the conservative and safer approach is to act on the clinically better validated assay result. A luminal A cancer with a recurrence score > 25 is treated with adjuvant chemotherapy, and a HER2-enriched but HER2- cancer would not qualify for HER2 targeted adjuvant therapy.

In summary, the discovery of intrinsic subtypes of breast cancer was paradigm shifting in that breast cancer is no longer viewed as a single disease with some heterogeneity in ER expression but rather a collection of molecularly and clinically distinct diseases that arise from breast epithelial cells. Different biomarkers and different treatment strategies are applied to the different molecular subtypes. All contemporary breast cancer clinical trials are subtype-specific, which is a major shift from 20 years ago when all breast cancers were included in a single study.

References

Agostinetto E, Rediti M, Fimereli D et al (2021) HER2-low breast cancer: molecular characteristics and prognosis. Cancers (Basel) 13:2824. https://doi.org/10.3390/cancers13112824

André F, Ciruelos EM, Juric D et al (2021) Alpelisib plus fulvestrant for PIK3CA-mutated, hormone receptor-positive, human epidermal growth factor receptor-2–negative advanced breast cancer: final overall survival results from SOLAR-1. Ann Oncol 32:208–217. https://doi.org/10.1016/j.annonc.2020.11.011

Andre F, Ismaila N, Allison KH et al (2022) Biomarkers for adjuvant endocrine and chemotherapy in early-stage breast cancer: ASCO guideline update. J Clin Oncol 40:1816–1837. https://doi.org/10.1200/JCO.22.00069

Barnard ME, Boeke CE, Tamimi RM (2015) Established breast cancer risk factors and risk of intrinsic tumor subtypes. Biochim Biophys Acta Rev Cancer 1856:73–85. https://doi.org/10.1016/j.bbcan.2015.06.002

Bazzi T, Al-husseini M, Saravolatz L, Kafri Z (2023) Trends in breast cancer incidence and mortality in the United States from 2004-2018: a surveillance, epidemiology, and end results (SEER)-based study. Cureus 2023:4–9. https://doi.org/10.7759/cureus.37982

Buonomo OC, Caredda E, Portarena I et al (2017) New insights into the metastatic behavior after breast cancer surgery, according to well-established clinicopathological variables and molecular subtypes. PLoS One 12:e0184680. https://doi.org/10.1371/journal.pone.0184680

Cardoso F, Kyriakides S, Ohno S et al (2019) Early breast cancer: ESMO clinical practice guidelines for diagnosis, treatment and follow-up. Ann Oncol 30:1194–1220. https://doi.org/10.1093/annonc/mdz173

Carey LA, Dees EC, Sawyer L et al (2007) The triple negative paradox: primary tumor chemosensitivity of breast cancer subtypes. Clin Cancer Res 13:2329–2334. https://doi.org/10.1158/1078-0432.CCR-06-1109

Cejalvo JM, De Dueñas EM, Galván P et al (2017) Intrinsic subtypes and gene expression profiles in primary and metastatic breast cancer. Cancer Res 77:2213–2221. https://doi.org/10.1158/0008-5472.CAN-16-2717

Chia SK, Bramwell VH, Tu D et al (2012) A 50-gene intrinsic subtype classifier for prognosis and prediction of benefit from adjuvant Tamoxifen. Clin Cancer Res 18:4465–4472. https://doi.org/10.1158/1078-0432.CCR-12-0286

Chung W, Eum HH, Lee H-O et al (2017) Single-cell RNA-seq enables comprehensive tumour and immune cell profiling in primary breast cancer. Nat Commun 8:15081. https://doi.org/10.1038/ncomms15081

Cortés J, Kim S-B, Chung W-P et al (2022) Trastuzumab Deruxtecan versus Trastuzumab Emtansine for breast cancer. N Engl J Med 386:1143–1154. https://doi.org/10.1056/NEJMoa2115022

Curigliano G, Mueller V, Borges V et al (2022) Tucatinib versus placebo added to trastuzumab and capecitabine for patients with pretreated HER2+ metastatic breast cancer with and without brain metastases (HER2CLIMB): final overall survival analysis. Ann Oncol 33:321–329. https://doi.org/10.1016/j.annonc.2021.12.005

Dowsett M, Sestak I, Lopez-Knowles E et al (2013) Comparison of PAM50 risk of recurrence score with Onco type DX and IHC4 for predicting risk of distant recurrence after endocrine therapy. J Clin Oncol 31:2783–2790. https://doi.org/10.1200/JCO.2012.46.1558

Dunbier AK, Anderson H, Ghazoui Z et al (2011) Association between breast cancer subtypes and response to neoadjuvant anastrozole. Steroids 76:736–740. https://doi.org/10.1016/j.steroids.2011.02.025

Ellis MJ, Tao Y, Luo J et al (2008) Outcome prediction for estrogen receptor-positive breast cancer based on postneoadjuvant endocrine therapy tumor characteristics. J Natl Cancer Inst 100:1380–1388. https://doi.org/10.1093/jnci/djn309

Ellis MJ, Suman VJ, Hoog J et al (2011) Randomized phase II neoadjuvant comparison between letrozole, anastrozole, and exemestane for postmenopausal women with estrogen receptor-rich stage 2 to 3 breast cancer: clinical and biomarker outcomes and predictive value of the baseline PAM50-based int. J Clin Oncol 29:2342–2349. https://doi.org/10.1200/JCO.2010.31.6950

Elloumi F, Hu Z, Li Y et al (2011) Systematic bias in genomic classification due to contaminating non-neoplastic tissue in breast tumor samples. BMC Med Genet 4:54. https://doi.org/10.1186/1755-8794-4-54

Falato C, Schettini F, Pascual T, Brasó-Maristany F, Prat A (2023) Clinical implications of the intrinsic molecular subtypes in hormone receptor-positive and HER2-negative metastatic breast cancer. Cancer Treat Rev 112:102496

Finn RS, Liu Y, Zhu Z et al (2020) Biomarker analyses of response to cyclin-dependent kinase 4/6 inhibition and endocrine therapy in women with treatment-Naïve metastatic breast cancer. Clin Cancer Res 26:110–121. https://doi.org/10.1158/1078-0432.CCR-19-0751

Gnant M, Filipits M, Dubsky P et al (2013) Predicting risk for late metastasis: the PAM50 risk of recurrence (ROR) score after 5 years of endocrine therapy in postmenopausal women with Hr+ early breast cancer: a study on 1,478 patients from the Abcsg-8 trial. Ann Oncol 24:iii29. https://doi.org/10.1093/annonc/mdt084.1

Goldhirsch A, Wood WC, Coates AS et al (2011) Strategies for subtypes—dealing with the diversity of breast cancer: highlights of the St Gallen International Expert Consensus on the Primary Therapy of Early Breast Cancer 2011. Ann Oncol 22:1736–1747. https://doi.org/10.1093/annonc/mdr304

Goldhirsch A, Winer EP, Coates AS et al (2013) Personalizing the treatment of women with early breast cancer: highlights of the st gallen international expert consensus on the primary therapy of early breast cancer 2013. Ann Oncol 24:2206–2223. https://doi.org/10.1093/annonc/mdt303

Gradishar WJ, Moran MS, Abraham J et al (2023) NCCN Guidelines® insights: breast cancer, version 4.2023. J Natl Compr Cancer Netw 21:594–608. https://doi.org/10.6004/jnccn.2023.0031

Harbeck N, Penault-Llorca F, Cortes J et al (2019) Breast cancer. Nat Rev Dis Prim 5:66. https://doi.org/10.1038/s41572-019-0111-2

Harbeck N, Rastogi P, Martin M et al (2021) Adjuvant abemaciclib combined with endocrine therapy for high-risk early breast cancer: updated efficacy and Ki-67 analysis from the monarchE study. Ann Oncol 32:1571–1581. https://doi.org/10.1016/j.annonc.2021.09.015

Herschkowitz JI, Simin K, Weigman VJ et al (2007) Identification of conserved gene expression features between murine mammary carcinoma models and human breast tumors. Genome Biol 8:R76. https://doi.org/10.1186/gb-2007-8-5-r76

Hu Z, Fan C, Oh DS et al (2006) The molecular portraits of breast tumors are conserved across microarray platforms. BMC Genom 7:1–12. https://doi.org/10.1186/1471-2164-7-96

Jung AY, Ahearn TU, Behrens S et al (2022) Distinct reproductive risk profiles for intrinsic-like breast cancer subtypes: pooled analysis of population-based studies. J Natl Cancer Inst 114:1706–1719. https://doi.org/10.1093/jnci/djac117

Kjällquist U, Acs B, Margolin S et al (2022) Real world evaluation of the Prosigna/PAM50 test in a node-negative postmenopausal Swedish population: a Multicenter study. Cancers (Basel) 14:2615. https://doi.org/10.3390/cancers14112615

Koboldt DC, Fulton RS, McLellan MD et al (2012) Comprehensive molecular portraits of human breast tumours. Nature 490:61–70. https://doi.org/10.1038/nature11412

Lin NU, Murthy RK, Abramson V et al (2023) Tucatinib vs placebo, both in combination with Trastuzumab and Capecitabine, for previously treated ERBB2 (HER2)-positive metastatic breast cancer in patients with brain metastases. JAMA Oncol 9:197. https://doi.org/10.1001/jamaoncol.2022.5610

Łukasiewicz S, Czeczelewski M, Forma A et al (2021) Breast cancer—epidemiology, risk factors, classification, prognostic markers, and current treatment strategies—an updated review. Cancers (Basel) 13:4287. https://doi.org/10.3390/cancers13174287

Masuda N, Lee S-J, Ohtani S et al (2017) Adjuvant capecitabine for breast cancer after preoperative chemotherapy. N Engl J Med 376:2147–2159. https://doi.org/10.1056/NEJMoa1612645

Modi S, Jacot W, Yamashita T et al (2022) Trastuzumab Deruxtecan in previously treated HER2-low advanced breast cancer. N Engl J Med 387:9–20. https://doi.org/10.1056/NEJMoa2203690

Modi S, Niikura N, Yamashita T et al (2023) Trastuzumab deruxtecan (T-DXd) vs treatment of physician's choice (TPC) in patients (pts) with HER2-low, hormone receptor-positive (HR+) unresectable and/or metastatic breast cancer (mBC): exploratory biomarker analysis of DESTINY-Breast04. J Clin Oncol 41:1020–1020. https://doi.org/10.1200/JCO.2023.41.16_suppl.1020

O'Meara T, Marczyk M, Qing T et al (2020) Immunological differences between immune-rich estrogen receptor–positive and immune-rich triple-negative breast cancers. JCO Precis Oncol 767–779. https://doi.org/10.1200/PO.19.00350

Parker JS, Mullins M, Cheang MCU et al (2009) Supervised risk predictor of breast cancer based on intrinsic subtypes. J Clin Oncol 27:1160–1167. https://doi.org/10.1200/JCO.2008.18.1370

Perou CM, Jeffrey SS, van de Rijn M et al (1999) Distinctive gene expression patterns in human mammary epithelial cells and breast cancers. Proc Natl Acad Sci U S A 96:9212–9217. https://doi.org/10.1073/pnas.96.16.9212

Perou CM, Sørlie T, Eisen MB et al (2000) Molecular portraits of human breast tumours. Nature 406:747–752. https://doi.org/10.1038/35021093

Perou CM, Parker JS, Prat A et al (2010) Clinical implementation of the intrinsic subtypes of breast cancer. Lancet Oncol 11:718–719. https://doi.org/10.1016/S1470-2045(10)70176-5

Piccart M, Hortobagyi GN, Campone M et al (2014) Everolimus plus exemestane for hormone-receptor-positive, human epidermal growth factor receptor-2-negative advanced breast cancer: overall survival results from BOLERO-2. Ann Oncol 25:2357–2362. https://doi.org/10.1093/annonc/mdu456

Prat A, Perou CM (2011) Deconstructing the molecular portraits of breast cancer. Mol Oncol 5:5–23. https://doi.org/10.1016/j.molonc.2010.11.003

Prat A, Parker JS, Fan C, Perou CM (2012) PAM50 assay and the three-gene model for identifying the major and clinically relevant molecular subtypes of breast cancer. Breast Cancer Res Treat 135:301–306. https://doi.org/10.1007/s10549-012-2143-0

Prat A, Carey LA, Adamo B et al (2014) Molecular features and survival outcomes of the intrinsic subtypes within HER2-positive breast cancer. JNCI J Natl Cancer Inst 106:1–8. https://doi.org/10.1093/jnci/dju152

Prat A, Brase JC, Cheng Y et al (2019) Everolimus plus exemestane for hormone receptor-positive advanced breast cancer: a PAM50 intrinsic subtype analysis of BOLERO-2. Oncologist 24:893–900. https://doi.org/10.1634/theoncologist.2018-0407

Prat A, Pascual T, De Angelis C et al (2020) HER2-enriched subtype and ERBB2 expression in HER2-positive breast cancer treated with dual HER2 blockade. J Natl Cancer Inst 112:46–54. https://doi.org/10.1093/jnci/djz042

Prat A, Chaudhury A, Solovieff N et al (2021) Correlative biomarker analysis of intrinsic subtypes and efficacy across the MONALEESA phase III studies. J Clin Oncol 39:1458–1467. https://doi.org/10.1200/JCO.20.02977

Pusztai L, Foldi J, Dhawan A et al (2019) Changing frameworks in treatment sequencing of triple-negative and HER2-positive, early-stage breast cancers. Lancet Oncol 20:e390–e396. https://doi.org/10.1016/S1470-2045(19)30158-5

Pusztai L, Yau C, Wolf DM et al (2021) Durvalumab with olaparib and paclitaxel for high-risk HER2-negative stage II/III breast cancer: results from the adaptively randomized I-SPY2 trial. Cancer Cell 39:989–998.e5. https://doi.org/10.1016/j.ccell.2021.05.009

Rakha EA, Reis-Filho JS, Ellis IO (2008) Basal-like breast cancer: a critical review. J Clin Oncol 26:2568–2581. https://doi.org/10.1200/JCO.2007.13.1748

Rouzier R, Perou CM, Symmans WF et al (2005) Breast cancer molecular subtypes respond differently to preoperative chemotherapy. Clin Cancer Res 11:5678–5685. https://doi.org/10.1158/1078-0432.CCR-04-2421

Schettini F, Martínez-Sáez O, Falato C et al (2023) Prognostic value of intrinsic subtypes in hormone-receptor-positive metastatic breast cancer: systematic review and meta-analysis. ESMO Open 8:101214. https://doi.org/10.1016/j.esmoop.2023.101214

Schmid P, Cortes J, Pusztai L et al (2020) Pembrolizumab for early triple-negative breast cancer. N Engl J Med 382:810–821. https://doi.org/10.1056/nejmoa1910549

Smid M, Wang Y, Zhang Y et al (2008) Subtypes of breast cancer show preferential site of relapse. Cancer Res 68:3108–3114. https://doi.org/10.1158/0008-5472.CAN-07-5644

Sørlie T, Perou CM, Tibshirani R et al (2001) Gene expression patterns of breast carcinomas distinguish tumor subclasses with clinical implications. Proc Natl Acad Sci U S A 98:10869–10874. https://doi.org/10.1073/pnas.191367098

Sørlie T, Tibshirani R, Parker J et al (2003) Repeated observation of breast tumor subtypes in independent gene expression data sets. Proc Natl Acad Sci U S A 100:8418–8423. https://doi.org/10.1073/pnas.0932692100

Tamimi RM, Colditz GA, Hazra A et al (2012) Traditional breast cancer risk factors in relation to molecular subtypes of breast cancer. Breast Cancer Res Treat 131:159–167. https://doi.org/10.1007/s10549-011-1702-0

Turner NC, Oliveira M, Howell SJ et al (2023) Capivasertib in hormone receptor–positive advanced breast cancer. N Engl J Med 388:2058–2070. https://doi.org/10.1056/NEJMoa2214131

von Minckwitz G, Untch M, Blohmer J-U et al (2012) Definition and impact of pathologic complete response on prognosis after Neoadjuvant chemotherapy in various intrinsic breast cancer subtypes. J Clin Oncol 30:1796–1804. https://doi.org/10.1200/JCO.2011.38.8595

von Minckwitz G, Huang C-S, Mano MS et al (2018) Trastuzumab Emtansine for residual invasive HER2-positive breast cancer. N Engl J Med. https://doi.org/10.1056/NEJMoa1814017

Vuong D, Simpson PT, Green B et al (2014) Molecular classification of breast cancer. Virchows Arch 465:1–14. https://doi.org/10.1007/s00428-014-1593-7

Weigelt B, Mackay A, A'hern R et al (2010) Breast cancer molecular profiling with single sample predictors: a retrospective analysis. Lancet Oncol 11:339–349. https://doi.org/10.1016/S1470-2045(10)70008-5

Weinstein JN, Collisson EA, Mills GB et al (2013) The cancer genome atlas pan-cancer analysis project. Nat Genet 45:1113–1120. https://doi.org/10.1038/ng.2764

Wu SZ, Al-Eryani G, Roden DL et al (2021) A single-cell and spatially resolved atlas of human breast cancers. Nat Genet 53:1334–1347. https://doi.org/10.1038/s41588-021-00911-1

Wuerstlein R, Harbeck N (2017) Neoadjuvant therapy for HER2-positive breast cancer. Rev Recent Clin Trials 12:81–92. https://doi.org/10.2174/1574887111266170202165049

Yao K, Goldschmidt R, Turk M et al (2015) Molecular subtyping improves diagnostic stratification of patients with primary breast cancer into prognostically defined risk groups. Breast Cancer Res Treat 154:81–88. https://doi.org/10.1007/s10549-015-3587-9

Yersal O (2014) Biological subtypes of breast cancer: prognostic and therapeutic implications. World J Clin Oncol 5:412. https://doi.org/10.5306/wjco.v5.i3.412

22 Targeting Oestrogen Receptor Signalling in Breast Cancer Therapy

Sacha J. Howell and Anthony Howell

Abstract

There has been over 130 years of research into the treatment of breast cancer using approaches that target oestrogen receptor signalling. Here, we summarise the development of the key pillars of such endocrine therapy, namely, oestrogen deprivation, achieved through ovarian suppression and/or aromatase inhibition, and oestrogen receptor blockade, through selective oestrogen receptor modulators, downregulators and novel compounds entering early phase development. The translation of these compounds from advanced to early breast cancer settings is discussed with a focus on the placebo-controlled breast cancer prevention studies to most accurately describe the side effect profiles of the main approaches.

Keywords

Oestrogen receptor · Endocrine therapy · Tamoxifen · Aromatase inhibitors · Selective estrogen receptor downregulator

S. J. Howell (✉) · A. Howell
Division of Cancer Sciences, University of Manchester, Manchester, UK

Manchester University NHS Foundation Trust, Manchester, UK

The Christie NHS Foundation Trust, Manchester, UK
e-mail: sacha.howell@nhs.net

Key Points

- The oestrogen receptor (ER) is expressed in approximately 70% of breast cancers, and the inhibition of oestrogen-ER signalling is a highly successful management approach, first recorded in 1896 through surgical removal of the ovaries.
- Surgical approaches are now rarely used since the advent of potent agents that can suppress the function of the ovaries in premenopausal women (gonadotropin-releasing hormone (GnRH) agonists) or block the conversion of androgens to oestrogens in postmenopausal women (aromatase inhibitors, AIs).
- Targeting the oestrogen receptor itself has been a highly fruitful therapeutic approach, initially with selective oestrogen receptor modulators (SERMs) such as tamoxifen. However, agonistic action on the ER complex can result in side effects such as cancer of the endometrium and venous thromboembolism, limiting their use in postmenopausal women in particular.
- Novel agents that target the ER for degradation (SERDs) hold great promise for the future, and multiple agents with diverse molecular mechanisms of action

T. Sørlie, R. B. Clarke (eds.), *A Guide to Breast Cancer Research*, Advances in Experimental Medicine and Biology 1464, https://doi.org/10.1007/978-3-031-70875-6_22

are currently in clinical development. These agents mostly show pure antagonistic activity and are particularly active in tumours with *ESR1* mutations that are resistant to other endocrine agents.
- ER-positive breast cancer can be prevented, in women at increased risk, through the use of SERMs and AIs. Future studies will undoubtedly test whether the novel SERDs are even more effective at preventing such cancers and further improving breast cancer mortality.

22.1 Introduction: The Evolution of Endocrine Therapy

Endocrine therapy has become an integral part of breast cancer therapy over the last century. In 1882 Nunn first reported the observation that breast cancers could regress after cessation of menstruation (Nunn 1882). Schinzinger proposed surgical oophorectomy as a treatment for breast cancer in 1889 (Schinzinger 1889), and the first recorded use of an endocrine approach was bilateral oophorectomy undertaken by the surgeon George Beatson in Glasgow in 1896 (Beatson 1896). Through his preclinical work in rabbits and sheep, the link between the ovaries and mammary glands was confirmed, and Beatson went on to remove both ovaries in three women with locally advanced breast cancer, two of whom responded to treatment. Remarkably, this was nearly 30 years before the discovery of oestrogen itself by Allen and Doisey (1923). With the development of radiotherapy, irradiation of the ovaries largely superseded oophorectomy, and bilateral ovarian irradiation was tested, and shown to be successful, in the first randomised adjuvant breast cancer trial, initiated in 1948 (Paterson and Russel 1959). Additional surgical approaches to breast cancer therapy, including adrenalectomy and hypophysectomy, demonstrated some success but are very rarely, if ever, performed today.

Following the discovery of oestrogen in 1923 (Allen and Doisy 1923), long-acting synthetic oestrogens were subsequently developed (Dodds et al. 1938; Robson et al. 1938). Stilboestrol and two analogues of triphenylethylene, trichlorophenylethylene (gynosome) and trimethylphenylethylene, entered clinical trials for advanced breast cancer in the early 1940s (Haddow et al. 1944). Stilboestrol became the mainstay of systemic therapy for advanced breast cancer until the development of the triphenylethylene tamoxifen 30 years later. The lead compound for tamoxifen development was found to be a mixture of cis and trans isomers (Harper and Walpole 1966). The cis isomer was found to be a pure oestrogen, whereas the trans isomer is a mixed oestrogen/anti-oestrogen, now in the clinic as tamoxifen (ICI 46,474). The further development of tamoxifen and its mechanism of action will be discussed in more detail below. It is interesting to note however that tamoxifen only superseded stilboestrol following clinical trials showing equivalent efficacy but reduced toxicity (Cole et al. 1971).

The demonstration that an anti-oestrogen resulted in improved outcomes for women with advanced breast cancer gave additional impetus to research efforts directed at inhibiting endogenous oestrogen production. In postmenopausal women oestrogen production is predominantly through the peripheral aromatisation of androgens to oestrogens. Inhibition of the aromatase enzyme was first shown to be effective in the treatment of advanced breast cancer with aminoglutethimide in 1967 (Cash et al. 1967); however, this drug was non-specific and required co-administration with corticosteroids. It was not until the development of the third-generation aromatase inhibitors (AIs; anastrozole, letrozole and exemestane) in the 1990s, which are highly selective and much better tolerated, that widespread use of this approach began. In premenopausal women the majority of endogenous oestrogen is produced in the ovaries in response to hypothalamic/pituitary gonadotrophins. Ovarian function suppression (OFS) using gonadotrophin-releasing hormone (GnRH) agonists (such as goserelin) was shown to be effective both as a single agent and in combination with tamoxifen in the 1980s (Klijn and de Jong 1982; Klijn et al. 1984; Williams et al. 1986). Subsequently the combination of GnRH analogues with tamoxifen or AIs has become standard of care for premenopausal women either with high-risk early breast cancer or advanced breast cancer.

Most recently the development of synthetic anti-oestrogens has focused on compounds that result in oestrogen receptor degradation. The first selective oestrogen receptor degrader (SERD) fulvestrant (ICI 182,780) was developed in the 1990s (DeFriend et al. 1994; Howell and Robertson 1995). Fulvestrant is given by intramuscular injection due to poor oral bioavailability. However, a raft of orally available compounds that downregulate the ER through varied mechanisms have been developed, and the first of these have very recently gained regulatory approval. These compounds also have a role in breast cancer harbouring *ESR1* gene mutations, which are rarely seen in primary breast cancers, but frequently emerge following therapeutic pressure from endocrine therapies, in particular the AIs (Will et al. 2023). The most clinically relevant *ESR1* mutations are in the ligand-binding domain of the ER and confer ligand-independent growth and resistance to SERMs. ER degraders show improved activity in the presence of certain *ESR1* mutations, and multiple clinical trials are now testing these molecules in this subset of patients (Rugo 2023; Turner et al. 2023). In addition to direct targeting of the oestrogen-ER alpha axis, multiple resistance-modifying agents have also been transitioned through preclinical to clinical testing and subsequently gained regulatory approval. These include the cyclin-dependent kinase 4/6 inhibitors (CDK 4/6i) palbociclib, ribociclib and abemaciclib (discussed in this Chap. 23) and agents that target the PI3K/AKT/mTOR pathway such as alpelisib, capivasertib and everolimus.

22.2 Selective Oestrogen Receptor Modulators

Oestrogen has important physiological effects on the growth and function of hormone-dependent reproductive tissues, including normal breast epithelium, uterus, vagina and ovaries, as well as preserving bone mineral density and reducing the risk of osteoporosis, protecting the cardiovascular system by reducing cholesterol levels and modulating cognitive function and behaviour. Thus, a strategy to antagonise oestrogen in an attempt to treat or prevent breast cancer may have a severe impact on a woman's health by interfering with normal oestrogen-regulated tissues.

The binding of oestradiol to the ligand-binding domain (LBD) of the ER initiates a series of events which include dissociation of heat-shock proteins and receptor dimerisation. Dimerisation facilitates the binding of the ER to specific sequences termed DNA oestrogen-response elements (EREs) in the vicinity of oestrogen-regulated genes (McGregor and Jordan 1998; Beato et al. 1989). The ER contains two activation functions: AF-1 towards the N-terminus affecting interaction with the ERE and AF-2 towards the C-terminus and in close proximity to the LBD and dimerisation domains. Full activation of gene transcription in response to oestradiol requires activation of both AF-1 and AF-2 (Grinshpun et al. 2023). Following oestradiol binding to the LBD, a conformational change in the LBD, involving the 12th α-helix, exposes the coactivator binding site in AF-2. In contrast, when the SERM tamoxifen binds to the LBD, helix-12 remains in apposition over AF-2, hindering both the binding of coactivators and the full activation of the receptor (Shiau et al. 1998). Tamoxifen does not affect AF-1 activity, however, leading to incomplete attenuation of transcription. Thus, the partial agonist activity of tamoxifen is attributed, in part, to its inability to inactivate AF-1.

This complex interplay between LBD and AF-1 and AF-2 explains why the SERMs are known as mixed agonists/antagonists. Attempts to harness ER transcription and optimise the balance between agonism and antagonism in different tissues have led to the development of a multitude of novel SERMs for various indications. Many of these agents have been tested in clinical trials of breast cancer treatment and prevention.

22.3 The Early Development of Tamoxifen and Other SERMs in Breast Cancer Therapy

Tamoxifen is a triphenylethylene (Fig. 22.1) derived from the lead molecule and parent compound trimethylphenylethylene by scientists at AstraZeneca (AZ; formerly ICI) in the 1960s. Originally tamoxifen was being developed in the AZ contraceptive programme but was found to stimulate rather than inhibit ovulation (Harper and Walpole 1967). The potential of the anti-oestrogenic cis isomer in the treatment of hormone-dependent tumours was recognised and a patent granted in 1965 (Harper and Walpole 1966). The first clinical trial of tamoxifen (then known as ICI 46,474) was initiated by Cole at The Christie Hospital, Manchester, UK, in 1969, and the results were published in 1971 (Cole et al. 1971). In this single-arm phase 2 study, 46 patients received tamoxifen, and 22% were assessed as responding to treatment. The response rates to tamoxifen were compared with the hospital records of 64 patients treated will stilboestrol, of which 16 (25%) responded, and 60 with high-dose androgens, of which 11 (18%) responded. The response rates of the compounds were, therefore, comparable, but major differences in toxicity profiles were reported (Cole et al. 1971).

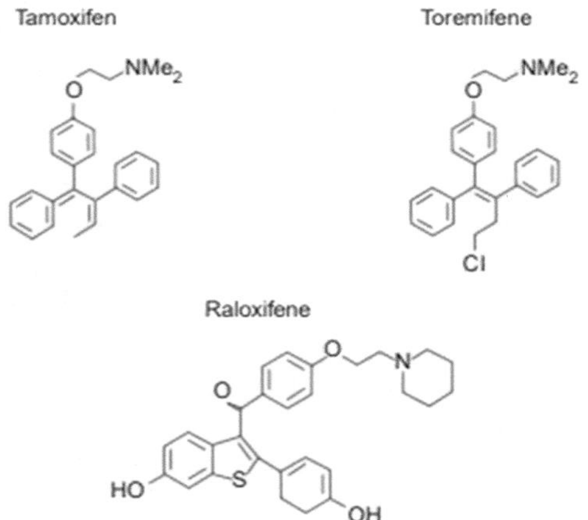

Fig. 22.1 Chemical structures of the SERMs: Tamoxifen, Toremifene and the 'fixed ring' compound raloxifene

Tamoxifen was then compared to multiple agents and approaches commonly in use at the time. These included stilboestrol, megestrol acetate, medroxyprogesterone acetate, fluoxymesterone, nandrolone, first- and second-generation aromatase inhibitors, surgical oophorectomy and adrenalectomy. A comprehensive review of all these trials reported no significant difference in survival (24 therapeutic comparisons, hazard ratio (HR) = 1.02) but a lower incidence of side effects with tamoxifen vs the 'standard of care', including fatigue, lethargy, congestive cardiac failure, alopecia and weight gain (Fossati et al. 1998). During this time there was considerable interest in the development of novel SERMs that could, potentially, improve on the anti-oestrogenic antitumour activity of tamoxifen whilst further improving its side effect profile.

Strategies employed to improve on tamoxifen have included its chemical modification, either by altering the side chains to produce new tamoxifen analogues such as toremifene (Fig. 22.1) or by altering the nonsteroidal triphenylethylene ring structure of tamoxifen to produce new nonsteroidal 'fixed ring' structures such as the benzothiophene derivative raloxifene (Fig. 22.1) or the benzopyran derivative acolbifene (not shown). However, toremifene was shown in a meta-analysis to have almost identical activity and safety profiles to tamoxifen in the first-line setting (Pyrhönen et al. 1999). Objective responses were seen in 24.0% and 25.3%, and median time to progression (TTP) was 4.9 and 5.3 months for toremifene (40–60 mg/day) and tamoxifen (20–40 mg/day), respectively (Pyrhönen et al. 1999). Toremifene was approved for use and was subsequently tested in a small adjuvant study in early breast cancer in a Japanese population (Tominaga et al. 2010). In this study toremifene and tamoxifen were shown to exert significant differences on serum lipid profiles, highlighting the tissue-specific sensitivity of the ligand-ER interaction given the similarities in their chemical structures (Fig. 22.1).

The two main side effects of concern with tamoxifen are venous thromboembolism and endometrial stimulation, the latter resulting in endometrial carcinoma in postmenopausal women. The fixed ring SERMs showed encouraging safety profiles, with reduced endometrial stimulation (Balfour and Goa 1998). However, despite encouraging preclinical and early clinical development, neither raloxifene nor arzoxifene (both fixed ring SERMs) was shown to be as effective as tamoxifen, and the development in breast cancer therapy ceased (Deshmane et al. 2007). Several of these agents have been tested in breast cancer prevention and will be discussed in greater detail in the section below.

22.4 Tamoxifen in Early Breast Cancer

Tamoxifen became the standard first-line therapy for advanced breast cancer due to its improved toxicity profile compared with other endocrine approaches available at the time. As with most cancer treatments, tamoxifen then progressed into the curative, adjuvant cancer setting (Fig. 22.2) and was tested in multiple clinical trials globally. By today's standards the initial studies used relatively short durations of tamoxifen treatment, but even these showed reduced recurrence rates and lead to successive iterations of clinical trials and longer durations of adjuvant endocrine therapy. Perhaps the most informative development in this setting was the establishment of the Early Breast Cancer Trialists' Collaborative Group (EBCTCG). Since 1985, the EBCTCG has been bringing together and analysing the evidence on the major questions in early breast cancer, including adjuvant tamoxifen therapy, through individual patient meta-analysis of almost all randomised trials conducted globally (EBCTCG website). Interestingly the perceived wisdom in the early days of tamoxifen therapy was that premenopausal women would be unlikely to benefit due to the high prevailing levels of oestrogen. Once studies in premenopausal women refuted this hypothesis and demonstrated comparable activity to the postmenopausal population, even more widespread adoption of tamoxifen ensued (Rydén et al. 2005).

The 2011 meta-analyses from EBCTCG, with a median of 13 years follow-up, demonstrated that 5 years of tamoxifen compared to none (usually placebo) reduced recurrence rates by almost

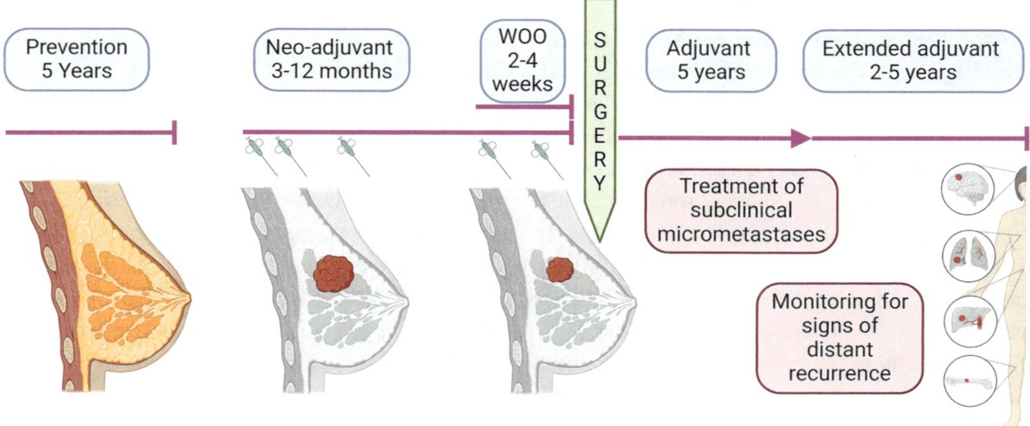

Fig. 22.2 Diagrammatic representation of the clinical stages of endocrine therapy from prevention on the left through to extended adjuvant therapy on the right. The approximate durations of therapy are given : tissue biopsy for response assessment through biomarker analyses. *WOO* window of opportunity. Created in BioRender. Harrison, H. (2024) BioRender.com/h00e807

half throughout the first 10 years (rate ratio 0.53 [standard error (SE) 0.03]) (EBCTCG 2011). Furthermore, the effect was durable with yearly breast cancer mortality reduced by approximately a third throughout the first 15 years (RR 0.70 [0.05], $p < 0.00001$). This led to 5 years of adjuvant tamoxifen becoming the standard of care in pre- and postmenopausal women with ER-positive early breast cancer.

This overview also explored the effect of ER level as measured by fmol/mg of cytosol protein on outcome. ER levels were shown to predict for tamoxifen efficacy, with benefit only being shown with ER levels of 10 fmol/mg of cytosol protein and above (EBCTCG 2011). More recently the cytosolic assay has been largely replaced by more accessible and reproducible immunohistochemical assays that also showed greater capacity to predict the benefit of tamoxifen (Harvey et al. 1999). However, IHC assays have also changed significantly over the ensuing years with the sensitivity driven up with advances in antigen retrieval and signal amplification techniques. Whereas 34% of tumours had low-positive oestrogen receptor Quick (Allred) scores of 3–5 in the original study report (Harvey et al. 1999), approximately 10% score 3–5 in more recent studies (Collins et al. 2005; Nadji et al. 2005; Sgroi et al. 2022). This has resulted in the weakening of the predictive capacity of the IHC ER assay (Kim et al. 2011; Sgroi et al. 2022). Retrospective analysis of the NSABP B14 trial showed quantitative oestrogen receptor mRNA expression to be linearly and positively related to the relative risk reduction of distant relapse by tamoxifen (Kim et al. 2011), and analyses of low ER-expressing tumours have, most recently, identified a high proportion to be of basal-like or HER2-enriched intrinsic subtypes, unlikely to benefit from single-agent endocrine approaches (Iwamoto et al. 2012; Schuster et al. 2023).

Subsequently two large studies have sought to explore whether extending adjuvant tamoxifen therapy to 10 years may add additional benefit. It must be noted that during the conduct of these trials, the third-generation aromatase inhibitors (AIs) demonstrated improved activity over tamoxifen and largely superseded extended adjuvant tamoxifen therapy in postmenopausal women—the AI studies are discussed further below. The two extended adjuvant tamoxifen studies were the ATLAS (Davies et al. 2013) and aTTom (Gray et al. 2013) trials. These studies both randomised women (pre- and postmenopausal) who had received 5 years of adjuvant tamoxifen to either no further treatment or an additional 5 years of tamoxifen. In the ATLAS study, in which 12,894 women were randomised, those allocated to continued tamoxifen had a significantly reduced risk of recurrence (RR 0.84, 95% CI 0.76–0.94; $p = 0.002$), breast cancer mortality (331 deaths with recurrence in women allocated to continue vs 397 in controls, $p = 0.01$) and all-cause mortality (639 deaths vs 722 deaths, $p = 0.01$) compared to women who discontinued tamoxifen at 5 years. Of note, the reduction in recurrence rate was more pronounced in the years after completion of extended tamoxifen treatment (Davies et al. 2013).

In the aTTom study which recruited 6953 women, those randomised to continue tamoxifen had a significant reduction in breast cancer recurrence (RR 0.85, 95% CI 0.76–0.95; $p = 0.003$), with an absolute difference of 4% at 15 years from randomisation. There was a non-significant reduction in breast cancer mortality (RR 0.88, 95% CI 0.77–1.01; $p = 0.06$), with an absolute difference of 3% at 15 years from randomisation.

22.5 Side Effect Profile of Tamoxifen

One of the key benefits to tamoxifen being 'first past the post' in early breast cancer trials was that it was tested against either placebo or no therapy in the majority. Such trials give us the strongest data on the side effect profiles of novel therapies, although in the context of breast cancer therapy, in which many women will also have undergone chemotherapy, radiotherapy and surgery prior to starting tamoxifen, discerning the precise aetiology of toxicities is more challenging. Tamoxifen is well known to cause menopause-like symptoms such as hot flushes, night sweats and vaginal dryness. These side effects will be discussed in more detail in the section on breast cancer prevention. However, the EBCTCG meta-analyses have focussed on potentially life-threatening side effects of tamoxifen, most notably the risks of endometrial cancer, venous thromboembolism (deep vein thrombosis (DVT) and/or pulmonary embolism (PE)) and cardiovascular events such as heart attacks and strokes. The risks of death from these events is particularly pertinent given that the treatment is intended to improve survival following an early breast cancer diagnosis from which the patient may not have succumbed.

In the 1998 EBCTCG meta-analysis, a highly statistically significant increase in the incidence of endometrial cancer was observed with a ratio of incidence rates of 2·58 [SD 0·35] comparing tamoxifen vs control ($2p < 0·00001$) (EBCTCG 1998). However, the absolute number of women developing endometrial cancer is small. Pooling the data for the three largest trials of 5 years tamoxifen vs none (Stockholm B, Scottish and NSABP B14 studies) demonstrated an absolute 10-year risk in the tamoxifen-treated women of 11 per 1000 compared with 3 per 1000 in controls (EBCTCG 1998). In terms of endometrial cancer mortality, the 10-year risk in those treated with tamoxifen was approximately 2 per 1000 compared with 0.4 per 1000 in controls. Although this is clearly an important issue, it must be put in context through analysis of the reduction in overall mortality with 5 years of tamoxifen. In EBCTCG 1998, 5 years of tamoxifen reduced overall mortality by 5.6% and 10.9% in women with lymph node negative and positive breast cancers, respectively, at 10 years of follow-up, dwarfing the increase in endometrial cancer mortality by a factor of about 28–55 (EBCTCG 1998). Updated meta-analysis confirmed this small increase in risk of death from endometrial cancer and a comparable relative risk increase in the risk of death from venous thromboembolism (VTE) (EBCTCG 2005). However, the absolute risks for VTE were even smaller than those for endometrial cancer.

The large extended adjuvant studies demonstrated ongoing increased risks of endometrial cancer with prolonged tamoxifen therapy. The relative risks (RR) of endometrial cancer were 1.74 (95% CI 1.30–2.34, $p = 0.0002$) and 2.20 (95% CI: 1.31–2.34, $p < 0.0001$) in ATLAS and aTTom, respectively, which translated to an increase in EC mortality of about 0.5% ($p = 0.02$) with 10 vs 5 years of tamoxifen (Davies et al. 2013; Gray et al. 2013). However, combining the ATLAS and aTTom data (a total of 17,477 patients), there was a statistically significant reduction in breast cancer mortality (RR 0.85; 95% CI 0.77–0.94; $p = 0.001$) and improvement in overall survival (RR 0.91; 95% CI 0.84–0.94; $p = 0.008$) with 10 years of tamoxifen. These results suggest that it is reasonable to continue tamoxifen to 10 years in women who remain premenopausal after 5 years of therapy, if the ongoing risk of the breast cancer outweighs these potentially serious, but relatively rare, side effects.

22.6 Tamoxifen and Other SERMs in Breast Cancer Prevention

In 1985 Cuzick and Baum published their observation from a UK clinical trial that tamoxifen used to reduce the recurrence of breast cancer as adjuvant treatment also reduced the incidence of contralateral breast cancer (Cuzick and Baum 1985). This finding was subsequently validated in the EBCTCG meta-analysis in which 1, 2 and 5 years of tamoxifen were shown to reduce the incidence of contralateral breast cancer by 13%, 26% and 47%, respectively, indicating that 5 years of tamoxifen approximately halved the annual incidence rate of contralateral disease. These data led to the design and conduct of four randomised placebo-controlled primary prevention trials of tamoxifen in women at increased risk of breast cancer (Cuzick et al. 2015; Fisher et al. 2005; Powles et al. 2007; Veronesi et al. 2007). These studies mainly recruited women at increased risk of breast cancer due to their family history or prior diagnosis of benign breast disease, except for the Italian study that recruited normal-risk women with prior hysterectomy (Veronesi et al. 1998). All four studies showed a reduction in the risk of invasive breast cancer with 5 years of tamoxifen treatment which on meta-analysis equated to a hazard ratio (HR) of 0.67 (95%CI; 0·59–0·76) over the 5 years of treatment and subsequent 5 years of follow-up

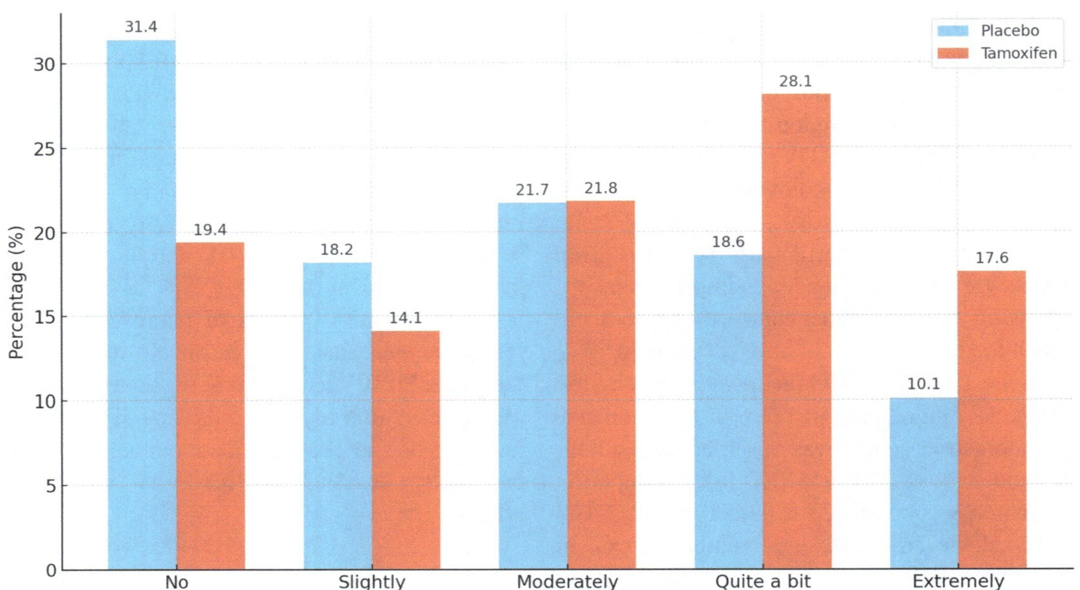

Fig. 22.3 Hot flush severity in the NSABP-P1 study of tamoxifen or placebo (Fisher et al. 1998)

(Cuzick et al. 2013). Importantly the risk reduction was only seen in ER-positive breast cancer with a HR 0·56 (0·47–0·67) for ER-positive disease and HR 1·13 (0·86–1·49) for ER-negative. This highlights the need for the personalisation of breast cancer primary prevention, and the identification of women at increased risk for ER-negative breast cancer is a priority, such that they can be offered alternate approaches (Couch et al. 2016; Milne et al. 2017).

Tamoxifen has subsequently been licensed for the indication of primary breast cancer prevention and approved for use in numerous countries. However, uptake of primary prevention is low with multiple contributory factors reported in the literature including the perceived impact of side effects and a lack of adequate information (Donnelly et al. 2014; Thorneloe et al. 2020). In addition, there is very limited understanding of therapeutic breast cancer prevention in primary care, often the primary source of medical information and prescribing in the community (Macdonald et al. 2021). The placebo-controlled trials of tamoxifen have led to a greater understanding of its side effects in women not previously treated for breast cancer. The most frequent side effects experienced by women receiving tamoxifen are gynaecological and vasomotor, which include hot flushes and night sweats. In the NSABP-P1 study that randomised 13,388 pre- and postmenopausal women to tamoxifen or placebo, there was a significant increase in vasomotor symptoms with tamoxifen although many women on placebo also experienced hot flushes presumably as part of their natural menopause, and many women taking tamoxifen had no or mild flushes only (Fig. 22.3).

In the IBIS-1 study, which randomised 7145 pre- and postmenopausal women to tamoxifen or placebo, the most common and more serious but rare side effects are presented in Table 22.1. The common side effect risks of gynaecological/vasomotor symptoms and the more serious VTE and endometrial cancer risks can be seen to be reduced with cessation of treatment. Interestingly both headaches and breast complaints were significantly reduced with tamoxifen therapy, and the reduction in breast complaints (including cysts and breast pain) persisted after cessation of therapy.

Table 22.1 More common and serious side effects of tamoxifen in the IBIS-1 study (Cuzick 2007). Column values represent the number of participants with % in parentheses. *RR* relative risk *CI* confidence interval

	During active treatment			During Follow up period		
Side effect	Placebo (n = 3575)	Tamoxifen (n = 3579)	RR (95% CI)	Placebo (n = 3489)	Tamoxifen (n = 3449)	RR (95% CI)
DVT/PE	23 (1.29)	52 (2.91)	2.26 (1.36 to 3.87)	14 (1.31)	16 (1.49)	1.14 (0.52 to 2.53)
Endometrial cancer	3	12	N/A	8	5	N/A
Gynecologic/ Vasomotor	1983 (55.5)	2389 (66.8)	1.20 (1.16 to 1.25)	1438 (41.2)	1508 (43.7)	1.06 (0.99 to 1.12)
Headaches	1030 (28.8)	878 (24.5)	0.85 (0.79 to 0.92)	343 (9.8)	386 (11.2)	1.14 (0.99 to 1.31)
All breast complaints	833 (23.3)	612 (17.1)	0.73 (0.67 to 0.81)	676 (19.4)	554 (16.1)	0.83 (0.75 to 0.92)

22.7 Other SERMs in Breast Cancer Prevention

Three other SERMs have been tested in large-scale randomised placebo-controlled trials in breast cancer prevention, namely, raloxifene, lasofoxifene and arzoxifene. The major results from these studies are reported in the meta-analysis from 2013 (Cuzick et al. 2013). In summary, the same pattern of reduction in ER-positive but not ER-negative breast cancer was seen across the board. Similarly, all of the SERMs increased the risk of VTE, but there were differences in the incidence of endometrial cancer, which was not increased in the studies with raloxifene or lasofoxifene. The initial study that randomised postmenopausal women with osteoporosis to raloxifene or placebo demonstrated impressive reductions in breast cancer incidence (Martino et al. 2004). This and the lack of endometrial agonism suggested that raloxifene may have a better benefit/risk profile than tamoxifen, and the only head-to-head prevention trial with cancer incidence as its primary endpoint was established. The STAR trial randomised 19,747 women to either tamoxifen 20 mg or raloxifene 60 mg daily for 5 years (Vogel et al. 2010). This updated analysis demonstrated that raloxifene was inferior to tamoxifen in reducing the incidence of invasive breast cancer (RR 1.24 (95% CI 1.05–1.47)) but induced significantly fewer endometrial cancers (RR 0.55 (95% CI, 0.36–0.83)) and VTEs (RR 0.75 (95% CI, 0.60–0.93)). Thus, raloxifene remains a valuable choice for postmenopausal women with an intact uterus who cannot tolerate or do not wish to pursue AI-based prevention. However, lasofoxifene and arzoxifene development has ceased in the breast cancer prevention field.

22.8 Oestrogen Deprivation Strategies

22.8.1 Ovarian Function Suppression

As noted previously the very first successful systemic therapeutic intervention in advanced breast cancer was oophorectomy (Beatson 1896). Surgical oophorectomy and later irradiation of both ovaries to stop oestrogen production (De Courmelles 1922) became standard approaches to manage advanced breast cancer until the development of the gonadotrophin-releasing hormone agonists. In premenopausal women ovarian production of oestrogen is under the control of the hypothalamic-pituitary axis. Gonadotrophin-releasing hormone (GnRH) is secreted from the hypothalamus and stimulates the release of follicle-stimulating hormone (FSH) and luteinising hormone (LH) from the anterior pituitary. Although initially developed as fertility-promoting agents, high doses of GnRH agonists were shown to result in the downregulation of gonadal gonadotropin receptors, decreased steroidogenesis and suppression of mammary tumour growth in preclinical studies (DeSombre et al. 1976; Maynard and Nicholson 1979). Successful treatment of premenopausal advanced breast cancer followed (Klijn and de Jong 1982), and several GnRH analogues subsequently entered clinical trials. Meta-analysis of the trials testing GnRH analogues with or without tamoxifen demonstrated the combination to be superior to GnRH agonist alone in premenopausal women with advanced breast cancer (Klijn et al. 2001).

These observations led to the establishment of multiple trials testing OFS in the adjuvant setting. Study designs differed widely, and the early studies were relatively small and statistically underpowered by today's standards. Premenopausal women who develop amenorrhoea with cytotoxic chemotherapy are known to have superior survival compared with those who do not (Pagani et al. 1998). Some early studies also showed that OFS was equivalent to chemotherapy in premenopausal women. Most recently two large studies examining the impact of cytotoxic chemotherapy in women with intermediate genomic risk scores have shown that the greatest benefit was in premenopausal women aged 40–50 years, who are most likely to develop permanent amenorrhea with treatment (Kalinsky et al. 2021; Sparano et al. 2019). This suggests that much of the benefit of chemotherapy in this population may be mediated through OFS.

The earlier results noted above led to the development of the Suppression of Ovarian Function Trial (SOFT) which began recruitment in 2003. This study randomised premenopausal women with confirmed premenopausal oestradiol levels if they had received cytotoxic chemotherapy, to tamoxifen alone, tamoxifen plus OFS or to the third-generation aromatase inhibitor exemestane plus OFS, each for 5 years. Updated results, after median follow-up of 8 years, showed that the addition of OFS to tamoxifen significantly improved disease-free and overall survival (Francis et al. 2018). The majority of the benefit was seen in women who had previously received cytotoxic chemotherapy and remained premenopausal. This may well have been due to the fact that the women without prior chemotherapy had better prognosis tumours with low recurrence rates, in whom single-agent tamoxifen may be the optimal therapy.

Contemporaneously with SOFT, the TEXT trial (Tamoxifen and Exemestane Trial) began recruitment and randomised premenopausal women to OFS in combination with either tamoxifen or exemestane for 5 years duration. The tamoxifen plus OFS and exemestane plus OFS arms of the SOFT and TEXT trials were combined in pre-planned analyses (Pagani et al. 2023). After a median follow-up of 13 years, distant recurrence-free but not overall survival (OS) was improved with the use of exemestane vs tamoxifen. However, subgroup analysis suggested clinically significant improvements in OS in high-risk patients, for example, those aged <35 years and those with at least T2 or grade 3 tumours. This has led to the development of a publicly available composite risk algorithm that can be used to guide physicians and their premenopausal patients on the absolute OS benefits of using OFS in combination with either tamoxifen or exemestane (https://rconnect.dfci.harvard.edu/ComposteRiskSTEPP/). This is important when considering the toxicities of OFS, which results in significant increases in hot flushes, vaginal dryness and loss of sexual interest, compared with tamoxifen or exemestane alone. The combination of OFS and exemestane also results in more vaginal dryness, loss of sexual interest and joint pain compared with OFS and tamoxifen (Bernard 2015; Ribi et al. 2016).

22.8.2 Aromatase Inhibition

At menopause oestrogen production in the ovaries ceases. However, the conversion of androgens to oestrogens by the aromatase enzyme in peripheral tissues, particularly abdominal adipose tissues, results in mean circulating oestradiol (E2) and oestrone (E1) levels of about 19.9 (SD 17.2) and 91.4 (SD 52.2) pmol/l, respectively (Richardson et al. 2020). The levels of oestrogen are strongly and positively associated with body mass index (BMI) with levels in those with a BMI >30 kg/m^2 approximately double those in women of normal BMI (<25 kg/m^2). The androgen precursor for oestrone is androstenedione, whereas for oestradiol it is testosterone. However, oestradiol is also derived from the conversion of oestrone by 17B-hydroxysteroid dehydrogenase. Both androstenedione and testosterone are primarily produced from cholesterol in the adrenal glands (Lønning 1996).

The first-generation aromatase inhibitor (AI) aminoglutethimide was initially developed to inhibit the production of adrenal steroids, resulting in a 'medical adrenalectomy'. This meant add-back glucocorticoids were required to prevent adrenal crisis and even then, the drug was poorly tolerated (Cash et al. 1967). Adrenal androgen levels were not reduced by aminoglutethimide, in contrast to oestrogen levels, suggesting the inhibition of aromatase activity in vivo (Santen et al. 1978; Samojlik et al. 1980). Although aminoglutethimide showed comparable clinical activity to tamoxifen, its toxicity profile was far inferior, and it was rapidly superseded by the SERMs (Smith et al. 1981).

The clinical activity of aminoglutethimide prompted extensive efforts to develop selective inhibitors of the aromatase enzyme. Several second-generation agents such as 4OH-androstenedione, formestane and fadrozole were developed, and although better tolerated than aminoglutethimide, their activity was not superior (reviewed in Lønning 2004). Three third-generation agents—anastrozole, letrozole and exemestane—were subsequently developed and remain in clinical practice to this day. These three inhibitors come from two classes, steroidal and nonsteroidal (Fig. 22.4). The steroidal AI exemestane is based on the four-ring chemical backbone of androstenedione and acts as a 'suicide' inhibitor of the aromatase enzyme, its metabolic intermediates then binding irreversibly to the active site. In contrast the nonsteroidal AIs bind reversibly, with high affinity, to the haem region of the active site (Howell 2005). All three agents inhibit total body aromatisation by at least 98% with profound suppression of oestradiol levels, which become undetectable even to supersensitive mass spectroscopy-based assays, in the majority of patients (Lønning and Eikesdal 2013).

The third-generation AIs have now been tested in all disease settings of breast cancer therapy (Fig. 22.2). A detailed review of trials in the advanced setting is beyond the scope of this chapter. However, we will review the adjuvant therapy data comparing the AIs to tamoxifen and the primary prevention trials since these are placebo controlled and provide the optimal data on AI toxicity.

22.8.3 Aromatase Inhibitors in Adjuvant Therapy

The three third-generation AIs are all approved for use in the early breast cancer setting, either as single agents in postmenopausal women or in combination with OFS in premenopausal women. When the adjuvant AI studies were designed, 5 years of tamoxifen was the standard of care. Some studies recruited patients who had already received 2–3 years of tamoxifen and randomised them to continue to 5 years or to switch over to a third-generation AI for the remainder of

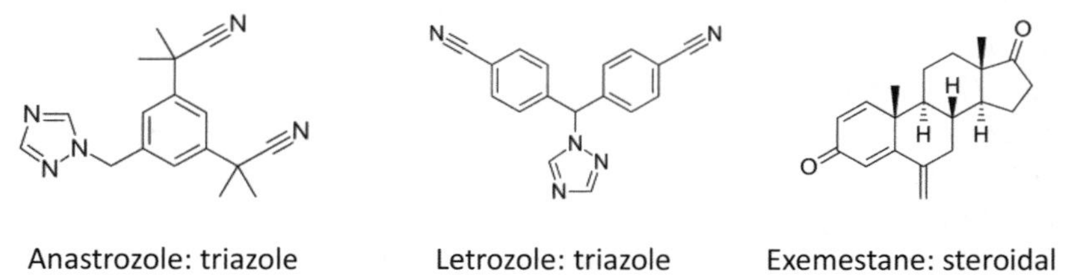

Fig. 22.4 Chemical structure of the three third generation aromatase inhibitors

Anastrozole: triazole

Letrozole: triazole

Exemestane: steroidal

the 5-year treatment period. These were called the 'switching' studies and would exclude women who relapsed in the first 2–3 years of tamoxifen therapy. In contrast, other studies randomised women to a sequence of tamoxifen then AI or the reverse with no prior endocrine therapy ET). These were known as the 'sequencing' studies and would include women likely to relapse early on tamoxifen who would have been excluded from the 'switching' studies. Several studies also tested the upfront use of AI vs tamoxifen alone for 5 years. Rather than consider each study individually, we will review the EBCTCG individual patient data meta-analysis of all available studies (EBCTCG 2015a). Only the Arimidex, Tamoxifen, Alone or in Combination (ATAC) study, compared tamoxifen and an AI in combination against each agent individually (Baum et al. 2002). ATAC was initially a three-arm study comparing tamoxifen vs anastrozole vs the combination. However, at the first review of the outcome data, the combination arm was shown to be inferior to anastrozole alone, and the Independent Data Monitoring Committee recommended that this arm be dropped from the trial.

The EBCTCG meta-analysis from 2015 synthesised the data from 35,129 patients randomised in 9 adjuvant trials testing aromatase inhibitors and tamoxifen as part of a 5 year course of adjuvant endocrine treatment (EBCTCG 2015a). Importantly the analysis was restricted to the 31,920 (91%) with ER-positive tumours. In view of the complexities of the different trial designs, five summary comparisons were presented in the final report: 5 years of AI vs 5 years of tamoxifen and then comparisons of the AI to tamoxifen sequence/switch vs 5 years of tamoxifen or 5 years of AI and of the reverse tamoxifen to AI sequence/switch vs 5 years of tamoxifen or 5 years of AI.

Two trials in the EBCTCG provided data on the AI vs tamoxifen for 5 years comparison, including 9885 patients. There were significant reductions in 10 year breast cancer recurrence (19·1% in the AI group versus 22·7% in the tamoxifen group, difference 3·6% (95% CI 1·7–5·4; $p < 0.00001$)) and improvements in breast cancer mortality (BCM; 12.1% vs 14.2%, difference 2.1% (95% CI 0.5–3.7; $p = 0.009$)) and all-cause mortality (ACM; 21.3% with AI vs 24.0% with tamoxifen, difference 2.7% (95% CI 0.1–4.7, $p = 0.01$)). Importantly there was an early separation of the recurrence curves after only 2 years of follow-up suggesting that starting with AI therapy is likely a superior approach to tamoxifen, possibly related to early tamoxifen resistance. In the second comparison, between 5 years of AI vs the tamoxifen to AI sequence, there was only a reduction in recurrence early in the treatment course resulting in small, non-statistically significant reductions in BCM and ACM. When comparing the reverse sequence of AI to tamoxifen vs 5 years of AI, there were no significant differences in any of the endpoints, again supporting the argument that early AI therapy offers advantages over starting with tamoxifen. Even 2 years of AI before switching to tamoxifen was superior to 5 years of tamoxifen in terms of ACM (gain at 7 years 2.0% (SE 1.1) $p = 0.05$), although only 3060 women were included in this analysis from 1 clinical trial (Regan et al. 2011).

Two large, randomised studies have also compared the aromatase inhibitors against each other. The open-label Femara (letrozole) versus Anastrozole Clinical Evaluation (FACE) trial (Smith et al. 2017) compared 5 years of anastrozole at a dose of 1 mg daily vs letrozole 2.5 mg daily. The 5-year estimated disease-free survival rate was 84.9% for letrozole vs 82.9% for anastrozole which was not statistically significant (hazard ratio, 0.93; 95% CI, 0.80–1.07; $P = 0.3150$). There were no differences in efficacy in any subgroups or between the treatment arms. In the second study (MA27), 7576 postmenopausal women were randomised to receive either exemestane 25 mg or anastrozole 1 mg daily for 5 years (Goss et al. 2013). No differences were seen in any of the efficacy endpoints. There were, however, differences in the side effect profiles with osteoporosis/osteopenia, hypertriglyceridaemia, vaginal bleeding and hypercholesterolaemia seen less frequently with exemestane, likely due to the steroidal structure of the parent drug and its metabolites. Vasomotor and musculoskeletal symptoms were comparable between the three AI arms. These data support the notion that the three third-generation AIs are largely interchangeable when it comes to their adjuvant activity and can be switched in individual patients to optimise tolerability and adherence.

The inclusion of the combination arm in ATAC and the conduct of the FACE and MA27 trials could potentially have been avoided if smaller biology-driven neoadjuvant studies had been employed to test the hypotheses. 3–4 months of AI treatment was shown to be associated with a greater suppression of Ki67 than tamoxifen in the neoadjuvant setting, with inferior suppression seen in the combination arm compared to anastrozole alone, mirroring the ATAC data (Ellis et al. 2003; Dowsett et al. 2005). More recently, the ACOSOG (American College of Surgeons Oncology Group) Z1031 trial randomised 380 women with ER-positive breast cancer to 16–18 weeks of therapy with anastrozole, exemestane or letrozole (Ellis et al. 2011). There were no significant differences in clinical or Ki67 response rates between the arms, suggesting that the neoadjuvant setting, utilising biological endpoints such as Ki67, has the capacity to accelerate drug development and reduce the size and cost of breast cancer trials.

When considering the differences in side effect profiles between AIs and tamoxifen in the EBCTCG meta-analysis, there were fewer uterine cancers and more bone fractures with aromatase inhibitors than with tamoxifen, reflecting their different mechanisms of action. Across all patients in the meta-analysis, the 10-year incidence of endometrial cancer was 0·4% in the aromatase inhibitor group versus 1·2% in the tamoxifen group (difference 0·8%, 95% CI 0·6–1·0; $p < 0{\cdot}0001$), which included 5 vs 9 deaths. There was no significant difference in incidence for any other cancer types, although the incidence of contralateral breast cancer was reduced in those receiving Ais, suggesting that AIs may be superior to tamoxifen in primary breast cancer prevention. In terms of bone fractures, the risk was higher in those randomised to AI during years 0–4 (RR 1·42, 95% CI 1·28–1·57; $p < 0{\cdot}0001$), and subsequently in years 5–9 (RR 1·29, 1·09–1·53; $2p = 0{\cdot}003$). The 5-year risk of a fracture was 8·2% with AI therapy vs 5·5% in the tamoxifen group (difference 2·7%, 95% CI 1·7–3·7). It is important to recognise that these differences will be a composite of improved bone health with tamoxifen and reduced bone health with AIs, with the true impact on fracture risk coming from the placebo-controlled extended adjuvant and prevention trials. There were no significant differences in mortality from cardiac, cerebrovascular or thromboembolic disease between the AI and tamoxifen groups.

22.8.4 Extended Adjuvant Aromatase Inhibitor Therapy

As discussed in the section on adjuvant tamoxifen therapy, extending treatment from 5 to 10 years has shown some benefits. The desire to consider extended therapy is driven by data demonstrating that late recurrence, beyond the 5 years of therapy, is common, particularly in patients with lymph node-positive disease (Pan et al. 2017). At least 12 studies of varied designs have now examined the role of extending adjuvant AI therapy beyond the initial 2–5 years of ET. There is some difficulty in interpreting these studies due to the variability in their designs, including the type and duration of ET that was allowed prior to randomisation and the subsequent duration of randomised AI therapy. The first extended therapy study to report was the MA17 trial from North America (Goss et al. 2003). This study randomised 5187 women who had completed 4.5–6 years of tamoxifen therapy to either letrozole for 5 years or placebo. However, after the first interim analysis, and a median follow-up of only 2.4 years, the independent data and safety monitoring committee recommended termination of the trial. Women randomised to letrozole had a 6% better disease-free survival (93% vs 87%; $p < 0.001$), although no significant difference was seen in overall survival (42 deaths on placebo and 31 on letrozole; $p = 0.25$) and longer-term follow-up was not possible due to the early closure of the study.

In women who did go on to complete 5 years of letrozole, a second randomisation was undertaken to continue for a further 5 years (total 10 years of AI and 15 of ET overall) vs placebo (5 years of Ai and 10 years of ET in total) (Goss et al. 2016). 1918 women were randomised, and there was a small but statistically significant improvement in 5-year disease-free survival rate between the groups (95% vs 91%; $p = 0.01$) after a median follow-up pf 6.3 years. However, of these DFS events there were only 11 fewer distant recurrences in the letrozole arm, most of which were in the bone (10/11) and could potentially have been prevented with bisphosphonate therapy that is now standard of care as adjuvant therapy in postmenopausal women at increased risk of recurrence (EBCTCG 2015a, b). This is particularly pertinent as bone-related toxic effects occurred more frequently in those receiving letrozole vs placebo, including bone pain, fractures and new-onset osteoporosis (Goss et al. 2016). Interestingly there were fewer contralateral BCs in the letrozole arm (13 vs 31), suggesting that longer-term ET is beneficial in preventing primary breast cancer despite the proven carry-over effect of 5 years of tamoxifen, as seen in the IBIS-1 study (Cuzick et al. 2015).

The other 10 extended AI studies randomised women to between 2.5–5 years of AI in the active arms and 0–3 years of AI in the control arms, after varied types and durations of preliminary ET (summarised in Petrelli et al. 2023). The individual results of these studies are mixed, and the follow-up remains relatively short. An independent (non-EBCTCG) meta-analysis of all 12 of these studies suggests that the optimal length of AI therapy in the adjuvant setting remains unknown (Petrelli et al. 2023). The risk-benefit ratio is in favour of limiting extended adjuvant AI to 2–3 years in those with axillary lymph node-negative disease. However, the risk of relapse remains high in women with node-positive disease, and more prolonged courses of AI are probably indicated in such cases. It must be noted, however, that the emergence of other targeted therapies such as the CDK4/6 inhibitor abemaciclib (and possibly ribociclib) has recently changed the treatment landscape for those with axillary lymph node-positive disease, meaning that the question of extended ET now needs to be re-evaluated in the post-CDK4/6i era (Rastogi et al. 2024).

22.8.5 Aromatase Inhibitors in Breast Cancer Prevention

Given the success of preventive tamoxifen therapy and the observation that AIs were superior to tamoxifen at preventing contralateral breast cancer in the adjuvant setting (EBCTCG 2015a, b), it was a logical step to test the AIs in primary prevention. To date only two of the third-generation AIs, exemestane and anastrozole, have undergone testing, in the MAP3 (Goss et al. 2011) and IBIS-II (Cuzick et al. 2014) studies, respectively. In the MAP3 trial, 4560 postmenopausal women with a median age of 62.5 years were randomised to exemestane 25 mg daily or placebo for 5 years. Women were eligible for the study if they had a 5 year risk of breast cancer of at least 1.66% (median across all participant 2.3%) or were aged at least 60 years. Approximately 10% of participants had had a prior diagnosis of atypical ductal hyperplasia (ADH), atypical lobular hyperplasia (ALH) or lobular carcinoma in situ (LCIS) or DCIS with mastectomy. Exemestane reduced the risk of breast cancer by 53% (hazard ratio, 0.47; 95% CI, 0.27 to 0.79; $P = 0.004$) after approximately 3 years of median follow-up, and the study was then closed with women on the placebo arm offered exemestane and no plans made for long-term follow-up.

In contrast the IBIS-II study recruited 3864 postmenopausal women with a median age of 59.5 years at study entry and has reported a median follow-up of 12 years currently (Cuzick et al. 2020) with ongoing publications planned. Women were randomised to anastrozole 1 mg daily or placebo for 5 years duration. Eligibility criteria were based on breast cancer risk and included women: aged 40–44 years who had a relative risk that was at least 4 times higher than the general population, aged 45–60 years who had a relative risk at least 2 times higher and aged 60–70 years at least 1·5 times higher. In the initial

Table 22.2 All grades of common and serious side effects in the two AI prevention trials vs placebo. * denotes statistically significant at $p < 0.05$ level

	MAP3		IBIS-II	
Toxicity	Exemestane $n = 2240$	Placebo $n = 2244$	Anastrozole $n = 1920$	Placebo $n = 1944$
Hot flushes	40.2*	31.9	56.8*	49.4
Vaginal Dryness	15.7	15.3	18.6*	16.6*
Diarrhoea	5.3*	3.3*	NR	NR
Hypertension	15.2	15.8	4.6*	2.8*
Cardiovascular events	NR	NR	2.6	3.3
Arthralgia	29.7*	27*	50.6*	46*
Fracture	6.7	6.4	8.5	7.7
New osteoporosis	1.7	1.3	NR	NR

report of IBIS-II, after a median follow-up of 5.0 years, anastrozole reduced the risk of breast cancer by 53% (hazard ratio 0·47, 95% CI 0·32–0·68, p < 0·0001) (Cuzick et al. 2014). In the second report with a median follow-up of 131 months (IQR 105–156), the overall reduction in breast cancer risk was 49% (HR 0·51, 95% CI 0·39–0·66, p < 0·0001). The reduction in incidence in the first 5 years of follow-up was 61% (0·39, 0·27–0·58, p < 0·0001), and a smaller but still significant 37% reduction (0·64, 0·45–0·91, p = 0·014) was seen in subsequent years, which was still larger than that seen for tamoxifen in previous trials (Cuzick et al. 2015).

As with the SERM prevention trials, MAP-3 and IBIS-II give us highly valuable data on the toxicity of the aromatase inhibitors compared to placebo in women who have not undergone the psychological and physical trauma of a breast cancer diagnosis. Table 22.2 shows the common and serious side effects of the AIs compared with placebo for the two trials. Although arthralgia is more common than placebo in both trials, there is a considerable level of arthralgia experienced by women in the placebo arms. However, in both trials the increase in arthralgia is with moderate to severe rather than mild symptoms, affecting about 1 in 20 to 1 in 30 women and often requiring cessation of therapy. In the updated analysis of IBIS-II, when all women had completed the 5 year treatment period, full 5 year adherence was 74·6% for anastrozole compared with 77·0% for placebo, a difference that was not statistically significant (HR 0·89, 95% CI 0·79–1·01, p = 0·081).

22.9 Selective Oestrogen Receptor Downregulators

22.9.1 Fulvestrant: The Prototypic SERD

Fulvestrant has an aromatised steroidal backbone and thus binds with high affinity to the ligand-binding domain of the ER (Parker 1993). The heavily fluorinated 7 alpha-alkylamide side chain results in targeting of the ER complex for ubiquitination and proteolysis (Long and Nephew 2006). Fulvestrant results in a reduction in the number of detectable ER molecules in the cell, both in vitro and in vivo, in contrast to the stable or increased levels of ER expression associated with tamoxifen and other SERMs (Pink and Jordan 1996). As resistance to SERMs can be mediated through agonistic actions, such as phosphorylation, on the persistent ER, this was recognised as a highly attractive mechanism of action. In vitro studies demonstrated that tamoxifen-resistant cell lines remained sensitive to growth inhibition by fulvestrant (Bunone et al. 1996; Hu et al. 1993), which also delayed the onset and suppressed the subsequent growth of ER-positive xenografts in vivo to a far greater extent than tamoxifen itself (Osborne et al. 1995).

Although these results were highly encouraging, fulvestrant had very poor oral bioavailability, necessitating intramuscular injection (im) and hampering its clinical development. Despite this obstacle fulvestrant was the first compound to be tested in window-of-opportunity (WOO) studies in the perioperative period (Fig. 22.1; DeFriend et al. 1994). Daily intramuscular injections of 6 mg or 18 mg doses in patients with ER-positive tumours resulted in significant reductions in ER, progesterone receptor (PR) and Ki67 expression. Fulvestrant was then formulated as a long-acting intramuscular injection and tested in a dose-finding WOO study at 50 mg, 125 mg and 250 mg im (single doses) against tamoxifen or placebo, both given daily for 14–21 days prior to breast surgery (Robertson et al. 2001). Fulvestrant reduced ER expression in a dose-dependent manner. In contrast to tamoxifen, which increased PR expression suggesting ER agonist activity, all doses of fulvestrant reduced tumour PR expression, confirming its lack of oestrogen-agonist activity.

Fulvestrant was then tested in two phase III studies in patients with advanced breast cancer who were randomised to receive the 250 mg dose of fulvestrant im monthly vs 1 mg daily of the AI anastrozole (Howell et al. 2002; Osborne et al. 2002). All patients had progressed on or after prior adjuvant endocrine therapy, almost all with tamoxifen. In both studies fulvestrant was at least as effective as anastrozole, with a longer duration of response in one trial (Osborne et al. 2002), confirming fulvestrant as an effective treatment in postmenopausal patients in this disease setting. In contrast, in a first-line study that tested fulvestrant (250 mg im every month) to tamoxifen, there was a significant difference for time-to-treatment failure in favour of tamoxifen ($P = 0.026$) with the median being 5.9 months for fulvestrant and 7.8 months for tamoxifen. The Kaplan-Meier curves separated early and was most pronounced at 3 months, suggesting a higher rate of early progressions in the fulvestrant group. Pharmacokinetic studies of fulvestrant had previously shown that accumulation of the drug occurs over the first 6 months of therapy and that it takes 3–6 months to reach steady-state plasma levels (Howell et al. 1996). These findings and the observation that the dose response had not been maximised in the WOO studies led to further dose-finding studies and the subsequent approval of 500 mg monthly (2 × 250mg im injections, one in each buttock) with an additional 500 mg loading dose at 2 weeks (Di Leo et al. 2010). A phase III study was subsequently undertaken in the first-line setting in women naïve to prior endocrine therapy, which demonstrated fulvestrant to be superior to anastrozole in terms of progression-free survival (fulvestrant median PFS 16·6 months (95% CI 13·83–20·99) vs anastrozole 13·8 months (11·99–16·59); HR 0·797, 95% CI 0·637–0·999, $p = 0{\cdot}049$)) (Robertson et al. 2016). However, the final overall survival results did not show an advantage for fulvestrant (HR, 0.97 [95% CI, 0.77–1.21]; $p = 0.7579$), and the protracted development meant it was not commercially viable to undertake large adjuvant studies. Of great translational importance, however, multiple oral SERDs were beginning to enter clinical testing during this time.

22.9.2 Oral Compounds that Downregulate the ER

Several approaches have been adopted in the search for oral agents that downregulate the ER, to mitigate mechanisms of resistance and enhance ET activity. Currently there are three classes of compounds that result in ER downregulation: oral SERDs (Selective Estrogen Receptor Degraders), CERANs (Complete ER ANtagonists) and PROTACs (PROteolysis-TArgeting Chimeras).

22.9.3 Oral SERDs

Oral SERDs share similarities in their mechanism of action with the prototypic SERD fulvestrant. Those that have made it into clinical development so far have nonsteroidal backbones with either an acrylic acid or, more recently, a basic amino-containing side chain. Only one acrylic acid containing oral SERD, rintodestrant (G1T48; Iqbal et al. 2023), remains in clinical development with all other agents (including GDC-810, LSZ102 and AZD9496), having their development ceased due to relatively poor efficacy and tolerability in early phase trials. These agents also had heterogenous ER degradation results between different cell lines. In contrast, the basic amino side chain compounds continue to be developed, with one, elacestrant, having been approved for routine clinical use in the advanced breast cancer setting and three, camizestrant, giredestrant and imlunestrant, entering the adjuvant early breast cancer setting (Fig. 22.2).

Elacestrant (RAD1901) is a SERM/SERD hybrid with ER antagonistic effects in breast and uterine tissues but agonism in the bone (Garner et al. 2015). Treatment of multiple patient-derived xenograft models demonstrated profound downregulation of the ER and superior activity compared with fulvestrant both alone and in combination with CDK4/6 and PI3K pathway inhibitors (Bihani et al. 2017). Promising activity was observed in phase I/II clinical studies in heavily pretreated populations, including patients with tumours harbouring *ESR1* mutations. This led to the phase 3 EMERALD trial which randomised patients with ER+/HER2- metastatic breast cancer (MBC), who had received treatment with at least one prior line of ET including a CDK4/6 inhibitor to either elacestrant or standard-of-care (SOC) ET (fulvestrant or a third-generation AI) (Bidard et al. 2022). In total 239 participants received elacestrant and 238 SOC, with ESR1 mutation detected in 47.8%. Elacestrant resulted in superior PFS in the whole cohort (HR 0.70; 95% CI, 0.55–0.88; $p = 0.002$) and in those with *ESR1* mutations (HR = 0.55; 95% CI, 0.39–0.77; $p = 0.0005$). The absolute values for median PFS were somewhat disappointing as approximately 50% of patients had cancer progression on their first on-treatment scan, likely reflecting the extensive pretreatment and ET resistance of this population. Landmark analyses at 6, 12 and 18 months all favoured elacestrant which gained FDA approval for the treatment of ER+/HER2- MBC with *ESR1* mutation on the back of these study data (Shah et al. 2024). A subsequent subgroup analysis by duration of prior CDK4/6 inhibitor therapy showed that elacestrant appeared particularly effective in patients who had *ESR1* mutations and had received a CDK4/6i to treat MBC for more than 12 months (median PFS elacestrant 8.6 months vs 1.9 months SOC; HR 0.41; 95%CI 0.26–0.63), presumably reflecting a more ET-sensitive subpopulation (Bardia et al. 2023). Although elacestrant is reasonably well tolerated, albeit with some gastrointestinal toxicity, and has shown some activity in early breast cancer in a small WOO study, there are currently no planned adjuvant studies (Bidard et al. 2022; Vidal et al. 2023).

Camizestrant (AZD9833) is a tricyclic indazole acid SERD that has been shown to suppress ER-regulated and G1-S phase transition gene signatures to a greater degree than either fulvestrant or elacestrant, with no recorded ER agonist activity (Lawson et al. 2023). Camizestrant reduces ER and PR levels in both ESR1wt and ESR1 mutant cell lines and patient-derived xenografts, albeit with somewhat reduced potency in ESR1 mutant models (Lawson et al. 2023). These encouraging preclinical data have seen camizestrant taken into clinical testing in the SERENA series of trials. SERENA-1 functioned as a platform study to evaluate single-agent camizestrant and combinations with CDK4/6 and PI3K pathway inhibitors (Turner et al. 2022). The phase 2 SERENA-2 trial was a head-to-head comparison between fulvestrant 500 mg and two doses of camizestrant, 75 mg and 150 mg daily (Oliveira et al. 2022). In the overall population, the median PFS with fulvestrant of 3.7 months (90%CI 2.0–6.0) increased significantly to 7.2 months (90%CI 3.7–10.9; $p = 0.012$) and 7.7 months (90%CI 5.5–12.9; $p = 0.016$) with the 75 mg and 150 mg doses, respectively. The effect was more marked in patients with tumours harbouring *ESR1* mutations (75 mg dose HR 0.33, 90% CI 0.18–0.58; median PFS of 6.3 versus 2.2 months and 150 mg dose HR 0.55, 90% CI 0.33–0.89; median PFS of 9.2 versus 2.2 months) compared with those with *ESR1* wild-type tumours (HR 0.78, 90% CI 0.50–1.22 and HR 0.76, 90% CI 0.48–1.20, respectively). Camizestrant is also being tested in the first-line MBC setting in combination with the CDK4/6i palbociclib (SERENA-4, NCT04964934) and in an interesting study in which participants who have already started first-line AI+CDK4/6i will be randomised to continue or switch to camizestrant 75 mg daily in combination with CDK4/6i but only if plasma ESR1 mutation becomes detectable (SERENA-6, NCT04964934). Results of these trials are expected in 2027/8.

In the SERENA-2 study, high-grade adverse events were more common in the 150 mg camizestrant arm, 21.9% of patients vs 12.2% with 75 mg and 13.7% with fulvestrant. Bradycardia and visual disturbances were notable dose-dependent side effects, and although these were of some concern initially, a well-conducted WOO study (SERENA-3) demonstrated equivalent suppression of ER (at day 5–7) and Ki67 (at day 12–15) with 75 mg, 150 mg and 300 mg dose levels (Robertson et al. 2023). This challenged the notion of maximum tolerated dose being desirable for late phase clinical testing and resulted in the 75 mg dose being taken forward in the adjuvant setting in the CAMBRIA studies as the optimal balance between efficacy and tolerability. In the CAMBRIA-1 study (NCT05774951), 4300 participants with early breast cancer who have already received 2–5 years of adjuvant ET will be randomised either to receive camizestrant 75 mg (+GnRH analogue if premenopausal) or to continue with SOC for a duration of 5 years. In contrast CAMBRIA-2 (NCT05952557) will adopt the same randomisation in 5500 participants who are yet to start adjuvant ET. Results are expected for these studies between 2027 and 2030.

Giredestrant (GDC-9545) was tested against fulvestrant, elacestrant and camizestrant during its preclinical development, demonstrating increased potency with reduced IC50s in multiple ER+/HER2- breast cancer cell line models (Liang et al. 2021). However, in the randomised phase 2 acelERA study, with a very similar design to the SERENA-2 and EMERALD studies, there was no significant improvement in median PFS in the overall population (giredestrant 30 mg 5.6 months vs standard of care 5.4 months; HR 0.81, 95%CI, 0.60–1.10), although a trend to improved PFS was seen in patients with ESR1 mutant tumours (HR 0.60, 95% CI, 0.35–1.03) (Jimenez et al. 2022). In the neoadjuvant coopERA study, giredestrant 30 mg in combination with the CDK4/6i palbociclib was tested against anastrozole and palbociclib (Fasching et al. 2022). At surgery the giredestrant combination resulted in superior suppression of proliferation with a reduction in Ki67 staining of −81% (95%CI: −86% to −75%) compared to the anastrozole plus palbociclib (−74% (95% CI −80% to −67%). However, no significant differences in the objective tumour response or complete pathological response rates were seen. Despite these somewhat mixed results, the lidERA randomised phase 3 adjuvant trial in the early breast cancer setting (NCT04961996) will randomise approximately 4200 patients to giredestrant 30 mg versus standard-of-care ET for 5 years in HR+/HER2- BC.

Imlunestrant (LY3484356) is less well described in the preclinical literature, and there remain comparatively few clinical data to this point. In the phase 1 EMBER trial, the 51 patients treated with the recommended phase 2 dose of 400 mg daily experienced a median PFS of 7.2 months (95% CI 3.7–8.3) overall and 7.1 months (95%CI 3.5–8.2) in the 26 patients who had received at least 2 lines of ET after CDK4/6i (Jhaveri et al. 2022). The EMBER-2 WOO study examined three dose levels of imlunestrant (200 mg, 400 mg and 800 mg) for approximately 15 days prior to definitive breast surgery (Neven 2023). All three doses resulted in significant downregulation of ER, PR and Ki67, and 400 mg was selected for the subsequent randomised phase 2 EMBER-3 study in AI pretreated MBC (NCT04975308) and the adjuvant EMBER-4 study (NCT05514054) with a comparable design to CAMBRIA-1 above.

22.9.4 Complete ER Antagonists (CERANs)

Palazestrant (OP-1250) is the first in class of the CERANs. Like SERMs and SERDs, CERANs bind to the ligand-binding domain of the ER. As discussed previously, whilst SERMs inhibit AF2, they may activate AF1, resulting in ER agonism. In contrast CERANs inhibit both AF1 and AF2, resulting in complete antagonism (Fanning et al. 2018; Parisian et al. 2023). Downregulation of the receptor ensues, but this is not absolutely required for ER antagonism (Wardell et al. 2011; Srinivasan et al. 2017). It is not yet certain that the proposed mechanism of action differentiates a separate class of drug, as the prototypic SERD fulvestrant induces similar ER conformational changes as the novel CERAN compounds (Fanning et al. 2018). Palazestrant showed comparable activity to imlunestrant and fulvestrant in the preclinical models presented to date (Parisian et al. 2023). Nevertheless, palazestrant has entered clinical testing and demonstrated clinical benefit in 40% (23/57) overall and 50% (11/22) in those with ESR1 mutant tumours as a single agent in pretreated MBC (NCT04505826; Lin et al. 2023). Good tolerability and activity have also been demonstrated in combination with the CDK4/6i palbociclib (NCT05266105), and a phase 3 study in the second-/third-line MBC (OPERA-01) has been launched which will randomise palazestrant against SOC fulvestrant or AI (NCT06016738).

22.9.5 PROteolysis-TArgeting Chimeras (PROTACs)

PROTACs are heterobifunctional small molecules that link an ER ligand with an E3 ligase that then induces ubiquitination and degradation of the ER complex by the proteasome (Chamberlain and Hamann 2019). The number of PROTACs proceeding through preclinical to clinical testing for multiple indications is rising rapidly (Wang et al. 2024). Two ER-targeting PROTACs, vepdegestrant (ARV-471) and AC0682, have so far entered clinical trials, but results are only available for vepdegestrant at present (Hamilton et al. 2022). Preclinically vepdegestrant showed superior potency to fulvestrant in ER degradation assays, including in ESR1 variants, Y537S and D538G, and demonstrated no agonist activity (Snyder et al. 2021). In a phase 1 dose escalation study, vepdegestrant was well tolerated, and there were no dose-limiting toxicities but promising activity in heavily pretreated patients (Hamilton et al. 2022). A phase 2 study tested vepdegestrant and showed comparable efficacy at 200 mg and 500 mg with approximately 71% suppression of ER expression. The 200 mg dose was thus taken forward and, in women with a median of 3 prior lines of ET, showed a median PFS of 3.5 months (95% CI 1.8–8.2) in ESR1wt and 5.7 months (95% CI 1.8–8.5) in ESR1 mutant tumours (VERITAC; NCT04072952; Campone et al. 2023). VERITAC-2 will test vepdegestrant 200 mg against fulvestrant 500 mg in ET-resistant MBC and VERITAC-3 (NCT05909397) the combination of vepdegestrant plus palbociclib against letrozole and palbociclib in the first-line setting.

22.10 Conclusions

Targeting oestrogen signalling to treat ER+ breast cancer has a long and distinguished history. Countless thousands, if not millions, of women have had their breast cancers prevented, cured or controlled for longer through manipulation of oestrogen production or its interaction with the ER. Over more than 100 years, the treatments available have become progressively more effective and, in general, better tolerated with fewer off-target effects. The future of ER targeting looks brighter than ever with the development of novel ER-degrading therapies which are orally bioavailable, potent and well tolerated. These agents will hopefully make further incremental steps in enhancing breast cancer survival. The challenges will be knowing how best to use them: in whom, for how long and in what combinations.

References

Allen E, Doisy E (1923) An ovarian hormone: preliminary report on its localisation, extraction and partial purification and action in test animals. JAMA J Am Med Assoc 81:819–821. https://doi.org/10.1001/jama.1923.02650100027012

Balfour JA, Goa KL (1998) Raloxifene. Drugs Aging 12:335–341

Bardia A, Bidard F, Neven P, Streich G, Montero AJ, Forget F, Mouret-Reynier M, Sohn JH, Taylor D, Harnden KK, Khong H, Kocsis J, Dalenc F, Dillon P, Babu S, Waters S, Deleu I, García-Sáenz A, Bria E, Cazzaniga ME, Aftimos P, Cortés J, Tonini G, Sahmoud T, Habboubi N, Grzegorzewski K (2023) Kaklamani V Abstract GS3-01: GS3-01 EMERALD phase 3 trial of elacestrant versus standard of care endocrine therapy in patients with ER+/HER2- metastatic breast cancer: Updated results by duration of prior CDK4/6i in metastatic setting. Cancer Res 83(5_Supplement):GS3-01

Baum M, Budzar AU, Cuzick J, Forbes J, Houghton JH, Klijn JG, Sahmoud T, ATAC Trialists' Group (2002) Anastrozole alone or in combination with tamoxifen versus tamoxifen alone for adjuvant treatment of postmenopausal women with early breast cancer: first results of the ATAC randomised trial. Lancet 359:2131–2139

Beato M, Chalepakis G, Schauer M, Slater EP (1989) DNA regulatory elements for steroid hormones. J Steroid Biochem 32:737–747

Beatson GT (1896) On treatment of inoperable cases of carcinoma of the mamma: suggestions for a new method of treatment with illustrative cases. Lancet 2:104–107

Bernhard J, Luo W, Ribi K, Colleoni M, Burstein HJ, Tondini C, Pinotti G, Spazzapan S, Ruhstaller T, Puglisi F, Pavesi L, Parmar V, Regan MM, Pagani O, Fleming GF, Francis PA, Price KN, Coates AS, Gelber RD, Goldhirsch A, Walley BA (2015) Patient-reported outcomes with adjuvant exemestane versus tamoxifen in premenopausal women with early breast cancer undergoing ovarian suppression (TEXT and SOFT): a combined analysis of two phase 3 randomised trials. Lancet Oncol 16:848–858

Bidard FC, Kaklamani VG, Neven P, Streich G, Montero AJ, Forget F, Mouret-Reynier MA, Sohn JH, Taylor D, Harnden KK, Khong H, Kocsis J, Dalenc F, Dillon PM, Babu S, Waters S, Deleu I, García Sáenz JA, Bria E, Cazzaniga M, Lu J, Aftimos P, Cortés J, Liu S, Tonini G, Laurent D, Habboubi N, Conlan MG, Bardia A (2022) Elacestrant (oral selective estrogen receptor degrader) versus standard endocrine therapy for estrogen receptor-positive, human epidermal growth factor receptor 2-negative advanced breast cancer: results from the randomized phase III EMERALD trial. J Clin Oncol 40:3246–3256

Bihani T, Patel HK, Arlt H, Tao N, Jiang H, Brown JL, Purandare DM, Hattersley G, Garner F (2017) Elacestrant (RAD1901), a selective estrogen receptor degrader (SERD), has antitumor activity in multiple ER+ breast cancer patient-derived xenograft models. Clin Cancer Res 23:4793–4804

Bunone G, Briand PA, Miksicek RJ, Picard D (1996) Activation of the unliganded estrogen receptor by EGF involves the MAP kinase pathway and direct phosphorylation. EMBO J 15:2174–2183

Campone M, Ma CX, De Laurentiis M, Iwata H, Hurvitz SA, Wander SA, Danso MA, Dongrui Ray L, Smith JP, Liu Y, Tran L, Anderson S, Hamilton EP (2023) VERITAC-2: a global, randomized phase 3 study of ARV-471, a proteolysis targeting chimera (PROTAC) estrogen receptor (ER) degrader, vs fulvestrant in ER+/ human epidermal growth factor receptor 2 (HER2)-advanced breast cancer. J Clin Oncol 41(16_suppl). https://doi.org/10.1200/JCO.2023.41.16_suppl.TPS118

Cash R, Brough AJ, Cohen M, Satoh PS (1967) Aminoglutethimide (Elipten-Ciba) as an inhibitor of adrenal steroidogenesis: mechanism of action and therapeutic trial. J Clin Endocrinol Metab 27:1239–1248

Chamberlain PP, Hamann LG (2019) Development of targeted protein degradation therapeutics. Nat Chem Biol 15:937–944

Cole MP, Jones CTA, Todd IDH (1971) A new anti-estrogenic agent in late breast cancer: an early clinical appraisal of ICI46474. Br J Cancer 25:270–275

Collins LC, Botero ML, Scnitt SJ (2005) Bimodal frequency distribution of estrogen receptor immunohistochemical staining results of 825 cases. Am J Clin Pathol 123:16–20

Couch FJ, Kuchenbaecker KB, Michailidou K et al (2016) Identification of four novel susceptibility loci for estrogen receptor negative breast cancer. Nat Commun 7:11375. https://doi.org/10.1038/ncomms11375

Cuzick J, Baum M (1985) Tamoxifen and contralateral breast cancer. Lancet 2:282. https://doi.org/10.1016/s0140-6736(85)90338-1

Cuzick J, Sestak I, Bonanni B, Costantino JP, Cummings S, DeCensi A, Dowsett M, Forbes JF, Ford L, LaCroix AZ, Mershon J, Mitlak BH, Powles T, Veronesi U, Vogel V, Wickerham DL (2013) SERM chemoprevention of breast cancer overview group. Selective oestrogen receptor modulators in prevention of breast cancer: an updated meta-analysis of individual participant data. Lancet 381(9880):1827–1834. https://doi.org/10.1016/S0140-6736(13)60140-3. Epub 2013 Apr 30. PMID: 23639488; PMCID: PMC3671272

Cuzick J, Sestak I, Forbes JF, Dowsett M, Knox J, Cawthorn S, Saunders C, Roche N, Mansel RE, von Minckwitz G, Bonanni B, Palva T, Howell A, IBIS-II investigators. (2014) Anastrozole for prevention of breast cancer in high-risk postmenopausal women (IBIS-II): an international, double-blind, randomised placebo-controlled trial. Lancet 383:1041–1048

Cuzick J, Sestak I, Cawthorn S, Hamed H, Holli K, Howell A, Forbes JF, IBIS-I Investigators (2015) Tamoxifen for prevention of breast cancer: extended long-term follow-up of the IBIS-I breast cancer prevention trial. Lancet Oncol 16:67–75. https://doi.org/10.1016/S1470-2045(14)71171-4

Cuzick J, Sestak I, Forbes JF, Dowsett M, Cawthorn S, Mansel RE, Loibl S, Bonanni B, Evans DG, Howell A, IBIS-II investigators. (2020) Use of anastrozole for breast cancer prevention (IBIS-II): long-term results of a randomised controlled trial. Lancet 395:117–122

Davies C, Pan H, Godwin J et al (2013) Adjuvant Tamoxifen: Longer Against Shorter (ATLAS) Collaborative Group. Long-term effects of continuing adjuvant tamoxifen to 10 years versus stopping at 5 years after diagnosis of estrogen receptor-positive breast cancer: ATLAS, a randomised trial. Lancet 381:805–816. https://doi.org/10.1016/S0140-6736(12)61963-1. Erratum in: Lancet 2013;381(9869):804

De Courmelles F (1922) La radiotherapie indirecte ou dirigee par les correlation organiques Arch. D'Electricite Med 32:264

DeFriend DJ, Howell A, Nicholson RI, Anderson E, Dowsett M, Mansel RE et al (1994) Investigation of a new pure antiestrogen (ICI 182780) in women with primary breast cancer. Cancer Res 54:408–414

Deshmane V, Krishnamurthy S, Melemed AS, Peterson P, Buzdar AU (2007) Phase III double-blind trial of arzoxifene compared with tamoxifen for locally advanced or metastatic breast cancer. J Clin Oncol 25:4967–4973

DeSombre ER, Johnson ES, White WF (1976) Regression of rat mammary tumors affected by a gonadoliberin analog. Cancer Res 36:3830–3833

Di Leo A, Jerusalem G, Petruzelka L, Torres R, Bondarenko IN, Khasanov R, Verhoeven D, Pedrini JL, Smirnova I, Lichinitser MR, Pendergrass K, Garnett S, Lindemann JP, Sapunar F, Martin M (2010) Results of the CONFIRM phase III trial comparing fulvestrant 250 mg with fulvestrant 500 mg in postmenopausal women with estrogen receptor-positive advanced breast cancer. J Clin Oncol 28:4594–4600

Dodds EC, Goldberg L, Lawson W, Robinson R (1938) Estrogenic activity of certain synthetic compounds. Nature 141:247–248. https://doi.org/10.1038/141247b0

Donnelly LS, Evans DG, Wiseman J et al (2014) Uptake of tamoxifen in consecutive premenopausal women under surveillance in a high-risk breast cancer clinic. Br J Cancer 110:1681–1687. https://doi.org/10.1038/bjc.2014.109

Dowsett M, Smith IE, Ebbs SR, Dixon JM, Skene A, Griffith C, Boeddinghaus I, Salter J, Detre S, Hills M, Ashley S, Francis S, Walsh G, Trialists IMPACT (2005) Short-term changes in Ki-67 during neoadjuvant treatment of primary breast cancer with anastrozole or tamoxifen alone or combined correlate with recurrence-free survival. Clin Cancer Res 11:951s–958s

Early Breast Cancer Trialists' Collaborative Group (1998) Tamoxifen for early breast cancer: an overview of the randomised trials. Lancet 351:1451–1467

Early Breast Cancer Trialists' Collaborative Group (EBCTCG) (2005) Effects of chemotherapy and hormonal therapy for early breast cancer on recurrence and 15-year survival: an overview of the randomised trials. Lancet 365:1687–1717. https://doi.org/10.1016/S0140-6736(05)66544-0

Early Breast Cancer Trialists' Collaborative Group (EBCTCG) (2015a) Aromatase inhibitors versus tamoxifen in early breast cancer: patient-level meta-analysis of the randomised trials. Lancet 386:1341–1352

Early Breast Cancer Trialists' Collaborative Group (EBCTCG) (2015b) Adjuvant bisphosphonate treatment in early breast cancer: meta-analyses of individual patient data from randomised trials. Lancet 386:1353–1361

Early Breast Cancer Trialists' Collaborative Group (EBCTCG); Davies C, Godwin J, Gray R, Clarke M, Cutter D, Darby S, McGale P, Pan HC, Taylor C, Wang YC, Dowsett M, Ingle J, Peto R (2011) Relevance of breast cancer hormone receptors and other factors to the efficacy of adjuvant tamoxifen: patient-level meta-analysis of randomised trials. Lancet 378:771–784

Ellis MJ, Coop A, Singh B, Tao Y, Llombart-Cussac A, Jänicke F, Mauriac L, Quebe-Fehling E, Chaudri-Ross HA, Evans DB, Miller WR (2003) Letrozole inhibits tumor proliferation more effectively than tamoxifen independent of HER1/2 expression status. Cancer Res 63:6523–6531

Ellis MJ, Suman VJ, Hoog J, Lin L, Snider J, Prat A, Parker JS, Luo J, DeSchryver K, Allred DC, Esserman LJ, Unzeitig GW, Margenthaler J, Babiera GV, Marcom PK, Guenther JM, Watson MA, Leitch M, Hunt K, Olson JA (2011) Randomized phase II neoadjuvant comparison between letrozole, anastrozole, and exemestane for postmenopausal women with estrogen receptor-rich stage 2 to 3 breast cancer: clinical and biomarker outcomes and predictive value of the baseline PAM50-based intrinsic subtype--ACOSOG Z1031. J Clin Oncol 29:2342–2349

Fanning SW, Hodges-Gallagher L, Myles DC, Sun R, Fowler CE, Plant IN, Green BD, Harmon CL, Greene GL, Kushner PJ (2018) Specific stereochemistry of OP-1074 disrupts estrogen receptor alpha helix 12 and confers pure antiestrogenic activity. Nat Commun 9:2368. https://doi.org/10.1038/s41467-018-04413-3

Fasching PA, Bardia A, Quiroga V, Park YH, Blancas I, Alonso JL, Vasilyev A, Adamchuk H, Salgado MRT, Yardley DA, Spera G (2022) Neoadjuvant giredestrant (GDC-9545) plus palbociclib (P) versus anastrozole (A) plus P in postmenopausal women with estrogen receptor–positive, HER2-negative, untreated early breast cancer (ER+/HER2–eBC): Final analysis of the randomized, open-label, international phase 2 coopERA BC study. J Clin Oncol 40(16_suppl):589

Fisher B, Costantino JP, Wickerham DL et al (1998) Tamoxifen for prevention of breast cancer: report of the National Surgical Adjuvant Breast and Bowel Project P-1 Study. J Natl Cancer Inst 90:1371–1388. https://doi.org/10.1093/jnci/90.18.1371

Fisher B, Costantino JP, Wickerham DL et al (2005) Tamoxifen for the prevention of breast cancer: current status of the National Surgical Adjuvant Breast and Bowel Project P-1 study. J Natl Cancer Inst 97:1652–1662. https://doi.org/10.1093/jnci/dji372

Fossati R, Confalonieri C, Torri V, Ghislandi E, Penna A, Pistotti V et al (1998) Cytotoxic and hormonal treatment for metastatic breast cancer: a systematic review of published randomized trials involving 31,510 women. J Clin Oncol 16:3439–3460

Francis PA, Pagani O, Fleming GF et al (2018) Tailoring adjuvant endocrine therapy for premenopausal breast cancer. New Engl J Med 379:122–137

Garner F, Shomali M, Paquin D, Lyttle CR, Hattersley G (2015) RAD1901: a novel, orally bioavailable selective estrogen receptor degrader that demonstrates antitumor activity in breast cancer xenograft models. Anti-Cancer Drugs 26:948–956

Goss PE, Ingle JN, Martino S, Robert NJ, Muss HB, Piccart MJ, Castiglione M, Tu D, Shepherd LE, Pritchard KI, Livingston RB, Davidson NE, Norton L, Perez EA, Abrams JS, Therasse P, Palmer MJ, Pater JL (2003) A randomized trial of letrozole in postmenopausal women after five years of tamoxifen therapy for early-stage breast cancer. N Engl J Med 349:1793–1802

Goss PE, Ingle JN, Alés-Martínez JE, Cheung AM, Chlebowski RT, Wactawski-Wende J, McTiernan A, Robbins J, Johnson KC, Martin LW, Winquist E, Sarto GE, Garber JE, Fabian CJ, Pujol P, Maunsell E, Farmer P, Gelmon KA, Tu D, Richardson H, NCIC CTG MAP.3 Study Investigators (2011) Exemestane for breast-cancer prevention in postmenopausal women. N Engl J Med 364:2381–2391

Goss PE, Ingle JN, Pritchard KI, Ellis MJ, Sledge GW, Budd GT, Rabaglio M, Ansari RH, Johnson DB, Tozer R, D'Souza DP, Chalchal H, Spadafora S, Stearns V, Perez EA, Liedke PE, Lang I, Elliott C, Gelmon KA, Chapman JA, Shepherd LE (2013) Exemestane versus anastrozole in postmenopausal women with early breast cancer: NCIC CTG MA.27--a randomized controlled phase III trial. J Clin Oncol 31:1398–1404

Goss PE, Ingle JN, Pritchard KI, Robert NJ, Muss H, Gralow J, Gelmon K, Whelan T, Strasser-Weippl K, Rubin S, Sturtz K, Wolff AC, Winer E, Hudis C, Stopeck A, Beck JT, Kaur JS, Whelan K, Tu D, Parulekar WR (2016) Extending aromatase-inhibitor adjuvant therapy to 10 years. N Engl J Med 375:209–219

Gray RG, Rea D, Handley K, Bowden SJ, Perry P, Earl HM, Poole CJ, Bates T, Chetiyawardana S, Dewar JA, Fernado IN, Grieve R, Nichol J, Rayter Z, Robinson A, Salman A, Yarnold J, Bathers S, Marshall A, Lee M, on behalf of the aTTom collaborative group (2013) Attom: Long term effects of continuing adjuvant tamoxifen to 10 years versus stopping at 5 years in 6953 women with early breast cancer. J Clin Oncol 2013:31(abstract 5)

Grinshpun A, Chen V, Sandusky ZM, Fanning SW, Jeselsohn R (2023) ESR1 activating mutations: From structure to clinical application. Biochim Biophys Acta Rev Cancer 1878:188830. https://doi.org/10.1016/j.bbcan.2022.188830

Haddow A, Watkinson JM, Paterson E, Koller PC (1944) Influence of synthetic estrogens on advanced malignant disease. BMJ 2:393–398. https://doi.org/10.1136/bmj.2.4368.393

Hamilton E, Vahdat L, Han HS, Ranciato J, Gedrich R, Keung CF, Chirnomas D, Hurvitz S (2022) First-in-human safety and activity of ARV-471, a novel PROTAC® estrogen receptor degrader, in ER+/HER2-locally advanced or metastatic breast cancer. Cancer Res 82(2022). https://doi.org/10.1158/1538-7445.SABCS21-PD13-08

Harper MJ, Walpole AL (1966) Contrasting endocrine activities of cis and trans isomers in a series of substituted triphenylethylenes. Nature 212:87. https://doi.org/10.1038/212087a0

Harper MJ, Walpole AL (1967) A new derivative of triphenylethylene: effect on implantation and mode of action in rats. J Reprod Fertil 13:101–119

Harvey JM, Clark GM, Osborne CK, Allred DC (1999) Estrogen receptor status by immunohistochemistry is superior to the ligand-binding assay for predicting response to adjuvant endocrine therapy in breast cancer. J Clin Oncol 17:1474–1481. https://doi.org/10.1200/JCO.1999.17.5.1474

Howell A (2005) New developments in the treatment of postmenopausal breast cancer. Trends Endocrinol Metab 16:420–428

Howell A, Robertson J (1995) Response to a specific antiestrogen (ICI 182780) in tamoxifen-resistant breast cancer. Lancet 345:989–990. https://doi.org/10.1016/S0140-6736(95)90739-4

Howell A, DeFriend DJ, Robertson JF, Blamey RW, Anderson L, Anderson E, Sutcliffe FA, Walton P (1996) Pharmacokinetics, pharmacological and anti-tumour effects of the specific anti-estrogen ICI 182780 in women with advanced breast cancer. Br J Cancer 74:300–308

Howell A, Robertson JF, Quaresma Albano J, Aschermannova A, Mauriac L, Kleeberg UR, Vergote I, Erikstein B, Webster A, Morris C (2002) Fulvestrant, formerly ICI 182,780, is as effective as anastrozole in postmenopausal women with advanced breast cancer progressing after prior endocrine treatment. J Clin Oncol 20:3396–3403

Hu XF, Veroni M, De Luise M, Wakeling A, Sutherland R, Watts CK, Zalcberg JR (1993) Circumvention of tamoxifen resistance by the pure anti-estrogen ICI 182,780. Int J Cancer 55:873–876

Iqbal R, Yaqub M, Bektas HO, Oprea-Lager DE, de Vries EGE, Glaudemans AWJM, Aftimos P, Gebhart G, Beelen AP, Schuit RC, Windhorst AD, Boellaard R, Menke-van der Houven van Oordt CW (2023) [18F] FDG and [18F]FES PET/CT imaging as a biomarker for therapy effect in patients with metastatic ER+ breast cancer undergoing treatment with Rintodestrant. Clin Cancer Res 29:2075–2084

Iwamoto T, Booser D, Valero V, Murray JL, Koenig K, Esteva FJ, Ueno NT, Zhang J, Shi W, Qi Y, Matsuoka J, Yang EJ, Hortobagyi GN, Hatzis C, Symmans WF, Pusztai L (2012) Estrogen receptor (ER) mRNA and ER-related gene expression in breast cancers that are 1% to 10% ER-positive by immunohistochemistry. J Clin Oncol 30:729–734. https://doi.org/10.1200/JCO.2011.36.2574

Jhaveri KL, Jeselsohn R, Lim E, Hamilton EP, Yonemori K, Beck JT, Kaufman PA, Sammons S, Bhave MA, Saura C, Calvo E (2022) A phase 1a/b trial of imlunestrant (LY3484356), an oral selective estrogen receptor degrader (SERD) in ER-positive (ER+) advanced breast cancer (aBC) and endometrial endometrioid cancer (EEC): Monotherapy results from EMBER. J

Clin Oncol 40:1021. https://doi.org/10.1200/JCO.2022.40.16_suppl.1021

Jimenez MM, Lim E, Mac Gregor MC, Bardia A, Wu J, Zhang Q, Nowecki Z, Cruz F, Safin R, Kim SB, Schem C (2022) Giredestrant (GDC-9545) vs physician choice of endocrine monotherapy (PCET) in patients (pts) with ER+, HER2–locally advanced/metastatic breast cancer (LA/mBC): primary analysis of the phase II, randomised, open-label acelERA BC study. Ann Oncol 33:S633–S634

Kalinsky K, Barlow WE, Gralow JR et al (2021) 21-Gene assay to inform chemotherapy benefit in node-positive breast cancer. N Engl J Med 385:2336–2347

Kim C, Tang G, Pogue-Geile KL, Costantino JP, Baehner FL, Baker J, Cronin MT, Watson D, Shak S, Bohn OL, Fumagalli D, Taniyama Y, Lee A, Reilly ML, Vogel VG, McCaskill-Stevens W, Ford LG, Geyer CE Jr, Wickerham DL, Wolmark N, Paik S (2011) Estrogen receptor (ESR1) mRNA expression and benefit from tamoxifen in the treatment and prevention of estrogen receptor-positive breast cancer. J Clin Oncol 29:4160–4167. https://doi.org/10.1200/JCO.2010.32.9615

Klijn JG, de Jong FH (1982) Treatment with a luteinising-hormone-releasing-hormone analogue (buserelin)in premenopausal patients with metastatic breast cancer. Lancet 319:1213–1216

Klijn JG, de Jong FH, Blankenstein MA, Docter R, Alexieva-Figusch J, Blonk-van der Wijst J, Lamberts SW (1984) Anti-tumor and endocrine effects of chronic LHRH agonist treatment (Buserelin) with or without tamoxifen in premenopausal metastatic breast cancer. Breast Cancer Res Treat 4(3):209–220

Klijn JG, Blamey RW, Boccardo F, Tominaga T, Duchateau L, Sylvester R, Combined Hormone Agents Trialists' Group and the European Organization for Research and Treatment of Cancer (2001) Combined tamoxifen and luteinizing hormone-releasing hormone (LHRH) agonist versus LHRH agonist alone in premenopausal advanced breast cancer: a meta-analysis of four randomized trials. J Clin Oncol 19:343–353

Lawson M, Cureton N, Ros S, Cheraghchi-Bashi A, Urosevic J, D'Arcy S, Delpuech O, DuPont M, Fisher DI, Gangl ET, Lewis H (2023) The next-generation oral selective estrogen receptor degrader camizestrant (AZD9833) suppresses ER+ breast cancer growth and overcomes endocrine and CDK4/6 inhibitor resistance. Cancer Res 83(23):3989–4004

Liang J, Zbieg JR, Blake RA, Chang JH, Daly S, DiPasquale AG, Friedman LS, Gelzleichter T, Gill M, Giltnane JM, Goodacre S, Guan J, Hartman SJ, Ingalla ER, Kategaya L, Kiefer JR, Kleinheinz T, Labadie SS, Lai T, Li J, Liao J, Liu Z, Mody V, McLean N, Metcalfe C, Nannini MA, Oeh J, O'Rourke MG, Ortwine DF, Ran Y, Ray NC, Roussel F, Sambrone A, Sampath D, Schutt LK, Vinogradova M, Wai J, Wang T, Wertz IE, White JR, Yeap SK, Young A, Zhang B, Zheng X, Zhou W, Zhong Y, Wang X (2021) GDC-9545 (Giredestrant): a potent and orally bioavailable selective estrogen receptor antagonist and degrader with an exceptional preclinical profile for ER+ breast cancer. J Med Chem 64:11841–11856

Lin NU, Borges VF, Patel MR, Okera M, Meisel J, Wesolowski J, Pluard T, Miller KD, McCarthy NJ, Conlin AK, Mahtani R, Sabanathan D, McCann KE, Roesch E, Mathauda-Sahota G, Schroeder J, Hamilton EP (2023) Updated results from the phase I/II study of OP-1250, an oral complete estrogen receptor (ER) antagonist (CERAN) and selective ER degrader (SERD) in patients (pts) with advanced or metastatic ER-positive, HER2-negative breast cancerAnnals of. Oncology 34(suppl_2):S334–S390. https://doi.org/10.1016/annonc/annonc1299

Long X, Nephew KP (2006) Fulvestrant (ICI 182,780)-dependent interacting proteins mediate immobilization and degradation of estrogen receptor-alpha. J Biol Chem 281:9607–9615

Lønning PE (1996) Aromatase inhibition for breast cancer treatment. Acta Oncol 35:38–43

Lønning PE (2004) Aromatase inhibitors in breast cancer. Endocr Relat Cancer 11:179–189

Lønning PE, Eikesdal HP (2013) Aromatase inhibition 2013: clinical state of the art and questions that remain to be solved. Endocr Relat Cancer 20:R183–R201

Macdonald C, Saunders CM, Keogh LA et al (2021) Breast cancer chemoprevention: use and views of australian women and their clinicians. Cancer Prev Res (Phila) 14:131–144. https://doi.org/10.1158/1940-6207.CAPR-20-0369

Martino S, Cauley JA, Barrett-Connor E et al (2004) Continuing outcomes relevant to Evista: breast cancer incidence in postmenopausal osteoporotic women in a randomized trial of raloxifene. J Natl Cancer Inst 96:1751–1761

Maynard PV, Nicholson RI (1979) Effects of high doses of a series of new luteinizing hormone-releasing hormone analogues in intact female rats. Br J Cancer 39:274–279

McGregor JI, Jordan VC (1998) Basic guide to the mechanisms of antiestrogen action. Pharmacol Rev 50:151–196

Milne RL, Kuchenbaecker KB, Michailidou K et al (2017) Identification of ten variants associated with risk of estrogen-receptor-negative breast cancer. Nat Genet 49:1767–1778. https://doi.org/10.1038/ng.3785

Nadji M, Gomez-Fernandez C, Ganjei-Azar P, Morales AR (2005) Immunohistochemistry of estrogen and progesterone receptors reconsidered: experience with 5993 breast cancers. Am J Clin Pathol 123: 21–27

Neven P, Stahl N, Vidal M, Pi A, Martín M, Harbeck N, Kaufman PA, Bidard F-C, Fasching PA, Aftimos P, Hamilton E, Carter S, Schmid P, Wheatley D, Bhave M, Hunt KK, Kulkarni SA, Ismail-Khan R, Karacsonyi C, Estrem ST, Ozbek U, Nguyen B, Ciruelos E (2023) A preoperative window-of-opportunity study of imlunestrant in estrogen receptor positive, HER2-negative early breast cancer: results from the EMBER-2 study. Cancer Res 83(5_Supplement):P6-10-06. https://doi.org/10.1158/1538-7445.SABCS22-P6-10-06

Nunn TW (1882) On Cancer of the Breast. J&A Churchill, London

Oliveira M, Pominchuck D, Nowecki Z, et al. GS3-02 - Camizestrant, a next generation oral SERD vs fulvestrant in postmenopausal women with advanced ER-positive HER2-negative breast cancer: Results of the randomized, multi-dose phase 2 SERENA-2 trial. SABCS 2022, San Antonio, TX

Osborne CK, Coronado-Heinsohn EB, Hilsenbeck SG, McCue BL, Wakeling AE, McClelland RA, Manning DL, Nicholson RI (1995) Comparison of the effects of a pure steroidal antiestrogen with those of tamoxifen in a model of human breast cancer. J Natl Cancer Inst 87:746–750

Osborne CK, Pippen J, Jones SE, Parker LM, Ellis M, Come S, Gertler SZ, May JT, Burton G, Dimery I, Webster A, Morris C, Elledge R, Buzdar A (2002) Double-blind, randomized trial comparing the efficacy and tolerability of fulvestrant versus anastrozole in postmenopausal women with advanced breast cancer progressing on prior endocrine therapy: results of a North American trial. J Clin Oncol 20:3386–3395

Pagani O, O'Neill A, Castiglione M et al (1998) Prognostic impact of amenorrhoea after adjuvant chemotherapy in premenopausal breast cancer patients with axillary node involvement: Results of the International Breast Cancer Study Group Trial VI. Eur J Cancer 34:632–640

Pagani O, Walley BA, Fleming GF, Colleoni M, Láng I, Gomez HL, Tondini C, Burstein HJ, Goetz MP, Ciruelos EM, Stearns V, Bonnefoi HR, Martino S, Geyer CE Jr, Chini C, Puglisi F, Spazzapan S, Ruhstaller T, Winer EP, Ruepp B, Loi S, Coates AS, Gelber RD, Goldhirsch A, Regan MM, Francis PA, SOFT and TEXT Investigators and the International Breast Cancer Study Group (a division of ETOP IBCSG Partners Foundation) (2023) Adjuvant exemestane with ovarian suppression in premenopausal breast cancer: long-term follow-up of the combined TEXT and SOFT trials. J Clin Oncol 41:1376–1382

Pan H, Gray R, Braybrooke J, Davies C, Taylor C, McGale P, Peto R, Pritchard KI, Bergh J, Dowsett M, Hayes DF, EBCTCG (2017) 20-year risks of breast-cancer recurrence after stopping endocrine therapy at 5 years. N Engl J Med 377(19):1836–1846. https://doi.org/10.1056/NEJMoa1701830. PMID: 29117498; PMCID: PMC5734609

Parisian AD, Barratt SA, Hodges-Gallagher L, Ortega FE, Peña G, Sapugay J, Robello B, Sun R, Kulp D, Palanisamy GS, Myles DC, Kushner PJ, Harmon CL (2023) Palazestrant (OP-1250), a complete estrogen receptor antagonist, inhibits wild-type and mutant ER-positive breast cancer models as monotherapy and in combination. Mol Cancer Ther. https://doi.org/10.1158/1535-7163.MCT-23-0351

Parker MG (1993) Action of "pure" antiestrogens in inhibiting estrogen receptor action. Breast Cancer Res Treat 26(2):131–137

Paterson R, Russel MH (1959) Clinical trials in malignant disease. Part II-breast cancer: value of irradiation of the ovaries. J Fac Radiol 10:130–133

Petrelli F, Cavallone M, Dottorini L (2023) 10 years or less of extended adjuvant endocrine therapy for postmenopausal breast cancer patients: a systematic review and network meta-analysis. Eur J Cancer 193:113322

Pink JJ, Jordan VC (1996) Models of estrogen receptor regulation by estrogens and antiestrogens in breast cancer cell lines. Cancer Res 56:2321–2330

Powles TJ, Ashley S, Tidy A, Smith IE, Dowsett M (2007) Twenty-year follow-up of the Royal Marsden randomized, double-blinded tamoxifen breast cancer prevention trial. J Natl Cancer Inst 99:283–290. https://doi.org/10.1093/jnci/djk050

Pyrhönen S, Ellmén J, Vuorinen J, Gershanovich M, Tominaga T, Kaufmann M, Hayes DF (1999) Meta-analysis of trials comparing toremifene with tamoxifen and factors predicting outcome of antiestrogen therapy in postmenopausal women with breast cancer. Breast Cancer Res Treat 56:133–143

Rastogi P, O'Shaughnessy J, Martin M, Boyle F, Cortes J, Rugo HS, Goetz MP, Hamilton EP, Huang CS, Senkus E, Tryakin A, Cicin I, Testa L, Neven P, Huober J, Shao Z, Wei R, André V, Munoz M, San Antonio B, Shahir A, Harbeck N, Johnston S (2024) Adjuvant abemaciclib plus endocrine therapy for hormone receptor-positive, human epidermal growth factor receptor 2-negative, high-risk early breast cancer: results from a preplanned monarchE overall survival interim analysis, including 5-year efficacy outcomes. J Clin Oncol:JCO2301994. https://doi.org/10.1200/JCO.23.01994

Regan MM, Neven P, Giobbie-Hurder A, Goldhirsch A, Ejlertsen B, Mauriac L, Forbes JF, Smith I, Láng I, Wardley A, Rabaglio M, Price KN, Gelber RD, Coates AS, Thürlimann B, BIG 1-98 Collaborative Group; International Breast Cancer Study Group (IBCSG) (2011) Assessment of letrozole and tamoxifen alone and in sequence for postmenopausal women with steroid hormone receptor-positive breast cancer: the BIG 1-98 randomised clinical trial at 8·1 years median follow-up. Lancet Oncol 12:1101–1108

Ribi K, Luo W, Bernhard J et al (2016) Adjuvant tamoxifen plus ovarian function suppression versus tamoxifen alone in premenopausal women with early breast cancer: patient-reported outcomes in the Suppression of Ovarian Function Trial. J Clin Oncol 34:1601–1610

Richardson H, Ho V, Pasquet R, Singh RJ, Goetz MP, Tu D, Goss PE, Ingle JN, MAP.3 Investigators (2020) Baseline estrogen levels in postmenopausal women participating in the MAP.3 breast cancer chemoprevention trial. Menopause 27:693–700

Robertson JF, Nicholson RI, Bundred NJ, Anderson E, Rayter Z, Dowsett M, Fox JN, Gee JM, Webster A, Wakeling AE, Morris C, Dixon M (2001) Comparison of the short-term biological effects of 7alpha-[9-(4,4,5,5,5-pentafluoropentylsulfinyl)-nonyl]estra-1,3,5, (10)-triene-3,17beta-diol (Faslodex) versus tamoxifen in postmenopausal women with primary breast cancer. Cancer Res 61:6739–6746

Robertson JFR, Bondarenko IM, Trishkina E, Dvorkin M, Panasci L, Manikhas A, Shparyk Y, Cardona-Huerta S, Cheung KL, Philco-Salas MJ, Ruiz-Borrego M, Shao Z, Noguchi S, Rowbottom J, Stuart M, Grinsted LM, Fazal M, Ellis MJ (2016) Fulvestrant 500 mg versus anastrozole 1 mg for hormone receptor-positive advanced breast cancer (FALCON): an international, randomised, double-blind, phase 3 trial. Lancet 388:2997–3005

Robertson J, Shao Z, Noguchi S, Singh S, Subramaniam S, Ellis MJ (2023) Final overall survival analysis for fulvestrant vs anastrozole in endocrine therapy (ET)-naïve, hormone receptor-positive (HR+) advanced breast cancer (FALCON). Ann Oncol 34:S334–S390

Robson JM, Schönberg A, Fahim HA (1938) Duration of action of natural and synthetic estrogens. Nature 142:292. https://doi.org/10.1038/142292a0

Rugo HS (2023) Addressing unmet need in the management of patients with ER+/HER2-, ESR1-mutated metastatic breast cancer: clinician's perspective. Clin Adv Hematol Oncol 21:623–632

Rydén L, Jönsson PE, Chebil G, Dufmats M, Fernö M, Jirström K, Källström AC, Landberg G, Stål O, Thorstenson S, Nordenskjöld B, South Swedish Breast Cancer Group; South-East Swedish Breast Cancer Group (2005) Two years of adjuvant tamoxifen in premenopausal patients with breast cancer: a randomised, controlled trial with long-term follow-up. Eur J Cancer 41:256–264. https://doi.org/10.1016/j.ejca.2004.06.030

Samojlik E, Veldhuis JD, Wells SA, Santen RJ (1980) Preservation of androgen secretion during estrogen suppression with aminoglutethimide in the treatment of metastatic breast carcinoma. J Clin Invest 65:602–612

Santen RJ, Santner S, Davis B, Veldhuis J, Samojlik E, Ruby E (1978) Aminoglutethimide inhibits extraglandular estrogen production in postmenopausal women with breast carcinoma. J Clin Endocrinol Metab 47:1257–1265

Schinzinger A. Ueber carcinoma mammae. In 18th congress of the German society for surgery 1889;16: 55–56

Schuster EF, Lopez-Knowles E, Alataki A, Zabaglo L, Folkerd E, Evans D, Sidhu K, Cheang MCU, Tovey H, Salto-Tellez M, Maxwell P, Robertson J, Smith I, Bliss JM, Dowsett M (2023) Molecular profiling of aromatase inhibitor sensitive and resistant ER+HER2- postmenopausal breast cancers. Nat Commun 14:4017. https://doi.org/10.1038/s41467-023-39613-z

Sgroi DC, Treuner K, Zhang Y, Piper T, Salunga R, Ahmed I, Doos L, Thornber S, Taylor KJ, Brachtel E, Pirrie S, Schnabel CA, Rea D, Bartlett JMS (2022) Correlative studies of the Breast Cancer Index (HOXB13/IL17BR) and ER, PR, AR, AR/ER ratio and Ki67 for prediction of extended endocrine therapy benefit: a TransaTTom study. Breast Cancer Res 24:90. https://doi.org/10.1186/s13058-022-01589-x. PMID: 36527133

Shah M, Lingam H, Gao X, Gittleman H, Fiero MH, Krol D, Biel N, Ricks TK, Fu W, Hamed S, Li F, Sun JJ, Fan J, Schuck R, Grimstein M, Tang L, Kalavar S, Abukhdeir A, Pathak A, Ghosh S, Bulatao I, Tilley A, Pierce WF, Mixter BD, Tang S, Pazdur R, Kluetz P, Amiri-Kordestani L (2024) US food and drug administration approval summary: elacestrant for estrogen receptor-positive, human epidermal growth factor receptor 2-negative, esr1-mutated advanced or metastatic breast cancer. J Clin Oncol JCO2302112. doi: https://doi.org/10.1200/JCO.23.02112

Shiau AK, Barstad D, Loria PM, Cheng L, Kushner PJ, Agard DA, Greene GL (1998) The structural basis of estrogen receptor/coactivator recognition and the antagonism of this interaction by tamoxifen. Cell 95:927–937

Smith IE, Harris AL, Morgan M, Ford HT, Gazet JC, Harmer CL, White H, Parsons CA, Villardo A, Walsh G, McKinna JA (1981) Tamoxifen versus aminoglutethimide in advanced breast carcinoma: a randomized cross-over trial. Br Med J (Clin Res Ed) 283:1432–1434

Smith I, Yardley D, Burris H, De Boer R, Amadori D, McIntyre K, Ejlertsen B, Gnant M, Jonat W, Pritchard KI, Dowsett M, Hart L, Poggio S, Comarella L, Salomon H, Wamil B, O'Shaughnessy J (2017) Comparative efficacy and safety of adjuvant letrozole versus anastrozole in postmenopausal patients with hormone receptor-positive, node-positive early breast cancer: final results of the randomized phase III femara versus anastrozole clinical evaluation (FACE) trial. J Clin Oncol 35:1041–1048

Snyder LB, Flanagan JJ, Qian Y, Gough SM, Andreoli M, Bookbinder M, Cadelina G, Bradley J, Rousseau E, Chandler J, Willard R, Pizzano J, Crews CM, Crew AP, Houston J, Moore MD, Peck R, Taylor I (2021) The discovery of ARV-471, an orally bioavailable estrogen receptor degrading PROTAC for the treatment of patients with breast cancer [abstract]. Cancer Res 81(13_Suppl):Abstract nr 44

Sparano JA, Gray RJ, Ravdin PM et al (2019) Clinical and genomic risk to guide the use of adjuvant therapy for breast cancer. N Engl J Med 380:2395–2405

Srinivasan S, Nwachukwu JC, Bruno NE, Dharmarajan V, Goswami D, Kastrati I, Novick S, Nowak J, Cavett V, Zhou HB, Boonmuen N, Zhao Y, Min J, Frasor J, Katzenellenbogen BS, Griffin PR, Katzenellenbogen JA, Nettles KW (2017) Full antagonism of the estrogen receptor without a prototypical ligand side chain. Nat Chem Biol 13(1):111–118. https://doi.org/10.1038/nchembio.2236

Thorneloe RJ, Hall LH, Walter FM, Side L, Lloyd KE, Smith SG, ENGAGE Investigators (2020) Knowledge of potential harms and benefits of tamoxifen among women considering breast cancer preventive therapy. Cancer Prev Res (Phila) 13:411–422. https://doi.org/10.1158/1940-6207.CAPR-19-0424

Tominaga T, Kimijima I, Kimura M, Takatsuka Y, Takashima S, Nomura Y, Kasumi F, Yamaguchi A, Masuda N, Noguchi S, Eshima N (2010) Effects of toremifene and tamoxifen on lipid profiles in postmenopausal patients with early breast cancer: interim results from a Japanese phase III trial. Jpn J Clin Oncol 40:627–633

Turner N, Vaklavas C, Calvo E, Garcia-Corbacho J, Incorvati J, Borrego MR, Twelves C, Armstrong A, Bermejo B, Hamilton E, Oliveira M (2022) SERENA-1: updated analyses from a Phase 1 study of the next generation oral selective estrogen receptor degrader camizestrant (AZD9833) combined with abemaciclib, in women with ER-positive, HER2-negative advanced breast cancer. SABCS. Abstract P3-07-28

Turner N, Huang-Bartlett C, Kalinsky K, Cristofanilli M, Bianchini G, Chia S, Iwata H, Janni W, Ma CX, Mayer EL, Park YH, Fox S, Liu X, McClain S, Bidard FC (2023) Design of SERENA-6, a phase III switching trial of camizestrant in ESR1-mutant breast cancer during first-line treatment. Future Oncol 19:559–573

Veronesi U, Maisonneuve P, Costa A et al (1998) Prevention of breast cancer with tamoxifen: preliminary findings from the Italian randomised trial among hysterectomised women. Italian Tamoxifen Prevention Study. Lancet 352:93–97

Veronesi U, Maisonneuve P, Rotmensz N, Bonanni B, Boyle P, Viale G, Costa A, Sacchini V, Travaglini R, D'Aiuto G, Oliviero P, Lovison F, Gucciardo G, del Turco MR, Muraca MG, Pizzichetta MA, Conforti S, Decensi A, Italian Tamoxifen Study Group (2007) Tamoxifen for the prevention of breast cancer: late results of the Italian randomized tamoxifen prevention trial among women with hysterectomy. J Natl Cancer Inst 99(9):727–737. https://doi.org/10.1093/jnci/djk154

Vidal M, Pascual T, Falato C, Sanchez-Bayona R, Muñoz M, Cerbrecos I, Gonzalez-Farré X, Cortadellas T, Margelí M, Luna MA (2023) Abstract PD13-01: PD13-01 Elacestrant in postmenopausal women with estrogen receptor positive and HER2-negative early breast cancer: primary efficacy and safety analysis of the preoperative, window of opportunity SOLTI-1905-ELIPSE trial. Cancer Res 83(Suppl. S5):PD13-01

Vogel VG, Costantino JP, Wickerham DL et al (2010) Update of the national surgical adjuvant breast and bowel project study of tamoxifen and raloxifene (STAR) P-2 trial: preventing breast cancer. Cancer Prev Res 3:696–706

Wang X, Qin ZL, Li N, Jia MQ, Liu QG, Bai YR, Song J, Yuan S, Zhang SY (2024) Annual review of PROTAC degraders as anticancer agents in 2022. Eur J Med Chem 267:116166. https://doi.org/10.1016/j.ejmech.2024.116166

Wardell SE, Marks JR, McDonnell DP (2011) The turnover of estrogen receptor alpha by the selective estrogen receptor degrader (SERD) fulvestrant is a saturable process that is not required for antagonist efficacy. Biochem Pharmacol 82:122–130

Will M, Liang J, Metcalfe C, Chandarlapaty S (2023) Therapeutic resistance to anti-oestrogen therapy in breast cancer. Nat Rev Cancer 23:673–685

Williams MR, Walker KJ, Turkes A, Blamey RW, Nicholson RI (1986) The use of an LH-RH agonist (ICI 118630, Zoladex) in advanced premenopausal breast cancer. Br J Cancer 53(5):629–636

23 CDK4/6 Inhibitor Resistance in ER+ Breast Cancer

Ilenia Migliaccio, Cristina Guarducci, and Luca Malorni

Abstract

The cyclin-dependent kinases 4 and 6 inhibitors are the mainstay of treatment for patients with hormone receptor-positive and HER2-negative breast cancer. The ability of these drugs to improve the outcome of patients both in the metastatic and the early setting has been largely demonstrated. However, resistance, either de novo or acquired, represents a major clinical challenge. In the past years, efforts have been made to identify biomarkers that might help in a better selection of patients or to unravel the mechanisms leading to resistance in order to develop new therapeutic strategies to overcome it. Alterations of cell cycle-related genes and proteins are among the best characterized markers of resistance, and pathways impacting the cell cycle, including nuclear and growth factor receptors signaling, have been thoroughly investigated. Despite this, to date, cyclin-dependent kinases 4 and 6 inhibitors are administered based only on the hormone receptor and HER2 status of the tumor, and patients progressing on therapy are managed with currently available treatments. Here we summarize present knowledge on the cyclin-dependent kinases 4 and 6 inhibitors' mechanisms of action, efficacy data, and mechanisms of resistance.

Keywords

CDK4/6 inhibitors · Resistance · Breast cancer · Cell cycle · Biomarkers

Key Points

- To understand the role of cyclin D-CDK4/6-Rb axis dysregulation in breast cancer
- To gain insight into the most relevant clinical data on CDK4/6 inhibitors in breast cancer
- To deepen the knowledge about selected mechanisms of resistance to CDK4/6 inhibitors in breast cancer
- To comprehend the importance of the identification of new biomarkers or targets for new therapies in the field of CDK4/6i research

I. Migliaccio · C. Guarducci · L. Malorni (✉)
Translational Research Unit, Hospital of Prato, AUSL Toscana Centro, Prato, Italy
e-mail: ilenia.migliaccio@uslcentro.toscana.it; cristina.guarducci@uslcentro.toscana.it; luca.malorni@uslcentro.toscana.it

T. Sørlie, R. B. Clarke (eds.), *A Guide to Breast Cancer Research*, Advances in Experimental Medicine and Biology 1464, https://doi.org/10.1007/978-3-031-70875-6_23

23.1 Introduction

In the past 10 years, the cyclin-dependent kinases (CDK) 4 and 6 inhibitors (CDK4/6i) palbociclib, ribociclib, abemaciclib, and more recently dalpiciclib have revolutionized the treatment of hormone receptor-positive and human epidermal growth factor receptor 2-negative (HR+/HER2-) breast cancer. These drugs are currently administered in combination with endocrine therapy (ET) in patients with advanced HR+/HER2- disease, both pretreated and untreated. In addition, abemaciclib might be administered as a single agent in heavily pretreated patients with HR+/HER2- metastatic breast cancer and has received the approval for the adjuvant setting, where it is indicated for 2 years in combination with ET in patients with early HR+/HER2- breast cancer at high risk of relapse. At present, dalpiciclib is approved for clinical use only in China.

Despite the great efficacy demonstrated by these agents, in the metastatic setting about 10–15% of patients recur early, demonstrating de novo resistance, and nearly all patients eventually progress, due to acquired resistance. Great efforts are being made to identify mechanisms underpinning both de novo and acquired resistance, in order to develop clinically useful biomarkers for patient stratification and efficacious treatment strategies for the resistant population.

In this chapter, we aim to give an overview of the role of CDK4/6 inhibitors in breast cancer and to provide an up-to-date revision of the resistance mechanisms with a special focus on those that might allow the identification of valuable biomarkers or be targets for innovative treatments.

23.2 Cell Cycle and the Role of Cyclin D-CDK4/6-Rb Axis

Cell cycle comprises a complex and organized series of biological processes that allow cells to grow, replicate, and divide. It proceeds through four phases: Gap1 (G1), during which the cell grows; synthesis (S), the phase of DNA replication; Gap2 (G2) in which the cell prepares to divide; and mitosis (M), the phase of the actual cell division (Vermeulen et al. 2003). Progression through the phases is tightly regulated at multiple checkpoints (G1, G2, and M checkpoints), with the G1 checkpoint, also called restriction point, being particularly critical, as it represents the irreversible commitment point for cell division (Vermeulen et al. 2003). Cell cycle is governed by cyclins, regulatory proteins whose levels fluctuate during cell cycle phases, that bind to and control the activity of a group of serine/threonine kinases, the cyclin-dependent kinases (CDKs). Among cyclins and CDKs, the D- (D1, D2, and D3) and E- (E1 and E2) type cyclins and CDK4, CDK6, and CDK2 are critical for the G1/S phase transition (Vermeulen et al. 2003). During the early G1 checkpoint, the levels of cyclin D rise and bind preferentially to CDK4/6. Cyclin D-CDK4/6 complex initiates the phosphorylation of the retinoblastoma susceptibility gene product (Rb), a negative regulator of the G1/S transition (Henley and Dick 2012). Rb and the other Rb family members, p107 and p130, in their hypo-phosphorylated status, bind to and inactivate the transcription factors of the E2F family (Henley and Dick 2012). During the late G1 checkpoint, the increased levels of cyclin E and the complete phosphorylation of Rb by the cyclin E-CDK2 complex induce the release of the E2F factors and the subsequent transcription of genes essential for the transition to the S phase (Henley and Dick 2012).

The cyclin D-CDK4/6-Rb axis is regulated at multiple levels, including transcription of cyclins and assembly, stability, subcellular localization, and phosphorylation status of the cyclin-CDK complexes. Additional regulation is provided by the association with specific inhibitory proteins, the CDK inhibitors (CKI) (Vidal and Koff 2000). These belong to two different families, the CIP-KIP family, including p21Cip1 (p21), p27Kip1 (p27), and p57Kip2 (p57), which preferentially inhibit CDK2-containg complexes, and the INK4 family, including p16Ink4a (p16), p15Ink4b (p15), p18Ink4c (p18), and p19Ink4d (p19), which mainly inhibit CDK4-associated activities (Vidal and Koff 2000). A variety of internal and external cues also insist on the cyclin D-CDK4/6-Rb axis and modulate its activity

(Lukas et al. 1996; Fu et al. 2004), including signals originating from nuclear receptors, growth factors and growth factor receptors, cytokines, cell-adhesion machinery, and extracellular matrix but also metabolic changes, DNA damage, and cell size sensors.

23.3 Cyclin D-CDK4/6-Rb Axis and Breast Cancer

In breast cancer, dysregulation of the cyclin D-CDK4/6-Rb axis plays a major role in tumor growth. Genetic alterations, including mutations, amplifications and deletions, and transcriptional modulations of the members of the cyclin D-CDK4/6-Rb axis are frequent findings in breast cancer (Koboldt et al. 2012). Cyclin D1 is overexpressed in 30–40% of breast cancer, often due to gene (*CCND1*) amplification, and gain of copy number of *CDK4* can also be observed, with both alterations being most frequently observed in luminal and HER2+ breast cancer. On the other hand, loss of *RB1*, the gene encoding for Rb, and overexpression of p16 are typically observed in basal-like breast cancers (Koboldt et al. 2012).

Many stimuli that impact the cyclin D-CDK4/6-Rb axis are well-recognized oncogenic drivers in breast cancer. *ERBB2* oncogene is overexpressed/amplified in 20–30% of breast cancers, and the cyclin D-CDK4/6-Rb axis has been shown essential for HER2-driven oncogenesis (Reddy et al. 2005; Nikolai et al. 2016). Amplification and/or overexpression of the proto-oncogene *MYC,* a transcription factor involved in cellular proliferation, is found in 15–40% of breast cancer (Xu et al. 2010). MYC was shown to regulate the expression of several cell cycle components, including CDK4 and cyclin D1 (Zafonte et al. 2000; Xu et al. 2010).

In breast cancer, estrogens and estrogen receptors (ER) are the major drivers of proliferation. ER favors G1/S transition by increasing the expression of cyclin D1 and MYC, both being ER-dependent genes, and by inducing the dissociation of p21 from the cyclin E-CDK2 complex (Saha et al. 2021). Of note, cyclin D1 can enhance ER-mediated transcription (Zwijsen et al. 1998). Breast cancers expressing ER respond to ET, including the selective ER modulator (SERM) tamoxifen, the selective ER degrader (SERD) fulvestrant, and the aromatase inhibitors (AI) anastrozole, letrozole, and exemestane. ET is highly effective, but resistance represents a major clinical hurdle. The cyclin D-CDK4/6-Rb axis has been implicated in ET resistance. *CCND1* overexpression/amplification has been linked to tamoxifen resistance (Stendahl et al. 2004; Jirström et al. 2005), and it was shown that the activation of ER induced by cyclin D1 is not inhibited by antiestrogens (Zwijsen et al. 1998). CDK6 overexpression might induce fulvestrant resistance (Giessrigl et al. 2013; Alves et al. 2016), and gene signatures of E2F activation have been associated with resistance to AI (Miller et al. 2011; Guerrero-Zotano et al. 2018). Breast cancers resistant to ET were shown to maintain high cyclin D1 levels and phosphorylation of Rb despite ER inhibition (Thangavel et al. 2011). FOXM1, a transcription factor involved in ET resistance (Millour et al. 2010), which is both a target and a regulator of ER (Sanders et al. 2013), was shown to be also regulated by CDK4/6 (Wierstra and Alves 2006; Anders et al. 2011).

These observations have suggested that cyclin D-CDK4/6 axis may represent an optimal target for the treatment of breast cancer, particularly the ER+ luminal subtype.

23.4 CDK4/6 Inhibitors (CDK4/6i) in Breast Cancer

Palbociclib, abemaciclib, ribociclib, and dalpiciclib are small-molecule, orally bioavailable, selective inhibitors of CDK4 and CDK6 which bind to the kinase ATP pocket and compete with its ligand, therefore preventing Rb phosphorylation and progression to the S phase. Despite a similar mechanism of action, slight differences in their structure, binding affinity, and profile exist, which might possibly explain some of the observed disparities in clinical activity, toxicity, and resistance mechanisms (Marra and Curigliano 2019; George et al. 2021; Grinshpun et al. 2023;

Johnston et al. 2023a). Palbociclib and ribociclib are more lipophilic and have different chemical structures from abemaciclib (Chen et al. 2016; Marra and Curigliano 2019). Palbociclib and dalpiciclib exert similar inhibition on both CDK4 and CDK6, while ribociclib and abemaciclib have a more potent effect on CDK4 than CDK6, with abemaciclib having the greatest CDK4/CDK6 inhibition ratio (Chen et al. 2016). In addition, abemaciclib was shown to exhibit inhibitory effects on other kinases, including CDK2 and CDK1 (Chen et al. 2016; Hafner et al. 2019). The main effect of CDK4/6i on cells is G1 arrest and senescence, a cellular state characterized by exit from cell cycle, associated with phenotypical, biochemical, and metabolic changes. However, G2 arrest and apoptotic and cytotoxic effects have been described for abemaciclib (Torres-Guzmán et al. 2017; Hafner et al. 2019). Another peculiarity of abemaciclib is the higher ability to cross the blood-brain barrier (Raub et al. 2015). Palbociclib, ribociclib, and dalpiciclib are administered once a day intermittently with a schedule of 21 days on and 7 days off, while abemaciclib, which has a shorter half-life, is administered twice a day, continuously. The reported side effects for palbociclib, ribociclib, and dalpiciclib are mainly hematological, with neutropenia being the most common adverse event (Finn et al. 2021; Burris et al. 2021). The most frequently reported adverse event with abemaciclib is diarrhea, while neutropenia is not common during abemaciclib treatment (Rugo et al. 2021a).

Multiple preclinical studies have demonstrated excellent activity of CDK4/6i in breast cancer models, particularly in the HR+/HER2- breast cancer subtype and in combination with ET (Finn et al. 2009; Thangavel et al. 2011; Torres-Guzmán et al. 2017; Long et al. 2019). The clinical development of these agents has followed mainly in the luminal breast cancer subtypes. In the metastatic setting, phase 3 randomized clinical trials investigating the clinical efficacy of the association of CDK4/6i with ET in HR+/HER2- advanced breast cancer demonstrated a significant improvement in progression-free survival (PFS) for the combination over ET alone, with very similar magnitude among the different CDK4/6i (Table 23.1). More recently, data on the overall survival (OS) became available and demonstrated a significant improvement for ribociclib and abemaciclib and a numerical improvement for palbociclib, particularly in the population that benefited from previous ET (Turner et al. 2018). Given the great efficacy of CDK4/6i in the advanced disease, trials are assessing the benefit of combining these drugs with ET in the adjuvant setting. Two trials on palbociclib and ET in an unselected (PALLAS) or high-risk population (i.e., residual invasive disease after neoadjuvant chemotherapy and CPS-EG score ≥ 3 or 2 and node positive, PENELOPE) with HR+/HER2- early breast cancer failed to demonstrate a statistically significant improvement in invasive disease-free survival (iDFS), the primary endpoint of the studies (Table 23.1). On the other hand, the MONARCHE trial showed a statistically significant improvement in iDFS for high-risk patients (i.e., 4 or more positive nodes or 1–3 nodes and either tumor size ≥ 5 cm, histologic grade 3, or central Ki-67 $\geq$ 20%) receiving abemaciclib and ET compared to those receiving ET alone. In addition, early data from the NATALEE trial with ribociclib and ET in stage II–III breast cancer demonstrated the superiority of the combination over ET alone (Table 23.1).

Discrepant OS and iDFS data among CDK4/6i might be explained by multiple factors, including the different populations and trial design, statistical power, crossover rate (for OS data), and possibly differences among the agents, but more data are needed to elucidate discrepancies.

23.5 Mechanisms of Resistance to CDK4/6 Inhibitors

In breast cancer, multiple mechanisms of resistance to CDK4/6i have been described. Some of these directly modify cell cycle-related genes and proteins, while others engage pathways that indirectly involve or impact the cyclin D-CDK4/6-Rb axis.

Table 23.1 Most relevant clinical trials of CDK4/6 inhibitors in HR+/HER2- breast cancer according to clinical setting

Trial name (NCT)	Phase/population	Primary endpoint	Treatments	Main results
Clinical setting: neoadjuvant				
neoMONARCH (NCT02441946) (Hurvitz et al. 2020)	2/stage I–IIIB	Change in Ki67 after 2 weeks	Abemaciclib vs abemaciclib + anastrozole vs anastrozole	91% abemaciclib 93% combination 63% anastrozole
NeoPalAna (NCT01723774) (Ma et al. 2017)	2/stage II–III	CCCA (Ki67 ≤ 2.7%)	Anastrozole → anastrozole + palbociclib → anastrozole	87% vs 26% after combination
Clinical setting: adjuvant				
PALLAS (NCT02513394) (Gnant et al. 2022)	3/stage II–III	iDFS	Palbociclib (2 yrs) + adjuvant ET vs adjuvant ET	84.2% vs 84.5% (HR 0.96, 95% CI 0.81–1.14
PENELOPE (NCT01864746) (Loibl et al. 2021)	3/high risk after neoadjuvant CHT	iDFS	Palbociclib (1 yr) + adjuvant ET vs placebo + adjuvant ET	81.2% vs 77.7% (HR 0.93, 95% CI 0.74–1.17
MONARCHE (NCT03155997) (Johnston et al. 2023b)	3/high risk	iDFS	Abemaciclib (2 yrs) + adjuvant ET vs adjuvant ET	85.8% vs 79.4% (HR 0.664, 95% CI 0.578-0.762)
NATALEE (NCT03701334) (Slamon et al. 2023)	3/stage II–III	iDFS	Ribociclib (3 yrs) + adjuvant ET vs adjuvant ET	90.4% vs 87.1% (HR 0.748, 95% CI 0.618–0.906)
Clinical setting: advanced				
DAWNA 1 (NCT03927456) (Xu et al. 2021)	3/second line	PFS	Dalpiciclib + fulvestrant vs placebo + fulvestrant	15.7 vs 7.2 months (HR 0.42, 95% CI 0.31–0.58)
DAWNA 2 (NCT03966898) (Zhang et al. 2023)	3/first line	PFS	Dalpiciclib + NSAI vs placebo + NSAI	30.6 vs 18.2 months (HR 0·51, 95% CI 0·38–0·69]
MONALEESA 2 (NCT01958021) (Hortobagyi et al. 2016)	3/first line	PFS	Ribociclib + letrozole vs placebo + letrozole	NR vs 14.7 months (HR 0.56, 95% CI 0.43–0.72)
MONALEESA 3 (NCT02422615) (Slamon et al. 2018)	3/first or second line	PFS	Ribociclib + fulvestrant vs placebo + fulvestrant	20.5 vs 12.8 months (HR 0.593, 95% CI 0.480–0.732) in the overall population
MONALEESA 7 (NCT02278120) (Tripathy et al. 2018)	3/first line, Premenopausal	PFS	Ribociclib + tamoxifen or NSAI + goserelin vs placebo + tamoxifen or NSAI + goserelin	23.8 vs 13.0 months (HR 0.55, 95% CI 0.44–0.69)
MONARCH 1 (NCT02102490) (Dickler et al. 2017)	2/CHT and ET pretreated	ORR	Abemaciclib	19.7%
MONARCH 2 (NCT02107703) (Sledge et al. 2017)	3/second line	PFS	Abemaciclib + fulvestrant vs placebo + fulvestrant	16.4 vs 9.3 months (HR 0.553, 95% CI 0.449–0.681)
MONARCH 3 (NCT02246621) (Goetz et al. 2017)	3/first line	PFS	Abemaciclib + NSAI vs placebo + NSAI	NR vs 14.7 months (HR 0.54, 95% CI 0.41–0.72

(continued)

Table 23.1 (continued)

Trial name (NCT)	Phase/population	Primary endpoint	Treatments	Main results
PALOMA-1 (NCT00721409) (Finn et al. 2015)	2/first line	PFS	Palbociclib + letrozole vs letrozole	20.2 vs 10.2 months (HR 0.488, 95% CI 0.319–0.748)
PALOMA-2 (NCT01740427) (Finn et al. 2016)	3/first line	PFS	Palbociclib + letrozole vs placebo + letrozole	24.8 vs 14.5 months (HR 0.58, 95% CI 0.46–0.72)
PALOMA-3 (NCT01942135) (Turner et al. 2015)	3/Second line	PFS	Palbocicib + Fulvestrant vs placebo + fulvestrant	9.2 vs 3.8 months (HR 0.42, 95% CI 0.32–0.56
TREND (NCT02549430) (Malorni et al. 2018)	2/ET pretreated	CBR	Palbociclib vs palbociclib + ET previous line	60% vs 54%

CCCA complete cell cycle arrest, *iDFS* invasive disease-free survival, *ET* endocrine therapy, *CHT* chemotherapy, *PFS* progression-free survival, *NR* not reached, *NSAI* nonsteroidal aromatase inhibitor, *ORR* objective response rate, *CBR* clinical benefit rate

23.5.1 Cell Cycle-Related Proteins

23.5.1.1 Rb and Rb/E2F Signaling

Rb is the main target of CDK4/6i. Rb expression was highlighted as a key determinant of sensitivity in the pivotal preclinical study on palbociclib in breast cancer (Finn et al. 2009). Since then, the role of Rb in determining resistance to CDK4/6i has been largely investigated in preclinical and clinical/translational studies. Rb expression levels were shown to contribute to de novo (Dean et al. 2012) and acquired resistance in preclinical studies using in vitro models of ER+ breast cancer (Dean et al. 2010; Yang et al. 2017; Guarducci et al. 2018; Ogata et al. 2021; Ono et al. 2021). In addition to Rb expression, *RB1* mutations and/or copy-number loss were described during acquired resistance to CDK4/6i in vitro and in vivo (Herrera-Abreu et al. 2016; Guarducci et al. 2018; Pancholi et al. 2020; Soria-Bretones et al. 2022; Palafox et al. 2022). In clinical studies, mutations in *RB1* were associated with de novo resistance to CDK4/6i (Li et al. 2018; André et al. 2023) and were also shown to be acquired during or after treatment (Condorelli et al. 2018; O'Leary et al. 2018a; Abu-Khalaf et al. 2022; Goetz et al. 2023; Park et al. 2023). However, in the pivotal study from Finn and colleagues, three cell lines retaining Rb expression were resistant to palbociclib (Finn et al. 2009), and Rb expression was not predictive of resistance to palbociclib in the PALOMA clinical trials (Finn et al. 2015, 2020; Turner et al. 2019). In addition, in the NeoPalAna trial (Ma et al. 2017), two patients with *RB1* mutated tumors still responded to palbociclib, and in MONARCH-3, abemaciclib improved survival regardless of *RB1* baseline genomic alterations (Goetz et al. 2023). These data suggest that, despite the central role of Rb, additional mechanisms of resistance/sensitivity are likely to be involved.

With the hypothesis that investigating the downstream signaling of Rb might better predict response or resistance, a signature of E2F activation has been developed, the RBsig (Malorni et al. 2016). This was able to discriminate palbociclib-sensitive versus resistant luminal breast cancer cell lines (Malorni et al. 2016) and was enriched in patients resistant to CDK4/6i in the neoMONARCH and NeoPalAna trials (Hurvitz et al. 2020; De Angelis et al. 2021). In line with this data, in the PALOMA-3 trial, a gene expression signature of E2F targets, the E2F regulon, was shown to be significantly associated with a lack of PFS improvement in patients treated with palbociclib (Turner et al. 2019). However, to date, the clinical utility of assessing the expression levels of Rb, the *RB1* status, or the downstream signaling remains to be demonstrated.

23.5.1.2 Cyclins and CDKs

Cyclin D, CDK4, and CDK6

Cyclin D1 is the principal partner for CDK4 and CDK6 and has been largely implicated in breast cancer progression, prognosis, and resistance to ET (Musgrove et al. 2011), but its role in CDK4/6i response has not been clarified yet. It was first demonstrated that, in breast cancer cell lines, high cyclin D1 expression is associated with sensitivity to palbociclib (Finn et al. 2009), and in line with this data, the clinical trial MONALEESA-7 showed a greater benefit from ribociclib in patients with *CCND1* alterations on circulating tumor DNA (ctDNA) (Bardia et al. 2021). Nevertheless, it was shown that ER+ breast cancer cells might quickly adapt to and circumvent CDK4/6 inhibition through a noncanonical cyclin D1-CDK2 signaling (Herrera-Abreu et al. 2016), and recent reports indicate that *CCND1* levels might be upregulated at the time of acquired resistance to CDK4/6i in breast cancer cell lines (Kharenko et al. 2022; Kumar et al. 2023). In addition, no predictive role has been demonstrated for cyclin D1 expression and/or *CCND1* amplification in the PALOMA and MONALEESA-2 trials (Finn et al. 2015, 2020; Hortobagyi et al. 2018; Turner et al. 2019).

Equally controversial are the data on CDK4, which is expressed at high levels in luminal cells sensitive to CDK4/6i (Li et al. 2022) and shown to be downregulated at the time of CDK4/6i resistance (Iida et al. 2019). Accordingly, high *CDK4* mRNA expression was associated with greater benefit from palbociclib in the PALOMA-2 trial (Finn et al. 2020) and high baseline *CDK4* mRNA levels, isolated from exosomes in patients with advanced breast cancer treated with fulvestrant and palbociclib, correlated with longer PFS (Del Re et al. 2019). Nevertheless, some preclinical models of palbociclib-resistant ER+ BC cell lines did show increased expression of *CDK4* (Pancholi et al. 2020; Kumar et al. 2023), and no interaction between *CDK4* and treatment was found in the PALOMA-3 trial (Turner et al. 2019). CDK4 can be activated by phosphorylation. It was shown that the presence of phosphorylated CDK4, or a surrogate gene expression signature, might predict sensitivity to palbociclib in breast cancer cells (Raspé et al. 2017); however, the predictive value of this signature in clinical trials with CDK4/6i has not been tested.

More consistent are the preclinical data on CDK6. Both amplification and increased expression of *CDK6* have been described in cellular models of CDK4/6i-resistant breast cancer and knockdown of *CDK6* was able to restore sensitivity (Yang et al. 2017; Cornell et al. 2019; Iida et al. 2019; Ogata et al. 2021; Ono et al. 2021; Kharenko et al. 2022; Al-Qasem et al. 2022; Kumar et al. 2023). *CDK6* upregulation may result from dysregulations of different pathways. Mutations inducing a loss of function of the tumor suppressor *FAT1* have been linked to resistance to CDK4/6i in metastatic breast cancer patients (Li et al. 2018). *FAT1* loss and genomic alterations in additional genes, including *PTEN* and *ARID1A* (Li et al. 2022), were shown to mediate resistance to CDK4/6i by converging on *CDK6* upregulation through a modulation of the Hippo pathway (Li et al. 2018, 2022). In addition, *CDK6* overexpression was shown to be dependent on the overexpression of miR-423-5p, induced by the suppression of the TGFβ signaling (Cornell et al. 2019). However, in the PALOMA-2 and PALOMA-3 trials, no predictive value was found for *CDK6* expression (Turner et al. 2019; Finn et al. 2020), and to date there is no evidence that testing for *CDK6* alone might help selecting patients for CDK4/6i treatment.

Cyclin E and CDK2

The cyclin E-CDK2 complex phosphorylates Rb and plays a key role in G1/S transition in addition to cyclin D-CDK4/6. Overexpression of *CCNE1*, often as a result of gene amplification, was demonstrated in preclinical models of breast cancer with acquired resistance to CDK4/6i (Herrera-Abreu et al. 2016; Yang et al. 2017; Guarducci et al. 2018; Pancholi et al. 2020; Freeman-Cook et al. 2021; Al-Qasem et al. 2022). Moreover, it was shown that CDK2 activity can compensate

CDK4/6 inhibition and that targeting CDK2 acts synergistically with CDK4/6i and could re-sensitize tumors to CDK4/6i in vitro and in vivo (Herrera-Abreu et al. 2016; Patel et al. 2018; Pandey et al. 2020; Freeman-Cook et al. 2021; Al-Qasem et al. 2022; Dietrich et al. 2023). Gene expression analyses from tissue samples obtained from patients enrolled in the PALOMA-3 trial demonstrated that *CCNE1* levels might predict resistance to palbociclib (Turner et al. 2019), and in the same trial, gain of *CCNE1* copy number on ctDNA samples was associated with PFS only in the palbociclib-treated but not in the placebo-treated patients (O'Leary et al. 2018a). In line with this data, high *CCNE1* expression was associated with worse outcome in the MONALEESA-2 trial and in patients treated with palbociclib and ET within the PEARL study, comparing palbociclib and ET versus the chemotherapeutic agent capecitabine (Formisano et al. 2019; Guerrero-Zotano et al. 2023). However, no association with outcome was found for *CCNE1* levels in PALOMA-2 (Finn et al. 2020). Further data are needed to validate the role of *CCNE1* and *CDK2* as biomarkers or targets for therapy in CDK4/6i-resistant patients.

Cell Cycle Inhibitors

Inhibitors of the INK4 family have been linked to CDK4/6i resistance in preclinical models. Levels of p16 were low in the breast cancer cells most sensitive to palbociclib (Finn et al. 2009), while p16 overexpression has been associated with reduced ribociclib activity in breast patients-derived xenograft (Palafox et al. 2022). It was also recently demonstrated that members of the INK4 family, particularly p18 and p15, bind to CDK6 in CDK6-overexpressing BC models resistant to CDK4/6i. The association of CDK6 with INK4 was able to reduce CDK4/6i binding, therefore inducing resistance; new compounds degrading CDK4 and CDK6 inhibited the growth of both CDK4/6i-sensitive and CDK4/6i-resistant in vitro and in vivo (Li et al. 2022).

Cyclin D-CDK4 stability and activity depend on the presence of a ternary complex with p27 that, in its phosphorylated form, is able to activate the complex. On the other hand, binding of p27 to cyclin E-CDK2 inhibits its activity. The ternary cyclin D-CDK4-p27 active complexes were shown not to be inhibited by CDK4/6i (Guiley et al. 2019). It was demonstrated that blocking p27 Y88 phosphorylation inhibited CDK4 activity and stabilized p27 with subsequent inhibition of CDK2. The dual inhibition of CDK4 and CDK2 was effective in inhibiting the growth of CDK4/6i-sensitive and CDK4/6i-resistant tumors in vivo and in vitro (Patel et al. 2018; Jilishitz et al. 2021). The expression of Y88 p27 might also represent a surrogate marker of CDK4 activity and potentially be used to predict response to CDK4/6i (Gottesman et al. 2019).

Despite the intriguing preclinical data, more evidence is needed to establish the role of the CIP-KIP and INK4 cell cycle inhibitors as potential targets or biomarkers for CDK4/6i treatment.

Other Cell Cycle-Related Genes

Drug and/or kinome knockdown screening highlighted the cyclin-dependent kinases *CDK7* and *CDK9*, and the *WEE1* G2 checkpoint kinase, as significant hits in CDK4/6i-resistant cells (Pancholi et al. 2020; Soosainathan et al. 2024). In addition, it was shown that circulating mRNA levels of *CDK9* were significantly increased in patients after 3 months of CDK4/6i treatment (Del Re et al. 2019). These kinases are particularly attractive targets as specific inhibitors are available and effective in preclinical studies on resistant cells (Pancholi et al. 2020; Fallah et al. 2021; Soosainathan et al. 2024). However clinical data in patients progressing on CDK4/6i are lacking.

23.5.2 Pathways Regulating Cyclin D-CDK4/6-Rb Axis

Alterations in membrane receptors and downstream signaling pathways converging on CDK4 and CDK6, including PI3K/AKT/mTOR signaling deregulations, *FGFR* overexpression/amplification, and *ERBB2* mutations, have been implicated in resistance to CDK4/6i.

23.5.2.1 PI3K/AKT/mTOR Signaling

The PI3K/AKT/mTOR pathway is an intracellular signaling pathway with a pivotal role in regulating proliferation, metabolism, and migration. PI3K, a heterodimeric enzyme comprising a catalytic and a regulatory subunit, is typically activated through phosphorylation by receptor tyrosine kinase (RTKs), such as HER2, EGFR, FGFR, and IGFR. PI3K catalyzes the conversion of the plasma membrane lipid phosphatidylinositol (3,4)-bisphosphate (PIP2) into the second messenger phosphatidylinositol (3,4,5)-trisphosphate (PIP3) which recruits 3-phosphoinositide-dependent kinase 1 (PDK1) and AKT to the cell membrane. At this site, PDK1 phosphorylates AKT, initiating a cascade that activates downstream proteins, including the mTORC1 complex. In physiological conditions, the activation of this pathway is controlled by feedback mechanisms and negative regulators, such as PTEN, a phosphatase that antagonizes the activity of PI3K by dephosphorylating PIP3 back to PIP2 (Mukherjee et al. 2021; Castel et al. 2021; Vasan and Cantley 2022).

Dysregulation of PI3K/AKT/mTOR is frequent in breast cancer. In CDK4/6i-resistant HR+ breast cancer, preclinical and clinical studies have shown that aberrant activation of the pathway might be due to activating mutations in *PIK3CA* and *AKT1*, increased expression and increased activity of PDK1, and *PTEN* loss (Herrera-Abreu et al. 2016; Jansen et al. 2017; O'Leary et al. 2018a, b; Wander et al. 2020; Costa et al. 2020; O'Brien et al. 2020; Li et al. 2022).

Amplification or activating mutations of *AKT1* have been identified as alterations associated with resistance to CDK4/6i in a study performed on tumors from patients treated with CDK4/6i and ET (Wander et al. 2020). Increased levels of PDK1 and phospho-PDK1 have been found associated to AKT activation in breast cancer cell lines with acquired resistance to ribociclib (Jansen et al. 2017). The specific contribution of *PIK3CA* mutations to CDK4/6i resistance is not yet fully understood. Mutations in *PIK3CA*, the PI3K catalytic subunit gene, have been identified both in patients sensitive and resistant to CDK4/6i (Wander et al. 2020). Moreover, in the PALOMA-3 trial, a small number of patients' tumors acquired mutations in *PIK3CA* at the time of progression, and these mutations were seen in both the palbociclib and the placebo arms (O'Leary et al. 2018a). However, preclinical studies have evidenced that targeting the PI3K/AKT/mTOR pathway with the PI3K inhibitor alpelisib overcomes resistance to palbociclib in both *PIK3CA* WT and mutant cell line xenograft models and reverts resistance to ribociclib in breast cancer cell lines with increased total and phospho-PDK1 (Jansen et al. 2017; O'Brien et al. 2020).

Loss of *PTEN* was identified as a possible mechanism of resistance to CDK4/6i in a study on serial biopsies from patients who progressed after treatment with ribociclib plus letrozole. Mechanistically, the loss of *PTEN* results in resistance to CDK4/6i by promoting AKT-dependent phosphorylation of p27, which leads to its nuclear exclusion and to decreased inhibition of cyclin E-CDK2 and by increasing the expression of CDK6 (Costa et al. 2020; Li et al. 2022). Of note, loss of *PTEN* is a mechanism of resistance not only to CDK4/6i but also to PI3K inhibitors, and therefore it has been suggested that this alteration may limit the efficacy of PI3K inhibitors after progression on CDK4/6i (Costa et al. 2020). Interestingly, both preclinical and clinical data have shown activity of the AKT inhibitor capivasertib in combination with fulvestrant in *PTEN*-reduced/*PTEN*-mutant breast cancer (Fu et al. 2014; Smyth et al. 2021), suggesting that AKT inhibition might be a preferred option for treating patients harboring such alterations.

In the last decade, a number of clinical trials have investigated the efficacy of drugs targeting the PI3K/AKT/mTOR signaling in patients who progressed on CDK4/6i. The phase 2 BYLieve trial (Rugo et al. 2021b) included only *PIK3CA*-mutant metastatic HR+/HER2- breast cancer patients who were treated with alpelisib in combination with ET. This study enrolled a subgroup of patients previously treated with CDK4/6i demonstrating clinical activity of alpelisib plus fulvestrant in this subgroup (Rugo et al. 2021b). The randomized phase 3 SOLAR-1 clinical trial enrolled patients with HR+/HER2- metastatic breast cancer, who had previously received ET, to receive alpelisib plus fulvestrant or placebo plus fulvestrant. This trial showed that, compared to the placebo arm, treatment with alpelisib and fulvestrant almost doubled the PFS of patients with mutant *PIK3CA* (11.0 months vs. 5.7 months; HR 0.65; 95% CI 0.50–1.25; $p < 0.001$). However, only 6% of patients with *PIK3CA*-mutant tumors had also previously been treated with a CDK4/6i in this trial, limiting the applicability of these results to a contemporary clinical scenario. For this reason, even if SOLAR-1 showed similar benefit from alpelisib in the CDK4/6i pretreated cohort compared to the overall population (André et al. 2019), the European Medicine Agency has limited the approval of alpelisib to patients pretreated with ET alone. On the contrary, the FDA approval of alpelisib includes patients who progressed on ET in combination with a CDK4/6i.

Targeting other downstream elements of the PI3K/AKT/mTOR pathway seems an attractive strategy in patients resistant to CDK4/6i. The CAPiTello-291 clinical trial tested the efficacy and safety of capivasertib in addition to fulvestrant in patients with HR+/HER2- metastatic breast cancer harboring PI3K/AKT-pathway gene alterations (in *PIK3CA*, *AKT1*, and *PTEN* genes) or not (WT), who progressed after treatment on ET with or without CDK4/6i. *PIK3CA* mutations represented >70% of the mutations in the PI3K/AKT pathway. In the overall population, the median PFS was significantly longer in patients receiving capivasertib compared to those receiving placebo (7.2 months vs. 3.6 months respectively; HR 0.60; 95% CI 0.51-0.71; $p < 0.001$). This benefit was irrespective of prior treatment with CDK4/6i but was largely driven by the population with PI3K/AKT altered tumors, being negligible in the PI3K/AKT non-altered group (when tumors with unknown status were excluded) (Turner et al. 2023). For these reasons, the FDA approval for capivasertib was restricted to patients harboring mutations in the PI3K/AKT/mTOR pathway. The mTOR inhibitor everolimus in combination with ET is a standard option for patients with endocrine-resistant disease in the metastatic setting. The effectiveness of everolimus plus ET in the CDK4/6i-resistant setting has been mainly explored in retrospective series and real-world studies. Therefore, at present there are limited data on the benefit of this combination (Turner et al. 2018; Dhakal et al. 2020; Sledge et al. 2020).

While preclinical data suggests that the triple combination of ET, CDK4/6i, and PI3K/AKT/mTOR inhibitors could be a successful treatment option to prevent or revert resistance (Herrera-Abreu et al. 2016), early clinical trials have shown high toxicity for these combinations. Therefore, more studies are needed to understand if they could represent a possible therapeutic strategy (Tolaney et al. 2021).

23.5.2.2 Growth Factors and Receptors

FGFR, EGFR, and HER2 are RTKs that upon dimerization activate downstream signaling cascades, including the PI3K/AKT/mTOR and Ras/MEK/ERK pathways, leading to cell cycle progression and proliferation. With the exception of HER2, which is a ligand orphan receptor, RTKs dimerization is induced by specific growth factor binding (Krook et al. 2021; Uribe et al. 2021; Schlam and Swain 2021).

In vitro studies on breast cancer models identified the amplification and the overexpression of *FGFR1* as a mechanism of resistance to CDK4/6i (Formisano et al. 2019). This finding has been supported by clinical data. Indeed, amplification or activating alterations in *FGFR1/2* have been detected in ctDNA or tumor biopsies of patients who progressed after treatment with CDK4/6i in combination with ET (Formisano et al. 2019; Wander et al. 2020; Goetz et al. 2023). Based on this evidence, preclinical studies have tested the addition of the FGFR inhibitor erdafitinib to palbociclib and fulvestrant in FGFR1-overexpressing patient-derived xenograft models and found that this combination suppressed tumor growth more effectively than palbociclib with or without fulvestrant, providing a potential combination treatment strategy to overcome resistance to CDK4/6i (Formisano et al. 2019).

Activating mutations in *ERBB2* have been implicated in resistance to CDK4/6i (Nayar et al. 2019; Wander et al. 2020). According to preclinical studies, resistance to CDK4/6i could be overcome by the addition of the HER2 tyrosine kinase inhibitor neratinib (Pancholi et al. 2020), and recently, the results of the phase 2 SUMMIT study have shown some activity of neratinib in combination with fulvestrant and trastuzumab for HR+ *ERBB2*-mutant metastatic breast cancer patients after progression on CDK4/6i (Jhaveri et al. 2023).

23.5.2.3 Estrogen and Progesterone Receptors

Currently, the expression of ER is the only biomarker indicated for the clinical use of any CDK4/6i in any setting. However, all the pivotal phase 3 trials investigating CDK4/6i in combination with ET have failed to demonstrate a predictive role of ER and PR levels, and current clinical guidelines indicate that CDK4/6i should be offered to patients independently of ER levels (Cristofanilli et al. 2016; Hortobagyi et al. 2018; di Leo et al. 2018; Turner et al. 2019; Finn et al. 2020). Similarly, the detection of *ESR1* mutations does not contraindicate the use of a CDK4/6i as none of the available data suggests a lesser effect of these agents in this context (Fribbens et al. 2016; Tolaney et al. 2022).

The ER and the cyclin D-CDK4/6-Rb axis are tightly linked by extensive cross-talk. While clinical trials have investigated CDK4/6i almost exclusively in combination with ET, preclinical studies using single-agent CDK4/6i have permitted to study how the ER pathway may be altered during the acquisition of resistance to these agents, even in the absence of ET. In an early report, acquired resistance to abemaciclib in vitro was associated with a reduction in ER and PR levels, possibly explained by transcriptional repression, as well as reduced ER pathway activity and reduced endocrine sensitivity (Yang et al. 2017). Subsequently, a wider in vitro study conducted in models resistant to either palbociclib, ribociclib, or abemaciclib, including both *ESR1* WT parental models and their derivatives with *D538G* or *Y537S* *ESR1* mutations, suggested that both ER levels and signaling, although variably affected by the different CDK4/6i, were generally maintained at resistance. Interestingly, the potent anti-estrogen elacestrant was effective in reducing cell proliferation and tumor growth of resistant models to all CDK4/6i, both with WT and mutant *ESR1* (Patel et al. 2019). Further to these observations, through ER-ChIP sequencing of endocrine and palbociclib dual-resistant models, Pancholi et al. found reduced ER binding to promoters of classical ER-dependent genes at time of resistance, with a reduced sensitivity to fulvestrant and tamoxifen. These data suggest that long-term treatment with CDK4/6i may drive chromatin remodeling, ER transcriptional reprogramming, and treatment resistance (Pancholi et al. 2020). These data collectively suggest that CDK4/6i resistance may be associated with a reduced but still active ER signaling that can be effectively targeted by potent endocrine agents. A reduction in ER and PR levels was also observed across paired clinical samples obtained before and after treatment with ribociclib or abemaciclib in combination with ET (Yang et al. 2017), and loss of ER expression was observed in about 7% of biopsies of patients with clinical resistance to CDK4/6i plus ET (Wander et al. 2020). In keeping with these data, clinical trials conducted in patients pretreated with CDK4/6i in the metastatic setting seem to indicate poor outcomes on ET-based approaches (Bidard et al. 2022). However, clinical characteristics indicative of endocrine sensitivity (such as a long duration of the treatment with CDK4/6i in the prior treatment line) have been associated with superior clinical activity of elacestrant versus ET of physician's choice in patients with *ESR1*-mutant disease (Bidard et al. 2022), suggesting that biomarkers of residual endocrine-sensitivity post-CDK4/6i may play an important role in identifying patients more likely to respond to potent-ER targeting in this setting. These biomarkers are currently not available, and future research is needed to identify patients who can be continued to be treated with endocrine-based approaches after progression on CDK4/6i, to spare them of the toxic effect of chemotherapy.

23.5.3 The Role of the Immune System

Alongside with the well-characterized effects on the cell cycle, multiple reports demonstrated that CDK4/6i also modulate the immune system by acting on both tumor cells and microenvironment.

Analyzing in vitro and in vivo models of breast cancer, it was demonstrated that abemaciclib stimulates the anti-tumor immunity by increasing antigen presentation and upregulating the expression of the interferon (IFN) signaling in breast cancer cells (Goel et al. 2017; Schaer et al. 2018). The upregulation of IFN signaling during treatment, confirmed also in tumor samples from patients with HR+/HER2- breast cancer receiving CDK4/6i (Goel et al. 2017; Hurvitz et al. 2020), was shown to be elicited by the decreased expression of *DNMT1*, an E2F target gene, induced by abemaciclib. *DNMT1* downregulation reduced the methylation of endogenous retroviral genes increasing the levels of intra-tumoral double-stranded RNA (dsRNA), therefore triggering the dsRNA response and IFN signaling genes (Goel et al. 2017). In colorectal and breast cancer cells, CDK4/6i treatment was also shown to increase the expression of the death receptor 5 (*DR5*), a receptor of the immune cytokine TRAIL, known to induce apoptosis in tumor cells (Von Karstedt et al. 2017). *DR5* upregulation was independent from *RB1* and *DNMT1* and mediated by reduced phosphorylation and nuclear translocation of p73, a transcription factor of the p53 family (Tong et al. 2022). On the other hand, it was shown both in vitro and in vivo that, upon CDK4/6i treatment, breast cancer cells upregulated the expression of the programmed death ligand 1 (*PD-L1*) (Zhang et al. 2018; Uzhachenko et al. 2021), which is known to block the activation of T cells and induce immune escape in tumor cells (Sun et al. 2018). Mechanistically, CDK4/6i were shown to phosphorylate SPOP, a component of the E3 ubiquitin-protein ligase complex involved in the proteasome-dependent degradation of PD-L1. The reduced phosphorylation of SPOP decreased its levels and increased *PD-L1* levels (Zhang et al. 2018).

Changes in tumor cells are accompanied by effects of CDK4/6i treatment on the tumor microenvironment which have been demonstrated in multiple tumor models. It was shown that CDK4/6i treatment alters the balance between cytotoxic and immune-suppressive T cells by increasing the CD4+ and CD8+ cytotoxic T cells and reducing the infiltration and proliferation of the T regulatory cells (Treg) (Goel et al. 2017; Deng et al. 2018; Schaer et al. 2018; Uzhachenko et al. 2021). In addition, CDK4/6i treatment might promote long-term anti-tumor immunity by increasing CD8+ memory-like T cells (Heckler et al. 2021; Lelliott et al. 2021). The downregulation of Treg during CDK4/6i treatment has also been demonstrated in blood samples obtained from patients with HR+/HER2- metastatic breast cancer (Peuker et al. 2022; Scirocchi et al. 2022).

CDK4/6i is known to induce senescence, which is characterized by alterations of cytokine and chemokine secretion, named the senescence-associated secretory phenotype (SASP). Two different reports failed to demonstrate an increased expression in genes encoding for canonical SASP factors during CDK4/6i treatment (Goel et al. 2017; Schaer et al. 2018); however, modulation of the cytokine profile of both tumor and inflammatory cells has been observed. Indeed, breast cancer cells treated with CDK4/6i showed increased expression and secretion of two T-cell chemoattractant chemokines, CCL5 and CXCL10, therefore promoting T cell infiltration into mammary tumors. This effect was dependent on Rb, but also on mTOR and PI3K, being abrogated by mTOR/PI3K inhibitors. Underlying mechanisms include an increase in the mTOR activity and a metabolic and oxidative stress induced by CDK4/6i (Uzhachenko et al. 2021). It was also demonstrated that CDK4/6i promote T cell activity through increased production of interleukin-2 (IL-2) mediated by the NFAT transcription factors, increased levels of CXCL9 and CXCL10, and reduced levels of T cell-suppressive IL-6, IL-10, and IL-23 (Deng et al. 2018).

Intriguingly, immune-system modulations have been implicated in the de novo or acquired resistance to CDK4/6i. It was shown, both in vitro and in vivo, that an increased IFN signaling in breast tumor cells was associated with CDK4/6i resistance, possibly favoring tumoral immune escape (Pandey et al. 2021; De Angelis et al. 2021; Gomes et al. 2023). Increased IFN was also observed in HER2+ in vivo models of breast cancer with acquired resistance to anti-HER2 therapies and palbociclib (Wang et al. 2019). In addition, resistant tumors were infiltrated by immature myeloid cells, suggesting an immunosuppressive microenvironment (Wang et al. 2019). In patients with HR+/HER2- breast cancer, the decrease in Treg upon treatment with CDK4/6i was more pronounced in responders versus nonresponders implying that lack of modulation might contribute to CDK4/6i resistance (Peuker et al. 2022; Scirocchi et al. 2022).

It has been hypothesized that strengthening the immune system through the rational combination of immune therapies and CDK4/6i might help overcome resistance and potentiate the effects of both treatments. Indeed, multiple reports in preclinical models demonstrated increased activity when CDK4/6i were administered together with agents targeting immune checkpoints (ICI) such as PD-L1 (Goel et al. 2017; Zhang et al. 2018; Schaer et al. 2018; Wang et al. 2019; Tong et al. 2022). Ongoing clinical trials are evaluating the combinations of CDK4/6i and ICI in patients with HR+/HER2- metastatic breast cancer, with preliminary reports indicating good clinical activity but also increased toxicity of the combination (Yuan et al. 2021; Rugo et al. 2022; Masuda et al. 2023). Therefore, thorough selection of patients more likely to respond is desirable.

23.6 Conclusion

CDK4/6i have reshaped the treatment paradigm for patients with HR+/HER2- breast cancer, and their use in combination with other therapies is likely to expand in the future. Despite this, some patients do not respond at all to CDK4/6i-based therapy, and nearly all patients eventually become refractory and progress.

In the last decade, multiple studies have started to shed light on the mechanisms of resistance to CDK4/6i in breast cancer. One major class of resistance mechanisms involves alterations in the cell cycle machinery, such as loss of Rb function, and amplification/overexpression of *CCNE1* and *CDK6*. In addition, deregulations of ER, RTKs, and PI3K/AKT/mTOR signaling and modulation of the immune system have also been found to confer resistance to these drugs.

Despite the number of published data, more studies are needed to identify new biomarkers predictive of response to CDK4/6i and alternative combinatorial or sequential therapeutic strategies to prevent or overcome CDK4/6i resistance.

To date, a common and clinically validated mechanism of resistance to CKD4/6i in breast cancer has yet to be identified, and the expression of ER remains the only biomarker to select patients that can be treated with these inhibitors. Although preclinical studies have unveiled various genomic and non-genomic mechanisms of resistance to these drugs, to date most of the clinical studies have relied solely on genomic data. This is a gap that might have limited the clinical validation of some preclinical findings. However, it is possible that future multiomic studies, integrating genomic, transcriptomic, and epigenomic data from clinical samples, will fill this gap, providing a more thorough understanding of the CDK4/6i resistance landscape in breast cancer.

Over the years it has become clear that different mechanisms of resistance to CDK4/6i can be observed among patients and coexist within the same tumor. Given this heterogeneity, current priorities include optimizing CDK4/6i-based treatment combinations and sequences and developing personalized strategies to overcome treatment resistance and maximize the efficacy of CDK4/6i.

References

Abu-Khalaf M, Wang C, Zhang Z et al (2022) Genomic aberrations in circulating tumor DNAs from palbociclib-treated metastatic breast cancer patients reveal a novel resistance mechanism. Cancers (Basel) 14. https://doi.org/10.3390/CANCERS14122872

Al-Qasem AJ, Alves CL, Ehmsen S et al (2022) Co-targeting CDK2 and CDK4/6 overcomes resistance to aromatase and CDK4/6 inhibitors in ER+ breast cancer. NPJ Precis Oncol 6. https://doi.org/10.1038/S41698-022-00311-6

Alves CL, Elias D, Lyng M et al (2016) High CDK6 protects cells from fulvestrant-mediated apoptosis and is a predictor of resistance to fulvestrant in estrogen receptor-positive metastatic breast cancer. Clin Cancer Res 22:5514–5526. https://doi.org/10.1158/1078-0432.CCR-15-1984

Anders L, Ke N, Hydbring P et al (2011) A systematic screen for CDK4/6 substrates links FOXM1 phosphorylation to senescence suppression in cancer cells. Cancer Cell 20:620–634. https://doi.org/10.1016/J.CCR.2011.10.001

André F, Ciruelos E, Rubovszky G et al (2019) Alpelisib for PIK3CA-mutated, hormone receptor–positive advanced breast cancer. N Engl J Med 380:1929–1940. https://doi.org/10.1056/nejmoa1813904

André F, Su F, Solovieff N et al (2023) Pooled ctDNA analysis of MONALEESA phase III advanced breast cancer trials. Ann Oncol 34:1003–1014. https://doi.org/10.1016/J.ANNONC.2023.08.011

Bardia A, Su F, Solovieff N et al (2021) Genomic profiling of premenopausal HR+ and HER2- metastatic breast cancer by circulating tumor DNA and association of genetic alterations with therapeutic response to endocrine therapy and ribociclib. JCO Precis Oncol 5:1408–1420. https://doi.org/10.1200/PO.20.00445

Bidard F-C, Kaklamani VG, Neven P et al (2022) Elacestrant (oral selective estrogen receptor degrader) versus standard endocrine therapy for estrogen receptor–positive, human epidermal growth factor receptor 2–negative advanced breast cancer: results from the randomized phase III EMERALD trial. J Clin Oncol 40:3246–3256. https://doi.org/10.1200/JCO.22.00338

Burris HA, Chan A, Bardia A et al (2021) Safety and impact of dose reductions on efficacy in the randomised MONALEESA-2, −3 and −7 trials in hormone receptor-positive, HER2-negative advanced breast cancer. Br J Cancer 125(5):679–686. https://doi.org/10.1038/s41416-021-01415-9

Castel P, Toska E, Engelman JA, Scaltriti M (2021) The present and future of PI3K inhibitors for cancer therapy. Nat Cancer 2:587–597. https://doi.org/10.1038/S43018-021-00218-4

Chen P, Lee NV, Hu W et al (2016) Spectrum and degree of CDK drug interactions predicts clinical performance. Mol Cancer Ther 15:2273–2281. https://doi.org/10.1158/1535-7163.MCT-16-0300

Condorelli R, Spring L, O'Shaughnessy J et al (2018) Polyclonal RB1 mutations and acquired resistance to CDK 4/6 inhibitors in patients with metastatic breast cancer. Ann Oncol 29:640–645. https://doi.org/10.1093/ANNONC/MDX784

Cornell L, Wander SA, Visal T et al (2019) MicroRNA-mediated suppression of the TGF-β pathway confers transmissible and reversible CDK4/6 inhibitor resistance. Cell Rep 26:2667–2680.e7. https://doi.org/10.1016/j.celrep.2019.02.023

Costa C, Ye W, Ly A et al (2020) Pten loss mediates clinical cross-resistance to CDK4/6 and PI3Kα inhibitors in breast cancer. Cancer Discov 10:72–85. https://doi.org/10.1158/2159-8290.CD-18-0830

Cristofanilli M, Turner NC, Bondarenko I et al (2016) Fulvestrant plus palbociclib versus fulvestrant plus placebo for treatment of hormone-receptor-positive, HER2-negative metastatic breast cancer that progressed on previous endocrine therapy (PALOMA-3): final analysis of the multicentre, double-blind, phase 3 randomised controlled trial. Lancet Oncol 17:425–439. https://doi.org/10.1016/S1470-2045(15)00613-0

De Angelis C, Fu X, Cataldo ML et al (2021) Activation of the IFN signaling pathway is associated with resistance to CDK4/6 inhibitors and immune checkpoint activation in ER-positive breast cancer. Clin Cancer Res. https://doi.org/10.1158/1078-0432.ccr-19-4191

Dean JL, Thangavel C, McClendon AK et al (2010) Therapeutic CDK4/6 inhibition in breast cancer: key mechanisms of response and failure. Oncogene 29:4018–4032. https://doi.org/10.1038/ONC.2010.154

Dean JL, McClendon AK, Hickey TE et al (2012) Therapeutic response to CDK4/6 inhibition in breast cancer defined by ex vivo analyses of human tumors. Cell Cycle 11:2756–2761. https://doi.org/10.4161/CC.21195

Del Re M, Bertolini I, Crucitta S et al (2019) Overexpression of TK1 and CDK9 in plasma-derived exosomes is associated with clinical resistance to CDK4/6 inhibitors in metastatic breast cancer patients. Breast Cancer Res Treat 178:57–62. https://doi.org/10.1007/s10549-019-05365-y

Deng J, Wang ES, Jenkins RW et al (2018) CDK4/6 inhibition augments antitumor immunity by enhancing T-cell activation. Cancer Discov 8:216–233. https://doi.org/10.1158/2159-8290.CD-17-0915

Dhakal A, Antony Thomas R, Levine EG et al (2020) Outcome of everolimus-based therapy in hormone-receptor-positive metastatic breast cancer patients after progression on palbociclib. Breast Cancer (Auckl) 14. https://doi.org/10.1177/1178223420944864

di Leo A, O'Shaughnessy J, Sledge GW et al (2018) Prognostic characteristics in hormone receptor-positive advanced breast cancer and characterization of abemaciclib efficacy. NPJ Breast Cancer 4(1):1–8. https://doi.org/10.1038/s41523-018-0094-2

Dickler MN, Tolaney SM, Rugo HS et al (2017) MONARCH 1, a phase II study of abemaciclib, a CDK4 and CDK6 inhibitor, as a single agent, n patients with refractory HR+/HER2- metastatic breast cancer. Clin Cancer Res 23:5218–5224. https://doi.org/10.1158/1078-0432.CCR-17-0754

Dietrich C, Trub A, Ahn A et al (2023) INX-315, a selective CDK2 inhibitor, induces cell cycle arrest and senescence in solid tumors. Cancer Discov. https://doi.org/10.1158/2159-8290.CD-23-0954

Fallah Y, Demas DM, Jin L et al (2021) Targeting WEE1 inhibits growth of breast cancer cells that are resistant to endocrine therapy and CDK4/6 inhibitors. Front Oncol 11. https://doi.org/10.3389/FONC.2021.681530

Finn RS, Dering J, Conklin D et al (2009) PD 0332991, a selective cyclin D kinase 4/6 inhibitor, preferentially inhibits proliferation of luminal estrogen receptor-positive human breast cancer cell lines in vitro. Breast Cancer Res 11. https://doi.org/10.1186/BCR2419

Finn RS, Crown JP, Lang I et al (2015) The cyclin-dependent kinase 4/6 inhibitor palbociclib in combination with letrozole versus letrozole alone as first-line treatment of oestrogen receptor-positive, HER2-negative, advanced breast cancer (PALOMA-1/TRIO-18): a randomised phase 2 study. Lancet Oncol 16:25–35. https://doi.org/10.1016/S1470-2045(14)71159-3

Finn RS, Martin M, Rugo HS et al (2016) Palbociclib and letrozole in advanced breast cancer. N Engl J Med 375:1925–1936. https://doi.org/10.1056/nejmoa1607303

Finn RS, Liu Y, Zhu Z et al (2020) Biomarker analyses of response to cyclin-dependent kinase 4/6 inhibition and endocrine therapy in women with treatment-naïve metastatic breast cancer. Clin Cancer Res 26:110–121. https://doi.org/10.1158/1078-0432.CCR-19-0751

Finn RS, Rugo HS, Gelmon KA et al (2021) Long-term pooled safety analysis of palbociclib in combination with endocrine therapy for hormone receptor-positive/human epidermal growth factor receptor 2-negative advanced breast cancer: updated analysis with up to 5 years of follow-up. Oncologist 26:e749–e755. https://doi.org/10.1002/ONCO.13684

Formisano L, Lu Y, Servetto A et al (2019) Aberrant FGFR signaling mediates resistance to CDK4/6 inhibitors in ER+ breast cancer. Nat Commun 10:1–14. https://doi.org/10.1038/s41467-019-09068-2

Freeman-Cook K, Hoffman RL, Miller N et al (2021) Expanding control of the tumor cell cycle with a CDK2/4/6 inhibitor. Cancer Cell 39:1404–1421.e11. https://doi.org/10.1016/J.CCELL.2021.08.009

Fribbens C, O'Leary B, Kilburn L et al (2016) Plasma ESR1 mutations and the treatment of estrogen receptor-Positive advanced breast cancer. J Clin Oncol 34:2961–2968. https://doi.org/10.1200/JCO.2016.67.3061

Fu M, Wang C, Li Z et al (2004) Minireview: Cyclin D1: normal and abnormal functions. Endocrinology 145:5439–5447. https://doi.org/10.1210/EN.2004-0959

Fu X, Creighton CJ, Biswal NC et al (2014) Overcoming endocrine resistance due to reduced PTEN levels in estrogen receptor-positive breast cancer by co-targeting mammalian target of rapamycin, protein kinase B, or mitogen-activated protein kinase kinase. Breast Cancer Res 16:1–17. https://doi.org/10.1186/S13058-014-0430-X/FIGURES/5

George MA, Qureshi S, Omene C et al (2021) Clinical and pharmacologic differences of CDK4/6 inhibitors in breast cancer. Front Oncol 11. https://doi.org/10.3389/FONC.2021.693104/FULL

Giessrigl B, Schmidt WM, Kalipciyan M et al (2013) Fulvestrant induces resistance by modulating GPER and CDK6 expression: implication of methyltransferases, deacetylases and the hSWI/SNF chromatin remodelling complex. Br J Cancer 109:2751–2762. https://doi.org/10.1038/BJC.2013.583

Gnant M, Dueck AC, Frantal S et al (2022) Adjuvant palbociclib for early breast cancer: the PALLAS trial results (ABCSG-42/AFT-05/BIG-14-03). J Clin Oncol 40:282–293. https://doi.org/10.1200/JCO.21.02554

Goel S, Decristo MJ, Watt AC et al (2017) CDK4/6 inhibition triggers anti-tumour immunity. Nature 548:471–475. https://doi.org/10.1038/nature23465

Goetz MP, Toi M, Campone M et al (2017) MONARCH 3: abemaciclib as initial therapy for advanced breast cancer. J Clin Oncol 35:3638–3646. https://doi.org/10.1200/JCO.2017.75.6155

Goetz MP, Hamilton EP, Campone M, et al (2023) Landscape of baseline and acquired genomic alterations in circulating tumor DNA with abemaciclib alone or with endocrine therapy in advanced breast cancer. Clin Cancer Res OF1–OF12. doi:https://doi.org/10.1158/1078-0432.CCR-22-3573

Gomes I, Gallego-Paez LM, Jiménez M et al (2023) Co-targeting RANK pathway treats and prevents acquired resistance to CDK4/6 inhibitors in luminal breast cancer. Cell Rep Med 4. https://doi.org/10.1016/J.XCRM.2023.101120

Gottesman SRS, Somma J, Tsiperson V et al (2019) Tyrosine phosphorylation of p27Kip1 correlates with palbociclib responsiveness in breast cancer tumor cells grown in explant culture. Mol Cancer Res 17:669–675. https://doi.org/10.1158/1541-7786.MCR-18-0188

Grinshpun A, Tolaney SM, Burstein HJ et al (2023) The dilemma of selecting a first line CDK4/6 inhibitor for hormone receptor-positive/HER2-negative metastatic breast cancer. NPJ Breast Cancer 9(1):1–4. https://doi.org/10.1038/s41523-023-00520-7

Guarducci C, Bonechi M, Benelli M et al (2018) Cyclin E1 and Rb modulation as common events at time of resistance to palbociclib in hormone receptor-positive breast cancer. NPJ Breast Cancer 4:38. https://doi.org/10.1038/s41523-018-0092-4

Guerrero-Zotano AL, Stricker TP, Formisano L et al (2018) ER+ breast cancers resistant to prolonged neoadjuvant letrozole exhibit an E2F4 transcriptional program sensitive to CDK4/6 inhibitors. Clin Cancer Res 24:2517–2529. https://doi.org/10.1158/1078-0432.CCR-17-2904

Guerrero-Zotano Á, Belli S, Zielinski C et al (2023) CCNE1 and PLK1 mediate resistance to palbociclib in HR+/HER2- metastatic breast cancer. Clin Cancer Res 29:1557–1568. https://doi.org/10.1158/1078-0432.CCR-22-2206

Guiley KZ, Stevenson JW, Lou K et al (2019) p27 allosterically activates cyclin-dependent kinase 4 and antagonizes palbociclib inhibition. Science 366. https://doi.org/10.1126/SCIENCE.AAW2106

Hafner M, Mills CE, Subramanian K et al (2019) Multiomics profiling establishes the polypharmacology of FDA-approved CDK4/6 inhibitors and the potential for differential clinical activity. Cell Chem Biol 26:1067–1080.e8. https://doi.org/10.1016/J.CHEMBIOL.2019.05.005

Heckler M, Ali LR, Clancy-Thompson E, et al (2021) Inhibition of CDK4/6 promotes CD8 T-cell memory formation. Cancer Discov candisc.1540.2020. doi:https://doi.org/10.1158/2159-8290.cd-20-1540

Henley SA, Dick FA (2012) The retinoblastoma family of proteins and their regulatory functions in the mammalian cell division cycle. Cell Div 7:10

Herrera-Abreu MT, Palafox M, Asghar U et al (2016) Early adaptation and acquired resistance to CDK4/6 inhibition in estrogen receptor-positive breast cancer. Cancer Res 76:2301–2313. https://doi.org/10.1158/0008-5472.CAN-15-0728

Hortobagyi GN, Stemmer SM, Burris HA et al (2016) Ribociclib as first-line therapy for HR-positive, advanced breast cancer. N Engl J Med 375:1738–1748. https://doi.org/10.1056/nejmoa1609709

Hortobagyi GN, Stemmer SM, Burris HA et al (2018) Updated results from MONALEESA-2, a phase III trial of first-line ribociclib plus letrozole versus placebo plus letrozole in hormone receptor-positive, HER2-negative advanced breast cancer. Ann Oncol 29:1541–1547. https://doi.org/10.1093/annonc/mdy155

Hurvitz SA, Martin M, Press MF et al (2020) Potent cell-cycle inhibition and upregulation of immune response with abemaciclib and anastrozole in Neomonarch, phase II neoadjuvant study in HR+/HER2- Breast cancer. Clin Cancer Res 26:566–580. https://doi.org/10.1158/1078-0432.CCR-19-1425

Iida M, Nakamura M, Tokuda E et al (2019) The p21 levels have the potential to be a monitoring marker for ribociclib in breast cancer. Oncotarget 10:4907–4918. https://doi.org/10.18632/ONCOTARGET.27127

Jansen VM, Bhola NE, Bauer JA et al (2017) Kinome-wide RNA interference screen reveals a role for PDK1 in acquired resistance to CDK4/6 inhibition in ER-positive breast cancer. Cancer Res 77:2488–2499. https://doi.org/10.1158/0008-5472.CAN-16-2653

Jhaveri K, Eli LD, Wildiers H et al (2023) Neratinib + fulvestrant + trastuzumab for HR-positive, HER2-negative, HER2-mutant metastatic breast cancer: outcomes and biomarker analysis from the SUMMIT trial. Ann Oncol 34:885–898. https://doi.org/10.1016/J.ANNONC.2023.08.003

Jilishitz I, Quiñones JL, Patel P et al (2021) NP-ALT, a liposomal:peptide drug, blocks p27Kip1 phosphorylation to induce oxidative stress, necroptosis, and regression in therapy-resistant breast cancer cells. Mol Cancer Res 19:1929–1945. https://doi.org/10.1158/1541-7786.MCR-21-0081

Jirström K, Stendahl M, Rydén L et al (2005) Adverse effect of adjuvant tamoxifen in premenopausal breast cancer with cyclin D1 gene amplification. Cancer Res 65:8009–8016. https://doi.org/10.1158/0008-5472.CAN-05-0746

Johnston S, Emde A, Barrios C et al (2023a) CDK4/6 inhibitors: existing and emerging differences. JNCI Cancer Spectr. https://doi.org/10.1093/JNCICS/PKAD045

Johnston SRD, Toi M, O'Shaughnessy J et al (2023b) Abemaciclib plus endocrine therapy for hormone receptor-positive, HER2-negative, node-positive, high-risk early breast cancer (monarchE): results from a preplanned interim analysis of a randomised, open-label, phase 3 trial. Lancet Oncol 24:77–90. https://doi.org/10.1016/S1470-2045(22)00694-5

Kharenko OA, Patel RG, Calosing C, van der Horst EH (2022) Combination of ZEN-3694 with CDK4/6 inhibitors reverses acquired resistance to CDK4/6 inhibitors in ER-positive breast cancer. Cancer Gene Ther 29:859–869. https://doi.org/10.1038/S41417-021-00375-9

Koboldt DC, Fulton RS, McLellan MD et al (2012) Comprehensive molecular portraits of human breast tumours. Nature 490:61–70. https://doi.org/10.1038/nature11412

Krook MA, Reeser JW, Ernst G et al (2021) Fibroblast growth factor receptors in cancer: genetic alterations, diagnostics, therapeutic targets and mechanisms of resistance. Br J Cancer 124:880–892. https://doi.org/10.1038/S41416-020-01157-0

Kumar B, Prasad P, Singh R et al (2023) Role of identified proteins in the proteome profiles of CDK4/6 inhibitor-resistant breast cancer cell lines. Mol Omics 19:404–417. https://doi.org/10.1039/D2MO00285J

Lelliott EJ, Kong IY, Zethoven M, et al (2021) CDK4/6 inhibition promotes anti-tumor immunity through the induction of T cell memory. Cancer Discov candisc.1554.2020. doi:https://doi.org/10.1158/2159-8290.cd-20-1554

Li Z, Razavi P, Li Q et al (2018) Loss of the FAT1 tumor suppressor promotes resistance to CDK4/6 inhibitors via the hippo pathway. Cancer Cell 34:893–905.e8. https://doi.org/10.1016/j.ccell.2018.11.006

Li Q, Jiang B, Guo J et al (2022) INK4 tumor suppressor proteins mediate resistance to CDK4/6 kinase inhibitors. Cancer Discov 12:356–371. https://doi.org/10.1158/2159-8290.CD-20-1726/674123/AM/INK4-TUMOR-SUPPRESSOR-PROTEINS-MEDIATE-RESISTANCE

Loibl S, Marmé F, Martin M et al (2021) Palbociclib for residual high-risk invasive HR-positive and HER2-negative early breast cancer—the penelope-B trial. J Clin Oncol 39:1518–1530. https://doi.org/10.1200/JCO.20.03639

Long F, He Y, Fu H et al (2019) Preclinical characterization of SHR6390, a novel CDK 4/6 inhibitor, in vitro and in human tumor xenograft models. Cancer Sci 110:1420–1430. https://doi.org/10.1111/CAS.13957

Lukas J, Bartkova J, Bartek J (1996) Convergence of mitogenic signalling cascades from diverse classes of receptors at the cyclin D-cyclin-dependent kinase-pRb-controlled G1 checkpoint. Mol Cell Biol 16:6917–6925. https://doi.org/10.1128/MCB.16.12.6917

Ma CX, Gao F, Luo J et al (2017) NeoPalAna: neoadjuvant palbociclib, a cyclin-dependent kinase 4/6 inhibitor, and anastrozole for clinical stage 2 or 3 estrogen receptor–positive breast cancer. Clin Cancer Res 23:4055–4065. https://doi.org/10.1158/1078-0432.CCR-16-3206

Malorni L, Piazza S, Ciani Y et al (2016) A gene expression signature of retinoblastoma loss-of-function is a predictive biomarker of resistance to palbociclib in breast cancer cell lines and is prognostic in patients with ER positive early breast cancer. Oncotarget 7:68012–68022. https://doi.org/10.18632/ONCOTARGET.12010

Malorni L, Curigliano G, Minisini AM et al (2018) Palbociclib as single agent or in combination with the endocrine therapy received before disease progression for estrogen receptor-positive, HER2-negative metastatic breast cancer: TREnd trial. Ann Oncol 29:1748–1754. https://doi.org/10.1093/annonc/mdy214

Marra A, Curigliano G (2019) Are all cyclin-dependent kinases 4/6 inhibitors created equal? NPJ Breast Cancer 5(1):1–9. https://doi.org/10.1038/s41523-019-0121-y

Masuda J, Sakai H, Tsurutani J et al (2023) Efficacy, safety, and biomarker analysis of nivolumab in combination with abemaciclib plus endocrine therapy in patients with HR-positive HER2-negative metastatic breast cancer: a phase II study (WJOG11418B NEWFLAME trial). J Immunother Cancer 11. https://doi.org/10.1136/JITC-2023-007126

Miller TW, Balko JM, Fox EM et al (2011) ERα-dependent E2F transcription can mediate resistance to estrogen deprivation in human breast cancer. Cancer Discov 1:338–351. https://doi.org/10.1158/2159-8290.CD-11-0101

Millour J, Constantinidou D, Stavropoulou AV et al (2010) FOXM1 is a transcriptional target of ERalpha and has a critical role in breast cancer endocrine sensitivity and resistance. Oncogene 29:2983–2995. https://doi.org/10.1038/ONC.2010.47

Mukherjee R, Vanaja KG, Boyer JA et al (2021) Regulation of PTEN translation by PI3K signaling maintains pathway homeostasis. Mol Cell 81:708–723.e5. https://doi.org/10.1016/J.MOLCEL.2021.01.033

Musgrove EA, Caldon CE, Barraclough J et al (2011) Cyclin D as a therapeutic target in cancer. Nat Rev Cancer 11:558–572

Nayar U, Cohen O, Kapstad C et al (2019) Acquired HER2 mutations in ER+ metastatic breast cancer confer resistance to estrogen receptor-directed therapies. Nat Genet 51:207–216. https://doi.org/10.1038/S41588-018-0287-5

Nikolai BC, Lanz RB, York B et al (2016) HER2 signaling drives DNA anabolism and proliferation through SRC-3 phosphorylation and E2F1-regulated genes. Cancer Res 76:1463. https://doi.org/10.1158/0008-5472.CAN-15-2383

O'Brien NA, McDermott MSJ, Conklin D et al (2020) Targeting activated PI3K/mTOR signaling overcomes acquired resistance to CDK4/6-based therapies in preclinical models of hormone receptor-positive breast cancer. Breast Cancer Res 22. https://doi.org/10.1186/S13058-020-01320-8

O'Leary B, Cutts RJ, Liu Y et al (2018a) The genetic landscape and clonal evolution of breast cancer resistance to palbociclib plus fulvestrant in the PALOMA-3 trial. Cancer Discov 8:1390–1403. https://doi.org/10.1158/2159-8290.CD-18-0264

O'Leary B, Hrebien S, Morden JP et al (2018b) Early circulating tumor DNA dynamics and clonal selection with palbociclib and fulvestrant for breast cancer. Nat Commun 9:896. https://doi.org/10.1038/s41467-018-03215-x

Ogata R, Kishino E, Saitoh W et al (2021) Resistance to cyclin-dependent kinase (CDK) 4/6 inhibitors confers cross-resistance to other CDK inhibitors but not to chemotherapeutic agents in breast cancer cells. Breast Cancer 28:206–215. https://doi.org/10.1007/S12282-020-01150-8

Ono M, Oba T, Shibata T, Ito K ichi (2021) The mechanisms involved in the resistance of estrogen receptor-positive breast cancer cells to palbociclib are multiple and change over time. J Cancer Res Clin Oncol 147:3211–3224. doi:https://doi.org/10.1007/S00432-021-03722-3

Palafox M, Monserrat L, Bellet M et al (2022) High p16 expression and heterozygous RB1 loss are biomarkers for CDK4/6 inhibitor resistance in ER+ breast cancer. Nat Commun 13. https://doi.org/10.1038/S41467-022-32828-6

Pancholi S, Ribas R, Simigdala N et al (2020) Tumour kinome re-wiring governs resistance to palbociclib in oestrogen receptor positive breast cancers, highlighting new therapeutic modalities. Oncogene 39:4781–4797. https://doi.org/10.1038/S41388-020-1284-6

Pandey K, Park N, Park KS et al (2020) Combined CDK2 and CDK4/6 inhibition overcomes palbociclib resistance in breast cancer by enhancing senescence. Cancers (Basel) 12:1–17. https://doi.org/10.3390/CANCERS12123566

Pandey K, Lee E, Park N et al (2021) Deregulated immune pathway associated with palbociclib resistance in preclinical breast cancer models: integrative genomics and transcriptomics. Genes (Basel) 12:1–14. https://doi.org/10.3390/GENES12020159

Park YH, Im SA, Park K et al (2023) Longitudinal multi-omics study of palbociclib resistance in HR-positive/HER2-negative metastatic breast cancer. Genome Med 15. https://doi.org/10.1186/S13073-023-01201-7

Patel P, Tsiperson V, Gottesman SRS et al (2018) Dual inhibition of CDK4 and CDK2 via targeting p27 tyrosine phosphorylation induces a potent and durable response in breast cancer cells. Mol Cancer Res 16:361–377. https://doi.org/10.1158/1541-7786.MCR-17-0602

Patel HK, Tao N, Lee K-M et al (2019) Elacestrant (RAD1901) exhibits anti-tumor activity in multiple ER+ breast cancer models resistant to CDK4/6 inhibitors. Breast Cancer Res 21:146. https://doi.org/10.1186/s13058-019-1230-0

Peuker CA, Yaghobramzi S, Grunert C et al (2022) Treatment with ribociclib shows favourable immunomodulatory effects in patients with hormone receptor-positive breast cancer-findings from the RIBECCA trial. Eur J Cancer 162:45–55. https://doi.org/10.1016/J.EJCA.2021.11.025

Raspé E, Coulonval K, Pita JM et al (2017) CDK4 phosphorylation status and a linked gene expression profile predict sensitivity to palbociclib. EMBO Mol Med 9:1052–1066. https://doi.org/10.15252/EMMM.201607084

Raub TJ, Wishart GN, Kulanthaivel P et al (2015) Brain exposure of two selective dual CDK4 and CDK6 inhibitors and the antitumor activity of CDK4 and CDK6 inhibition in combination with temozolomide in an intracranial glioblastoma xenograft. Drug Metab Dispos 43:1360–1371. https://doi.org/10.1124/DMD.114.062745

Reddy HKDL, Mettus RV, Rane SG et al (2005) Cyclin-dependent kinase 4 expression is essential for neu-induced breast tumorigenesis. Cancer Res 65:10174–10178. https://doi.org/10.1158/0008-5472.CAN-05-2639

Rugo HS, Huober J, García-Sáenz JA et al (2021a) Management of abemaciclib-associated adverse events in patients with hormone receptor-positive, human epidermal growth factor receptor 2-negative advanced breast cancer: safety analysis of MONARCH 2 and MONARCH 3. Oncologist 26:e53–e65. https://doi.org/10.1002/ONCO.13531

Rugo HS, Lerebours F, Ciruelos E et al (2021b) Alpelisib plus fulvestrant in PIK3CA-mutated, hormone receptor-positive advanced breast cancer after a CDK4/6 inhibitor (BYLieve): one cohort of a phase 2, multicentre, open-label, non-comparative study. Lancet Oncol 22:489–498. https://doi.org/10.1016/S1470-2045(21)00034-6

Rugo HS, Kabos P, Beck JT et al (2022) Abemaciclib in combination with pembrolizumab for HR+, HER2- metastatic breast cancer: phase 1b study. NPJ Breast Cancer 8. https://doi.org/10.1038/S41523-022-00482-2

Saha S, Dey S, Nath S (2021) Steroid hormone receptors: links with cell cycle machinery and breast cancer progression. Front Oncol 11:620214. https://doi.org/10.3389/FONC.2021.620214/BIBTEX

Sanders DA, Ross-Innes CS, Beraldi D et al (2013) Genome-wide mapping of FOXM1 binding reveals co-binding with estrogen receptor alpha in breast cancer cells. Genome Biol 14:1–16. https://doi.org/10.1186/GB-2013-14-1-R6/FIGURES/7

Schaer DA, Beckmann RP, Dempsey JA et al (2018) The CDK4/6 inhibitor abemaciclib induces a T cell inflamed tumor microenvironment and enhances the efficacy of PD-L1 checkpoint blockade. Cell Rep 22:2978–2994. https://doi.org/10.1016/j.celrep.2018.02.053

Schlam I, Swain SM (2021) HER2-positive breast cancer and tyrosine kinase inhibitors: the time is now. NPJ Breast Cancer 7. https://doi.org/10.1038/S41523-021-00265-1

Scirocchi F, Scagnoli S, Botticelli A et al (2022) Immune effects of CDK4/6 inhibitors in patients with HR+/HER2- metastatic breast cancer: Relief from immunosuppression is associated with clinical response. EBioMedicine 79. https://doi.org/10.1016/J.EBIOM.2022.104010

Slamon DJ, Neven P, Chia S et al (2018) Phase III randomized study of ribociclib and fulvestrant in hormone receptor-positive, human epidermal growth factor receptor 2-negative advanced breast cancer: MONALEESA-3. J Clin Oncol 36:2465–2472. https://doi.org/10.1200/JCO.2018.78.9909

Slamon DJ, Stroyakovskiy D, Yardley DA, et al (2023) Ribociclib and endocrine therapy as adjuvant treatment in patients with HR+/HER2- early breast cancer: primary results from the phase III NATALEE trial. doi:https://doi.org/10.1200/JCO.2023.41.17_SUPPL.LBA500

Sledge GW, Toi M, Neven P et al (2017) MONARCH 2: abemaciclib in combination with fulvestrant in women with HR+/HER2-advanced breast cancer who had progressed while receiving endocrine therapy. J Clin Oncol 35:2875–2884. https://doi.org/10.1200/JCO.2017.73.7585

Sledge GW, Toi M, Neven P et al (2020) The effect of abemaciclib plus fulvestrant on overall survival in hormone receptor-positive, ERBB2-negative breast cancer that progressed on endocrine therapy - MONARCH 2: a randomized clinical trial. JAMA Oncol 6:116–124. https://doi.org/10.1001/jamaoncol.2019.4782

Smyth LM, Batist G, Meric-Bernstam F et al (2021) Selective AKT kinase inhibitor capivasertib in combination with fulvestrant in PTEN-mutant ER-positive metastatic breast cancer. NPJ Breast Cancer 7(1):1–7. https://doi.org/10.1038/s41523-021-00251-7

Soosainathan A, Iravani M, El-Botty R et al (2024) Targeting transcriptional regulation with a CDK9 inhibitor suppresses growth of endocrine- and palbociclib-resistant ER+ breast cancers. Cancer Res 84. https://doi.org/10.1158/0008-5472.CAN-23-0650

Soria-Bretones I, Thu KL, Silvester J et al (2022) The spindle assembly checkpoint is a therapeutic vulnerability of CDK4/6 inhibitor-resistant ER+ breast cancer with mitotic aberrations. Sci Adv 8. https://doi.org/10.1126/SCIADV.ABQ4293

Stendahl M, Kronblad À, Rydén L et al (2004) Cyclin D1 overexpression is a negative predictive factor for tamoxifen response in postmenopausal breast cancer patients. Br J Cancer 90:1942. https://doi.org/10.1038/SJ.BJC.6601831

Sun C, Mezzadra R, Schumacher TN (2018) Regulation and function of the PD-L1 checkpoint. Immunity 48:434–452. https://doi.org/10.1016/J.IMMUNI.2018.03.014

Thangavel C, Dean JL, Ertel A et al (2011) Therapeutically activating RB: reestablishing cell cycle control in endocrine therapy-resistant breast cancer. Endocr Relat Cancer 18:333–345. https://doi.org/10.1530/ERC-10-0262

Tolaney SM, Im YH, Calvo E et al (2021) Phase Ib study of ribociclib plus fulvestrant and ribociclib plus fulvestrant plus PI3K inhibitor (alpelisib or buparlisib) for HR+ advanced breast cancer. Clin Cancer Res 27:418–428. https://doi.org/10.1158/1078-0432.CCR-20-0645

Tolaney SM, Toi M, Neven P et al (2022) Clinical significance of PIK3CA and ESR1 mutations in circulating tumor DNA: analysis from the MONARCH 2 study of abemaciclib plus fulvestrant. Clin Cancer Res 28:1500–1506. https://doi.org/10.1158/1078-0432.CCR-21-3276/678415/AM/CLINICAL-SIGNIFICANCE-OF-PIK3CA-AND-ESR1-MUTATIONS

Tong J, Tan X, Song X et al (2022) CDK4/6 inhibition suppresses p73 phosphorylation and activates DR5 to potentiate chemotherapy and immune checkpoint blockade. Cancer Res 82:1340–1352. https://doi.org/10.1158/0008-5472.CAN-21-3062

Torres-Guzmán R, Calsina B, Hermoso A et al (2017) Preclinical characterization of abemaciclib in hormone receptor positive breast cancer. Oncotarget 8:69493–69507. https://doi.org/10.18632/ONCOTARGET.17778

Tripathy D, Im SA, Colleoni M et al (2018) Ribociclib plus endocrine therapy for premenopausal women with hormone-receptor-positive, advanced breast cancer (MONALEESA-7): a randomised phase 3 trial. Lancet Oncol 19:904–915. https://doi.org/10.1016/S1470-2045(18)30292-4

Turner NC, Ro J, André F et al (2015) Palbociclib in hormone-receptor–positive advanced breast cancer. N Engl J Med 373:209–219. https://doi.org/10.1056/nejmoa1505270

Turner NC, Slamon DJ, Ro J et al (2018) Overall survival with palbociclib and fulvestrant in advanced breast cancer. N Engl J Med 379:1926–1936. https://doi.org/10.1056/nejmoa1810527

Turner NC, Liu Y, Zhu Z et al (2019) Cyclin E1 expression and palbociclib efficacy in previously treated hormone receptor-positive metastatic breast cancer. J Clin Oncol 37:1169–1178

Turner NC, Oliveira M, Howell SJ et al (2023) Capivasertib in hormone receptor-positive advanced breast cancer. N Engl J Med 388:2058–2070. https://doi.org/10.1056/NEJMOA2214131

Uribe ML, Marrocco I, Yarden Y (2021) EGFR in cancer: signaling mechanisms, drugs, and acquired resistance. Cancers (Basel) 13. https://doi.org/10.3390/CANCERS13112748

Uzhachenko RV, Bharti V, Ouyang Z et al (2021) Metabolic modulation by CDK4/6 inhibitor promotes chemokine-mediated recruitment of T cells into mammary tumors. Cell Rep 35. https://doi.org/10.1016/J.CELREP.2021.108944

Vasan N, Cantley LC (2022) At a crossroads: how to translate the roles of PI3K in oncogenic and metabolic signalling into improvements in cancer therapy. Nat Rev Clin Oncol 19:471–485. https://doi.org/10.1038/S41571-022-00633-1

Vermeulen K, Van Bockstaele DR, Berneman ZN (2003) The cell cycle: a review of regulation, deregulation and therapeutic targets in cancer. Cell Prolif 36:131–149

Vidal A, Koff A (2000) Cell-cycle inhibitors: three families united by a common cause. Gene 247:1–15. https://doi.org/10.1016/S0378-1119(00)00092-5

Von Karstedt S, Montinaro A, Walczak H (2017) Exploring the TRAILs less travelled: TRAIL in cancer biology and therapy. Nat Rev Cancer 17:352–366. https://doi.org/10.1038/NRC.2017.28

Wander SA, Cohen O, Gong X et al (2020) The genomic landscape of intrinsic and acquired resistance to cyclin-dependent kinase 4/6 inhibitors in patients with hormone receptor–positive metastatic breast cancer. Cancer Discov 10:1174–1193. https://doi.org/10.1158/2159-8290.CD-19-1390

Wang Q, Guldner IH, Golomb SM et al (2019) Single-cell profiling guided combinatorial immunotherapy for fast-evolving CDK4/6 inhibitor-resistant HER2-positive breast cancer. Nat Commun 10:3817. https://doi.org/10.1038/S41467-019-11729-1

Wierstra I, Alves J (2006) Transcription factor FOXM1c is repressed by RB and activated by cyclin D1/Cdk4. Biol Chem 387:949–962. https://doi.org/10.1515/BC.2006.119

Xu J, Chen Y, Olopade OI (2010) MYC and breast cancer. Genes Cancer 1:629–640. https://doi.org/10.1177/1947601910378691

Xu B, Zhang Q, Zhang P et al (2021) Dalpiciclib or placebo plus fulvestrant in hormone receptor-positive and HER2-negative advanced breast cancer: a randomized, phase 3 trial. Nat Med 27(11):1904–1909. https://doi.org/10.1038/s41591-021-01562-9

Yang C, Li Z, Bhatt T et al (2017) Acquired CDK6 amplification promotes breast cancer resistance to CDK4/6 inhibitors and loss of ER signaling and dependence. Oncogene 36:2255–2264. https://doi.org/10.1038/ONC.2016.379

Yuan Y, Lee JS, Yost SE et al (2021) Phase I/II trial of palbociclib, pembrolizumab and letrozole in patients with hormone receptor-positive metastatic breast cancer. Eur J Cancer 154:11–20. https://doi.org/10.1016/J.EJCA.2021.05.035

Zafonte BT, Hulit J, Amanatullah DF et al (2000) Cell-cycle dysregulation in breast cancer: breast cancer therapies targeting the cell cycle. Front Biosci 5:938–961. https://doi.org/10.2741/ZAFONTE/PDF

Zhang J, Bu X, Wang H et al (2018) Cyclin D-CDK4 kinase destabilizes PD-L1 via cullin 3-SPOP to control cancer immune surveillance. Nature 553:91–95. https://doi.org/10.1038/nature25015

Zhang P, Zhang Q, Tong Z et al (2023) Dalpiciclib plus letrozole or anastrozole versus placebo plus letrozole or anastrozole as first-line treatment in patients with hormone receptor-positive, HER2-negative advanced breast cancer (DAWNA-2): a multicentre, randomised, double-blind, placebo-controlled, phase 3 trial. Lancet Oncol 24:646–657. https://doi.org/10.1016/S1470-2045(23)00172-9

Zwijsen RML, Buckle RS, Hijmans EM et al (1998) Ligand-independent recruitment of steroid receptor coactivators to estrogen receptor by cyclin D1. Genes Dev 12:3488–3498. https://doi.org/10.1101/GAD.12.22.3488

HER2-Positive Breast Cancer Treatment and Resistance

24

Jamunarani Veeraraghavan, Carmine De Angelis, Carolina Gutierrez, Fu-Tien Liao, Caroline Sabotta, Mothaffar F. Rimawi, C. Kent Osborne, and Rachel Schiff

Abstract

HER2-positive (+) breast cancer is an aggressive disease with poor prognosis, a narrative that changed drastically with the advent and approval of trastuzumab, the first humanized monoclonal antibody targeting HER2. In addition to another monoclonal antibody, more classes of HER2-targeted agents, including tyrosine kinase inhibitors, and antibody-drug conjugates were developed in the years that followed. While these potent therapies have substantially improved the outcome of patients with HER2+ breast cancer, resistance has prevailed as a clinical challenge ever since the arrival of targeted agents. Efforts to develop new treatment regimens to treat/overcome resistance is futile without a primary understanding of the mechanistic underpinnings of resistance. Resistance could be attributed to mechanisms that are either specific to the tumor epithelial cells or those that emerge through changes in the tumor microenvironment. Reactivation of the HER receptor layer due to incomplete blockade of the HER receptor layer or due to alterations in the HER receptors is one of the major mechanisms. In other instances, resistance may occur due to deregulations in key downstream signaling such as the PI3K/AKT or RAS/MEK/ERK pathways or due to the emergence of compensatory pathways such as ER, other RTKs, or metabolic pathways. Potent new targeted agents and approaches to target key actionable drivers of resistance have already been identified, many of which are in early clinical development or under preclinical evaluation. Ongoing and future translational research will

J. Veeraraghavan · M. F. Rimawi
Lester & Sue Smith Breast Center, Baylor College of Medicine, Houston, TX, USA

Dan L. Duncan Comprehensive Cancer Center, Baylor College of Medicine, Houston, TX, USA

Department of Medicine, Baylor College of Medicine, Houston, TX, USA

C. De Angelis · C. Gutierrez · F.-T. Liao
Lester & Sue Smith Breast Center, Baylor College of Medicine, Houston, TX, USA

Dan L. Duncan Comprehensive Cancer Center, Baylor College of Medicine, Houston, TX, USA

C. Sabotta
Department of Molecular and Cellular Biology, Baylor College of Medicine, Houston, TX, USA

C. K. Osborne · R. Schiff (✉)
Lester & Sue Smith Breast Center, Baylor College of Medicine, Houston, TX, USA

Dan L. Duncan Comprehensive Cancer Center, Baylor College of Medicine, Houston, TX, USA

Department of Medicine, Baylor College of Medicine, Houston, TX, USA

Department of Molecular and Cellular Biology, Baylor College of Medicine, Houston, TX, USA
e-mail: rschiff@bcm.edu

T. Sørlie, R. B. Clarke (eds.), *A Guide to Breast Cancer Research*, Advances in Experimental Medicine and Biology 1464, https://doi.org/10.1007/978-3-031-70875-6_24

continue to uncover additional therapeutic vulnerabilities, as well as new targeted agents and approaches to treat and/or overcome anti-HER2 treatment resistance.

Keywords

HER2 · HER2-targeted therapy · Treatment resistance · Estrogen receptor · Growth factor receptors · Receptor cross talk · Genetic aberrations

Key Points

- HER2+ breast cancer, which overexpresses the HER2 protein largely via gene amplification, accounts for 15–20% of all breast cancers. It is an aggressive subtype with increased metastatic tropism to the brain.
- The advent of several potent HER2-targeted therapies with different mechanisms of action over the past two decades has revolutionized the outcome of patients with HER2+ breast cancer.
- About half of HER2+ breast tumors also express the estrogen receptor (ER) wherein the treatment strategy is to simultaneously block both ER and HER2.
- Despite effective HER2-targeted therapies, disease recurrence due to treatment resistance prevails and presents a major clinical challenge.
- Understanding the molecular complexity of the resistance mechanisms is crucial to developing new effective and tailored treatment strategies to treat and/or overcome resistance.
- The continued development of new targeted treatment strategies and modalities, including efforts of treatment de-escalation, continues to reshape the treatment landscape of HER2+ breast cancer and improve patient outcome.

24.1 Introduction

Breast cancer is a clinically and pathologically heterogeneous disease comprised of different subtypes originally classified mainly based on the immunohistochemical presence of estrogen receptor (ER), progesterone receptor (PR), and the human epidermal growth factor receptor 2 (HER2; also known as ERBB2) (Blows et al. 2010). Breast tumors that express ER and/or PR are classed as ER-positive (+) or hormone receptor-positive (HR+), while tumors overexpressing HER2 are termed HER2+. Triple-negative breast cancer (TNBC), as the name suggests, lacks the expression of ER, PR, and HER2. A molecular classification, however, profiled breast cancer at the gene expression (transcriptomic) level into five major intrinsic subtypes – luminal A, luminal B, HER2-enriched, basal-like, and normal-like – though additional new subtypes have also been proposed (Perou et al. 2000; Sorlie et al. 2001; Curtis et al. 2012). A more detailed description of the different molecular subtypes of breast cancer is presented in Chaps. 11 and 21. Adding to this molecular complexity, breast cancers, both across and within each subtype, portray distinct histopathological and molecular features and outcomes, suggesting that breast cancer is in fact a collection of diseases. Treatment approaches vary according to the subtype with the more common therapies being targeted treatments in the form of endocrine therapy (block estrogen signaling) for ER+ disease or anti-HER2 therapy for HER2+ disease, as well as chemotherapy which is used in certain patients.

Characterized by overexpression of HER2, largely via gene amplification, the HER2+ subtype accounts for 15–20% of all breast cancers, with about half of them also expressing ER. Being a major oncogenic driver of the growth and aggressiveness of tumors that overexpress it, HER2 is both a biomarker of tumor aggressiveness and a therapeutic vulnerability. Despite the arsenal of potent HER2-targeted agents at our disposal that revolutionized the outcome of patients with HER2+ breast cancer, treatment resistance prevails as a subset of the tumors still show intrinsic resistance or relapse after initial response, posing major challenges in the clinical management of HER2+ breast cancer. In the evolving landscape of HER2-targeted therapies, gaining a better understanding of the mechanism of action of different targeted agents and that of treatment resistance that either pre-exist at the time of treatment (intrinsic) or emerge under treatment pressure (acquired) is key to finding effective treatment strategies to overcome them. Over the past several years, numerous studies have reported varied mechanisms of anti-HER2 treatment resistance and the identification of new actionable targets, as well as the discovery of novel treatment strategies targeting HER2. In this chapter, we offer a brief overview of the biology of the HER2 pathway and a summary of the key recent findings with a particular focus on currently approved HER2-targeted therapies, key molecular mechanisms of anti-HER2 treatment resistance, and new emerging treatment strategies and approaches for patients with HER2+ breast cancer.

24.2 HER2-Positive Breast Cancer and the HER Pathway

Tumor HER2 Status The HER2 status of a tumor is assessed and diagnosed by routine (Food and Drug Administration) FDA-approved immunohistochemistry (IHC) for membrane HER2 staining or fluorescent in situ hybridization (FISH) for HER2 gene levels through which a tumor is designated HER2-positive, HER2-negative, or equivocal (Fig. 24.1). The American Society of Clinical Oncology (ASCO) and College of American Pathologists (CAP) HER2 testing guidelines define HER2 positivity as HER2 FISH ratio ≥ 2, *HER2* gene copy number (CN) ≥ 6.0, or a strong complete immunohistochemical membrane staining (i.e., score 3+) in ≥10% of invasive tumor cells (Wolff et al. 2018) to predict sensitivity to adding HER2-targeted agents to chemotherapy. Importantly, in the recent years, a new subset of breast tumors termed HER2-low, defined as tumors with HER2 IHC 1+ by itself or 2+ and *HER2* gene amplification-negative by ISH, have been identified, mostly due to their sensitivity to the new class of HER2-targeted agents, the antibody drug conjugates (ADCs) (Modi et al. 2022). However, a detailed discussion of this subset of HER2-low breast cancer is beyond the scope of this chapter. Finally, heterogeneity in HER2 levels, defined as varying expression levels or amplification of HER2 in different regions of the same tumor (intratumor heterogeneity) or in tumors from different patients (inter-tumor heterogeneity), has been shown to contribute to resistance to multiple HER2-targeted therapies (*see Sect. 24.4 for more details*) (Hamilton et al. 2021).

The HER Pathway HER2 is a key member of the receptor tyrosine kinase family comprised of four HER receptors: HER1 (also known as EGFR), HER2, HER3, and HER4. Briefly, the HER receptors are transmembrane proteins with an extracellular ligand-binding domain, a transmembrane domain, and an intracellular tyrosine kinase domain. They are expressed as monomers on the cell surface. Upon ligand binding to the extracellular domain, the HER receptors undergo conformational change, which allows homo-/heterodimerization of the receptors and the activation of their kinase domains, except in the case of HER3, which possesses an inactive kinase domain. HER2, on the other hand, lacks a known ligand and exists in an already open conformation and is activated either by heterodimerization with other ligand-bound HER members or by homodimerization when overexpressed. Dimerization of HER receptors leads to autophosphorylation or transphosphorylation of the tyrosine residues in the cytoplasmic domain of the dimers and the subsequent initiation of a cascade of signaling pathways. The HER family of receptors govern a highly redundant and complex signaling network via key downstream pathways, primar-

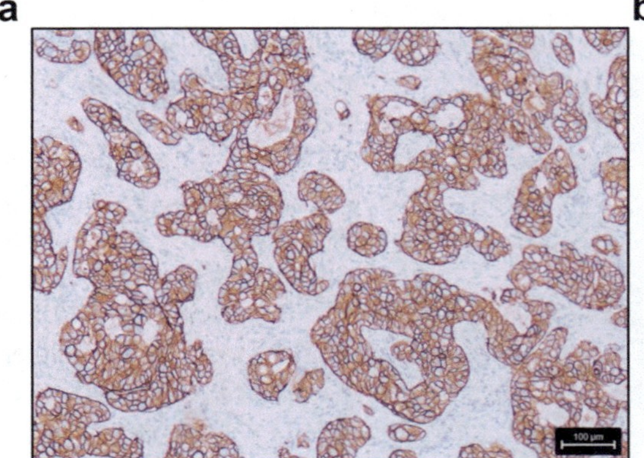

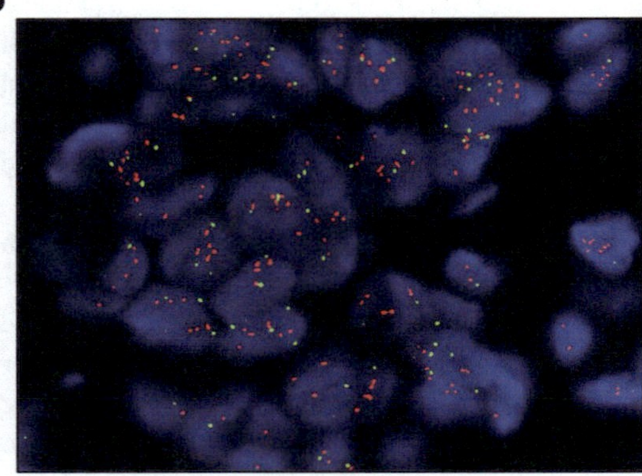

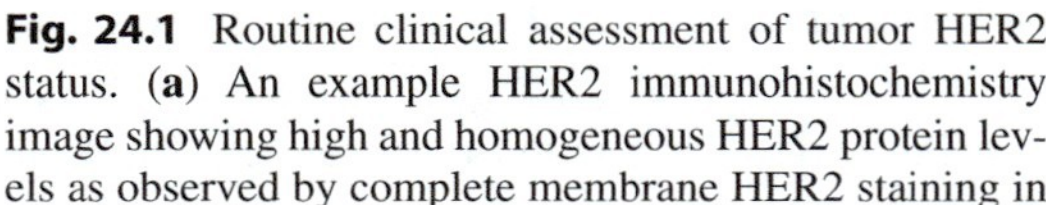

Fig. 24.1 Routine clinical assessment of tumor HER2 status. (**a**) An example HER2 immunohistochemistry image showing high and homogeneous HER2 protein levels as observed by complete membrane HER2 staining in brown. (**b**) An example HER2 fluorescence in situ hybridization (FISH) image of a HER2-amplified tumor assessed using probes to the HER2 locus (red) and the chromosome 17 centromere (green). Scale bar: 100 μm

ily the phosphatidylinositol-4,5-bisphosphate 3-kinase (PI3K)/AKT/mTOR and RAS/mitogen-activated protein kinase (MAPK)/ERK pathways to promote cell proliferation and survival, resulting in tumor growth and metastasis (Fig. 24.2a) (Rimawi et al. 2015a; Gutierrez and Schiff 2011).

Prognosis and Treatment Strategies HER2+ breast cancer is an aggressive subtype with poor prognosis and increased metastatic tropism to the brain (Swain et al. 2023). The advent of the HER2-targeted humanized monoclonal antibody trastuzumab, a pioneering targeted therapy for HER2+ breast cancer, was a remarkable success story that altered the face of HER2+ breast cancer from being a dreaded diagnosis to one with better prognosis. This successful strategy also offered hope and headlined the insight that a tumor biology-centered treatment approach is the way forward. Ever since the breakthrough approval of trastuzumab more than two decades ago, several new classes of HER2-targeted agents have been developed and approved for clinical use, which are discussed in detail in Sect. 24.3. With the advent of several potent HER2-targeted agents through the years, there has been a marked improvement in patient outcome, with survival rates exceeding 90% in the early setting when patients are treated with dual anti-HER2 therapy and chemotherapy (von Minckwitz et al. 2017). Emerging treatment approaches are also taking the biology and heterogeneity of HER2+ breast cancers into consideration and are attempting to reduce the treatment-associated adverse effects through personalized strategies discussed in further detail in Sect. 24.5. However, with up to ~50% of patients with HER2+ metastatic breast cancer developing brain metastases during the course of the disease (Gabos et al. 2006; Dong et al. 2019), one of the key prevailing challenges is the clinical management of HER2+ brain metastasis (Swain et al. 2023). This problem is further complicated by the presence of the blood-brain/tumor barrier (BBB) that regulates drug distribution and prevents active agents from entering the brain. While great strides have been made in treating systemic HER2+ disease, a parallel paradoxical increase in brain-only recurrences has been observed, perhaps because the monoclonal antibodies which are effective outside the brain do not effectively cross the BBB (Chiu et al. 2019). Importantly, the prognosis of HER2+ breast cancer after recurrence in the central nervous system is dismal with poor survival rates (Pestalozzi et al. 2006). The trajectory of this scenario, however, is changing due to the recent development of potent small-molecule tyrosine kinase inhibitors (TKIs) as well as new ADCs that can effectively cross the BBB and

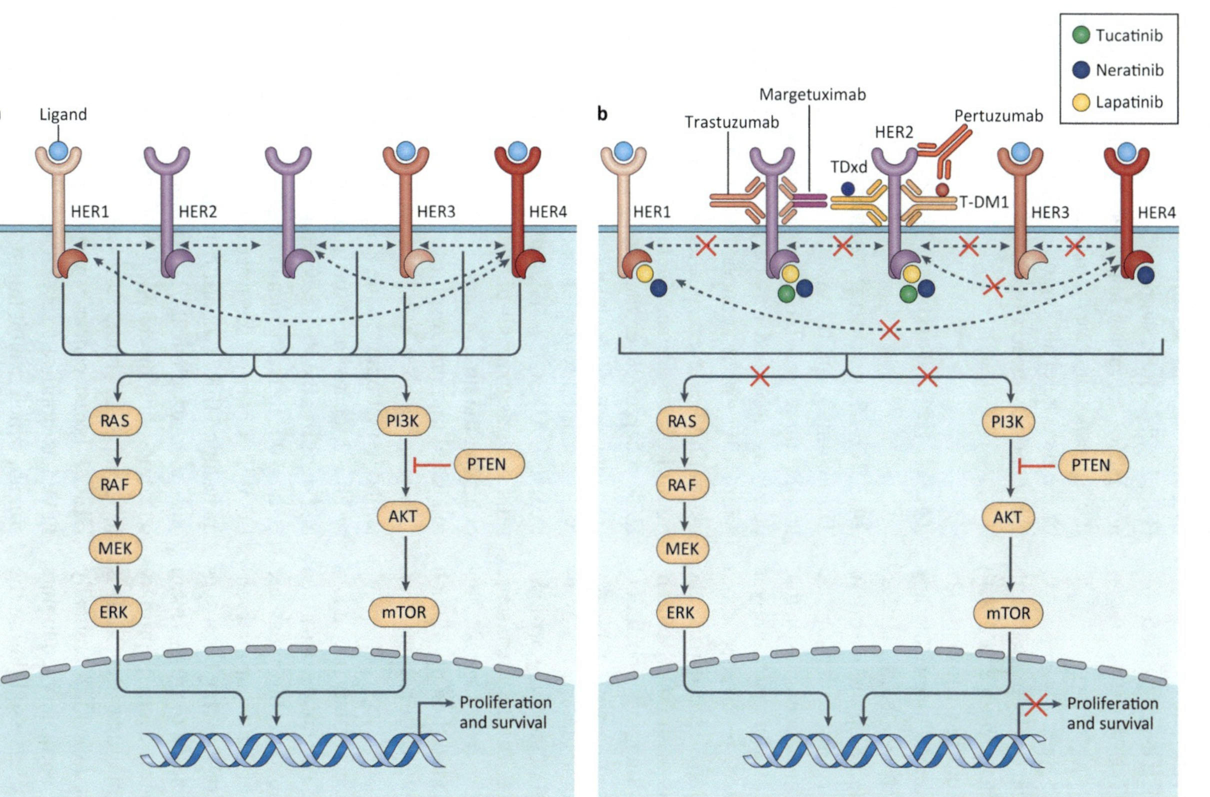

Fig. 24.2 Signaling by HER2 and other HER family members and the clinically approved HER2-targeted agents. (**a**) The HER family of receptor tyrosine kinases consists of four receptors: EGFR (HER1), HER2, HER3, and HER4. Activation of signaling through all HER proteins, except HER2, is induced by ligand binding. Upon ligand binding, these receptors undergo conformational changes, leading to the formation of homodimers or heterodimers. HER2 lacks any known ligand but has a conformation that is conducive to dimerization and can thus be activated through homodimerization, when it is overexpressed, or heterodimerization with other ligand-bound members of the HER family. Dimerization of HER protein results in transphosphorylation of specific tyrosine residues in their intracellular domains, which in turn activates downstream signaling cascades, including the PI3K/AKT and MEK/ERK pathways. These signaling pathways mediate diverse cellular activities, including those controlled by transcription factors that regulate the transcription of multiple genes associated with survival and proliferation. (**b**) Eight HER2-targeted agents are currently approved for the treatment of patients with HER2+ breast cancer, which are categorized as monoclonal antibodies (trastuzumab, pertuzumab, and margetuximab), small-molecule tyrosine kinase inhibitors (TKIs) (lapatinib, neratinib, and tucatinib), or antibody-drug conjugates (ADCs) (trastuzumab emtansine (T-DM1) and trastuzumab deruxtecan (T-Dxd)). *Figure adapted from Goutsouliak et al., Nat Rev Clin Oncol 17, 233–250 (2020) and modified in part using* Biorender.com

therefore demonstrated to be more effective against metastatic lesions in the brain, as discussed further in Sect. 24.3.2.

24.3 The Major Classes of Approved HER2-Targeted Therapies and Treatment Strategies

Clinically, HER2+ breast cancer is treated with systemic HER2-targeted therapy together with chemotherapy. In the early setting when there are no obvious metastases, neoadjuvant therapy refers to administration of systemic HER2-targeted therapy with chemotherapy to shrink or eliminate the primary tumor prior to its surgical removal and to eliminate micrometastases that may be present. Postoperative adjuvant therapy is intended to prevent disease recurrence from micrometastases that may have spread from the primary tumor to other parts of the body but are not detectable by routine imaging or clinical methods. In the advanced setting with clinically detectable metastases, systemic therapy is administered with the primary goal of stopping or slowing the growth and spread of the metastatic disease in other organs. These treatment settings and the recommended systemic therapy in each setting are discussed in more detail in *Sect. 24.3.2*.

In clinical research trials, endpoints play a key role in determining the success or failure of a given trial. Endpoints are specific outcomes that are measured to determine the effect of an intervention, such as, in the context of this chapter, a specific cancer treatment regimen. There are two main types of endpoints in a clinical trial: (i) primary endpoint (the main outcome that the trial is designed to measure and often the most clinically relevant endpoint) and (ii) secondary endpoints (other outcomes that are also assessed during the trial but are of lesser importance compared to the primary endpoint). The specific primary and secondary endpoints assessed in a trial depend on the phase of the trial (phase I, II, or III) or the treatment setting (adjuvant, neoadjuvant, or metastatic).

The three major classes of anti-HER2 therapies include monoclonal antibodies and TKIs directed against the extracellular and intracellular domains of HER2, respectively, and the HER2-targeting ADCs that use HER2 to deliver potent cytotoxic agents selectively to the tumor cells (Fig. 24.2b). Here, we provide an overview on the anti-HER2 therapies approved by the FDA and the corresponding key clinical trials and list some of the most relevant ongoing clinical trials in the early and advanced disease settings (Table 24.1).

24.3.1 HER2-Targeted Therapies

24.3.1.1 Monoclonal Antibodies

Trastuzumab, pertuzumab, and margetuximab are the three anti-HER2 monoclonal antibodies currently approved for the treatment of patients with HER2+ breast cancer. Anti-HER2 monoclonal antibodies exert anti-tumor activity through multiple mechanisms including inactivation of HER receptor layer and associated downstream signaling pathways and induction of apoptosis, as well as antibody-dependent cell mediated cytotoxicity (ADCC), a mechanism that targets and kills the trastuzumab-bound tumor cells through engaging the host immune system to elicit a cell-mediated immune response.

Trastuzumab is a fully humanized monoclonal antibody that binds to the extracellular domain IV of HER2 located near the transmembrane domain and stabilizes the HER2-containing dimers (Molina et al. 2001). Trastuzumab was approved by the FDA in 1998 for the treatment of patients with metastatic HER2+ breast cancer. Since then, several landmark clinical trials demonstrated superior outcomes with the addition of trastuzumab to chemotherapy in both early-stage and metastatic HER2+ breast cancer. Over the past decade, the FDA has approved several biosimilars of trastuzumab, which exhibit highly similar structural and functional properties to the original trastuzumab (Goutsouliak et al. 2020; Triantafyllidi and Triantafillidis 2022). Additionally, a subcutaneous form of trastuzumab (trastuzumab-hyaluronidase-oysk) has been developed as an alternative to intravenous trastuzumab (Duco et al. 2020).

Table 24.1 Selected randomized clinical trials of HER2-targeted therapies for patients with HER2+ breast cancer

			Treatment arms		Improved outcomes
	Setting	Patients (n)	Experimental arm	Control arm	
Monoclonal antibodies					
APHINITY	Adjuvant	4805	Chemotherapy + Trastuzumab + Pertuzumab	Chemotherapy + Trastuzumab + Placebo	iDFS
NEOSPHERE	Neoadjuvant	417	Chemotherapy + Trastuzumab + Pertuzumab Chemotherapy + Pertuzumab Trastuzumab + Pertuzumab	Chemotherapy + Trastuzumab	pCR
CLEOPATRA	Metastatic	808	Chemotherapy + Trastuzumab + Pertuzumab	Chemotherapy + Trastuzumab + Placebo	PFS and OS
PERTAIN	Metastatic	258	Endocrine therapy + Trastuzumab + Pertuzumab	Endocrine therapy + Trastuzumab + Placebo	PFS
SOPHIA	Metastatic	536	Chemotherapy + Margetuximab	Chemotherapy + Trastuzumab	PFS
Antibody drug conjugates					
KATHERINE	Post-neoadjuvant	1486	T-DM1	Trastuzumab	DFS and OS
EMILIA	Metastatic	991	T-DM1	Lapatinib + Capecitabine	PFS and OS
DESTINY-Breast03	Metastatic	524	T-DXd	T-DM1	PFS
DESTINY-Breast02	Metastatic	608	T-DXd	TPC	PFS and OS
Tyrosine kinase inhibitors					
EXTENET	Adjuvant	2840	Neratinib	Placebo	iDFS
PHOEBE	Metastatic	267	Capecitabine + Pyrotinib	Capecitabine + Lapatinib	PFS and OS
HER2CLIMB	Metastatic	612	Trastuzumab + Capecitabine + Tucatinib	Trastuzumab + Capecitabine + Placebo	PFS and OS
NALA	Metastatic	621	Capecitabine + Neratinib	Capecitabine + Lapatinib	PFS

Abbreviations: *iDFS* invasive disease-free survival, *OS* overall survival, *pCR* pathologic complete response, *PFS* progression-free survival, *TPC* treatment of physician's choice

Pertuzumab is a humanized monoclonal antibody with a mechanism of action that is complementary to that of trastuzumab since it binds and blocks the extracellular domain II responsible for heterodimerization of HER2 with other HER family members (Franklin et al. 2004; Badache and Hynes 2004). Though pertuzumab alone has shown only modest anti-tumor activity, it has proven to be synergistic when combined with trastuzumab in preclinical models (Nahta et al. 2004). In patients with HER2+ breast cancer, dual HER2 blockade with trastuzumab plus pertuzumab together with chemotherapy demonstrated better outcomes than trastuzumab plus chemotherapy in the metastatic (Baselga et al. 2012a; Swain et al. 2015), adjuvant (von Minckwitz et al. 2017; Piccart et al. 2021), and neoadjuvant (Gianni et al. 2016) settings leading to FDA approval. A subcutaneous formulation of a fixed dose of pertuzumab and trastuzumab with recombinant human hyaluronidase (Pertuzumab-trastuzumab-hyaluronidase-zzxf) achieved complete response rates comparable to intravenous pertuzumab plus trastuzumab in patients with HER2+ early breast cancer treated with neoadjuvant therapy, supporting the FDA approval (DuMond et al. 2021).

Margetuximab is a chimeric antibody that shares epitope specificity with trastuzumab and incorporates an engineered fragment crystallizable (Fc) region to increase binding affinity for the activating Fcγ receptor (CD16A) and to decrease binding affinity for the inhibitory Fcγ receptor (CD32B) expressed on immune effector cells to increase the ADCC activity. The FDA granted regulatory approval for margetuximab plus chemotherapy for the treatment of metastatic HER2+ breast cancer based on the results from the phase III SOPHIA study demonstrating a marginal progression-free survival (PFS) benefit but no significant overall survival (OS) improvement with margetuximab over trastuzumab plus chemotherapy in patients with metastatic HER2+ breast cancer who had previously received ≥2 HER2-targeted treatments. Of note, compared to trastuzumab, margetuximab has also been suggested to have improved binding affinity for the polymorphic allelic variants 158V or 158F of the activating Fcγ receptor CD16A. Indeed, an exploratory analysis of treatment efficacy in relation to CD16A receptor genotypes suggested a potential higher benefit of margetuximab versus trastuzumab in CD16A-158FF patients (Rugo et al. 2023).

24.3.1.2 Tyrosine Kinase Inhibitors

Small-molecule TKIs that target the intracellular catalytic kinase domain of HER2 and other HER family members and compete with ATP represent an alternative mechanism to suppress HER2 downstream signaling. Compared with monoclonal antibodies, HER2 TKIs have the advantages of oral administration, a better blood-brain barrier penetration, and lower cardiac toxicity.

Lapatinib is a dual reversible inhibitor of EGFR (also known as HER1) and HER2 that demonstrated clinical activity in trastuzumab-resistant HER2+ breast cancer models (Xia et al. 2002; Nahta et al. 2007). In patients with advanced HER2+ breast cancer who had progressed after treatment with trastuzumab, the addition of lapatinib to capecitabine demonstrated superior efficacy compared to capecitabine alone (Geyer et al. 2006). Additionally, lapatinib plus the aromatase inhibitor letrozole that inhibits the estrogen-receptor pathway was found to be more effective than letrozole alone in HR+/HER2+ metastatic disease (Johnston et al. 2009), resulting in regulatory approval for these combination therapies. Several trials have evaluated the activity of lapatinib alone or in combination with trastuzumab with or without chemotherapy in the neoadjuvant setting. Collectively, in these trials, the addition of lapatinib to trastuzumab yielded superior pathologic complete response (pCR) rates, a clinical endpoint and surrogate marker defined as the absence of residual invasive cancer cells in the resected breast tissue and regional lymph nodes. This difference, however, did not translate to significant improvement of event-free survival (EFS). Similarly, the large phase III ALTTO trial failed to demonstrate the superiority of adjuvant dual HER2 blockade with lapatinib plus trastuzumab and chemotherapy over trastuzumab plus chemotherapy in terms of disease-free survival (DFS) or OS (Moreno-Aspitia et al. 2021).

Neratinib is a second-generation irreversible pan-HER TKI that targets EGFR, HER2, and HER4. In the preclinical setting, neratinib proved to be more effective than trastuzumab and pertuzumab in HER2+ breast cancer xenograft models and inhibited the growth of trastuzumab-resistant cell lines (Rabindran et al. 2004; Veeraraghavan et al. 2021). The combination of neratinib and capecitabine versus lapatinib+capecitabine significantly improved PFS in patients with HER2+ metastatic breast cancer progressing after ≥2 lines of HER2-directed treatment offering an alternative treatment option for these patients (Saura et al. 2020). In the early-stage setting, neratinib given for 1 year after standard neoadjuvant and adjuvant chemotherapy plus trastuzumab improved invasive disease-free survival (iDFS) in patients with HER2+ breast cancer, especially in patients with HR+ disease (Martin et al. 2017; Chan et al. 2021). However, no statistically significant improvement in mortality was observed with neratinib compared with placebo after 8 years follow-up (Holmes et al. 2023).

Pyrotinib is an irreversible pan-HER TKI targeting EGFR, HER2, and HER4. Based on the results from the phase III PHOEBE trial, pyrotinib was approved by the Chinese regulatory authority in combination with capecitabine for patients with HER2+ metastatic breast cancer treated with trastuzumab and taxanes (Xu et al. 2021), and it is currently undergoing further clinical evaluation in this setting.

Tucatinib is a potent, highly selective inhibitor of the kinase domain of HER2 with minimal inhibition of EGFR (Moulder et al. 2017), thus sparing some side effects associated with EGFR inhibition such as diarrhea and skin toxicity. Similar to other TKIs, tucatinib showed higher antitumor activity, especially when combined with trastuzumab and demonstrated BBB penetration in xenograft models. The pivotal HER2CLIMB trial showed that tucatinib plus capecitabine-trastuzumab significantly improved PFS and OS versus trastuzumab and capecitabine in metastatic HER2+ breast cancer previously treated with anti-HER2 therapies. Of note, around half of the patients enrolled into the HER2CLIMB trial had stable or active brain metastases (Lin et al. 2023). In these patients, the addition of tucatinib to trastuzumab-capecitabine significantly improved the intracranial objective response rates, PFS, and OS while reducing the risk of developing new brain lesions (Lin et al. 2023). Tucatinib was FDA approved in April 2020 for the treatment of HER2+ MBC, including patients with brain metastases. Ongoing trials are evaluating tucatinib plus trastuzumab and pertuzumab as maintenance therapy for metastatic HER2+ breast cancer (HER2CLIMB05) and tucatinib plus T-DM1 in patients with residual HER2-positive invasive breast cancer after neoadjuvant chemotherapy combined with HER2-directed treatment (compassHER2 RD).

24.3.1.3 Antibody-Drug Conjugates (ADCs)

ADCs are a novel rapidly growing class of cancer therapeutics designed to deliver potent cytotoxic drugs selectively to the tumor cells expressing a specific target protein (Tarantino et al. 2022). An ADC is composed of a monoclonal antibody directed against a tumor-associated antigen and a cytotoxic payload connected via a synthetic linker. Upon binding to their target antigens expressed on the tumor cell surface, the ADCs are internalized into the cell and processed by the endo-lysosomal system. The linker connecting the antibody and the cytotoxic drug is then cleaved, and the payload is released into the cytoplasm where it induces apoptotic cell death. Some cytotoxic payloads can diffuse across the target cell membrane to the extracellular space leading to the death of neighboring cells, the so-called bystander effect. Although this effect may increase the off-target toxicity of ADCs, it can be beneficial when tackling solid tumors with heterogeneous expression of the target antigen (Tarantino et al. 2022).

Trastuzumab emtansine (T-DM1) was the first ADC developed to target the HER2 receptor. T-DM1 is comprised of trastuzumab conjugated by a non-cleavable linker to the maytansine derivative and microtubule inhibitor DM1, with a drug-to-antibody ratio (DAR) of ~3.5. Based on the significant improvement in response and survival outcomes over capecitabine plus lapatinib reported in the EMILIA trial (Table 24.1), T-DM1 gained FDA approval for patients with metastatic HER2+ breast cancer who progressed on prior trastuzumab-based chemotherapy (Verma et al. 2012). An exploratory analysis of the KAMILLA trial also showed that T-DM1 was active and well tolerated in patients with brain metastases (Montemurro et al. 2020). Of note, T-DM1 reduced the risk of recurrence of invasive breast cancer by half and also improved OS compared with trastuzumab in patients with HER2+ early breast cancer who had residual invasive disease after completion of neoadjuvant therapy (von Minckwitz et al. 2019; Hurvitz et al. 2023a).

Trastuzumab deruxtecan (T-DXd) is a third-generation ADC that consists of trastuzumab conjugated by a cleavable tetrapeptide linker with the topoisomerase 1 inhibitor payload derivative of exatecan (DXd), with a high DAR of 8:1 (Tamura et al. 2019). The linker of DXd is stable in plasma and undergoes selective cleavage by lysosomal cathepsins, which are upregulated in cancer cells, limiting the systemic exposure of the cytotoxic payload. In addition, DXd is also cell membrane permeable resulting in a potent bystander effect. The phase II DESTINY-

Breast01 study showed the remarkable antitumor activity of T-DXd in heavily pretreated patients with advanced HER2+ breast cancer leading to its accelerated FDA approval (Modi et al. 2020). The subsequent phase III DESTINY-Breast03 trial demonstrated that T-DXd significantly improved PFS and OS compared with T-DM1 in patients with HER2+ breast cancer who had previously received trastuzumab and a taxane for metastatic disease (Hurvitz et al. 2023b). Notably, while HER2-targeting monoclonal antibodies showed only modest activity against brain metastases due to their limited ability to cross the blood-brain barrier, T-DXd yielded encouraging intracranial responses in patients with HER2+ breast cancer brain metastases (Modi et al. 2020; Perez-Garcia et al. 2023). Ongoing phase III clinical trials are comparing T-DXd with or without pertuzumab versus the standard of care pertuzumab, trastuzumab, and chemotherapy in first-line metastatic setting (DESTINY-Breast09); T-DXd versus T-DM1 in patients with residual invasive disease following neoadjuvant therapy (DESTINY-Breast05); and neoadjuvant T-DXd alone or followed by paclitaxel, trastuzumab, and pertuzumab (THP) compared with standard-of-care doxorubicin and cyclophosphamide followed by THP in patients with early-stage breast cancer (DESTINY-Breast11). The results of these pivotal trials, if promising, may lead to a paradigm shift in the treatment of HER2+ disease.

Trastuzumab duocarmycin (T-Duo) is a HER2-targeted ADC based on trastuzumab that is bound to the DNA alkylating agent duocarmazine with a protease-cleavable linker. A phase III trial randomly assigned patients with HER2+ locally advanced or metastatic breast cancer who had previously received at least two therapies or T-DM1 in the metastatic setting to T-Duo or physician's choice of chemotherapy plus anti-HER2 therapy. T-Duo showed a meaningful improvement in PFS but a statistically non-significant improvement in OS compared to treatment of physician's choice (Aftimos et al. 2023). In July 2022, the FDA approved T-Duo for use in patients with HER2+ advanced breast cancer; however, given the remarkable efficacy of T-DXd and tucatinib in the second and third lines of therapy, it appears that the utilization of T-Duo may be restricted to later lines of treatment.

24.3.2 Systemic Therapy for Patients with HER2+ Breast Cancer: The Current Practice

The primary objective of systemic therapy is to minimize the risk of recurrence and mortality associated with the newly diagnosed, non-metastatic HER2+ breast cancer. Patients undergoing initial surgery to remove the primary tumor should receive adjuvant chemotherapy in combination with HER2-directed therapy and endocrine therapy if HR+. The use of a de-escalated regimen consisting of weekly paclitaxel and trastuzumab (Tolaney et al. 2015) has been demonstrated to be a viable therapeutic option for patients with tumors measuring less than 2 cm in diameter and no involved lymph nodes (stage I). For patients diagnosed with lymph node-positive breast cancer, the standard-of-care treatment is the combination of pertuzumab with trastuzumab, with either anthracycline-based or anthracycline-free chemotherapy regimens. For patients with tumors greater than 2 cm or positive node status (stage II–III), neoadjuvant systemic therapy is the preferred approach. This therapeutic intervention aims to minimize the extent of the surgical procedure and enable the implementation of individualized adjuvant therapy. In this setting, dual HER2 blockade with trastuzumab and pertuzumab in combination with anthracycline-based or anthracycline-free regimens increases the rate of pCR compared with trastuzumab alone and potentially translates into improved long-term outcomes (Gianni et al. 2016). Patients who achieved pCR have a lower risk of disease recurrence compared to those who did not and should continue anti-HER2 therapy for a total of 1 year. On the contrary, patients who have residual invasive breast cancer after receiving neoadjuvant chemotherapy plus HER2-targeted therapy have a worse prognosis and should receive adjuvant T-DM1 for up to 14 cycles. In selected patients with high-risk HR-positive tumors, the duration of adjuvant treatment with trastuzumab may be extended with an additional year of neratinib as per the ExteNET trial (Chan et al. 2021).

Some patients with early-stage HER2+ breast cancer treated with HER2-directed therapy will eventually relapse in distant sites (stage IV). Distant metastases are found at time of diagnosis in a significant proportion of patients with HER2+ disease (de novo). Interestingly, patients with de novo HER2+ breast cancer experienced better outcomes than those with recurrent breast cancer (Tripathy et al. 2020). Local therapies such as stereotactic radiosurgery (SRS) and whole-brain radiation therapy (WBRT) are the primary treatment modalities for patients with metastatic HER2+ breast cancer who develop brain metastases during their disease (Pestalozzi et al. 2006). Standard first-line treatment for patients with metastatic HER2+ breast cancer is pertuzumab plus trastuzumab in combination with a taxane for at least six cycles, if tolerated, followed by maintenance pertuzumab plus trastuzumab until disease progression. A less toxic chemotherapy or a chemo-free anti-HER2 therapy may be considered in case of comorbidities or patient preferences. In case of patients with HR+/HER2+ disease that are not suitable for chemotherapy, endocrine therapy plus single or dual HER2-targeted therapy could be considered. T-DXd is the preferred second-line therapy after progression on a taxane and trastuzumab. Tucatinib-capecitabine-trastuzumab or T-DXd may be used in the second-line setting in selected patients with brain metastasis, especially when a local intervention is not indicated. The choice of treatment for the third line and beyond depends on prior therapies, patient comorbidities, and performance status, as well as treatment toxicity profile and availability. Continuing HER2-targeted treatment is the prevailing clinical approach for individuals diagnosed with HER2+ tumors. Tucatinib, T-DXd, and T-DM1 are the most active treatment options in the third-line setting. Other options include lapatinib, neratinib, margetuximab, and rechallenge with trastuzumab if other anti-HER2 therapies have been exhausted.

24.4 Mechanisms of Resistance to HER2-Targeted Therapy

Resistance to HER2-targeted therapies is a complex and multifaceted phenomenon, one that is determined largely by the nature and biology of the targeted agent and the overall genomic/molecular makeup of the tumor. In general, resistance could be attributable to mechanisms that are either prevalent at time of initial treatment (*intrinsic resistance*) or emerge under treatment pressure through selection of rare pre-existing or newly acquired resistant subclones (*acquired resistance*). Through the past several decades, studies have uncovered many such potential mechanisms that occur often at the level of the tumor, though the tumor microenvironment (TME), as well as its interaction with the tumor epithelial cells, has also been implicated in resistance, and such studies have gained traction in the recent years (Fig. 24.3). The tumor cell-specific mechanisms of resistance can be grouped into two major categories: (i) reactivation of the HER pathway either due to incomplete therapeutic inhibition of the redundant HER receptor layer resulting in continued transmission of the survival signals or due to alterations in HER2 itself or in other HER receptors and (ii) alterations in key HER2 downstream components or the emergence of alternate survival signaling pathways to bypass complete and sustained blockade of the HER receptor layer. More recently, studies have reported that the TME, particularly the host immune system, plays a crucial role in determining the response of a tumor to targeted therapy and in conferring resistance (Savas et al. 2016; Luen et al. 2017). Of note, other major constraints in the effective management of HER2+ breast cancer are decrease in HER2 expression levels and intra- and inter-tumoral heterogeneity in HER2 levels (Marchio et al. 2021). Downregulation in HER2 levels has been reported post HER2-targeted therapy, particularly ADCs, and such downregulation is potentially associated with cross-resistance to other ADCs (Morganti et al. 2022a). In addition, intra-tumor heterogeneity of HER2 expression has also been associated with poor patient outcome and inferior response to HER2-

targeted therapy (Marchio et al. 2021; Filho et al. 2021). Such tumors may therefore need to be deemed a distinct subset of the HER2+ disease that necessitate a different treatment approach since the subset of tumor epithelial cells lacking HER2 expression may be driven by other oncogenic signaling mechanisms (Filho et al. 2021). Aside from HER2 heterogeneity and downregulation in HER2 expression levels, detailed below are some of the major modules and their key elements that determine response and resistance to HER2-targeted therapy in HER2+ breast cancer, and the same are also depicted in orange boxes in Fig. 24.3.

24.4.1 Tumor Epithelial Cell-Specific Mechanisms of Anti-HER2 Treatment Resistance

24.4.1.1 Reactivation of the HER Receptor Layer

At the outset, one of the major determinants of a HER2+ tumor's response to HER2-targeted therapy is HER2 addiction, a measure of the extent of functional and survival dependence of the tumor on HER2 signaling. However, some tumors, despite being HER2-addicted, could exhibit resistance to anti-HER2 agents. This could potentially be either due to (i) incomplete blockade of the functionally redundant HER receptor layer resulting in compensatory survival signaling emanating from the unblocked HER receptor; (ii) genetic/epigenetic alterations in the HER2 receptor itself, which might essentially compromise the binding or the inhibitory activity of anti-HER2 agents to the receptor, thereby impairing their therapeutic efficacy; or (iii) genetic alterations in key downstream components of the HER signaling pathway (e.g., PI3K/AKT, MAPK/ERK pathway) that render the pathway hyperactive and bypass effective blockade of the upstream HER receptor layer.

Incomplete Blockade of the HER Receptor Layer One of the key, yet generally overlooked, mechanisms of resistance to anti-HER2 therapy is the failure to achieve a comprehensive blockade of the entire HER receptor layer. The functional redundancy of the HER signaling network is evident at multiple levels, including (i) at the level of the multiple HER ligands with shared or overlapping receptor specificities and (ii) at the level of the different HER receptors with multiple homodimers and heterodimers, as well as shared downstream signaling pathways. This redundancy coupled with compensatory signaling originating from the HER receptor left uninhibited was the fundamental cause for strategies to ensure more complete therapeutic blockade of the entire HER receptor layer and not just HER2. Along this line, studies have shown that a dual HER2 blockade approach using agents with complementary mechanism of action and blocking beyond HER2 alone has superior antitumor efficacy compared to single-agent therapy (von Minckwitz et al. 2017; Swain et al. 2015; Baselga et al. 2012b). Further, the complex and redundant nature of the HER2 signaling network has also influenced the recent development of new anti-HER2 agents with broader target specificity profile such as the pan-HER TKIs neratinib and poziotinib. Another potential mechanism that renders inhibition of HER2 challenging is the masking of the trastuzumab binding site on the extracellular domain of HER2 through overexpression of membrane-associated glycoprotein mucins (Chen et al. 2012). In particular, mucin 4 (MUC4) (Giugliano et al. 2023; Miranda et al. 2022), which can interact with the HER receptors, has very recently been shown to be associated with an immunosuppressive tumor microenvironment in HER2+ BC (Schillaci et al. 2022). Furthermore, MUC1, another member of the mucin family, has also been implicated in trastuzumab resistance when overexpressed as a cleaved form (Fessler et al. 2009).

Alterations in the HER Receptor Layer Genetic or epigenetic alterations in HER2, particularly *HER2* mutations and splice variants, have been long reported in breast cancer and is a highly invested area of research that spans decades. Being the predominant alteration observed in HER2 beyond amplification, *HER2* mutations are reported in ~3% of all breast can-

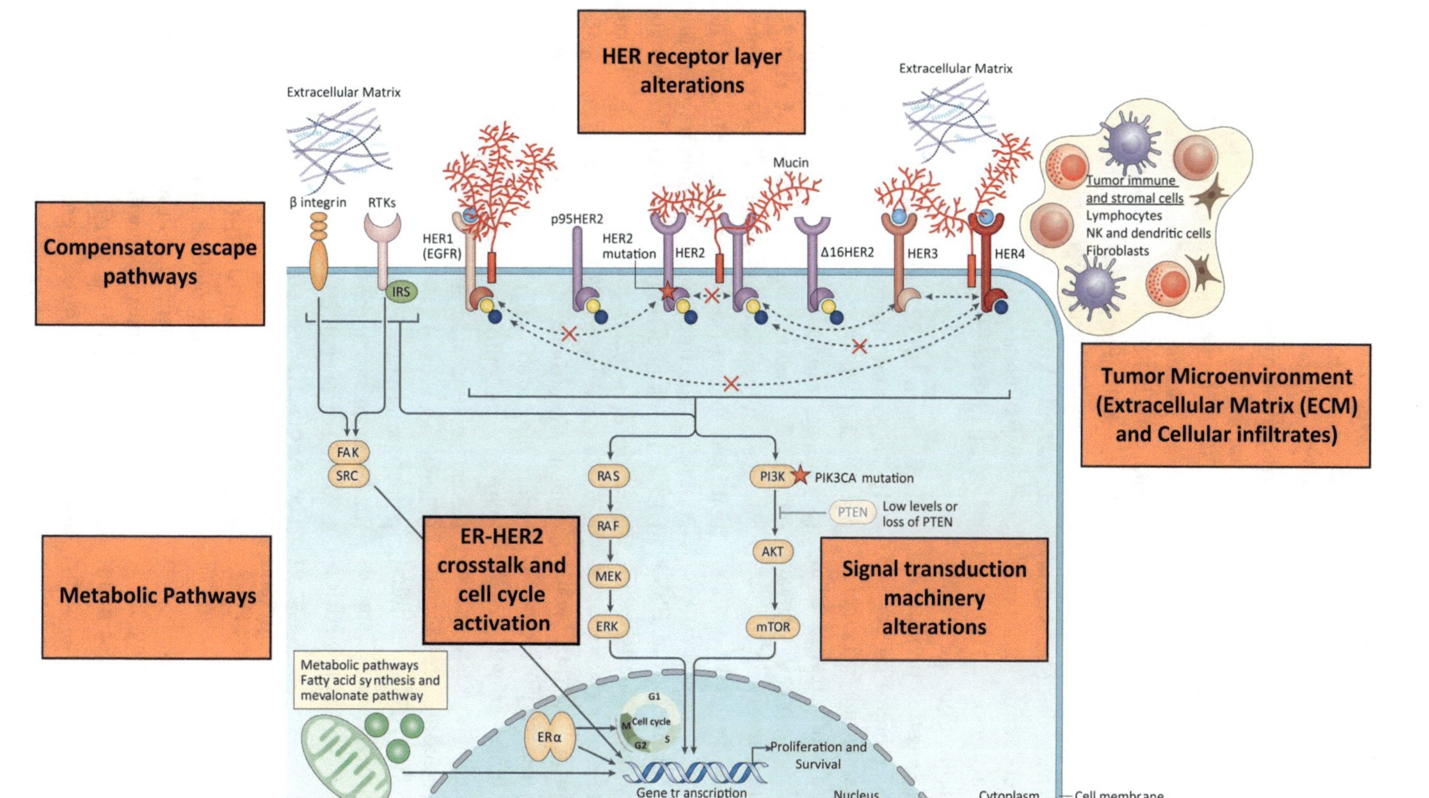

Fig. 24.3 Major mechanisms of resistance to HER2-targeted therapy. In tumors with homogeneous HER2-amplification, resistance can arise owing to failure to achieve complete blockade of the entire HER receptor layer, alterations in the HER signaling pathway itself, or the activation of alternative bypass signaling pathways supporting cell survival or proliferation. When the HER receptor network is effectively inhibited, resistance can arise due to the emergence of several other genomic and adaptive "escape" mechanisms, including via cross talk of HER2 with transcription factors and receptor tyrosine kinases (RTKs) or β-integrin, alterations in components of downstream signaling pathways such as SRC and FAK, or via metabolic pathways. Finally, the tumor microenvironment, primarily composed of the extracellular matrix and cellular infiltrates including immune cells and fibroblasts, could also modulate responses and resistance to HER2-targeted therapy. Orange boxes denote the major modules of resistance to HER2-targeted therapy in HER2+ breast cancer, with each major module comprising multiple elements that determine treatment response and resistance. *Figure adapted from Goutsouliak et al., Nat Rev Clin Oncol 17, 233–250 (2020) and modified in part using* Biorender.com

cers (TCGA; cBioPortal), but are not necessarily associated with HER2 amplification (Cerami et al. 2012; Gao et al. 2013). When present ab initio or acquired, activating *HER2* mutations either activate or reactivate, under the pressure of anti-HER2 therapy, the HER2 pathway in HER2 non-amplified or HER2-amplified tumors, respectively, and present a distinct therapeutic vulnerability. In ER+/HER2 non-amplified tumors, *HER2* mutations are acquired mostly under the pressure of targeted therapy for ER+/HER2- tumors and are observed to be enriched in the metastatic setting, wherein they hyperactivate the PI3K/AKT/mTOR axis via HER2 activation and lead to subsequent endocrine resistance (Croessmann et al. 2019; Nayar et al. 2019). The incidence and clinical implications of *HER2* mutations arising under the selection pressure of anti-HER2 therapy in HER2+ breast cancer are analogous to that of *ESR1* mutations that emerge under endocrine therapy and confer resistance to endocrine therapy in ER+ breast cancer (Jeselsohn et al. 2015). Interestingly, in the setting of metastatic ER+/HER2- breast cancer, *HER2* mutations represent a mechanism of acquired resistance that is distinct from ESR1 mutations, as evidenced by the mutually exclusivity of these two key alterations (Nayar et al. 2019). In the HER2-amplified setting, while HER2 amplification and overexpression continue to be the major drivers of tumor growth, *HER2* mutations could either be present to begin with or be acquired under the selection pressure of HER2-targeted therapy. In the HER2-amplified setting, *HER2* mutations reactivate HER2 signaling to diminish the efficacy of several key HER2-targeted treatments and confer resistance to subsequent lines of HER2-targeted therapy and are associated with poor prognosis (Boulbes et al. 2015; Wen et al. 2015; Xu et al. 2017). Further, enrichment of *HER2* mutations is also observed in the HER2+ metastatic setting, highlighting the clinical importance of *HER2* mutations irrespective of the subtype (Zuo et al. 2016). One of the key clinical challenges in the setting of HER2-amplified breast cancer, however, is the detection of *HER2* mutations, since not all HER2 copies in a HER2-amplified tumor are endogenously mutated. Further, unlike *HER2* amplification, *HER2* mutations are not part of routine clinical testing. Notably, however, irrespective of the subtype and HER2 amplification status, breast tumors harboring *HER2* mutations may benefit from new-generation pan-HER TKIs such as neratinib and poziotinib that can bind to and better inhibit the activity of mutant *HER2* (Cocco et al. 2018; Hyman et al. 2018; Robichaux et al. 2019). In addition, newer more potent targeted agents with better activity against *HER2* mutations are fast emerging and are currently either under preclinical evaluation (Irie et al. 2019; Son et al. 2022; Wilding et al. 2022; Zhao et al. 2023) or in early clinical development (Ma et al. 2023), including in breast cancer.

Apart from *HER2* mutations, other therapeutically important alterations in HER2 include p95HER2 (Anido et al. 2006) and Δ16HER2 (Kwong and Hung 1998; Castiglioni et al. 2006). p95HER2, reported in about 30% of HER2+ tumors, is a truncated form of the HER2 receptor that lacks the extracellular domain (Molina et al. 2002) and therefore loses the ability to bind anti-HER2 agents targeting the extracellular domain (Scaltriti et al. 2007; Arribas et al. 2011) but remains sensitive to TKIs that target the kinase domain (Scaltriti et al. 2010). While a previous report suggested that p95HER2 is generated by matrix metalloproteases-mediated cleavage of the extracellular domain of the full-length HER2 (Christianson et al. 1998), more recent studies point to alternative initiation of translation of the transcript encoding the full-length receptor as the cause (Arribas et al. 2011; Rius Ruiz et al. 2018). The Δ16HER2 variant, on the other hand, is devoid of a small exon 16 coded region in the extracellular domain of HER2 but retains the trastuzumab-binding epitope in the extracellular domain and is associated with stabilization of the HER2 homodimers and constitutive HER2 signaling (Castagnoli et al. 2019). Tumors expressing Δ16HER2 are more aggressive (Castiglioni et al. 2006; Mitra et al. 2009), which could potentially be attributed to its signaling either through direct coupling with the Src kinase (Castagnoli et al. 2014; Turpin et al. 2016) or through the

NOTCH signaling pathway (Castagnoli et al. 2017). The Δ16HER2 variant was long thought to confer resistance to trastuzumab. This notion, however, was upended by a recent study, which showed that tumors harboring Δ16HER2 express elevated levels of pSRC and an activated Δ16HER2–SRC signaling axis and, more importantly, are sensitive to trastuzumab (Castagnoli et al. 2014; Volpi et al. 2019). Of note, Δ16HER2 may also modulate the immune microenvironment of the tumor by activating ectonucleotide pyrophosphatase/phosphodiesterase 1 (ENPP1) and rendering the tumor immune cold with low immune infiltrates and altered cytokine profile (Attalla et al. 2023). Finally, the presence of amplification or overexpression of other HER receptors, particularly HER1 (EGFR) (Ritter et al. 2007) and HER3 (Sergina et al. 2007), has been shown to be associated with resistance to HER2-targeted therapy, further underscoring the functional redundancy of the HER receptor layer.

24.4.1.2 Alterations in Downstream Signaling Components

Being the two major downstream pathways that are modulated by HER2, the extent of inhibition of the PI3K/AKT/mTOR and RAS/MAPK/ERK pathways is one of the signaling read-outs for the efficacy of HER2-targeted agents. Evidently, deregulation of these downstream effector pathways (Sanchez-Vega et al. 2018), via mutations in key components of these pathways, has major implications in the response of a tumor to effective HER2-targeted therapy, as discussed below.

PI3K/AKT/mTOR Pathway Alterations in key components of the PI3K/AKT/mTOR pathway, including activating mutations in *PIK3CA*, MTOR, RICTOR, TSC2, and AKT3; loss of low levels of the tumor suppressor PTEN; and loss of tumor suppressor inositol polyphosphate-4-phosphatase, type II (INPP4B), among others, are observed in HER2+ breast cancer with potential therapeutic implications (Andre et al. 2016; Rexer and Arteaga 2012). Activating mutations in *PIK3CA*, the gene encoding the p110α catalytic subunit of PI3K, or low levels of PTEN, a tumor suppressor and a negative regulator of the PI3K/AKT pathway, are among the most common deregulations leading to constitutive activation of the PI3K/AKT pathway (Veeraraghavan et al. 2019; Rimawi et al. 2018; Chandarlapaty et al. 2012). *PIK3CA* mutations are frequently observed in multiple tumor types, including in ~25% of HER2+ breast cancers (Loi et al. 2013; Loibl et al. 2016), with 80% of the mutations occurring in exon 9 (helical domain) and exon 20 (kinase domain) (Cancer Genome Atlas N 2012; Hoadley et al. 2014). In HER2+ breast cancer, *PIK3CA* mutations have historically been known to be associated with poor response to anti-HER2 therapies in both early and metastatic setting (Loibl et al. 2016; Baselga et al. 2014; Zagami et al. 2023). Alpelisib (BYL719) is an α-specific PI3K inhibitor and was the first of its kind to be approved for use in *PIK3CA*-mutated ER+/HER2-negative metastatic breast cancer. In the HER2+ setting, a phase I trial demonstrated the safety and efficacy of this drug in combination with T-DM1 for patients with metastatic HER2+ breast cancer that progressed on trastuzumab, suggesting the potential for further clinical development (Jain et al. 2016). However, amid concerns of toxicity associated with alpelisib, the field has witnessed the advent of more potent and less toxic PI3KCA mutant-specific inhibitors (Verret et al. 2019), some of which are in early clinical development.

Loss or low levels of PTEN leading to hyperactivation of the PI3K pathway is observed in about 20–25% of HER2+ breast cancers (Fujita et al. 2006; Nagata et al. 2004). Unlike the clear therapeutic importance of *PIK3CA* mutations in resistance, evidence regarding the association of PTEN levels with anti-HER2 treatment resistance is murky. Clinically, while some studies observed an association of PTEN levels with trastuzumab resistance (Nagata et al. 2004; Pandolfi 2004; Rimawi et al. 2015b), several others in the neoadjuvant, adjuvant, and metastatic settings failed to do so (reviewed in (Veeraraghavan et al. 2017)). This could be, in part, due to challenges associated with the quantification of PTEN owing to varied cutoffs for PTEN expression across different studies, as well as due to lack of standardized methods to quantify PTEN levels. Interestingly, a preclinical study suggested that activation of the PI3K/AKT pathway, via *PIK3CA* mutations or low levels of PTEN, was associated with resistance to trastuzumab but was predictive of response to lapatinib due to better inhibition of the p-MAPK and p-AKT levels by lapatinib (Dave et al. 2011), a finding that warrants additional investigation. Additionally, correlative analysis of a cohort of clinical metastatic HER2+ breast tumors revealed that ~47% of the tumors exhibited hyperactive pathway (i.e., *PIK3CA* mutations or low PTEN levels), 40% of the tumors harbored aberrations in the PI3K-AKT-mTOR pathway, and patients harboring tumors with these alterations benefited from the addition of everolimus, an mTOR inhibitor (Andre et al. 2016).

RAS/MEK/ERK Pathway In an interesting early study in HER2+ breast cancer, loss of the tumor suppressor PTEN was observed to cause noncanonical activation of the MAPK pathway and upregulation of the PI3K/AKT pathway, which contributed to aggressive tumor growth (Ebbesen et al. 2016). Of therapeutic relevance, however, was a preclinical study that reported the role of MAPK signaling in aggressiveness and trastuzumab resistance in HER2+ breast cancer cells (Donnelly et al. 2014). Further, while mutations in the MAPK pathway in HER2+ tumors were reported before (Sinkala et al. 2021; Chen et al. 2019), a recent study showed enrichment of mutations in the RAS/MEK/ERK signaling pathway, including in NF1, KRAS, and BRAF, in metastatic HER2+ breast tumors previously treated with anti-HER2 therapies (Smith et al. 2021). This study further uncovered that these RAS/MAPK pathway mutations led to activation of the MAPK pathway and promote resistance to anti-HER2 therapies through a signaling rewiring that causes the tumors to switch from being highly dependent on the PI3K/AKT pathway to instead rely on the MEK/ERK pathway via loss of neurofibromatosis 1 (NF1), a negative regulator of RAS. Moreover, depletion of the tumor suppressor NF1 in HER2-positive breast cancer cell lines was observed to promote resistance to the TKIs lapatinib, neratinib, and tucatinib (Smith et al. 2021). Barring the small sample size, a recent study, however, showed that patients with tumors harboring loss-of-function NF1 mutations had better progression-free survival on TDM1 than those with wild-type NF1 (Duso et al. 2022). Nevertheless, patients with MAPK pathway-altered tumors may benefit from a MEK/ERK inhibitor-containing treatment regimen.

24.4.1.3 Emergence of Alternate Survival Signaling Pathways

The signaling networks in a tumor cell are highly dynamic and evolve extensively under treatment, including acts of modulation of the pathway dependency of a tumor to ensure sustained proliferation and tumor growth. When HER2 does remain sustainably inhibited by potent HER2-targeted therapy, the tumors undergo potential rewiring of the signaling networks, both at the level of the signaling input and at the level of the downstream molecular cascade, to either activate new drivers/pathways or use already partially active signaling pathways as compensatory mechanisms to evade HER2 blockade and to sustain cell proliferation and survival. Such compensatory mechanisms function either autonomously or through cross talk with the HER receptors and their signaling network to drive resistant tumor growth.

The Role of ER Activation of ER, a key driver of tumor growth and survival in breast cancer, is particularly important in HER2+ tumors that also express ER, which constitute about 60–70% of all HER2+ breast cancers (Pegram et al. 2023). The ER+ and ER- subsets of HER2+ breast cancer are two different diseases, and the co-expression of these two receptors has impacts on the clinical behavior of the tumor as well as its response to both HER2-targeted and endocrine therapy (Llombart-Cussac et al. 2017; Vaz-Luis et al. 2013). The extensive bidirectional cross talk between ER and HER2 and the ensuing signaling compensation between these two key receptors have long been implicated in treatment resistance, both to endocrine and HER2-targeted therapy (Pegram et al. 2023; Giuliano et al. 2013;

Nardone et al. 2015). In the ER+ HER2 non-amplified setting, under the pressure of endocrine therapy, tumors either activate HER1/2 expression or acquire *HER2* mutations, which all lead to activation of the HER2 pathway and endocrine resistance (Razavi et al. 2018; Massarweh and Schiff 2007). In the HER2-amplified setting, the ER receptor when left uninhibited upfront (in HER2+/ER+ tumors) or when re-expressed and/or reactivated under treatment pressure (in HER2+/ER- tumors), could transmit alternative proliferative and survival signals to evade sustained HER2 blockade (Llombart-Cussac et al. 2017; Carey et al. 2016; Wang et al. 2011; Giuliano et al. 2015). Indeed, preclinical studies have shown complete tumor eradication upon concurrent blockade of the HER2 and ER receptors in HER2+/ER+ tumor models (Wang et al. 2011; Rimawi et al. 2011; Arpino et al. 2007). Consistently, across multiple clinical trials, HR-positive tumors had inferior response rates compared to HR-negative tumors using mono and dual anti-HER2 therapy in patients with HER2+ breast cancer, which could at least partly be mitigated by adding endocrine therapy (reviewed in (Veeraraghavan et al. 2017).

Further, several clinical trials observed switching of a substantial percentage (~30–67%) of baseline HER2-enriched tumors to luminal subtypes post anti-HER2 therapy, suggesting reactivation of the classic ER signaling in the presence of potent HER2 inhibition (Llombart-Cussac et al. 2017; Carey et al. 2016; Braso-Maristany et al. 2020). Of note, a recent study showed that this subtype switch is apparent in the HR+ subset of the HER2+ disease. Further, while this switch is reversible upon stopping anti-HER2 therapy, the luminal tumors that evolved under anti-HER2 therapy are more sensitive to CDK4/6 inhibition (Braso-Maristany et al. 2020). Indeed, CDK4/6 inhibitors, targeting the G1/S cell cycle check point that is also regulated by ER, have proven to be highly effective and are now the standard of care in patients with HR+/HER2- breast cancer. CDK4/6 inhibition is also emerging as a promising targeted treatment strategy in HER2+ breast cancer, which is discussed in more detail in Sect. 24.5.3.

Activation of Other Compensatory Pathways Activation of additional alternative bypass signaling mechanisms is another effective way to evade HER2 blockade causing resistance. Over the years, several studies have documented the significance of other cellular or receptor tyrosine kinases (RTKs), outside of the HER family of receptors, as a mechanism of resistance to potent HER2 blockade, either through transactivation of HER2 to escalate the downstream signaling cascade or through their own downstream signaling pathway. The insulin-like growth factor receptor (IGF1R), when overexpressed, could cross talk with HER2 and potentially form heterodimer complexes with HER2 and HER3 to activate the PI3K/AKT signaling and confer resistance (Lu et al. 2001; Nahta et al. 2005; Huang et al. 2010). Similarly, activation of the FGFR pathway, through amplification of FGFR1 or FGF3, is associated with intrinsic and acquired resistance to therapeutic HER2 blockade (Hanker et al. 2017a). An additional different RTK that has been implicated in anti-HER2 treatment resistance is MET. Overexpression of MET together with its ligand, HGF, was observed in HER2+ patients who failed to respond to chemotherapy plus trastuzumab (Shattuck et al. 2008). Src has been documented as a key modulator of anti-HER2 response (Liang et al. 2010; Zhang et al. 2011), and its inhibition has been reported to re-sensitize trastuzumab-resistant cells to trastuzumab (Zhang et al. 2011). Further, amplification of Yes1, a member of the Src family and a proto-oncogene, was observed in the trastuzumab+lapatinib-resistant cells, and, more importantly, Yes1 inhibition re-sensitized the resistant cells to trastuzumab (Takeda et al. 2017). The integrins are a group of transmembrane receptors that regulate multiple cellular processes including cell proliferation, survival, and tumor progression (Huck et al. 2010; Guo et al. 2006). While the cross talk of the integrin family of cell adhesion receptors with HER receptors possesses substantial therapeutic implications (Campbell et al. 2016), β1, β3, and β4 integrins, in particular, have been well documented to promote tumor aggressiveness and resistance to HER2-targeted therapy (Hanker et al. 2017b; Nagpal et al. 2023; Huang et al.

2011). Overexpression of the RTK AXL and its heterodimerization with HER2 resulting in activation of the PI3K/AKT and MAPK pathways is another potential mechanism of resistance to trastuzumab (Adam-Artigues et al. 2022).

Other compensatory processes that cross talk with HER2 and emerge in response to potent HER2 blockade are metabolic pathways, including the cholesterol biosynthetic mevalonate pathway (Sethunath et al. 2019), and other lipid metabolic pathways such as fatty acid synthesis, uptake, and storage (Feng and Kurokawa 2020). A recent study reported that activation of the mevalonate pathway and its signaling through the yes-associated protein (YAP)/transcriptional coactivator with PDZ-binding motif (TAZ) and mTORC1 is associated with resistance in models of anti-HER2 treatment resistance (Sethunath et al. 2019). Further, altered lipid metabolism through key molecules such as the fatty acid synthase (FAS) or the fatty acid transporter CD36 (Feng et al. 2019) has also been implicated in acquired resistance to HER2-targeted therapies in breast cancer (Feng and Kurokawa 2020; Feng et al. 2019; Blancafort et al. 2015). Finally, cell survival and DNA repair pathways have long been reported to contribute to breast cancer drug resistance in general. In the past few years, they have also emerged as potential mechanisms of resistance to HER2-targeted therapy in particular (Koirala et al. 2022; Lee et al. 2023).

24.4.2 Tumor Microenvironment in Anti-HER2 Treatment Resistance

The role of tumor microenvironment (TME) in anti-HER2 treatment resistance has been a topic of extensive investigation in the recent past. The TME is comprised primarily of the extracellular matrix (ECM) and immune and other cellular infiltrates. Depending on the composition, the TME, in general, holds the power to play both a tumor-promoting and a tumor-suppressing role (Schreiber et al. 2011). In HER2+ breast cancer, the role of TME is even more substantial considering the fact that HER2-targeted agents, particularly antibody-based therapies, confer tumor-suppressing effect not just by inhibiting HER2 signaling but also by engaging the host immune system to elicit ADCC, as discussed earlier (Savas et al. 2016). Therefore, it is not surprising that the cellular composition of the TME has implications on the treatment outcome of HER2+ breast cancer.

24.4.2.1 The TME ECM Compartment

The ECM of a tumor is composed of proteins such as collagen, the most abundant component of the ECM, as well as fibronectin, elastin, and laminin, among others. Several studies have documented the potential role of ECM in resistance, including to HER2-targeted therapy. Interestingly, one study reported the specific involvement of collagen I and II in anti-HER2 treatment resistance through integrin β1/Src signaling (Hanker et al. 2017b). Further, significant upregulation of ECM genes such as collagen, integrin, and laminin was noted in HER2+ PIK3CA-mutant tumors with acquired resistance to HER2/PI3K inhibitors. In addition to the role of specific components of the ECM, the rigidity of ECM, in general, also promotes resistance to anti-HER2 therapy likely through YAP/TAZ-dependent mechanism (Lin et al. 2015).

24.4.2.2 The TME Cellular Component

Immune cells and other stromal cells are the two major constituents of the cellular compartment of the TME. The host immune system plays a key role in breast cancer pathogenesis and progression (Savas et al. 2016). The immune system's cells can exhibit a dual behavior, either fostering an antitumor response or, conversely, triggering chronic inflammation that accelerates disease progression (Savas et al. 2016; Salgado et al. 2015). This duality is significantly influenced by the immune cell infiltrate present within the tumor and the interactions that immune cells engage in with the tumor cells (Savas et al. 2016; Salgado et al. 2015). Compared with HR+/HER2- subtype, HER2+ breast cancer is characterized by high tumor mutational burden and extensive immune infiltrate and is therefore considered a more immunogenic tumor (Bianchini and Gianni 2014). Tumor-infiltrating lymphocytes (TILs) consist of various subsets, including CD8+ and CD4+ effector T cells, regulatory T cells (Tregs), B cells, natural killer cells, and macrophages (Savas et al. 2016; Salgado et al. 2015). Typically, TILs are examined using hematoxylin and eosin (H&E)-stained slides and identified based on their morphological features or by using additional immune markers (Salgado et al. 2015; Dieci et al. 2018). Intratumoral TILs are defined as lymphocytes that come into direct contact with the tumor epithelial cells, while stromal (s-) TILs are lymphocytes that are situated throughout the stroma without any direct interaction with the cancer cells (Dieci et al. 2018) and reported as a percentage of stromal area occupied by mononuclear inflammatory cells over the total stromal area within the tumor (Dieci et al. 2018). Over the past decade, several studies have demonstrated a significant association between elevated levels of s-TILs and higher pCR rates following neoadjuvant treatment, as well as improved survival outcomes for patients with HER2+ breast cancer (Luque et al. 2022). Besides the mere count of lymphocytic infiltration, the phenotypic characteristics of the lymphocytes may also dictate the clinical outcome of HER2+ breast cancer patients, as every immune subset has a specific role in cancer development with a predominant contribution to either pro- or anti-tumor activities (Luque et al. 2022). As an example, increased levels of the immune effector CD8+ and CD4+ T cells have been associated with increased response to anti-HER2 therapy and reduced risk of recurrence or death in patients with HER2+ breast cancer (De Angelis et al. 2020; Mahmoud et al. 2011). B cells play a crucial role in regulating the immune system by producing antibodies and cytokines, presenting antigens to other cells, and supporting mononuclear cells. Additionally, they also contribute to inflammatory pathways. Tumor-infiltrating B cells have been associated with the presence of both CD4+ and CD8+ T cells, higher tumor grades and proliferation rates, and negative hormone receptor status (Garaud et al. 2019). Interestingly, high levels of CD20+ B cells were associated with a higher chances of achieving pCR following neoadjuvant anti-HER2 therapy with (Brown et al. 2014) or without chemotherapy in patients with early-stage HER2+ breast cancer (De Angelis et al. 2020). The impact of the additional components of the immune infiltrate such as CD4+ Tregs, NK cells, and tumor-associated macrophages (TAM) on anti-HER2 therapy efficacy and patient outcome is still controversial (Luque et al. 2022).

Employing quantitative assessment of the immune infiltrate by multiplexed immunofluorescence, researchers identified a distinct immune cell profile (characterized by elevated levels of CD4+, CD8+, and CD20+ s-TILs, as well as increased CD20+ intratumoral TILs) that displayed a significant association with improved pCR rates in patients with HER2+ breast cancer who received a chemotherapy-free neoadjuvant treatment with lapatinib plus trastuzumab (Andersson et al. 2021). Interestingly, a multiplexed imaging assay for immune contexture analysis revealed a strong association between response to neoadjuvant anti-HER2 treatment and the spatial interaction of immune cells with tumor epithelial cells (Griguolo et al. 2021). Several immune-related gene expression signatures, in particular the immunoglobulin G (IgG) signature, have also been associated with higher pCR rates and prolonged survival in patients with early-stage HER2+ breast cancer (Fumagalli et al. 2017; Chumsri et al. 2022). Notably, a recent analysis from two neoadjuvant trials of anti-HER2 therapy, one with and another without chemotherapy, suggests that the prognostic and predictive value of RNA sequencing-based immune signatures is superior to that of TILs evaluated by H&E in patients with early-stage HER2+ breast cancer (Fernandez-Martinez et al. 2023).

The non-immune stromal cells in the TME are yet another key contributor of resistance in HER2+ breast cancer (Rivas et al. 2022). In particular, the cancer-associated fibroblasts (CAFs) are one of the major cellular components of the stroma, and they help promote cell survival, tumor growth, and aggressiveness through different mechanisms. Some studies have shown that CAFs promote tumor growth and anti-HER2 treatment resistance through the secretion of growth factors such as fibroblast growth factor (FGF) or the insulin-like growth factor 1 (IGF-1) (Balkwill et al. 2012; Fernández-Nogueira et al. 2020). A recent study further demonstrated that CAFs confer resistance to trastuzumab through expression of neuregulin-1 (NRG1), a HER3 ligand, which however was overcome by the addition of pertuzumab (Guardia et al. 2021).

24.5 Next-Generation Therapies for HER2+ Breast Cancer

Recent advances in engineering technology, coupled with a more profound understanding of the complex biology of the HER2+ disease and the various mechanisms of resistance to current HER2-targeted agents, are fueling the rapid development of new drugs to further expand the arsenal of targeted treatment agents. In addition to the advent of innovative new classes of therapies, newer more potent therapies within the previously discussed classes of agents that target the HER2 signaling pathway (*see Sect. 24.3*) and harness the immune system are also being developed (Swain et al. 2023). A few key examples of these new emerging therapies that are already under clinical evaluation are briefly discussed below.

24.5.1 Bispecific Antibodies

Bispecific antibodies are a class of engineered antibodies with binding sites directed at two different antigens or two different epitopes on the same antigen [recently reviewed in Lan et al. (2023)]. One such drug is zanidatamab, a humanized monoclonal antibody against domains II and IV of HER2. Zanidatamab has shown superior in vivo anti-tumor activity compared to trastuzumab monotherapy and trastuzumab+pertuzumab in HER2-overexpressing tumors (Weisser et al. 2023). A phase I study demonstrated its promising anti-tumor activity and a manageable safety profile in multiple HER2-expressing or HER2-amplified diseases (Meric-Bernstam et al. 2022). Ongoing trials are investigating zanidatamab in combination with endocrine therapy plus CDK4/6 inhibitor in metastatic HR+/HER2+ breast cancer (NCT04224272) or as a neoadjuvant monotherapy in early HER2+ breast cancer (NCT05035836). KN026 is another bispecific antibody that targets domains II and IV of HER2 and is potentially more effective than trastuzumab and pertuzumab in HER2+ tumor cell lines and has a growth inhibitory effect in trastuzumab-resistant models. The encouraging efficacy and acceptable safety profile of KN06 from early-phase clinical trials (Zhang et al. 2022; Wu et al. 2023) warrant further investigation in patients with HER2+ breast cancer. Bispecific T cell engagers (BiTEs) bind to CD3 on T cells and HER2 on cancer cells to recruit and activate cytotoxic T cells and kill the HER2-expressing cancer cells (Yu et al. 2019). The bispecific killer cell engagers (BiKEs), another type of bispecific antibody, bind to CD16 on natural killer (NK)/monocytic cells and HER2 on tumor cells and elicit ADCC (Nikkhoi et al. 2022).

24.5.2 Antibody-Drug Conjugates

Zanidatamab zovodotin (ZW49) is a novel ADC comprised of a HER2-targeting bispecific antibody directed against the domains II and IV of HER2 coupled via a protease-cleavable linker to a proprietary auristatin toxin. ZW49 exhibited increased lysosomal trafficking and internalization compared to HER2-targeted monospecific ADC and was effective in inhibiting the growth of both low and high HER2-expressing breast cancer preclinical models (Hamblett et al. 2019). A first-in-human phase 1 trial showed encouraging responses and a manageable toxicity profile for ZW49 monotherapy in heavily pretreated patients with HER2+ solid cancers, including breast cancer (Jhaveri et al. 2022). Disitamab vedotin (RC48-ADC) comprises the humanized antibody disitamab targeting different epitopes of HER2 combined with the cytotoxic agent monomethyl auristatin E (MMAE) by a cleavable linker. Preclinical data showed anti-tumor activity and a robust bystander effect in HER2+ preclinical models, and multiple clinical trials are ongoing in solid tumors including breast and gastric cancer. In addition, ongoing clinical trials are exploring the potential benefits of combining HER2-targeting ADCs with immune-checkpoint inhibitors and other targeted therapies, such as HER2 TKIs, with the goal of enhancing patient outcomes (von Arx et al. 2023).

24.5.3 Cell Cycle Inhibitors

Three CDK4/6 inhibitors (palbociclib, ribociclib, and abemaciclib) are currently approved by the FDA for the treatment of endocrine-sensitive and endocrine-resistant HR+/HER2- advanced or metastatic breast cancer. Recently, adjuvant treatment with abemaciclib or ribociclib has demonstrated to significantly reduce the risk of recurrence in patients with early-stage HR+/HER2- breast cancer, making it the new standard of care in this setting (O'Sullivan et al. 2023). Targeting the cell cycle machinery is emerging as a promising therapeutic approach also for HR+/HER2+ breast cancer. In patients with HR+/HER2+ early-stage breast cancer, substantial reduction of cell proliferation measured by KI67 and a pCR of 27% were achieved with the neoadjuvant combination of trastuzumab, pertuzumab, palbociclib, and the ER degrader fulvestrant (Gianni et al. 2018). In the metastatic setting, abemaciclib significantly improved PFS but not OS when compared to chemotherapy plus trastuzumab, thereby offering a potential chemotherapy-free option for patients with pretreated HR+/HER2+ advanced breast cancer (Tolaney et al. 2020, 2024). Interestingly, an exploratory analysis of tumor transcriptomic profiles within this HR+/HER2+ patient cohort revealed that luminal A and luminal B intrinsic subtypes were associated with longer PFS and OS compared with non-luminal subtypes (Tolaney et al. 2024). Several ongoing clinical trials are examining the potential of combining CDK4/6 inhibition together with endocrine therapy and anti-HER2 treatment in patients with metastatic HR+/HER2+ breast cancer (NCT02947685; NCT02344472).

24.5.4 Immune Checkpoint Inhibitors

Immune checkpoint inhibitors (ICIs) are monoclonal antibodies that promote anticancer immune responses by targeting immunologic inhibitory receptors on T-lymphocytes or their ligands on cancer cells. ICIs targeting either the programmed death-ligand 1 (PD-L1) or its receptor programmed cell death protein 1 (PD-1) have been evaluated in combination with HER2-targeted agents in patients with previously treated metastatic HER2+ breast cancer. Early-phase clinical trials of ICIs alone or in combination with trastuzumab or T-DM1 have shown modest anti-tumor activity, mainly in patients with PD-L1+ tumors (Emens et al. 2020; Loi et al. 2019). Ongoing trials are evaluating T-DM1 in combination with the anti-PD-L1 atezolizumab in metastatic HER2+/PD-L1+ breast cancer (NCT04740918) or in patients with HER2+ breast cancer and residual disease after neoadjuvant systemic therapy (NCT04873362).

24.5.5 Cancer Vaccines and CART Cells Targeting HER2

Cancer vaccines are an attractive strategy to engage the host immune system and to induce durable immunological memory. Different methods have been explored to develop anti-HER2 vaccines. These include B or T cell peptide-based vaccines, matured dendritic cells loaded with tumor-associated antigens (TAA) or tumor-specific antigens (TSA), and DNA vaccination using plasmids delivering genes encoding the TAA or TSA (Al-Hawary et al. 2023; Tobias et al. 2022). HER2-derived peptides demonstrated to elicit specific T cell and humoral immunity are in the late stage of clinical development. Among them, nelipepimut-S (NeuVax) is a major histocompatibility class (MHC) I vaccine that consists of a nine-amino-acid immunogenic peptide derived from the extracellular domain of HER2 (E75) combined with a granulocyte-macrophage colony-stimulating factor (GM-CSF). In phase I/II studies, nelipepimut-S (NP-S) plus GM-CSF vaccine was well tolerated and effectively raised HER2-specific immunity in patients with breast cancer; however, no significant difference in DFS was observed between NP-S and placebo in the phase III confirmatory trial (Mittendorf et al. 2019). GP2 is a biologic nine-amino-acid peptide of HER2 delivered in combination with GM-CSF (GLSI-100) that showed remarkable results in HLA-A*02-positive patients with early-stage HER2+ breast cancer. A phase III trial (NCT05232916) is assessing the safety and efficacy of GLSI-100 in HER2+ breast cancer patients who are HLA-A*02-positive following adjuvant anti-HER2 therapy. The utilization of advanced delivery methods, including lipid-based systems, virus-like particles, and polymeric particles, in conjunction with mRNA technology, holds great promise for enhancing vaccine effectiveness and optimizing patient outcomes. Finally, based on promising preclinical data suggesting HER2 as a potential target for CAR-T cell therapy [reviewed in Yang et al. (2022)], a near-future clinical development of HER2-CAR-T cells targeting HER2 as a new treatment module for HER2+ breast cancer is anticipated.

24.5.6 Escalating and De-escalating Therapy for HER2+ Breast Cancer

Identifying patients with HER2+ breast cancer who may require additional therapy beyond standard treatments and those who could benefit from less toxic regimens is crucial for the implementation of personalized therapy. In this context, considerable efforts have been dedicated to optimizing treatments for early-stage HER2+ breast cancer by exploring various escalation and de-escalation approaches. One potential strategy to treatment de-escalation is to shorten the duration of therapy. Multiple adjuvant studies have investigated shorter durations of trastuzumab treatment, producing varied outcomes (Morganti et al. 2022b). A recent meta-analysis of five randomized trials failed to demonstrate non-inferiority for the shorter duration (9 weeks and 6 months) versus 12-month adjuvant trastuzumab in reducing the risk of recurrence in patients with HER2+ early breast cancer (Earl et al. 2021). Therefore, 1-year trastuzumab remains the standard treatment option. However, a shorter trastuzumab treatment duration for patients who are at low risk of recurrence and/or high risk of cardiac side effects may be considered. Additional de-escalation approaches include reducing the intensity or omitting the chemotherapy backbone. De-escalation of adjuvant chemotherapy using anthracycline-free regimens is a viable alternative with excellent outcomes and lower toxicity, including cardiotoxicity, for patients with stage I HER2+ breast cancer (Tolaney et al. 2015, 2021). In addition, the use of anti-HER2 agents in combination with chemotherapy regimens that do not include anthracycline has yielded similar pCR rates to those achieved with anthracycline-based chemotherapy in the neoadjuvant setting (van Ramshorst et al. 2018; Nitz et al. 2022). Ongoing clinical trials are exploring the most effective approach to de-escalate chemotherapy while maintaining favorable results (NCT04266249, NCT04675827). Interestingly, a series of three phase II trials investigated the efficacy of neoadjuvant dual HER2 blockade in the absence of chemotherapy in patients with HER+ breast cancer. Overall, these trials indicated that approximately 20–30% of patients with early-stage HER2+ breast cancer can be effectively treated without chemotherapy and thus be spared from chemotherapy-associated toxicities (Goutsouliak et al. 2020). Building on these findings, a recent correlative study developed a multiparameter molecular classifier to differentially identify patients whose HER2+ tumors are highly addicted to HER2, as measured by high and homogeneous levels of HER2, wild-type PIK3CA, and HER2-enriched subtype, and may therefore benefit from HER2-targeted therapy alone without chemotherapy (Veeraraghavan et al. 2023). Of note, patients with HER2+ tumors that harbor mutant PIK3CA may still be able to benefit from a de-escalated strategy using potent mutant PIK3CA inhibitors in combination with HER2-targeted therapy, a strategy that is currently under clinical evaluation (NCT05306041). Collectively, a growing body of evidence suggests that predictive biomarkers derived from the molecular characterization of tumor and immune microenvironment are indispensable for identifying patients who could benefit from chemotherapy-free anti-HER2 therapy (Veeraraghavan et al. 2017, 2023).

However, treatment escalation may still be essential for some patients who have a higher risk of disease recurrence and death, such as those with large tumor and/or nodal involvement or with residual disease after neoadjuvant treatment. Despite extending the duration of adjuvant trastuzumab to 2 years beyond the standard 1-year duration, no significant benefits have been demonstrated for patients with HER2+ breast cancer (Cameron et al. 2017). On the other hand, 1 year of neratinib following standard chemotherapy and trastuzumab has shown a modest but statistically significant benefit, particularly in patients with four or more positive lymph nodes and those with HR+ tumors (Martin et al. 2017). The addition of pertuzumab to trastuzumab and chemotherapy represents the gold standard for patients with HER2+ breast cancer for neoadjuvant systemic therapy. In addition, this approach is recommended for patients undergoing primary surgery and presenting with node-positive disease (von Minckwitz et al. 2017). Patients with invasive residual disease after neoadjuvant chemotherapy plus HER2-targeting monoclonal antibodies benefit from switching postoperative therapy to T-DM1. Currently, clinical trials are evaluating the efficacy of novel HER2-targeting ADCs or their combination with targeted therapies (i.e., tucatinib) or immunotherapies in patients with high-risk HER2+ breast cancer who have residual invasive disease following neoadjuvant therapy (Dowling et al. 2023).

24.6 Conclusions

The approach of therapeutically targeting HER2 in breast tumors that overexpress it to selectively target and kill the tumor cells and its phenomenal success in improving patient outcome paved the way for successful tumor biology-based treatment approaches in the decades that followed. Since then, numerous therapeutic approaches to target HER2 have stemmed leading to the development and approval of several classes of HER2-targeted agents, including monoclonal antibodies, small-molecule tyrosine kinase inhibitors, and, more recently, the antibody-drug conjugates. Collectively, these agents have substantially improved the outcome of patients with HER2+ breast cancer. Despite such improvements, some tumors either fail to respond to these agents or show initial response but eventually become resistant due to the emergence of adaptive or compensatory mechanisms. Treatment resistance, in its entirety, is one of the key and prevailing challenges in the clinical management of HER2+ breast cancer. The field has dedicated huge efforts toward understanding the mechanistic insights of such resistance and, as a result, has uncovered several major modules of resistance mechanisms and the key elements each module is comprised of, which are briefly discussed in this chapter. For the most part, resistance is either tumor epithelial cell-specific or is the result of changes in the microenvironment that the tumor grows in and the interaction of the tumor epithelial cells with this microenvironment. Many studies have, in the process of understanding treatment resistance, identified several key actionable drivers of resistance, therapeutic targeting of which holds the potential to overcome resistance. Multiple new agents that belong to already existing classes of therapy, as well as altogether new classes of targeted agents, including immunotherapy, cell cycle checkpoint inhibitors, and HER2 vaccines, have also been added to the arsenal of HER2-targeted therapy. A plethora of ongoing clinical trials are testing the efficacy and safety of these new agents, either alone or in combination, including with already approved HER2-targeted agents, in multiple treatment settings of HER2+ breast cancer. In addition, some new agents are in the stages of preclinical testing, and many more are still in their infancy. Evidently, the forthcoming decades will witness the addition of multiple new targeted agents to the ever-evolving treatment landscape of HER2+ breast cancer. A recent new paradigm in the management of HER2+ breast cancer is treatment de-escalation, especially for patients who are being overtreated and may benefit from less chemotherapy or no chemotherapy, thereby sparing them from the unnecessary toxicity, an approach that is gaining momentum in this era of personalized medicine. Resistance is an ever-evolving phenomenon and thus will remain a field of continued interest in the decades to come with additional new mechanisms of resistance to both existing and emerging HER2-targeted therapy being uncovered. Building on the emerging new findings of the mechanistic underpinnings of anti-HER2 treatment resistance, new more potent and less toxic targeted agents will continue to be developed. Ongoing and future studies will thus continue to follow the cycle of development of new targeted therapy, understanding treatment resistance that may ensue, and the identification of new regimens to overcome such resistance.

References

Adam-Artigues A, Arenas EJ, Martinez-Sabadell A et al (2022) Targeting HER2-AXL heterodimerization to overcome resistance to HER2 blockade in breast cancer. Sci Adv 8:eabk2746

Aftimos PG, Turner N, O'Shaughnessy J et al (2023) 386MO Trastuzumab duocarmazine versus physician's choice therapy in pre-treated HER2-positive metastatic breast cancer: final results of the phase III TULIP trial. Ann Oncol 34:S340–S341

Al-Hawary SIS, Saleh EAM, Mamajanov NA et al (2023) Breast cancer vaccines; A comprehensive and updated review. Pathol Res Pract 249:154735

Andersson A, Larsson L, Stenbeck L et al (2021) Spatial deconvolution of HER2-positive breast cancer delineates tumor-associated cell type interactions. Nat Commun 12:6012

Andre F, Hurvitz S, Fasolo A et al (2016) Molecular alterations and everolimus efficacy in human epidermal growth factor receptor 2-overexpressing metastatic breast cancers: combined exploratory biomarker analysis from BOLERO-1 and BOLERO-3. J Clin Oncol 34:2115–2124

Anido J, Scaltriti M, Bech Serra JJ et al (2006) Biosynthesis of tumorigenic HER2 C-terminal fragments by alternative initiation of translation. EMBO J 25:3234–3244

Arpino G, Gutierrez C, Weiss H et al (2007) Treatment of human epidermal growth factor receptor 2-overexpressing breast cancer xenografts with multiagent HER-targeted therapy. J Natl Cancer Inst 99:694–705

Arribas J, Baselga J, Pedersen K, Parra-Palau JL (2011) p95HER2 and breast cancer. Cancer Res 71:1515–1519

Attalla SS, Boucher J, Proud H et al (2023) HER2Delta16 engages ENPP1 to promote an immune-cold microenvironment in breast cancer. Cancer Immunol Res 11:1184–1202

Badache A, Hynes NE (2004) A new therapeutic antibody masks ErbB2 to its partners. Cancer Cell 5:299–301

Balkwill FR, Capasso M, Hagemann T (2012) The tumor microenvironment at a glance. J Cell Sci 125:5591–5596

Baselga J, Cortes J, Kim SB et al (2012a) Pertuzumab plus trastuzumab plus docetaxel for metastatic breast cancer. N Engl J Med 366:109–119

Baselga J, Bradbury I, Eidtmann H et al (2012b) Lapatinib with trastuzumab for HER2-positive early breast cancer (NeoALTTO): a randomised, open-label, multicentre, phase 3 trial. Lancet 379:633–640

Baselga J, Cortes J, Im SA et al (2014) Biomarker analyses in CLEOPATRA: a phase III, placebo-controlled study of pertuzumab in human epidermal growth factor receptor 2-positive, first-line metastatic breast cancer. J Clin Oncol 32:3753–3761

Bianchini G, Gianni L (2014) The immune system and response to HER2-targeted treatment in breast cancer. Lancet Oncol 15:e58–e68

Blancafort A, Giró-Perafita A, Oliveras G et al (2015) Dual fatty acid synthase and HER2 signaling blockade shows marked antitumor activity against breast cancer models resistant to anti-HER2 drugs. PLoS One 10:e0131241

Blows FM, Driver KE, Schmidt MK et al (2010) Subtyping of breast cancer by immunohistochemistry to investigate a relationship between subtype and short and long term survival: a collaborative analysis of data for 10,159 cases from 12 studies. PLoS Med 7:e1000279

Boulbes DR, Arold ST, Chauhan GB et al (2015) HER family kinase domain mutations promote tumor progression and can predict response to treatment in human breast cancer. Mol Oncol 9:586–600

Braso-Maristany F, Griguolo G, Pascual T et al (2020) Phenotypic changes of HER2-positive breast cancer during and after dual HER2 blockade. Nat Commun 11:385

Brown JR, Wimberly H, Lannin DR et al (2014) Multiplexed quantitative analysis of CD3, CD8, and CD20 predicts response to neoadjuvant chemotherapy in breast cancer. Clin Cancer Res 20:5995–6005

Cameron D, Piccart-Gebhart MJ, Gelber RD et al (2017) 11 years' follow-up of trastuzumab after adjuvant chemotherapy in HER2-positive early breast cancer: final analysis of the HERceptin Adjuvant (HERA) trial. Lancet 389:1195–1205

Campbell MR, Zhang H, Ziaee S et al (2016) Effective treatment of HER2-amplified breast cancer by targeting HER3 and beta1 integrin. Breast Cancer Res Treat 155:431–440

Cancer Genome Atlas N (2012) Comprehensive molecular portraits of human breast tumours. Nature 490:61–70

Carey LA, Berry DA, Cirrincione CT et al (2016) Molecular heterogeneity and response to neoadjuvant human epidermal growth factor receptor 2 targeting in CALGB 40601, a randomized phase III trial of paclitaxel plus trastuzumab with or without lapatinib. J Clin Oncol 34:542–549

Castagnoli L, Iezzi M, Ghedini GC et al (2014) Activated d16HER2 homodimers and SRC kinase mediate optimal efficacy for trastuzumab. Cancer Res 74:6248–6259

Castagnoli L, Ghedini GC, Koschorke A et al (2017) Pathobiological implications of the d16HER2 splice variant for stemness and aggressiveness of HER2-positive breast cancer. Oncogene 36: 1721–1732

Castagnoli L, Ladomery M, Tagliabue E, Pupa SM (2019) The d16HER2 splice variant: a friend or foe of HER2-positive cancers? Cancers (Basel):11

Castiglioni F, Tagliabue E, Campiglio M et al (2006) Role of exon-16-deleted HER2 in breast carcinomas. Endocr Relat Cancer 13:221–232

Cerami E, Gao J, Dogrusoz U et al (2012) The cBio cancer genomics portal: an open platform for exploring multidimensional cancer genomics data. Cancer Discov 2:401–404

Chan A, Moy B, Mansi J et al (2021) Final efficacy results of neratinib in HER2-positive hormone receptor-positive early-stage breast cancer from the phase III ExteNET trial. Clin Breast Cancer 21:80–91 e87

Chandarlapaty S, Sakr RA, Giri D et al (2012) Frequent mutational activation of the PI3K-AKT pathway in trastuzumab-resistant breast cancer. Clin Cancer Res 18:6784–6791

Chen AC, Migliaccio I, Rimawi MF et al (2012) Upregulation of mucin4 in ER-positive/HER2-overexpressing breast cancer xenografts with acquired resistance to endocrine and HER2-targeted therapies. Breast Cancer Res Treat 134:583–593

Chen Z, Zhang Y, Zhao J et al (2019) Molecular features of refractory metastatic breast cancer. Cancer Res 79:1697–1697

Chiu JW, Leung R, Tang V et al (2019) Changing pattern of recurrences in patients with early HER2-positive breast cancer receiving neoadjuvant chemotherapy in the era of dual anti-HER2 therapy. Postgrad Med J 95:155–161

Christianson TA, Doherty JK, Lin YJ et al (1998) NH2-terminally truncated HER-2/neu protein: relationship with shedding of the extracellular domain and with prognostic factors in breast cancer. Cancer Res 58:5123–5129

Chumsri S, Li Z, Serie DJ et al (2022) Adaptive immune signature in HER2-positive breast cancer in NCCTG (Alliance) N9831 and NeoALTTO trials. NPJ Breast Cancer 8:68

Cocco E, Javier Carmona F, Razavi P et al (2018) Neratinib is effective in breast tumors bearing both amplification and mutation of ERBB2 (HER2). Sci Signal 11:eaat9773

Croessmann S, Formisano L, Kinch LN et al (2019) Combined blockade of activating ERBB2 mutations and ER results in synthetic lethality of ER+/HER2 mutant breast cancer. Clin Cancer Res 25:277–289

Curtis C, Shah SP, Chin SF et al (2012) The genomic and transcriptomic architecture of 2,000 breast tumours reveals novel subgroups. Nature 486:346–352

Dave B, Migliaccio I, Gutierrez MC et al (2011) Loss of phosphatase and tensin homolog or phosphoinositol-3 kinase activation and response to trastuzumab or lapatinib in human epidermal growth factor receptor 2-overexpressing locally advanced breast cancers. J Clin Oncol 29:166–173

De Angelis C, Nagi C, Hoyt CC et al (2020) Evaluation of the predictive role of tumor immune infiltrate in patients with HER2-positive breast cancer treated with neoadjuvant anti-HER2 therapy without chemotherapy. Clin Cancer Res 26:738–745

Dieci MV, Radosevic-Robin N, Fineberg S et al (2018) Update on tumor-infiltrating lymphocytes (TILs) in breast cancer, including recommendations to assess TILs in residual disease after neoadjuvant therapy and in carcinoma in situ: a report of the International Immuno-Oncology Biomarker Working Group on Breast Cancer. Semin Cancer Biol 52:16–25

Dong R, Ji J, Liu H, He X (2019) The evolving role of trastuzumab emtansine (T-DM1) in HER2-positive breast cancer with brain metastases. Crit Rev Oncol Hematol 143:20–26

Donnelly SM, Paplomata E, Peake BM et al (2014) P38 MAPK contributes to resistance and invasiveness of HER2- overexpressing breast cancer. Curr Med Chem 21:501–510

Dowling GP, Keelan S, Toomey S et al (2023) Review of the status of neoadjuvant therapy in HER2-positive breast cancer. Front Oncol 13:1066007

Duco MR, Murdock JL, Reeves DJ (2020) Trastuzumab/hyaluronidase-oysk: a new option for patients with HER2-positive breast cancer. Ann Pharmacother 54:254–261

DuMond B, Patel V, Gross A et al (2021) Fixed-dose combination of pertuzumab and trastuzumab for subcutaneous injection in patients with HER2-positive breast cancer: a multidisciplinary approach. J Oncol Pharm Pract 27:1214–1221

Duso BA, Dorronzoro EG, Tini G et al (2022) Abstract P5-13-04: NF1 mutations render HER2+ breast cancer highly sensitive to T-DM1 by altering microtubule dynamics. Cancer Res 82:P5-13-04-P15-13-04

Earl HM, Hiller L, Dunn JA et al (2021) LBA11 Individual patient data meta-analysis of 5 non-inferiority RCTs of reduced duration single agent adjuvant trastuzumab in the treatment of HER2 positive early breast cancer. Ann Oncol 32:S1283

Ebbesen SH, Scaltriti M, Bialucha CU et al (2016) Pten loss promotes MAPK pathway dependency in HER2/neu breast carcinomas. Proc Natl Acad Sci USA 113:3030–3035

Emens LA, Esteva FJ, Beresford M et al (2020) Trastuzumab emtansine plus atezolizumab versus trastuzumab emtansine plus placebo in previously treated, HER2-positive advanced breast cancer (KATE2): a phase 2, multicentre, randomised, double-blind trial. Lancet Oncol 21:1283–1295

Feng WW, Kurokawa M (2020) Lipid metabolic reprogramming as an emerging mechanism of resistance to kinase inhibitors in breast cancer. Cancer Drug Resist 3:1–17

Feng WW, Wilkins O, Bang S et al (2019) CD36-mediated metabolic rewiring of breast cancer cells promotes resistance to HER2-targeted therapies. Cell Rep 29:3405–3420. e3405

Fernandez-Martinez A, Pascual T, Singh B et al (2023) Prognostic and predictive value of immune-related gene expression signatures vs tumor-infiltrating lymphocytes in early-stage ERBB2/HER2-positive breast cancer: a correlative analysis of the CALGB 40601 and PAMELA Trials. JAMA Oncol 9:490–499

Fernández-Nogueira P, Mancino M, Fuster G et al (2020) Tumor-associated fibroblasts promote HER2-targeted therapy resistance through FGFR2 activation. Clin Cancer Res 26:1432–1448

Fessler SP, Wotkowicz MT, Mahanta SK, Bamdad C (2009) MUC1* is a determinant of trastuzumab (Herceptin) resistance in breast cancer cells. Breast Cancer Res Treat 118:113–124

Filho OM, Viale G, Stein S et al (2021) Impact of HER2 heterogeneity on treatment response of early-stage HER2-positive breast cancer: phase II neoadjuvant clinical trial of T-DM1 combined with pertuzumab. Cancer Discov 11:2474–2487

Franklin MC, Carey KD, Vajdos FF et al (2004) Insights into ErbB signaling from the structure of the ErbB2-pertuzumab complex. Cancer Cell 5:317–328

Fujita T, Doihara H, Kawasaki K et al (2006) PTEN activity could be a predictive marker of trastuzumab efficacy in the treatment of ErbB2-overexpressing breast cancer. Br J Cancer 94:247–252

Fumagalli D, Venet D, Ignatiadis M et al (2017) RNA sequencing to predict response to neoadjuvant anti-HER2 therapy: a secondary analysis of the NeoALTTO randomized clinical trial. JAMA Oncol 3:227–234

Gabos Z, Sinha R, Hanson J et al (2006) Prognostic significance of human epidermal growth factor receptor positivity for the development of brain metastasis after newly diagnosed breast cancer. J Clin Oncol 24:5658–5663

Gao J, Aksoy BA, Dogrusoz U et al (2013) Integrative analysis of complex cancer genomics and clinical profiles using the cBioPortal. Sci Signal 6:pl1

Garaud S, Buisseret L, Solinas C et al (2019) Tumor infiltrating B-cells signal functional humoral immune responses in breast cancer. JCI Insight:5

Geyer CE, Forster J, Lindquist D et al (2006) Lapatinib plus capecitabine for HER2-positive advanced breast cancer. N Engl J Med 355:2733–2743

Gianni L, Pienkowski T, Im YH et al (2016) 5-year analysis of neoadjuvant pertuzumab and trastuzumab in patients with locally advanced, inflammatory, or early-stage HER2-positive breast cancer (NeoSphere): a multicentre, open-label, phase 2 randomised trial. Lancet Oncol 17:791–800

Gianni L, Bisagni G, Colleoni M et al (2018) Neoadjuvant treatment with trastuzumab and pertuzumab plus palbociclib and fulvestrant in HER2-positive, ER-positive breast cancer (NA-PHER2): an exploratory, open-label, phase 2 study. Lancet Oncol 19:249–256

Giugliano F, Carnevale Schianca A, Corti C et al (2023) Unlocking the resistance to Anti-HER2 treatments in breast cancer: the issue of HER2 spatial distribution. Cancers (Basel):15

Giuliano M, Trivedi MV, Schiff R (2013) Bidirectional crosstalk between the estrogen receptor and human epidermal growth factor receptor 2 signaling pathways in breast cancer: molecular basis and clinical implications. Breast Care (Basel) 8:256–262

Giuliano M, Hu H, Wang YC et al (2015) Upregulation of ER signaling as an adaptive mechanism of cell survival in HER2-positive breast tumors treated with anti-HER2 therapy. Clin Cancer Res 21:3995–4003

Goutsouliak K, Veeraraghavan J, Sethunath V et al (2020) Towards personalized treatment for early stage HER2-positive breast cancer. Nat Rev Clin Oncol 17:233–250

Griguolo G, Serna G, Pascual T et al (2021) Immune microenvironment characterisation and dynamics during anti-HER2-based neoadjuvant treatment in HER2-positive breast cancer. NPJ Precis Oncol 5:23

Guardia C, Bianchini G, Arpi LO et al (2021) Preclinical and clinical characterization of fibroblast-derived neuregulin-1 on trastuzumab and pertuzumab activity in HER2-positive breast cancer. Clin Cancer Res 27:5096–5108

Guo W, Pylayeva Y, Pepe A et al (2006) β4 integrin amplifies ErbB2 signaling to promote mammary tumorigenesis. Cell 126:489–502

Gutierrez C, Schiff R (2011) HER2: biology, detection, and clinical implications. Arch Pathol Lab Med 135:55–62

Hamblett K, Barnscher S, Davies R et al (2019) Abstract P6-17-13: ZW49, a HER2 targeted biparatopic antibody drug conjugate for the treatment of HER2 expressing cancers. Cancer Res 79:P6-17-13-P16-17-13

Hamilton E, Shastry M, Shiller SM, Ren R (2021) Targeting HER2 heterogeneity in breast cancer. Cancer Treat Rev 100:102286

Hanker AB, Garrett JT, Estrada MV et al (2017a) HER2-overexpressing breast cancers amplify FGFR signaling upon acquisition of resistance to dual therapeutic blockade of HER2. Clin Cancer Res 23:4323–4334

Hanker AB, Estrada MV, Bianchini G et al (2017b) Extracellular matrix/integrin signaling promotes resistance to combined inhibition of HER2 and PI3K in HER2(+) breast cancer. Cancer Res 77:3280–3292

Hoadley KA, Yau C, Wolf DM et al (2014) Multiplatform analysis of 12 cancer types reveals molecular classification within and across tissues of origin. Cell 158:929–944

Holmes FA, Moy B, Delaloge S et al (2023) Overall survival with neratinib after trastuzumab-based adjuvant therapy in HER2-positive breast cancer (ExteNET): a randomised, double-blind, placebo-controlled, phase 3 trial. Eur J Cancer 184:48–59

Huang X, Gao L, Wang S et al (2010) Heterotrimerization of the growth factor receptors erbB2, erbB3, and insulin-like growth factor-i receptor in breast cancer cells resistant to herceptin. Cancer Res 70:1204–1214

Huang C, Park CC, Hilsenbeck SG et al (2011) beta1 integrin mediates an alternative survival pathway in breast cancer cells resistant to lapatinib. Breast Cancer Res 13:R84

Huck L, Pontier S, Zuo D, Muller W (2010) β1-integrin is dispensable for the induction of ErbB2 mammary tumors but plays a critical role in the metastatic phase of tumor progression. Proc Natl Acad Sci 107:15559–15564

Hurvitz S, Loi S, O'Shaughnessy J et al. HER2-CLIMB-02: randomized, double-blind, phase 3 trial of tucatinib and trastuzumab emtansine for previously treated HER2-positive metastatic breast cancer. San Antonio Breast Cancer Symposium 2023a; Abstract GS01-10

Hurvitz SA, Hegg R, Chung WP et al (2023b) Trastuzumab deruxtecan versus trastuzumab emtansine in patients with HER2-positive metastatic breast cancer: updated results from DESTINY-Breast03, a randomised, open-label, phase 3 trial. Lancet 401:105–117

Hyman DM, Piha-Paul SA, Won H et al (2018) HER kinase inhibition in patients with HER2-and HER3-mutant cancers. Nature 554:189–194

Irie H, Ito K, Fujioka Y et al (2019) TAS0728, a covalent-binding, HER2-selective kinase inhibitor shows potent antitumor activity in preclinical models. Mol Cancer Ther 18:733–742

Jain S, Nye LE, Santa-Maria CA et al (2016) Phase I study of alpelisib and T-DM1 in trastuzumab-refractory HER2-positive metastatic breast cancer. J Clin Oncol 34:588–588

Jeselsohn R, Buchwalter G, De Angelis C et al (2015) ESR1 mutations-a mechanism for acquired endocrine resistance in breast cancer. Nat Rev Clin Oncol 12:573–583

Jhaveri K, Han H, Dotan E et al (2022) 460MO Preliminary results from a phase I study using the bispecific, human epidermal growth factor 2 (HER2)-targeting antibody-drug conjugate (ADC) zanidatamab zovodotin (ZW49) in solid cancers. Ann Oncol 33:S749–S750

Johnston S, Pippen J Jr, Pivot X et al (2009) Lapatinib combined with letrozole versus letrozole and placebo as first-line therapy for postmenopausal hormone receptor-positive metastatic breast cancer. J Clin Oncol 27:5538–5546

Koirala N, Dey N, Aske J, De P (2022) Targeting cell cycle progression in HER2+ breast cancer: an emerging treatment opportunity. Int J Mol Sci 23

Kwong KY, Hung MC (1998) A novel splice variant of HER2 with increased transformation activity. Mol Carcinog 23:62–68

Lan HR, Chen M, Yao SY et al (2023) Bispecific antibodies revolutionizing breast cancer treatment: a comprehensive overview. Front Immunol 14:1266450

Lee J, Kida K, Liu H et al. (2023) The DNA repair pathway as a therapeutic target to synergize with trastuzumab deruxtecan in HER2-targeted antibody-drug conjugate–resistant HER2-overexpressing breast cancer

Liang K, Esteva FJ, Albarracin C et al (2010) Recombinant human erythropoietin antagonizes trastuzumab treatment of breast cancer cells via Jak2-mediated Src activation and PTEN inactivation. Cancer Cell 18:423–435

Lin C-H, Pelissier FA, Zhang H et al (2015) Microenvironment rigidity modulates responses to the HER2 receptor tyrosine kinase inhibitor lapatinib via YAP and TAZ transcription factors. Mol Biol Cell 26:3946–3953

Lin NU, Murthy RK, Abramson V et al (2023) Tucatinib vs placebo, both in combination with trastuzumab and capecitabine, for previously treated ERBB2 (HER2)-positive metastatic breast cancer in patients with brain metastases: updated exploratory analysis of the HER2CLIMB randomized clinical trial. JAMA Oncol 9:197–205

Llombart-Cussac A, Cortés J, Paré L et al (2017) HER2-enriched subtype as a predictor of pathological complete response following trastuzumab and lapatinib without chemotherapy in early-stage HER2-positive breast cancer (PAMELA): an open-label, single-group, multicentre, phase 2 trial. Lancet Oncol 18:545–554

Loi S, Michiels S, Lambrechts D et al (2013) Somatic mutation profiling and associations with prognosis and trastuzumab benefit in early breast cancer. J Natl Cancer Inst 105:960–967

Loi S, Giobbie-Hurder A, Gombos A et al (2019) Pembrolizumab plus trastuzumab in trastuzumab-resistant, advanced, HER2-positive breast cancer (PANACEA): a single-arm, multicentre, phase 1b-2 trial. Lancet Oncol 20:371–382

Loibl S, Majewski I, Guarneri V et al (2016) PIK3CA mutations are associated with reduced pathological complete response rates in primary HER2-positive breast cancer: pooled analysis of 967 patients from five prospective trials investigating lapatinib and trastuzumab. Ann Oncol 27:1519–1525

Lu Y, Zi X, Zhao Y et al (2001) Insulin-like growth factor-I receptor signaling and resistance to trastuzumab (Herceptin). J Natl Cancer Inst 93:1852–1857

Luen SJ, Savas P, Fox SB et al (2017) Tumour-infiltrating lymphocytes and the emerging role of immunotherapy in breast cancer. Pathology 49:141–155

Luque M, Sanz-Alvarez M, Morales-Gallego M et al (2022) Tumor-infiltrating lymphocytes and immune response in HER2-positive breast cancer. Cancers (Basel):14

Ma F, Li Y, Yao H et al (2023) Preclinical and early clinical data of ZN-1041, a best-in-class BBB penetrable HER2 inhibitor to treat breast cancer with CNS metastases. J Clin Oncol 41:1040–1040

Mahmoud SM, Paish EC, Powe DG et al (2011) Tumor-infiltrating CD8+ lymphocytes predict clinical outcome in breast cancer. J Clin Oncol 29:1949–1955

Marchio C, Annaratone L, Marques A et al (2021) Evolving concepts in HER2 evaluation in breast cancer: heterogeneity, HER2-low carcinomas and beyond. Semin Cancer Biol 72:123–135

Martin M, Holmes FA, Ejlertsen B et al (2017) Neratinib after trastuzumab-based adjuvant therapy in HER2-positive breast cancer (ExteNET): 5-year analysis of a randomised, double-blind, placebo-controlled, phase 3 trial. Lancet Oncol 18:1688–1700

Massarweh S, Schiff R (2007) Unraveling the mechanisms of endocrine resistance in breast cancer: new therapeutic opportunities. Clin Cancer Res 13:1950–1954

Meric-Bernstam F, Beeram M, Hamilton E et al (2022) Zanidatamab, a novel bispecific antibody, for the treatment of locally advanced or metastatic HER2-expressing or HER2-amplified cancers: a phase 1, dose-escalation and expansion study. Lancet Oncol 23:1558–1570

Miranda F, Prazeres H, Mendes F et al (2022) Resistance to endocrine therapy in HR + and/or HER2 + breast cancer: the most promising predictive biomarkers. Mol Biol Rep 49:717–733

Mitra D, Brumlik MJ, Okamgba SU et al (2009) An oncogenic isoform of HER2 associated with locally disseminated breast cancer and trastuzumab resistance. Mol Cancer Ther 8:2152–2162

Mittendorf EA, Lu B, Melisko M et al (2019) Efficacy and safety analysis of nelipepimut-S vaccine to prevent breast cancer recurrence: a randomized, multicenter, phase III clinical trial. Clin Cancer Res 25:4248–4254

Modi S, Saura C, Yamashita T et al (2020) Trastuzumab deruxtecan in previously treated HER2-positive breast cancer. N Engl J Med 382:610–621

Modi S, Jacot W, Yamashita T et al (2022) Trastuzumab deruxtecan in previously treated HER2-low advanced breast cancer. N Engl J Med 387:9–20

Molina MA, Codony-Servat J, Albanell J et al (2001) Trastuzumab (herceptin), a humanized anti-Her2 receptor monoclonal antibody, inhibits basal and activated Her2 ectodomain cleavage in breast cancer cells. Cancer Res 61:4744–4749

Molina MA, Saez R, Ramsey EE et al (2002) NH(2)-terminal truncated HER-2 protein but not full-length receptor is associated with nodal metastasis in human breast cancer. Clin Cancer Res 8:347–353

Montemurro F, Delaloge S, Barrios CH et al (2020) Trastuzumab emtansine (T-DM1) in patients with HER2-positive metastatic breast cancer and brain metastases: exploratory final analysis of cohort 1 from KAMILLA, a single-arm phase IIIb clinical trial(☆). Ann Oncol 31:1350–1358

Moreno-Aspitia A, Holmes EM, Jackisch C et al (2021) Updated results from the international phase III ALTTO trial (BIG 2-06/Alliance N063D). Eur J Cancer 148:287–296

Morganti S, Ivanova M, Ferraro E et al (2022a) Loss of HER2 in breast cancer: biological mechanisms and technical pitfalls. Cancer Drug Resist 5:971–980

Morganti S, Bianchini G, Giordano A et al (2022b) How I treat HER2-positive early breast cancer: how long adjuvant trastuzumab is needed? ESMO Open 7:100428

Moulder SL, Borges VF, Baetz T et al (2017) Phase I study of ONT-380, a HER2 inhibitor, in patients with HER2(+)-advanced solid tumors, with an expansion cohort in HER2(+) metastatic breast cancer (MBC). Clin Cancer Res 23:3529–3536

Nagata Y, Lan KH, Zhou X et al (2004) PTEN activation contributes to tumor inhibition by trastuzumab, and loss of PTEN predicts trastuzumab resistance in patients. Cancer Cell 6:117–127

Nagpal A, Needham K, Lane DJR et al (2023) Integrin alphavbeta3 is a master regulator of resistance to TKI-induced ferroptosis in HER2-positive breast cancer. Cancers (Basel):15

Nahta R, Hung MC, Esteva FJ (2004) The HER-2-targeting antibodies trastuzumab and pertuzumab synergistically inhibit the survival of breast cancer cells. Cancer Res 64:2343–2346

Nahta R, Yuan LX, Zhang B et al (2005) Insulin-like growth factor-I receptor/human epidermal growth factor receptor 2 heterodimerization contributes to trastuzumab resistance of breast cancer cells. Cancer Res 65:11118–11128

Nahta R, Yuan LX, Du Y, Esteva FJ (2007) Lapatinib induces apoptosis in trastuzumab-resistant breast cancer cells: effects on insulin-like growth factor I signaling. Mol Cancer Ther 6:667–674

Nardone A, De Angelis C, Trivedi MV et al (2015) The changing role of ER in endocrine resistance. Breast 24(Suppl 2):S60–S66

Nayar U, Cohen O, Kapstad C et al (2019) Acquired HER2 mutations in ER(+) metastatic breast cancer confer resistance to estrogen receptor-directed therapies. Nat Genet 51:207–216

Nikkhoi SK, Li G, Eleya S et al (2022) Bispecific killer cell engager with high affinity and specificity toward CD16a on NK cells for cancer immunotherapy. Front Immunol 13:1039969

Nitz U, Gluz O, Graeser M et al (2022) De-escalated neoadjuvant pertuzumab plus trastuzumab therapy with or without weekly paclitaxel in HER2-positive, hormone receptor-negative, early breast cancer (WSG-ADAPT-HER2+/HR-): survival outcomes from a multicentre, open-label, randomised, phase 2 trial. Lancet Oncol 23:625–635

O'Sullivan CC, Clarke R, Goetz MP, Robertson J (2023) Cyclin-dependent kinase 4/6 inhibitors for treatment of hormone receptor-positive, ERBB2-negative breast cancer: a review. JAMA Oncol 9:1273–1282

Pandolfi PP (2004) Breast cancer--loss of PTEN predicts resistance to treatment. N Engl J Med 351:2337–2338

Pegram M, Jackisch C, Johnston SRD (2023) Estrogen/HER2 receptor crosstalk in breast cancer: combination therapies to improve outcomes for patients with hormone receptor-positive/HER2-positive breast cancer. NPJ Breast Cancer 9:45

Perez-Garcia JM, Vaz Batista M, Cortez P et al (2023) Trastuzumab deruxtecan in patients with central nervous system involvement from HER2-positive breast cancer: the DEBBRAH trial. Neuro-Oncology 25:157–166

Perou CM, Sorlie T, Eisen MB et al (2000) Molecular portraits of human breast tumours. Nature 406:747–752

Pestalozzi BC, Zahrieh D, Price KN et al (2006) Identifying breast cancer patients at risk for Central Nervous System (CNS) metastases in trials of the International Breast Cancer Study Group (IBCSG). Ann Oncol 17:935–944

Piccart M, Procter M, Fumagalli D et al (2021) Adjuvant pertuzumab and trastuzumab in early HER2-positive breast cancer in the APHINITY trial: 6 years' follow-up. J Clin Oncol 39:1448–1457

Rabindran SK, Discafani CM, Rosfjord EC et al (2004) Antitumor activity of HKI-272, an orally active, irreversible inhibitor of the HER-2 tyrosine kinase. Cancer Res 64:3958–3965

Razavi P, Chang MT, Xu G et al (2018) The genomic landscape of endocrine-resistant advanced breast cancers. Cancer Cell 34:427–438 e426

Rexer BN, Arteaga CL (2012) Intrinsic and acquired resistance to HER2-targeted therapies in HER2 gene-amplified breast cancer: mechanisms and clinical implications. Crit Rev Oncog 17:1–16

Rimawi MF, Wiechmann LS, Wang YC et al (2011) Reduced dose and intermittent treatment with lapatinib and trastuzumab for potent blockade of the HER pathway in HER2/neu-overexpressing breast tumor xenografts. Clin Cancer Res 17:1351–1361

Rimawi MF, Schiff R, Osborne CK (2015a) Targeting HER2 for the treatment of breast cancer. Annu Rev Med 66:111–128

Rimawi MF, De Angelis C, Schiff R (2015b) Resistance to anti-HER2 therapies in breast cancer. Am Soc Clin Oncol Educ Book:e157–e164

Rimawi MF, De Angelis C, Contreras A et al (2018) Low PTEN levels and PIK3CA mutations predict resistance to neoadjuvant lapatinib and trastuzumab without chemotherapy in patients with HER2 overexpressing breast cancer. Breast Cancer Res Treat 167: 731–740

Ritter CA, Perez-Torres M, Rinehart C et al (2007) Human breast cancer cells selected for resistance to trastuzumab in vivo overexpress epidermal growth factor receptor and ErbB ligands and remain dependent on the ErbB receptor network. Clin Cancer Res 13:4909–4919

Rius Ruiz I, Vicario R, Morancho B et al (2018) p95HER2-T cell bispecific antibody for breast cancer treatment. Sci Transl Med:10

Rivas EI, Linares J, Zwick M et al (2022) Targeted immunotherapy against distinct cancer-associated fibroblasts overcomes treatment resistance in refractory HER2+ breast tumors. Nat Commun 13:5310

Robichaux JP, Elamin YY, Vijayan RSK et al (2019) Pan-cancer landscape and analysis of ERBB2 mutations identifies poziotinib as a clinically active inhibitor and enhancer of T-DM1 activity. Cancer Cell 36:444–457 e447

Rugo HS, Im SA, Cardoso F et al (2023) Margetuximab versus trastuzumab in patients with previously treated HER2-positive advanced breast cancer (SOPHIA): final overall survival results from a randomized phase 3 trial. J Clin Oncol 41:198–205

Salgado R, Denkert C, Demaria S et al (2015) The evaluation of tumor-infiltrating lymphocytes (TILs) in breast cancer: recommendations by an International TILs Working Group 2014. Ann Oncol 26:259–271

Sanchez-Vega F, Mina M, Armenia J et al (2018) Oncogenic signaling pathways in the cancer genome atlas. Cell 173:321–337 e310

Saura C, Oliveira M, Feng YH et al (2020) Neratinib plus capecitabine versus lapatinib plus capecitabine in her2-positive metastatic breast cancer previously treated with >/= 2 HER2-directed regimens: phase III NALA trial. J Clin Oncol 38:3138–3149

Savas P, Salgado R, Denkert C et al (2016) Clinical relevance of host immunity in breast cancer: from TILs to the clinic. Nat Rev Clin Oncol 13:228–241

Scaltriti M, Rojo F, Ocana A et al (2007) Expression of p95HER2, a truncated form of the HER2 receptor, and response to anti-HER2 therapies in breast cancer. J Natl Cancer Inst 99:628–638

Scaltriti M, Chandarlapaty S, Prudkin L et al (2010) Clinical benefit of lapatinib-based therapy in patients with human epidermal growth factor receptor 2-positive breast tumors coexpressing the truncated p95HER2 receptor. Clin Cancer Res 16:2688–2695

Schillaci R, Bruni S, Mauro F et al (2022) Abstract P5-13-32: Mucin 4 expression in high risk breast cancer: predicting and overcoming resistance to immunotherapy. Cancer Res 82:P5-13-32-P15-13-32

Schreiber RD, Old LJ, Smyth MJ (2011) Cancer immunoediting: integrating immunity's roles in cancer suppression and promotion. Science 331:1565–1570

Sergina NV, Rausch M, Wang D et al (2007) Escape from HER-family tyrosine kinase inhibitor therapy by the kinase-inactive HER3. Nature 445:437–441

Sethunath V, Hu H, De Angelis C et al (2019) Targeting the mevalonate pathway to overcome acquired anti-HER2 treatment resistance in breast cancer. Mol Cancer Res 17:2318–2330

Shattuck DL, Miller JK, Carraway KL 3rd, Sweeney C (2008) Met receptor contributes to trastuzumab resistance of Her2-overexpressing breast cancer cells. Cancer Res 68:1471–1477

Sinkala M, Nkhoma P, Mulder N, Martin DP (2021) Integrated molecular characterisation of the MAPK pathways in human cancers reveals pharmacologically vulnerable mutations and gene dependencies. Commun Biol 4:9

Smith AE, Ferraro E, Safonov A et al (2021) HER2 + breast cancers evade anti-HER2 therapy via a switch in driver pathway. Nat Commun 12:6667

Son J, Jang J, Beyett TS et al (2022) A novel HER2-selective kinase inhibitor is effective in HER2 mutant and amplified non-small cell lung cancer. Cancer Res 82:1633–1645

Sorlie T, Perou CM, Tibshirani R et al (2001) Gene expression patterns of breast carcinomas distinguish tumor subclasses with clinical implications. Proc Natl Acad Sci USA 98:10869–10874

Swain SM, Baselga J, Kim SB et al (2015) Pertuzumab, trastuzumab, and docetaxel in HER2-positive metastatic breast cancer. N Engl J Med 372:724–734

Swain SM, Shastry M, Hamilton E (2023) Targeting HER2-positive breast cancer: advances and future directions. Nat Rev Drug Discov 22:101–126

Takeda T, Yamamoto H, Kanzaki H et al (2017) Yes1 signaling mediates the resistance to Trastuzumab/Lap atinib in breast cancer. PLoS One 12:e0171356

Tamura K, Tsurutani J, Takahashi S et al (2019) Trastuzumab deruxtecan (DS-8201a) in patients with advanced HER2-positive breast cancer previously treated with trastuzumab emtansine: a dose-expansion, phase 1 study. Lancet Oncol 20:816–826

Tarantino P, Carmagnani Pestana R, Corti C et al (2022) Antibody-drug conjugates: Smart chemotherapy delivery across tumor histologies. CA Cancer J Clin 72:165–182

Tobias J, Garner-Spitzer E, Drinic M, Wiedermann U (2022) Vaccination against Her-2/neu, with focus on peptide-based vaccines. ESMO Open 7:100361

Tolaney SM, Barry WT, Dang CT et al (2015) Adjuvant paclitaxel and trastuzumab for node-negative, HER2-positive breast cancer. N Engl J Med 372: 134–141

Tolaney SM, Wardley AM, Zambelli S et al (2020) Abemaciclib plus trastuzumab with or without fulvestrant versus trastuzumab plus standard-of-care chemotherapy in women with hormone receptor-positive, HER2-positive advanced breast cancer (monarcHER): a randomised, open-label, phase 2 trial. Lancet Oncol 21:763–775

Tolaney SM, Tayob N, Dang C et al (2021) Adjuvant Trastuzumab emtansine versus paclitaxel in combination with trastuzumab for stage I HER2-positive breast cancer (ATEMPT): a randomized clinical trial. J Clin Oncol 39:2375–2385

Tolaney SM, Goel S, Nadal J et al (2024) Overall Survival and Exploratory Biomarker Analyses of Abemaciclib plus Trastuzumab with or without Fulvestrant versus Trastuzumab plus Chemotherapy in HR+, HER2+ Metastatic Breast Cancer Patients. Clin Cancer Res 30:39–49

Triantafyllidi E, Triantafillidis JK (2022) Systematic review on the use of biosimilars of trastuzumab in HER2+ breast cancer. Biomedicines:10

Tripathy D, Brufsky A, Cobleigh M et al (2020) De novo versus recurrent HER2-positive metastatic breast cancer: patient characteristics, treatment, and survival from the SystHERs registry. Oncologist 25:e214–e222

Turpin J, Ling C, Crosby EJ et al (2016) The ErbB2ΔEx16 splice variant is a major oncogenic driver in breast cancer that promotes a pro-metastatic tumor microenvironment. Oncogene 35:6053–6064

van Ramshorst MS, van der Voort A, van Werkhoven ED et al (2018) Neoadjuvant chemotherapy with or without anthracyclines in the presence of dual HER2 blockade for HER2-positive breast cancer (TRAIN-2): a multicentre, open-label, randomised, phase 3 trial. Lancet Oncol 19:1630–1640

Vaz-Luis I, Winer EP, Lin NU (2013) Human epidermal growth factor receptor-2-positive breast cancer: does estrogen receptor status define two distinct subtypes? Ann Oncol 24:283–291

Veeraraghavan J, De Angelis C, Reis-Filho JS et al (2017) De-escalation of treatment in HER2-positive breast cancer: determinants of response and mechanisms of resistance. Breast 34(Suppl 1):S19–S26

Veeraraghavan J, Angelis CD, Mao R et al (2019) A combinatorial biomarker predicts pathologic complete response to neoadjuvant lapatinib and trastuzumab without chemotherapy in patients with HER2+ breast cancer. Ann Oncol 30:927–933

Veeraraghavan J, Gutierrez C, Sethunath V et al (2021) Neratinib plus trastuzumab is superior to pertuzumab plus trastuzumab in HER2-positive breast cancer xenograft models. NPJ Breast Cancer 7:63

Veeraraghavan J, Gutierrez C, De Angelis C et al (2023) A multiparameter molecular classifier to predict response to neoadjuvant lapatinib plus trastuzumab without chemotherapy in HER2+ breast cancer. Clin Cancer Res 29:3101–3109

Verma S, Miles D, Gianni L et al (2012) Trastuzumab emtansine for HER2-positive advanced breast cancer. N Engl J Med 367:1783–1791

Verret B, Cortes J, Bachelot T et al (2019) Efficacy of PI3K inhibitors in advanced breast cancer. Ann Oncol 30(Suppl 10):x12–x20

Volpi CC, Pietrantonio F, Gloghini A et al (2019) The landscape of d16HER2 splice variant expression across HER2-positive cancers. Sci Rep 9:3545

von Arx C, De Placido P, Caltavituro A et al (2023) The evolving therapeutic landscape of trastuzumab-drug conjugates: Future perspectives beyond HER2-positive breast cancer. Cancer Treat Rev 113:102500

von Minckwitz G, Procter M, de Azambuja E et al (2017) Adjuvant pertuzumab and trastuzumab in early HER2-positive breast cancer. N Engl J Med 377:122–131

von Minckwitz G, Huang CS, Mano MS et al (2019) Trastuzumab Emtansine for Residual Invasive HER2-Positive Breast Cancer. N Engl J Med 380:617–628

Wang YC, Morrison G, Gillihan R et al (2011) Different mechanisms for resistance to trastuzumab versus lapatinib in HER2-positive breast cancers--role of estrogen receptor and HER2 reactivation. Breast Cancer Res 13:R121

Weisser NE, Sanches M, Escobar-Cabrera E et al (2023) An anti-HER2 biparatopic antibody that induces unique HER2 clustering and complement-dependent cytotoxicity. Nat Commun 14:1394

Wen W, Chen WS, Xiao N et al (2015) Mutations in the kinase domain of the HER2/ERBB2 gene identified in a wide variety of human cancers. J Mol Diagn 17:487–495

Wilding B, Scharn D, Bose D et al (2022) Discovery of potent and selective HER2 inhibitors with efficacy against HER2 exon 20 insertion-driven tumors, which preserve wild-type EGFR signaling. Nat Cancer 3:821–836

Wolff AC, Hammond MEH, Allison KH et al (2018) HER2 testing in breast cancer: American Society of Clinical Oncology/College of American pathologists clinical practice guideline focused update summary. J Oncol Pract 14:437–441

Wu J, Yang B, Ma L et al (2023) Abstract OT2-16-04: KN026 in combination with docetaxel as neoadjuvant treatment for HER2-positive early or locally advanced breast cancer: a single arm, multicenter, phase 2 study. Cancer Res 83:OT2-16-04-OT12-16-04

Xia W, Mullin RJ, Keith BR et al (2002) Anti-tumor activity of GW572016: a dual tyrosine kinase inhibitor blocks EGF activation of EGFR/erbB2 and downstream Erk1/2 and AKT pathways. Oncogene 21:6255–6263

Xu X, De Angelis C, Burke KA et al (2017) HER2 reactivation through acquisition of the HER2 L755S mutation as a mechanism of acquired resistance to HER2-targeted therapy in HER2(+) breast cancer. Clin Cancer Res 23:5123–5134

Xu B, Yan M, Ma F et al (2021) Pyrotinib plus capecitabine versus lapatinib plus capecitabine for the treatment of HER2-positive metastatic breast cancer (PHOEBE): a multicentre, open-label, randomised, controlled, phase 3 trial. Lancet Oncol 22:351–360

Yang YH, Liu JW, Lu C, Wei JF (2022) CAR-T cell therapy for breast cancer: from basic research to clinical application. Int J Biol Sci 18:2609–2626

Yu S, Zhang J, Yan Y et al (2019) A novel asymmetrical anti-HER2/CD3 bispecific antibody exhibits potent cytotoxicity for HER2-positive tumor cells. J Exp Clin Cancer Res 38:355

Zagami P, Fernandez-Martinez A, Rashid NU et al (2023) Association of PIK3CA mutation with pathologic complete response and outcome by hormone receptor status and intrinsic subtype in early-stage ERBB2/HER2-positive breast cancer. JAMA Netw Open 6:e2348814

Zhang S, Huang WC, Li P et al (2011) Combating trastuzumab resistance by targeting SRC, a common node downstream of multiple resistance pathways. Nat Med 17:461–469

Zhang J, Ji D, Cai L et al (2022) First-in-human HER2-targeted bispecific antibody KN026 for the treatment of patients with HER2-positive metastatic breast cancer: results from a phase I study. Clin Cancer Res 28:618–628

Zhao C, Kulyk L, Botrous I et al (2023) Abstract 4034: a potent and highly selective irreversible HER2 inhibitor for treating HER2-driven cancers. Cancer Res 83:4034–4034

Zuo WJ, Jiang YZ, Wang YJ et al (2016) Dual characteristics of novel HER2 kinase domain mutations in response to HER2-targeted therapies in human breast cancer. Clin Cancer Res 22:4859–4869